# Mayes' Midwifery

For Elsevier

Commissioning Editor: *Mairi McCubbin*
Development Editor: *Sheila Black*
Project Manager: *Glenys Norquay*
Designer: *Charles Gray*
Illustration Manager: *Gillian Richards*
Illustrator: *Cactus*

# Mayes' Midwifery

FOURTEENTH EDITION


**Edited by**

**Sue Macdonald** MSc PGCEA ADM RM RN ILTM FETC

Education and Research Manager and Lead Midwife for Education, Learning, Research and Practice Development Department International Office, Royal College of Midwives, London, UK

**Julia Magill-Cuerden** MA PhD DN DipEd MTD NTF FRCM RM RN

Emeritus Scholar of Thames Valley University, Formerly Principal Lecturer and Senior Research Fellow, Thames Valley University, London, UK

**Foreword by**

**Cathy Warwick** Professor, CBE, General Secretary of the Royal College of Midwives, London, UK

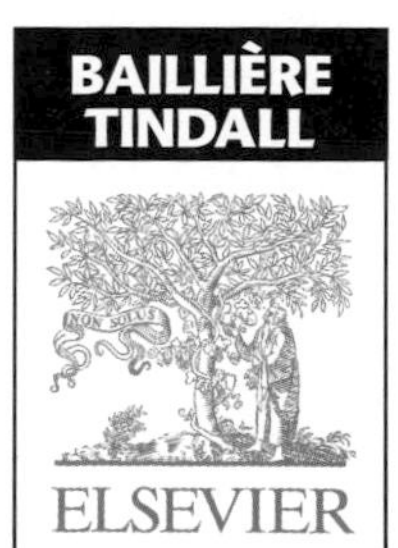



Edinburgh London New York Oxford Philadelphia St Louis Sydney Toronto 2010

BAILLIÈRE
TINDALL
ELSEVIER

Baillière Tindall, an imprint of Elsevier Ltd



Twelfth edition 1997
Thirteenth edition 2004
Fourteenth edition 2011
Reprinted 2011
ISBN 978-0-7020-3105-2

**British Library Cataloguing in Publication Data**
A catalogue record for this book is available from the British Library

**Library of Congress Cataloging in Publication Data**
A catalog record for this book is available from the Library of Congress

**Notice**

Knowledge and best practice in this field are constantly changing. As new research and experience broaden our knowledge, changes in practice, treatment and drug therapy may become necessary or appropriate. Readers are advised to check the most current information provided (i) on procedures featured or (ii) by the manufacturer of each product to be administered, to verify the recommended dose or formula, the method and duration of administration, and contraindications. It is the responsibility of the practitioner, relying on their own experience and knowledge of the patient, to make diagnoses, to determine dosages and the best treatment for each individual patient, and to take all appropriate safety precautions. To the fullest extent of the law, neither the Publisher nor the Editor assumes any liability for any injury and/or damage to persons or property arising out of or related to any use of the material contained in this book.

The Publisher



The publisher's policy is to use **paper manufactured from sustainable forests**

Printed in Italy

# Contents

# Contributors

**Belinda Ackerman** **MA PGDip PGCEA ADM HV RM RN**
Consultant Midwife, Guy's and St Thomas' Foundation Trust St Thomas's Hospital, Women's Services Directorate, London, UK
*Chapter 3 Statutory Framework for Practice*
*Chapter 43 Infant feeding*

**Luisa Acosta** **BSc(Hons) MSc PGDip**
Senior Lecturer, School of Nursing, Midwifery and Healthcare, Faculty of Health and Human Sciences, Thames Valley University, London, UK
*Chapter 68 Complications of the third stage of labour*

**Debbie Barber** **BSc(Hons) MSc PGDE PGCMU DipCouns RGN RM NT**
Nurse Consultant, Oxford Fertility Unit, John Radcliffe Hospital; Honorary Lecturer, Oxford Brookes University and Guilford University, Oxford, UK
*Chapter 28 Infertility and assisted conception*

**Maria Barrell** **MA PhD PGDip CertEd ADM RMT RM RN**
Principal Lecturer, School of Health, Community and Education Studies, Northumbria University, Newcastle Upon Tyne, UK
*Chapter 6 Leadership and management in midwifery*

**Cecelia M. Bartholomew** **BSc(Hons) MSc PGDip RM RN**
Senior Lecturer, Thames Valley University, London, UK
*Chapter 38 Pain, labour and women's choice of pain relief*
*Chapter 53 Nausea and vomiting*

**Carol Bates** **MA PGCEA ADM RN RM**
Midwifery Education and Practice Consultant, Harpenden, UK
*Chapter 47 Infection*
*Chapter 48 Congenital anomalies, fetal and neonatal surgery, and pain*
*Chapter 49 Metabolic and endocrine disorders*

**Christine A. Bewley** **BEd MSc PhD ADM RN RM**
Head of Department, Midwifery, Child Health and Primary Care; Lead Midwife for Education, Middlesex University, London, UK
*Chapter 55 Medical disorders of pregnancy*
*Chapter 56 Hypertensive disorders of pregnancy*

**Kuldip Kaur Bharj** **OBE RM RN MTD DN (London) IHSM RSACounsSkills**
Senior Lecturer, School of Healthcare, University of Leeds, Leeds, UK
*Chapter 32 Confirming pregnancy and care of the pregnant woman*

**Jane Bott** **MSc PGCEA ADM RN RM**
Senior Lecturer in Midwifery, Faculty of Health and Social Care Sciences, Kingston University and St George's Hospital Medical School, London, UK
*Chapter 57 Sexually transmitted infections*

**Maureen Boyle** **MSc PGCEA ADFM RN RM**
Midwife Teacher, Thames Valley University, London, UK
*Chapter 33 Antenatal investigations*

**Margaret Brock** **PGCEA SCM ADM SRN**
Senior Midwife and Manager, Delivery Suite, John Radcliffe Hospital, Women's Centre, Oxford, UK
*Chapter 65 Disproportion, obstructed labour and uterine rupture*

**Gill Brook** **MCSP**
Physiotherapy Co-ordinator, Bradford Teaching Hospitals NHS Foundation Trust, Bradford, UK; Secretary of the International Organization of Physical Therapists in Women's Health
*Chapter 22 Physical preparation for childbirth and beyond, and the role of physiotherapy*

**Barbara Burden** **MSc PhD PGCEA ADM RN RM**
Head of Community Services and Lead Midwife for Education, University of Bedfordshire, Luton, UK
*Chapter 15 Legal frameworks for the care of the child*
*Chapter 20 Preconception care*
*Chapter 24 Anatomy of male and female reproduction*
*Chapter 30 The fetal skull*

**Joan Cameron** **MSc RGN RM**
Senior Lecturer and Lead Midwife for Education, School of Nursing and Midwifery, University of Dundee, Dundee, UK
*Chapter 45 Respiratory and cardiac disorders*

# Contributors

**Sarah Church** **MSc PhD PGDE CertRes RGN RM ENB997**
School of Health, University College Northampton, UK
*Chapter 63 Rhythmic variations of labour*

**Terri Coates** **MSc ADM DipEd RM RN CIMI**
Clinical Midwife, Salisbury NHS Trust, Salisbury, UK
*Chapter 66 Shoulder dystocia*

**Margie Davies** **RGN RM**
Midwifery Liaison Officer, Queen Charlotte's and Chelsea Hospital, London, UK
*Chapter 59 Multiple pregnancy*

**Tandy Deane-Gray** **BSc MA PGCEA ADM RGN RM**
Senior Lecturer Midwifery, University of Hertfordshire, Hatfield, UK
*Chapter 21 Education for parenthood*

**Jane Denton** **RGN RM**
Director, Multiple Births Foundation, Queen Charlotte's and Chelsea Hospital, London, UK
*Chapter 59 Multiple pregnancy*

**Bridgit Dimond** **MA LLB DSA AHSM**
Barrister-at-law; Emeritus Professor, University of Glamorgan, Pontypridd, UK
*Chapter 9 Law and the midwife*

**Jean Donnison** **BA(Oxon) PhD**
Formerly Senior Lecturer, Department of Social Policy and Administration, University of East London, London, UK
*Chapter 2 A history of the midwifery profession in the United Kingdom*

**Soo Downe** **BA(Hons) MSc PhD RM**
Professor of Midwifery Studies, University of Central Lancashire, Preston, UK
*Chapter 37 Care in the second stage of labour*

**Jacqueline Dunkley-Bent** **MSc PGCEA ADM MRIPH RGN RM**
Professor of Midwifery, London South Bank University, London, UK
*Chapter 19 Health promotion and education*

**Kathryn Eglinton** **BSc(Hons) RN**
Clinical Facilitator, Neonatal Intensive Care Unit, The Whittington Hospital, London, UK
*Chapter 44 The preterm baby and the small baby*

**Liz Gale** **BSc(Hons) PP PGDipHE RGN RM**
Senior Lecturer (Midwifery), University of Greenwich, School of Health and Social Care, London, UK
*Chapter 11 Social, cultural and spiritual context of childbearing*
*Chapter 34 The choice agenda and place of birth and care*

**Anna Gaudion** **BSc(Hons) MA RM RN**
Project Lead, Health Equity Audit of Access to Maternity Services, South East London; Consultant,The Polyanna Project, London, UK
*Chapter 23 Vulnerable women*

**Kathryn Gutteridge** **MSc(Couns&Psych) PGDip SRN RM SoM**
Consultant Midwife, City Hospital, Birmingham, UK
*Chapter 69 Maternal mental health and psychological problems*

**Tina Harris** **BA(Hons) PhD SRN SCM ADM**
Senior Lecturer in Midwifery, De Montfort University, Leicester, UK
*Chapter 39 Care in the third stage of labour*

**Anne-Marie Henshaw** **MMid RM RGN**
Lecturer, Midwifery and Women's Health Group; Supervisor of Midwives, The School of Health Care, University of Leeds, Leeds, UK
*Chapter 32 Confirming pregnancy and care of the pregnant woman*

**Tina Heptinstall** **BSc(Hons) MSc PGCEA ADM RN RM**
Addenbrookes Hospital, Cambridge, UK
*Chapter 11 Social, cultural and spiritual context of childbearing*
*Chapter 34 The choice agenda and place of birth and care*

**Simon Hettle** **BSc(Hons) PhD CSci MIBMS FHEA**
Lecturer, Biological Sciences, School of Science, Faculty of Science and Technology, University of the West of Scotland, Paisley, UK
*Chapter 26 Genetics*

**Tracey Hodgson** **MSc PGCEA ADM SRN RM**
Principal Lecturer – Lead Midwife for Education, University of Northampton, Northampton, UK
*Chapter 63 Rhythmic variations of labour*

**Claire Homeyard** **BSc(Hons) MSc RM RN**
Consultant Midwife (Public Health) and Supervisor of Midwives, Barking, Havering and Redbridge NHS Trust, London; Consultant, The Polyanna Project, London, UK
*Chapter 23 Vulnerable women*

**Amanda Hutcherson** **MA DipHEMid PGCE**
Lecturer in Midwifery, City University London, London, UK
*Chapter 54 Bleeding in pregnancy*

**Karen Jackson** **BSc(Hons) RGN RN**
Midwife Teacher, Midwifery Education Department, Queen's Medical Centre, Nottingham, UK
*Chapter 13 Sexuality*

**Patricia Jackson** **BA(Hons) MA MTD RN RM**
Senior Lecturer, University of Greenwich, London, UK
*Chapter 51 Content and organization of postnatal care*
*Chapter 52 Morbidity following childbirth*

**Gail Johnson** **MA DPSM DipAdultEd RGN RM**
Education and Professional Development Advisor, Royal College of Midwives, London, UK
*Chapter 50 Sudden infant death syndrome*

**Patricia Jones** **BA(Hons) RN RM**
Antenatal Screening Co-ordinator, Fetal Medicine Unit, Elizabeth Garrett Anderson Hospital and University College Hospital, London, UK
*Chapter 20 Preconception care*

**Shirley R Jones** **MA ADM CertEd(FE) ILT RGN RM SoM**
Emeritus Professor of Midwifery, Birmingham City University, Birmingham, UK
*Chapter 8 Ethics and midwifery practice*

**Sue Jordan** **MBBCh PhD PGCE(FE) FHEA**
Reader, School of Human and Health Sciences, Swansea University, Swansea, UK
*Chapter 10 Pharmacology and the midwife*

**Tara Kaufmann** **BA**
Change Manager, Service Transformation Team, Barts and the London NHS Trust, London, UK
*Chapter 14 The health service context and midwifery*

**Chris Kettle** **PhD DM SCM SRN**
Professor of Women's Health, University Hospital of North Staffordshire, Academic Unit of Obstetrics and Gynaecology, Stoke-On-Trent, UK
*Chapter 40 The pelvic floor*

**Paul Lewis** **BSc(Hons) MSc DipN PGCEA ADM RM RN RMN FHEA(Hon) FRCM**
Professor of Midwifery Practice and Development; Associate Dean – Midwifery, Rehabilitation and Health Sciences, Bournemouth University, UK
*Chapter 64 Malpositions and malpresentations*

**Patricia Lindsay** **RN RM ADM PGCEA MSc DHC**
Lecturer, Florence Nightingale School of Nursing and Midwifery, King's College, London, UK
*Chapter 58 Abnormalities of the genital tract*
*Chapter 67 Presentation and prolapse of the umbilical cord*

**Sue Macdonald** **MSc PGCEA ADM RM RN ILTM FETC**
Education and Research Manager and Lead Midwife for Education, Learning, Research and Practice Development Department International Office, Royal College of Midwives, London, UK
*Chapter 4 The midwife as a lifelong learner*

**Gaynor D. MacLean** **MBE BA PhD MTD RN RM**
International Midwifery Consultant, Safe Motherhood and Reproductive Health, Swansea, UK
*Chapter 1 The global midwife*

**Julia Magill-Cuerden** **MA PhD DN DipEd MTD NTF FRCM RM RN**
Emeritus Scholar of Thames Valley University, Formerly Principal Lecturer and Senior Research Fellow, Thames Valley University, London, UK
*Chapter 5 Evidence-based practice and research for practice*
*Chapter 71 Midwifery for the 21st century*

**Pat McGeown** **MSc RGN RM SoM**
Head of Midwifery, Perinatal Institute, Birmingham, UK
*Chapter 62 Induction of labour and post-term pregnancy*

**Mary McNabb** **BA BSc MSc PGCEA ADM RN RM**
Educational Consultant, School of Midwifery, Faculty of Health and Social Care Sciences, Kingston University/St George's University of London, London, UK
*Chapter 25 Female reproductive physiology*
*Chapter 29 Fertilization, embryonic, fetal and placental development*
*Chapter 31 Maternal and fetal responses to pregnancy*
*Chapter 35 Physiological changes from late pregnancy until the onset of lactation*

**Stephanie Meakin** **BA MA RN RM**
Head of Midwifery Education, School of Nursing and Midwifery, University of Southampton, Southampton, UK
*Chapter 61 Procedures in obstetrics*

**Maggie Meeks** **MBChB MD DipEd FRCPCH**
Consultant Neonatologist, Christchurch Women's Hospital, Christchurch, New Zealand
*Chapter 46 Neonatal jaundice*

**Stephanie Michaelides** **ADM PGCEA RN RM**
Senior Lecturer, Middlesex University, School of Health and Social Sciences, London, UK
*Chapter 41 Physiology, assessment and care*
*Chapter 42 Thermoregulation*
*Chapter 46 Neonatal jaundice*

**Carol Paeglis** **BHSc MA ADM ENB997 RN RM SoM**
LSA Midwifery Officer, Yorkshire and the Humber Local Supervising Authority, NHS Yorkshire and the Humber, Leeds, UK
*Chapter 7 Governance in midwifery*

**Michael Preston-Shoot** **BA(Hons) PhD CQSW PGDipSW PGDipPsych**
Dean, Faculty of Health and Social Sciences, University of Bedfordshire, Luton, UK
*Chapter 15 Legal frameworks for the care of the child*

**Jean Rankin** **BSc(Hons) MSc PhD RM RGN RSCN PGCert**
Academic Director (Midwifery), University of the West of Scotland, Paisley, UK
*Chapter 26 Genetics*

## Contributors

**Susan Sapsed** **BPS BA(Hons) MPhil ADM NTD RN RM**
Senior Lecturer, Midwifery and Women's Health, Education Centre, University of Luton, Luton and Dunstable NHS Trust Hospital, Luton, UK
*Chapter 30 The fetal skull*

**Mary Sidebotham** **MA PhD DPSM RM RGN**
Midwifery Lecturer, Griffith University, Queensland, Australia
*Chapter 16 Epidemiology*

**Maria Simons** **BSc RN RM**
Midwife, Maternity Department, Milton Keynes General NHS Trust, Milton Keynes, UK
*Chapter 24 Anatomy of male and female reproduction*

**Lynne T. Spencer** **MA MSc ADM PGCEA PGDip(Couns) ADip PGCert DipSup RN RM**
Visiting Lecturer, School of Health and Social Care and School of Education, Campus of Student Affairs Medway, University of Greenwich, Chatham, Kent, UK
*Chapter 12 Psychological context*

**Jenni Thomas** **OBE NNEB DipCouns DipHumPsychol HonDUniv**
Founder and former President, The Child Bereavement Trust, High Wycombe, UK
*Chapter 70 Grief and bereavement*

**Denise Tiran** **MSc PGCEA ADM RM RGN**
Director, Expectancy Ltd., Kent, UK
*Chapter 17 Nutrition*
*Chapter 18 Complementary therapies in maternity care: responsibilities of midwives*

**Rosemary Towse** **BA(Hons) MSc DipN MTD RN RM**
Tutor (Midwifery), Faculty of Health and Medical Sciences, University of Surrey, UK
*Chapter 27 Fertility and its control*

**Nicola Wales** **BSc MA**
Practice Development Midwife, Northwick Park Hospital, North West London NHS Trust, London, UK
*Chapter 60 Pre-term labour*

**Denis Walsh** **MA PhD DPSM RM**
Associate Professor in Midwifery, University of Nottingham, Nottingham, UK
*Chapter 36 Care in the first stage of labour*

**Teresa Walsh** **MSc RM RN**
Research Midwife, Australia and New Zealand Stillbirth Alliance, Mater Medical Research Institute, Brisbane; Caseload Midwife, "My Midwives" Midwifery Group Practice, Ipswich, Australia
*Chapter 16 Epidemiology*

**Margaret Yerby** **MSc ADM C&G730 PGCEA RN RM**
Senior Lecturer (Midwifery), Wolfson Institute of Health Sciences, Thames Valley University, London, UK
*Chapter 38 Pain, labour and women's choice of pain relief*

# Foreword

It is a pleasure to write the Foreword for the fourteenth edition of *Mayes' Midwifery*. The text has been further revised to bring the contents up to date and to ensure that Mayes' Midwifery retains its place as a key midwifery text for student midwives and qualified midwives. The text is written by an even more diverse range of authors than contributed to past editions and each chapter is supported by a list of references that allows further in-depth study of any one of the subjects covered. The reader cannot but be impressed by the number of midwifery researchers who now contribute to the text alongside researchers from other related disciplines.

This is a difficult time in which to be a midwife. I write this at a point in our history when we are faced by extreme economic uncertainty in the developing world and the reality that expenditure on health services cannot continue at its previous level. At the same time the childbearing population both in the developed and in the developing world has an ever-increasing need for high-quality maternity care that is both physically safe and emotionally satisfying. Finding a way to balance these two opposing forces is not going to be easy.

We also live in a society which is increasingly conscious of risk and are becoming increasingly aware that maternity services provision could easily become dominated by an approach to risk that fails to take into account the individual woman and her needs and wishes. Another balancing act is essential if midwives are to ensure maternity services are risk aware as opposed to risk averse. If midwives are to play their part in ensuring success in meeting these two major challenges, it is critical that we have an educated, thoughtful and flexible workforce that is prepared to consider its practice to ensure that it delivers the very highest quality of service to women, achieves the best outcomes for mothers and babies and makes effective use of our limited resources.

Whilst the fundamentals of childbirth do not change, our understanding of the physiology of pregnancy and birth continues to develop as does our knowledge of the complex interplay of physical, emotional and social processes that contribute to the overall needs and experience of each woman, her baby and their family. More than ever before midwives must work as part of a network of maternity professionals and service provision and interact continuously with service users. It is essential that today's student midwives and midwives are helped to keep up to date and to modify their practice in the light of the latest knowledge and evidence.

*Mayes' Midwifery* is a vital resource for all of those working in the midwifery profession who are determined to make progress in meeting the broader political and social challenges that we face, whilst ensuring that they provide every individual with the highest quality of care. I believe that this text is an invaluable resource and commend it to you.

Professor Cathy Warwick CBE

# Preface

## to Mayes fourteenth edition

The transition to a multi-author and multi-expert resource for the midwife, developing a strong international reputation, began with the two previous editions of *Mayes' Midwifery*. Since the thirteenth edition, viewed positively by its student and midwife readers, the editors have further developed the text, aiming for a more concise style, with a smaller book. An extensive on-line resource supports the textbook, and includes additional reference material, explanatory sections and multiple choice quizzes, to enable readers to test their learning.

The aim has been to provide extensive research and evidence-based knowledge and information to support contemporary midwifery practice, in its myriad settings. This edition reflects the nature of midwifery today, and the needs of those who work globally, from highly technical settings to areas with minimal facilities. Ultimately, this should facilitate the knowledge, confidence and competence of the midwives, and improve care to women, babies and their families.

The concept described by François de la Rochefoucauld in the 17th century that 'The only thing constant in life is change' has underpinned the book and its accompanying web-site. This is illustrated by the stream of policy drivers, national and international reports and, above all, the changing needs of women and their families. Life has become more complex and thus maternity care has had to adapt and develop. Students and qualified midwives need knowledge, tools and resources that will support them in working with these changes, to be proactive rather than reactive and able to provide high quality, evidence-based, culturally sensitive and, above all, kind care to the woman and her family.

The foundations set by the *Winterton Report* (1992) and *Changing Childbirth* (1994) in England, have been and continue to be built upon. All four UK countries introduced policies for maternity services to work towards providing a more individualized and responsive service for women and their families, built on explicit and informed choice about all aspects of their care (Department of Health, 2004, 2007; Department of Health and Social Services Northern Ireland, 2004; Scottish Office, 2004; Welsh Office, 2004).

The World Health Organization initiative *Making Pregnancy Safer* and the *Global strategy for women and children's health* (2010) address international issues for midwifery, emphasizing the need for skilled and competent care as part of national policy initiatives. UK government policies have focused on guaranteeing choice on access to maternity care, place of birth, midwife-led care and the type of antenatal and postnatal care. Professional bodies, working alongside consumer pressure groups, have developed strategies and standards such as the Maternity Care Working Party joint statement *Making normal birth a reality* and the Royal College of Obstetricians and Gynaecologists, Royal College of Midwives, Royal College of Anaesthetists, Royal College of Paediatrics and Child Health (RCOG/RCM, RCA & RCPCH) *Standards for Maternity Care Report of a Working Party* (2008); and the *RCM Birth Centre Standards* (2009) and *Birth Centre Resources* (RCM 2010). These strategies have then led to initiatives such as the Scottish government's *Keeping Childbirth Natural and Dynamic* programme, the Royal College of Midwives' *Campaign for Normal Birth* and the development of midwife-led units and birth centres.

A crucial part of service provision has been finding out what service users think about the service. Recent reports include the Audit Commission's *Recorded delivery* (2007) and the Healthcare Commission's *Towards better births, A review of maternity services in England* (2009) which have highlighted some less-positive feelings about current maternity services, and in particular, postnatal care, oft quoted as the Cinderella of the maternity service.

The most recent joint work towards *Midwifery 2020*, a UK-wide document, has provided a strategic education and career pathway for midwives in the coming years, which should influence the education, continuing professional development and practice of midwives and supporting staff. This, alongside changes within the NHS and in the Higher Education sector, will impact on the role of the midwife. The role and sphere of practice is enshrined in statute within the UK, but can never be taken for granted. Midwives must continue to be prepared to practise to that role as autonomous, skilled practitioners, capable of developing and challenging their practice and working to the highest possible standard of care, and with the ability to work alongside the wider multidisciplinary healthcare team.

All of these developments provide challenges, new perspectives and opportunities, and underpin the development of this text; background rationale and application will be found in individual chapters. Whilst the text should, therefore, continue to be a key professional source, it will, with the secondary resources of the website, enable the reader to understand the context of care, and act as a signpost to gaining further information or knowledge.

We appreciate that to enable midwives to be effective, the initial pre-registration programme, now at degree level, has to be built upon, and this requires a constant process of updating, and refining one's personal store of professional knowledge. Knowing where to seek information and how to assimilate and question knowledge should be enhanced through the shape and structure of this book.

The book and web resource continue to have a strong physiological basis. There are chapters focusing on maternal, fetal and neonatal physiology and others, such as the chapters dealing with care in labour and the care of the newborn, weave physiology into applied practice. All chapters are fully referenced and well supported by research and evidence. Different approaches and perspectives appear throughout the text, making it an interesting and challenging resource for all of those interested in women's health and childbirth – both qualified and student readers.

The overall design of the chapters has been retained and further developed, with 'Learning outcomes' at the beginning of each chapter and 'Key points' at the end, to highlight the most important parts. Figures, diagrams and illustrations have been reviewed and added to, enhancing a strong visual impact. While a range of 'Reflective activities' have been retained within each chapter, there are further activities on the website that provide opportunities for the reader to consider how theories may be applied in practice. This should encourage readers to question practice and ask women about their experiences, helping midwives and potential midwives to make the maternity services safer and more user-friendly. The website provides an additional source of references and further reading, websites and electronic resources. All appropriate chapters have a number of multiple choice questions that the reader may use as self-testing/assessment to identify whether further study might be required.

In this exciting new edition, we had the challenge of producing a text that reflects the changes over the last 10 years as well as horizon scanning to identify possible further changes. We have been delighted to work with many of the original authors and welcome new contributors. All authors are experts and leaders in their field and have been enthusiastic and fully commited to developing their chapters and the online material. All have worked incredibly hard to produce a dynamic and accessible text, both for the book and the online resources. Many have taken a fresh approach, introducing new thinking and new ideas, which has made the task a real labour of love, and we hope the result will be useful, interesting and challenging to the readers.

The textbook will undoubtedly raise many questions, stimulate debate and hopefully encourage a spirit of enquiry. We see it as a stepping-stone for readers to explore beyond its pages to look at new evidence and the care we give as our knowledge expands, bearing in mind that evidence includes women's and midwives' experiences, as well as research.

We hope you enjoy using the 14th edition of *Mayes' Midwifery*. If you have any comments about the book we would be delighted to hear from you.

Sue Macdonald
Julia Magill-Cuerden
London, January 2011

## REFERENCES


Audit Commission: *First Class Delivery: improving maternity services in England and Wales*, Abingdon: 1997, Audit Commission.

Department of Health: *Maternity Matters: Choice, access and continuity of care in a safe service*, London, 2007, DH.

Department of Health: *Making it better: For mother and baby*, London, 2007, DH.

Department of Health: *National Service Framework for Children, Young People and Maternity Services: standard 11*, London, 2004, DH.

Department of Health: *Changing Childbirth. Report of the Expert Maternity Group (Cumberlege Report)*, London, 1993, HMSO.

Department of Health and Social Services Northern Ireland: *Delivering Choice: the report of the Northern Ireland Maternity Unit Study Group*, Belfast, 1994, DHSS.

Delivering the best: midwives' contribution to the NHS Plan http://www.dh.gov.uk/en/Publicationsandstatistics/Publications/PublicationsPolicyAndGuidance/DH_4128157 (accessed Jan 2011).

DHSS: *Report of the Northern Ireland. Maternity Group: Delivering Choice*, Belfast, 1994, DHSS.

Healthcare Commission: *Towards better births: a review of maternity services in England*, London, 2008, Healthcare Commission.

Healthcare Inspectorate Wales: *Maternity services in Wales – findings and themes from the All Wales Review*, Caerphilly, 2007, Healthcare Inspectors Wales.

Ladipo D, Reed H, Wilkinson F: *Changing Midwifery: working conditions and the quality of care*. Cambridge, 1999, ESRC Centre for Business Research, University of Cambridge.

Maternity Care Working Party Consensus statement from the Maternity Care Working Party: *Making normal birth a reality*, London, NCT.

National Childbirth Trust: *Ten Point Plan for Maternity Care*, London, 1998, NCT.

NCT: *Left to your own devices: The postnatal care experiences of 1260 first-time mothers*, London, 2010, NCT.

NCT: Postnatal care – still a Cinderella story? 2010.

National Perinatal and Epidemiology Unit: *Recorded delivery: a national survey of women's experience of maternity care*, Oxford, 2007, NPEU.

NICE: *Antenatal care: Routine care for the healthy pregnant woman*, London, 2008, NICE.

RCM: *Vision 2000*, London, 2000, RCM.

RCM: *Socioeconomic value of the midwife*, London, 2010, RCM.

RCOG/RCM: *Safer childbirth: Minimum Standards for the Organisation and delivery of care in labour*, London, 2007, RCOG Press.

Scottish Executive: *A framework for maternity services in Scotland*, Edinburgh, 2001, Scottish Executive.

Scottish Programme for Clinical Effectiveness in Reproductive Health: *Maternity Care Matters: an audit of maternity services in Scotland*, Edinburgh, 1999, SPCERH.

SEHD: A Framework for Maternity Services: Scotland, 2001.

Scottish Governnment: Implementing A Framework for Maternity Services in Scotland: Overview Report of the Expert Group on Acute Maternity Services, 2003.

Scottish Government: Keeping Childbirth Natural and Dynamic (KCND) programme, 2009.

Scottish Office Home and Health Department: *Provision of Maternity Services in Scotland: A Policy Review*, Edinburgh, 1993, HMSO.

Singh D, Newburn M: *Access to maternity information and support: the experiences and needs of women before and after giving birth London*, London, 2000, National Childbirth Trust.

Standing Nursing and Midwifery Advisory Committee: *Midwifery: delivering our future*, London, 1998, Department of Health.

Welsh Assembly Government: *Delivering the future in Wales: a framework for realising the potential of midwives in Wales*, Cardiff, 2002, Welsh Assembly Government.

Welsh Health Planning Forum: *Protocol for investment in the health gain: maternal and early health*, Cardiff, 1991, WHPF.

World Health Organization: *Having a Baby in Europe. Public Health in Europe 26*, Copenhagen, 1985, WHO.

World Health Organization, Maternal and Newborn Health/Safe Motherhood Unit: *Care in Normal Birth: a practical guide*, Geneva, 1996, WHO.

World Health Organization: Making Pregnancy Safer website 2010. http://who.int/making_pregnancy_safer/en/

World Health Organization: *Global Strategy for Women's and Children's Health Making Pregnancy Safer* (website). http://who.int/making_pregnancy_safer/en/. Accessed 2010.

# Acknowledgements

Many people have contributed to and supported the development of this textbook, with its online resources, throughout its long gestation. Most importantly, we wish to sincerely thank our many authors, all busy and expert practitioners, who have worked so incredibly hard on both the book and the online material, coping with the deadlines, and thinking creatively to make the content alive and contemporary for the reader. We also thank the many contributors to previous editions, whose work has been the foundation for the development of this edition. Without the input from so many midwife and professional authors who have been concerned to ensure current evidence for practice, this edition would not have achieved its current quality.

We would also like to thank our organisations, Thames Valley University and the Royal College of Midwives, who remained supportive to both of us.

As always, however, it is our friends and families who have had less of our time and attention, and who have been unfailingly supportive and generous in enabling us both to live transfixed to computers, websites and mountains of proofs. A special thank you again goes to Alison Macdonald for providing particular expert advice and information.

Without our colleagues Sheila Black, Mairi McCubbin and, latterly, Glenys Norquay at Elsevier, who have seen this edition through from its inception, and who have provided us with guidance on the publishing processes, we could not have completed this text and its resources. Our thanks go to them for their continued support.

# Part 1

# The midwife in context

Chapter | 1 |

# The global midwife

Gaynor D. Maclean

## LEARNING OUTCOMES

After reading this chapter, you will be able to:

- gain insight into critical issues affecting maternal and newborn health worldwide
- consider the Millennium Development Goals (MDGs) relevant to midwifery practice and reflect on their significance
- identify the major causes of maternal death historically and geographically, exploring predisposing factors
- consider the role of international organizations
- reflect on your place as a midwife in the global context.

## CHALLENGES IN GLOBAL MIDWIFERY FOR THE 21ST CENTURY

Midwives originating from the West will hold very different perspectives of childbirth and midwifery practice compared with colleagues from other countries, especially those classified as less and least developed (WHO 2007). Midwives worldwide aim to provide a safe environment for birth. However, countless women in today's world are forced to experience childbirth, not as a fulfilling experience, but as one fraught with fear and danger. In the 21st century, a majority of women still cannot dissociate birth from death. Consequently, midwives are challenged to play a leading part in making childbirth safer. Of the 130 million babies born worldwide each year, it is estimated that almost 8 million die before their first birthday, 4 million in the first month of life (WHO 2006a).

The Millennium Development Goals (MDGs) (see website) include efforts to improve the health of both women and children, particularly in the context of poverty and disease (Box 1.1). Making pregnancy safer challenges not only health professionals, but also technical experts, including water engineers, road builders, telecommunication experts and vehicle mechanics. Community mobilization even in the farthest reaches of the globe needs to find resonance in political will at the highest levels.

## CONTRASTS AND INEQUALITIES

It has been stressed that one of the most striking measurable contrasts between industrialized and developing countries becomes evident in examining maternal mortality ratios. The 2005 estimates confirm the highest figures in sub-Saharan Africa followed by South Asia (Table 1.1). Globally, the maternal mortality ratio (MMR) (see Ch. 16) reduction has proceeded on average by 1% between 1990 and 2005. MMR, as a key indicator for MDG 5 (Box 1.1), needs to decrease at a much faster rate if this goal is to be met (WHO 2007).

On a global scale, it is estimated that every minute of every day, a woman dies of pregnancy-related complications; the massive death toll exceeds half a million each year (WHO 2008a); 99% of these deaths occur in developing countries, figures varying considerably (Table 1.1). Motherless newborns are between 3 and 10 times more likely to die than those whose mothers survive (UNICEF 2008a).

### Causes of maternal death

#### Main causes

In developing countries, maternal death is the second most common cause of death after HIV/AIDS. There are five main obstetric causes of maternal death worldwide: haemorrhage, infection, unsafe abortion, hypertensive disorders and obstructed labour (WHO 2008a). Haemorrhage accounts for around a quarter of deaths globally.

However, the leading cause of death tends to vary with the region (see Table 1.2). In many countries, adolescent mothers are twice as likely to die as other pregnant women (WHO 2008a) (see Ch. 16).

**Box 1.1 The millennium development goals**

1. Eradicate extreme poverty and hunger
2. Achieve universal primary education
3. Promote gender equality and empower women
4. Reduce child mortality
5. Improve maternal health
6. Combat HIV/AIDS, malaria and other diseases
7. Ensure environmental sustainability
8. Develop a global partnership for development

Source: UN 2008

## Predisposing factors

Maternal death is influenced by numerous factors. The reasons why women die have been described as 'many layered' (AbouZahr & Royston 1991). These layers include *social, cultural* and *political* factors that determine crucial issues including the *status of women, women's health* and *fertility*, and their *'health-seeking behaviour'*. *Failures in healthcare systems* and *transportation* add to the problems.

One of the issues confronting an estimated 100–140 million women and girls each year is *female genital mutilation* (FGM) (see website and Ch. 58). The United Nations agencies are committed to addressing this practice which violates the human rights of a person (WHO 2008a).

Although sub-Saharan Africa accommodates just over 10% of the world population, 63% of all *HIV infections* are evident there (UNAIDS/WHO 2006). Linkage between HIV and maternal mortality has been established in the

**Table 1.1 Maternal and neonatal mortality across the globe**

| UN region | Maternal mortality ratio 2005[1] | No of maternal deaths 2005[1] | Lifetime risk of maternal death 2005[1] | Neonatal mortality rate (per 1000 live births) 2000[2] |
|---|---|---|---|---|
| World | 400 | 536,000 | 1 in 92 | 30 |
| Developed regions | 9 | 960 | 1 in 7300 | 5 |
| Developing regions | 450 | 533,000 | 1 in 75 | Less developed = 33<br>Least developed = 42 |
| Commonwealth of Independent States | 51 | 1800 | 1 in 1200 | – |
| Africa | 820 | 276,000 | 1 in 26 | 41 |
| Northern Africa | 160 | 5700 | 1 in 210 | 22 |
| Sub-Saharan Africa | 900 | 270,000 | 1 in 22 | Eastern = 42<br>Middle = 26<br>Southern = 23<br>Western = 49 |
| Asia | 330 | 241,000 | 1 in 120 | 32 |
| Eastern Asia | 50 | 9200 | 1 in 1200 | 21 |
| Southern Asia | 490 | 188,000 | 1 in 61 | 43 |
| SE Asia | 300 | 35,000 | 1 in 130 | 19 |
| Western Asia | 160 | 8300 | 1 in 170 | 28 |
| Latin America & Caribbean | 130 | 1500 | 1 in 290 | 15 |
| Oceania | 430 | 890 | 1 in 62 | 26 |

Sources: [1]WHO 2007; [2]WHO 2006a
Japan, Australia and New Zealand have been excluded from the regional figures and included in the 'developed regions'

**Table 1.2 Maternal mortality causes per UN region**

| Cause of death | Africa | Asia | Latin America | Developed countries |
|---|---|---|---|---|
| Haemorrhage | ***33.9%*** | ***30.8%*** | ***20.8%*** | ***13.4%*** |
| Anaemia | 3.7% | ***12.8%*** | 0.1% | 0 |
| Obstructed labour | 4.1% | 9.4% | ***13.4%*** | 0 |
| HIV/AIDS | 6.2% | 0 | 0 | 0 |
| Sepsis | 9.7% | ***11.6%*** | 7.7% | 2.1% |
| Abortion | 3.9% | 5.7% | ***12%*** | 8.2% |
| Hypertensive disorders | 9.1% | 9.1% | ***25.7%*** | ***16.1%*** |
| Embolism | 2% | 0.4% | 0.6% | ***14.9%*** |
| Ectopic pregnancy | 0.5% | 0.1% | 0.5% | 4.9% |
| Other direct causes* | 4.9% | 1.6% | 3.8% | ***21.3%*** |
| Other indirect causes** | ***16.7%*** | ***12.5%*** | 3.9% | ***14.4%*** |
| Unclassified deaths | 5.4% | 6.1% | ***11.7%*** | 0 |

*'Other direct causes' include operative and anaesthetic complications
**'Other indirect causes' include malaria and heart disease
Leading causes of death in each region (>10%) are indicated in bold italics
Sources: WHO 2005

region (DFID 2005). *Malaria* kills more than a million each year and pregnant women and their unborn children are particularly vulnerable, placing them at risk for low birthweight and anaemia (UNICEF 2007). HIV is thought to increase the susceptibility of multigravid women to pregnancy-associated malaria (Keen et al 2007).

In addition to the 1500 women who die daily due to pregnancy-related causes, 10,000 newborn babies die, and it is estimated that most of these deaths could be prevented through skilled care during childbirth and the management of life-threatening complications (WHO 2008b). Whereas more than 99% of births are attended by skilled personnel in the most developed countries, this reduces to 59% and 34% respectively in the less and least developed countries (WHO 2007). It is estimated that mortality and morbidity in the perinatal and neonatal periods are caused mainly by preventable or treatable conditions (WHO 2006a). Infections, including pneumonia and neonatal tetanus, asphyxia, preterm birth and congenital anomalies contribute to 36% of the global deaths in children under 5 years (UNICEF 2007).

## Maternal morbidity

*Morbidity* is less easily measurable. It is estimated that of the 136 million women who give birth each year, 20 million suffer pregnancy-related illness (WHO 2008a). The term 'severe acute maternal morbidity' (SAMM) has recently entered obstetric literature, several definitions include the concept of 'near-miss' and a situation where pregnancy-related complications lead to the failure of body organs. Utilizing the latter concept, it has been estimated that 4–8% of women in resource-poor areas will experience SAMM, compared with 1% in more developed areas (WHO 2005). Horrific injuries such as obstetric fistulae (see website), stigmatizing women in their families and communities, have been described as one of the most visible indicators of the massive gaps in maternal healthcare between the developing and developed world (WHO 2006b). Other morbidities include anaemia, infertility and depression.

## Inequalities associated with being a mother

The experience of childbearing can be vastly different depending on the country of residence. Comparisons of data in Tables 1.3 and 1.4 provide insight into some of the major factors affecting women in the 21st century.

The *highest numbers* of women and children who die are evident in India, Nigeria and Pakistan, and the 10 countries listed in Table 1.5 contribute to the majority of global maternal and neonatal deaths.

**Table 1.3** The top ten *best* places to be a mother

| Rank[1] – from best | Country | MMR (2005)[2] | Lifetime risk of dying in pregnancy (2005)[2] | Female life expectancy at birth (years)[1] | Maternity leave benefits[1] | |
|---|---|---|---|---|---|---|
| | | | | | Length | % of wages paid* |
| 1 | Sweden | 3 | 1 in 17,400 | 83 | 14 weeks | 80–100 |
| 2 | Iceland | 4 | 1 in 12,700 | 83 | 3 months | 80 |
| 3 | Norway | 4 | 1 in 7700 | 82 | 42–52 weeks | 80–100 |
| 4 | New Zealand | 9 | 1 in 5900 | 82 | 14 weeks | 100 |
| 5 | Australia | 4 | 1 in 13,300 | 83 | 52 weeks | 0 |
| 6 | Denmark | 3 | 1 in 17,800 | 80 | 18 weeks | 90 |
| 7 | Finland | 7 | 1 in 8500 | 82 | 105 days | 100 |
| 8 | Belgium | 8 | 1 in 7800 | 83 | 15 weeks | 83 |
| 9 | Spain | 4 | 1 in 16,400 | | | |
| 10 | Germany | 4 | 1 in 19,200 | 82 | 14 weeks | 100 |

Skilled attendance at delivery reported consistently at >99% in this group
*These figures provide a rough guide in some cases; payment may vary, for example, before and after birth or over time
Sources: [1]SC 2007; [2]WHO 2007

**Table 1.4** The top ten *worst* places to be a mother

| Rank[1] – from worst | Country | MMR (2005)[2] | Lifetime risk of dying in pregnancy (2005)[2] | Skilled attendance at delivery 2000–2006[2] | Female life expectancy at birth (years)[1] | Expected no of years of formal schooling for girls[1] | % women using modern contraception[1] |
|---|---|---|---|---|---|---|---|
| 1 | Niger | 1800 | 1 in 7 | 15.7% (2000) | 45 | 3 | 4 |
| 2 | Sierra Leone | 2100 | 1 in 8 | 41.7% (2000) | 43 | 4 | 6 |
| 3 | Yemen | 430 | 1 in 39 | 21.6% (1997) | 63 | 7 | 10 |
| 4 | Chad | 1500 | 1 in 11 | 14.4% (2000) | 54 | 4 | 2 |
| 5 | Guinea Bissau | 1100 | 1 in 13 | 34.7% (2000) | 47 | 4 | 4 |
| 6 | Angola | 1400 | 1 in 12 | 47.1% (2000) | 43 | 3 | 5 |
| 7 | Eritrea | 450 | 1 in 44 | 28.2% (2003) | 57 | 5 | 5 |
| 8 | Ethiopia | 720 | 1 in 27 | 5.6% (2000) | 49 | 5 | 6 |
| 9 | Burkina Faso | 700 | 1 in 22 | 56.5% (2003) | 49 | 4 | 9 |
| 10 | Djibouti | 650 | 1 in 35 | 60.6% (2003) | 55 | 3 | – |

[1]SC 2007
[2]WHO 2007

**Table 1.5 The top ten countries* with the highest *numbers* of maternal and child deaths (representing approximately 60% of the global MMR & NMR totals)**

| Country | Number of maternal deaths[1] | Maternal mortality ratio (MMR) (2005)[2] | Number of child deaths[1] (under 5 years) | Neonatal mortality rate (2000)[3] | Life expectancy at birth (male + female) (2006)[3] | Lifetime risk of dying in pregnancy 2005[3] | Skilled attendance at delivery 2000–2006[3] |
|---|---|---|---|---|---|---|---|
| 1. India | 136,000 | 450 | 1,929,000 | 43 | 64 years | 1 in 70 | 47% |
| 2. Nigeria | 37,000 | 1100 | 1,043,000 | 53 | 47 years | 1 in 18 | 35% |
| 3. Pakistan | 26,000 | 320 | 473,000 | 57 | 65 years | 1 in 74 | 31% |
| 4. DR Congo | 24,000 | 1100 | 589,000 | 47 | – | 1 in 13 | 61% |
| 5. Ethiopia | 24,000 | 720 | 509,000 | 51 | 39 years | 1 in 27 | 6% |
| 6. Afghanistan | 20,000 | 1800 | 370,000 | 60 | 43 years | 1 in 8 | 14% |
| 7. Bangladesh | 16,000 | 570 | 274,000 | 36 | 43 years | 1 in 51 | 20% |
| 8. China | 11,000 | 45 | 467,000 | 21 | 52 years | 1 in 1300 | 98% |
| 9. Angola | 11,000 | 1400 | 199,000 | 54 | 42 years | 1 in 12 | 45% |
| 10. Uganda | 10,000 | 550 | 200,000 | 32 | 50 years | 1 in 25 | 42% |

*Ranked in order of the ten countries demonstrating the highest numbers of maternal deaths. Where two countries display the same number of maternal deaths, the country with the higher number of child deaths is ranked higher.
Sources: [1]SC 2007; [2]WHO 2007; [3]UNICEF 2007

Survival of women at risk is extremely precarious in countries where health services are inaccessible, inadequate or non-existent. Risk is not eliminated in the West; vulnerable women still face enormous challenges to achieving safe childbirth wherever they struggle to exist.

## THE SAFE MOTHERHOOD INITIATIVE

It was estimated that 88–98% of all maternal deaths could 'probably have been avoided' (WHO 1986). Consequently, the *Safe Motherhood Initiative* was inaugurated in 1987 with the aim of reducing maternal mortality and morbidity by 50% by 2000 (SMI 1987).

Action messages agreed by Safe Motherhood Partners in 1997, setting priorities for the next decade (Box 1.2), find resonance today in the MDGs, including the current emphasis on safe motherhood and human rights. In order to work towards the MDGs (Box 1.1), many governments have committed to reducing poverty and promoting human rights when providing aid to the developing world (DFID 2006, Sveriges Riksdag 2005).

**Box 1.2 Action messages for the next decade for the Safe Motherhood Initiative**

1. Advance safe motherhood through human rights
2. Empower women; ensure choices
3. Perceive safe motherhood as a vital social and economic investment
4. Delay marriage and first birth
5. Acknowledge that every pregnancy faces risks
6. Ensure skilled attendance at delivery
7. Improve access to quality maternal health services
8. Prevent unwanted pregnancy; address unsafe abortion
9. Measure progress
10. Utilize the power of partnership

Source: FCI 1997

**Reflective activity 1.1**

Consider the Millennium Development Goals (Box 1.1).

- How do these goals challenge your current midwifery practice?
- What challenges do you think midwives working in the least developed countries face in trying to achieve these goals?
- How may midwives in industrialized countries co-operate with them in this challenge?

## THE IMPACT OF MODERNIZATION AND DEVELOPMENT

The process of modernization and development is inextricably linked with numerous health issues. Undoubtedly, as countries develop, childbirth becomes safer. This is a complex issue and the reader would do well to explore it further (Fig. 1.1). Progress of modernity tends to be inversely related to the lifetime risk of dying in childbirth. The website section entitled 'The significance of historical issues' offers explanations of how historical use of data has significance in understanding relationships between

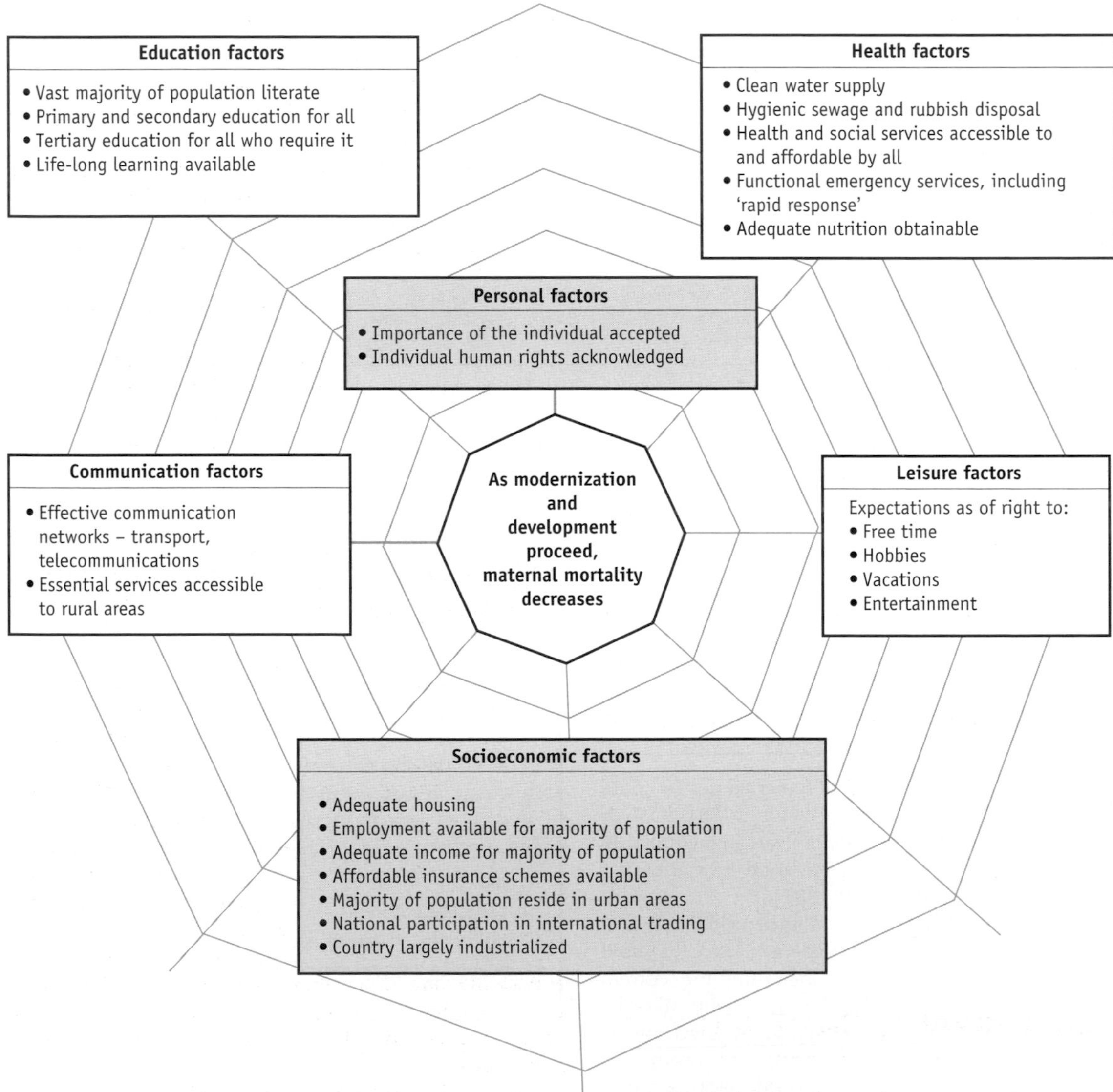


**Figure 1.1** Modernity and mortality: a complex web of 'interrelated developmental factors'.

developments in maternity care and its practice influencing the safety of birth.

## ENSURING SKILLED CARE DURING CHILDBIRTH

During the second decade of the Safe Motherhood Initiative, focus moved towards a new era in promoting the concept of skilled care at every delivery. The term 'skilled attendant' refers exclusively to people with midwifery skills who have been 'trained to proficiency' in the necessary skills to enable them to 'manage normal deliveries and diagnose, manage or refer complications'. These may be doctors, midwives or nurses but do not include traditional birth attendants (WHO 2000). The skilled attendant at delivery is regarded as a 'reproductive health indicator' (WHO 2006c) and as such is considered a proxy for a healthcare provider who can provide skilled care throughout pregnancy, labour and the postnatal period.

Political commitment has been historically and contemporarily associated with successful MMR reduction. Cuba, Malaysia, Sri Lanka, and Thailand were amongst the countries that made earlier progress in reducing MMR and political commitment was critical to this (WHO 1998).

## EPIDEMIOLOGICAL FACTORS

If skilled attendance during childbirth were the only issue claiming association with significant MMR reduction, cause and effect, process and outcome may be easier to define and declare. However, socioeconomic and demographic indicators have been associated with safer childbirth internationally. These include female literacy rate, total fertility rate and urban population (see website for definitions).

Women living in rural areas are least likely to have access to skilled care, since the majority of the health services are habitually situated in urban areas. This issue is compounded by problems of transport and communication. Skilled attendants without access to essential equipment and a functional referral chain will be limited in their ability to save life, therefore the 'enabling environment' forms an essential component of promoting safer childbirth (WHO 2004, WHO 2008b). In countries with high MMRs there is often poverty, illiteracy, malnutrition and a low social status of women (Hafez 1998).

## INTERNATIONAL ORGANIZATIONS

International organizations may comprise governmental, intergovernmental or non-governmental organizations. There are also voluntary organizations, both religious and secular. Currently, there is an explosion of international aid sweeping into a volatile world economy, with an apparent movement of wealth from rich to poor nations. However, the reality is more complex. Issues surrounding aid and trade between governments and the role of such giant organizations as the World Bank have long raised ethical queries concerning who really benefits from some aid schemes (Juva 1994, Madeley et al 1994). The reader may find it instructive to consider the role of governments as well as international organizations in the context of poverty relief and debt repayment.

Without underestimating the valuable contribution of numerous others, some of the important organizations for international developments in maternity care are, for example:

- International organizations:
  The World Health Organization
  United Nations Children's Fund (UNICEF)
- Midwifery organizations:
  The International Confederation of Midwives (ICM)
  Africa Midwives Research Network (AMRN)
- Other important international organizations:
  The Partnership for Maternal, Newborn and Child Health (PMNCH)
  The White Ribbon Alliance for Safe Motherhood (WRA)
- European Committees relevant to midwifery:
  The European Midwives Association (EMA)
  Action for Global Health (AfGH).

Brief descriptions of each of these organizations are given on the website.

## THE PLACE OF THE MIDWIFE IN THE GLOBAL CONTEXT

In the 21st century the world is increasingly described as a global village. Communications expedite both travel and news. Increased awareness should assist the global battle to combat the ever-present dangers and death associated with giving birth in the less developed areas of the world. Midwives, similar to other professionals, are likely to travel to other countries for study or work temporarily or permanently. The migration of workers from east to west has caused much heart searching in recent years. Migration rates of health workers trained in countries across Africa vary between 8% and 60% (Sambo 2007). There is an ethical dilemma associated with the *'brain drain'* that saps poor countries struggling with massive health issues to supplement relative shortages in the wealthier western hemisphere.

Overall, Africa faces a shortage of 800,000 doctors and nurses and it is estimated that only 10–30% of the required skilled health workers are trained. It is from this situation that 20,000 skilled health professionals are lost each year through migration (Bruntland & Robinson 2008). Yet the right of individuals to improve their own career prospects and lift their families out of poverty is also an issue.

In order to identify situations in which the health-related MDGs, including MDG 5, are very unlikely to be achieved, WHO has indicated a *workforce density threshold*. Currently, 57 countries fall below this threshold and are classified as suffering a critical shortage of health workers. Thirty-six of these 57 countries are in Africa. This represents a global deficit of 2.4 million doctors, nurses and midwives. The greatest proportional shortfalls are reported in sub-Saharan Africa and enormous deficits related to population size exist in SE Asia (WHO 2006d). Not surprisingly, such statistics are commonly associated with countries reporting high maternal and child mortality figures (Tables 1.1, 1.4 and 1.5; see website).

Amongst the factors underlying the critical shortages in Africa, poverty and weak planning without appropriate motivation and retention schemes have been identified. In some countries, more physicians than midwives are being trained (Sambo 2007). It is estimated that between 2008 and 2015, another 330,000 midwives are required to achieve universal skilled care during childbirth (WHO 2008a).

To try to redress this crisis, international agreements have been formulated. These include a joint investment in research and information systems; agreements on ethical recruitment of, and working conditions for, migrant health workers; plus international planning of health workforces for humanitarian emergencies and global health threats. A commitment from donor countries to assist crisis countries in efforts to improve and support the health workforce has also been agreed (WHO 2006d).

**Reflective activity 1.2**

Think about the concept of 'skilled attendance during childbirth'.

- How would you define 'skilled'?
- What national and local policies aim to ensure skilled attendance for every woman in your area of practice?
- What issues need to be addressed in order to ensure that midwives in your country acquire, retain and can utilize the clinical skills that you consider critical to promoting safe childbirth?

## IMPORTANT CONSIDERATIONS FOR MIDWIVES INTENDING TO WORK OVERSEAS

In the context of promoting safer childbirth worldwide (MDG 5), midwives may find that they are increasingly in demand for short-term or long-term assignments in countries struggling to address these critical issues. Some may also travel to more developed countries for study tours or personal professional advancement. Midwives practising in any country other than that in which they were educated must adapt to vastly differing situations.

*Midwives who have been educated in an industrialized country* intending to work in a less developed country need to have considerable experience and be conversant with relevant and current evidence-based practice. It can be helpful to learn some advanced clinical skills where practicable; for example, vacuum extraction, suturing cervical and vaginal tears, manual removal of placenta, neonatal intubation, inserting intrauterine contraceptive devices. Regulations may restrict midwives from acquiring some of these skills in the UK, but policy and tradition can sometimes be overcome in consultation with obstetricians and supervisors of midwives willing to arrange suitable learning opportunities. Short courses in tropical medicine and health can be most valuable. Discussions with persons experienced in the intended country of practice can be invaluable.

National authorities will specify their own country's priorities in health. Increasingly, needs are expressed for midwives with expertise in education or management, but all midwives must be clinically skilled, able and willing to adapt to local needs. Ability to speak another language or a willingness to learn is an asset, and respect for different cultures and religions crucial. It is important for any expatriate workers to appreciate that they will never know, nor understand, many things in another country and that change must come from *within* a country. They must appreciate that 'experts' from another country can best help colleagues by demonstrating appropriate knowledge, skills and attitudes with sensitivity. Midwives practising in cross-cultural situations need an acute sense of awareness, and an attitude of humility and willingness to learn. In a developing country, they need to be able to empathize with colleagues working in very different situations, exercise patience and cope using extremely limited resources.

*Midwives who have been educated in less developed countries* intending working or studying in industrialized countries will find more advanced technology in use than experienced at home. There may also be more emphasis on informed choice for women and partnership in care. They may be migrating to a society that is very litigation conscious and so will find that medico-legal issues impact upon midwifery and medical practice. Midwives therefore need a good understanding of current issues and popular demands, and may need to undertake an orientation programme. They must constantly update their knowledge and practice by critically evaluating research. There are benefits and hazards associated with both technology and freedom of choice demanding consideration. In returning to developing countries, indigenous midwives, as do expatriates, need to evaluate new practices in the light of local situations, available resources and national priorities, before attempting to transfer them from one country to another.

Midwives who have practised in countries where resources are scarce may be skilled at improvising and can sometimes share innovations with colleagues who face different, though significant, resource limitations. Midwives who have practised in regions remote from medical services can share with colleagues their experience of complications rarely seen in the West. It is salutary for all midwives to appreciate the consequences of delayed referral and intervention; the reality of, for example, obstructed labour and ruptured uterus, as inevitable consequences of cephalopelvic disproportion, and the frightening speed with which septicaemia can occur. Such complications will, of course, result in maternal death anywhere in the world unless there is appropriate and skilled intervention.

## CONCLUSION

Issues relating to global midwifery have now become an essential component of the body of knowledge owned by midwives working in the West. In less developed countries, safer childbirth continues to receive increasing attention with the advent of the MDGs (Box 1.1). Safety is at the heart of every midwife's practice, and whilst tragedies associated with childbirth are not observed on such a great scale in the West, experiences from the rest of the world can provide salutary lessons about fundamentals of midwifery care. Assertions that 'that could never happen here' must find evidence in reality. Safety needs to continue to be a priority in every country, including the UK. Historically, midwives have played a critical part and the concept of promoting maternal and neonatal health still falls naturally into the midwife's domain. It is midwives who make their profession what it is today and what it will be tomorrow, globally. This warrants critical evaluation and constant reappraisal of essential professional issues, including midwifery curricula, standards of practice, protocol and policy, professional politics and practice ethics. These must reflect safety as a priority. Other issues, whilst important, will always be secondary.

During the first decade of the 21st century it has been recognized that 'the main obstacle to progress towards better health for mothers is the lack of skilled care' (WHO 2008a). Midwives represent a large part of the solution to this dilemma. The global midwife holds the key to a chance of life instead of death for the world's childbearing women. Obstetric and paediatric colleagues form essential links in the life-saving chain that can bring hope to women, families and their communities in the most desperate need. The right to live is the most fundamental human right and midwives across the globe need to meet the challenge of the coming decades with superlative skills, infinite commitment and an enduring determination.

## KEY POINTS

- MMRs vary enormously across the globe, with large discrepancies between industrialized and least developed countries; hence the rationale for activities directed at promoting maternal and neonatal health. Midwives play a key role in working towards the Millennium Development Goals (MDGs).
- There are five major causes of maternal death worldwide, predisposed to by numerous and complex factors. The World Health Organization estimates that most of these deaths are avoidable. Promoting safer childbirth embraces health, education, socioeconomic and political issues. Skilled attendance during childbirth is a key indicator for MDG 5. Numerous international organizations exist giving priority to promoting maternal and child health.
- Migration of skilled health workers severely compromises critical human resources in many developing countries where maternal and newborn mortality remain high.
- Historical experience of MMR reduction in the West offers some inspiration in world regions where risks associated with childbirth remain as high in the 21st century as they were in the West more than a century ago.
- Internationally, high female literacy rates, low total fertility rates and large urban population ratios have been associated with MMR reduction.
- A midwife intending to work internationally needs special preparation, but considering her role as a global midwife should enrich personal professional development wherever she chooses to practise.

## REFERENCES


AbouZahr C, Royston E, editors: *Maternal mortality: a global factbook*, Geneva, 1991, WHO.

Bruntland GH, Robinson M: *Advancing global health: a shared responsibility* (website). www.everyhumanhasrights.org. 2008. Accesssed August 21, 2008.

Department for International Development (DFID): *DFID's maternal health strategy, reducing maternal deaths: evidence and action*, 1st Progress Report, December 2005, London, 2005, DFID.

Department for International Development (DFID): *Eliminating world poverty. Making governance work for the poor*, London, 2006, DFID.

Family Care International (FCI): *The Safe Motherhood Action Agenda: priorities for the next decade*. Report on the Safe Motherhood Technical Consultation, 18–23 October 1997, Colombo, Sri Lanka, New York, 1997, FCI.

Hafez G: Maternal mortality: a neglected and socially unjustifiable tragedy, *Eastern Mediterranean Health Journal* 4(1):7–10, 1998.

Juva M: The roots of development co-operation. In Lankinen KS, Bergstrom S, Makela PH, et al, editors: *Health and disease in developing countries*, London, 1994, Macmillan.

Keen J, Serghides L, Ayi K, et al: HIV impairs opsonic phagocytic clearance of pregnancy-associated malaria parasites, *Plos Medicine* 4(5):e181, 2007.

Madeley J, Sullivan D, Woodroffe J: *Who runs the world?* London, 1994, Christian Aid.

Safe Motherhood Initiative (SMI): *Preventing the tragedy of maternal deaths*. A report of the International Safe Motherhood Conference, Nairobi, Kenya, February 1987, Geneva, 1987, WHO.

Sambo LG: Message of the Regional Director on the occasion of World Health Day 2006, *African Health Monitor* 7(1):1–3, 2007.

Save the Children (SC): *The state of the world's mothers 2007 – saving the lives of children under 5*, Connecticut, 2007, Save the Children.

Sveriges Riksdag (Swedish Parliament): *Sweden's new policy for global development*, Stockholm, 2005, The Swedish Parliament.

UN: *Millennium Development Goals* (website). www.un.org/millenniumgoals/. 2008. Accessed August 5, 2008.

UNAIDS/WHO: *Fact Sheet 06. Sub-Saharan Africa*. Last updated December 2006. Geneva, 2006, WHO.

United Nations Children's Fund (UNICEF): (2007) *The state of the world's children*, New York, 2007, UNICEF.

UNICEF: *99%: the proportion of maternal deaths that occur in developing countries* (website). www.unicef.org/factoftheweek/index_39707.html. 2008a. Accessed August 28, 2008.

World Health Organization (WHO): Maternal mortality: helping women off the road to death, *WHO Chronicle* 40(5):175–183, 1986.

World Health Organization (WHO): *Country profiles of reproductive health indicators*, Updated November 1998, Geneva, 1998, WHO.

World Health Organization (WHO): *Update of statement on the 'skilled attendant at delivery' in WHO (1999) Reduction of maternal mortality. A ioint statement WHO/UNFPA/UNICEF/World Bank*, Geneva, 2000, WHO.

World Health Organization (WHO): *Making pregnancy safer, the critical role of the skilled attendant. A joint statement by WHO, ICM & FIGO*, Geneva, 2004, WHO.

World Health Organization (WHO): Systematic review reveals main causes of maternal mortality and morbidity, *Progress in Reproductive Health Research* 71:5–7, 2005.

World Health Organization (WHO): *Neonatal and perinatal mortality: country, regional and global estimates*, Geneva, 2006a, WHO.

World Health Organization (WHO): *Obstetric fistula. Guiding principles for clinical management and programme development*, Geneva, 2006b, WHO.

World Health Organization (WHO): *Reproductive health indicators. Guidelines for their generation, interpretation and analysis for global monitoring*, Geneva, 2006c, WHO.

World Health Organization (WHO): *WHO fact sheet No 301. Migration of health workers*, Geneva, 2006d, WHO.

World Health Organization (WHO): *Maternal mortality estimates in 2005 developed by WHO, UNICEF, ENFPA & the World Bank*, Geneva, 2007, WHO.

World Health Organization (WHO): *Ten facts on maternal health* (website). www.who.int/features/factfiles/maternal_health/en/index.html. 2008a. Accessed August 27, 2008.

World Health Organization (WHO): Department of Making Pregnancy Safer Annual Report 2007, Geneva, 2008b, WHO.

Chapter | 2 |

# A history of the midwifery profession in the United Kingdom

*Jean Donnison*

**LEARNING OUTCOMES**

After reading this chapter, you should be able to appreciate:

- the significance of socioeconomic factors in the development of an occupation
- the extent to which ruling ideas about women's abilities and social status have affected the occupation of midwife in the UK
- the innate power of healthy women, except in a small minority of cases, to give birth safely without intervention
- the importance of clarity and rigour in the use of concepts like 'normality' and 'risk'
- the necessity for persistence, patience, pugnacity and organization among midwives to the continuance of the midwifery profession as guardians of normal childbirth.

## THE OFFICE OF MIDWIFE: A FEMALE DOMAIN

The office of midwife is a truly ancient calling. Sculptures of midwives attending birth date back at least 8000 years and the old Egyptian fertility goddess, Hat-hor, was frequently portrayed in this role. Midwives appear, too, in the Old Testament; the quick-witted Shiprah and Puah outmanoeuvre Pharaoh, and the birth of Tamar's twins testifies to the midwife's resourcefulness and skill.

Until early modern times, childbirth was considered a female province, of which women alone had special understanding. No word existed in any language to signify a *male* birth attendant, and when these appeared in the late 16th century, new terms had to be created. The Anglo-Saxon 'midwife', or 'with-woman', denotes the office of *being with* the labouring woman. Other titles like the old French *'leveuse'* and the German *'hebamme'* imply her function of *receiving the child.* The later French usage, *'sage-femme'* (wise-woman), implies wider concerns and, indeed, midwives were commonly consulted on matters of fertility, female ailments, and care of the newborn.

Occasionally, when instruments were necessary to extract the child, a man might be called in. Traditionally, their use belonged to surgeons, who, with the increasing exclusion of women from medicine and surgery from the 1300s, were overwhelmingly men. Yet the surgeon's scope was limited. Using hooks and knives, he might extract piecemeal an infant presumed dead or, hoping to save its life, swiftly perform a caesarean section on the newly dead mother. Hence a man's advent into the birth chamber usually presaged the death of mother or child, or both. Where surgeons were not available, however, midwives themselves might undertake such operations. In wealthy households, a physician (a university-educated practitioner of internal medicine), whose midwifery knowledge came from classical writings rather than practical experience, might be called to prescribe medicines judged necessary for mother or child.

### What manner of women were midwives?

Little is known about individual European midwives before the 16th century. As later, they would be married women or widows, generally of middle age or older. Most would have given birth, since until the late 1700s this experience, except for daughters following their mothers into the work, was usually considered essential. What formally educated midwives there were came generally from the artisan class or lower gentry. Such women invested time and money in several years' apprenticeship to a senior midwife, and by the 17th century most would be literate. These midwives would mostly be found in towns, where there was sufficient prosperity to make their outlay worthwhile. Most would start by practising among the poor, possibly acquiring a more affluent clientèle as their reputation grew. Town midwives engaged by country nobility or gentry would arrive well beforehand, and stay several days or weeks afterwards, being recompensed accordingly. Attendance on royalty was the greatest prize. In 1469, Margaret Cobb, midwife to Edward IV's queen, received in addition to her fee a life pension of £10 a year, as did Alice Massey, who attended Elizabeth of York in 1503. Mme Peronne, who in 1630 travelled from France to attend Charles I's French queen, was paid £300, with £100 for her expenses.

These midwives, however, were in a minority. Inevitably the rest attended only the poor (the majority of the population), many living in rural, perhaps isolated, places. Such women would learn their midwifery through their own and their neighbours' birthing experiences, undertaking the work by virtue of their seniority or the large number of children they had borne (McMath 1694; Siegemundin 1690, preface). Their work might entail travelling long distances on foot to outlying habitations, for a few pence or a small payment in kind. Many such women took up the work from necessity, eking out a poor living with sick nursing and laying out the dead, as did their successors until the early 20th century.

## Midwifery knowledge

Before the 16th century, most midwifery knowledge, like knowledge in other fields, would be transmitted by word of mouth and by example. The first midwifery manual printed in English appeared in 1540 – *The Byrth of Mankynde*, translated via Latin from a 1513 German work by Eucharius Roesslin, City Physician of Wurms. Drawn largely from ancient and mediaeval texts, the *Byrth* included many of their errors, thus demonstrating the ignorance of practical midwifery then general among physicians. Yet it contained much good sense on the care of the labouring woman, together with directions for managing abnormal cases, including delivery of the infant by the feet, instrumental removal of the dead fetus and caesarean section on the dead mother. However, although addressed to pregnant women and midwives, the work could only benefit the literate minority who could afford to buy it.

### 'In the straw'

Generally, birth took place at home, poorer women typically delivering in the communal room, before the hearth, the floor covered with straw which would later be burnt. Usually the birth chamber was darkened, windows and doors sealed, with a fire kept burning for several days. These precautions were taken lest the woman took 'cold' (developed the possibly lethal 'childbed fever'), and in more superstitious households for fear that malevolent spirits might gain entrance, harming mother or infant (Gélis 1996:97, Thomas 1973:728–732). Care was taken, too, that the afterbirth and its attachments (all credited with powerful magical properties) were disposed of safely, lest they be used in spells to harm the family. These beliefs were still current in remote parts of Europe in the early 20th century.

To hasten matters on in early labour the parturient would periodically be encouraged to walk, supported by two sturdy women, her strength sustained by warm broth or spicy drinks. The midwife, sharing the universal and time-honoured belief that the *child* provided the motive power for its birth, would follow ancient practice in greasing and stretching the woman's genitalia and dilating the cervix to 'help' the infant emerge. Hence the 'ideal' midwife possessed, along with appropriate qualities of character, small hands with long tapering fingers (Temkin 1956).

The second stage of labour usually took place, as for millennia, with the woman in an upright or semi-upright position (Kuntner 1988). In rich households a birth chair might be used, but more commonly the parturient sat on a woman's lap. Some women knelt or stood, leaning against a support; some adopted a half-sitting, half-lying posture, with a solid object to push their feet against during contractions, while others delivered on all fours (Blenkinsop 1863:8,10,73, Gélis 1996:21–36). As labour progressed, the woman would instinctively change position, 'as shall seeme commodious and necessarye to the partie', as the *Byrth* put it, urging the midwife to comfort her with refreshments and encourage her with 'swete wurdes' (see Fig. 2.1). Following delivery, the mother would be put to bed to 'lie in' – rich women for up to a month, the poor for days at most. The infant would be washed, then swaddled to 'straighten' its limbs, and if circumstances permitted, an all-woman celebration of this female life event would ensue.

## THE MIDWIFE, THE CHURCH AND THE LAW

The midwife's duties did not end with the birth, however. In pre-Reformation times, she carried heavy responsibilities for the salvation of the infant's soul, being required to take weakly infants directly to the priest for baptism. If death seemed imminent, she should perform the ceremony herself, taking care on pain of severe punishment to use only the Church's prescribed words. If the woman died undelivered, she was immediately to open the body,

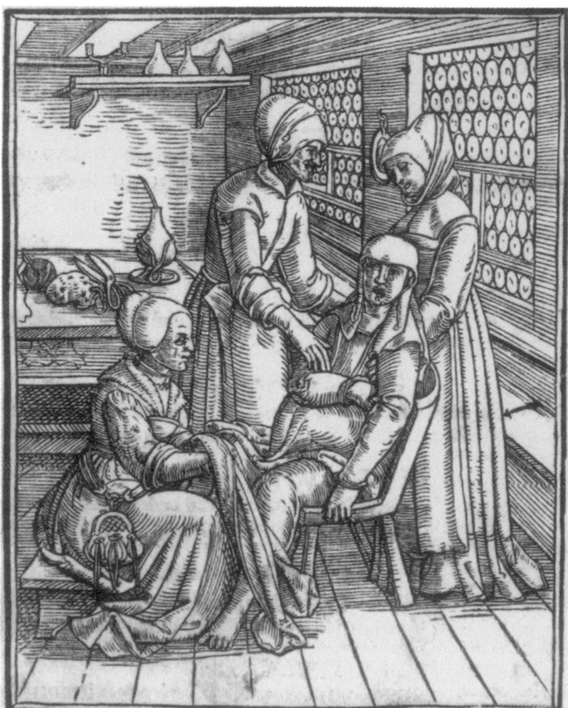

**Figure 2.1** Midwife attending a labouring woman seated on a birth chair. Two women hold her shoulders firmly while the midwife carries on with her work. The midwife's sponge, with scissors and thread for cutting and tying the cord, lie in readiness by the rear wall. *(From Rueff, Iacobus:* Ein schön lustig Trostbüchle von den Empfengknussen und Geburten der Menschen, *Zurich, 1554 (Wellcome Library, London).)*

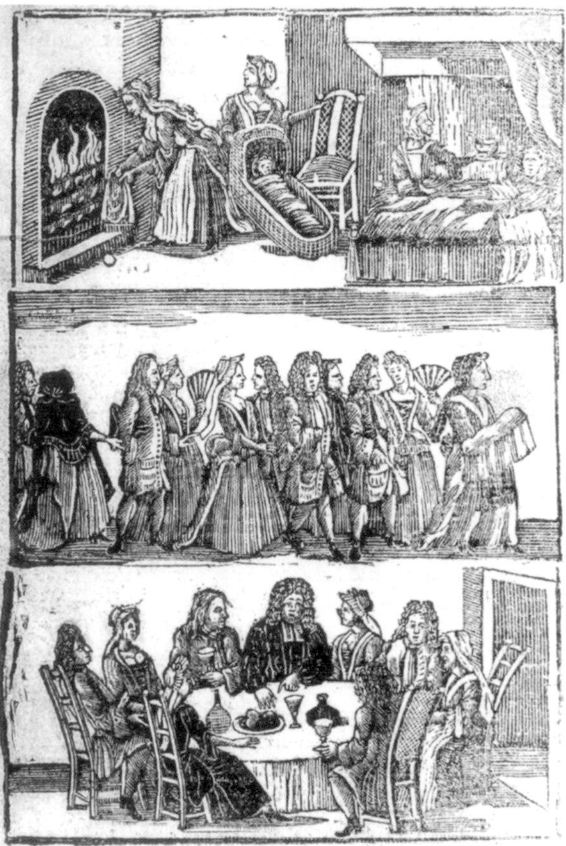

**Figure 2.2** Frontispiece from Jane Sharp's *Compleat Midwife's Companion,* 1724, showing the midwife handing the mother a bowl of broth following the birth; later, infant in arms, she heads the christening procession to the church, subsequently appearing as a guest at the christening feast where she will receive substantial tips from the assembled company. The mother is not present, being still in seclusion in the lying-in room until her churching some weeks later. *(Wellcome Library, London)*

and if the infant were alive, to baptise it. Stillborn infants, in their unhallowed state unfit for Christian burial, she was to bury in unconsecrated ground, safely and secretly, where neither man nor beast would find them. Baptism would generally take place within a week of birth, and the midwife, infant in arms, headed the procession to the church, the mother remaining in seclusion until she had been 'churched'. The midwife enjoyed an honoured place at post-christening celebrations and in prosperous households would be liberally tipped by family and friends (see Fig. 2.2). Later, after the lying-in period, she would accompany the mother to her 'churching' – originally a 'purification' ceremony, but under Protestantism merely one of maternal thanksgiving.

The midwife also had an important role in legal matters. Where a woman condemned to death pleaded pregnancy in the hope of postponing or mitigating punishment, a panel of midwives would be summoned to examine her, though some post-execution dissections demonstrated these examinations' unreliability (Pechey 1696:55–56). Midwife panels were also called to examine unmarried women alleging rape, women accused of aborting themselves or of concealing the birth (and possible murder) of an unwanted infant, or determine the alleged prematurity of infants born within less than 9 months of marriage. Midwives attending an unmarried woman were also expected to make her name the father, lest he escape the Church's punishment for fornication and his responsibility to the parish for the child's upkeep.

## Governing the midwife

In view of these religious and legal duties, the midwife's character and religious orthodoxy were inevitably of concern to the Church. In 1481, Agnes Marshall of Emeswell, Yorkshire, was 'presented' at the Bishop's Court, not because she lacked skill in midwifery, but because she used (pagan) 'incantations' to 'help' the labour. Midwives were suspect, too, because of their access to stillbirths, allegedly used in devil-worship. In 1415, a successful Parisian midwife, Perette, was turned in the pillory and banned from practice for supplying a tiny fetus used, unbeknownst to her, in sorcery. On account of her great skill, however, she was restored to practice by order of the King.

Probably the first system of compulsory midwife licensing in Europe was instituted in the city of Regensberg in Bavaria in 1452, a system gradually emulated in other European cities. Applicants for a licence were commonly examined by a panel of physicians, who, innocent of practical midwifery, based their examination on classical texts. Generally, midwives were required to send for a physician or surgeon in difficult cases, and in Strasbourg, midwives were prohibited from using hooks or sharp instruments on pain of corporal punishment. Many cities appointed midwives to serve the poor, supplementing their remuneration with payment in kind and providing financial aid in old age or disability (Gélis 1988:25, Wiesener 1993:78–84).

In England, the first arrangements for formal control of midwives were made under the 1512 Act for regulating physicians and surgeons. The Act's aim was to limit unskilled practice and prevent the use of 'sorcery' and 'witchcraft' in medicine. It therefore provided for Church Courts to license practitioners able to produce testimony to their skill and religious orthodoxy, and to prosecute the rest. A midwife applying for a licence would normally bring to the Court a reference from the local parson, together with 'six honest matrons' she had delivered, to testify to her competence. There was, however, no *formal* examination on this point as existed under Continental schemes.

Successful applicants swore a long and detailed oath, promising 'faithfully and diligently' to help childbearing women, to serve 'as well poor as rich', not to charge more than the family could afford, nor divulge private matters. They swore not to use 'sorcery' to shorten labour; to use only prescribed words when christening infants; and to bury as directed all stillborn children. They undertook not to procure abortion nor connive at child destruction, false attribution of paternity or substitution of infants. Neither were they to allow any woman to be delivered secretly, and always, if possible, see that lights were available and 'two or three honest women' present, a requirement clearly aimed at preventing the speedy suffocation of an unwanted child.

## ADVENT OF THE MAN-MIDWIFE

Around the mid-16th century came other changes laden with import for midwives, as surgeons, inspired by the new Renaissance spirit of enquiry, turned their attention to the anatomy of childbirth. Outstanding in this field was the French barber-surgeon Ambroise Paré (1510–1590), notable for his description in his 1549 *Briefve Collection* of the use of podalic version in malpresentation cases. The success of men like Paré was to encourage the extension of male attendance from 'extraordinary' to routine cases. This development gradually spread throughout Europe, being recognized around 1600 in Britain with the new term 'man-midwife', and in France that of 'accoucheur'.

The centrality of anatomical knowledge to good midwifery was well understood by leading practitioners, men and women. The London midwife Jane Sharp began her 1671 '*Midwives Book*' by deploring 'the many Miseries' women endured at the hands of midwives who practised 'without any skill in Anatomy...merely for Lucres sake'. Her contemporary, the Derbyshire man-midwife Willughby, concurred, finding that many country midwives could not manage malpresentations, however also condemning inexperienced young surgeons and ill-prepared apothecaries, whose 'fatal bunglings' deserved the branding-iron or the hangman's noose.

## Maternal mortality

Given the general lack of statistics, the extent of contemporary maternal mortality (calculated as death at or within the month after the birth) is impossible to discover. However, in his 1662 study of the London Bills of Mortality, John Graunt estimated maternal mortality in London at about 15 per 1000 births. Those dying from the 'hardness' of their labour, as distinct from other causes, he put at *less than 1 in 200* (5 per 1000). Significantly, along with other authorities, Graunt believed that poor hard-working countrywomen did best in childbirth. The celebrated Dr Harvey went further. Challenging the general practice of dilating the parturient's vulva and *os uteri,* he argued that women delivering unattended fared best, since Nature, escaping the midwife's interventions, was allowed unhindered to take her course. His friend Willughby confessed himself converted to this view, condemning interference in all but abnormal cases, as always harmful

Interestingly, Willughby also links such interference with the woman 'taking cold' (Blenkinsop 1863:6), a likely reference to 'puerperal' fever, not so named, but recognized under 'fevers' and 'agues' occurring after childbearing. Following ancient humoral theory, the condition was ascribed to a bodily 'humours' imbalance (Jonas 1540: xxxiii, Sharp 1671:243–250) and was probably then, as later, the chief single cause of maternal death. Not until the late 18th century was it publicly proposed that this deadly malady might be carried to the woman on the attendants' clothing or unwashed hands (Gordon 1795:98–99), a view not completely accepted, even in medical circles, until the 1940s.

## Midwives under threat

When urging midwives to study anatomy, Jane Sharp had recognized that women's exclusion from the universities and 'schools of learning', where this was taught, disadvantaged them compared with men. Girls were barred, too, from grammar schools, which taught Latin, knowledge of which was the mark of an educated person and which was still used for many medical texts. Leading male practitioners therefore enjoyed higher social status than midwives, however successful. Although in 1762 Mrs Draper delivered the future George IV, with Dr Hunter and the surgeon Caesar Hawkins waiting elsewhere, Hunter's diary makes their relative ranking clear (Stark 1908). Moreover, the distinction of great 18th-century practitioners like Manningham, Ould, Hunter and Smellie was to reflect credit on every man-midwife, deserved or not.

However, it was probably the general introduction in the 1720s of the midwifery forceps that precipitated the rapid acceleration of the existing trend. The forceps enabled the delivery of live infants where previously child or mother might have been lost, and the shortening of tedious labour. Since custom discouraged use of instruments by midwives, this development further enhanced the position of men and many surgeon-apothecaries, taking up midwifery, became general practitioners in fact if not yet in name. Some men-midwives, too, saw childbirth as a *mechanical* process and themselves, with their right to use instruments, as better suited to preside over it. Indeed, for many, the educated male practitioner represented the new enlightened age, while midwives, whose ranks included many ignorant, illiterate and superstitious women, appeared relics of a benighted past.

Keenly aware of the threat to their livelihood, midwives fought back, supported in books and pamphlets by both medical and lay sympathizers. For reasons of modesty, these argued, many women would not send for a man, nor would their husbands allow it. Many could not afford men's fees, and male assistance, especially in the country, was commonly unavailable. Men-midwives, it was contended, resorted to unnecessary use of instruments in order to save their time and increase their fees, and were thus responsible for increased maternal and infant mortality. Furthermore, they exaggerated the dangers of childbirth, frightening women into believing that extraordinary measures, and therefore male attendance, were more necessary than they actually were. Also, by insisting on being called to every 'trifling' difficulty, men were reducing midwives to 'mere nurses', while taking every opportunity to denigrate their competence and blame them, however unjustly, for any mishap, even if caused by themselves.

## Lying-in hospitals and 'out-door' charities

One champion of the midwives' cause was the London surgeon John Douglas. Writing in 1736 to rebut men-midwives' claims that difficult births were beyond female capacities, he instanced the career of Mme du Tetre, lately Head Midwife at the great Paris hospital the Hôtel-Dieu. Douglas maintained that if English midwives had the same opportunities as Frenchwomen (the Hôtel-Dieu had trained midwives since 1631), they could reach equally high standards. British counterparts of such hospitals had been abolished in Henry VIII's dissolution of the monasteries, and Douglas, seeing lying-in hospitals as essential to improved midwife instruction, demanded their establishment in all the principal English cities. The first such permanent foundation, however, was the Dublin 'Rotunda', established in 1745. Two lying-in wards were created in the Middlesex Hospital in 1747, and four (tiny) lying-in hospitals opened in London shortly afterwards. Similar institutions appeared in major provincial cities as the century progressed.

These hospitals, like others founded at the time, were charitable institutions, funded by the subscriptions of the wealthy for the benefit of the poor (in this case 'respectable' poor married women), and run by voluntary lay boards. Hospitals were a mixed blessing for the women attended there. Outbreaks of puerperal fever, a regular feature until the adoption of antiseptic practice in the late 19th century (and occurring sporadically even in the 1930s), boosted death rates and necessitated closure for weeks on end. Safer and cheaper were 'out door' charities, such as the Royal Maternity Charity, London (founded 1757). These provided poor women with midwife attendance at home, with designated medical assistance as necessary, and probably trained far more midwives than the tiny hospitals. There was, however, no move in England from government, central or local, on this vital matter of midwife instruction. By this time, Bishops' licensing – which although no great guarantee of skill, and never properly enforced, had given the licensed midwife some status – was generally defunct.

## Continental comparisons

Meanwhile, on the Continent, state control in matters perceived to be in the public interest, including midwife instruction and regulation, grew ever stronger. Many German towns had midwife schools and 'midwife-masters' to teach midwives. In 1759 the French King sent the eminent midwife Mme du Coudray around the country to lecture to midwives and surgeons, and to found lying-in hospitals. Educated English midwives, realizing that lack of official instruction and regulation at home was hastening the midwife's decline, called vainly for

Continental-style systems in England. Scotland, where Continental influence was stronger, was different. In 1694 Edinburgh Town Council had established a system of midwife regulation and in 1726 appointed an honorary Professor of Midwifery, Joseph Gibson, for their instruction. In 1740 the Glasgow Faculty of Physicians and Surgeons instituted a similar system for the city and surrounding counties, which, like Edinburgh's, appears to have operated throughout the century.

## 'Towards a complete new system of midwifery'

By the mid-18th century, male practitioners, disdaining the familiar 'man-midwife', began to adopt the French term 'accoucheur', as conveying greater status. Their approaches to delivery varied, however. Some still dilated the cervix and the labia vulvae, practices continuing among the more ignorant at the century's close (Clarke 1793:21). Some extracted the placenta immediately after delivery by introducing the hand into the uterus, while others roundly condemned this (Smellie 1752–64:238–239). The general trend, however, was towards less intervention. This development stemmed from the new realization that it was not exertions by the child but uterine muscular action that provided the necessary expulsive force (ibid. 202). Significantly, Smellie (since regarded as the 'father of British obstetrics') concluded from his vast experience that, out of 1000 parturients, 990 would be safely delivered 'without any other than common assistance' (ibid. 195–196).

Though ambulation in the first stage was still encouraged, women's freedom to choose their delivery position was gradually being curtailed. Earlier authorities, male and female, had encouraged women to adopt the position most comfortable to them as facilitating the best outcome for mother and infant. Smellie underlined the advantages of upright positions in furthering labour, partly through gravity, and partly through the 'equalisation of the uterine force', recommending them for 'tedious labours' (ibid. 202). Yet, along with other authorities, Smellie generally advised delivery in bed (half-sitting, half-lying) for fear that otherwise the woman might take 'cold', and hence develop 'childbed fever' (ibid. 204). Others, like Dr John Burton of York, favoured the 'dorsal' and 'left lateral' positions as 'easiest for the Patient and most convenient for the Operator' (Burton 1751:106–107). Indeed, sitting by the edge of the bed, his hand concealed under the sheet, was less tiring and less undignified for men hoping for recognition of their art as part of medicine proper, than was crouching at the woman's knees on the midwife's low stool (see Fig. 2.3).

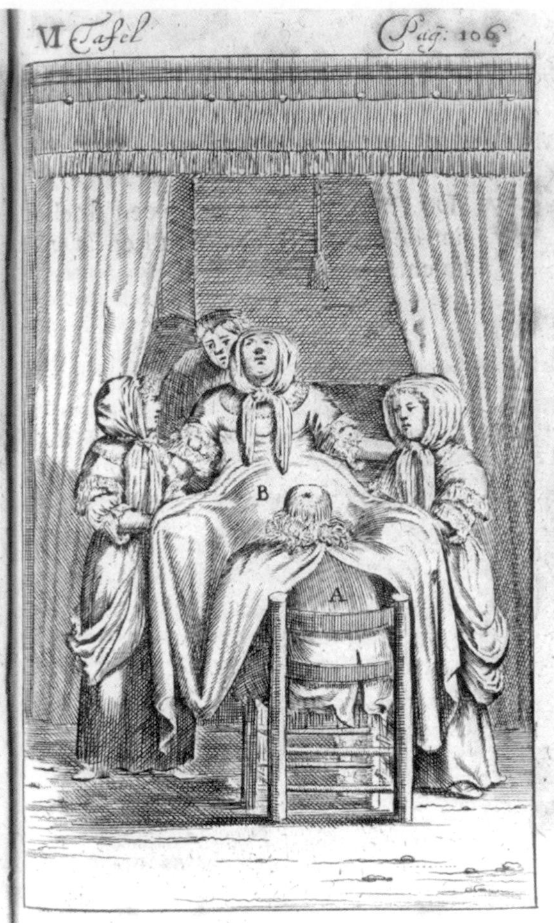


**Figure 2.3** A man-midwife attends a birth in Holland. The parturient is now labouring in bed. Although in a semi-upright position she has lost some of the benefits of being fully upright, with her feet on the floor, in aiding her expulsive efforts. She holds on to her attendants' shoulders while they push against her feet to give her some purchase for her pushing. To protect the woman's modesty the corners of a sheet are pinned around the man-midwife's neck so that he perforce works blind, a situation that sometimes led to error. *(From S. Janson,* Korte en Bonding verbandeling, van de voortteelingen't Kinderbaren, *Amsterdam 1711 (Wellcome Library, London))*

Recumbent delivery positions gradually became the norm for 'civilised' practice. Although delivery out of bed was to continue in rural areas into the 20th century, it was generally considered low class, if not inhumane. Significantly, the parturient's transfer to bed, together with her increasing designation as a 'patient' (a word originally used only of the sick), indicated her transition from an active to a passive role in this important life-event, and, implicitly, the growing medicalization of childbirth itself.

## THE DECLINE OF THE MIDWIFE

By the early decades of the 19th century the midwife's situation had deteriorated still further. Growing prudery, largely the result of the Evangelical movement, had rendered reference to childbirth, and even the word 'midwife', taboo in polite society. Together with the male capture of the wealthier private practice and the growing reluctance of the middle classes to allow their women to work, this prudery meant that fewer educated women were entering midwifery, leaving many who wanted skilled assistance in childbirth forced to send for a man. Midwife supporters argued that midwives' instruction (where it existed) had not kept pace with men's and increasingly calls arose for the better education of female practitioners to the highest professional standards, in midwifery and women's diseases. The medical response was predictable. Women were unfitted by nature for 'scientific mechanical employment' (which midwifery was), and could never use obstetrical instruments with 'advantage or precision', even if presumptuous enough to try. Such remarks, together with allegations that midwives were generally abortionists, prompted one midwife supporter to remark that 'the greatest slanders against the moral and intellectual characters of women have been uttered by practitioners of man-midwifery'.

This animosity towards midwives arose partly from men-midwives' generally low status within the medical profession. Their specialty was not officially recognized as part of medicine and no official qualification existed in England to distinguish men with midwifery training from those with none. Hence men seeking such qualifications were forced to go to Scotland or the Continent. For decades leading accoucheurs had requested the English chartered medical corporations to establish such a qualification, but had been repeatedly rebuffed. Many leading medical figures viewed attendance on childbirth as 'women's work', and below the dignity of professional men. In 1827 Sir Anthony Carlisle (later President of the Royal College of Surgeons) denounced man-midwifery as a 'dishonorable vocation', whose practitioners from financial motives sought to turn a natural process into a 'surgical operation'. It was 1852 before the College established its Midwifery Licence and 1888 before such qualification was required for admission to the Medical Register kept by the General Medical Council, the doctors' regulatory body established in 1859. Thenceforth midwifery was formally recognized in the UK as part of medicine.

### Maternal mortality and the State

From 1839 maternal mortality statistics became available from the newly created Registrar-General's Office for Births, Marriages and Deaths. The Office's Statistical Superintendent, Dr W Farr, deplored the high loss of maternal life represented by the estimated rate for 1841 of nearly 6 maternal deaths per 1000 live births. Looking wistfully at Continental legislation for midwife regulation, Farr concluded that comparable arrangements at home were ruled out by British suspicion of State direction combined with general prudery concerning childbirth. Yet with better-instructed midwives, Farr declared, the annual 3000 maternal deaths could be reduced by a third. That some midwives were incompetent was demonstrated in press reports on those who had pulled out the womb or torn the child's body from its head. Such disasters were paralleled, however, in accounts of ignorant male practitioners cutting out the womb or part of the intestines with scissors or knife. Some of these men (graphically described in the *London Medical Gazette* in 1845 as 'disembowelling accoucheurs') were regularly qualified medical men; others chemists, but in neither case was instruction in midwifery required by law.

### The end of the midwife?

The midwife's image had not been helped by Charles Dickens' caricature in *Martin Chuzzlewit* (1844) of the unsavoury 'Mrs Gamp', a poor widow who, like so many over the centuries, earned her living by practising midwifery, sick and 'monthly' nursing, and laying out the dead. A blowsy, tippling, unscrupulous character, Mrs Gamp soon became the stereotypical midwife (see Fig. 2.4). But although along with Farr some medical men advocated the replacement of such midwives by respectable, trained women, certain accoucheurs, seeking a male monopoly of midwifery (achieved in North America by

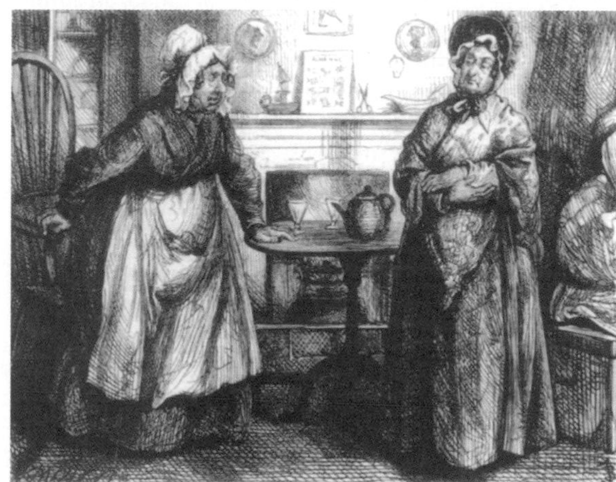

**Figure 2.4** Dickens' Mrs Gamp quarrels with her friend and colleague, Betsy Prig, a nurse from St. Bartholomew's Hospital, London, both being the worse for drink. C. Dickens, *Martin Chuzzlewit*, 1844.

the 1950s), were pressing for the midwife's total abolition. 'All midwives are a mistake', Tyler Smith told his students at the Hunterian Medical School in 1847, 'and it should be the aim of every obstetric practitioner to discourage their employment'. Furthermore, because of its origin, the word 'midwifery' should no longer be used to describe male attendance on childbirth, being replaced by the new construct 'obstetrics'. Here Smith well understood that a term of Latin origin, even if derived actually from the Latin for 'midwife' ('obstetrix'), had a snob value which would further elevate men above their female competitors. This substitution of 'obstetrics' for 'midwifery' in male practice was, however, not fully achieved until after World War II.

## The Royal Maternity Charity and maternal mortality

Directly in Smith's line of fire was the 98-year-old Royal Maternity Charity. The Charity's employment of midwives, however well instructed, Smith contended, was 'degrading' to 'obstetrics' and harmful to its clients, who instead should be attended by 'educated' practitioners. Yet the Charity's statistics, published annually by the eminent medical men supervising its work, repeatedly disproved these allegations. Serving only poor women, many undernourished and living in unhealthy conditions, the Charity (and similar foundations) consistently demonstrated death rates of less than half the Registrar-General's current rates for England and Wales.

A further onslaught on such charities came in 1870 from the obstetrician Matthews Duncan in his *Mortality of Childbed*. Dismissing the charities' results as an impossibility since 'educated accoucheurs', in [affluent] private practice, lost five times as many women, Duncan postulated an 'irreducible minimum' of at least 8 per 1000, an admission, in fact, suggesting that the rich might indeed fare worse in childbirth than the poor.

Despite this obvious inference, the anti-midwife faction had an answer. The cause of higher mortality among wealthier women lay not with their medical attendants but with their own 'artificial ' way of life, which disabled them for parturition. *Increased* (medical) vigilance was therefore necessary in attending them, not less. The degree to which childbirth among the prosperous was progressively viewed as pathology was evident in Chavasse's 1842 *Advice to a wife*. While declaring childbirth a natural event, Chavasse required the 'pregnant female' to rest for 2 to 3 hours daily, while the post-parturient was to keep to a meagre diet, lying flat on her back for 10 to 14 days lest she should faint, haemorrhage, or suffer a prolapsed womb.

This invalidization of pregnancy and childbirth naturally implied more medical attention and higher fees, catching women in a double bind. Not only were they regarded as physically, intellectually and morally incapable of undertaking the ancient female duty of attendance on childbirth, but were also increasingly seen as requiring male assistance to give birth at all.

## THE MIDWIVES INSTITUTE, MIDWIFE REGISTRATION AND MATERNAL MORTALITY

Accepting this reality, in 1880 three educated midwives, together with Louisa Hubbard, a wealthy pioneer in women's employment, formed the Matrons Aid Society, later to become the Midwives Institute and ultimately the Royal College of Midwives (RCM) (Fig. 2.5).

The Society's avowed aim was the improvement of midwife practice, and, by implication, a reduction in maternal mortality. This was to be achieved through a registration Act similar to other professional legislation, as was the rehabilitation of midwifery as a respectable profession for educated women. Realizing that general

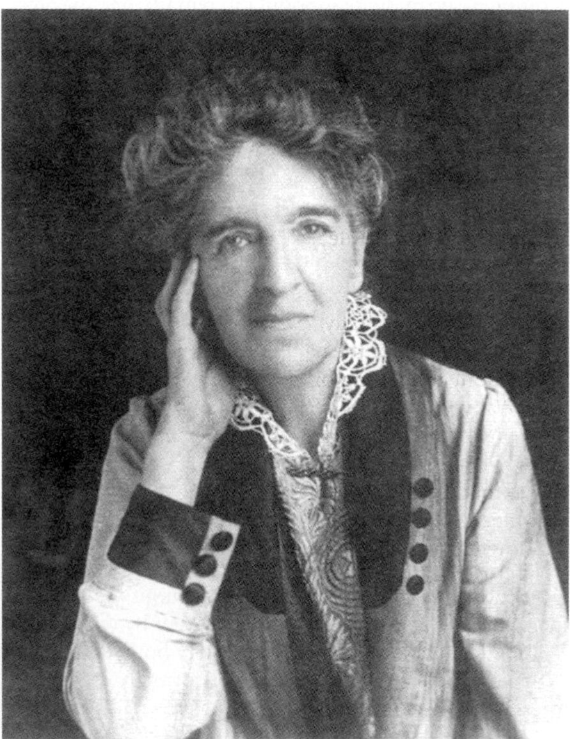

**Figure 2.5** Rosalind Paget (1855–1948). Trained in nursing and midwifery, Miss Paget joined the Midwives Institute in 1886, in 1887 financing the establishment of the Institute's journal, *Nursing Notes*. Also prominent in the Queen's Nursing Institute, she was for 20 years its representative on the Central Midwives Board. *(Royal College of Midwives)*

practitioners might view registered midwives as competitors for their better-paying cases, the Institute argued that midwives would attend only women too poor to pay doctors' fees and would not encroach on medical ground by acting in abnormal labour.

Yet what proportion of annual maternal mortality (still around 5 per 1000 live births) could be laid at the midwife's door? The obstetrician Dr Aveling, when pressing for midwife registration before the 1892 Commons' Select Committee, had implied that untrained midwives were responsible for most of the annual 3000 or so maternal deaths in England and Wales. Since there was as yet no notification of births, nor any system of identifying the birth attendant, this could only be guesswork. Indeed, WC Grigg, Physician to Queen Charlotte's Hospital, concluded in 1891 that more cases of 'injury and disaster' resulted from the imprudent use of forceps and turning by doctors than from the negligence and ignorance of midwives.

## The Midwives Act 1902

But how was a registration Act to be obtained? Despite continued strengthening of Continental midwife legislation, home governments, still heavily imbued with 'laissez-faire' ideology, declined to intervene. The Midwives Institute therefore began seeking friendly medical and Parliamentary support for the promotion of a Private Member's Bill, a difficult task when women did not have the vote, there were no women MPs, and matters regarding childbirth were not discussed in polite circles. For 20 years, this handful of voteless women struggled against indifference and ridicule from an all-male Parliament and, latterly, bitter opposition from among general practitioners, their professional associations and the General Medical Council. Finally, however, possibly as a result of growing concern for the national welfare following revelations about the falling birthrate and poor health among Boer War volunteers, the first State registration measure in modern England for an all-female occupation became law. However, fierce medical opposition to registration had meant that the status of the new registered English midwife was much lower than that of her counterparts in leading Continental countries. Similar legislation for Scotland and Ireland (with the difference that new entrants must also be qualified nurses) followed in 1915 and 1918 respectively.

## The Central Midwives Board

The Act established a midwives' regulatory authority, the Central Midwives Board (CMB), with responsibility for keeping a 'Roll' of 'certified' midwives. In recognition of midwives' general poverty, this regulatory machinery would be largely financed from public funds. Moreover, unlike doctors and chemists, midwives were not to be self-regulating. The Bill's promoters, in order to keep their medical allies' support, had been forced to concede that the Board should be in medical hands. The additional requirement of Local Government supervision through the agency of the (possibly hostile) Medical Officers of Health, meant that at both national and local level midwives would be regulated by a competing profession. There was a further burden: midwives, uniquely for a nationally regulated profession, were liable to erasure from the register (and subsequent loss of livelihood) for 'misconduct' in their *private*, as well as in their professional, life.

In 1905, the first year of enrolment, over 22,308 midwives registered. Of these, less than half held relevant certificates of competence, the remaining 12,521 registering as midwives in 'bona fide' practice. Five years' grace was allowed for unregistered women to continue to practise, but after 1910 such activity became a criminal offence. For new entrants to the profession, 3 months' approved training was required prior to taking the Board's examination (doubled to 6 months in 1916 for non-nurse-trained applicants, in 1926 to 1 year, and in 1938 to 2 years). The Board's rules limited midwives to attendance on natural labour (which included twin and breech deliveries), and required them to send for a doctor in difficult cases. Significantly, it forbade them to lay out the dead, traditionally an important part of poorer midwives' work. Detailed directions also governed their daily practice, extending to their clothing, their equipment and their record-keeping; breaches of the rules could be punished by erasure from the Roll.

## 'Certified Midwife'

Despite these restrictions on midwives' independence, the Act worked gradually to raise the occupation's status, consequently preventing the disappearance from the UK (as virtually happened in North America) of this ancient female calling. The requirement of hospital training and examination for new entrants, however, brought changes in the occupation's social composition as younger, single women entered its ranks. Meanwhile, the poorer, older working-class women who had for centuries delivered their neighbours were prevented by the cost of training, books and examination fees from becoming registered midwives, being allowed to act as maternity nurses only (Leap & Hunter 1993:44–47).

As always, life could be very arduous for midwives attending women at home. This was especially so in the country, where long distances would be travelled in all weathers, on foot or by bicycle, possibly through difficult terrain. Fees were low (possibly 30 shillings to £2 per case) and generally paid in instalments during the pregnancy, though some payment might be in kind. In 1929, a few midwives with extensive practices were found to be earning over £275 annually, but many practising full time earned only £90–£100. Salaries for nursing association work in rural areas could also be low, the life very lonely and hardly supportable without private means. Hours worked could be very long, some midwives delivering 90–100 women a year. A Portsmouth midwife recalled how, when in independent practice, she once went without sleep for 4 days while single-handedly conducting seven deliveries, one of a 12½ lb baby, finally going home to sleep the clock around twice (Leap & Hunter 1993:50–56,63–68).

Domiciliary midwife practice appears to have followed guidelines laid down in contemporary obstetricians' textbooks. Though allowed by the CMB to give mild analgesics (only doctors were allowed to give chloroform), some midwives employed warm baths and back-rubbing to ease pain. It was not until the 1940s that the self-operated *Minnit inhalation analgesic apparatus* became available in portable form for carriage on the midwife's bicycle. In difficult cases midwives were required to send for medical help, but if this were delayed they would have to manage the emergency themselves, and if the doctor were inexperienced they might help him put on the forceps (ibid. 56–58,176–178). Midwife–doctor relations varied, but, as in earlier centuries, some doctors sought to blame midwives for their own incompetence (ibid. 56–58). After delivery, the mother was to lie flat for at least a day, staying in bed for 10 to 14 days for fear of uterine prolapse (ibid. 143,164–171,179). As tradition prescribed, she was kept, officially at least, on a meagre diet, a regimen that, as contemporary midwifery manuals show, only began to change in the 1950s.

## The continuing problem of maternal mortality

When the 1902 Act was passed, it was expected that maternal mortality would fall as untrained midwives, known to be chary of sending for medical help in difficult cases, were gradually replaced by their formally trained successors. Instead, the rate remained puzzlingly stable. Worse still, from 1928 it had shown a significant rise, climbing to exceed 4 per 1000 live births in 1930. Interestingly, enquiries by the Ministry of Health showed that maternal mortality was lower among the poor, many of whom had poor health and lived in insanitary conditions, than among the better-off, who generally had medical attendance. Allegations of fatal abuse of instruments had followed male practitioners for over two centuries. Even now, reported an editorial in *The Lancet* (Anon 1929), many GPs confessed to routinely using instruments, solely to save time, maintaining that they could not afford to do otherwise. Another factor, contended Eardley Holland, President of the new College of Obstetricians and Gynaecologists, was the increasing tendency among GPs, despite warnings from leading obstetrics teachers, to view childbirth as pathology; consequently, they widened their indications for intervention, with catastrophic results (Holland 1935). Significantly, charitable and municipal outdoor midwife services for the poor consistently returned a maternal death rate of half the Registrar-General's national figure, and lower than rates in more affluent areas where medical attendance predominated.

## State midwifery

With continuing worries about the falling birth rate and high maternal mortality, Parliament's response was the 1936 Midwives Act. This required County and County Borough Councils to provide for a whole-time midwife service adequate to local needs and free or at reduced cost to poorer women. Thenceforward, the majority of midwives would be salaried, uniformed, pensioned professionals, with time off and annual leave, offering a more complete service and receiving official recognition of their contribution to national wellbeing. Many of those not selected for the new service were bought out of their practices and those considered unfit compulsorily retired. Further, unregistered women were no longer permitted to act as maternity nurses. The Act passed without adverse comment from the medical press, probably because of general practitioners' improved financial security (largely consequent on the 1911 National Insurance panel system), and GPs were now content to leave 'cheap midwifery' to the midwife. However, although municipal midwives were better off, broken nights followed by a full working day remained a feature of domiciliary practice (see Fig. 2.6).

# THE NATIONAL HEALTH SERVICE, MATERNITY CARE AND THE MIDWIFE

Twelve years later, in 1948, under the free and comprehensive National Health Service (NHS) established by the 1945 Labour Government as part of the new Welfare State, midwife, general practitioner and hospital services were provided free to all women, irrespective of income. A great expansion of professional education also took place and, at last, midwife training was free. Yet continuing prejudice was directed against non-nurse midwives. Indeed, the upper-middle-class ladies who had led the Midwives' Institute to victory had come into midwifery *from nursing*, already made 'respectable' by Florence Nightingale and others. By being nurses first, they had cast a cloak of respectability over midwifery and established an ethos which was to prevail for over 80 years. Midwives lacking the sanitizing badge of a nurse qualification were treated as if carrying the lingering taint of 'Mrs Gamp', and

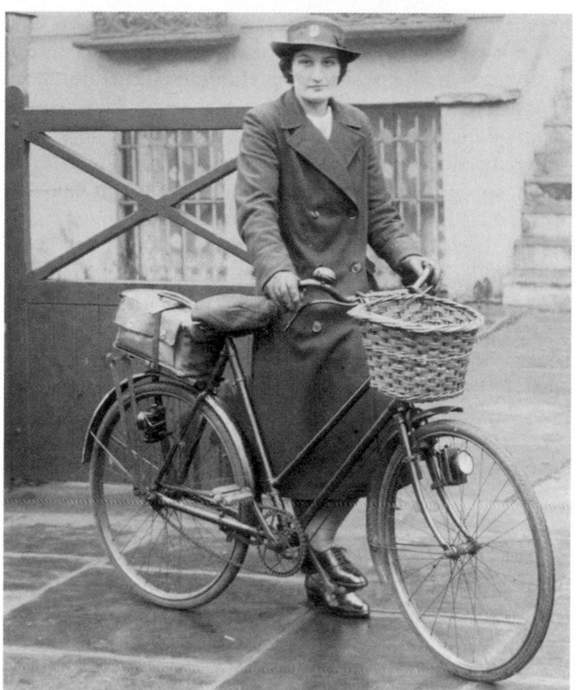

**Figure 2.6** A London County Council domiciliary midwife prepares to go on a call. *(London Metropolitan Archives)*

although many such midwives had more midwifery experience than those holding nurse qualifications, midwifery promotion invariably went to the latter (Radford & Thompson 1988). Furthermore, the Scottish and Irish registration Acts had required all midwife pupils to be qualified nurses and over time English 'direct-entry' midwifery courses were officially discouraged, until by 1980 only one such school remained. Yet many nurses qualifying in midwifery never practised it, whereas the great majority of direct-entry midwives stayed in the work.

## Place of birth

By the 1950s, the long-sought fall in maternal mortality had arrived. Sulphonamide drugs had appeared in 1936, followed a decade later by antibiotics. Together with stricter attention to asepsis and antisepsis in delivery and puerperium, these drugs had virtually eliminated puerperal sepsis, in 1930 still responsible for around 40% of maternal deaths. By 1945 the 1931–35 figure of 4 deaths per 1000 live births had been halved and by 1950 halved again. A crucial factor in this continued decline, however, as McKeown noted in relation to other health problems (McKeown 1976), has been the generally improved standard of living, resulting, in particular, in a dramatic reduction in rachitic pelves and anaemia (Worth 2002).

Despite these advances and the excellent results consistently achieved by domiciliary midwives, the trend to (more expensive) hospital delivery was officially encouraged, on obstetricians' advice, as being safer for mother and baby in *all* cases, a view subsequently challenged by independent statistical analysis (Tew 1978). By 1958, 64% of births took place in hospital, many in general practitioner units (GPUs), smaller and more local than consultant-led units (CUs). With estimated maternal mortality rates (now more widely defined as deaths from causes attributed to pregnancy and childbirth per 1000 total live and stillbirths) as low as 0.18 for England and Wales in 1968 (DHSS 1975, Table 1.3) and 0.14 for 1969 in Scotland (Macfarlane et al 2000, II, Tables A 3.3.2, A 10.2.1), attention had turned increasingly to perinatal mortality. Defined as stillbirth and infant death within the first week, and standing at over 23 per 1000 births, this was higher in low-income groups (where maternal health was poorer) than among the better-off.

In 1970, the Health Department's Maternity Advisory Committee, chaired by Sir John Peel, President of the Royal College of Obstetricians and Gynaecologists (RCOG), presented its recommendations for remedial measures. These were based (unscientifically, in the absence of impartial statistical analysis) on the facile but erroneous equation between the falling perinatal mortality rate (PMR) and increasing hospitalization. Ignoring substantial general practitioner and midwife opinion to the contrary, the Committee recommended the transfer of home midwifery services to hospital control, effected in 1974 with their removal from elected local councils to the new unelected, hospital-dominated Area Health Authorities. Hospital delivery was now over 80% and, expecting this soon to reach 100%, the Committee pronounced 'academic' any discussion of their scheme's advantages or disadvantages. The consultant-led 'obstetric team' (to include general practitioners and midwives) should therefore undertake the 'education' of the community on the 'benefits' of the reorganization.

Most obvious were the benefits to obstetricians' status and career prospects, with increased resources directed to CUs at the expense of home midwifery and GPUs. Equally clear were the drawbacks for midwives and mothers. Midwives, who had successfully looked after women throughout pregnancy, labour and puerperium, enjoying independence and variety in their duties, and receiving recognition and respect in their localities, were forced into the impersonal hospital ward to work under the direction of the obstetrician, or restricted to community postnatal care. Women's choice of place of delivery under the NHS was also disappearing. Many had preferred the familiarity of home, with the attention of a known midwife; others had chosen the local GPU, again with attendants known to them. Increasingly, however, they were to be compelled, possibly with children in tow, to make time-consuming visits to the large central district hospital for antenatal care, and to deliver in stark, impersonal surroundings among strangers. In many areas, women insisting on home birth or other non-interventionist care have since made private arrangements with a midwife or doctor at their own expense.

## Pathways to abnormality: the 'new obstetrics'

Perinatal mortality was considered further by the 1980 Commons' Social Services Committee (the Short Committee). Despite hospital births now standing at 98%, and despite preferential allocation of medical resources to less favoured regions, the gap between perinatal mortality rates for wealthier areas, as compared with poorer areas, had widened. While admitting that some procedures employed in intrapartum care had never been scientifically evaluated, the Committee nevertheless accepted its medical advisers' view that it was 'reasonable' to believe that 'professional' intervention could substantially lower the PMR. It therefore recommended further increases in consultant obstetrician posts with even greater concentration of births in large CUs and further restriction of home birth. Furthermore, wholly accepting the view of childbirth as pathology, its report demanded its routine management on a par with acute illness, in conditions of 'intensive care'.

This was already the case in many CUs. Here, older obstetricians' 'watchful expectancy' in normal birth had been superseded by the current North American doctrine of 'active management'. With the synthesis in the late 1950s of *oxytocin* as '*Syntocinon®*' had come a more reliable means of induction of labour. Hitherto, induction had generally been employed only in instances of fetal postmaturity and maternal pre-eclampsia; thenceforth, however, its use escalated, rising from 13% in 1958 to nearly 40% in 1974, and to 75% with particular consultants. Significantly, fewer births took place on weekends or Bank Holidays. Syntocinon® could also be used to accelerate labour already ongoing and to shorten it to conform to new restricted definitions of 'normal labour' derived from the arithmetical averages of the new 'partograms', rather than the limits of healthy experience.

Yet none of these procedures, observed critics, was wholly benign. Instead they led to a 'cascade of interventions' as obstetricians, many apparently still infected with the ancient Aristotelian notion of the female body as defective (Barnes 1984:1144) and hence requiring correction, persuaded themselves that techniques helpful in abnormal labour would assuredly benefit *all* cases. No birth therefore could be viewed as normal except in retrospect. Indeed, with multiple interventions, fewer births were truly normal. Syntocinon® infusions, together with continuous electronic fetal monitoring (which carries a high false positive rate and is associated with higher caesarean section rates), both inhibited mobility, for centuries valued as facilitating labour. Contractions were more violent and more painful than in natural labour, with greater danger of uterine rupture.

Enhanced pain required stronger pain relief, progressively supplied with new drugs and lumbar epidural analgesia. Epidurals diminish uterine activity, tending to hinder the natural rotation and descent of the fetus and inhibit the urge to push, thus prolonging labour, with the risk also of maternal circulatory collapse. More malpresentations and forceps deliveries resulted, with attendant risk to the child, and the discomfort of episiotomy, with possible lasting adverse sequelae for the mother (Wagner 2001). If the epidural were mismanaged, permanent paralysis, coma or even death could ensue (May 1994). Episiotomy became routine, mistakenly justified as preventing serious perineal tears and pelvic floor damage, and by 1980 being used on average in 52% of cases in England and Wales (Tew 1995:165). Dorsal delivery (the legs possibly raised in stirrups) replaced left lateral delivery, becoming the standard delivery position. Though it was known to be more painful for the woman and problematic for the fetus, it was praised in a leading midwives' manual as more 'comfortable,' and as facilitating pushing (Myles 1981:309).

Moreover, as 'failure to progress' (defined by the strict timetables routinely now governing labour) increasingly resulted in caesarean section (CS), rates for this major operation rose rapidly. This fact alone led to further intervention – the prohibition or restriction of nutrition to *every* parturient to fit her for general anaesthesia in case a caesarean should be performed. Clearly such debilitating deprivation at a time when women need all their physical and mental strength – a deprivation now officially advised against but still imposed in some UK hospitals (NICE 2007:18) – is itself likely to contribute to 'failure to progress'. Growing use of analgesic drugs, too, had consequences for the baby. Crossing the placenta, these have a depressing effect on the fetus, which may result in protracted difficulties in breathing and sucking, necessitating time in the (expensive) neonatal care unit.

## Responses of the midwifery profession

Although the Peel and Short Committees had both recommended that full use should be made of midwives' expertise, their recommendations pointed in the opposite direction. The disappearance of home midwifery and increased medicalization of hospital birth meant that midwives, officially excluded by the 1902 Act from attending abnormal labour, were now losing their role as guardians of normal birth. Midwifery skills were devalued in favour of interventionist methods that midwives themselves, many unwillingly, and against their professional judgement, were required to adopt (Reid 2002). Moreover, experienced midwives were increasingly required to defer to senior house officers who, despite their designation, were merely junior doctors doing their 6 months' obstetric training. Further, hospital midwives' work was increasingly compartmentalized into antenatal, intrapartum or postnatal care, some midwives seldom delivering a baby and practically none following a pregnancy through to labour and delivery.

For domiciliary midwives whose long years of low pay and broken nights had nonetheless given them the immense satisfaction of delivering women successfully in their own homes, the condemnation of home midwifery, despite excellent safety records, as 'unsafe' was tantamount to the negation of their life's work. For many, the experience was traumatic and retirement could not come too soon (Allison 1996:ix–x). Others tolerated the transfer to hospital as bringing shorter, more convenient hours, less responsibility and improved career opportunities. Nor did the RCM seriously oppose this transformation of the midwife's work. Overcome by the confidence with which obstetricians, generally male, and of superior educational and social status, put their case to Government, the College merely acquiesced as the ancient office of midwife was increasingly eroded, and its own avowed purpose, 'the advancement of the art and science of midwifery', effectively abandoned. Signalling its acceptance of the total hospitalization of birth in 1974, it abolished its long-standing Domiciliary Midwives Council. Some leading midwives expressed regret at these changes; others espoused them whole-heartedly, seeing reliance on technology as increasing midwives' status, rather than, in fact, reducing it. Here was no sympathy for midwives seeking to undertake home delivery; and women desiring this, or intervention-free hospital care, were to be bullied into acceptance of what was now NHS policy.

Especially striking was the turnabout demonstrated in the 1975, 1981 and 1987 editions of Margaret Myles' *Textbook for Midwives,* a standard work used in many midwifery schools since 1953. Hitherto, Myles, herself a midwife, had spoken of home as the 'ideal' place of delivery, affirming Nature's power in the vast majority of cases to complete childbirth successfully unaided, and warning against the dangers of 'meddlesome midwifery'. Yet these later editions dismissed the older philosophy of 'watchful expectancy' in labour as 'negative', applauding instead the 'modern concept' of 'active management', with its 'planned positive approach'. The management of 'normal' labour now included routine interventions, justified as ensuring greater maternal and fetal safety, while psychophysical methods of pain management were dismissed in favour of drugs. Midwives must accept 'modern ideas', working to secure the compliance of the 'misinformed' minority of expectant mothers who demanded intervention-free birth and 'outmoded' continuity of carer. Hospital delivery was strongly advocated: indeed, for a midwife to take sole charge of a woman, depriving her of the 'scientific expert care' of the 'obstetric team', would be a retrograde step. Midwives should relish their new, more fulfilling role as technically qualified members of the medically controlled 'team' (as 'mini-obstetricians' is implied) rather than seeing themselves as clinically independent practitioners as sanctioned by the Midwives Acts. Not all midwives approved of these developments. Some, the Association of Radical Midwives, decided to fight the trend from within the NHS; others left the service in order to practise privately as independent practitioners, offering home delivery and choice of birth positions.

## User protest and the 'Active Childbirth' Movement

Protests came, too, from among childbearing women themselves, their complaints supported by healthcare user organizations forming part of the post-war consumer movement. Among these were the National Childbirth Trust (NCT) and the increasingly assertive Association for Improvements in the Maternity Services (AIMS). AIMS demanded more sympathetic maternity care, including choice of home birth, of intervention-free care and of birthing positions, ideas generally dismissed in medical circles as the fads of a misguided middle-class minority. Such women, wrote one obstetrician, were too ignorant or selfish to accept their role as 'patients', even for their infants' safety. Clearly viewing the womb as a railway engine, he censured complainants for 'dictating their treatment', thus relegating professionals 'from the signal-box to the footplate' (namely, from their *rightful position of controlling labour* to one of merely *observing* it). Moreover, despite radiological evidence that squatting enlarged the pelvic outlet by almost 30% compared with the generally used supine position (Russell 1982), upright delivery was condemned as too 'primitive' (outdated) or too 'innovative' (untested). Furthermore, the 'bizarre' positions 'professionals' would have to adopt would adversely affect their 'sense of security' in their work.

## NURSES, MIDWIVES AND HEALTH VISITORS ACT, 1979

Meanwhile, midwives faced other problems following the implementation in 1983 of the Government-sponsored Nurses, Midwives and Health Visitors Act, 1979. This replaced the different regulatory machinery for these three professions in England, Wales, Scotland and Northern

Ireland with one umbrella organization, the United Kingdom Central Council (UKCC). Following representations to Government by a re-invigorated RCM, the midwife's distinctive nature was recognized with the establishment of a statutory Standing Midwifery Committee to consider all 'matters relating to midwifery'. However, since the Committee was subordinate to the nurse-dominated UKCC, midwives were no more a self-regulating profession than under the CMB.

Nurses' lack of empathy for midwifery matters was especially manifest in *Project 2000*, the UKCC's 1986 proposal for combining the basic education of the three professions in one 2-year nursing programme followed by a year's specialization, with midwifery as one of the 'specialties'. Midwifery education for students taking such courses would thus be reduced to 1 year. Opposing strongly, the RCM argued that midwives' clinical responsibilities clearly distinguished them from nurses, and that to cut midwife education would demote midwifery to a branch of nursing (RCM 1986). Moreover, the proposal contravened the 1980 European Community requirements for UK midwives wishing to practise in EC countries, where midwives, as in former times, had longer midwifery training and generally were not nurses. Faced with this reality, the Council yielded. An interesting turnabout then took place. Direct-entry midwifery courses, instead of being phased out, were to be expanded and given higher status, thus reversing a century-old trend and preventing official downgrading of midwifery to obstetric nursing.

## Finding a new voice

A further sign of a more vigorous, enterprising stance among midwives was the 1989 edition of *Myles' Textbook*, now under new authorship. The new edition contrasted sharply with previous ones, with their authoritarian celebration of interventionist obstetrics. In an entirely new departure for a midwifery manual, it emphasized the midwife's duty to accommodate, where feasible, women's choice of labour and delivery positions, forms of pain relief and so on. Midwives should also strive to make this normal but critical life event as happy as possible for mother, partner and family. Another 'first' was the referencing of the text, along with suggested further reading, indications of a new vision among midwife educators, now holding up the ideal of the midwife as a life-long learner in a 'research-based' profession. Significantly, similar emphases characterized the corresponding edition of *Mayes' Midwifery*, the other standard textbook in the field. Further noteworthy professional developments arising from the ranks were the foundation in 1986 of MIDIRS, a midwife-run quarterly critical digest of recent literature and research in maternity care. This, together with the arrival in 1993 of the *British Journal of Midwifery*, soon followed by other midwife-led publications, was to present a serious challenge to the staid *Midwives' Chronicle*, official journal of the RCM, ultimately forcing it also to adopt a more proactive stance.

## 'Choice in childbirth'

In 1991, on the initiative of Audrey Wise, MP, who wished to know why young women she knew were finding childbirth so traumatic, maternity services were again studied, this time by the Commons' Health Committee (Chairman Nicholas Winterton, MP). Unlike previous enquiries appointed by the Health Department, the Committee did not start from the negative standpoint of childbirth as an inevitably hazardous enterprise needing medical management, but as a normal physiological function that healthy women could generally perform successfully unaided. For the first time, too, midwives were included among the advisers, and submissions, written and oral, invited from service users as well as providers. Again unlike previous Committees, Winterton placed more credence on impartial statistical analyses than on the unproven assertions of obstetricians.

Moreover, since evidence on safety did not support the policy of 100% consultant unit (CU) delivery, the Committee argued for wider choice of place of birth (House of Commons Health Committee 1992:xlviii). GP units, rural or urban, offered a compromise between home birth and delivery in a CU and their closure on presumptive grounds of safety or cost should be abandoned forthwith (ibid. lxv). Taking maternal satisfaction with maternity services as its criterion of success, the Committee condemned the current professional choice of the PMR as the sole yardstick of the performance of maternity services, arguing rather for these to be audited in terms of *maternal morbidity* (ibid. 1992:lxii).

Like other medical specialties, the Committee observed, obstetrics had been subject to fashion, procedures introduced merely because they were available, and used routinely without consideration of possible adverse maternal consequences (ibid. xlviii–xlix). Women should therefore be given the option of refusing interventions, including induction, electronic fetal monitoring, epidurals and episiotomies, rather than having to undergo them as routine (ibid. xxiii). They should also be enabled to feel in control of their labours, to adopt positions of choice (ibid. lxix) and to be attended throughout labour by the same midwife. The Committee summed up its philosophy under the tenets, 'Choice, Continuity and Control'. Significantly, it concluded that essential to the development of the more user-friendly maternity services, was a re-assessment of the midwife's role. Calling for the restoration of midwives' former clinical responsibilities, the Committee condemned current use of midwives as 'a scandalous waste of money' (ibid. lxxxi).

The Government's response, *'Changing childbirth'* (DH 1993), accepted Winterton's philosophy of 'woman-centred' care, suggesting 5-year targets towards the implementation of its recommendations. However, this document was merely consultative and lacked the 'teeth' necessary to enforce any widespread change. Women seeking home birth still reported GPs threatening to strike them off their NHS lists, while many Health Authorities refused them on grounds of midwife shortages. Where they existed, midwife-run units, despite their recorded low intervention rates and increased maternal satisfaction, remained on sufferance, Health Authorities resenting the expense of maintaining these 'experiments' in addition to their ordinary hospital establishment (Lee 2001).

## Whose choice in childbirth?

Responding to '*Changing childbirth*', the RCOG qualified its acceptance of the ideal of 'woman-oriented care', invoking considerations of 'safety', a veiled justification of current interventionist practice. Significantly, it also argued for 'equal attention' to be paid to the welfare of the fetus, '*the other important person*' in the case (RCOG 1993). For centuries, English law had not recognized the unborn child as a 'person' (the principle underlying current abortion law). Yet in 1992, obstetricians from a London hospital had obtained a court order for a forced caesarean on a mother refusing her consent on religious grounds. Similar orders followed, all granted *without* maternal representation in court, until in May 1998 the Appeal Court ruled illegal the forcible invasion of a competent adult's body, even if a woman's life *or* that of her fetus depended on it. The fetus was *not* a separate person from its mother and its medical needs could not override her rights to self-determination. Notwithstanding this definitive judgement, many obstetricians persist in a curious doublethink. This allows them to view the aborted fetus (up to term if handicapped) as a *non-person*, but to describe the fetus of the pregnant mother who may resist intervention as a 'patient', thus, illogically and incorrectly, endowing it with *full-person* status with rights equal to, or overriding, those of the mother (RSM 2002).

Apart from the Appeal Court's clear-cut confirmation of the parturient's legal autonomy, how has user choice fared in general? For true choice to be exercised, full and unbiased information on available options is essential (see Ch. 34). However, a recent assessment of hospital antenatal information-giving showed that in some units choice was limited. In effect, women were steered towards acceptance of obstetrician-determined technological intervention through information that minimized its risks and exaggerated the potential harm of doing without (Stapleton et al 2002). Moreover, intervention was actually coming to be represented as part of normal birth. Indeed, a 2001 study in the Trent region demonstrated that in over 60% of the 956 deliveries recorded as 'normal' or 'spontaneous' (that is, excluding instrumental or CS deliveries), interventions had in fact occurred. These included amniotomy, induction, augmentation of labour, episiotomy and epidural anaesthesia. In about a third, induction or augmentation of labour had taken place, while 89% of amniotomies were performed before the cervix was fully dilated (Downe 2001, Downe et al 2001).

## Childbirth a 'surgical operation?'

Given this high level of intervention, it was unsurprising that the 2001 Scottish Expert Advisory Group reported that Scotland's caesarean rate (CSR) approached 20%, while the National Sentinel Audit revealed even higher rates in England, Wales and Northern Ireland. Moreover, remarkable variations in CSRs existed between regions and between hospitals. These disparities were inexplicable by reference to case-mix, as were variations in CS percentages ascribed to different primary indications, clearly demonstrating the absence of any agreed objective criteria of 'need'. Disturbingly, while half the obstetricians responding to the enquiry considered existing rates too high, 21% did not. Furthermore, in private hospitals, where obstetricians are paid by item-of-service, much larger fees are paid for this invasive procedure than for the oversight of vaginal delivery. Here, the CSR has been much higher, in some over 40% (Churchill et al 2006:54). Yet the 1985 Consensus Conference of the World Health Organization (WHO) concluded that no improvement in outcomes could be expected from a CSR exceeding 10–15%, a rate maintained by Holland and the Scandinavian countries, which have some of the world's lowest maternal and perinatal mortality rates (Wagner 2000). Nor, declared Wagner, WHO's former Director of Women's and Children's Health, was there any evidence for obstetricians' claims that CS reduced perinatal mortality (ibid.).

Though the direct financial inducements that may influence obstetricians' CS decisions in private hospitals do not apply in the NHS, the system of *payment by results* (PBR) has created perverse incentives for hospital trusts to favour elective CS (Baldwin et al 2007). Other factors include 'daylight obstetrics' to suit the obstetrician's convenience (Brown 1996, Gans et al 2007), fear of litigation, and repeat CS (around 14% of the total [Churchill et al 2006:88]), thus further augmenting the CSR. Another element in the rise in CS is the 7% or so of cases recorded by obstetricians as responses to 'maternal request'. Some women requesting CS are motivated by previous negative experience of vaginal birth; others are possessed by a general fear of childbirth generated by today's culture, especially by TV (Baxter 2007, Gould 2007). Some have been persuaded that CS is safer for the baby (NICE 2004, Weaver & Statham 2005), an opinion the 2001 Sentinel Audit found was held by half of its obstetrician respondents. The Audit also found that obstetricians probably under-estimated how far women 'choosing' CS were in fact influenced by the advice they themselves had given. Obstetricians may also argue that they have no time to give women full and unbiased information on what is known about CS (Wagner 2000) and, as women's testimony demonstrates, some obstetricians believe that *women do not need this knowledge* (Barbieri 2006).

Certainly, recent research suggests that a significant proportion of women who have had CS have not understood the reason for it (Baldwin et al 2007, Baxter 2007) and some complain that they have been brow-beaten into having caesareans they did not want (Weaver & Statham 2005). Indeed, AIMS reports that they are contacted almost daily by women desperate to avoid a caesarean (Beech 2006). Constituting 24% or so of all births for 2005/06, CS deliveries accounted for over 40% of delivery spending, at a cost of £2 billion a year to the NHS (NHS Institute for Innovation and Improvement 2006).

## Governmental views

This financial burden on the NHS was duly noted in the 2004 CS guidelines from the National Institute for Clinical Excellence (NICE), in the hope of reducing the ever-rising CSR (Scotland has similar guidelines). Risks to mother and infant of both methods of delivery were compared and CS discouraged where any supposed benefits over vaginal delivery were uncertain, while maternal request for CS was not automatically considered adequate grounds. Though many obstetricians regard the CSR as too high, others celebrate its increase, and the guidelines ('this edict') came under immediate attack from two London obstetricians. Invoking the Winterton principle of 'Choice in childbirth', they declared CS the safest method of delivery for the mother and (especially) the baby, insisting that 'most' obstetricians shared this view (Fisk & Paterson Brown 2004).

Yet repeatedly the International Federation of Gynaecology and Obstetrics (FIGO) has declared normal vaginal delivery to be safer both in the short and long term for both mother and child, and CS for non-medical reasons ethically unjustified (FIGO 1999, 2003, 2008). Significantly, also, in 2002 the leading private health insurance firm AXA-PPP ceased paying for CS because it was becoming increasingly difficult for them to distinguish between medically necessary sections and those that were a matter of personal choice (BBC 2002).

FIGO's stance on the overall greater safety of vaginal over caesarean delivery is supported by the recent multicentre prospective cohort study (part of a WHO global survey) of 97,095 births. The study concluded that the increased CSR at an institutional level over recent years was not associated with any clear overall benefit for mother or baby, but linked with greater morbidity for both (Villar et al 2007).

Other negative effects may include emergency hysterectomy, reduced fertility, an increased rate of unexplained stillbirths, iatrogenic prematurity, fetal laceration, perforation of the maternal bowel and sepsis of the genital tract (Langdana et al 2001; Robinson 2004/5; Smith et al 1997, 2003a, 2003b; Wagner 2000). Indeed, two female London obstetricians propose that in the absence of medical indications CS should be performed only with a confirmatory second opinion (Bewley & Cockburn 2002).

## 'Choice, Continuity and Control'?: Winterton revisited

Three years after the publication of its CS guidelines, NICE offered 'best practice advice' on the care of healthy labouring women and their babies (NICE 2007). Echoing Winterton, the guidelines stipulated that care should be 'woman-and-baby centred', women being treated with kindness and respect and given enough information to make their own informed decisions, including choice of birth at home (Fig. 2.7) or in a midwife-led unit. Mobility during labour should be encouraged to hasten the process, as it had traditionally been before the advent of the 'new obstetrics' in the 1970s, together with the adoption of birthing positions most comfortable to the individual parturient. Strikingly, supine or semi-supine delivery postures (part and parcel of the 'new obstetrics') were strongly discouraged as more uncomfortable and less conducive to the infant's expulsion and, if all was progressing well, clinical interventions (such as amniotomy or oxytocin) should be neither offered nor advised.

How far, however, does this counsel of perfection square with current realities? Home births, currently

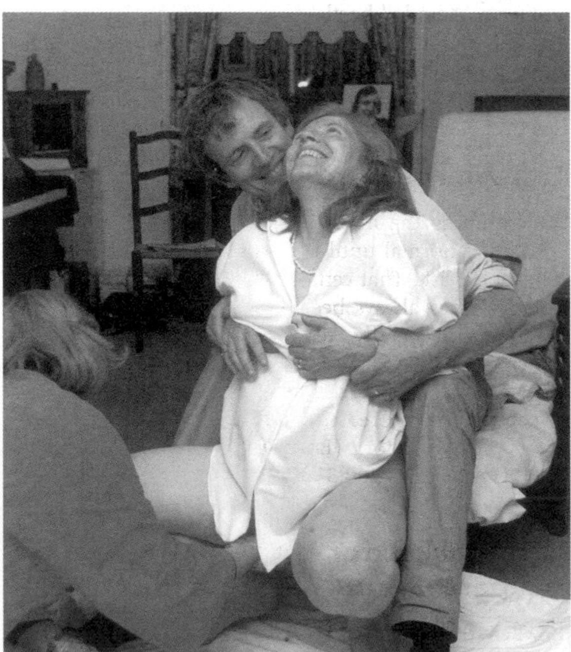

**Figure 2.7** A modern home birth. *(Sally and Richard Greenhill Photographic Library)*

averaging 2.5% of the total in England (less in Scotland, more in Wales), are actively discouraged by most obstetricians, general practitioners, and, indeed, midwives, whose general lack of experience of such birth leads them to fear it (Edwards 2005, 2008). Even where home birth has been agreed, it may not happen for lack of midwives. Moreover, midwife-led units provide for a mere 5% of total births. Significantly, despite their consistently good results (Rowbotham & Hunt 2006), government support for such centres is condemned by some obstetricians as a 'cheese-paring' move to substitute an 'inferior' service for that of the obstetrician-led CU (Carlisle 2007).

Women's own views of their birth experiences were recently recorded by the Healthcare Commission's (HCC) nationwide survey of 26,000 respondents giving birth early in 2007. Nearly a quarter of these women considered they had *not* been treated with kindness or respect, and around 30% that they had been excluded from decision-making during labour or delivery (HCC 2007). Only 61% had been able to choose their most comfortable position during the greater part of their labour, and despite the known links between continuous fetal monitoring and increased intervention (including CS) 45% of respondents suffered this (HCC 2008:41). Of those delivering vaginally, 12% exercised choice of birthing position, giving birth standing, squatting or kneeling. A quarter reported giving birth 'sitting in bed' (semi-supine), while as many as 57% delivered on their backs (supine), a position condemned by leading obstetricians 10 years ago (Steer & Flint 1999). Worse still, 27% of these delivered in the infamous 'stranded beetle' position with their feet in stirrups (HCC 2007). Continuous care by the same midwife throughout labour was enjoyed by only 20%, while 26% were left alone at a time of anxiety to them (ibid.).

## Can we measure 'risk'?

Underpinning the much-used obstetricians' dictum that no birth is normal until it is over is the now ubiquitous concept of 'risk'. That certain risks exist in pregnancy and childbirth has always been known, the most serious of which are generally readily recognizable by expert clinicians. Yet difficulties in 'risk factor' definition and quantification render risk-scoring 'systems' highly suspect, and their predictive values, positive and negative, have proved poor (Enkin et al 2000:49–51; Tew 1995:110–111,256–268,330–338).

## Strait-jacket for labour: the partogram

So where does this medically inspired preoccupation with 'risk' leave midwives, the supposed guardians of normal (intervention-free) birth? Nowadays, except when they attend home births or work in freestanding midwife-led birth centres, their practice is generally governed by obstetrician-determined protocol, usually based on each unit's particular partogram, or pictorial representation of labour progress. Most of these incorporate an 'action [intervention] line' (drawn 2, 3, or 4 hours to the right of a previous 'alert' line) which determines the 'need' for intervention, ranging from amniotomy through to caesarean section, with the aim of hastening the delivery. Yet different units vary widely in their partogram format and the data they base it on. A survey by Lavender et al (2008) found that most do not define the start of active labour. The rate of progress, too, was usually not reported, and when it was, some units specified 'normal' progress as cervical dilation of 0.5 cm an hour, others as 1 cm an hour, or *twice* as much. Interestingly, only seven units used different partograms for multiparous and primiparous women (Lavender et al 2008).

Are there any advantages, then, to be derived from forcing these rigid frameworks on labouring women? Clearly the practice benefits obstetricians, since on this is built their lucrative routine control of the highly individual process of childbirth. As for midwives, some may view the partogram's built-in directives as a severe constraint on the exercise of their professional judgement, while others consider it a 'useful tool' (Lavender et al 2008). To these it may give a sense of security, acting as a 'concrete' guide for the timing of the routine interventions characterizing the assembly-line style practice so general today (Osbourne & Lavender 2005). So far, however, there appears to be no evidence that partogram use has contributed to improved maternal and fetal outcomes (Lavender et al 2008).

In fact, recent research suggests that the very reverse may be true (Albers 2001). A recent randomized controlled trial of 3000 low-risk primigravidae in spontaneous labour showed that earlier intervention simply increased total obstetric interventions, neither reducing the CS rate nor improving maternal satisfaction. Moreover, the assessment of 51% of a sample of healthy women as in 'prolonged' labour suggests that current expectations of progressive cervical dilation of 1 cm an hour are unrealistic and that such progress *may not be linear* (Lavender et al 2006). Clearly, women come in different shapes, sizes, ages, parity and heredity, differing also in length of menstrual cycle and of gestation. It would therefore seem logical to expect each woman to have her particular inherited blueprint for the length and speed of her labour, rather than speak of 'inefficient' uteri, and 'deviations' from some externally imposed medically derived standard. One midwife, reflecting on her own long but totally successful labour, suggested, '... was this simply *normal for me*?' (Davies 2008, emphasis mine). In other words, women's individual differences make standardized guidance for labour progress inappropriate (Lavender et al 2006).

Yet we are informed, somewhat fatalistically, that tools such as the partogram are 'entrenched' in the system

(Lavender et al 2008). Such situations, however, are not new. In former times, childbearing women and their infants suffered from currently accepted medical interventions and proscriptions, also presented as vital to their wellbeing, and equally based on the false premise that Nature *routinely* needs help, control and correction. Among many such discarded 'best' medical practices have been 'prophylactic' blood-letting in pregnancy, labour and miscarriage; routine purging of newborns and substitution of indigestible artificial foods for the 'harmful' colostrum; and for post-parturient women the mandatory semi-starvation diet and prolonged bedrest, these last, indeed, persisting till after World War II (Donnison 2007).

## HAS THE MIDWIFE A FUTURE?

As already stated, the future of midwives proper (as opposed to those acting under medical direction in interventionist birth, in fact, as maternity nurses) is bound up with normal birth. However, except for births at home or in midwife-led units, normal births are nowadays in a minority. Some women planning home birth view NHS midwives as too controlling, hiring instead an independent midwife; others decide to give birth on their own (Cooper & Clarke 2008, Walsh 2008). Moreover, as in Willughby's day, some hide their pregnancies, giving birth silently in secret, leaving the child to be found by strangers. Lest any doubt the continuing and awesome power of Nature, they need only recall Sophia Pedro, who in March 2000, after four days in a tree surrounded by the swirling floodwaters of the Limpopo River, gave birth there to a healthy daughter before her helicopter rescue (Daniel 2008, NPR 2000).

Of recent years, government has demonstrated an unprecedented interest in NHS maternity care services, publishing evidence-based guidelines for practitioners and sponsoring research into user opinion, the latter giving rise to *Maternity matters* (DH 2007). This proposes that by end-2009, pregnant women should be able to refer themselves to a midwife or GP, as preferred; to choose birth at home or a birth centre rather than hospital; and to receive individual midwife attendance throughout labour and birth. Yet allocation of NHS funds still favours interventionist over non-interventionist care (O'Sullivan & Tyler 2007), contributing to the persistent midwife shortages hampering provision of midwife attendance in the home and continuity of care in hospital. Though many midwives are devoted to their calling, long hours (some possibly unpaid) and insufficient staffing result in a constant drain of qualified midwives from the workforce. Additionally, many are disillusioned by the gulf between their aspirations to be *true* midwives, or 'with-women', and the hurried reality of care ruled by medical direction and managerial imperative (Ball et al 2006, Curtis et al 2006, Kirkham 2007). Unsurprisingly, critics argue that the goals of *Maternity matters* are unlikely to be realized in time for the target date (ARM 2007, Clift-Matthews 2009).

### A leadership for our times?

Ahead of the pioneers of the tiny Midwives Institute stretched a long hard road, before, in 1902, they achieved their aim of a midwives registration Act. Equally onerous was their successors' struggle for the acceptance of midwifery as a profession, only achieved with the Institute's official elevation in 1941 to a 'College', and the granting of a Royal Charter in 1947. Since then, however, the centralization of maternity care in hospitals and the development of the 'new obstetrics' have bid fair to eradicate normal birth and with it the art of midwifery itself. Although recent government support for midwife-conducted birth has encouraged the RCM to speak of a 'renaissance' in midwifery (Davis 2005), this rebirth will not come of itself. First and foremost, it will require the active and enthusiastic leadership of a College committed to the purpose stated in its Royal Charter, namely, the furtherance of the 'art and science of midwifery'. Secondly, it will need, through cooperation with user groups and wider women's organizations, to make allies of the women it aims to serve (Savage 2007:176). Thirdly, if its 'campaign' for normal birth is to succeed, the College, like its Victorian founders, must continue to use political skills and combative determination necessary to hand down to posterity, as they did, the ancient office of midwife.

## KEY POINTS

When considering the history of midwives and of midwifery we need to recognize:

- that until relatively recently much of this was written by male practitioners, members of a dominant and rival group, many of whom, confident in their male superiority, looked forward to the total abolition of the midwife
- that many of these medical writers displayed a clear misogynistic prejudice, or at best a belittling condescension towards midwives, however skilled these were, and in fact towards childbearing women themselves
- that these lessons from the past have real relevance for the present organization of maternity care, and indeed for that of the future as well.

## REFERENCES


Unless otherwise referenced, material in this chapter is taken from Jean Donnison, *Midwives and medical men: a history of the struggle for the control of childbirth*, London, 1988, Historical Publications.

Allison J: *Delivered at home*, London, 1996, Chapman and Hall.

Anon: Editorial, *The Lancet* 1:507, 1929.

Association of Radical Midwives (ARM): Maternity Matters report – ARM's response, *Midwifery Matters* 113, Summer 2007.

Baldwin J, Brodrick A, Mason N, et al: Focus on normal birth and reducing caesarean section rates, *MIDIRS Midwifery Digest* 17(2):279, 2007.

Ball L, Curtis P, Kirkham M: Management and morale: challenges in contemporary maternity care, *British Journal of Midwifery* 14(2):100–103, 2006.

Barbieri A: Yes, we need to know, *The Guardian* 31, September 11, 2006.

Barnes J, editor: The complete works of Aristotle: the revised Oxford translation, vol 1, Bollingen Series, LXXI, 2,

Princeton, 1984, Princeton University Press, p. 1114.

Baxter J: Do women understand the reasons given for their caesarean sections? *British Journal of Midwifery* 15(9):536, 2007.

BBC Health News, November 2, 2002, http//news.bbc.co.uk/1/hi/health/2391843.stm.

Beech B: Defining and recording normal birth, *AIMS Journal* 18(4):3–4, 2006.

Bennett VR, Brown LK: *Myles textbook for midwives*, ed 11, London, 1989, Churchill Livingstone.

Bewley S, Cockburn J: The unfacts of 'request' caesarean section, *British Journal of Obstetrics and Gynaecology* 109(6):597–605, 2002.

Blenkinsop H, editor: *Observations in midwifery by Percival Willughby*, Warwick, 1863.

Brown HS: Physician demand for leisure: implications for cesarean section rates, *Journal of Health Economics* 15(2):233–242, 1996.

Burton J: *An essay towards a complete new system of midwifery*, London, 1751, James Hodges.

Carlisle D: Safe in their hands? *MIDIRS Midwifery Digest* 17(2):288, 2007.

Chamberlain G, Steer P: The ABC of labour care: labour in special circumstances, *British Medical Journal* 318(7191):1124–1127, 1999.

Churchill H, Savage W, Francome C: *Caesarean birth in Britain: a book for health professionals and parents*, Enfield, 2006, Middlesex University Press.

Clarke J: *Practical essays on the management of pregnancy and labour*, London, 1793.

Clement C: Amniotomy in spontaneous, uncomplicated labour at term, *British Journal of Midwifery* 9(10):629–634, 2001.

Clift-Matthews V: Assessing progress in Maternity Matters, *British Journal of Midwifery* 12(1):4, 2009.

Cooper T, Clarke P: Home alone: a concerning trend? *Midwives* June-July pp. 34–35 and Aug-Sep pp. 34–35, 2008.

Curtis P, Ball L, Kirkham M: Why do midwives leave? (Not) being the kind of midwife you want to be, *British Journal of Midwifery* 14(1):27–31, 2006.

Daniel L: There's no place like home, *British Journal of Midwifery* 16(12):819, 2008.

Davies S: Home birth and normality, *AIMS Journal* 20(3), 2008.

Davis K: Leading the midwifery renaissance, General Secretary's address to the RCM Annual Conference, Harrogate, *Midwives* 8(6):264–268, 2005.

Department of Health (DH): *Changing childbirth: report of the Expert Maternity Group*, London, 1993, HMSO.

Department of Health (DH): *Maternity matters: choice, access and continuity of care in a safe service*, London, 2007, Department of Health.

Department of Health and Social Security (DHSS): *Report on Confidential Enquiries into Maternal Deaths in England and Wales for 1970–1972 (Reports on Health and Social Subjects, No. 11)*, London, 1975, HMSO.

Donnison J: Sworn Midwife: Mistress Katherine Manley of Whitby, her work and world, *MIDIRS* 17(1):25–34, 2007.

Downe S: Active birth, active management, *RCM Midwives Journal* 4(7):228–230, 2001.

Downe S, McCormick C, Beech BL: Labour interventions associated with normal birth, *British Journal of Midwifery* 9(10):602–606, 2001.

Edwards N: *Birthing autonomy: women's experiences of planning home births*, Abingdon, 2005, Routledge.

Edwards N: Negotiating a normal birth, *AIMS Journal* 20(3):3–8, 2008.

Enkin M, Keirse MJNC, Neilson J, et al: *A guide to effective care in pregnancy and childbirth*, Oxford, 2000, OUP.

Fisk N, Paterson Brown S: The doctor's tale, *The Observer* 18, May 2, 2004.

Gans JS, Leigh A, Varganova E: *Minding the shop: the case of obstetrics conferences*, Centre for Economics Policy Research Discussion Paper 55, 2007, Australian National University.

Gélis J: *La sage-femme ou le médecin: une nouvelle conception de la vie*, Paris, 1988, Fayard.

Gélis J: *History of childbirth (trans. Morris R)*, Cambridge, 1996, Polity Press.

Gordon A: *A treatise on the epidemic puerperal fever of Aberdeen*, London, 1795.

Gould D: Rising caesarean rates: the power of mass suggestion, *British Journal of Midwifery* 15(7):398, 2007.

Healthcare Commission (HCC): *Women's experiences of maternity care in the NHS in England: key findings from a survey of NHS trusts carried out in 2007*, London, 2007, HCC.

Healthcare Commission (HCC): *Towards better births: a review of maternity services in England*, London, 2008, Commission for Healthcare Audit and Inspection.

Holland E: *The Lancet* 1:936, 1935.

House of Commons Health Committee (chaired by N Winterton): *Second Report: Maternity Services*, vol 1, London, 1992, HMSO.

International Federation of Gynaecology and Obstetrics (FIGO): *Recommendations on ethical issues in obstetrics and gynaecology by the FIGO*, London, 1999, 2003, 2008, Committee for the Ethical Aspects of Human Reproduction and Women's Health.

Jonas R: *The Byrth of Mankynde*, London, 1540.

Kirkham M: Retention and return in the NHS in England, *Midwives* 10(5):224–226, 2007.

Kuntner L: *Die Gebährung der Frau: Schwangerschaft und Geburt aus geschichtlicher, völkerkundlicher und medizinischer Sicht*, Munich, 1988, Marseille Verlag.

Langdana M, Geary W, Haw D, et al: Peripartum hysterectomy in the 1990s: any new lessons? *Journal of Obstetrics and Gynaecology* 21(2):121–123, 2001.

Lavender T, Alfrevic Z, Walkinshaw S: Effect of different action lines on birth outcomes: a randomized controlled trial, *Obstetrics and Gynaecology* 108(2):295–302, 2006 (authors' abstract, and MIDIRS' comments, see Caine D: *MIDIRS Midwifery Digest* 17(1):78–79)

Lavender T, Tsekiri E, Baker L: Recording labour: a national survey of partogram use, *British Journal of Midwifery* 16(6):359–362, 2008.

Leap N, Hunter B: *The midwife's tale: an oral history from handywoman to professional midwife*, London, 1993, Scarlet Press.

Lee B, editor: Big is policy: small is beautiful: the amalgamation of maternity units, *RCM Midwives' Journal* 4(1):12–13, 2001.

Macfarlane A, Mugford M, Henderson J: *Birth counts: statistics of pregnancy and childbirth*, London, 2000, HMSO.

McKeown T: *The role of medicine: dream, mirage or nemesis?* Oxford, 1976, Blackwell.

McMath J: *The expert mid-wife: a treatise of the diseases of women with child and in childbed*, Edinburgh, 1694.

May A: *Epidurals for childbirth*, Oxford, 1994, OUP.

Myles M: *Textbook for midwives*, eds 8 & 9, London, 1975 & 1981, Churchill Livingstone.

NHS Institute for Innovation and Improvement: *Focus on Caesarean Section*, London, 2006, NHS III.

National Institute for Clinical Excellence (NICE): *Caesarean section*, NICE Clinical Guideline 13, London, 2004, NICE.

National Institute for Clinical Excellence (NICE): *Intrapartum care: care of healthy women and their babies during childbirth*, NICE Clinical Guideline 55, London, 2007, NICE.

NPR News: Music cues: Rosetta Pedro was born this week, out of a biblical swirl of flood waters, NPR News Weekend Edition, March 4, 2000, www.npr.org/programs/wesat/000304.floods.html.

Osbourne A, Lavender T: Partograms are not needed in birth centres, *British Journal of Midwifery* 13(10):618–619, 2005.

O'Sullivan S, Tyler S: Payment by results: speaking in code, *RCM Midwives* 10(5):241, 2007.

Pechey J: *A general treatise of the diseases of maids, big-bellied women, child-bed women, and widows*, London, 1696.

Radford N, Thompson A: *Direct entry: a preparation for midwifery practice*, Guildford, 1988, University of Surrey.

Reid L: Turning tradition into progress: moving midwifery forward, *RCM Midwives' Journal* 5(8):250–254, 2002.

Robinson J: Why are more mothers dying? *AIMS Journal* 16(4):1–5, 2004/5.

Rowbotham M, Hunt S: Birth centre closures: avoiding long-term costs for short-term savings? *British Journal of Midwifery* 14(6):376–377, 2006.

Royal Society of Medicine: *The fetus as a patient*, Meeting of Obstetrics and Gynaecology Section Programme, November 11, 2002.

Royal College of Midwives (RCM): *Project 2000: Comments of the Royal College of Midwives*, London, 1986, RCM.

Royal College of Obstetrics and Gynaecology (RCOG): *Response to the report of the Expert Maternity Group: Changing childbirth*, London, 1993, RCOG.

Russell JGB: The rationale of primitive delivery positions, *British Journal of Obstetrics and Gynaecology* 89:712–715, 1982.

Savage W: *Birth and power: a Savage enquiry revisited*, London, 2007, Middlesex University Press.

Sharp J: *'The midwives book'*, London, 1671.

Siegemundin J: *Die königliche Preussische und Chur-Brandenburgische Hof-Wehe-Mutter, Das ist, Ein höchstnötiger Unterricht von schweren und unrechtstehenden Geburthen*, Coln an der Spree, 1690.

Smellie W: *Treatise on the theory and practice of midwifery*, London, 1752–64.

Smith JF Hernandez C, Wax J: Fetal laceration at cesarean delivery, *Obstetrics and Gynecology* 90(3):344–346, 1997.

Smith G, Pell J, Dobbie R: Caesarean section and risk of unexplained stillbirth, *The Lancet* 362(9398):1779–1784, 2003a.

Smith G, Pell J, Dobbie R: Interpregnancy interval and risk of preterm birth and neonatal death: retrospective cohort study, *British Medical Journal* 327(7410):313–316, 2003b.

Stapleton H, Kirkham M, Thomas G: Qualitative study of evidence based leaflets in maternity care, *British Medical Journal* 324(7338):639–643, 2002.

Stark JN, editor: An obstetric diary of William Hunter 1762–1765, *Glasgow Medical Journal* 70:167–177, 1908.

Steer P, Flint C: ABC of labour care: physiology and management of normal labour, *British Medical Journal* 318(7186):793–796, 1999.

Temkin O, editor: *Soranus' gynecology*, Baltimore, 1956, John Hopkins University Press.

Tew M: The case against hospital deliveries: the statistical evidence. In Kitzinger S, Davis J, editors: *The place of birth*, Oxford, 1978, OUP.

Tew M: *Safer childbirth? A critical history of maternity care*, London, 1995, Chapman and Hall.

Thomas K: *Religion and the decline of magic*, London, 1973, Penguin.

Villar J, Carroli G, Zavaleta N, et al; World Health Organization 2005 Global Survey of Maternal and Perinatal Health Research Group: Maternal and neonatal individual risks and benefits associated with caesarean delivery: multicentre prospective study, *British Medical Journal* 335(7628):1025, 2007.

Wagner M: Choosing caesarean section, *Lancet* 356(9242):1677–1680, 2000.

Wagner M: Fish can't see water: the need to humanize birth, *International Journal of Gynaecology and Obstetrics* 75(Suppl 1):S25–S37, 2001.

Walsh D: Free-birthing and the midwifery services, *British Journal of Midwifery* 16(11):702, 2008.

Weaver J, Statham H: Wanting a caesarean: the decision-making process, *British Journal of Midwifery* 13(6):370–373, 2005.

Wiesener M: The midwives of South Germany and the public/private dichotomy. In Marland H, editor: *The art of midwifery: early modern midwives in Europe*, London, 1993, Routledge.

Worth J: District midwifery in the 1950s, *MIDIRS Midwifery Digest* June 174–175, 2002.

# Chapter 3

# Statutory framework for practice

Belinda Ackerman

## LEARNING OUTCOMES

After reading this chapter, you will be able to:

- understand the legislation surrounding midwifery practice
- appreciate the role and functions of the Nursing and Midwifery Council (NMC)
- be conversant with the midwives' rules and standards, the code, and the midwife's statutory responsibilities for clinical practice
- be familiar with the role of the Local Supervising Authority Midwife
- have a working knowledge of the role of the Supervisor of Midwives
- understand the importance of the midwife in maintaining individual PREP and portfolio requirements.

## INTRODUCTION

This chapter provides an overview of the history of midwifery regulation, midwifery legislation ensuring protection of the public, and the rules and codes by which midwives are supported. The role of midwifery supervision is discussed, as well as how this differs from but works in conjunction with midwifery management, and is an integral component of clinical governance.

It is vital that midwives grasp the fundamentals of the unique professional support provided by midwifery supervision and use it to improve the quality of care given to women and their babies.

## LEGISLATION REGULATING THE MIDWIFERY PROFESSION

### Historical background

The first Midwives Act in 1902 sanctioned the establishment of a statutory body, the Central Midwives' Board for England and Wales (CMB), prescribed its constitution and laid down statutory powers. This Act was amended in 1918, 1926, 1934, 1936 and 1950. The Midwives Act of 1951 consolidated all previous Acts.

The Nurses, Midwives and Health Visitors Act of 1979 set up the United Kingdom Central Council (UKCC) and four country boards and established a combined statutory structure for nursing, midwifery and health visiting in the UK. It established a register of the three professions, containing 15 parts, to include the different specialities of nursing. Midwives registered on Part 10. This was the first time midwives were amalgamated in law with other professional groups.

A separate Midwifery Committee was set up in Statute following protests from the Royal College of Midwives (RCM) and Assocation of Radical Midwives (ARM) that midwives would be over-ruled by nurses (Jowitt & Kargar 1997).

However, in 1987, professional-specific education officers were replaced by *generic* education officers. Despite protest from members at the time, the Midwifery Committee was overruled on this matter.

Ten years later, an external review of the 1979 Act was commissioned by the Health Department. This resulted in a smaller, directly elected, central council with smaller appointed national boards. The responsibility for funding nursing and midwifery education was removed and delegated to regional health authorities. National boards remained responsible for course validation and accreditation only.

Government proposals that followed in Working Paper 10 (DH 1989) suggested setting up the purchaser–provider model – hospitals would contract with education providers for the requisite number of places to fulfil local workforce planning. These recommendations were accepted by the Government (DH 1991, Northern Ireland Office 1991, Scottish Office 1991) and were incorporated into the 1992, Nurses, Midwives and Health Visitors Act, including the revised structure of the UKCC and national boards. Consolidation of the 1979 and 1992 Acts, incorporating all the reforms, was made in the 1997 Nurses, Midwives and Health Visitors Act.

## Reform of the health professions

The drive to strengthen control of the healthcare professions followed several scandals involving the nursing (Clothier et al 1994) and medical professions (DH 2002a). In 1997, a further review of nursing and midwifery legislation was commissioned by the four UK health departments and complete reform of the UKCC and four national boards was recommended (JM Consulting 1998).

In February 1999, the government response accepted the need for new regulation of the 'various health professions' and proposed an amendment to the new Health Bill in progress at the time 'to make provision to repeal the Nurses, Midwives and Health Visitors Act 1997' (NHS Executive 1999).

Replacement legislation, by Order, regulating the professions was to be made subject to full consultation and publication of the Order in Draft. The Regulation of Health Care and Associated Professions under Clause 47(2) and Schedule 3.1 of the Health Bill clearly stated the scope of the Secretary of State's powers of regulation via an 'Order' following a period of 3 months' consultation.

The haste to replace primary legislation and substitute it with a Statutory Instrument by 'Order' for Nursing and Midwifery was a departure from the normal practice of parliamentary procedure customary during the previous century. Nursing and midwifery legislation had previously been subject to professional scrutiny throughout all the earlier stages, including publication of Green and White Papers. The midwifery protests to the restrictions of the legislation went unheeded.

## Current legislation regulating midwifery

### Health Act 1999 (Section 60) (DH 1999)

The current legislation for midwives drawn up under Section 62(9) of the Health Act 1999 (DH 1999) set out the Order for the establishment of the Nursing and Midwifery Council (NMC).

### Modernising regulation – the new Nursing and Midwifery Council – a consultation document (NHS Executive 2000)

This consultation document proposed the new structure of the UK body: the Nursing and Midwifery Council (NMC). It recommended a smaller, more transparent Council with equal representation of elected nurses, midwives and health visitors from each country. In addition, it proposed lay membership that would be almost equal numerically to the professional membership, with a lay chair. Partnership with the public was important to reduce concern about safety issues with self-regulation.

### Establishing the new Nursing and Midwifery Council (DH 2001a)

The Government drafted new legislation, with the NMC directly responsible to the independent Privy Council rather than the Secretary of State, thus removing a possible source of bias as the main employer of nurses and midwives.

### Modernising regulation in the health professions – NHS consultation document (DH 2001b)

The NHS Plan (DH 2000) proposed the establishment of a *UK Council of Health Regulators* to act as a forum and coordinate complaints from all the professions and their regulatory bodies.

This framework was also suggested in the Kennedy report on the Bristol Royal Infirmary Inquiry (DH 2002a). This Council would be independent of the State and accountable to Parliament, as would all the professional regulatory bodies, through the new Council. This, in turn, would have the power to require changes to the regulatory framework. It would not have the power to take over or intervene in individual fitness-to-practise cases.

### Nursing and Midwifery Order 2001 Statutory Instrument 2002 No. 253 (DH 2002b)

The Orders to establish the Nursing and Midwifery Council were set out in Draft and laid before Parliament in October 2001 for approval under Section 62(9) of the Health Act 1999. Royal Assent was given in February 2002. The Nursing and Midwifery Order 2001 came into force and the UK Nursing and Midwifery Council commenced office on 1 April 2002.

Part III set up Registration. Three parts of the Register were opened from August 2004:

- Nurses
- Midwives

- Specialist community public health nurses (that is: health visitors, school nurses, occupational health nurses, sexual health nurses, and health promotion nurses).

Part IV set up Education and Training.
Part V set up Fitness to Practise.
Part VIII related to Midwifery.

Midwifery-specific articles set out the following:

Article 41 – Establishment of the Midwifery Committee
Article 42 – Rules as to midwifery practice
Article 43 – Regulation of the LSA and supervisors of midwives
Article 45 – Regulation of attendance in childbirth.

### Trust, assurance and safety – the regulation of health professionals in the 21st century CM 7013 (DH 2007a)

This White Paper set out a major reform of the UK health professions following two reviews of professional regulation, 'The regulation of non-medical healthcare professions' (DH 2006a) and 'Good doctors, safer patients' (DH 2006b), and recommendations of the Fifth Report of the Shipman Inquiry (HM Government 2004) and recommendations of the Ayling, Neale and Kerr/Haslam Inquiries (HM Government 2007a, 2007b). It changed several areas:

- the Council structure of all professional regulators to parity of membership between lay and professional members
- independent appointment of professional members
- the criminal standard of proof to the civil standard of proof
- improving fitness to practise through standards (doctors to re-validate every 5 years) and required greater accountability to Parliament.

It included changes to the size and membership of the Council for Healthcare Regulatory Excellence (CHRE), established in 2003 (DH 2002c) to promote best practice in regulating health professionals.

In response to a request for the CHRE to expedite its annual performance review by the Minister of State for Health in March 2008, a special report identifed areas of weakness in the management of fitness to practise by the NMC, and other issues related to approval of education provision and governance (CHRE 2008).

Recommendations were made resulting in improvements in processing cases in a timely fashion using an integrated IT case-management system, improved training of panellists on child protection issues, and improved governance with greater transparency to stakeholders. The report included referral to the Charity Commission as the NMC is a registered charity.

The Health and Social Care Act (DH 2008a) later extended CHRE's powers to include reviewing fitness to practise where health is an issue and set up the Care Quality Commission.

**Box 3.1 Committee structure of the NMC**

**Four statutory committees**

1. Midwifery Committee
2. Investigating Committee*
3. Health Committee*
4. Conduct and Competence Committee*

**Five non-statutory committees**

1. Appointments Board
2. Audit, Risk and Assurance
3. Business, Planning and Governance
4. Fitness to Practise
5. Professional Practice and Registration

*The Investigating, Health, and Conduct and Competence Committees consist of pools of panellists and never meet.

### The Nursing and Midwifery (Amendment) Order 2008 (DH 2008b)

This amended Paragraphs 16, 17 and 18 of Schedule 1 of the Nursing and Midwifery Order 2001 in direct response to the DH White Paper 'Trust, assurance and safety' (DH 2007a) and the Health and Social Care Act (DH 2008a). It updated the size and membership of the NMC Council, the Midwifery Committee and Practice Committees (Box 3.1) and came into force in January 2009.

**Reflective activity 3.1**

Look on the Department of Health website and find the legislation that currently regulates your practice.

## NURSING AND MIDWIFERY COUNCIL

### Core functions

The primary function of the NMC is as a regulator of the professions, thereby safeguarding the public, through:

1. Establishment and maintenance of a register of all nurses, midwives and health visitors.
2. Setting standards for the education and practice of all nurses, midwives and health visitors.
3. Regulating fitness to practise, conduct and performance through rules and codes.

The Council has the power to remove a person from the Register, thus preventing the individual from practising as a nurse, midwife or health visitor. It also has a statutory duty to inform and educate registrants and to inform the public about its work.

## Membership

The Council consists of 14 members (seven registrants and seven lay members) appointed by the Appointments Commission on behalf of the Privy Council.

## Role and functions of the NMC Statutory Committees

### 1. Midwifery Committee

The Midwifery Committee advises the NMC on *any matter affecting midwifery practice* (including midwives' rules and standards), education (development of standards and guidance for pre- and post-registration midwifery education) and statutory supervision of midwives (standards for local supervising authorities and supervisors of midwives). It responds to policy trends, research and ethical issues and conducts consultations on behalf of the Council. It operates under the NMC Standing Orders 2009 (NMC 2010a).

**Membership:** five midwives and five lay members (at least one from each of the UK countries).

### 2. Investigating Committee

Panels of the Investigating Committee are responsible for considering any allegations of 'unfitness to practise' referred to the NMC.

A registered medical practitioner will be present if the registrant's health is in question. These deliberations take place in private and the panel decides whether there is a case to answer. If there is, referral is made to the Health Committee or the Conduct and Competence Committee (DH 2002b). The Panel may refer immediately to an Interim Orders hearing if the registrant is thought to be an immediate threat to the public. The panel can then impose the following:

a) An 'interim suspension' order – registration is suspended. This prevents registrants from working during investigation of the case. This can be imposed for up to 18 months but must be reviewed after 6 months and thereafter every 3 months. This would be used in cases such as rape, to protect the public.
b) An 'interim conditions of practice' order – an alternative to postponing judgement where the registrant agrees to be bound by a set of agreed conditions. It can be revoked, modified or replaced with a different order according to circumstances.

In addition, a 'removal' from the Register can be authorised by the Investigating Committee to correct an incorrect or fraudulent entry (NMC 2008a).

### 3. Health Committee

The Panel's role is to consider: 'any allegation referred to it by the Investigating Committee or the Conduct and Competence Committee and any application for restoration referred by the Registrar' (DH 2002b).

### 4. Conduct and Competence Committee

The Panel's role is to consider any allegations referred to it by the Investigating Committee or the Health Committee. Hearings are held in public but parts of the case may be held in private to protect the identity of the person or confidential medical evidence (NMC 2008a). A panel must consist of at least three people, and must include a lay person and a 'due regard' (that is, someone from the same speciality as the professional being investigated).

### Conduct and Competence Committee and Health Committee Panels' sanctions

The Conduct and Competence Committee Panel and Health Committee Panel establish, in cases referred to them, whether fitness to practise is impaired by any of the following:

- misconduct
- lack of competence
- a criminal offence
- mental or physical health
- a determination by a health professions body in the UK that fitness to practise is impaired (NMC 2008a).

All decisions are based on evidence presented at the hearing of the case. The panel will only hear information about the previous history of the 'respondent' and any evidence in mitigation prior to making a final decision (NMC 2010d).

The range of powers it holds in relation to sanctions are as follows:

They may decide on no further action; or make one of the following orders to the Registrar:

a) a 'striking-off' order – this removes the registrant's name from the Register for a minimum of 5 years; this prevents individuals from employment requiring registration and will probably be implemented for cases of misconduct
b) a 'suspension' order – not exceeding 1 year; this is more in respect of lack of competence (LOC) and health
c) a 'conditions of practice' order – not exceeding 3 years; this also is more in respect of LOC and health
d) a 'caution' order – not less than 1 year and not more than 5 years; the practitioner works normally and

the caution remains on the register entry for the prescribed period. Future employers will be alerted to the caution and will be informed as to why it was imposed.

An appeal may be made by the registrant within 28 days of a committee's decision.

### Restoration to the Register of practitioners who have been struck off

An application may be made before the end of 5 years, or in any period of 12 months in which an application for restoration to the Register has already been made, by the person who has been struck off. The application for restoration to the Register is made via the Registrar and is forwarded to the relevant Committee that made the 'striking-off' order. If the Committee is satisfied that the registrant has achieved the additional education or training or experience required, then the registration fee is paid and the practitioner is restored to the Register.

If an application is unsuccessful, an appeal may be made within 28 days of the decision date. If a second or subsequent application is made while a striking-off order is in force and is rendered unsuccessful, the Committee may direct that the person be suspended indefinitely (DH 2001a).

## Other requirements

The NMC are required to appoint legal assessors, medical assessors and registrant assessors to advise the Council or its committees as appropriate.

## Civil Standard of Proof

The 'Civil Standard of Proof' was brought into force on 16th October 2008 following the DH White Paper (DH 2007a) and Health and Social Care Act 2008 (Commencement No. 3) Order 2008 (SI 2008/2717 [C. 120]) (DH 2008a). All NMC hearings have used this standard since 3rd November 2008. This means that evidence is based on the 'balance of probabilities' rather than the previously used 'Criminal Standard of Proof', where facts needed to be proved 'beyond reasonable doubt'.

## Role and functions of the NMC Non-Statutory Committees

### 1. Appointments Board

This board deals with the appointment, development and appraisal of Fitness to Practice panellists and processing applicants for non-Council membership of committees and local supervising authority (LSA) reviewers. It ensures relevant academic or clinical expertise on a committee and also advises Council on removal of panellists from office.

### 2. Audit, Risk and Assurance

This committee ensures that the business of Council is conducted with integrity and probity. It agrees internal and external auditing arrangements and management of risk. It also ensures the quality and standards for education and training are being met and approval of training institutions and programmes by monitoring the UK Quality Assurance framework contract.

### 3. Business Planning and Governance

This committee advises Council on all matters relating to the management of resources and the maintenance of good governance standards throughout the NMC. It appoints members to the Council, recommends any amendments to the Standing Orders or code of conduct for members, and the development, performance and appraisal of Council members (NMC 2010e).

### 4. Fitness to Practise

This is a strategic committee separate from the three practice committees. It advises Council on matters related to standards, conduct, performance and ethics expected of registrants (and students who are prospective registrants). It also advises on the requirements as to good character and good health expected of registrants and ensures protection of the public where fitness to practise is impaired (NMC 2004a, 2009a).

### 5. Professional Practice and Registration

This Committee advises on all matters relating to nursing and community public health nursing such as standards of education and training and practice guidance (midwifery standards and guidance are dealt with by the Midwifery Committee).

In addition, it advises on all aspects of registration and renewal of registration (NMC 2010f).

## FUNCTIONS OF THE NMC

## Function 1: The Register

The Register is divided into parts determined by the Privy Council. There are currently three parts to the Register:

1. Nurses
2. Midwives
3. Specialist Community Public Health Nurses (Health Visitors).

The Council determines the fee to be charged and coordinates initial registration or renewal to the Register. Visiting European Union nurses or midwives are deemed registered and can practise in the UK subject to knowledge of English and comparable qualifications (see website).

## Function 2: Setting standards for education and practice

### Pre-registration midwifery

The NMC is charged with establishing the pre-registration standards of education and training, including requirements for good health and good character. It ensures standards of education programmes remain high through a network of heads of midwifery education called Lead Midwives for Education (LMEs) (NMC 2010g).

It appoints 'visitors' to visit institutions and report back on the nature and quality of the instruction given, including facilities provided. The NMC visitors are trained for their role and are midwives drawn from the profession. Visitors are not allowed to be NMC employees or employees of the universities being visited or anyone who has a close connection with the university through, for example, lecturing. Visitors are required to complete a report summarizing the information gained and are reimbursed by the NMC for expenses incurred. If the Council is of the opinion that the standards established under Article 15(1) are not met, it may refuse to approve, or withdraw approval from, the particular institution (DH 2002b); therefore, a university would be unable to continue to teach students undertaking professional programmes until approval had been reinstated.

Institutions are required to provide information to the Council about all the programmes they offer for registration to the different parts of the Register.

### Pre-registration midwifery standards and fitness to practise

A review of pre-registration midwifery education was carried out on behalf of the NMC in 2006 (Burke & Saldanha 2006). As a result, a minimum academic level of a degree for midwifery programmes was recommended by the Midwifery Committee (NMC 2007a). Other recommendations were:

- practice/theory ratio – no less than 50% practice and no less than 40% theory
- clinical practice to be included as part of the academic award and therefore graded
- students to take on a small caseload of women to provide antenatal, intrapartum and postnatal care during their training.

Supporting birthing women in a variety of settings, such as home births and birth centres, was also recommended (NMC 2007b).

The second edition of standards to support learning and assessment in practice was published in 2008 (NMC 2008b). This ensured students were to be supported and assessed by mentors who had met the additional sign-off criteria. Sign-off mentors are now to make the final assessment of practice and confirm that the required proficiences for practice have been achieved (NMC 2008b). A triennial review of mentors and practice teachers is required to be maintained on a local register and all mentors must have completed an NMC-approved mentorship or teacher preparation (NMC 2009a&b).

Standards for pre-registration midwifery education were updated in 2009 (NMC 2009c). The length of the programmes are set at 3 years (156 weeks) and 18 months (78 weeks) for registered nurses.

The NMC set competencies required by students to achieve the standards, which are divided into four domains:

- Effective midwifery practice
- Professional and ethical practice
- Developing the individual midwife and others
- Achieving quality care through evaluation and research.

*Essential skills clusters*, including communication, initial consultation between the woman and midwife, normal labour and birth, initiation and continuance of breastfeeding, and medicines management, are also required (NMC 2009c).

Declaration of good health and good character of each midwifery student must be made by the LME at the education institution on successful completion of the programme 'in order to satisfy the Registrar that an applicant is capable of safe and effective practice as a nurse or midwife' [Article 5(2)(b)] Nursing and Midwifery Order 2001 (NMC 2008c).

## Function 3: Regulating Fitness to Practise, Conduct and Performance

This function is supported by the NMC rules, standards and advice publications set out by the NMC practice committees (see Box 3.2). In midwifery, audit and monitoring of compliance is carried out by the local supervising authorities and supervisors of midwives (NMC 2009d).

**Box 3.2 Rules and standards**

**Rules:** rules are established through legislation set out in the Order and are requirements for registration and practice (NMC 2004b).

**Standards:** the NMC is required by the Nursing & Midwifery Order 2001 to establish standards of proficiency to be met by applicants to the register [Article 5 (2)(a)].

The practice committees ensure non-compliance to the rules and standards is reviewed and individual cases are investigated.

A synopsis of the NMC rules and codes are listed below (see www.nmc-uk.org).

## Midwives rules and standards (NMC 2004b)

The midwives rules and standards are currently under review and awaiting public consultation but will remain in effect until the end of 2011.

There are 16 rules.

**Rule 1** is a citation of when the Rules came into force in August 2004 and **Rule 2** is an interpretation of the definitions.

Rules relating to midwifery practice are in Table 3.1 and rules relating to statutory supervision and local supervising authority midwives in Table 3.2.

**Table 3.1 Midwives rules relating to midwifery practice**

| Rule | Title | Practice issues |
|---|---|---|
| Rule 3 | Notification of intention to practise (ITP) | If a midwife practises clinically or holds a post for which midwifery is a required qualification, a midwife must notify the Local Supervising Authority, through her Supervisor of Midwives. This is required annually (usually by 31st March) or within 48 hours of care given in an emergency |
| Rule 6 | Responsibility and sphere of practice | A practising midwife is responsible for providing care to both a woman and baby and must refer to the relevant practitioner in an emergency if the situation deviates from the norm. The midwife must not give care unless she is trained to do so unless it is during an emergency |
| Rule 7 | Administration of medicines | A midwife shall supply and administer drugs only for which she has been trained and she must abide by drugs regulations |
| Rule 8 | Clinical trials | A practising midwife may only participate in clinical trials if there is a protocol approved by a relevant ethics committee |
| Rule 9 | Records | A practising midwife must keep contemporaneous records, detailed observations and a record of any medications administered to a woman or baby. It also includes arrangements for storage with the employer or LSA |
| Rule 10 | Inspection of premises and equipment | A practising midwife must allow her supervisor or the LSA access to monitor her records and equipment |

## Confidentiality (NMC 2006a)

This advice covers all aspects of information about patients and clients and laws covering access to records.

## Gifts and gratuities (NMC 2008e)

Gifts or hospitalities should be refused if they are interpreted as an attempt to gain preferential treatment.

## Environment of care (NMC 2008f)

It is the responsibility of registrants to practise in a safe environment and to report concerns if problems in the environment are putting people at risk.

## Accountability (NMC 2008g)

Registrants are reminded that they are professionally accountable to the NMC, accountable to the law, as well as having a contractual accountability to their employer. They must act in the best interests of the person in their care at all times.

## The PREP handbook (NMC 2008h)

This comprises post-registration education and practice (PREP) guidance to ensure registrants remain updated in their field of practice. Practising for a minimum of 450 hours and maintenance of continuing professional development over the 3-year registration period must be completed. Guidance is given for returning to practice if registration has lapsed.

## The code (NMC 2008i)

This includes advice regarding treating people with dignity and respect, consent, maintaining professional boundaries, working as part of a team, delegation, keeping skills up to date, using best available evidence, maintaining clear, accurate records, acting with integrity and upholding the reputation of the profession.

## Standards for medicines management (NMC 2008j)

Twenty-six standards are listed under the following sections: supply and administration; dispensing; storage and transportation; practice of administration; delegation; disposal; unlicensed medicines; complementary and alternative therapies; managing adverse events; and controlled

**Table 3.2 Midwives rules relating to statutory supervision and local supervising authority midwives (NMC 2004b)**

| Rule | Title | Statutory supervision and LSA issues |
|---|---|---|
| Rule 4 | Notifications by local supervising authority (LSA) | The LSA is required to publish the name of the LSA officer, the date by which all ITPs should be submitted, receive the ITPs and notify the NMC annually. This is a means to ensuring a complete list of practising midwives is submitted by each LSA midwife |
| Rule 5 | Suspension from practice by a local supervising authority | Invests the power and authority to suspend a midwife from practice in order to protect the public if the midwife poses an immediate danger and is reported to the NMC. This would be progressed to an interim suspension order pending the outcome of an investigation |
| Rule 11 | Eligibility for appointment as a supervisor of midwives (SOM) | A midwife needs to be a practising midwife with 3 years' experience and have completed a *programme for a supervisor of midwives as agreed by the NMC and maintain updated, as required of a supervisor. |
| Rule 12 | The supervision of midwives | A practising midwife shall have a SOM appointed by the LSA covering her main area of practice. The LSA must ensure that each midwife has a named SOM and meets her at least once annually to review her practice and identify her training needs. The SOM must maintain a record of all meetings. Midwives must have 24-hour access to a SOM |
| Rule 13 | The local supervising authority midwifery officer | Each LSA shall appoint an LSA midwifery officer (LSAMO). The LSAMO must be a practising midwife and meet the standards of experience and education set by the NMC |
| Rule 14 | Exercise by a local supervising authority of its functions | Where an LSA has concerns about whether an LSAMO or a SOM meets the Council's standards, the Council should discuss their concerns |
| Rule 15 | Publication of local authority procedures | Each LSA shall publish the name and address of the LSAMO and procedure for reporting all adverse incidents relating to midwifery practice or impaired fitness to practise and how it will investigate such reports. In addition, how it will deal with complaints against LSAMOs or SOMs within its area |
| Rule 16 | Annual report | The LSA must submit an annual report to the NMC every year |

*Amendment to Rule 11– NMC (Midwives) (Amendment) Rules 2007 (SI2007/1887) – March 2008 NMC Circular 04/2008 (NMC 2008d) *'If the programme was completed more than 5 years ago without appointment, the knowledge and experience gained is no longer valid and a new programme of preparation must be undertaken'*

drugs. A CD-ROM is also provided which includes the relevant legislation.

## Record keeping: guidance for nurses and midwives (NMC 2009e)

The principles and purpose of record-keeping are discussed, including confidentiality, access to records, and disclosure, and relevant Acts are listed.

## Guidance on professional conduct for nursing and midwifery students (NMC 2010h)

This guidance covers all aspects of fitness to practise and behaviour expected of a student, including areas of concern such as cheating and plagiarism.

## Raising and escalating concerns: guidance for nurses and midwives (NMC 2010b)

This draft guidance states that raising a concern should be made in a timely manner in order to safeguard the public. Examples include: a danger or risk to health and safety; issues regarding care delivery; issues relating to the environment of care, such as staffing problems; issues related to the health of a colleague; and issues related to misuse or unavailability of medical equipment. The guidance suggests contacting a supervisor of midwives, mentor or university tutor and relevant contact organizations are listed. Consultation with both the public and professionals is completed and awaiting publication in late Autumn 2010.

### Advice and information for employers of nurses and midwives (NMC 2010c)

Responsibilities as an employer and recognition of misconduct, lack of competence, bad character and poor health are discussed in this guidance and how to investigate and refer to the NMC.

## Midwifery supervision

Statutory supervision of midwives supports protection of the public by promoting best practice and excellence in care; preventing poor practice and intervening in unacceptable practice (NMC 2006b).

### History of midwifery supervision

Statutory supervision of midwives was enshrined in the 1902 Midwives Act which set up the Central Midwives Board (CMB). Initially, the board had a medical majority and was required to discipline midwives who disobeyed or ignored the Rules or who were guilty of negligence, malpractice or misconduct (personal or professional). The CMB delegated supervision and monitoring to local supervising authorities, then under the control of county councils and county borough councils, until 1973 when they came within the NHS.

The 1936 Midwives Act empowered the CMB to make rules relating to the qualifications of medical and non-medical supervisors of midwives. It required non-medical supervisors to be practising midwives. In 1937, a Ministry of Health letter was released expanding on the detail of the 1936 Act, stating that inspectors of midwives were now to be known as supervisors of midwives; and most importantly that the supervisor should act as a 'counsellor and friend'.

The 1973 NHS Reorganisation Act abolished LSAs under borough councils and nominated regional health authorities as LSAs. The delegation of duties to supervisors of midwives was nominated by district health authorities. The 1977 Statutory Instrument (SI) No. 1850 eradicated the role of 'medical supervisor' and removed the words 'non-medical' from the title of supervisor.

Since 1996, employment of LSA officers has been devolved to Strategic Health Authorities (SHAs). The LSA officer was now required to be a practising midwife in line with the DH document *Managing the new NHS* (DH 1994).

The Nursing and Midwifery Order 2001 (DH 2002b) sets out the current responsibility of the LSA for the function of statutory supervision of midwives and this is enshrined in the midwives rules and standards (NMC 2004b) (see Table 3.2).

### Education and training for supervisors of midwives

In 1978 the CMB introduced courses of instruction for supervisors, initially for those in post since 1974. These courses later became mandatory before or immediately after appointment as a supervisor (UKCC 1986 44(2)). A formal open learning programme and training package 'Preparation for supervisors of midwives' was first developed at diploma level in 1992 by the English National Board (ENB 1992) and successful completion of the programme was required prior to being nominated to become a supervisor. UK standards for the preparation and practice of supervisors of midwives (NMC 2006b) now set out the standards of competence required in accordance with the midwives rules and standards, Rule 11 (NMC 2004b). Programmes of education are delivered by HEIs and approved and monitored annually by the NMC (NMC 2006b).

### The Local Supervising Authority Midwifery Officer (LSAMO)

The LSAMO is appointed by the Strategic Health Authority in England (Health Boards in Scotland, Health Inspectorate in Wales and the Public Health Agency in Northern Ireland) and is responsible for the provision of statutory midwifery supervision on behalf of the NMC (DH 2002b, NMC 2004b).

The LSA sets standards for statutory supervision of midwives and carries out an annual audit of the standards of midwifery practice locally. This includes receipt of the annual intention to practise data from supervisors, evidence of liaison with services users, engagement with HEIs, and any investigations of misconduct or lack of competence undertaken.

The LSAMO is responsible for suspension of midwives from practice (NMC 2004b: Rule 5), ensuring a full investigation is carried out and advising the investigating supervisor of midwives (SOM) if a period of supervised practice is required (NMC 2007c).

An annual report is submitted to the NMC about the standards, local activities, good practice and trends affecting the maternity service within its area (NMC 2004b: Rule 16).

The NMC reviews the LSA profiles annually using a risk assessment approach (NMC 2009d). Based on this, a decision is made to carry out a formal review of selected LSAs to verify if they are meeting the standards and a panel is appointed by the NMC Appointments Board.

The NMC produces an analysis of all the LSAs in the form of an annual report with recommendations on the 10 standards (NMC 2009f) (Table 3.3).

### The Supervisor of Midwives (SOM)

The role of the Supervisor of Midwives is unique in its protection of the public and support to midwives by providing a high standard of care to women and their babies. Supervisors provide leadership and guidance to midwives, including the provision of a 24-hour service for midwives and women (LSAMO National Forum 2009, NMC 2007c).

**Table 3.3 Rule 16 standards (NMC 2004b)**

| Number | Standard |
|---|---|
| 1. | Each LSA will ensure their report is made available to the public |
| 2. | Numbers of supervisors of midwives appointments, resignations and removals |
| 3. | Details of how midwives are provided with continuous access to SOMs |
| 4. | Details of how the practice of midwives is supervised |
| 5. | Evidence that services users have been involved in monitoring supervision of midwives and assisting the LSAMO with the annual audits |
| 6. | Evidence of engagement with HEIs in relation to supervisory input into midwifery education |
| 7. | Details of any new policies related to the supervision of midwives |
| 8. | Evidence of developing trends that may impact on the practice of midwives in the LSA |
| 9. | Details of the number of complaints regarding the discharge of the supervisory function |
| 10. | Reports on all LSA investigations undertaken during the year |

Supervision provides support for parents regarding choice for place of birth, concerns regarding midwifery care and maintenance of safety, for example, at a home birth (NMC 2009g). The midwife has a duty of care to the woman, as well as a contractual duty to the employer, and she may need to seek advice from her supervisor should any conflict arise.

Statutory supervision combines *professional* and *practice* responsibilities for challenging inferior practice and setting required standards, as well as carrying out clinical audit. Supervisors ensure that midwives have access to the statutory NMC rules, codes and standards and access to local clinical guidelines.

Supervision involves administrative and education tasks, including receipt of a midwife's annual notification of intention to practise. Supervisors audit records, arrange regular meetings with individual midwives, at least once annually, and work with them to identify areas of practice requiring development (LSAMO National Forum 2009). They monitor staffing levels and skill-mix in relation to safe practice, and notify senior management when there is a shortfall. They contribute to risk management and clinical governance within the NHS, investigate any allegations of professional misconduct and report upwards to the LSA (see Fig. 3.1).

Every midwife should have a named supervisor of her or his choosing. Supervisors have a responsibility to provide support to all midwives outside the NHS, including the private sector, higher education institutions (HEIs), prisons, independent midwives and GP practice midwives (NMC 2007b, 2007c). The ratio of supervisors to midwives should be 1 : 15 (NMC 2004a).

**Reflective activity 3.2**

Have you been allocated a named supervisor? What is the ratio of midwives to supervisors in your locality?

## Statutory supervision and management

Statutory supervision and management are distinct and separate from each other but must liaise, especially regarding allegations of unfitness to practise. Midwives should be appraised of the difference, and given access to a named supervisor who is not their manager, so that the roles are not confused.

## Statutory supervision and clinical governance

Statutory supervision is a vital component of leadership and clinical governance within the maternity services (see Ch. 7), supporting clinical risk management by monitoring service developments and reconfigurations to identify trends, provide a framework for continuous improvement and ensure that safety and quality is assured (DH 2007b).

It provides a proactive service and can limit the volume of *serious adverse incidents* within an organization by the very nature of its practice and education support to every individual midwife in the UK. Specifically, supervisors can work with midwives and risk managers to carry out the recommendations of the most recent clinical guidelines, such as the NICE guidelines (NICE 2004, 2006, 2007, 2008).

Supervision can support standards for staffing maternity units, such as those identified in *Safer childbirth* (RCOG 2007) and those of the Health Care Commission (HCC 2008), King's Fund (King's Fund 2008) review of the maternity services that recommended improved staffing, training and communication skills and the RCM publication specifying the ratio of midwives to women and babies to provide safety of practice (RCM 2009). The more recent project on *Safer births* (NPSA 2009) is actively supported by statutory supervision.

Delivering high-quality midwifery care (DH 2009) calls for further work to be carried out on the aspects of supervision that are most effective. It challenges supervisors to include feedback from women as part of their annual review and can only serve to strengthen supervision.

Finally, the supervisor must ensure that midwives are aware of national and local safeguarding policies and are

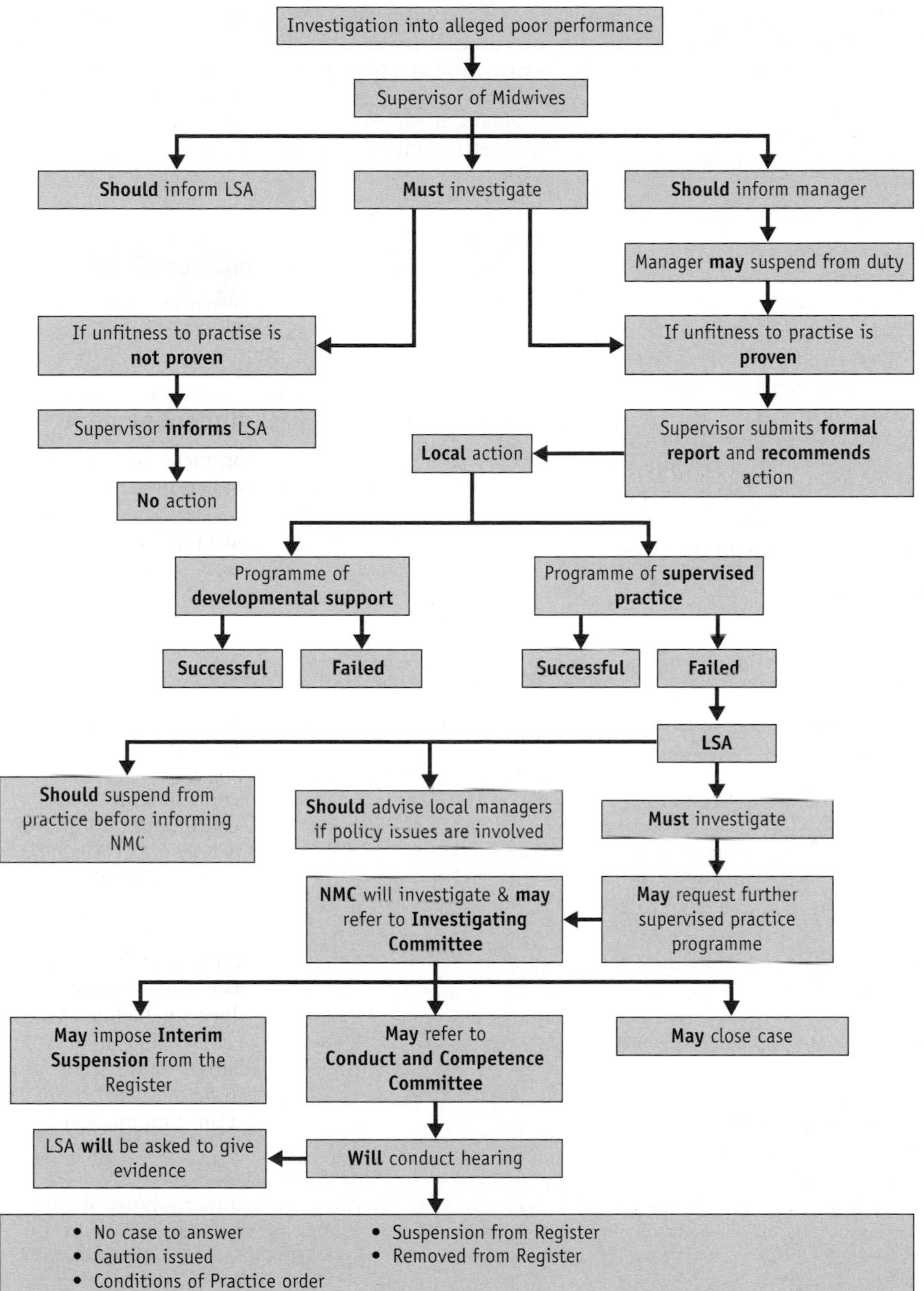


**Figure 3.1** Flow chart regarding allegations of unfitness to practise (NMC 2007b).

supported in their practice during any involvement in child protection cases. Multidisciplinary training can be arranged jointly by the supervisor and risk manager.

## CONCLUSION

Midwifery legislation has provided over 100 years of statutory supervision, and protection of the public has been upheld through its quality and standards. The number of midwifery registrants referred to the regulating body for professional misconduct has remained insignificant, demonstrating a mature forward-thinking approach to continuing professional development.

Midwives have always worked closely with the users of the service throughout their history. Recent revision of the Nursing and Midwifery Order (DH 2008b) to provide parity between lay and professional members of Council is a welcome move towards greater transparency in regulation of the professions.

The formation of a UK LSAMO's forum will provide additional support to supervisors and strengthen statutory supervision by working together to set standards and audit practice.

Finally, the revision of the *Midwives Rules and Standards* in 2011 should be a positive move in uniting the midwifery profession under improved regulation and alignment with other professions.

### KEY POINTS

- The statutory framework provides safety of practice for women and their families.
- Midwives must be knowledgeable about the statutory framework within which they practise, which includes familiarity with the rules and standards.
- Midwifery supervision is an important component of clinical risk management in improving care for mothers and babies, and supporting and developing midwifery practice.

## REFERENCES


Burke A, Saldanha M: *NMC consultation on a review of pre-registration midwifery education. Final report*, London, 2006, NMC.

Clothier C, Macdonald CA, Shaw DA: *The Allitt Enquiry*, London, 1994, The Stationery Office.

Council for Healthcare Regulatory Excellence (CHRE): *Special report to the Minister of State for Health on the Nursing and Midwifery Council*, London, 2008, CHRE.

Department of Health (DH): *Working for patients: education and training*. Working Paper 10, London, 1989, The Stationery Office.

Department of Health (DH): *Statement by the Secretary of State for Health on nursing, midwifery and health-visiting education and the future role and structure of the statutory bodies*, London, 1991, The Stationery Office.

Department of Health (DH): *Managing the new NHS*, London, 1994, The Stationery Office.

Department of Health (DH): *Health Act 1999*, London, 1999, The Stationery Office.

Department of Health (DH): *The NHS plan. A plan for investment. A plan for reform*. CM 4818-4811, London, 2000, The Stationery Office.

Department of Health (DH): *Establishing the new Nursing and Midwifery* Council, London, 2001a, The Stationery Office.

Department of Health (DH): *Modernising regulation in the health professions – NHS Consultation Document*, London, 2001b, DH. Available at: www.doh.gov.uk/modernisingregulation.

Department of Health (DH): *Learning from Bristol: The Department of Health's response to the report of the public inquiry into children's heart surgery at the Bristol Royal Infirmary 1984–1995. Executive summary*, London, 2002a, The Stationery Office.

Department of Health (DH): *Nursing and Midwifery Order 2001 Statutory Instrument 2002 No. 253*, London, 2002b, The Stationery Office.

Department of Health (DH): *NHS Reform and Health Care Professions Act*, London, 2002c, The Stationery Office.

Department of Health (DH): *The regulation of non-medical healthcare professions: a review by the Department of Health*, London, 2006a, The Stationery Office.

Department of Health (DH): *Good doctors, safer patients: proposals to strengthen the system to assure and improve the performance of doctors and to protect the safety of patients. A report by the Chief Medical Officer*, London, 2006b, The Stationery Office.

Department of Health (DH): *Trust, assurance and safety – the regulation of health professionals in the 21st century*, CM 7013, London, 2007a, The Stationery Office.

Department of Health (DH): *Maternity matters: choice, access and continuity of care in a safe service*, London, 2007b, DH.

Department of Health (DH): *The Health and Social Care Act*, London, 2008a, The Stationery Office.

Department of Health (DH): *The Nursing and Midwifery Council (Constitution) Order 2008 No. 2553*, London, 2008b, The Stationery Office.

Department of Health (DH): *Delivering high quality midwifery care: the priorities, opportunities and challenges for midwives*, London, 2009, DH.

English National Board (ENB): *Preparation of supervisors of midwives, Module 1–4*, London, 1992, ENB.

Healthcare Commission (HCC): *Towards better births: a review of maternity services in England*, London, 2008, HCC.

HM Government: *The Shipman Inquiry- safeguarding patients: lessons from the past, proposals for the future*, London, 2004, The Stationery Office.

HM Government: *Safeguarding patients: the Government's response to the recommendations of Shipman Inquiry's Fifth Report and to the recommendations of the Ayling, Neale and Kerr/Haslam Inquiries*, London, 2007a, The Stationery Office.

HM Government: *Learning from tragedy, keeping patients safe*, CM7014, London, 2007b, The Stationery Office.

JM Consulting: *Regulation of nurses, midwives and health-visitors. Report on a review of the Nurses, Midwives and Health-Visitors Act 1997*, Bristol, 1998, JM Consulting.

Jowitt M, Kargar I: *Radical midwifery. Celebrating 21 years of ARM*, Lancashire, 1997, Association of Radical Midwives.

King's Fund: *Safe births: everybody's business*, London, 2008, King's Fund.

LSAMO National Forum (UK): *Modern supervision in action*, London, 2009, NMC.

National Patient Safety Agency (NPSA): *Safer births: supporting maternity services to improve safety*, London, 2009, NPSA.

National Institute for Clinical Excellence (NICE): *Caesarean section*, London, 2004, NICE.

National Institute for Clinical Excellence (NICE): *Postnatal care: routine postnatal care of women and their babies*, London, 2006, NICE.

National Institute for Clinical Excellence (NICE): *Intrapartum care: care of healthy women and their babies during birth*, London, 2007, NICE.

National Institute for Clinical Excellence (NICE): *Antenatal care: routine care for the healthy pregnant woman*, London, 2008, NICE.

NHS Executive: *Review of the Nurses, Midwives and Health Visitors Act*, Health Service Circular HSC 1999/030, Leeds, 1999, DH.

NHS Executive: *Modernising regulation – the new Nursing and Midwifery Council: a consultation document*, London, 2000, NHS.

Northern Ireland Office: *Statement by the Secretary of State for Northern Ireland on Peat Marwick McClintock Review of Statutory Nursing Bodies*, London, 1991, HMSO.

Nursing and Midwifery Council (NMC): *Rule 9 (3) (Fitness to Practise) Rules Order of Council*, London, 2004a, NMC.

Nursing and Midwifery Council (NMC): *Midwives rules and standards*, London, 2004b, NMC.

Nursing and Midwifery Council (NMC): *Confidentiality – Advice sheet*, London, 2006a, NMC.

Nursing and Midwifery Council (NMC): *Standards for the preparation and practice of supervisors of midwives*, London, 2006b, NMC.

Nursing and Midwifery Council (NMC): *Review of pre-registration midwifery education-decisions made by the Midwifery Committee 12th May 2007 14/NMC Circular*, London, 2007a, NMC.

Nursing and Midwifery Council (NMC): *Standards for the supervised practice of midwives*, Annexe 1 to the NMC Circular 32/2007 September, London, 2007b, NMC.

Nursing and Midwifery Council (NMC): *Statutory supervision of midwives. A resource for midwives and mothers*, London, 2007c, Quay Books.

Nursing and Midwifery Council (NMC): *Fitness to practise annual report 2007–2008*, London, 2008a, NMC.

Nursing and Midwifery Council (NMC): *Standards to support learning and assessment in practice*, 2nd ed, London, 2008b, NMC.

Nursing and Midwifery Council (NMC): *Good health and good character: guidance for educational institutions*, London, 2008c, NMC.

Nursing and Midwifery Council (NMC): *Amendment to Rule 11- Eligibility for appointment as a supervisor of midwives*, NMC Circular 04/2008, London, 2008d, NMC.

Nursing and Midwifery Council (NMC): *Gifts and gratuities – advice sheet*, London, 2008e, NMC. Available at: www.nmc-uk.org/aDisplayDocument.aspx?documentID=4176.

Nursing and Midwifery Council (NMC): *Environment of care – advice sheet*, London, 2008f, NMC. Available at: www.nmc-uk.org/aArticle.aspx?ArticleID=4013.

Nursing and Midwifery Council (NMC): *Accountability*, London, 2008g, NMC. Available at: www.nmc-uk.org/aDisplayDocument.aspx?documentID=4018.

Nursing and Midwifery Council (NMC): *The PREP handbook*, London, 2008h, NMC. Available at: www.nmc-uk.org/DisplayDocument.aspx?documentID=4340.

Nursing and Midwifery Council (NMC): *The code*, London, 2008i, NMC. Available at: www.nmc-uk.org/Publications/Standards. Accessed October 2010.

Nursing and Midwifery Council (NMC): *Standards for medicines management*, London, 2008j, NMC. Available at: http://www.nmc-uk.org/Publications/Standards. Accessed October 2010.

Nursing and Midwifery Council (NMC): *Operational guidance for sharing fitness to practise information*, London, 2009a, NMC.

Nursing and Midwifery Council (NMC): *Additional information to support implementation of NMC standards to support learning and assessment in practice*, London, 2009b, NMC.

Nursing and Midwifery Council (NMC): *Standards for pre-registration midwifery education*, London, 2009c, NMC.

Nursing and Midwifery Council (NMC): *NMC framework for reviewing local supervising authorities*, London, 2009d, NMC.

Nursing and Midwifery Council (NMC): *Record keeping: guidance for nurses and midwives*, London, 2009e, NMC. Available at: www.nmc-uk.org/Publications/Guidance. Accessed October 2010.

Nursing and Midwifery Council (NMC): *Supervision, support and safety: analysis of the 2008–2009 LSA Annual Reports to the NMC*, London, 2009f, NMC. Available at: www.nmc-uk.org/Publications/Midwifery-Supervision. Accessed October 2010.

Nursing and Midwifery Council (NMC): *Support for parents leaflet*, London, 2009g, NMC.

Nursing and Midwifery Council (NMC): *NMC Standing Orders 2009*, London, 2010a, NMC.

Nursing and Midwifery Council (NMC): *Raising and escalating concerns: guidance for nurses and midwives*, London, 2010b, NMC. Awaiting publication. Consultation closed March 2010.

Nursing and Midwifery Council (NMC): *Advice and information for employers of nurses and midwives*, London, 2010c, NMC. Available at: www.nmc-uk.org/Publications/Information-for-employers. Accessed October 2010.

Nursing and Midwifery Council (NMC): *Conduct and Competence Committee*, London, 2010d, NMC. Available at: www.nmc-uk.org/Hearings/How-the-process-works/adjudication/Fitness-to-Practise-committees/conduct-and-competence-committee. Accessed October 2010.

Nursing and Midwifery Council (NMC): *Business Planning and Governance Committee*, London, 2010e, NMC. Available at: www.nmc-uk.org/About-us/The-Council/Committees-of-the-Council/Business-Planning-and-Governance-Committee. Accessed October 2010.

Nursing and Midwifery Council (NMC): *Professional Practice and Registration Committee*, London, 2010f, NMC. Available at: www.nmc-uk.org/About-us/The-Council/Committees-of-the-Council/Professional-Practice-and-Registration-Committee. Accessed October 2010.

Nursing and Midwifery Council (NMC): *Lead midwives for education (LMEs)*, London, 2010g, NMC. Available at: www.nmc-uk.org/Nurses-and-midwives/Midwifery/Midwifery-Education-and-Practice/Lead-Midwives-for-Education-LMEs. Accessed October 2010.

Nursing and Midwifery Council (NMC): *Guidance on professional conduct for nursing and midwifery students*, ed 2, London, 2010h, NMC. Available at: www.nmc-uk.org/Publications/Guidance. Accessed October 2010.

Royal College of Obstetricians (RCOG), Royal College of Midwives (RCM), Royal College of Anaesthetists (RCA) and Royal College of Paediatrics and Child Health (RCPCH): *Safer childbirth*, London, 2007, RCOG.

Scottish Office: *Statement by the Secretary of State for Scotland on policy review of the statutory nursing bodies and the future funding and management of nursing, midwifery and health-visiting education*, London, 1991, HMSO.

United Kingdom Central Council for Nursing, Midwifery and Health Visiting (UKCC): *Midwives rules*, London, 1986, UKCC.

Chapter | 4 |

# The midwife as a lifelong learner

Sue Macdonald

## LEARNING OUTCOMES

After reading this chapter, you will:

- have an understanding of the development of pre- and post-registration education for midwives in the UK, including educational and academic structures
- be conversant with your own learning style and be able to consider your education and development needs and how these might best be met
- have a framework within which to effectively reflect on practice, and use this knowledge to guide future practice
- have commenced a portfolio which demonstrates achievements so far, utilizes your learning needs and helps you plan your future development
- be able to utilize the clinical area fully, whether community or hospital based, as a learning environment, and facilitate the learning and development of those with whom you work.

## INTRODUCTION

One of the strengths of UK midwifery has been that midwives have had control of their education. This chapter includes an overview of the recent history of midwifery education, in the context of some of the policy and practice issues which have shaped and influenced the provision of pre- and post-registration education in the UK. To understand midwifery education in the UK now, and to think about the future direction it will take, it is helpful to appreciate some of the influencing factors and history of midwifery. Education and learning will also be explored in a broader sense, and how both may be utilized by midwives in their present and future practice.

## LIFELONG LEARNING

Lifelong learning is about holding a view that the pre-registration education is a springboard for future practice with the clinical area a place of learning and development (see website). This approach encourages a dynamic and enriching process, for midwives to think and reflect on their practice, to learn from each experience, refining and improving their knowledge and skills and imparting this philosophy to their clients and students. This creative and positive approach, where the health service is a learning organization, able to learn and develop from positive events and mistakes, can provide a high quality of service to women and their babies.

In reality, this must be more than 'paying lip service'. The pace of change and of the development of knowledge means that midwives must continually be updating their knowledge and skills in order to provide a safe and effective level of care.

## MIDWIFERY EDUCATION

Midwifery traditionally emerged from an apprenticeship model of education (Leap & Hunter 1993). Generally, women had personal experience of pregnancy and childbirth and would literally 'learn by Nellie' by accompanying a midwife in her daily work. The 'education' of midwives was, therefore, variable as regards the quality of experience to which a learner midwife could be exposed, and limited by the difficulty of accessing scientific information which would have been available to their male counterparts (Donnison 1988 and Ch. 2). Education and practice reflected the society of the time, often guided by superstition, custom and practice.

Many years of campaigning by the Midwives Institute (later to become the Royal College of Midwives) and its redoubtable members, including Rosalind Paget and Louisa Hubbard, supported by a small number of powerful politicians, achieved the Midwives Act of 1902. The primary purpose of the legislation was to *safeguard the public* from the practices of uneducated and untrained women, who assisted those who were too poor to pay for medical care during childbirth. Midwives were amongst the first to achieve professional regulation and were set on the pathway to standardized education, training and practice. Other parts of the UK attained registration of midwifery practice at a later date: Scotland in 1915 and Ireland in 1918. The Nurses Registration Act (1919), set up the General Nursing Council, brought nursing training and standards along similar lines to those of midwives.

The Central Midwives' Board (CMB), established by the 1902 Act, was charged by Government with responsibility for training midwives and conducting their examinations. The educational programmes developed accordingly, as shown in Table 4.1 and Figure 4.1.

By the late 1980s, there was increasing concern within the profession about both the direction midwifery education was taking and reduced recruitment into the profession. By 1988, only one school in England provided a 'direct entry' programme, though it was believed that this route could be more cost-effective and a more health-focused way of training midwives.

Acting on the findings of an ENB/DH-funded study (Radford & Thompson 1988), the Department of Health supported seven pilot schools to develop direct entry programmes, generally at DipHE level, linked to higher education institutions (HEIs). The success of these programmes was such that by 2000, three-quarters of midwives qualifying had been trained through the direct entry route (UKCC 1999). Though there is some debate about whether the shortened course for nurses should be retained, this route is still supported by midwives, and its retention recommended by the UKCC Commission for Education (1999) and currently by commissioners (see website).

## Moving into higher education

The last 30 years have been a time of tremendous change, from a scenario where midwifery education was provided locally, managed by the head of midwifery in the hospital, funded from the maternity care budget, to being absorbed into schools of nursing and midwifery, then colleges of health and/or nursing, and the final move into universities, with more complex funding streams controlled through strategic health authorities.

*Project 2000* (UKCC 1986) recommended that nursing and midwifery education have an 18-month shared core, followed by an 18-month 'branch' in midwifery, children's nursing, mental health, acute care or learning disabilities; that students be supernumerary, and courses be offered in higher education (HE) at diploma or degree level. Midwives overwhelmingly rejected this model for midwifery education, choosing to retain the direct entry route or 18-month programme, generally keeping control over their curriculum, though midwifery education moved, like nursing, into higher education. It is possible that this rejection avoided some of the problems experienced in nursing as described in the Peach Report (UKCC Commission for Education 1999).

It has been suggested that the move into higher education, which coincided with Project 2000 development, impacted on the student experience and the development of clinical expertise and confidence. Contributory factors were larger class sizes and geographical move from hospitals and clinical areas (Bower 2002). Though some midwives worked closely with their nursing colleagues to the extent of sharing elements of their programmes, others retained their midwifery identity, preferring to develop shared learning between the direct entry and 18-month route (Eraut et al 1995).

The RCM Education Strategy (RCM 2003) highlighted actions to redress the balance and align education more closely with clinical practice. Some recommendations, such as the development of a national midwifery curriculum, are straightforward, especially given the development of a national curriculum in children's education. Others, including the recommendation that students undertake at least five home births, two births within a birth centre setting, complete at least two experiences of physiological third stage, and have experience in a variety of settings, are more challenging. Utilizing the strategy could assist students and midwives to move clinical practice towards normality and community settings.

This strategy also recommends that educationalists spend a minimum of 20% of their time within the clinical area; that clinical managers seek to find a space for educators, and work to mitigate negative effects of geographical separation. Presently, the MINT project is exploring the clinical role of the midwife teacher (see website).

> *There may be midwives who seek the academic ivory towers, but there are also a significant number of midwives locked in the turret!*
>
> (RCM 2003:9)

Regional shortages of midwives mirror a corresponding shortage of educationalists. The proliferation of different roles, such as practice facilitator, clinical facilitator and practice development midwives, may, in part, replace the

**Table 4.1 The development of midwifery education courses in the UK**

| Year | Awarding Body | Length Of Course | Examination | Award (Level) | Comments |
|---|---|---|---|---|---|
| Late 19th century | London Obstetrical Society | 3 months | None formal | Certificate of proficiency | Small number of students meant impact on practice negligible |
| 1902–1915 | Central Midwives Board (CMB) | 3 months | 3-hour written examination<br>15-minute viva conducted by an obstetrician | Certificate | Focus on labour and postnatal care |
| 1916 | CMB | 6 months (2-month exemption for nurses) | | Certificate | |
| 1926 | CMB | 1 year for non-nurses | | | |
| 1938 | CMB | Part 1: 12 months for non-nurses; 6 months for nurses<br>Part 2: 6 months for all | Practical assessment and submission of set number of case histories | Certificate | Midwifery and obstetric theory and hospital-based practice<br>Clinical experience based in community and some lectures from the local Medical Officer of Health |
| 1968 | CMB | 1 year for nurses<br>2 years for direct entrants | Two 3-hour written examinations<br>Viva voce | Certificate | Normal midwifery and complicated obstetrics and neonatal care |
| 1980 | CMB | 18 months for nurses<br>3 years for direct entrants | Two 3-hour written examinations<br>Viva voce | Certificate | Normal midwifery and complicated obstetrics and neonatal care + new technologies (i.e. CTGs, inductions, etc.) – some doctors' lectures |
| 1990s | UKCC/National Boards – registration<br>College/University – academic qualification | 18 months for nurses<br>3 years for direct entrants | Development of continuous assessment processes and devolvement of assessment | Diploma of Higher Education (DipHE)<br>Degrees in Midwifery | Increased focus on psychology, sociology, physiology and social policy |
| 2000s | Nursing and Midwifery Council (NMC) – registration<br>University – academic qualification | 18 months for nurses<br>3 years for direct entrants<br>Some variation in programmes i.e. 20 months for nurses and 4 years for degree | Continuous assessment theory and practice<br>Use of mentors as assessors | All at university degree level – BSc/BA (Hons) | Most programmes in modular form<br>Credit accumulation and transfer possible<br>Minimum 50% practice<br>Grading of clinical practice<br>Increased emphasis on importance of knowledge and skills in normal practice |

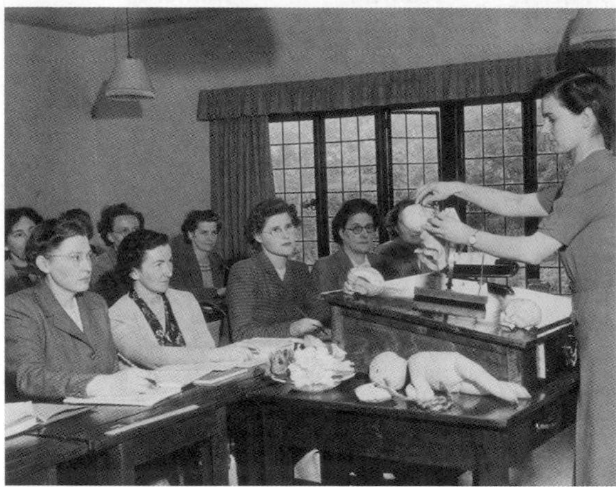

**Figure 4.1** Midwifery education in the 1950s. *(Courtesy of the Royal College of Midwives.)*

traditional role of the midwife teacher, but removes a potentially valuable resource from students and qualified staff. Midwifery teachers are usually highly experienced in clinical practice and thoroughly grounded in the theory of advanced midwifery, enhanced by a knowledge of the principles and practice of the education of adults. This level of knowledge and skills is a significant investment, and makes the educationalist a useful member of the maternity services, if fully involved and utilized.

## Diplomas, degrees and scholarship

Two programmes are available to the person wishing to enter midwifery in the UK: either a 3-year direct entry programme, or an 18-month shortened programme for those who have completed nursing. Both are at degree level. Figure 4.2 illustrates the educational system in the UK.

Courses are designed around the key competencies and clinical experience as laid down by the EC Midwives Directives (EC 1983, 2005) and Nursing and Midwifery proficiencies (NMC 2009). Clinical practice is a crucial part of the programme, and includes students working a variety of shifts (including weekends). Courses include 'self-directed study time', and a variety of different learning and teaching methods to enhance learning. Students are often mature people, sometimes on their second or third career, and possibly the family breadwinner; with different stressors from those of traditional university students.

There is a debate about whether qualifications make the practitioner a better midwife (Bower 2002). Research into nursing graduate practitioners demonstrated that 6 months after qualification, given appropriate support, practitioners had reached a similar point to those who had followed a less academic path. Graduate practitioners tend to remain in practice (Bircumshaw & Chapman 1988); demonstrate the ability to problem-solve and have a similar level of competence to their diplomate colleagues (Bartlett et al 2000, While et al 1998); and are more likely to be motivated to undertake continuing professional education (CPE) than are diplomates (Dolphin 1983).

As a graduate profession, practitioners should be equipped with analytical thinking and reflective skills, supporting practical skills. Though the academic requirements may discourage some people from pursuing midwifery, strategies are in place to provide additional academic and pastoral support for people with non traditional qualifications.

Practitioners who have completed midwifery programmes in the past, or who have completed a diploma, can apply to 'top up' to BSc (Hons) level. Most universities stipulate a total of 360 credits to gain an honours degree – usually consisting of 120 credits at each of levels 1, 2 and 3 (Fig. 4.3).

The RCM strategy (2003) proposed a continuum of midwifery, from a 'pre-midwifery' programme, through pre-registration training, to the different pathways of consultant midwife, educationalist or manager, always with a firm foundation of clinical practice. The process of moving along the continuum of midwifery illustrates that practitioners often start at different points and have enormous potential for professional and personal growth, and reiterates the commitment to continuing professional education (see Fig. 4.4).

*Continuing professional development/education* (CPD/E) forms a crucial and enduring part of the midwife's role, and has been part of midwifery practice since the 1936 Midwives Act, requiring midwives to undertake periodic refreshment in order to be able to continue practising. The Post-Registration Education and Practice (PREP) Project (UKCC 1990) brought these principles to nursing and health visiting, requiring practitioners to complete 5 days every 3 years with a professional portfolio illustrating self-assessment, development plan and reflective activities.

The PREP standard presently requires that practitioners complete a minimum of 450 hours of practice and 35 hours of study during the 3 years prior to renewal of registration, and those holding dual qualifications must demonstrate 900 hours of practice in nursing *and* midwifery (NMC 2008).

## 'PREP', portfolios and practice

Nurses and midwives are required as part of their PREP requirements to maintain a personal profile. The purpose of this is to record their learning activity for re-registration purposes. A profile is a personal document. It does not belong to the NMC or to the nurse or midwife's employer (NMC 2008).

The PREP (NMC 2008) requirement to keep a professional 'profile' (or portfolio) has resulted in structured approaches to recording learning and development. It is

| Higher education qualifications within each level | FHEQ level (UK) | Corresponding FQ-EHEA cycle |
|---|---|---|
| Doctoral degrees (eg, PhD/DPhil (including new-route PhD), EdD, DBA, DClinPsy) | 8 | Third cycle **(end of cycle)** qualifications |
| Master's degrees (eg, Masters in Philosophy (MPhil), MLitt, MRes, MA, MSc) | 7 | Second cycle **(end of cycle)** qualifications |
| Integrated master's degrees (eg, MEng, MChem, MPhys, MPharm) | | |
| Postgraduate diplomas | | |
| Postgraduate Certificate in Education (PGCE) | | |
| Postgraduate certificates | | |
| Bachelor's degrees with honours (eg, BA/BSc Hons) | 6 | First cycle **(end of cycle)** qualifications |
| Bachelor's degrees | | |
| Professional Graduate Certificate in Education (PGCE) | | |
| Graduate diplomas | | |
| Graduate certificates | | |
| Foundation Degrees (eg, FdA, FdSc) | 5 | Short cycle **(within or linked to the first cycle)** qualifications |
| Diplomas of Higher Education (DipHE) | | |
| Higher National Diplomas (HND) | | |
| Higher National Certificates (HNC) | 4 | |
| Certificates of Higher Education (CertHE) | | |
| AS levels; A levels and AVCE/Scottish Higher/NVQ/SVQ/\|National Certificate and National Diploma Level | Levels 1/2/3 | |

**Figure 4.2** Typical higher education qualifications at each level of the frameworks for higher education qualifications (FHEQ) and the corresponding cycle of the Framework for Qualifications of the European Higher Education Area (FQ-EHEA). For more information, see website. *(Adapted from* The framework for higher education qualifications in England, Wales and Northern Ireland*, August 2008. © The Quality Assurance Agency for Higher Education, 2008. www.qaa.ac.uk. Reproduced with permission.)*

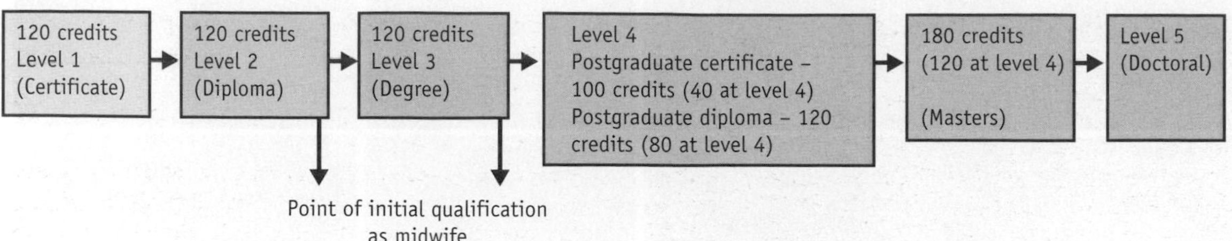


**Figure 4.3** Credit accumulation.

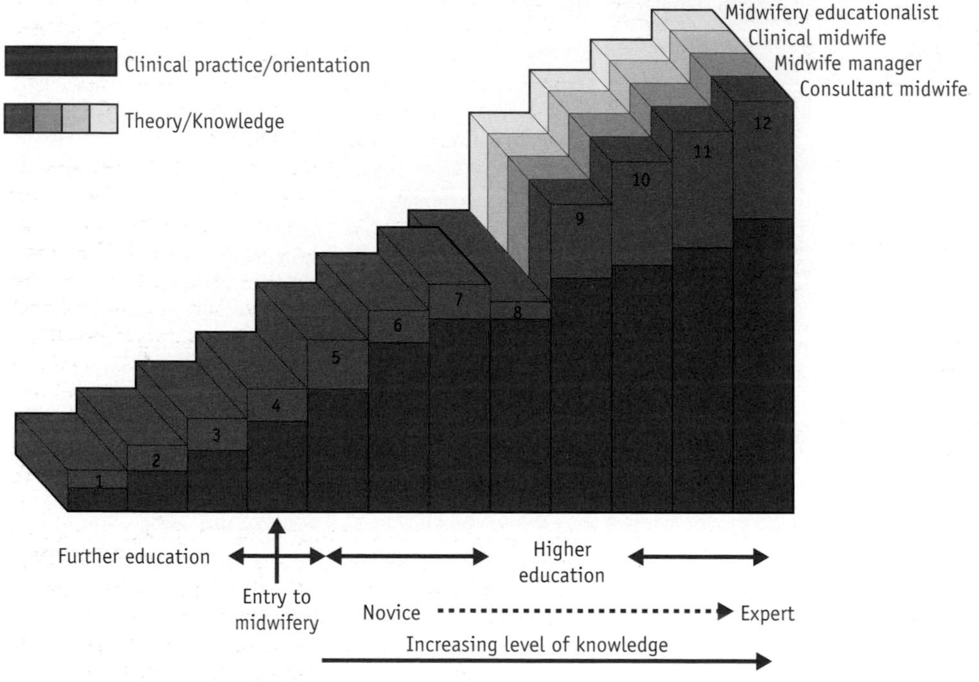


**Figure 4.4** The professional escalator for midwives (RCM 2003:4).

important to consider the 'shape' of the portfolio – moving from a view of a portfolio as a collection of certificates from different study days to a more dynamic tool allowing the practitioner to record activities, reflect on practice, and consider learning and development in the past, present and future, as a development plan. The latter approach includes a curriculum vitae (CV), and, indeed, one way of seeing the portfolio is to think of it as a dynamic CV.

There are several guidance publications available to guide portfolio development (NMC 2008, RCM 2000). The practitioner can choose to use a commercially produced portfolio, loose-leaf binder, computer, or even a personal digital assistant (PDA) unit to record learning and experience (Fig. 4.5) (see website).

Updating can include study days, conferences, working in different practice areas, or private study, such as undertaking a literature review. The important element is identifying the **learning** resulting from the activity, maximizing its effect.

If a literature search or reading activity is used as an updating activity, rigour needs to be used to ensure that the work is focused and applied to the individual's practice. This makes **active reading** critical (see website).

**Reflective activity 4.1**

After your next study day, spend some time afterwards thinking about it. What were the key elements of the day? Were there any keynote speakers who had an impact on you? Did you learn anything new? If not, why not? Write this down – perhaps using the framework in Box 4.1. Record at least one thing that you learned that you could bring into practice.

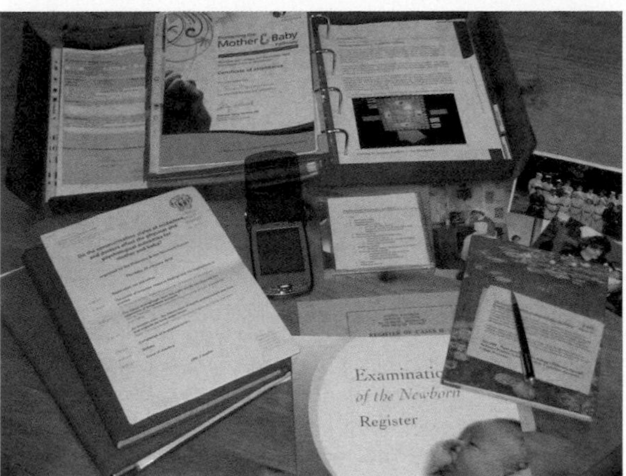


**Figure 4.5** Midwifery portfolio.

> Box 4.1 **Recording continuing education/development**
>
> You need to include:
>
> **Date, time and place**
>
> **Where learning took place**
>
> Conference centre/ward or community area/library
>
> **A review of your current role**
>
> **The learning activity:**
>
> - Why did you choose the particular topic/activity?
> - How did you plan this activity?
> - How many hours did you study/work?
> - Briefly describe the learning activity (i.e. reading a relevant clinical article; attending a course; observing practice)
> - Were there any disappointments or difficulties you had to face?
> - What was the best part of the learning for you?
>
> **Learning outcomes:**
>
> - What were the key aspects of the learning for you?
> - How will you put this into practice?
> - What sort of learning plans do you have for the future?

## FUTURE DEVELOPMENTS: DEGREES, MASTERS AND PhDS/APEL/APL

A plethora of choice exists for midwives wishing to develop their knowledge and skills. A decade ago, diplomas were the highest qualification available for the majority of practitioners, and a midwife wanting a Masters degree had to settle for a Masters in Social Science, Psychology, Nursing or Education. Now, most universities offer degree studies from Bachelors to Masters level studies in Midwifery Studies or Science.

A growing number of midwives are undertaking doctoral studies (PhD) and/or clinical doctorates (DClinPrac). Figure 4.2 illustrates the academic hierarchy, with the Master in Philosophy (MPhil) and PhD considered the pinnacle of study, requiring the practitioner to learn the knowledge and skills of research, and then apply them to a research project. As the number of midwives holding these higher degrees grows, the status of, and internal belief in, midwifery will increase, though it will be important to ensure that at the heart of what is studied is knowledge pertinent and applicable to midwives, midwifery, and, above all, to women and their babies.

*Work-based learning* (WBL) may include elements of *accreditation of prior learning* (APL) or *accreditation of prior experiential learning* (APEL). This can involve guided study within the clinical area, practical sessions or activity. Some programmes include work-based learning to denote the practical part of the course, either self-assessed or under the supervision of the course tutor or suitably qualified colleagues. Students are provided with a workbook or logbook, and this forms part of the reflection and recording necessary for demonstrating their progress.

WBL is sometimes viewed as a way of providing practitioners with learning experience, without 'losing them' while they go elsewhere for study. It enables learning to be applied and placed firmly within the practitioner's own workplace, and can contribute to the concept of the learning organization (ENB 1995). A learning organization is a dynamic one that can adapt and change as required, and which enables its workers to participate at all levels in the organization (ENB 1995, Jarvis 1992, Marsick 1987) (see website). This requires a cultural and psychological shift in ensuring that there are appropriate opportunities for utilizing the principles of experiential learning, and providing adequate opportunities for review and reflection.

APEL and APL present exciting possibilities for midwives, and are increasingly being used as a means to validate and add value to clinical practice. It is necessary to enrol in a university or further education college, and formally apply to have academic credit applied to clinical practice and learning in that practice. Time must be spent in preparing a professional portfolio documenting clinical activities, including evidence of critical reflection and a 'claim' for the academic credits appropriate to the clinical learning and development achieved.

### Computers, e-learning and the Net

The development of computer-assisted learning and the growth of the Internet have revolutionized learning and information retrieval, and shortened the 5-year 'sell-by date' of knowledge. Midwives need to become comfortable using computers, and retrieving information through varied databases (see Ch. 5). Courses and programmes such as the European Computer Driving Licence (ECDL) can direct learning a variety of computer skills, including word processing and spreadsheet utilization (Jacob 1999).

Increasingly, modules and programmes of learning are available in electronic form (Jordan 1999, RCM 2010) (see website) and *WebCT* (web course tools) are being developed to support different facets of learning, offering notice boards, chat rooms and a range of guided learning facilities. Research suggests that students like the variety this offers, though the development of electronic packages is time hungry (Wilson & Mires 1998), and that students need different skills to work with e-learning (Valaitis et al 2005). The way in which learning takes place using e-learning and internet tools is different – even verging on the chaotic as the learner 'surfs' into different sites (Savin–Baden & Wilkie 2006) sometimes at considerable speed.

The Internet also offers other activities such as social networking possibilities, including 'Facebook' and 'YouTube,' which provide links with others, and access to PowerPoint presentations and video clips that can assist understanding of theory such as physiology (see website)

The NHS has provided information and resources to practitioners within the workplace. Initiatives include the National Knowledge Service (NKS) (NHS 2010), which covers clinical practice, healthcare, social care, and public health; providing a website of portals into databases and evidence-based resources, and can be utilized by patients and the public, clinicians, managers, and public health professionals. The aim of the NKS is to facilitate co-coordinating of a range of publicly funded activities that generate, procure, organize, mobilize, localize or promote the use of knowledge. NKS projects are currently being conducted for tuberculosis, oral health, diabetes, breast cancer and congestive heart failure. Other useful sources include the National Institute for Clinical Excellence (NICE) and the Scottish Intercollegiate Guidelines Group (SIGN) (see website).

## New approaches in education

Midwifery education links with other professions in interprofessional education, which can aid interprofessional working and understanding. Examples of this include the Advanced Life Support in Obstetrics (ALSO) and Neonatal Life Support (NLS) courses. Some pre-registration courses include interprofessional components in an effort to improve learning and working. Problem- and inquiry-based learning also provides an approach which is congruent with adult learning philosophy, enabling students to develop higher-level problem-solving and critical skills (McCourt & Thomas 2001, McNiven et al 2002, Savin–Baden & Wilkie 2006).

# LEARNING AND DEVELOPMENT

By the time students and qualified midwives have begun studying, they have gone through positive and negative experiences of educational activities. These include experiences of rote learning, tests and examinations, and inevitably some failures. Often, early negative experiences can colour people's approach to learning and to their self-image.

There are many different models and theories around learning styles, and several questionnaires and quizzes which can be used to identify a person's learning style. One is that proposed by Honey and Mumford (1992), based on work by Kolb, which suggested that people fit into one of four main groups:

- *Pragmatist* – practical and keen to try out new ideas.
- *Reflector* – prefers to observe, think and gather information before making a judgement.
- *Theorist* – likes to tease out and think through information in a systematic way.
- *Activist* – likes to be active, and moves straight into experimentation on learning something new.

One study identified that teaching reflection included a model incorporating surface, impersonal to deep personal, then surface personal and deep personal approaches (Miller et al 1994) (see website for more information).

# LEARNING

The complex nature of learning has been explored extensively (Bloom 1956, Boud et al 1988, Bruner 1977, Freire 1972, Jarvis 1983, Mezirow 1981). The sheer breadth and depth of previous work within this area precludes more than an overview within this chapter.

There are many approaches: behaviourist, humanistic, the cultural environs, cognitive, through the spectrum to radical and emancipatory learning and education. Most of the earlier experiments and research into learning in humans were based on experiments with animals – even birds. Only during the development of 'progressive' education did research into human learning begin to be carried out. When looking at children's and adult education broadly, there is evidence of a complex interplay of many of these different theories and approaches, and, indeed, in most situations, experience and how learning is approached are similarly complex.

Some learning theories, such as, *conditioning*, can be applied to simple learning, and applies in many situations – for example, in how individuals learn fear and develop phobias, as in Box 4.2, and how these might be diminished.

**Box 4.2 Learning fear – applied to midwifery**

Vaginal examination (VE) during labour – woman anxious, midwife perhaps does not realize the woman's anxiety:

VE acutely painful (unconditioned stimulus) → pain/fear (unconditioned response)

Suggestion that VE is required (conditioned stimulus) + VE painful (unconditioned stimulus) → pain/fear (unconditioned response)

Suggestion that VE is required (conditioned stimulus) → fear (conditioned response)

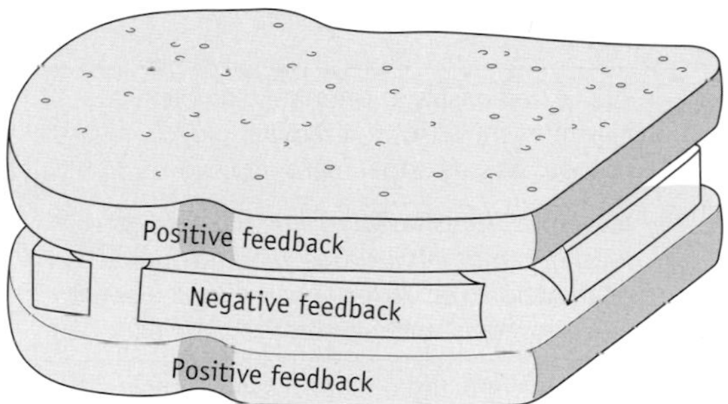


**Figure 4.6** The 'Skinner sandwich'.

This example illustrates that it is possible to develop fear and anxiety from one or two negative experiences, leading to anxiety and panic at the thought of the examination, or even the sight of the midwife preparing the pack. This theory was reinforced by work by Dick-Read (1986), who advocated that those supporting women in childbirth needed to address the fear–tension–pain cycle, and this knowledge should inform the midwife's support and education approach. This means providing a safe environment for the woman, sensitively identifying her previous experiences, fears and anxieties, and then planning how best to aid understanding and learning.

*Behaviourist learning* translates to providing feedback to the person learning – which might be yourself, the student you are working with, or the woman and family. Praise and criticism are substituted for food or electric shocks as used in behaviourist experiments, remembering that *positive* rewards are more effective than negative reactions (see Fig. 4.6).

Positive feedback is provided first: 'You did x really well ...'; followed by the negative criticism: 'This needed to be done differently ... because ...'; and the feedback is completed with another positive comment: 'This was really an excellent approach.' The person is then left with a clear idea of what needs to be improved, but is not swamped by thinking that nothing that was done was right or good.

*Trial and error learning* can be understood by knowing that the theory suggests that the individual may try out different approaches to solve a problem, and then use that solution when faced with the same or a similar problem in the future (see website).

*Cognitive Gestalt theory: Gestalt* means pattern, shape or form, and describes the individual's need to make sense of what is being seen and learned and put this into a 'whole'. This problem-solving aptitude helps the individual gain insight into learning – the 'Aha' experience. Gestalt includes concepts such as insightful learning, the nature versus nurture debate, and field theory.

The individual's natural tendency to seek understanding needs to be supported, though some gaps in knowledge may act as an impetus for learning. In teaching, this can be used to help make sense of what is being learned – perhaps planning a learning activity in which some information is provided and some not, so that the learner is encouraged to develop *closure* in composing the whole problem, and gets the experience of elements of *discovery learning*. Gestalt provided the tools for discovery learning and for the spiral curriculum which was taken forward by Gagne, in which new learning is linked with existing information.

This was developed in Bloom's *taxonomy of learning*, which included three *domains* or categories of educational activities: cognitive (mental skill), affective (growth in feelings), and psychomotor (practical and physical skills). These domains are still used to set learning objectives, and in assessment (see Table 4.2). The taxonomy did not include the psychomotor domain; and therefore the experience of working with practical skills was limited (Bloom 1956), which echoes the difficulty experienced in healthcare settings of appropriately identifying and assessing practical skills and abilities.

The spiral curriculum, used extensively in education, is a way of increasing depth of learning, built upon the importance of structure; readiness for learning; intuition as a productive but neglected area; and the importance of climate and teacher. The words: 'teaching is a superb way of learning' (Bruner 1977:88), and '[the] teacher is not only a communicator but a model' (Eraut 1994:90), are useful things for midwives to think in their day-to-day life, in their own learning, and in teaching women and students.

The *humanist theorists* Carl Rogers and Malcolm Knowles are probably the most influential adult education theorists in relation to midwifery. Rogers proposed that students be given intellectual freedom, allowing them to direct their own studies (Rogers 1969, Rogers & Freiberg 1994). This manifested on midwifery education as the inclusion of self-directed sessions and negotiated programmes. The freedom concept cannot be wholly subscribed to, given the limited training time in which to learn and to be assessed as competent in certain skills in order to be deemed safe to practise (EC 1980, 2005, NMC 2008).

**Table 4.2 Taxonomy of educational objectives within the cognitive domain.**

| Competence | Skills | Descriptive terms used |
|---|---|---|
| **Knowledge:**<br>• of specifics<br>• of terminology<br>• of specific facts<br>• of theories and structure | • Observation and recall of information – facts or theories<br>• Knowledge of dates, events, places<br>• Knowledge of major ideas<br>• Mastery of subject matter | List, define, tell, describe, identify, show, label, collect, examine, tabulate, quote, name, who, when, where, etc.<br>**Example:** *The student will list the major landmarks of the pelvis and fetal skull* |
| **Comprehension:**<br>• understanding (lowest level)<br>• translation<br>• interpretation<br>• extrapolation | • Understanding information<br>• Grasp meaning<br>• Translate knowledge into new context<br>• Interpret facts, compare, contrast<br>• Order, group, infer causes<br>• Predict consequences | Summarize, describe, interpret, contrast, predict, associate, distinguish, estimate, differentiate, discuss, extend<br>**Example:** *The student will describe the significance of the major landmarks of the pelvis and fetal skull* |
| **Application** | • Use information<br>• Use methods, concepts, theories in new situations<br>• Solve problems using required skills or knowledge<br>• Ability to predict possible effects of a change | Apply, demonstrate, calculate, complete, illustrate, show, solve, examine, modify, relate, change, classify, experiment, discover<br>**Example:** *The student will demonstrate the mechanism of labour describing the interaction of the fetal skull with the pelvis, and is able to teach students and women the basic principles* |
| **Analysis**<br>Of:<br>• elements<br>• relationships<br>• organizational principles | • Seeing patterns<br>• Organization of parts<br>• Recognition of hidden meanings<br>• Identification of components | Analyse, separate, order, explain, connect, classify, arrange, divide, compare, select, explain, infer<br>**Example:** *The student will be able to discuss the greater significance of different variations of shapes and sizes of pelves, and the effect on the mechanism of labour and outcomes. She may question the sources of this knowledge* |
| **Synthesis**<br>Production of a<br>• unique communication<br>• plan or proposed set of operations<br>• a set of abstract relations | • Use old ideas to create new ones<br>• Generalize from given facts<br>• Relate knowledge from several areas<br>• Predict, draw conclusions | Combine, integrate, modify, rearrange, substitute, plan, create, design, invent, what if?, compose, formulate, prepare, generalize, rewrite<br>**Example:** *The student will be able to assess pelvic capacity and identify women who may have assisted labour difficulties. She may consider the effect of posture, mobilization and link research to this aspect of midwifery* |
| **Evaluation:**<br>• Making judgements using internal and external evidence and criteria | • Compare and discriminate between ideas<br>• Assess value of theories, presentations<br>• Make choices based on reasoned argument<br>• Verify value of evidence, recognize subjectivity | Assess, decide, rank, grade, test, measure, recommend, convince, select, judge, explain, discriminate, support, conclude, compare, summarize<br>**Example:** *The student is able to merge her knowledge of the anatomy and physiology, with the research from major studies, and also the evidence of her own practice to provide the woman with unbiased choices, and aid her own process of problem solving and decision making* |

Adapted from Bloom (1956) and Bloom et al (1964)

Knowles believed that the education of adults required a different approach to that of children, suggesting that *pedagogy* – the science of teaching – was no longer appropriate. He analysed this concept, which he initially viewed as appropriate only for children, and presented a new word – *andragogy* – *the art and science of helping adults learn* (Knowles 1973, 1980) (see Table 4.3).

*Andragogy* was seen as a polar opposite to *pedagogy*, and it was presumed that it was inappropriate to use pedagogy for a group of adult learners (Knowles 1973). Later, he suggested that *andragogy* and *pedagogy* could be viewed as two 'extremes on a spectrum', used according to the needs of the student group of the time (Knowles 1980). This theory has been criticized for its assumption that adults are more self-directing than children (Tennant 1986), that adults differ from children in their 'reservoir' of experience (Jarvis 1983) and the different motivation and readiness to learn of the two groups (Tennant 1986).

Andragogy has been adopted almost completely by midwifery, as well as by nursing and other streams of education involving adults, though some aspects do conflict with the current directive to be cost-effective, reduce teacher–student contact time, and increase the student–teacher ratio. As well as philosophical differences, andragogical approaches require different classroom settings – desks and chairs arranged in semicircles or circles; more experiential learning; negotiated sessions where students set the agenda; and an increase in self-directed provision.

Teachers (or facilitators) used Knowles' assumptions and processes in the delivery of sessions, and in designing programmes of learning which incorporated a process model (as in Fig. 4.7), in which the starting point is an environment which is conducive to learning, and the end point is an evaluation of the learning that has taken place, and identification of the next step required.

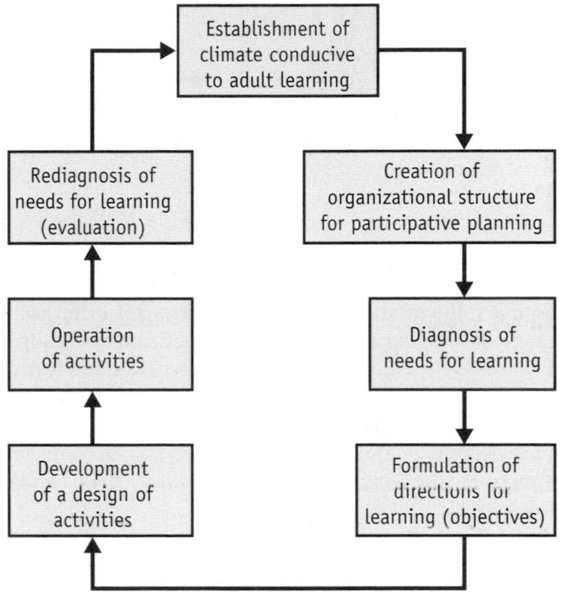


**Figure 4.7** The process of facilitating learning. *(Adapted from Knowles 1973.)*

**Table 4.3 Comparisons of pedagogy and andragogy**

| | Pedagogy | Andragogy |
|---|---|---|
| Definition | Educating children in a didactic fashion – to lead | The art and science of helping adults learn |
| Learner | Dependent | Deep need to be self-directing<br>Occasionally dependent |
| Learner's previous experience | Limited<br>Of little worth | Rich reservoir of experience – resource for learning |
| Learner's readiness to learn | When society says | When the individual feels ready – 'need to know' |
| Learner's orientation to learning | Subject-orientated | Problem-solving<br>Developing full potential |
| Teacher | Holds the knowledge<br>In control of what and how learning takes place | Is a co-learner<br>Facilitator of learning experiences rather than teacher |
| Practical implications | Fixed set of knowledge to be learned, though with time and societal changes this alters | Need self-directed opportunities<br>Problem-based enquiry<br>Need to review previous experience (may prevent further learning)<br>Need to explicitly value previous experience |

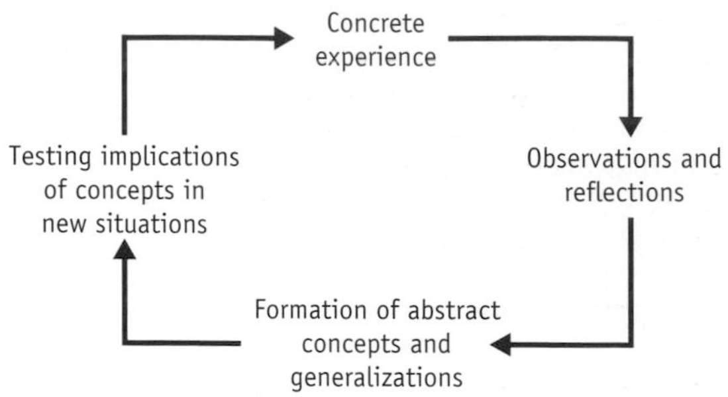

Concrete experience → Observations and reflections → Formation of abstract concepts and generalizations → Testing implications of concepts in new situations → Concrete experience

**Figure 4.8** The Lewinian experiential model (Kolb 1984:21).

## From andragogy to reflection

Another influential stream of theory emerged from Kolb (1984) developing experiential learning, which included reflection as the crucial link between experience and learning (Fig. 4.8). This was also incorporated into midwifery education – through increased use of experiential learning and reflection – and reflective practice has become an important component of the midwife's daily work (Box 4.3).

Kolb's work proposed that people fit into one of four main groups having a matching learning style, linked closely with the experiential learning cycle. The preference an individual has is congruent with their personalities, educational preparation, chosen career, or role function of the time (Kolb 1984) (see website).

Kolb viewed learning as a dynamic and fluid process, in which the experience and outcome are different for each person, and emphasized that, rather than being an empty vessel to be filled, the student enters learning with a range of learning and experience, and needs to 'relearn' rather than learn 'from scratch'. The teacher therefore assists individuals to modify or dispose of old ideas and change their belief system (see website).

*Experiential learning* is an important tool in developing learning, in which more effective interaction with the concepts being taught is achieved, as the person is encouraged in a lesser or greater degree to actually sense what the concept would feel like. An example in midwifery would be students learning how to give 'bad news' to women and their families. This could be achieved by practising in a classroom setting what it feels like from the perspective of both the mother and midwife, and what words, body language or strategies are most caring and effective. A crucial part of this exercise is the debriefing and reflective phase that follows, during which all participants can present their perspective, and explore events and strategies together.

This type of learning is not always as easy as it might appear. To tell individuals just 'to act it out' does not provide enough guidance, and may result in limited learning or, in the worst case scenario, entering uncharted and unsupported territory.

If the midwife uses role play, either with student midwives or with women (such as during antenatal education), it is important to have a structure for the session (see website).

**Box 4.3 Practical illustration of reflective cycle**

Normally, the cycle starts with the experience (at a concrete level) as something tangible to the senses of the individual. This might be the experience of a practical event such as witnessing a normal delivery. It might be that this delivery is a student's first experience of witnessing a birth, and the woman in labour may react as some labouring women do, by being quite noisy, but as she enters transition becomes centred on herself. The baby is delivered, and it is a huge emotional experience. The student notes that the baby looks pink, but has blue extremities. She observes and reflects as she is part of this experience. The result is a sorting out in her own mind of the practical experience and her previous knowledge plus her 'classroom knowledge', and she begins to add to her personal knowledge bank. Each component of the experience may be processed separately according to her knowledge. If we look at one aspect, say the colour of the baby, she may make sense of it by thinking that this is the way babies are, and initially this simple acceptance might serve as a temporary working knowledge. Taking this to the next step of the cycle, she will then perhaps be expecting a pink baby with blue extremities at the next birth.

However, as she becomes more experienced and, hopefully, begins to learn more about neonatal physiology, she will appreciate that this is a visual illustration of the transitional effects of birth. She will also begin to understand the individuality of the experience, for the mother, midwife and indeed the baby.

## Reflection and reflective practice

*The Reflective Practitioner* (Schon 1983) described the crisis of the professions, popularizing reflection. Reflection was discussed by Aristotle, and later by Dewey (1933). Schon brought it to the attention of professions such as nursing, midwifery and social work. This book valued intuition and a more qualitative approach to problem-solving in practice, providing a means of understanding how practitioners make sense of and add to their repertoire of knowledge. Becoming a reflective practitioner has since become an ideal to which many practitioners aspire (Brockbank & McGill 1998, Driscoll 1994). Schon's work describes a practitioner who chooses to utilize a technical rationality model and work logically to address the problems of the 'high, hard ground where practitioners can make effective use of research-based theory and technique', or alternatively take a more intuitive path through the 'swampy lowland where situations are confused "messes" incapable of technical solutions' (Schon 1983:42). Schon suggested that clients were more likely to have the sort of problems which required the more creative and holistic approach, and, in a period of time when nursing and midwifery in common with other emerging professions wished to develop their professional standing, this supported the more feminine, tacit nature of clinical practice.

Certainly, clients often present with a combination of risk factors, clinical and psychosocial problems, presenting a profile more akin to the swampy lowlands than those high hard grounds, and therefore this viewpoint is seductive. Though Schon described several 'exemplars' of teachers working with students to develop reflective practice, there was not really a clear tool available to assist a practitioner in developing the skills. Since that time, however, several other writers have published tools and frameworks to guide reflection.

It is often helpful to try out some of the many reflective tools to explore whether they can assist in making sense of experiences, and develop learning (see Box 4.4). This triggers questions to facilitate thinking about an experience or an area of practice, and develop it into learning (Atkins & Murphy 1993, Benner 1984, Driscoll 1994, Johns 1995). This includes *critical incident analysis* (see website), a term for an incident during which something went wrong, a crisis or a situation recorded for risk-management purposes, and also used in research and increasingly in the field of reflective practice to denote a variety of situations.

If truly subscribed to, reflective practice can be a potent model for the practitioner to audit day-to-day practice, and continue learning and development from the complex digestion and assimilation of theory and practice (James 2009). It is not without problems and requires significant time and energy investment, plus support (Macdonald 2002). It is seldom highlighted that reflection can be difficult, which means that many people will avoid thinking beyond the most obvious. It may also be uncomfortable as areas of practice are revisited – some long forgotten and some more enduring. Reflection needs therefore to carry something of a 'health warning', and an understanding that it is not always possible to reflect on all areas of practice all of the time (see website).

There is some evidence that just thinking about the individual's philosophy generates some reflection (Kottkamp 1990) (see website for reflective activity). This is a useful means of articulating what is personally believed in as a midwife, and sharing this with colleagues. It is important to acknowledge at this point that reflection is an individual activity, and it is not possible to reflect for another person.

**Reflective activity 4.2**

Use the tool in Box 4.4 to reflect on an aspect of your practice – perhaps how you conduct a 'booking interview'. You may wish to do this with a peer, or write it down as a reflective piece for your professional portfolio.

### Reflection for you ... and others

Others in the maternity service will be learners, who will need to be assisted through the reflective cycle, in order to make sense of their experiences. Student midwives usually have a clinical record and a clinical assessment tool in which they may be required to illustrate some critical reflection on their practice. They will, therefore, value working with midwives who are familiar with the terminology, and will also find it helpful to have a chance to reflect on different experiences and issues in practice. Sharing reflective incident analysis can be interesting and bring different perspectives, serving as an illustration to the student of how practitioners utilize reflection in day-to-day practice.

Perhaps most fundamentally, women themselves need to reflect. It is clearly not practical to ask women to complete pages of reflective accounts of their experiences, though some women may find this beneficial. It is good practice to review aspects of the woman's experience with her, at a point where she has had time to consider events, and has begun to question what happened and why. The midwife can give the woman a unique opportunity for reflection on the whole continuum of pregnancy and childbirth. In reflecting with women, it is important to remember that, as in all reflections, she has to reflect on her own experience. Some trigger questions (Box 4.5) and a focus on her as the key player can be helpful, just providing information and clarification when asked to do so. Counselling skills (i.e. learning not to be quick to give a neatly packaged answer) are really helpful at this stage.

Issues around debriefing may need more skilled support, and it is not unusual during the 'routine' reflections to identify a woman who may require additional counselling support.

## Mentorship and the midwife as a role model

An important part of developing learning and practice is through interaction with others, and a powerful way in which humans learn physical, communication and caring skills is through the medium of role modelling. This allows absorption of the culture of the service (Hindley 1999), which may be negative as well as positive learning (Kirkham 1999), and even different parts of the service

**Box 4.4 A reflective model**

### Prior to the event/experience

How did you prepare for the incident/experience? Were you prepared?

Is this an issue that you have considered/thought about recently? Why?

What was in your mind prior to the event?

Did you have any worries/concerns about it? How did you address them?

### The incident/experience

Describe what happened (no analysis at this stage):

- Who said/did what?
- Record the wheres and hows
- Were your feelings:
  - discomfort?
  - troubled?
  - very positive?
- What other aspects affected your handling of the situation, i.e. busyness of ward/community, other stressors?
- What knowledge did you use (was this from textbook/research or from colleagues/routine practice)?

### Analysis stage

What were you trying to achieve?

Why did you respond to the situation/event in the way you did?

What was the outcome for:

- you?
- the woman and baby?
- your colleagues?
- your student?

How did others feel about what happened:

- the woman and baby?
- your colleagues?
- your student?

And how do you know:

- from assessing body language/posture?
- from what was said to you?

Was this similar to previous responses from other similar situations/events?

What were the main thoughts/concerns in your mind at the time?

Thinking about the knowledge you were using, was it based on:

- training/text book?
- research?
- evidence?
- your assumptions?

Were there any tensions or difficulties which arose from the knowledge you were using?

Was this knowledge appropriate to the situation, and were you conscious of any gaps in your knowledge?

### The 'what if' stage – alternatives and choices

How could you have dealt with this differently?

Would this have changed what happened – and how?

Were you in a position to actually influence this?

Would you do the same things if this situation happened again?

- If so, why?
- If not, why not?

### Plan of action

What did you learn from this – good and bad? (Don't forget your personal Skinner sandwich.)

What element of practice, or what you did, did you feel was special and needs to be celebrated?

Will you use this in your future practice?

How will you share this with colleagues?

If you do not want to share with your colleagues, why not? What does that tell you, and how do you deal with it?

What do you need to update yourself or find out next:

- theory?
- practical skills?
- research?

What is your personal calendar for this – tonight, tomorrow or next week?

If you are not sure of what you have to learn, whom do you use to help you find out? And why?

- supervisor of midwives?
- link teacher?
- consultant midwife?
- doctor?
- colleague?

### Evaluation

When will you review this reflection?

With whom will you share this (supervisor/mentor or colleague)?

### Perspective – suspended judgement

At this point, what are your views on this event/experience?

How have you incorporated this into your personal knowledge store?

Box 4.5 **Trigger questions for assisting the woman to reflect**

- Having booked to have your baby here ... how did you feel when you first met your midwives ... do you feel that account was taken of your individual needs? (antenatal, labour and/or postnatal)
- How do you feel that the labour and birth were for you? Were they how you thought they would be?
- Did you feel you had sufficient information and support about becoming a mother? (postnatal)

Box 4.6 **The student learns ...**

Midwife X sees Mrs Brown, who is 32 weeks' pregnant, with student midwife A. On examining Mrs Brown, the midwife feels that the fetus is not growing perhaps as fast as she would expect. She asks Mrs Brown about her nutrition patterns, and whether she smokes, drinks alcohol, etc. She provides the appropriate advice, but decides to ask Mrs Brown to attend antenatal clinic the following week. She therefore makes the appointment and records this in the notes.

Student A works in the clinic a couple of weeks later, and is encouraged by midwife Y to undertake the examination and the 'talking' under her supervision. Mrs Clarke is 32 weeks' pregnant, and her observations are all within normal parameters – her fetus is growing well. Student midwife A makes an appointment for the following week.

Midwife Y is completely confused ... surely this is not what they teach in the university these days! She challenges the student, and is actually a little sharp with her.

may have a different approach to mentoring (Kroll et al 2009). It may also lead to tensions for students when mentors are not practising in an evidence-based way, or contradicting what students are being taught in university (Armstrong 2010).

As a practitioner, it is important to be aware that actions, attitudes and demeanour may be perceived in different ways by students, other practitioners, women and their families and friends. Students, especially, are observant of their mentors, and may emulate their attitudes, though they tend to prefer the woman-centred and flexible rather than prescriptive approach (Bluff 2002). It is crucial to share the way decisions and judgements are made with junior colleagues – demonstrating how the very complex process that takes place during the woman's care in the context of the service can be learned (see Box 4.6).

Not to share this process robs the student and practitioner of a valuable learning experience. This process of talking through what is being done and why – almost reflecting 'on your feet', which Loughran describes – can help students understand the thought processes an experienced practitioner has, and illustrates the complexities of those processes (Loughran 1996, 2000).

Students learn theory (and some practice) in the university setting, and the real world practice is learned from their mentors in practice (see website).

## CONCLUSION

In considering aspects of learning and education, midwives must be aware of their own learning patterns, and be willing to review their own learning history. This will assist in planning education and development activities, and, more importantly, will assist them in analysing the learning and development needs of the women with whom they are working, and the students for whom they are responsible. The good teacher should be able to plan and assess learning, and this includes an analysis – even unlearning – of things that have been learned before; or unpicking and addressing assumptions that others may have about learning, or about the whole experience of pregnancy, childbirth and motherhood.

An important part of practice is to have a framework and tools which can assist in critically reflecting and assessing the effects of that practice. However, this requires the skills described many years ago of open-mindedness, wholeheartedness and responsibility (Dewey 1933). This does carry a health warning, in that truly reflecting on practice brings new challenges and perspectives which may not always be comfortable.

This chapter has reviewed the multifaceted nature of learning, education and development. As midwifery faces new challenges and different ways of working, it is paramount that midwives continue to learn and develop. To do so well will certainly benefit the profession and the individual midwife both professionally and personally. Most importantly of all it will benefit the care provided to women, their babies and families, and thus society as a whole.

## KEY POINTS

- An understanding of the structure of general education and professional education pathways is useful in viewing the opportunities which are available to those in the healthcare setting.
- Midwives should be aware of the impact of learning on themselves, their colleagues, students and the women with whom they work.

- An understanding of learning theory assists midwives in their professional and personal development and enables them to facilitate the learning of others.
- Understanding and using the principles of reflection enables the midwife to consider and improve her practice, assist students to develop their reflective skills and provides an opportunity for the woman to reflect on her pregnancy and childbirth experience.
- The clinical area is a learning environment for midwives, students and women and families.
- There are a wide variety of educational and development opportunities available to practitioners, often accessible locally.

## REFERENCES


Armstrong N: Clinical mentors' influence on student midwives' clinical practice, *British Journal of Midwifery* 18(2):114–117, 119–123, 2010.

Atkins S, Murphy M: Reflection: a review of the literature, *Journal of Advanced Nursing* 18:1188–1192, 1993.

Bartlett HP, Simonite V, Westcott E, et al: A comparison of the nursing competence of graduates and diplomates from UK nursing programmes, *Journal of Clinical Nursing* 9(3):369–379, 2000.

Benner P: *From novice to expert: excellence and power in clinical nursing practice*, California, 1984, Addison-Wesley.

Bircumshaw D, Chapman CM: A follow-up of the graduates of the 3-year post-registration Bachelor of Nursing degree course in the University of Wales, *Journal of Advanced Nursing* 13(4):520–524, 1988.

Bloom BS, editor: *A taxonomy of educational objectives. Handbook I: Cognitive domain*, New York, 1956, David McKay.

Bloom BS, Engelhart MD, Furst EJ, et al, editors: *A taxonomy of educational objectives. Handbook II: Cognitive domain*, New York, 1964, David McKay.

Bluff R: The midwife as role model. *International Confederation of Midwives. Midwives and Women Working Together for the Family of the World*, ICM proceedings Vienna, The Hague, 2002, International Confederation of Midwives.

Boud D, Keogh R, Walker D, editors: *Reflection: turning experience into learning*, London, 1988, Kogan Page.

Bower H: Educating the midwife. In Mander RF, Fleming V, editors: *Failure to progress: the contraction of the midwifery profession*, London, 2002, Routledge, Taylor and Francis.

Brockbank A, McGill I: *Facilitating reflective learning in higher education*, Buckingham, 1998, Society for Research into Higher Education and Open University Press.

Bruner J: *The process of education*, Cambridge, Massachusetts, 1977, Harvard University Press.

Dewey J: *How we think*, London, 1933 (reprinted 1960), DC Heath.

Dick-Read G: *Childbirth without fear: the original approach to natural childbirth*, New York, 1986, Harper & Row.

Dolphin N: Why do nurses come into continuing education programs? *Journal of Continuing Education in Nursing* 14(4):8–16, 1983.

Donnison J: *Midwives and medical men*, London, 1988, Heinemann.

Driscoll J: Reflective practice for practise, *Senior Nurse* 13(7):47–50, 1994.

English National Board for Nursing, Midwifery and Health Visiting (ENB): *Creating lifelong learners: partnerships for care*, London, 1995, ENB.

Eraut M: *Developing professional knowledge and competence*, London, 1994, Falmer Press.

Eraut MA, Alderton J, Boylan A, et al: *Learning the use of scientific knowledge in nursing and midwifery education*, London, 1995, ENB.

European Economic Community: *European Community Directive 80/155/EEC*, Article 4. Brussels, 1980, European Economic Community.

EC Directive 2005/36/EC of the European Parliament and of the Council of 7 September 2005 on the recognition of professional qualifications, Article 40. http://ec.europa.eu/internal_market/qualifications/future_en.htm

Freire P: *Pedagogy of the oppressed*, Harmondsworth, 1972, Penguin.

Hindley C: An assessment of clinical competency on an undergraduate midwifery programme: midwives' and students' experiences, *Journal of Clinical Excellence* 1(3):157–162, 1999.

Honey P, Mumford A: *The manual of learning styles*, Maidenhead, 1992, Peter Honey Publications.

Jacob S: Union learning fund supporting information technology training, *RCM Midwives Journal* 2(8):254, 1999.

James J: Using a reflective model to aid professional development: reactions and responsibilities in management of a major postpartum haemorrhage, *MIDIRS Midwifery Digest* 19(4):534–539, 2009.

Jarvis P: *Adult and continuing education: theory and practice*, London, 1983, Croom Helm.

Jarvis P: Quality in practice: the role of education, *Nurse Education Today* 12(3):3–10, 1992.

Johns C: Framing learning through reflection within Carpers's fundamental ways of knowing in nursing, *Journal of Advanced Nursing* 22:226–234, 1995.

Jordan G: The use of communications and information technologies (C&ITS) as a tool for continuing professional development (CPD): a case study, *CTI Nursing and Midwifery Newsletter* 4(3):5–6, 1999.

Kirkham M: The culture of midwifery in the National Health Service in England, *Journal of Advanced Nursing* 30(3):732–739, 1999.

Knowles MS: *The adult learner: a neglected species*, Houston, 1973, Gulf Publishing.

Knowles MS: *The modern practice of adult education: from pedagogy to andragogy*, revised edition, Chicago, 1980, Association Press.

Kolb DA: *Experiential learning: experience as the source of learning and development*, New Jersey, 1984, Prentice Hall.

Kottkamp RB: Means for facilitating reflection, *Education and Urban Society* 22(2):182–203, 1990.

Kroll D, Ahmed S, Lyne M: Student midwives' experiences of hospital-based postnatal care, *British Journal of Midwifery* 17(11):690–697, 2009.

Leap N, Hunter B: *The midwife's tale*, London, 1993, Scarlet Press.

Loughran J: *Developing reflective practice: learning about teaching and learning through modelling*, London, 1996, Falmer Press.

Loughran J: Effective reflective practice. *Making a difference through reflective practice: values and actions*, Reflective Practice Conference, University College, Worcester, July 2000, pp 38–44.

McCourt C, Thomas BG: Evaluation of a problem-based curriculum in midwifery, *Midwifery* 17(4):323–331, 2001.

Macdonald SE: *Reflecting on reflection*. ICM 26th Triennial Congress Vienna, April 2002, pp 1–19.

McNiven P, Kaufman K, McDonald H: A problem-based learning approach to midwifery, *British Journal of Midwifery* 10(12):751–755, 2002.

Marsick VJ, editor: *Learning in the workplace*, London, 1987, Croom Helm.

Mezirow J: A critical theory of adult learning and education, *Adult Education* 32(1):3–24, 1981.

Miller C, Tomlinson A, Jones M: *Learning styles and facilitating reflection*, London, 1994, English National Board (ENB).

National Health Service (NHS): *The National Knowledge Service* (website). www.nks.nhs.uk. 2010.

Nursing and Midwifery Council (NMC): *The PREP handbook*, London, 2008, NMC.

Nursing and Midwifery Council (NMC): *Standards for pre-registration midwifery education*, London, 2009, NMC.

Radford N, Thompson A: *Direct entry – a preparation for midwifery practice*, Guildford, 1988, University of Surrey.

Rogers CR: *Freedom to learn: a view of what education might become*, Columbus, Ohio, 1969, Charles E Merrill Publishing.

Rogers CR, Freiberg JM: *Freedom to learn*, ed 3, London, 1994, Prentice Hall.

Royal College of Midwives (RCM): *Portfolio development series*, London, 2000, RCM.

Royal College of Midwives (RCM): *Valuing practice: a springboard for midwifery education*, London, 2003, RCM.

Royal College of Midwives (RCM): *RCM I-Learn Learning Suite*, 2010. www.rcm.org.uk

Savin-Baden M, Wilkie K: *Problem based learning on line*, Milton Keynes, 2006, Open University.

Schon DA: *The reflective practitioner: how professionals think in action*, USA, 1983, Basic Books.

Tennant M: An evaluation of Knowles' theory of adult education, *International Journal of Lifelong Education* 5(2):113–122, 1986.

United Kingdom Central Council for Nursing, Midwifery and Health Visiting (UKCC): *Project 2000: a new preparation for practice*, London, 1986, UKCC.

United Kingdom Central Council for Nursing, Midwifery and Health Visiting (UKCC): *The report of the Post-Registration and Practice Project (PREPP)*, London, 1990, UKCC.

UKCC Commission for Education: *Fitness for practice*, London, 1999, UKCC.

United Kingdom Central Council for Nursing and Midwifery (UKCC): *Statistical Analysis of the Register, 1 April 2001 to 31 March 2002*, London, 2002, UKCC.

Valaitis RK, Sword W A, Jones B, et al: Problem based learning online: perceptions of health science students, *Advances in Health Sciences Education* 10(3):231–252, 2005.

While AEF, Fitzpatrick JM, Roberts JD: An exploratory study of similarities and differences between senior students from different pre-registration nurse education courses, *Nurse Education Today* 18(3):190–198, 1998.

Wilson TM, Mires G: Teacher versus the computer for instruction: a study, *British Journal of Midwifery* 6(10):655–658, 1998.

# Chapter 5

# Evidence-based practice and research for practice

*Julia Magill-Cuerden*

## LEARNING OUTCOMES

After reading this chapter and using the website, you will be:

- aware of the range of sources of evidence and research which may inform midwifery decisions and practice, and some of their strengths and limitations
- able to frame a question on the basis of a clinical encounter and initiate a search for relevant evidence
- aware of the need to critically appraise research evidence prior to making use of it in practice
- able to recognize some of the complexities of the process of translating research findings into practice
- able to appreciate the contexts within which midwives might apply and contribute to the development of research and evidence-based practice.

## INTRODUCTION

An essential skill for all professionals is using evidence in practice. Being able to determine the quality of research or information upon which evidence is based is a necessary skill for all midwives. Evidence-based healthcare should be the foundation for all policy decisions made within the health service and by midwives (DH 1997,1999; 2008). Having the appropriate knowledge to evaluate research and evidence to assist in decision-making with women and families, appropriate to their individual needs, requires development of knowledge and skills with understanding of information, resources and women's views.

## DEFINITION

At its most descriptive level, an evidence-based approach to healthcare involves basing decisions and actions on the best available evidence. Evidence-based healthcare (EBHC) can be viewed as a strategy, using a set of tools that enable practitioners to be aware of and locate the available evidence, judge its strength and soundness and be in a position to apply it in practice.

Central to the whole enterprise of EBHC is the concept of 'evidence'; however, the term itself is confounded by complexity through different interpretations of its meaning.

## WHAT IS EVIDENCE?

Evidence is a familiar concept within a legal context, where it has been defined as information which may be presented to a court of law, in order for a decision to be made about the *probability* that a claim is true. In other words, it is the information on the basis of which facts are proved or disproved (Keane 2008), where evidence is sought for the basis of clinical decision-making.

Judging what constitutes 'sound evidence' in healthcare can be problematic. Evidence can be drawn from a variety of sources:

- from one's own personal experience (personal testimony)
- from the reported experience of others (expert testimony)
- from systematic research (forensic evidence).

While each of these may give rise to evidence which is adequate for making decisions in practice, they also have their limitations. Sources of evidence for practice are examined for their strengths and limitations.

Evidence used by a professional influences their decision-making in practice. The foundation for all decisions is the knowledge base of that professional. For forms of knowledge used in midwifery, see website. The knowledge base of a society is influenced by experts in the field (see website for expert opinions).

## Research

All rigorous research is designed to produce evidence which gains strength because built into the research process are mechanisms that act as internal challenges to address some of the shortcomings identified above. This is true of both *quantitative* and *qualitative* research approaches, although they vary in the challenges they pose (Bryman 1992). The research process is systematic and logical with strategies to:

- investigate questions
- gather data
- analyse data
- validate findings, which can then be accepted as credible beyond the limits of the particular study.

In designing and reporting research, it is essential to be clear in:

- stating explicitly and publicly the basis for the research design
- explaining how the study was conducted
- demonstrating how conclusions were drawn from the data.

*Quantitative* studies will effectively:

- answer questions or hypotheses posed
- indicate how the study is valid and reliable
- consider the results can be generalized to a wider population.

*Qualitative* research must fulfil similar criteria, although the terminology used differs, arising from different assumptions about the nature of investigation that may arise from a problem or a research question (Denzin & Lincoln 2005). Researchers in this field will present support for:

- trustworthiness
- authenticity
- dependability
- replicability
- credibility, and
- auditability of their results (Lincoln & Guba 1985).

Discussion of the above should be presented in the methodological descriptions in a research report that gives the research question, sampling strategy, data collection, tools, and analytical and ethical processes.

The research process is undertaken in a specific context and is shaped by the values and beliefs of those carrying out the study. Implicit judgements underpin all research activity. These include:

- the judgement of what is a worthwhile question to ask
- the way in which the question is posed or the problem is to be addressed
- decisions about what data are worth including
- tests applied to judge the soundness of the conclusions drawn.

The decisions at each stage of the research process are generated within, and selected by, individuals whose worldview and values have been shaped within a particular social and professional context. Thus, knowledge is shaped by its social context (Davis-Floyd & Sargent 1997, Downe & McCourt 2008, Jordan 1993). In this sense, there can be no 'absolute truth'. An awareness of this can be a fruitful basis for generating new questions which reflect and incorporate wider perspectives than just those of the medical or other professions.

However, even in its own terms, research cannot offer finality or certainty in its investigation of the world (Downe & McCourt 2008). Research studies can only present a **partial perspective** on the questions investigated:

- the focus of the investigation
- decisions regarding the form of investigation
- the process of analysis
- presentation of the data.

All are subject to a variety of constraints, including the beliefs and values of the investigator. A study will be influenced by:

- perspectives of funding bodies
- decisions of where the study is conducted
- personnel involved
- autonomy of research participants
- rigour of data collection and analysis
- dissemination of findings
- debate generated by the publication of the study.

Even when these factors have been well considered and addressed within the research design and interpretation of findings, the applicability of results to wider spheres may be affected by small sample size, contextual factors or the acceptance of the study findings (see Downe & McCourt 2008) – for example, the series of studies carried out to investigate active management of the third stage of labour, in which selection of subjects, preparation of midwives and interpretation of data have all given rise to questions affecting the translation of research findings into practice.

Particular problems are encountered when a number of studies addressing the same issue present apparently conflicting results (see website for evidence dichotomies in interpretation of evidence in use for: steroids in preterm labour, the term breech trial and third stage management).

Limitations can be addressed in a number of ways. For a single research report, applying a strategy for rigorous critical appraisal (CASP 2010, Greenhalgh 2006) can enable the practitioner to distinguish between findings that are sound and those that are not.

**Systematic review:** Techniques such as *systematic review* attempt to address the limitations of single studies and the ambiguity of study findings. This strategy involves systematically searching for a comprehensive sample of studies on a particular issue, including a wide range of publications and the so-called 'grey literature' of unpublished studies. It is an analytical tool to synthesize information (Brownson et al 2003).

Studies can then be selected for inclusion in the review, on the basis of explicit criteria applied to research method, and their evidence is evaluated.

A systematic review is a rigorous way of examining the methodology and findings of individual studies in order to overcome the limitations discussed above – for example, the problems of generalizing from small local samples or evaluating conflicting results. By validating study methodology and findings, the systematic review identifies those that can be confidently applied in guiding practice (Mulrow 1994).

**Meta-analysis:** This further development of systematic review involves grouping similar studies and systematically applying particular research questions, as identified by a systematic review, and subjecting those data to further statistical analysis (see Enkin et al 2005, Olsen 1997, Olsen & Jewell 1998).

Whilst these strategies for comprehensive analysis can offer guidance for evidence, they are not without limitations (see Trinder & Reynolds 2000). It may be difficult to source the full range of information about a particular topic for study – for example, obtaining all sources, as a result of language differences, variations in the forms of study, or dissimilar inclusion and/or exclusion criteria. Furthermore, applying generalizable conclusions to a whole population may be neither individualized nor culturally or socially appropriate. However, the experience of dexamethasone demonstrates another obstacle to an evidence-based approach: 'Despite repeated randomised trials in 1987 providing incontrovertible evidence in favour of antenatal corticosteroid therapy, obstetricians all over the world have been slow to adopt this treatment. The cause of this reluctance is unclear …' (Crowley 2001) (see website for further debate).

Evidence derived from current literature, primary research studies, systematic reviews and meta-analyses or in-depth literature reviews (Gray 2001, Hart 1998) are not the only form available to practitioners. Practice guidelines, issued by local NHS standard-setting committees, by the Royal Colleges with joint statements on best practice, government recommendations or WHO initiatives, when they are based on critically appraised evidence and referenced as such, present evidence in a form which is easily accessible and applicable to practitioners (see website for sources).

## HIERARCHY OF EVIDENCE

The preceding section has considered the sources of evidence and knowledge forms (see website) used to inform clinical practice, indicating strengths and limitations of approaches.

The literature promoting an evidence-based approach to healthcare (see Gray 2001, Greenhalgh 2006, Sackett et al 2000, amongst others) suggests a hierarchical order of value for different sources of evidence. This places a hierarchy in order of:

- meta-analysis
- systematic review
- a single well-conducted randomized controlled trial
- cohort studies
- case reports.

Methods at the 'top end' of the above hierarchy are valued more highly because they have mechanisms built into them which are intended to counter bias (Fig. 5.1).

However, it needs to be remembered that no one method is free from bias and therefore all evidence must be examined in a critical way before it can be used. Whilst personal experiences and knowledge are additional sources of evidence which should inform practice and research at every level, all evidence needs to be judicious in its use for each woman and baby and their individual context (Sackett et al 2000). Many issues requiring clinical decisions have not yet been studied in a systematic way and therefore personal experience and case reports remain important and essential in clinical decision-making (Walsh 2008).

## WHAT STIMULATES THE SEARCH FOR EVIDENCE TO USE IN PRACTICE?

The search for evidence may be generated when practitioners or service users try to challenge the perpetuation of traditional practices. Early research pioneers in midwifery used their findings to change practice and challenge traditions (Romney 1980, Romney & Gordon 1981, Sleep et al 1984). This may stem from the desire to confirm and disseminate personal approaches to clinical care

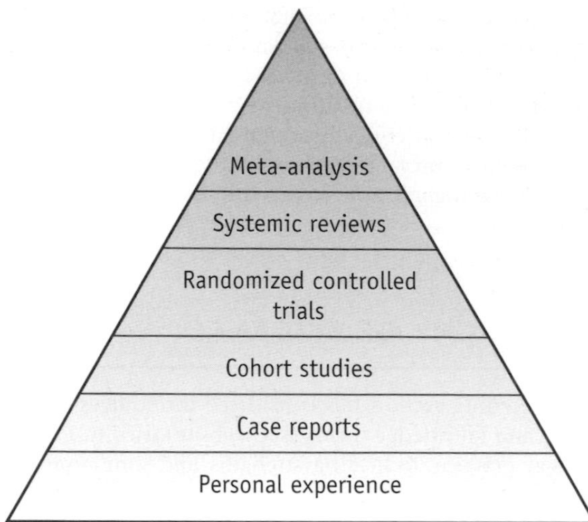


**Figure 5.1** 'Hierarchy' of evidence. *(Adapted from Greenhalgh 2006)*

(McCandlish et al 1998). Whilst it may arise from an interest in investigating the nature of midwifery practice, it may also be stimulated by the numerous debates that surround the provision of maternity care – such as antenatal care (Sikorski et al 1996), place of birth (Olsen 1997), nutrition in labour (Scrutton et al 1999), or midwifery-led care (Hatem et al 2008).

The two activities – conducting primary research to generate knowledge and critically appraising existing research findings – are closely linked. The further development of midwifery practice and care women receive depends on practitioners applying both of these activities in their professional lives with recurrent self-questioning of use of evidence to answer clinical questions.

**Reflective activity 5.1**

Reflect on your own experience and think of a question you may wish to ask yourself about current practice and whether this practice conflicts with evidence. Examples could be:

Antenatally – Do you measure height and weight of women?

Intranatally – Do you use alternative ambulatory methods, such as beanbags, balls and floor mats and rocking chairs?

Postnatally – What advice is given to women about babycare when they go home?

When you have decided your questions, use the guidelines below to find out the evidence.

Box 5.1 **Moving from clinical practice to the literature and back (adapted from Sackett et al 2000)**

1. Describing a clinical encounter
2. Posing or framing an answerable question
3. Searching for evidence
4. Critically appraising and validating the evidence
5. Implementing and evaluating the findings in practice

## WHY SEARCH FOR EVIDENCE?

A midwife may begin a search for evidence to apply to practice for a number of reasons. The search may start with a question raised by:

- a client or family's wishes for care or answers to questions
- a student or another colleague
- research findings in other fields raising questions about present or past practice
- media or ethical debates
- where tensions exist between a practitioner's experience and rituals and traditions in theory or practice.

It may be helpful to think about the process as consisting of a series of steps that can take the individual from a clinical question or problem, to finding, appraising and applying evidence that will help to answer it. The steps taken in developing the process of investigation for evidence are in Box 5.1 and will now be considered using a familiar clinical situation as a case study.

### Resumé of case scenario

The case scenario concerns a midwife who is caring for a woman in normal labour in a hospital where there is a policy for limited eating and drinking in labour. (Full information may be found on the website.)

### Framing an answerable question

The NHS Executive (1998,1999) commented that *defining the question* is the starting point of evidence-based practice, and that once healthcare practitioners are clear about the question, this will help in locating the evidence needed to discover answers to the problem. (For developing research questions, see website for Case scenario.) A guide for designing an evidence-based question is suggested by Sackett et al (2000) (Box 5.2).

This format would not be suitable for *every* question generated by clinical practice, and other formats should

**Box 5.2 Elements in framing a question for a healthcare intervention**

A question about a healthcare intervention contains four elements. These are:

- the client population
- the intervention being considered
- the comparison or alternative intervention
- the outcome or outcomes the healthcare practitioner is interested in.

**Box 5.3 Elements recommended for constructing an answerable question (adapted from Sackett 2000) with examples relating to case scenario under discussion**

**Client population**

Labouring women during the first stage of uncomplicated labour

**The intervention being considered**

Fasting in labour

**Alternative intervention**

Eating and drinking in labour

**The outcomes of interest**

Maternal and fetal hazards/risks:

- prolonged labour
- increased need for pain relief
- fetal distress

be considered when appropriate, such as where the questions relate to prognosis (Laupacis et al 1994), economic evaluation (Drummond et al 1997), and guideline evaluation (Oxman et al 2006).

Box 5.3 summarizes the elements recommended for constructing an answerable question and how they have been applied to the scenario.

### Composing an answerable question

After identifying the key elements of the scenario (see website for details), the next step is to formulate a question that can be phrased from the above parts.

## Searching for the evidence

The process of tracking evidence in the databases is not as simple as it sounds on paper. It requires skills to navigate through the many different systems to find credible and trustworthy sources that have rigour. All healthcare professionals are now required to develop their Information Technology (IT) skills, to use the internal and external internet, databases and retrieve information. Computer literacy skills are necessary in all aspects of work (see website).

It is important to learn to navigate use of local guidelines and policies and ensure access to email so that you are kept up to date. Whilst there are a number of areas for which evidence exists to support sound decision-making, there are many clinical questions which still require evidence of good quality to be generated; this discovery in itself should be seen as a positive finding if it leads to further research. Clients, such as women and their families, may be more skilled at searching for information than are professionals but may not be able to discern the quality of research and evidence; therefore, sharing information with women is essential to assist them with participating in their care and decisions for their health and wellbeing. There is a case for involving women in developing the evidence and questions for practice (Soltani 2007).

**Box 5.4 Processes used in searching skills**

Make a record of all details
Clarify the topic area and its parameters
Define the research question or problem
Identify key words and your search strategy
Decide the selection criteria and search limits
Decide where to search

- Define types of journals
- Decide time spans, year dates for search
- Which databases
- What journals need to be hand-searched

Search words to be used (combinations) – phrases
Narrowing or broadening the search

### The searching process

When undertaking a search, you will need to go through the steps in Box 5.4. (Refer to website for more detailed information and full explanations for Box 5.4.)

### Some helpful hints in undertaking a search

If the search question relates to an intervention and its effects on outcomes, begin with a search of the Cochrane Database (see website). Cochrane will enable location of any relevant systematic reviews or references of trials relating to the question listed in the Cochrane Controlled Trials Register. It may be that the answer to the question

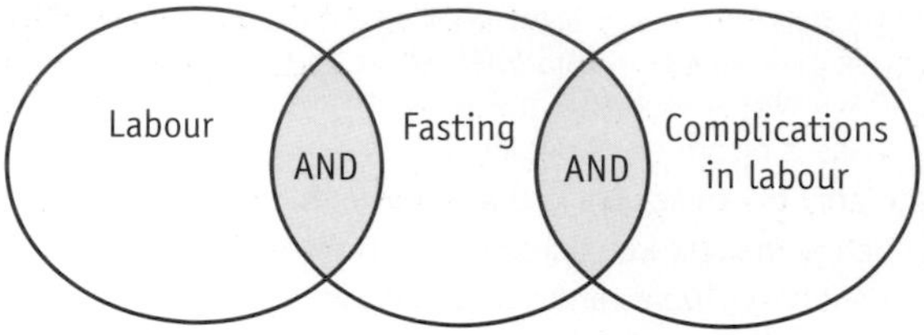

**Figure 5.2** Step-by-step searching.

is already available in the findings of a systematic review and further searching will not be necessary.

A search may work most efficiently if it is built up step by step, including new search terms one at a time (Fig. 5.2) (see website).

## Judging the evidence

It may be tempting to look only at the findings of research studies or guideline recommendations relying on these to influence practice. However, it is necessary to exercise critical skills, even when the source of the evidence can be expected to have applied rigorous standards in its preparation.

Judgement can be exercised and developed by making use of the range of general and specific appraisal guides in order to validate the available research evidence, for example, Greenhalgh (2006) or Sackett et al (2000). A critical guide enables a systematic approach to appraisal, ensuring that attention is given to all elements of the research process, guarding against 'snap' decisions and ensuring that judgements are well grounded.

It is impossible to offer a comprehensive list of appraisal guides, as it is a rapidly developing area of literature (see website for references to guides). However, some resources that may be useful to develop a global way of appraising a research study include Rees (2003), Cluett and Bluff (2006), and Rudestam and Newton (2007), each of which provides a strategy for analysing and critiquing research reports. It is important, however, that you choose the appropriate guide for the question, topic and the form of report that you are appraising.

Some appraisal guides are developed specifically to examine clinical and related studies according to the specific research problem under investigation and/or the study design. Thus, there are guides specific to examining a clinical trial, a systematic review or a qualitative study of client experience. You will need a different set of criteria for qualitative and quantitative reports, as you will for appraising policy or other documents such as narrative enquiry.

Whatever the design of the study being appraised, it is helpful to use a tool specially designed for the purpose, which enables the important characteristics of the study to be examined.

Once the evidence is validated, the next issue to consider is how it is put into practice.

## Contexts for implementing the evidence

The 'practice' of midwifery does not happen only when the midwife is 'with woman', and the application of evidence to midwifery can be regarded as happening at several levels of practice:

- *Individual*: the decision-making that occurs at the time of giving care to an individual client.
- *Collective*: the consensus expressed in the guidelines and protocols agreed within a collaborative setting, for example, an NHS trust or a group midwifery practice.
- *Professional*: the body of knowledge and the implications for practice which emerge from it, as reflected, for example, in Royal College of Midwives' Position Papers (RCM 2010) and Nursing and Midwifery Council (NMC) standard setting, rules and codes of practice (NMC 2008a,b). In addition, professional knowledge (see website) is developed, debated and published at conferences and in peer-reviewed journals.
- *Societal/public debates and consensus:* as expressed in Department of Health recommendations, government policy, for example, *The new NHS: modern and dependable* (DH 1997), Clinical Governance (NHS Executive 2000).

It is important for midwives to contribute to and engage in debates at all these levels in order to provide rational, justifiable, equitable and good-quality care for childbearing women.

Whilst at an individual level, it may seem relatively easy to implement change based on evidence – for example, individual midwives might examine and alter their usual practice – changing evidence-based practice is difficult when working in a context where practice is not consistently informed by good evidence. Thus, for example, many midwives face the difficulty of working in an environment where continuous electronic fetal monitoring is used in the care of most women, in spite of the absence of evidence to support this (Thacker et al 2001). This 'evidence–practice gap' is demonstrated in the case scenario about offering nutrition to women in normal labour (Scrutton et al 1999). So, consistent application of evidence to practice depends on more than the good intentions of individual practitioners.

Care for women and babies is delivered by many professional groups and individuals. In this respect, a 'collective' approach to evidence-based practice is essential. Implementation of evidence in practice is inextricably linked to the mechanisms for quality standards, risk management stategies and change within an organization. There are a variety of multidisciplinary activities, such as risk management groups, guideline and policy development initiatives, audit activities, and meetings looking at maternal and neonatal morbidity and mortality, where midwives have to play a key role (see Ch. 7). Consultant midwives and practice development midwives make vital contributions in this sphere.

Midwives' practice and use of evidence and research is shaped by influences beyond the local sphere and practice within a national professional framework (NMC 2004).

Supervision of midwives (NMC 2007) has a special and unique contribution to make in facilitating the development of an EBHC culture. An annual meeting with a supervisor (see Ch. 3) may assist in assessing the needs of a midwife's development of knowledge and skills. Annual organizational audits for supervision of midwives may demonstrate practices that are poorly supported by evidence with action for change initiated.

A range of influences at the social level has relevance for creating a climate and context for evidence-based practice. In maternity care, multiprofessional critical appraisal of adverse events or client pressure, expressed through a range of user groups, has been pivotal in compelling professionals to re-examine the evidence base for practices. Such groups include the National Childbirth Trust (NCT), Association for Improvements in Maternity Services (AIMS), Active Birth Movement, Stillbirth and Neonatal Death Society (SANDS), and many others.

The National Institute for Health and Clinical Excellence (NICE) was set up in April 1999 with the aim of providing 'patients, health professionals and the public with authoritative, robust and reliable guidance on current "best practice"', underpinned by review of the available evidence. All midwives must be conversant with the publication of guidelines (see website). The NICE guidelines are based on a review panel of a multidisciplinary team, evidence-based and referenced with the aim to achieve consistency of practice nationally (NICE 2010). Midwives will also find helpful the RCOG Green-top guidelines that provide systematically developed practice recommendations (RCOG 2010).

Another initiative, which bridges the gap between service user and professional practice, is the DISCERN, a resource questionnaire that enables consumers to evaluate the quality of the information offered to them as part of their care (DISCERN 2010).

## Evidence in practice for individual women

Publications by women's organizations, such as the MIDIRS information leaflets (AIMS 2010, Birthchoice UK 2010, NCT 2010), all provide information for women. Furthermore, many women themselves have access to the internet and can manage to find their own information, though this may not always be based on evidence. Research reports are also published in the media and so keeping up to date with information in the public domain assists with discussing current anxieties that women may have. It is therefore essential that midwives fully discuss all evidence clearly so that women are fully informed to make choices and decisions with the midwife in their own best interest. The future will be to involve women in review of evidence for policy making (DH 2004).

## Getting research into practice

The discussion of implementation of evidence-based practice can hardly be complete without considering the complexity of the process whereby evidence is translated into practice. Individual and organizational behaviours are important elements in the translation of research into practice. Two influences in a maternity setting are the commitment of all staff to policy and guidelines and the responses to the management of change (Bury & Mead 2000, Evans & Haines 2000, Haines & Donald 1998, Kanter et al 1992, NHS Scotland 2010, Sanders & Heller 2006). Without an active multiprofessional group to commit to revising guidelines and policies as new evidence becomes available, relevant to local needs and maternity philosophy, and reliable, there is little commitment to respond to change. It is suggested that it is essential to understand the characteristics of change and its impact on organizational activity, when embarking on implementation of evidence into practice (CASP 2010). Not to be forgotten is that evidence itself is subject to change. With further research and changing technology, the knowledge base for practice may alter very rapidly, so the search for evidence must be a continuing process.

A number of studies have examined the effectiveness of different strategies for disseminating and implementing research findings into practice. Bero et al (1998) conducted an overview of systematic reviews on interventions for the implementation of findings. Gawlinski and Rutledge (2008) suggest there is no one model for implementing research evidence in practice but offer a guide on a way to implement a change in practice. Kitson et al (1998) suggest the need to go beyond these linear representations of change, presenting a multidimensional model which takes into consideration three elements:

- the nature of the evidence
- the environment into which it is being introduced
- the process for facilitating its introduction.

Each of these elements may be more or less favourable to the change process. Kitson et al (1998) propose that the model may be applied diagnostically to help in planning the implementation of change. The case studies they analyse suggest that facilitation of change is the key element to successful implementation. In the light of this suggestion, consultant or practice development midwives are strong candidates for initiating and sustaining research-based changes in practice.

**Reflective activity 5.2**

Rohini is 36 weeks' pregnant. She has one son, Kishan. Kishan was born by emergency caesarean section for fetal distress at 38 weeks, 3 years ago. Rohini's pregnancy has been uncomplicated. She is attending for her antenatal appointment today and asks you what her chances are of a vaginal birth this time around.

Consider what question you would ask prior to tracking the evidence for the above scenario.

Compare your question with our suggested one on the website.

## Evaluating the implementation of evidence in practice

Like all change, the change process involved when evidence is translated into practice needs to be evaluated. A plan for evaluation may be part of the implementation process, or data may be collected through on-going audit activity (see Ch. 7), but there must be some thought given to measuring the impact of clinical change on client outcomes, organizational processes and staff activity.

Gray (2001) proposes an 'evidence-driven audit cycle'. This is a useful model because of the way in which it integrates the search for evidence, translation of evidence into practice and measurement of its impact using audit tools. A question is generated within clinical practice, which stimulates the search for evidence. Changes in practice can be implemented on the basis of relevant evidence and the results of such changes monitored through audit activity. Evidence is made use of by being the basis for the audit standards against which practice is measured and a means by which further questions can be generated.

## CONCLUSION

All midwives are required to use evidence-based practice (NMC 2008a and b). Whilst some midwives will apply bodies of evidence as interpreted in pre-appraised resources, such as *The Cochrane Library* and *NICE*, or in locally developed practice guidelines, others will take a more active part by contributing to the development of evidence-based guidelines. However, each professional is expected to use skills for searching and appraising current research evidence. Midwives may use research and appraisal strategies to challenge and change practice and some will engage directly in the research process: designing and conducting primary research, participating in systematic reviews and meta-analyses. Whilst each of these activities requires different levels of expertise in the skills for EBHC, all of them require a basic knowledge of the research and appraisal process. The aim of using evidence-based practice in midwifery is to ensure women receive the care that offers the the best possible outcome for themselves and their babies.

**KEY POINTS**

- Evidence may derive from personal experience, expert knowledge or systematic investigation.
- Midwives need to be able to discern strengths and limitations of different sources of evidence and seek to strengthen the evidence base for their own practice.
- A number of tools and strategies exist, with which the practitioner should become familiar.
- A strategy for posing questions about clinical practice and searching for evidence can be a tool for challenging existing practice, revealing gaps in available evidence and developing the evidence base for practice.
- It is important that midwives gain skills, including IT skills, in order to contribute to and engage at the individual, collective, professional and public levels in debates about the evidence for practice and the best means for using evidence to improve the care of mothers and babies.

## REFERENCES


Association for Improvement of Maternity Services (AIMS): Information and home page available at: www.aims.org.uk. Accessed April 2010.

Bero L, Grilli R, Grimshaw JM, et al: Closing the gap between research and practice: an overview of systematic reviews of interventions to promote the implementation of research findings, *British Medical Journal* 317(7156):465–468, 1998.

Birthchoice UK: MIDIRS Informed choice leaflets available at: www.birthchoiceuk.com/BirthChoiceUKFrame.htm?http://www.birthchoiceuk.com/InformedChoice.htm. Accessed April 2010.

Brownson RC, Baker EA, Leet TL, et al: *Evidence based public health*, Oxford, 2003, Oxford University Press.

Bryman A: *Quantity and quality in social research*, London, 1992, Routledge.

Bury T, Mead J: *Evidence-based healthcare*, London, 2000, Butterworth Heinemann.

Cluett R, Bluff R: *Principles and practice of research in midwifery*, ed 2,

Edinburgh, 2006, Elsevier Health Sciences.

Critical Appraisal Skills Programme (CASP): NHS Public Health Resource Unit. www.phru.nhs.uk/pages/PHD/CASP.htm. Accessed April 2010.

Crowley P: Prophylactic corticosteroids for preterm birth (Cochrane Review), *The Cochrane Library*, Issue 2, Oxford, 2001, Update Software.

Davis-Floyd R, Sargent C: *Childbirth and authoritative knowledge: cross cultural perspectives*, Los Angeles, 1997, University of California Press.

Denzin NK, Lincoln YS, editors: *The Sage handbook of qualitative research*, ed 3, Thousand Oaks, 2005, Sage.

Department of Health (DH): *The new NHS: modern and dependable*, London, 1997, The Stationery Office.

Department of Health (DH): *Making a difference*, London, 1999, DH.

Department of Health (DH): *Patient and public involvement in health: the evidence for policy implementation*, London, 2004, DH.

Department of Health (DH): *High Quality Care For All. NHS Next Stage Review Final Report*. The Stationery Office, 2008. www.tsoshop.co.uk http://www.dh.gov.uk/prod_consum_dh/groups/dh_digitalassets/@dh/@en/documents/digitalasset/dh_085828.pdf. Accessed May 2010.

DISCERN: Website and on-line information available at: www.discern.org.uk. Accessed April 2010.

Downe S, McCourt C: From being to becoming: reconstructing childbirth knowledges. In Downe S, editor: *Normal childbirth: evidence and debate*, London, 2008, Churchill Livingstone.

Drummond MF, Richardson WS, O'Brien BJ, et al: Users' guides to the medical literature: how to use an article on economic analysis of clinical practice, *Journal of the American Medical Association* 277(19):1552–1557, 1997.

Enkin M, Kierse MJN, Renfrew M, et al: *A guide to effective care in pregnancy & childbirth*, ed 2, Oxford, 2005, Oxford University Press.

Evans D, Haines A, editors: *Implementing evidence-based changes in healthcare*, Abingdon, 2000, Radcliffe Medical.

Gawlinski A, Rutledge D: Selecting a model for evidence-based practice changes: a practical approach, *Advanced Critical Care* 19(3):291–300, 2008.

Gray M: *Evidence-based health care*, Edinburgh, 2001, Churchill Livingstone.

Greenhalgh T: *How to read a paper: the basics of evidence based medicine*, ed 3, London, 2006, Wiley Blackwell.

Haines A, Donald A, editors: *Getting research findings into practice*, London, 1998, BMJ Press.

Hart C: *Doing a literature review*, London, 1998, Sage.

Hatem M, Sandall J, Devane D, et al: Midwife-led versus other models of care for childbearing women, *Cochrane Database of Systematic Reviews* (4):CD004667, 2008.

Jordan B: *Birth in four cultures: a crosscultural investigation of childbirth in Yucatan, Holland, Sweden, and the United States*, rev. ed. expanded by R. Davis-Floyd, Prospect Heights, IL, 1993, Waveland Press.

Kanter RM, Stein B, Jick TD: *The challenge of organisational change*, New York, 1992, Free Press.

Keane A: *The modern law of evidence*, ed 7, Oxford, 2008, Oxford University Press.

Kitson A, Harvey G, McCormack B: Enabling the implementation of evidence-based practice: a conceptual framework, *Quality in Health Care* 7(3):149–158, 1998.

Laupacis A, Wells G, Richardson WS, et al: Users' guides to the medical literature: how to use an article about prognosis, *Journal of the American Medical Association* 272(3):234–237, 1994.

Lincoln YS, Guba EG: *Naturalistic inquiry*, London, 1985, Sage.

McCandlish R, Bowler U, van Asten H, et al: A randomised controlled trial of care of the perineum during second stage of normal labour, *British Journal of Obstetrics and Gynaecology* 105(12):1262–1272, 1998.

Mulrow C: Rationale for systematic reviews, *British Medical Journal* 308(6954):597–599, 1994.

National Childbirth Trust (NCT): Information and leaflets available at: www.nctpregnancyandbabycare.com/press-office/background-information/nct-facts. Accessed April 2010.

National Insititute for Health and Clinical Excellence (NICE): Website: www.nice.org.uk. Accessed April 2010.

NHS Executive: *A first class service*, London, 1998, 1999, DH.

NHS Executive: *Building the information core: implementing the NHS plan*, London, 2000, DH.

NHS Scotland: *Educational resources: clinical governance* (website). www.clinicalgovernance.scot.nhs.uk/section6/implement.asp. Accessed April 2010.

Nursing and Midwifery Council (NMC): *Midwives rules and standards*, London, 2004, NMC.

Nursing and Midwifery Council (NMC): *Standards for supervision of midwives*, London, 2007, NMC.

Nursing and Midwifery Council (NMC): *The code: standards of conduct, performance and ethics for nurses and midwives*, London, 2008a, NMC.

Nursing and Midwifery Council (NMC): *Standards 2007, 2008, 2009* (website). www.nmc-uk.org/aArticle.aspx?ArticleID=2596. 2008b.

Olsen O: Metaanalysis of the safety of home birth, *Birth* 24(1):4–13, discussion 14–16, 1997.

Olsen O, Jewell MD: Home versus hospital birth (Cochrane Review), *The Cochrane Library*, Issue 2, Oxford, 1998, Update Software.

Oxman AD, Schünemann HJ, Fretheim A: Improving the use of research evidence in guideline development. 16. Evaluation, *Health Research Policy and Systems* 1006 4:28, 2006.

Rees C: *An introduction to research for midwives*, Edinburgh, 2003, Elsevier.

Romney M: Predelivery shaving: an unjustified assault? *Journal of Obstetrics and Gynaecology* 1(1):33–35, 1980.

Romney M, Gordon H: Is your enema really necessary? *British Medical Journal (Clinical Research Edition)* 282(6272):1269–1271, 1981.

Royal College of Midwives (RCM): Position Papers, available at: www.rcm.org.uk/college/standards-and-practice/position-papers. Accessed April 2010.

Royal College of Obstetricans and Gynaecologists (RCOG): Green top guidelines, available at: www.rcog.org.uk/womens-health/guidelines?filter0%5B%5D=12. Accessed April 2010.

Rudestam EK, Newton RR: *Surviving your dissertation: a comprehensive guide to content and process*, ed 3, Thousand Oaks, 2007, Sage.

Sackett DL, Richardson WS, Rosenberg W, et al: *Evidence-based medicine (multimedia): how to practise and teach EBM*, ed 2, Edinburgh, 2000, Churchill Livingstone.

Sanders J, Heller R: Improving the implementation of evidence-based practice: a knowledge management perspective, *Journal of Evaluation in Clinical Practice* 12(3):341–346, 2006.

Scrutton MJ, Metcalfe GA, Lowy C, et al: Eating in labour: a randomised controlled trial assessing risks and benefits, *Anaesthesia* 54(4):329–334, 1999.

Sikorski J, Wilson J, Clement S, et al: A randomised controlled trial comparing two schedules of antenatal visits: the antenatal care project, *British Medical Journal* 312(7030):546–553, 1996.

Sleep J, Grant A, Garcia J, et al: The West Berkshire perineal management trial, *British Medical Journal* 289:587–590, 1984.

Soltani H: Women's involvement in healthcare: a practical model for maternity services. In Richens Y, editor: *Challenges for midwives*, London, 2007, Quay Books.

Thacker SB, Stroup D, Chang M: Continuous electronic fetal heartrate monitoring for fetal assessment during labour (Cochrane Review), *The Cochrane Library*, Issue 3, Oxford, 2001, Update Software.

Trinder L, Reynolds S: *Evidence-based practice: a critical appraisal*, Oxford, 2000, Blackwell Science.

Walsh D: Research evidence and clinical expertise, *British Journal of Midwifery* 16(8):498, 2008.

Chapter | 6 |

# Leadership and management in midwifery

Maria Barrell

## LEARNING OUTCOMES

By the end of this chapter, you will be able to:

- recognize the knowledge and skills required to develop expertise for management and leadership of resources in maternity care
- consider the application of effective leadership in supporting, enabling and valuing staff in their professional and personal development
- critically evaluate the strengths and weaknesses of a range of contemporary leadership and management theories and their application to midwifery and maternity services
- determine an appropriate personal leadership style that will enhance and further develop midwifery practice, education and research
- complete a 5-year plan of measurable and time-limited personal and professional leadership goals that will drive change, support innovation, and manage resources effectively in the development of quality maternity services at both a local and national level.

## INTRODUCTION

Government strategies for maternity services focus on the premise that all women and their families will have access to quality maternity services, designed to meet their individual needs (DH 2004, Scottish Office NHSiS 2001, Welsh Assembly 2005). The Maternity Services Survey (DH 2007c) revealed that 80% of women were satisfied with care they received during pregnancy and childbirth. Women also stated their preference for more choice regarding their care. In response, the Government published *Maternity matters: choice, access and continuity of care* (DH 2007b) with a renewed focus to improve the quality of maternity services. Safety, quality of care, choice and satisfaction are recognized as the key priorities for women and their families during their pregnancy, childbirth and postnatal experience (DH 2007b). To support its commitment to women, the Government has underpinned its strategy with a guarantee to all women regarding the quality of the care they will receive. Women will be offered choices in:

- access to maternity care
- model of antenatal care
- place of birth.

The key features of government policy are shown in Figure 6.1.

The key to the successful implementation of the government strategy is through effective dissemination across health authorities and with stakeholders who will engage with a commitment to operationalize the strategy. Consequently, midwives need to be aware of developments in their local maternity services (DH 2007b). In order for plans to be fully implemented, resourced, sustained, monitored and evaluated, effective midwifery leadership is fundamental for this agenda for change (Scottish Office NHSiS 2001). Additionally, the financial cost of maternity services must be accurately and realistically assessed so that resources may be provided for effective and efficient management (DH 2007b). In order to assess resources, each episode of maternity care – for example, an antenatal visit, delivery by caesarean section or normal postnatal inpatient care over a 24-hour period – is allocated a specific cost (tariff), thereby influencing the funding of resources (Fig. 6.2). The cost may be allocated regardless

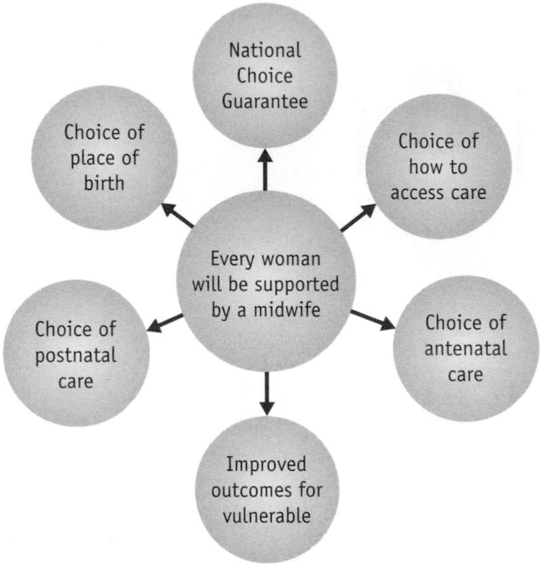

National Choice Guarantee

Choice of place of birth

Choice of how to access care

Every woman will be supported by a midwife

Choice of postnatal care

Choice of antenatal care

Improved outcomes for vulnerable

**Figure 6.1** Maternity matters: choice, access and continuity of care (DH 2007b), indicating all choices are available to women.

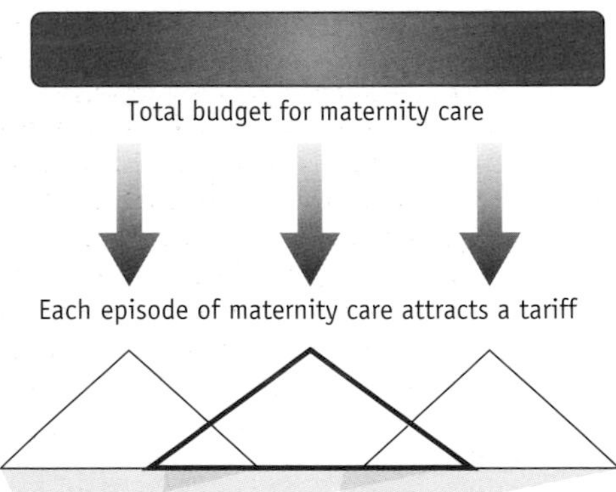


Tariffs establish a realistic costing for maternity care

**Figure 6.2** Maternity matters: choice, access and continuity of care (DH 2007b).

of geographical location but will need to take account of social issues that affect the resources required by women in the maternity services.

Whilst leadership and management of maternity services have been devolved, there are developments for national standards and objective monitoring frameworks to ensure quality of care and equity of provision for all women across the United Kingdom (DH 2007b). Improving the care given to women and their families is through preparation of the maternity services workforce, with investment in staff development and education (DH 2007b, Scottish Office NHSiS 2001). Midwife leaders and

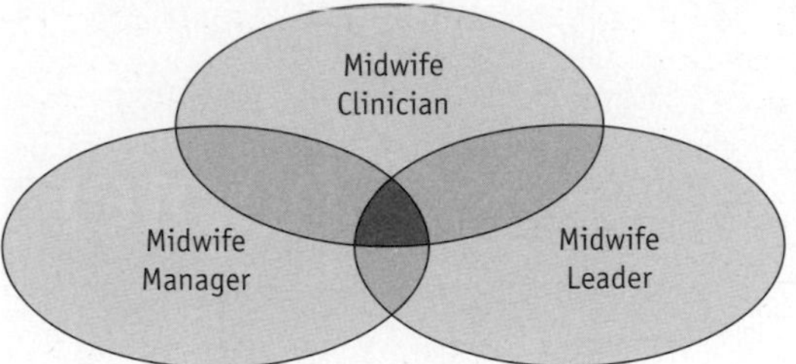


**Figure 6.3** The midwife as clinician, manager and leader.

managers at each health service level are required and need to be prepared for their roles in management and leadership.

Whilst their role, responsibility and accountability is to ensure the quality and safety of care for women during pregnancy, childbirth and the postnatal period, midwives require leadership and management skills as key aspects of their role (Fig. 6.3). Midwives need to develop a critical insight and understanding of the theory and practice of leadership and management and its application to their practice, regardless of whether their practice is in the health service or independent sector. Acquiring leadership and management knowledge and skills will enhance effectiveness in the development of quality maternity services and the progression of the midwifery profession in the 21st century and beyond. Figure 6.3 shows how the functions within their role overlap.

A range of leadership theories will be explored, including examples of traditional and alternative approaches. Consideration is given to the application of appropriate theories and experiences in leadership and resource management to develop quality maternity services and sustain a workforce that feels valued, motivated and committed to the delivery of quality care.

## THE DEVELOPMENT OF LEADERSHIP AND MANAGEMENT THEORY

In leadership and management, there are variations in use and application of terminology. There are examples of literature where the terms management and leadership are used synonymously (Buchko 2007, Manning 2002, Muldoon & Miller 2005, Nienaber & Roodt 2008), and where the term *management* is used primarily with some reference to *leadership* (Ollila 2008, Ozcelik et al 2008, Pounder & Coleman 2002, Prosen 2008, Sadler-Smith & Shefy 2006), and where the term leadership is used predominantly. These sources identify the role of the leader as having primacy, with need for additional skill development in the management of resources (Buchanan et al 2007, Greenfield 2007, Guillory 2007a, Guillory 2007b, Hammett 2008, Turner & Mavin 2007, Wood & Winston

2007). Ackloff (1981) argues that the principles of leadership and management are interwoven, proposing an effective leader has to gain legitimacy, which is acquired through previous resource management success. A further degree of clarification is offered by French et al (2008), who suggest a simple distinction between management and leadership. The role of a *manager* within an organization is concerned primarily with ensuring stability and enabling the organization to run effectively. The role of a *leader* within an organization is to inspire the workforce and promote innovation and long-term change.

In making distinctions between the role of leader and manager, French et al (2008) indicate that the senior person is identified as leader. This distinction is useful in concepts for strategic and operational leadership and management terminology, for example, the strategic leader is considered the visionary and the most senior post, the operational manager ensures the effective utilization of resources to sustain the business. However, it is important to acknowledge that size and complexity in organizations may determine their leadership and management roles and responsibilities.

The terms *strategic* and *operational* appear to be widely utilized by organizations in determining a leadership and management hierarchy. Nonetheless, the roles of leader and manager are neither distinct nor clearly demarcated, and overlaps between the two are perhaps inevitable and unavoidable (Adair 2006). As the understanding of leadership and management has developed, it is increasingly acknowledged that the role of manager requires leadership skills regardless of the level of the management role within an organization (Adair 2006).

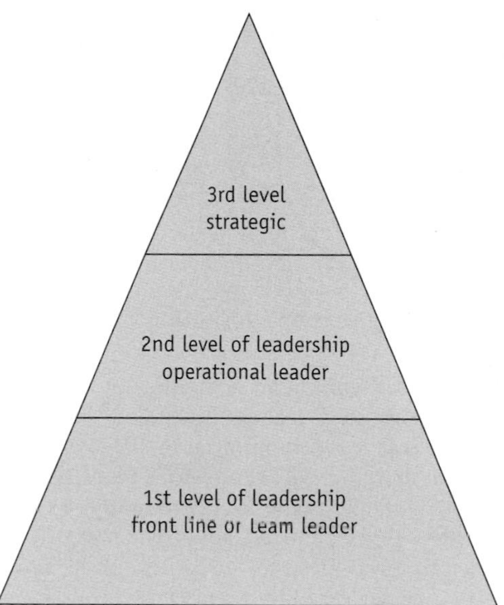


**Figure 6.4** Levels of leadership (Adair 2006).

## LEADERSHIP

Adair (2006) advocates the use of the term leadership and suggests there are three levels of leadership (Fig. 6.4):

- *First level – the front-line or team leader:* This leader creates specific outcomes or goals for the team that reflect the business of the organization, which are achieved within a determined timescale using agreed allocated resources.
- *Second level – the operational leader:* This leader is responsible for ensuring a stable culture within the workplace, resulting in effective, efficient and productive working practices.
- *Third level – the strategic leader:* This leader is responsible for the creation of the vision and long-term goals of the organization and the effective communication of the vision and goals to both the workforce and the customer.

Whilst leadership theory has evolved since the beginning of the 20th century (Yukl 2005) and effective leadership is a key facet of an organization's success, there is lack of clarity regarding what is an effective leader; however, what is clear is that there is no single style of leadership that works in **all** situations. Growing organizational complexity necessitates alternative leadership strategies to gain insight into the management of understanding and the principles of effective leadership (Ackloff 1981, Yukl 2005). Ackloff (1981) coined the term 'contextual mess' to describe the increasing complexity of work environments. Within an organization's contextual mess and the complexity of health services, maternity services leaders and managers are faced with multifaceted challenges which appear to be underpinned by ambiguity, uncertainty and shifting priorities.

## TRADITIONAL THEORIES OF LEADERSHIP

### Trait theory

Trait theory is considered the earliest documented approach of the study of leadership and can be plotted back to the early 20th century (French et al 2008). This theory attempts to capture the traits of recognized leaders in history, for example Napoleon and Churchill, and apply these traits to identify future leaders. Stogdill (1974) argued that there are specific identifiable traits which are linked to leadership success. These specific traits can be identified in leaders working within a wide range of professions and disciplines, including military services, law, business organizations and politics. Whilst research

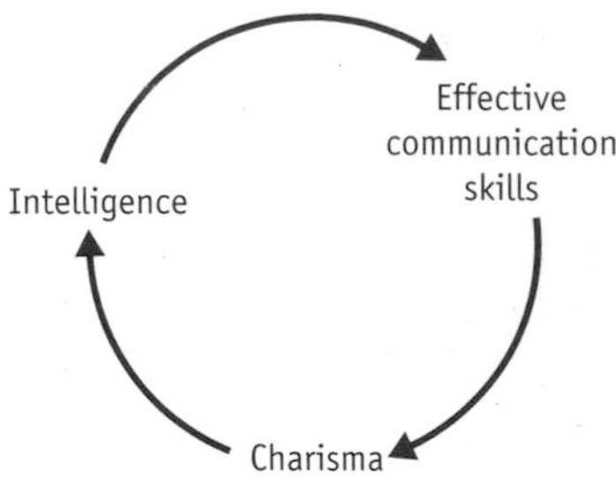


**Figure 6.5** Examples of leadership traits (Stogdill 1974).

succeeded in the recognition of a number of common behaviours of established leaders, including charisma, intelligence and effective communication skills, it failed to recognize that there were also exceptions to the possession of these identified traits to be found amongst other successful leaders (Bass 1990, Stogdill 1974) (Fig. 6.5). Little consideration was given to the context of the situation in which a leader may find themselves, for example the difference between leading an independent midwifery group practice and a midwife leading/managing a maternity unit of over 9000 deliveries per annum. The skills of a leader may be situation- or context-specific.

## Behavioural theory

In the 1950s, theorists considered a behavioural approach to leadership, through studying behaviours demonstrated by recognized leaders (French et al 2008). The theory suggested that an effective leader demonstrates specific behaviours and that leadership and effective resource management were central to maintenance and development of a successful organization. This could be applied to leadership and management in midwifery. Two research studies revealed two key behaviours of effective leadership (Bass 1990, Likert 1961):

- the leader who focuses on the *task*
- the leader who focuses on the *people* or the *workforce*.

Research into leadership identified that a distinct leadership style was of an employee-centred approach, and a second a production-centred approach. Effective performing organizations demonstrated high levels of employee-centred leadership. Leaders who were employee-centred demonstrated a higher level of production with a greater degree of employee satisfaction and positive morale (Likert 1961). Leadership behaviours were considered in terms of 'human-relations-orientated' or 'task-orientated' (Likert 1961). It was not clear from the results whether any of the organizations examined demonstrated leaders utilizing **both** distinct behaviours simultaneously or separately within the same organization and the potential impact on either employee or production.

An Ohio State University research study examined perceptions of leadership styles amongst the most senior organization staff. It revealed that leaders who were considerate to the feelings of employees or junior staff were deemed to be the more successful leaders. Those leaders who were orientated to the achievement of the task were less popular and did not maintain staff morale. The research later concluded that the most successful leaders demonstrated both behaviours, they were considerate of the workforce and their needs and also remained task-focused (Bass 1990).

It appears that a successful leader within an organization demonstrates in equal portions a concern for the workforce and concern for production. In midwifery, this would apply to leaders having a central concern for care of women and working within the team for the quality of service. Trait and behavioural theories may fail to recognize the potential conflicts that can arise between the workforce and production and how a leader deals effectively with conflict situations. If a successful business organization is faced with a downturn in the economy, the potential impact will be reduced production and a loss of revenue. In this circumstance, a leader may have to decide to reduce the workforce in order for the organization to survive. Therefore, in an economic crisis, priority will be given to sustained production, leading to conflict between the workforce and the service.

### Behavioural theory and the midwife leader

In a healthcare setting, an effective midwife leader may find that restricted financial resources may result in an overstretched workforce, which leads to feelings of anxiety and being devalued. In addition, midwives and their colleagues may express concern that the quality of care may be compromised, leading to the additional dissatisfaction of women regarding their care. In a crisis situation, leaders increasingly find their skills and effectiveness being tested. Theoretical approaches to leadership may not be effective for a health service meeting changes.

# ALTERNATIVE LEADERSHIP STYLES

## Transformational leadership

Transformational leadership is determined by a leader demonstrating key characteristics, including charisma, and the ability to inspire and motivate staff in the achievement of a shared vision or goal. Through these characteristics, a leader will gain the trust and confidence of employees. Successful transformational leadership ensures the organization benefits from enhanced employee commitment and performance. Transformational leadership creates changes in an organization which can present the greatest challenges as the outcome of change cannot be fully predicted (Ackerman 1986). In a transformational

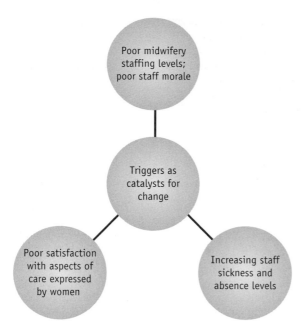


**Figure 6.6** Triggers as catalysts for change.

change, reciprocal levels of trust and confidence are required between the workforce and the leader (Jick 1993). Therefore, leading changes in maternity services involves teamwork and staff participation.

Implementing transformational leadership may highlight a range of issues, such as unpredicted emotional behaviours, which challenges a leader's self-awareness and the prospect of failure (Mitki et al 2008). Early recognition of unpredicted or adverse outcomes such as resistance of staff or the effects of changing a rostering pattern on part-time staff need to be addressed during a change process. The transformational process can be effective as it facilitates the leader's positive influence over colleagues (Bass 1998). If managed effectively, change can result in individual and team performances beyond expectation with recognition by colleagues of effective transformational leadership in both the management of resources and productivity.

The effectiveness of sustained transformational leadership may be underpinned by robust trigger identification (Mitki et al 2008). Triggers in a maternity service are problem areas that require intervention, such as poor morale or complaints from women or families about the service (Fig. 6.6). Recognition of triggers in the workplace becomes a precursor for change and development. Triggers can also alert a leader to a potential conflict that, with prompt action, could be avoided. Transformational leaders will identify the need for alternative strategies and ways of working and support the workforce through change (Ackloff 1981, Mitki et al 2008). Nadler (1998) argues that a leader must recognize the potential

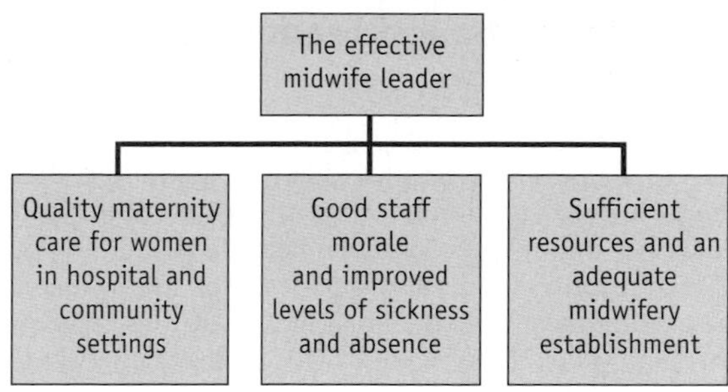


**Figure 6.7** Effective midwifery leadership approaches.

magnitude of a trigger event in assisting colleagues to conceptualize and understand change, adapt to changing working patterns and recognize the need to change or redefine roles and responsibilities and so involve the staff in their development and to seek answers for change.

Ensuring all staff or those involved in the process learn about a change that is to take place is a key point to its successful outcome. Effective leaderships will create a responsive climate to changes (Fig. 6.7). The capacity to learn and the establishment of a learning process are critical during a transformation process and the key element to determining successful outcome (Mitki et al 2008) – for example, all staff understanding new implementation of polices in relation to a change in care for women in labour. Careful attention to the learning process and support of colleagues' needs will underpin the successful implementation of new structures, changing working patterns and the development of leadership styles (Mitki et al 2008, Senge 1990). For transformational leadership to be successful it is essential that leaders monitor colleagues' understanding of the change and encourage their contribution to the process.

## Transformational leadership in contemporary midwifery practice

There is a place for transformational leadership to bring about effective implementation of government strategies and quality, safe maternity services (DH 2007a), as well as maintaining a motivated workforce. Midwives possess a shared vision; they aim to support women in their choice of care, and midwife leaders must work with Government, and stakeholders, such as local commissioners and providers of healthcare, to ensure that maternity services are fully resourced to meet the government's guarantees to women (DH 2007a). Midwife leaders in clinical practice can initiate and motivate midwives to change, by demonstrating transformational leadership characteristics. With expertise and experience, they recognize triggers for change (Fig. 6.6), including poor staffing levels, increasing staff sickness and absence, poor staff morale and poor satisfaction of aspects of maternity care expressed by women and their families.

## Competence-based leadership and supervision

Leadership and resource management involves a complicated mechanism of human and social interactions that requires an understanding of human relationships and conflicts as well as problem-solving skills (Ollila 2008). An organization's leadership and resource management strategies are most effective when human actions are supported and valued (Sveiby 1990). The success of an organization is primarily the outcome of human actions that include motivation, ability and commitment. In addition to the establishment of leadership and management strategies, Sveiby (1990) suggests there are three key factors underpinning an organization's effectiveness:

- *Human capital* emerges from an organization's shared knowledge and competence, effective communication, ongoing learning and support for innovation.
- *Social capital* is supported by human capital and demonstrates a shared organizational viewpoint in relationship to the organization's customers, interest groups and standards and the organization's leadership and management strategies.
- *Structural capital* is the data that belong to the organization, including its procedures, systems and technology.

When these three factors work in harmony underpinned by effective leadership and resource management strategies, then an organization is able to develop and deal with change (Sveiby 1990). The future of healthcare services is dependent on effective leadership and resource management in order to achieve the government healthcare agenda and to develop and utilize competence and skills in order to improve the quality of healthcare, including maternity services.

Sanchez & Heene (2004) and Sanchez (2004) suggest strategic leadership and resource management is established on the premise that there is a possibility for change. Change initiates an appraisal of the competencies that exist within an organization and a consideration of the competencies that need to be acquired in order to meet the strategic goals for change and development. Durand (2000) suggests competence comprises a range of skills an individual utilizes to complete a given task. Competence is based upon knowledge, skills and attitudes and forms the cornerstone to a successful organization.

Competence-based resource management focuses on the recognition of knowledge and skills, and the refocusing of this knowledge and skills to meet the organization's goals and aspirations, for example training the workforce in new techniques for antenatal screening. A leader must recognize the need for established competencies within the organization and also anticipate the requirement to develop new competencies to move the organization forward (Fig. 6.8) (Ollila 2008, Sanchez 2004). Utilization of a competence-based management structure is central to the maintenance, continuous assessment, evaluation and redefinition of the organization's core competencies to ensure continued success (Ollila 2008, Sanchez 2004).

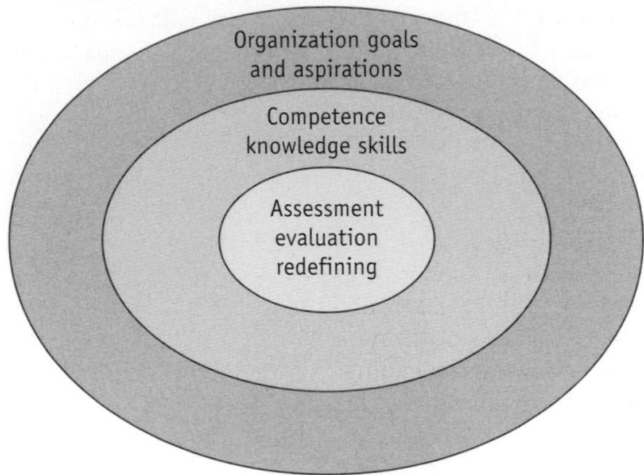


**Figure 6.8** Competence-based leadership.

## Statutory midwifery supervision

In the UK, supervision is central to effective leadership and competence-based resource management (Ollila 2008), enabling support for strategic development of roles within any organization (Sanchez & Heene 2004). Without supervision, leaders face dissatisfaction with their role, incompetence and eventual burnout. Organizations should consider the role of supervision as both preventative of leader burnout and effective in maintaining the wellbeing and efficiency of leaders and managers (Ollila 2008). Supervision within an organization can ensure that leadership and management strategies are common across the organization, reinforcing the vision, goals and direction.

Through a process of supervision, working practices can be viewed, human behaviours interpreted and better understood, policies evaluated in action, resource management broadened and the role of leader strengthened and developed (Ollila 2008).

## Leadership of self, failure, self-efficacy and emotional intelligence

The successful critical leadership of self predisposes to broadening of skills in the leadership of others that includes colleagues, clients and the organizations in the workplace. When considering leadership it is appropriate to consider ourselves, as individuals, and the individual strategies required for managing personal development, goal achievement and failure. Success and failure are experienced by all to a greater or lesser degree throughout life's journey, within an individual's personal, educational and career experiences. Individuals may choose to give up after the first experience of failure and function within the comfort zone, resulting in disillusionment, dissatisfaction and dreams of early retirement. For the majority, failure can also be the determinant of future success.

Boss & Sims (2008) argue that through the process of living everyone must experience failure. Failure can manifest itself in a number of guises – it may be small and personal or large and public, exposed to scrutiny and debate. If failure is common to all, then the reaction to failure can vary depending on the individual and the personal circumstances, leading to different personal strategies:

- failure determines future action taken
- recovery from the failure with little reflection on the process
- pain which, after a short interval, is rationalized.

Allowing failure to affect self-esteem and confidence may lead to a downward spiral. Failure can be perceived as a stepping-stone to eventual success; the only real failure being ceasing to aspire to individual goals, and can be managed as an impetus to encourage further development and aspirations. Insight and reflection on personal and organizational failure, utilizing acquired knowledge and skills in emotional intelligence, efficacy and leadership can provide essential personal experience in the development of an effective strategy (Fig. 6.9) (Boss & Sims 2008).

Self-efficacy is an individual's own judgement regarding how they are able to lead a situation. It is not about the skills possessed but what the individual believes they are capable of achieving. If personal judgement results in failure, then there is also doubt in self-efficacy skills (Bandura & Locke 2003, Judge et al 1997). An example to demonstrate the impact of self-efficacy may well be useful to explain its potential significance. If a midwife's time has been spent in leading a project to its fruition whilst demonstrating effective and efficient management of allocated resource, a failure to achieve success in the project can lead to doubt regarding judgement or self-efficacy. The impact of failure can therefore affect the individual, colleagues, clients and the organization.

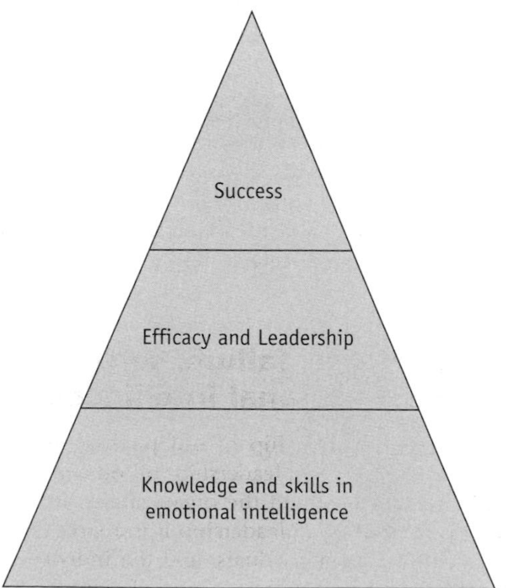


**Figure 6.9** Steps to success of self, others and the organization.

- *Emotional leadership* and management in decision making, negotiations and interpersonal behaviour has been recognized in recent years. Emotional leadership forms a significant element of emotional intelligence (Salovey & Mayer 1990).
- *Emotional intelligence* impacts upon an individual's insight and management of self and also on the emotional insight and intelligence of others. The emotional reaction to a situation conveys messages.

The ability to read an individual's emotions can build a body of intelligence which may be utilized in the leadership strategies employed and management of resources (Salovey & Mayer 1990). Emotional intelligence demonstrates the ability to identify, express, assimilate, regulate and manipulate emotions in both self and others, whether positively or negatively (Zeidner et al 2004). With the possession of emotional intelligence, emotions can be managed. It is possible for a leader to manipulate and regulate individual and group emotion, creating either a positive or negative working environment (Salovey & Mayer 1990).

Emotional regulation and control are associated with both leadership and self-efficacy and knowledge of the human resource (Boss & Sims 2008). Emotional recognition and regulation deals with the subjective and can be difficult to measure (Goleman 1995, 1998). Goleman (1995, 1998) suggests emotion deals with thoughts which enable understanding, whilst leadership deals with cognitive skill and the organization of thought and action into measurable outcomes. Leadership is the influence individuals use to control their behaviours and thoughts in order to increase personal effectiveness and performance (Frese & Fay 2001, Sims & Manz 1996). Emotional intelligence can also be utilized as an effective facet of leadership, though the skill in managing and controlling emotion may be difficult to measure objectively and therefore must be considered sensitively.

## Emotional Intelligence and the midwife leader

A midwife leader working with a team of staff in a clinical environment will, over a period of time, get to know each member of staff. Midwives working in clinical situations inevitably will demonstrate some emotional reaction in caring for women and their families. Leaders can build emotional intelligence of individual and groups of staff. This intelligence can be used positively as a management strategy; for example, a midwife who has dealt with a particularly difficult clinical situation may need a less difficult workload when next on duty. Alternatively, emotional intelligence can have a negative impact; for example, a midwife may not be asked to deal with a particular situation because of a previous emotional reaction. A number of variables can affect an individual emotional reaction in a particular situation. The midwife leader may gain emotional intelligence regarding her colleagues, but there needs to be a recognition that this intelligence is subjective and should be used with caution. However, midwifery is a caring profession where emotions may surface and effective leadership involves a degree of care and consideration of colleagues including valuing their emotional investment in the care of women and their families.

## Authentic leadership

Traditional leadership theories are not sufficient to prepare future leaders for the contemporary workplace (Turner & Mavin 2007). Authentic leadership focuses upon the individual's own life experiences, journeys and reflections rather than the application of established theoretical models of leadership (Cameron et al 2003, Lord & Brown 2004, Turner & Mavin 2007). Authentic leadership has been described as the process of owning one's individual experiences through self-awareness and self-acceptance (Cameron et al 2003) and authentic leaders are portrayed as being self-aware with clearly defined and articulated values (Shamir & Eilam 2005). In addition, authentic leaders demonstrate a motivation towards realistic goal achievement and they possess the ability to attract followers (Fig. 6.10) (Cameron et al 2003, Luthans & Avolio 2003).

Authentic leaders can be seen as genuine in that they do not aspire to a leadership role for individual reward, but their actions are based upon their personal values and convictions (Shamir & Eilam 2005). They also recognize the areas in which they are vulnerable and are willing to share and discuss those vulnerabilities with colleagues, basing their values upon their own life experiences, and this shapes their authentic and individual leadership style (Shamir & Eilam 2005). Gardner et al (2005) consider triggers and life events to be key aspects of the development of an authentic leadership style through an understanding of self. This can comprise both positive and negative experiences which trigger changes in an individual's self-identity (Lord & Brown 2004). Interpreting life experiences with application and adaptation of this experiential knowledge to leadership situations is part of authentic leadership (Luthans & Avolio 2003). If this application of life experience is undertaken with honesty and integrity and a clear insight into areas of vulnerability, then this leadership style can prove to be effective. Individuals therefore face different life experiences which build a body of knowledge and self-awareness. The authentic leader may present an eclectic style of leadership with a range of knowledge and skills being applied effectively in similar situations. It may be concluded that it is the *application* of life experience to a situation that provides authentic leadership effectiveness, **not** the possession of a particular set of learned skills or theoretical approach.

Kernis (2003) suggests that to behave in an authentic manner means personal values are reflected in actions. This means that actions taken by an authentic leader are not demonstrated merely to respond to another's needs. An authentic leader does not support instant decision making or decisions that ensure personal reward and this reflects personal values based on perceptions of fairness. Therefore, the values held by an authentic leader are not necessarily those thought to be acceptable to the organization (Kernis 2003).

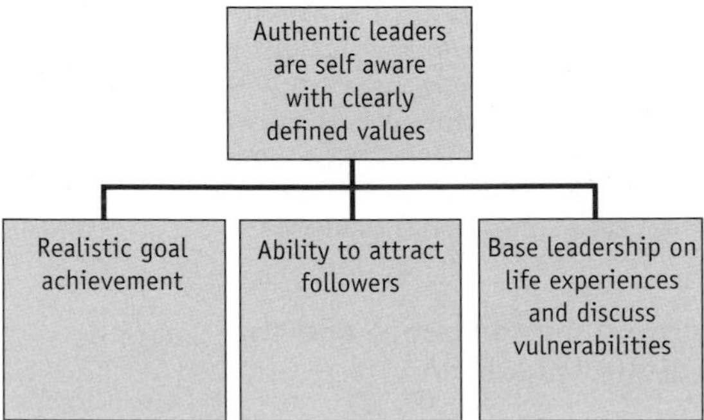


**Figure 6.10** Attributes of the authentic leader.

### Reflective activity 6.1

- Do you feel that you possess leadership skills? If so, identify these skills.
- Reflect on any recent situations in your current role where you feel you have demonstrated effective leadership.
- Now you have increased your knowledge and insight of a range of leadership theories, critically consider which style you would apply to your role and why.

The traditional theories of leadership imply that successful leaders do not display emotional behaviours, retaining objectivity in leadership situations (Likert 1961). Behaviourist theory recognizes the importance of employee wellbeing but this does not necessitate a leader sharing personal emotional experiences. Conversely, authentic leadership supports a leader bringing more of themselves to the workplace, which may include personal emotional experiences where these are deemed to be appropriate However, it is crucial that the authentic leader minimizes the sharing of inappropriate or potentially damaging personal emotional experiences which may compromise their position (Gardner et al 2005).

The role of leader can create negative emotional experiences, including anxiety and feelings of vulnerability and underachievement of goals (Turner & Mavin 2007). For many leaders and managers, emotional reactions to pressures of role and responsibilities are hidden beneath the surface. These hidden emotions may manifest themselves in different guises, including poor communication with colleagues, underachievement and sickness. There is a dichotomy for a leader between the control of emotions (Likert 1961) and the expression of emotions within a leadership role (Gardner et al 2005). An empirical study of senior leaders suggested that the sharing of personal life experiences through narrative stories might enable senior leaders to reflect upon their values and further develop and grow (Turner & Mavin 2007). However, these authors highlight that expression of emotion by senior leaders is restricted by personal regulation or control in order to maintain the impression of the leader not being personally exposed, thus creating personal boundaries.

Authentic leadership advocates experiential learning and development as opposed to the application of theoretical approaches where the endpoint is the goal, not the experiences gained throughout a process or journey. The sharing of an authentic leader's life experiences predisposes to the development of values, self-awareness, fairness and motivation. However, it may be problematic to those potential leaders who wish to adopt an authentic leadership style if it is perceived personal life experiences are limited.

**Reflective activity 6.2**

- Consider your current role in midwifery and identify three situations where you have utilized resource management skill and competence.
- For each of the three situations you have identified, reflect on the skills you applied and how effective you were.
- Now you have increased your knowledge and insight into the management of resources, critically consider how you would effectively apply this knowledge to your present role.

## Authentic leadership in midwifery

It is probable that authentic leadership is evident in midwifery. Midwife leaders will share a number of personal experiences with the women for whom they care and their midwifery colleagues. Many midwives have personally experienced childbirth and all have practised midwifery. Midwife leaders possess experiential learning experiences that can prove useful in leadership roles. The values, self-awareness and motivation they demonstrate are usually constructed from their own experiences. Subjectivity may be the result of personal experiences of childbirth and clinical midwifery practice; therefore, it is appropriate that both an authentic experience and knowledge of leadership theory are combined to ensure the development of a midwife leader's objective style.

## CONCLUSION: LEADERSHIP AND MANAGEMENT WITHIN CONTEMPORARY MIDWIFERY

Through supervision of midwives or promotion of midwives within an organizational structure, midwife leaders and managers have emerged at different levels of the health service. Midwives have often been appointed to leadership and management posts because they are recognized for their exceptional skills in midwifery practice. However, they may not have been adequately prepared for this leadership and management role. Some leaders and managers are effective in their role, respected by colleagues for their skills and expertise. Others may be left feeling unsupported and dissatisfied and consequently their emotions can be cascaded to their colleagues, affecting the morale of staff and subsequently the quality of care.

Midwives are ideally placed at the centre of the government's strategy to support the agenda of change and improve the quality of contemporary maternity services. Midwives have emerged as valuable members of the multiprofessional team, sharing their knowledge and expertise with and learning from fellow professionals with a shared aim to provide holistic care in a range of health and social care settings. Therefore, all midwives require knowledge and skills for leadership and management.

**Reflective activity 6.3**

- Consider your career goals and aspirations for the next 5 years.
- Identify the goals you need to set in order to achieve your aspirations.
- What continuing professional development would you require in order to achieve your career aspirations and goals?
- Develop a written plan which identifies your career plan and the goals you need to achieve (example of template below in Table 6.1).

Women trust midwives to deliver the care they require. However, midwives can be stretched to capacity with poor

Table 6.1 Example of a career plan template

| Career aspirations for 5 years | Goals to achieve aspirations | Professional development plan |
|---|---|---|
| **Current role (2010)**<br>e.g. Clinical Midwife | – Ensure experience and competence gained in all aspects of midwifery practice | – Contemporary knowledge of evidenced-based midwifery practice<br>– Mentorship preparation |
| **Aspired role (2015)**<br>e.g. Supervisor of Midwives,<br>Consultant Midwife,<br>Clinical Midwifery Lead,<br>Risk Manager (Maternity Services),<br>Director of Midwifery,<br>Local Supervising Authority Midwifery Officer,<br>Midwifery Lecturer,<br>Lead Midwife in Education,<br>Midwifery Researcher | – To demonstrate safe and competent care of women and their babies during pregnancy, childbirth and the postnatal period<br>– To work effectively as member of a team<br>– To teach and support student midwives and newly qualified staff<br>– To demonstrate leadership and management skills of both staff and resources<br>– To acquire the knowledge, skill and competence to fulfil a senior role in midwifery | – Achievement of graduate status<br>– Postgraduate studies in, for example, Supervisor of Midwives, Research, Advanced Clinical Practice, Quality Assurance, Risk Management, Leadership and Management, Teaching and Education |

strategic leadership by those with little insight into the roles and responsibilities of midwives, or the needs of women and their families. Poor strategic leadership leads invariably to poor resource management including limited financial investment to realistically sustain and develop strategy for maternity services and a national shortage of practising registered midwives.

Midwives work in a range of environments and contexts where leadership and management of resources will depend on a number of variables, including the environment, the team, the skill mix, the available budget, the workload and the nature of a project. These areas of leadership and management will affect the delivery of services to women and their families. With knowledge and insight into theories of leadership and management of resources a midwife may consider one particular leadership approach suitable to their practice or may reflect that an eclectic approach where elements of a number of approaches is applicable. The acquisition of leadership and management knowledge and skills is critical to the recognition and progression of a contemporary midwifery profession continuing to deliver expert care to women and their families.

## REFERENCES


Ackerman L: Development, transition or transformation: the question of change in organizations, *Organization Development Practitioner* 18(1):1–8, 1986.

Ackloff RL: *Creating the corporate future*, New York, 1981, John Wiley.

Adair J: *Effective leadership*, London, 2006, Chartered Institute of Personnel and Development.

Bandura A, Locke EA: Negative self-efficacy and goal effects revisited, *Journal of Applied Psychology* 88:1.87–99, 2003.

Bass BM: *Bass and Stodgill's handbook of leadership*, New York, 1990, Free Press.

Bass BM: *Transformational leadership*, Mahwah, NJ, 1998, Lawrence Erlbaum.

Boss AD, Sims HP Jr: Everyone fails! *Journal of Management Psychology* 23(2):135–150, 2008.

Buchko AA: The effect of leadership on values-based management, *Leadership and Organizational Development Journal* 28(1):36–50, 2007.

Buchanan D, Caldwell R, Meyer J, et al: Leadership transmission: a muddled metaphor? *Journal of Health Organization and Management* 21(3):246–258, 2007.

Cameron KS, Dutton JE, Quinn RE, editors: *Positive organizational scholarship: foundation of a new discipline*, San Francisco, 2003, Barret-Koehler.

Denning S: How leaders can use powerful narratives as change catalysts, *Strategy and Leadership* 36(2):11–15, 2008.

Department of Health: *National service framework for children, young people and maternity services*, London, 2004, HMSO.

Department of Health: *Making it better for mother and baby*, London, 2007a, HMSO.

Department of Health: *Maternity matters: choice, access and continuity of care*, London, 2007b, HMSO.

Department of Health: *Maternity services survey*, London, 2007c, HMSO.

Durand T: Forms of incompetence. In Sanchez R, Heene A, editors: *Theory development for competence-based management*, Greenwich, 2000, JAI Press.

French R, Rayner C, Rees G, et al: *Organizational behaviour*, West Sussex, 2008, Wiley.

Frese M, Fay D: Personal initiative: an active performance concept for work in the 21st century, *Research in Organizational Behaviour* 23:133–187, 2001.

Gardner WL, Avolio BJ, Luthans F, et al: Can you see the real me? A self based model of authentic leader and follower development, *Leadership Quarterly* 16:343–372, 2005.

Goleman D: *Emotional intelligence: why it can matter more than IQ*, New York, 1995, Bantam Books.

Goleman D: *Emotional intelligence*, New York, 1998, Bantam Books.

Greenfield D: The enactment of dynamic leadership, *Leadership in the Health Service* 8(3):159–166, 2007.

Guillory WA: The future perfect organization: leadership for the twenty-first century – Part 1, *Industrial and Commercial Training* 39(1):52–58, 2007a.

Guillory WA: The future perfect organization: leadership for the twenty-first century – Part 2, *Industrial and Commercial Training* 39(2):91–97, 2007b.

Hammett P: The paradox of gifted leadership: developing the generation of leaders, *Industrial and Commercial Training* 40(1):3–9, 2008.

Jick TD: *Managing change*, Burr Ridge, 1993, Irwin.

Judge TA, Locke EA, Durham CC: The dispositional causes of job satisfaction: a core evaluations approach, *Research in Organizational Behaviour* 19:151–188, 1997.

Keating P: 9 January, Time, cited Jay A (2007) *Oxford Book of Political Quotations*, Oxford, 1955, Oxford University Press.

Kernis MH: Toward a conceptualisation of optimal self-esteem, *Psychological Inquiry* 14(1):1–26, 2003.

Likert R: *New patterns of management*, New York, 1961, McGraw-Hill.

Lord RG, Brown DJ: *Leadership processes and follower self identity*, Mahwah, NJ, 2004, Erlbaum.

Luthans F, Avolio BJ: Authentic leadership: a positive developmental approach. In Cameron KS, Dutton JE, Quinn RE, editors: *Positive organizational scholarship*, San Francisco, 2003, Barrett-Koehler, pp 241–262.

Manning TT: Gender, managerial level, transformational leadership and work satisfaction, *Women in Management Review* 17(5):207–216, 2002.

Mitki Y, Shani AB, Stjernberg T: Leadership, development and learning mechanisms, *Leadership and Organization Development Journal* 29(1):68–84, 2008.

Muldoon SD, Miller S: Leadership: interpreting life patterns and their managerial significance, *Journal of Management Development* 24(2):132–144, 2005.

Nadler D: *Champions of change*, San Francisco, 1998, Jossey-Bass.

Nienaber H, Roodt G: Management and leadership: buccaneering or science? *European Business Review* 20(1):36–50, 2008.

Nursing and Midwifery Council (NMC): *Standards for the preparation and practice of supervisors of midwives*, London, 2006, NMC.

Ollila S: Strategic support for managers by management supervisor, *Leadership in Health Services* 21(1):16–27, 2008.

Ozcelik H, Langton N, Aldrich H: Doing well and doing good, *Journal of Managerial Psychology* 23(2):186–203, 2008.

Pounder JS, Coleman M: Women – better leaders than men? In general educational management it still 'all depends', *Leadership and Organization Development Journal* 23(3):122–133, 2002.

Prosen B: Leadership that works (website). www.kisstheorygoodbye.com/blog/2008/03/22/leadership-that-works/. Accessed March 25, 2008.

Sadler-Smith E, Shefy E: Applying holistic principles in management development, *Journal of Management Development* 25(4):368–385, 2006.

Salovey P, Mayer JD: Emotional intelligence, *Imagination, Cognition and Personality* 9(3):185–211, 1990.

Sanchez R, Heene A: *The new strategic management: organization, competition and competence*, New York, 2003, John Wiley.

Sanchez R: Understanding competence-based management: identifying and managing five modes of competence, *Journal of Business Research* 57(5):518–532, 2004.

Scottish Office NHSiS: *A framework for maternity services in Scotland*, Edinburgh, 2001, ISD Publications.

Senge P: *The fifth discipline*, New York, 1990, Doubleday.

Shamir B, Eilam G: 'What's your story?' A life-stories approach to authentic leadership development, *Leadership Quarterly* 16(3):395–417, 2005.

Sims HP, Manz CC: *Company of heroes: unleashing the power of self-leadership*, New York, 1996, Wiley.

Stogdill RM: *Handbook of leadership*, New York, 1974, Free Press.

Sveiby KE: *The power and management in an expert organization*, Jtvaskyla, 1990, Gummerus Kirjapaino.

Turner J, Mavin S: Exploring individual leadership journeys through authentic leadership theory, *8th International Conference on HRD Research and Practice Across Europe*, Oxford, 2007, Oxford Brookes University.

Welsh Assembly: *National Service Framework (NSF) for children and young people in Wales*, Cardiff, 2005, Welsh Assembly.

Wood JA, Winston BE: Development of three scales to measure leader accountability, *Leadership and Organization Development Journal* 28(2):167–185, 2007.

Yukl G: *Leadership in organizations*, Thousand Oaks, CA, 2005, Prentice Hall.

Zeidner M, Matthews G, Roberts RD: Emotional intelligence in the workplace: a critical review, *Applied Psychology – An International Review* 53(3):371–399, 2004.

Chapter 7

# Governance in midwifery

Carol Paeglis

## LEARNING OUTCOMES

After reading this chapter, you will be able to:

- describe governance in the UK National Health Service
- discuss the relevance of governance in maternity services
- highlight issues that need to be addressed in midwifery in order to continually improve care
- describe ways of improving quality in midwifery.

## INTRODUCTION

This chapter will initially focus on systems of governance within the NHS, primarily in England though the importance of governance in healthcare systems is highlighted in the World Health Organization (WHO) and European Health Observatory (for example, WHO 1997). This chapter intentionally provides a broad perspective on governance, because to improve midwifery care, midwives need to be politically astute and be aware of quality improvement practices both within and outside midwifery. For the purposes of this chapter, integrated governance, which encompasses both financial and clinical governance, is defined as:

> *'systems, processes and behaviours by which trusts lead, direct and control their functions in order to achieve organisational objectives, safety and quality of service and in which they relate to patients and carers, the wider community and partner organisations'*
>
> (DH 2006:11).

Good governance in healthcare is considered essential by the Council of Europe, which sets standards for health policy and considers the inclusion of ethics and human rights as essential within the framework of good governance (Council of Europe 2009).

## NHS GOVERNANCE SYSTEMS

The governance of maternity care is measured by outcomes for mothers and babies, particularly in relation to morbidity and mortality and, importantly, the satisfaction for women and their families with the service (see Ch. 16). Whilst governance encompasses quality, overall governance is reflected in the outcomes of providing a service that meets the needs of the population it serves and achieved within budgetary systems. Governance includes planning, strategic development, policy and guidance for practice with standards, audit and measurement linked to governmental strategic goals of the healthcare service and for maternity care, being mindful of the ethical nature of care. This includes clinical governance (see website).

## THE NHS

### The NHS management and governance

The UK Health Departments are accountable to Parliament for the management of the public money invested in health and social care (DH 2008a) (see website for further information) and the work includes setting national standards, shaping the direction of the NHS and social care services, and promoting healthier living. Figure

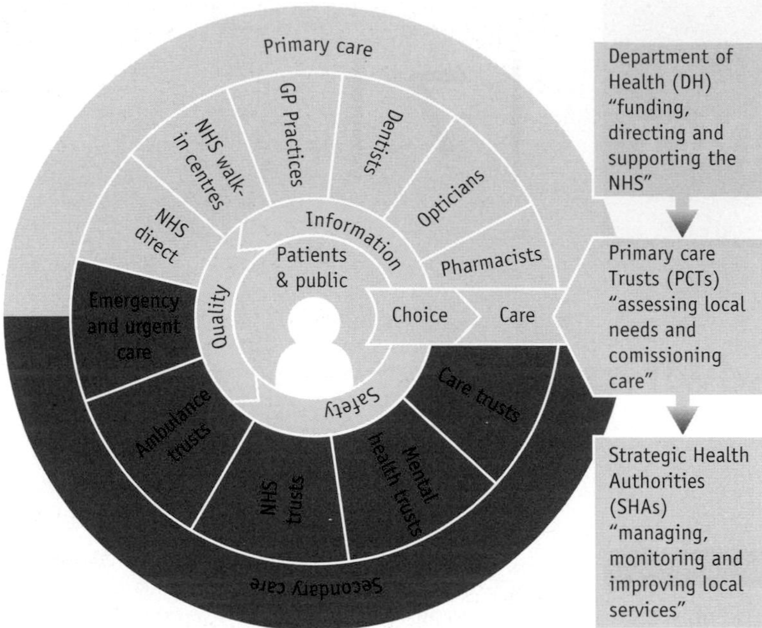


**Figure 7.1** NHS structure. (NHS structures are due to change in 2012/3.) *(Courtesy of NHS Choice website: www.nhs.uk/aboutnhs/howthenhsworks/pages/nhsstructure.aspx. Reproduced with permission.)*

> Box 7.1 **The Quality Framework**
>
> The components of the Quality Framework include:
> - bringing clarity to quality
> - measuring quality
> - publishing on quality
> - rewarding quality
> - raising standards
> - safeguarding quality
> - staying ahead
>
> Summarized from DH 2010a:34

7.1 provides an outline of the different levels and networks of the NHS structure, some of which are referred to in this chapter and website.

The Department of Health outlines the Government's national priorities for the NHS and social care services through the annual publication of an 'Operating framework' (DH 2008b) (see Box 7.1). Each of these components of quality is expanded into activities, for example the NICE guidelines (NICE 2004, 2008), and includes the collaboration of other agencies in the quality of healthcare discussed later in this chapter.

Maternity care is one of the priority areas for the NHS, with an emphasis on normal birth (DH 2010a), particularly in relation to the reduction of health inequalities. Midwives need to be aware of the midwifery-related NHS priorities or Public Service Agreements (PSA), for example 'reduce health inequalities by 10 per cent by 2010', and their relevant measurements, such as 'infant mortality and life expectancy at birth' (DH 2008c:24) as money follows them. Funding and economic management are central to the governance of an institution (see website for Payment by results [PBr] and Ch. 14).

## Strategic health authorities (see website)

The Government's commitment to de-centralize its control of the NHS led to the establishment of the 28 strategic health authorities (SHAs) in 2002. SHAs have acted as the regional headquarters on behalf of the Secretary of State and their number was reduced to 10 in 2006 to deliver stronger commissioning functions. SHAs will be abolished in 2012/3 but in the meantime will lead and provide transition advice (DH 2010d). Key functions of the SHAs were strategic leadership, and organizational and workforce development, ensuring that local health and social care systems operate effectively and deliver improved performance.

## Multi-agency bodies

Multi-agency bodies (MABs) are also termed 'arms' length bodies' (ALBs). These regulate the health and social care

**Box 7.2 A maternity-related priority within the NHS Operating Framework for 2007–08 (DH 2008b)**

Primary Care Trusts do the preparatory work to support the achievement of the Government's commitment that by the end of 2009 there will be a choice for:

- how to access maternity care
- type of antenatal care
- place of birth – depending upon circumstances
- place of postnatal care

Source: DH 2008b:16

system and establish national standards to protect patients and the public and provide central services to the NHS (see website). These are stand-alone bodies that support the Department of Health in its function. These may be classified into the following: Regulatory ALBs, Standard ALBs, Public Welfare ALBs, and Central services to the NHS. The bodies within these MABs/ALBs are given as examples (see website, also for other countries). MAB/ALB-style agencies are an important feature of other major health systems around the world, particularly in relation to regulation for health, such as hospitals and pharmacology. In the UK, MABs operate in three key areas:

- regulating the health and social care system and workforce
- establishing national standards and protecting patients and the public
- providing central services to the NHS (DH 2010b).

They should also contribute and influence their work to enhance care and services for mothers and babies. Therefore, midwives should be aware of these bodies. By being aware of current evidence, research and women's views, midwives can contribute towards policies that affect their practice.

## NHS AND QUALITY

The Department of Health has set out its framework for quality in its 'operating framework' (DH 2010a) (see Box 7.2).

The National Health Service is divided into different areas for care, with the woman and family being central to the services provided. Figure 7.1 reflects the range of services involved that need to work collaboratively with each other and with the woman and her family. Whilst services in midwifery are integrated between primary and secondary care, in other areas of the health service there are two different arrangements for governance of the primary and secondary healthcare services (see website).

**Box 7.3 The National Health Service Constitution: seven key principles**

Seven key principles guide the NHS in all it does:

1. The NHS provides a comprehensive service, available to all.
2. Access to NHS services is based on clinical need, not an individual's ability to pay.
3. The NHS aspires to high standards of excellence and professionalism.
4. NHS services must reflect the needs and preferences of patients, their families and their carers.
5. The NHS works across organizational boundaries and in partnership with other organizations in the interest of patients, local communities and the wider population.
6. The NHS is committed to providing best value for taxpayers' money and the most effective and fair use of finite resources.
7. The NHS is accountable to the public, communities and patients that it serves.

Source: DH 2010c:2,3

**Box 7.4 Rights and pledges for patients covering the seven key areas of the NHS Constitution**

- Rights and pledges for access to health services
- Rights and pledges for quality of care and environment
- Rights and pledges relating to nationally approved treatments, drugs and programmes
- Rights and pledges covering respect, consent and confidentiality
- Rights and pledges for informed choice
- Rights and pledges relating to involvement in your own healthcare and in the NHS
- Rights and pledges for complaint and redress

Source: DH 2009a

Other types of NHS trusts are Acute trusts that may offer tertiary care, which manage hospitals, Ambulance trusts, Care trusts and Mental health trusts (see website). The majority of midwives are employed by either foundation or acute hospital trusts and are bound by their governance systems.

Additionally, the first-ever NHS Constitution has been published, with quality as a central tenet (Boxes 7.3 and 7.4) (DH 2009a, 2010c). The ethos of the NHS Constitution is respect, dignity and compassion, quality care, improving lives, with everyone being valued and working together for patients. The NHS Constitution makes national and local accountability clear by publishing what individuals can expect from the NHS, who is responsible for what, and how decisions about the NHS will be made. The Constitution applies to all those employed within the NHS, but regardless of employment within an organization or being self-employed, all midwives are governed by the rules, standards and codes of the UK regulatory body for nurses and midwives, the Nursing and Midwifery Council (NMC 2008).

**Reflective activity 7.1**

How are respect, dignity and the compassion of care provided to women and their families in your maternity services measured, reported and acted upon?

Sixty years after the NHS was established, the full national Quality Framework will be in place (DH 2009a). The drive for quality healthcare was a founding principle of the NHS. Within the document *High care quality for all,* produced by the Department of Health (2008a), quality was defined as safety, effectiveness and patient experience. From April 2010, NHS care providers will produce annual 'Quality accounts' to provide the public with information on the quality of care they provide (DH 2008a). Along with a statement on the quality of care offered by the provider organization and a description of the priorities for quality improvement, Quality accounts report on locally selected indicators that will cover patient safety, clinical effectiveness and patient experience (DH 2009b). Some indicators for quality improvement (IQI) are published by the NHS Information Centre (2010) and others are being developed under the headings of effectiveness, patient experience and safety. Though there are limited maternity-related indicators to date, they will increase each year and currently include:

- deliveries (births) at home or midwifery unit
- % caesarean deliveries
- unplanned births to hospital (NHS Information Centre 2010).

A limited range of patient-reported outcome measures (PROMs) have been introduced from April 2009 to measure outcomes as assessed by patients themselves (DH 2009c). Whilst not yet applying to midwifery care, PROMs are measures – typically short, self-completed questionnaires – which assess the patients' health status or health-related quality of life at a single point in time, that is, effectiveness of care from the patient's perspective (DH 2009c).

Now for the first time, a National Commissioning Board has been established to bring together all those with an interest in improving quality to align and agree what the quality goals of the NHS should be, whilst respecting the independent status of participating organizations. It will have responsibility for commissioning maternity services (DH 2010d).

## DEVELOPING A VISION AND STRATEGY

In 2008, the strategic health authorities published their 10-year 'visions' for the delivery of regional services within eight care pathways, one of which was for maternity and the newborn. Local NHS organizations are supported by SHAs to implement these 'visions' and midwives and supervisors of midwives will be instrumental in embedding the 'visions' in practice to ensure optimal midwifery care for mothers and babies. The final report of the Next Stage Review (DH 2008a) collated the visions of the 10 SHAs and provided the national picture of quality healthcare services fit for the future (DH 2008a).

The four themes underpinning the vision for the healthcare system are that it is:

- fair
- personalized
- effective
- safe (DH 2008a).

Midwives need to influence the development of a vision for their own service and the measurement methods of the standards that will apply to midwifery care.

(Examples of SHA visions are referred to on the website.)

## QUALITY IN MATERNITY CARE

Quality may be considered in terms of effectiveness, patient focus, timeliness, efficiency and equity. Poor quality, at times, may still be considered safe, but unsafe care can never be considered of good quality (Kings Fund 2008). High-quality care is delivered through clinical effectiveness, risk management, research, effective communication, lifelong learning, supervision and effective leadership, strategic planning and the efficient use of resources. Bevan (2008) supports this integrated approach and, additionally, purports that leadership and human dynamics are the key determinants to successful governance (see Chs 3 and 6). More national tools now focus on improving quality in maternity care. Some are included in Table 7.1 below.

### Clinical governance

Over the last decade, a raft of piecemeal complex governance systems, procedures, reporting frameworks, standards and inspection requirements have been implemented to provide reassurance on financial, safety and service quality

| Table 7.1 National tools to aid quality improvement in maternity services |
|---|
| Focusing on normal birth and reducing LSCS rates tool (NHS Institute for Innovation and Improvement) http://www.institute.nhs.uk/quality_and_value/high_volume_care/focus_on:_caesarean_section.html |
| Implementation of the Productive Ward for maternity (NHS Institute for Innovation and Improvement) http://www.institute.nhs.uk/quality_and_value/productive_ward.html |
| UNICEF's Baby Friendly Initiative (BFI) http://www.babyfriendly.org.uk/ |
| NPSA's Intrapartum Scorecard http://www.nrls.npsa.nhs.uk/resources/?EntryId45=66358 |
| RCOG's Maternity Dashboard http://www.rcog.org.uk/womens-health/clinical-guidance/maternity-dashboard-clinical-performance-and-governance-score-card |
| Heath Innovation and Education Clusters (HIEC) High Impact Actions: Promoting normality (NHS Institute for Innovation and Improvement) http://www.institute.nhs.uk/building_capability/hia_supporting_info/promoting_normal_birth.html |

(DH 2006). Since the 1999 Act (DH 2006) the corporate responsibility for quality and the first use of the term 'clinical governance', the aim of integrated governance has evolved to mainstream clinical governance as an internal planning, decision-making and monitoring activity for Health Boards on a par with money, probity and meeting national targets, with an increased priority on patient safety (DH 2006). Clinical governance is an umbrella under which come evidence-based practice, clinical audit, risk management, education, clinical or statutory supervision of midwives, research and partnership with users working together to continuously improve care. As part of implementing clinical governance, two government-appointed bodies were established to produce standards and guidelines to provide a national framework for standardizing and improving clinical practice – the National Institute for Health and Clinical Excellence (NICE) and National Commissioning Board, a peer and lay body for assessing quality. At the local level, the essence of clinical governance is a partnership between women and professionals. Maternity networks provide an excellent forum for service users; that is, women and their partners to work with healthcare providers and commissioners to enhance multi-professional working, communication and collaboration for a united approach to clinical governance and practice, that are framed by the local guidelines, policies and standards. Although providing guidance, their importance is at the interface of the service between professional groups and women and their families. The responsibility is for midwives, medical staff and other professionals to collaborate to provide a service in which the same standard is met by all professionals caring for women.

Joint statements by professional bodies are aimed to assist professionals to work and collaborate in providing safe and effective care (RCOG RCM 2006, RCM RCOG RCP 2006, RCM RCOG NCT 2007) (see website for examples). Good practice requires that these statements are used by groups of professionals in maternity units to discuss and see where local developments and changes need to be made when determining local policy (see RCM RCOG 2007).

## Policies, guidelines and standards

Each healthcare provider, and therefore every maternity unit, is required to have guidelines, policies and standards for the safe, effective delivery of care (see website). While *National Service Frameworks* (NSF) (DH 2004) are being implemented to introduce national standards for specific services or care groups, such as women, their partners and babies, clinical practice guidelines underpin the national standards. Both must be interpreted locally to provide quality to meet the needs of the geographic and demographic populations: an ideal forum being the maternity networks.

*NICE* provides patients, health professionals and the public with authoritative, robust and reliable guidance on current best practice. For example, it has produced guidelines such as NICE 2004, 2006a&b, 2007a&b, 2008. The Royal College of Obstetricians' evidence-based guidelines, for example RCOG 2008, are also useful. All guidelines and associated standards of practice are required to be based on best evidence. An example of use of evidence and research is given on the website (and see Ch. 5).

Midwives must ensure that they articulate the benefits of the current research and evidence when discussing midwifery care and when services are commissioned; for example, a recently published Cochrane review concluding that evidence of improved outcomes, with no adverse outcomes, indicates that all women should be offered midwife-led models of care, as opposed to medical or shared-care models of care (Hatem et al 2008) (see website).

Guidelines and standards act as performance indicators against which progress is measured within an agreed timescale. Standards are objective assessments against which measurements of effectiveness may be made through the processes of audit.

**Reflective activity 7.2**

What standards are routinely measured in your maternity services?

## Audit

Audit in maternity care has many forms (see website). Audits are undertaken clinically to measure standards of practice against national benchmarks, for example in perinatal and maternal morbidity and mortality statistics (see Ch. 16). Surveys take place to audit patient satisfaction (see website for the national study by Green et al 2003). Each maternity unit should undertake regular satisfaction surveys of all areas of midwifery care to assess women's view of the care they receive and if these achieve the expected standards. These audits will also demonstrate areas for improvement.

Each maternity unit will publish its local statistics and monitor, through the local NHS trust, generic indicators of effectiveness and efficiency of the health service, such as measurements of infection rates, health and safety issues, sickness and absence rates. Maternity indicators of health, such as rates of breastfeeding, midwife-led care, normal births, one-to-one care in labour, reducing anaemia and smoking in pregnancy, provide an indication of the quality of care in a maternity unit. Audit extends to reviews of both qualitative and quantitative measurements. Both measurements can be advised to demonstrate quality of care. Audit of risk factors over a shift and over monthly time-spans are utilised in the NPSA Intrapartum Scorecard and the RCOG Maternity Dashboard. These nationally recommended tools benchmark the acuity and outcomes of maternity units to present contemporary data to act as 'flags' to Trust Boards to ensure that resources provided to maternity units are sufficient to enhance good outcomes.

## Management of risk

Managing risk is a fundamental element of clinical governance. Risk is where there is perceived harm or injury that may occur as a result of care. Managing risk is aimed at preventing and reducing risk that may occur as a result of care which is below an acceptable standard.

Risk management aims to improve the quality of care, prevent occurrences which may harm clients or staff, reduce the risks of adverse events and reduce costs to healthcare providers. The aim of managing risk is to minimize adverse outcomes. This process begins by identifying and assessing risks, such as poor outcomes and 'near-misses', through critical incident reporting which is followed by prompt, open investigation. Why something went (or nearly went) wrong is established, not to apportion blame, but so that processes can be put into place to prevent recurrence. Poor performance is addressed and other lessons learned, with the overall aim of improving care and reducing complaints and litigation.

Whilst the aim is to improve maternal and perinatal outcomes, it is important that the processes do not ignore the individual choices and preferences for care that women may make. The midwife must be clear of her role and accountability in supporting women. In this a midwife needs to keep herself infomed of current developments and evidence and ensure her own education (see Ch. 4).

## When standards are not met – learning from failures ...

In recent years, concerns have been expressed about the quality and safety of some services, including maternity (Healthcare Commission 2008a, Kings Fund 2008). Also, concerns about individual practitioners and institutional management (see website) have led to a review of medicines laws, the White Paper on the self-regulation of healthcare professionals (DH 2007, 2008d), and organizations such as the National Patient Safety Agency, a body with a remit focused primarily on safety.

Poor leadership has been implicated in a number of Healthcare Commission investigations into poor-quality services, including maternity services. The Care Quality Commission is the independent single regulator for health and social care (CQC 2010). It provides validation of provider and commissioner performance, using indicators of quality agreed nationally with the Department of Health. It publishes an assessment of their comparative performance in the annual healthcheck and has made commitments in a 5-year plan to focus more improvement and monitoring work on maternity services (CQC 2010) (see website).

Box 7.5 indicates common themes that occur within the investigatory work of the Healthcare Commission (Healthcare Commission 2008b). The failings reiterate everyone's roles and responsibilities in relation to integrated

**Box 7.5 Common themes within the investigatory work of the Healthcare Commission**

- Deficiencies in Board leadership
- Discontinuity of leadership
- Lack of team-working
- Autocratic management styles restricting organizations' ability to learn from failure
- Inadequate governance and use of data
- Mergers and organizational changes
- Institutional abuse or poor-quality care of the vulnerable
- Poorly performing maternity services
- Poor infection control
- Poor mental health services

Source: Healthcare Commission 2008b

governance, from individual clinicians, to managers, Trust Boards, commissioners, regulators, and strategic health authorities (DH 2009a).

Additionally, it is important to recognize that NHS staff who 'whistle-blow' on aspects of safety, have full protection under the Public Interest Disclosure Act. Employers have a duty to support staff in doing so and midwives have the accountability to do so within their Code (NMC 2010a&b).

Within a maternity unit, failures are identified through the incident review and management procedures, with regular reports and analysis of incidents and near-misses. It is good practice to review regularly good and problem case scenarios in an environment that is without blame, bringing together all multi-professional groups. This should be an educative process, sensitively managed by each profession involved, to ensure that no individual is targeted for fault but rather the systems, and areas for improvement and lessons to be learned to improve collaborative practice are identified.

Defective practice, lack of knowledge and poor communication are commonly found to be causes of avoidable maternal and perinatal mortality and morbidity. Whilst these problems may never be completely eliminated, much can be done to improve care by evidence-based practice which is regularly and rigorously audited and acted upon by addressing deficiencies and 'near-misses' through management or statutory supervision of midwives.

## The role of supervision of midwives

The Kings Fund acknowledge that maternity services have:

> *'a strong tradition of championing safety, of pioneering quality initiatives (such as the drives for woman- or family-centred and evidence-based care) and of using women's views to inform service planning'*
>
> (Kings Fund 2008:14)

The Kings Fund also recognize that supervisors of midwives have a key leadership role in the safety of maternity services and that whilst safe healthcare is often linked with quality, the relationship between safety and quality do get confused. They outline that quality of care critically encompasses safety.

All practising midwives have a named supervisor of midwives to support them in their practice. Midwives would risk breaching their accountability by not upholding their Code if they were complacent within an organization whose governance was not optimal, or if their own practice was not of a high standard (Box 7.6). Statutory supervision of midwives supports midwives in practice to protect mothers and babies. Established as an inspectorial function to lower maternal mortality rates, it has evolved to:

> *'support protection of the public by promoting best practice, preventing poor practice and intervening in unacceptable practice'*
>
> (NMC 2007)

The roles and responsibilities of supervisors are, amongst others, to monitor standards of midwifery practice, contribute towards risk management and clinical audit, investigate critical incidents, and provide leadership which supports and empowers good practice through women-centred evidence-based decision-making (NMC 2007). Working effectively, statutory supervision of midwives contributes significantly towards clinical governance in producing first-class maternity services.

**Box 7.6 Principles of the Nursing and Midwifery Council Code (2008)**

The people in your care must be able to trust you with their health and wellbeing. To justify that trust, you must:

- make the care of people your first concern, treating them as individuals and respecting their dignity
- work with others to protect and promote the health and wellbeing of those in your care, their families and carers, and the wider community
- provide a high standard of practice and care at all times
- be open and honest, act with integrity, and uphold the reputation of your profession

Source: NMC 2008

**Reflective activity 7.3**

What one change to midwifery care could you discuss with your named supervisor of midwives that would have the potential to increase the quality or safety for women and their families?

## FUTURE QUALITY ISSUES

Two reports commissioned by the Department of Health explored the future funding issues faced by the NHS (Wanless 2002, 2004). The reports articulate resources required for the NHS to cope with increasing expectations, an ageing population, a rise in lifestyle disease, and the

**Table 7.2 The Institute for Health Care Improvement (IHI ) ten rules**

| The old rules | The new rules |
|---|---|
| Care is based on visits | Care is based on continuous healing relationships |
| Professional autonomy drives variability | Care is customized according to patient needs and values |
| Professionals control care | The patient is the source of control |
| Information is a record | Knowledge is shared and information flows freely |
| Decision-making is based on training and experience | Decision-making is evidence-based |
| Do no harm is an individual responsibility | Safety is a system property |
| Secrecy is necessary | Transparency is necessary |
| The system reacts to needs | Needs are anticipated |
| Cost reduction is sought | Waste is continuously decreased |
| Preference is given to professional roles over the system | Cooperation among clinicians is a priority |

Source: IHI 2008

cost of new treatments and technologies (DH 2008a). The Institute for Healthcare Improvement (IHI), an independent non-profit organization working to improve healthcare throughout the world, argues that 21st century healthcare should adopt new 'rules' (Table 7.2). Its ethos of *'all teach, all learn'* brings together committed individuals and organizations, recognizing that more healthcare improvements can be achieved collectively than individually (IHI 2008).

The latest Operating Framework (DH 2010a) makes moral and financial arguments for optimizing the health of newborn babies to reduce the demand for neonatal care, thereby realizing health, wellbeing and cost benefits in the future. It recommends tools now available to support the NHS in improving maternity and neonatal services (see website). This will be even more challenging as the transition towards structural reforms occurs which highlights the important roles of midwives in driving the quality within maternity services (DH 2010e, DH 2010f).

## WHAT GOVERNANCE MEANS FOR MIDWIVES

Midwives need to be innovative, to build on existing structures and processes and develop new ones in order to embed excellent practice. It is vital to have midwifery representation in the decision-making processes involving procurement of systems and to ensure that systems are flexible enough to introduce developments which can improve care and be audited easily (preferably by a clinician) to monitor standards of care. Midwives also need to be aware of and act upon the views of women and families regarding the maternity services. Midwives need to be knowledgeable and adapt their care for and argue on behalf of women for the care required within the local community.

Computers are increasingly being used to store clinical data, replacing paper-based records and documentation. Electronic materials such as antenatal bookings can be utlized for clinical audit and financial purposes – for example, data for Payment by Results processes. Midwives need to seize opportunities to use these systems to improve care. Flexible clinical computer systems lend themselves extremely well to incorporating prompts and audit tools which appear on screen under specific conditions, taking little time to complete and, with appropriate software, being easy to audit. Successful innovations in this and other areas should be shared through publication, conferences, and other local and national forums.

In all areas of governance, ethical considerations are paramount, as maternity care involves people (women, babies and families) and harm may arise when any system of governance changes unless consideration is given to the outcomes of this change (Walsh 2003). Ethical issues will continue to challenge midwives as economic constraints change the way we practise and new developments, such as advanced and comprehensive screening tests, become ever-more sophisticated.

Whilst midwives will focus on the care of women, this should not be only on the narrow issues of providing individualized, quality care to women, babies and their families. Midwives do not practise in a vacuum but in a local context, with their peers, obstetricians, paediatricians, anaesthetists, GPs and paramedical staff. They need to be aware of their contribution to wider public health issues that impinge upon maternity care, such as mental health, social inequality, or disability care. Over the last few years, midwives have at times retreated into their world of midwifery and have sometimes minimized or even dismissed the contribution of their professional colleagues. Midwives need to contribute meaningfully to multidisciplinary policies, protocols and guidelines in order to improve standards of care and universalize good practice, whilst retaining their unique and distinctive role.

Midwives have an important part to play and their impact should not be underestimated. Reducing smoking in pregnancy, cot death, teenage conceptions; promoting breastfeeding, healthy diet, parentcraft education; and meeting the needs of socially deprived women are just some of the issues on which midwives can and do have enormous influence, not only on women, but also on their partners, families and beyond. Auditing and monitoring these areas may contribute to wider public health knowledge. Nationally, midwives need to be at the forefront of policy-making processes around maternity care, such as contributing to Midwifery 2020 (NHS et al 2009). At a national level, midwives should grasp opportunities to work more closely on policy.

## CONCLUSION

Quality of care in midwifery is that which demonstrates competent caring, tailored to individual women. It aims to involve the woman and her family so that she experiences as positive and safe and normal a pregnancy, delivery and puerperium as possible. The midwife whose practice is woman centred and evidence based, working cooperatively with her peers in her local situation and being aware of her unique role and contribution in the wider context of society, is ideally placed to have an impact on both the short-term and long-term health and wellbeing of mothers, babies and their families.

## KEY POINTS

- All midwives should recognize the importance of governance in the NHS and the relevance of midwifery leadership in ensuring quality, innovation, productivity and prevention in managing the maternity services.
- Midwives need to be politically astute and recognize that their contributions are essential in formulating plans and policies for maternity care.
- Developing strategic plans and a vision for maternity care, together with policies, protocols, guidelines and standards, requires multi-professional collaboration to ensure safe teamworking and to provide an environment that supports women's choices.
- The development of quality in midwifery is a responsiblity of each midwife and within their communications with other staff and women. It is enhanced by their personal reflective practice to improve outcomes and care for women.
- Clinical governance is a framework which midwives can use to continuously improve the quality of their care through clinical audit and other processes such as risk management, professional regulation, education, research and statutory supervision of midwives.
- Care for women should ensure equity, ethical principles and the rights of individuals to participate in their care.

## REFERENCES


Bevan H: Foreword. In Broaden R, Harvey G, Moxham C, et al, editors: *Quality improvement: theory and practice in healthcare*, Coventry, 2008, NHS Institute for Innovation and Improvement.

Care Quality Commission (CQC): *Position statement and action plan for children, young people and maternity services* (website). www.cqc.org.uk/aboutcqc/whatwedo.cfm. 2010.

Council of Europe: *Good governance in health care* (website). www.coe.int/t/dg3/health/goodgov_en.asp. 2009.

Department of Health (DH): *Maternity module of the NSF for children, young people and maternity services* (website). www.dh.gov.uk/en/publicationsandstatistics/. 2004.

Department of Health (DH): Integrated governance handbook. A handbook for executives and non-executives in healthcare organizations (website). www.dh.gov.uk/prod_consum_dh/groups/dh_digitalassets/@dh/@en/documents/digitalasset/dh_4129615.pdf. 2006.

Department of Health (DH): *White Paper. Trust, assurance and safety: the regulation of health professionals in the 21st century*, London, 2007, The Stationery Office.

Department of Health (DH): *High quality care for all. NHS Next Stage Review final report* (website). www.dh.gov.uk/prod_consum_dh/groups/dh_digitalassets/@dh/@en/documents/digitalasset/dh_085828.pdf. 2008a.

Department of Health (DH): *High quality care for all. The operating framework 2009–10. High quality care throughout the NHS* (website). www.lp-publicservices.org.uk/News.aspx?title=NHS%20Operating%20Framework%202009-10&ID=36. 2008b.

Department of Health (DH): *Department of Health: Departmental Report 2008* (website). www.dh.gov.uk/en/Publicationsandstatistics/Publications/AnnualReports/DH_084908. 2008c.

Department of Health (DH): *The future regulation of health and adult social care in England*, London, 2008d, DH.

Department of Health (DH): *NHS 2010–2015: from good to great. Preventative, people-centred, productive* (website). www.dh.gov.uk/prod_consum_dh/groups/dh_digitalassets/@dh/@en/@ps/@sta/@perf/documents/digitalasset/dh_109887.pdf. 2009a.

Department of Health (DH): *The NHS performance framework: implementation guidance* (website). www.dh.gov.uk/prod_consum_dh/groups/dh_digitalassets/documents/digitalasset/dh_098526.pdf. 2009b. Accessed May 2010.

Department of Health (DH): *Guidance on the routine collection of Patient Reported Outcome Measures (PROMs)* (website). www.dh.gov.uk/en/Publicationsandstatistics/Publications/PublicationsPolicyAndGuidance/DH_092647. 2009c. Accessed June 2009.

Department of Health (DH): *The operating framework for the NHS in England 2010–2011* (website). www.dh.gov.uk/prod_consum_dh/groups/dh_digitalassets/@dh/@en/@ps/@sta/@perf/documents/digitalasset/dh_110159.pdf. 2010a. Accessed May 2010.

Department of Health (DH): Arms length bodies webpage on DH website. www.dh.gov.uk/en/Aboutus/OrganisationsthatworkwithDH/Armslengthbodies/index.htm. 2010b. Accessed April 2010.

Department of Health (DH): *The NHS Constitution: the NHS belongs to us all* (website). www.dh.gov.uk/prod_consum_dh/groups/dh_digitalassets/@dh/@en/@ps/documents/digitalasset/dh_113645.pdf. 2010c. Accessed May 2010.

Department of Health (DH): *Equity and excellence: liberating the NHS*, London, 2010d, DH.

Department of Health (DH): *Frontline care: the future of nursing and midwifery in England. Prime Ministers Commission for England*, London, 2010e, DH.

Department of Health (DH): *Midwifery 2020: delivering expectations*, London, 2010f, DH. www.midwifery2020.org

Green J, Baston H, Easton S, et al: *Greater expectations? Summary report* (website). www.york.ac.uk/healthsciences/miru/greaterexpdf.pdf. 2003.

Hatem M, Sandall J, Devane D, et al: Midwife-led versus other models of care for childbearing women, *Cochrane Database of Systematic Reviews* 2008;(4)CD004667, 2008.

Healthcare Commission: *Learning from investigations*, London, 2008a, Commission for Healthcare Audit and Inspection.

Healthcare Commission: *Towards better births – a review of maternity services in England*, London, 2008b, Healthcare Commission.

Institute for Healthcare Improvement (IHI): *Quality rules* (website). www.IHI.org. 2008.

Kings Fund: *Safe births: everybody's business* (website). www.kingsfund.org.uk/publications. 2008.

National Health Service (NHS), Northern Ireland Health Service (HSC), NHS Scotland, NHS Wales (GIG): *Midwifery 2020* (website). www.midwifery2020.org/. 2009.

NHS Choices website: www.nhs.uk/NHSEngland/thenhs/about/Pages/nhsstructure.aspx. Accessed April 2010.

NHS Information Centre website: https://www.mqi.ic.nhs.uk/. Accessed May 2010.

National Institute for Health and Clinical Excellence (NICE): *Caesarean section*, London, 2004, NICE.

National Institute for Health and Clinical Excellence (NICE): *Postnatal care: routine postnatal care of women and their babies*, London, 2006a, NICE.

National Institute for Health and Clinical Excellence (NICE): *Postnatal care: routine postnatal care of women and their babies*, London, 2006b, NICE.

National Institute for Health and Clinical Excellence (NICE): *Antenatal and postnatal mental health: clinical management and service guidance*, London, 2007a, NICE.

National Institute for Health and Clinical Excellence (NICE): *Intrapartum care: care of healthy women and their babies during birth*, London, 2007b, NICE.

National Institute for Health and Clinical Excellence (NICE): *Antenatal care: routine care for the healthy pregnant woman*, London, 2008, NICE.

Nursing and Midwifery Council (NMC): *Standards for the supervised practice of midwives*, London, 2007, NMC.

Nursing and Midwifery Council (NMC): *The code: standards of conduct, performance and ethics for nurses and midwives*, London, 2008, NMC.

Nursing and Midwifery Council (NMC): *Advice and information for employers of nurses and midwives* (website). www.nmc-uk.org. 2010a.

Nursing and Midwifery Council (NMC): *Raising and escalating concerns: guidance for nurses and midwives*, London, 2101b, NMC.

Royal College of Midwives (RCM), Royal College of Obstetricians and Gynaecologists (RCOG): *Home births – Joint statement* (website). www.rcog.org.uk/index.asp?PageID=81. 2007.

Royal College of Midwives (RCM), Royal College of Obstetricians and Gynaecologists (RCOG), National Childbirth Trust (NCT): *Making normal birth a reality: consensus statement from the Maternity Care Working Party* (website). www.rcog.org.uk/index.asp?PageID=81. 2007.

Royal College of Midwives (RCM), Royal College of Obstetricians and Gynaecologists (RCOG), Royal College of Physicians (RCP): *Training and maintenance of skills for professionals responsible for resuscitation of babies at birth – Joint statement* (website). www.rcog.org.uk/index.asp?PageID=81. 2006.

Royal College of Obstetricians and Gynaecologists (RCOG): *Guidelines for induction of labour: national evidence-based guidelines*, London, 2008, RCOG.

Royal College of Obstetricians and Gynaecologists (RCOG), Royal College of Midwives (RCM): *Immersion in water during labour and birth – Joint statement No. 1* (website). www.rcog.org.uk/index.asp?PageID=81. 2006.

Walsh D: Birth as a risky behaviour: reflections on risk management, *MIDIRS Midwifery Digest* 13(4):545–549, 2003.

Wanless D: *Securing our future health: taking a long-term view*, London, 2002, The Stationery Office.

Wanless D: *Securing good health for the whole population: final report*, London, 2004, The Stationery Office.

World Health Organization (WHO): *Health system governance for improving health system performance: report of the WHO Global Consultation, Cairo Egypt, 7–9 November 2007* (website). gis.emro.who.int/HealthSystemObservatory/PDF/Publications/Reports%20of%20Workshops%20and%20Meetings/PHP043healthsystemgovernancefinal.pd. 1997.

Chapter | 8 |

# Ethics and midwifery practice

*Shirley R. Jones*

## LEARNING OUTCOMES

At the end of this chapter, the reader should be:

- aware of the difference between morality and ethics
- aware of the three areas of ethics and their applicability to practice
- able to recognize the importance of ethics in midwifery practice
- familiar with the difference between moral conflicts and dilemmas
- able to distinguish between the various normative ethical theories and their tenets
- able to apply certain pluralist duties within the duty of care
- able to recognize the need to uphold the principle of women's autonomy in practice
- able to reflect on the ethical aspects of their practice
- able to follow up on principles and issues by further reading.

Ethics is now recognized as a major part of both midwifery education and practice; it permeates all professional relationships. Many childbearing women are no longer willing to be passive recipients of care; they expect to be fully informed of all aspects of their care so that they, rather than the professionals, make informed decisions, thereby retaining their autonomy and control. Knowledge of ethics will enable midwives to have a clear understanding of issues related to their practice and, in particular, of their role in empowering women to achieve a pleasurable, fulfilling experience of childbirth.

## WHAT IS ETHICS?

Ethics is basically moral philosophy, or at least the vehicle by which we transport moral philosophy into practical, everyday situations. There is a tendency to consider 'moral' to be related to matters of sexuality; however, here it relates to the 'rights and wrongs' or the 'oughts and ought nots' of any situation. There are three levels to ethics:

1. *Meta-ethics* involves the deeper philosophy of examining everything in abstract; for instance, what we mean by 'right' and 'wrong'. In everyday situations, we do not have time for this level of consideration.
2. *Ethical theory* aims to create mechanisms for problem solving, much as mathematicians created formulae for solving problems related to their field. Whether such theories are of use to midwives will be discussed later.
3. *Practical ethics*, as the term suggests, is the active part where the work of the moral philosophers is put into practice. It is also the area on which this chapter will generally concentrate.

In everyday life, morality underpins our actions; particularly those that involve other people and their possessions. It is translated into our thoughts and actions by principles and concepts that we have learned since early childhood, such as truth telling. This clearly should start within the family but there are outside influences: educational and religious institutions, the media and peer groups. This is not to say that all adults will behave within a given moral code. As is all too obvious, there are those who never receive the principles and concepts in the first place and others who choose to take a different path. However, these individuals will still be judged according to the code which is generally accepted by society at the time of the incident, and which underpins our civil law. Everyone has the right to expect that moral principles will be upheld; these, therefore, become 'moral rights'. As professionals in healthcare, it is important that midwives have a deeper understanding of morality than do members of the public. This depth of understanding is achieved by education regarding relevant moral principles, concepts and theories; by analysing real-life situations and posed dilemmas; by evaluation of the actions of ourselves and others. In this way, we move from morality into ethics.

There are numerous principles, concepts and doctrines, some of which are listed here. Further reading in relation to these principles, concepts and doctrines is suggested, sources for which are included at the end of this chapter, as they cannot all be discussed in depth here. However, autonomy will be discussed later in the chapter.

- Accountability
- Beneficence
- Non-maleficence
- Confidentiality
- Justice
- Autonomy
- Paternalism
- Consent
- Value of life
- Quality of life
- Sanctity of life
- Status of the fetus
- Acts and omissions
- Killing or letting die
- Ordinary or extraordinary means
- Double effect
- Truth telling.

## WHY IS ETHICS IMPORTANT IN MIDWIFERY?

Women do not surrender their moral rights once they seek care; these rights have to be observed within their new experience, in any setting. In midwifery, care is very intimate – from the handling of personal information through the spectrum of physical, psychological, social and educational care. Added to this there is another dimension: there is no other field of human care where there is one person at the first point of contact and more than one at the end (obstetrics is considered with midwifery here). This transition itself is the source of great complexity when decisions have to be made. An understanding of ethics not only will assist the carer to make decisions, it will also help with the empowerment of the woman to make informed decisions and assist the carer in understanding the basis of those decisions. There are ethical issues (i.e. debate or concern regarding the right and wrong actions) in all areas of midwifery. It is fairly easy to construct a list of the various areas from preconception care, through fertility and screening issues, to the end of the puerperium. Most people's lists would consist mainly of the highly emotive areas, which gain media coverage, but there are many issues involved in the care of 'normal' pregnancy, labour, puerperium and the neonatal period. Where there are ethical issues, there is the potential for conflicts and dilemmas to occur.

### Moral conflict

A moral conflict could be considered to be a show of strength within a moral principle, for instance the autonomy of the woman versus that of the midwife or, more commonly, the autonomy of two or more professionals. A conflict could also arise between two or more different principles. On closer examination of the conflict, one side becomes a clear winner. Consider the following case.

**Reflective activity 8.1**

On immediate visual examination, a neonate is thought to have Down syndrome and the mother's first question is: 'Is he alright?' Should the midwife protect the mother (non-maleficence) by answering 'yes', on the grounds that the Apgar scores were good and chromosome studies need to be performed for confirmation? Alternatively, should the midwife tell the truth and explain that tests are required to confirm the suspicion?

Ethically, telling the truth wins. The mother has the right to know, especially as a positive test will indicate to her that she was initially deceived and this could affect her ability to trust the midwives, or other healthcare professionals, in future encounters. Added to which, the mother's permission should be sought regarding tests to be performed on her baby; she cannot consent unless she has the information. It is hoped that the reader can see, from this example, that a conflict is logical in resolution once thought through properly. It is also acknowledged that in some units, in circumstances similar to this example, not all practitioners take this particular action; they obviously find that their clear solution is to protect the mother.

### Moral dilemma

When examination of an apparent conflict between principles indicates two or more options, none of which is morally ideal, then this is a dilemma, such as the following case.

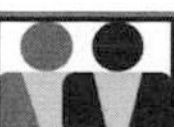

**Case scenario 8.1**

A primiparous woman is admitted in established labour. She has a birth plan which states that under no circumstances will she give consent to an episiotomy. During the second stage of labour, progress is slow but positive; however, the perineum remains thick and rigid. The situation is explained to the woman but she maintains her position regarding episiotomy. As time progresses, the fetal heart shows signs of slight distress, to the point where most midwives would consider episiotomy to be the action of choice, but still the woman withholds consent. The midwife could either continue, hoping that the fetus will survive (obviously notifying appropriate personnel), or she could perform the procedure without consent, in order to protect the fetus. If she carries out the episiotomy without consent, she could face a claim of battery against her. Neither is the ideal solution. (Jones 2000)

*The Code: Standards of conduct, performance and ethics for nurses and midwives* (NMC 2008:4) states that you must 'make the care of [women] your first concern, treating them as individuals and respecting their dignity.' What the woman feels is in her best interests may not correspond with the midwife's view; it could be considered detrimental to the woman's condition, or that of her fetus. However, where at one time paternalism was virtually encouraged, The Code now states: 'You must respect and support people's rights to accept or decline treatment and care' (NMC 2008:4).

## HOW ARE DILEMMAS SOLVED?

This is where level two of ethics is required – ethical theory. There are possibly nearly as many theories as there are philosophers, as they will all have their own particular stance, but generally speaking their views fit broadly into major theories. Two such theories of normative ethics, at either end of the spectrum, are utilitarianism and deontology.

### Utilitarianism

Utilitarianism is a consequentialist theory, where possible actions are considered in terms of their probable consequences. The original aim was for all actions to create the greatest happiness for the greatest number of people. Current thinking would probably use the term benefit rather than happiness, which would describe the essential outlook of those managing the National Health Service (NHS). It would also describe the intentions of Hitler in the Second World War, with his views of improving the human race, as, unfortunately, a belief within this theory is 'the end justifies the means'.

There are two forms of the theory: act-utilitarianism and rule-utilitarianism. The first is the purer form, developed in the 18$^{th}$ and 19$^{th}$ centuries by Bentham, Mill and Sidgwick, which expects every potential action to be assessed according to its predicted outcomes in terms of benefit. The second form does not look directly at the actual benefit of each act, rather it considers moral rules which are intended to ensure the greatest benefit, and each act is assessed as to its conformity to the rules.

Using in-vitro fertilization (IVF) as an example, a technique initially researched in the concentration camps of the Second World War, it can be shown how these two schools of thought differ. Act-utilitarians would view the actions taken in light of the anticipated outcomes: many people today benefit from IVF, therefore, they may believe that this beneficial consequence justifies the research methods used. Rule-utilitarians, however, would want the benefit but would consider whether society would accept the means by which it was achieved. It is likely that they would want to find a more acceptable method of achieving the outcome.

### Deontology

Deontology is a duty-based theory. Consequences are not considered, as deontologists believe that what is good in the world is brought about by people doing their duty. This theory divides into three schools of thought, each competing with the others as well as with utilitarianism. A well-known name in philosophy is Immanuel Kant. He developed rational monism which he believed was how people already thought – that one's actions should be rational and stem from 'good will'; he believed in duty for its own sake – the 'categorical imperative'. He used two tests for the moral value of an action. The first was whether it would be suitable if universalized, i.e. if everyone was to do it. The second test involved whether the act would use anybody as a means to an end, which would not be acceptable, or as an end in himself, which would be acceptable as this is the basis of autonomy, which was paramount. For instance, in a healthcare research project, is the research to benefit the individual (i.e. treating him as an end in himself), or to benefit others – e.g. treatment of future patients; achievement of academic acclaim for the researcher; making a profit for a company (i.e. in each case, a means to someone else's end)?

The second school is *traditional deontology*; this is firmly seated in a belief in God and the sanctity of life. Each religion has its own model for behaviour; for instance, Christians have the Ten Commandments. With this system there is little room for conflict as it is possible to carry out all the commands at one time.

The third form is *intuitionistic pluralism*, where it is believed that there are a number of moral rules which are of equal importance; unfortunately, the possibility of rule conflict exists. To minimize this, Ross considered seven *prima facie* duties which he felt were reasonable for people to abide by:

1. Duty of fidelity – involves keeping promises, being loyal and not deceiving.
2. Duty of beneficence – the obligation to help others.
3. Duty of non-maleficence – not harming others; which is more stringent than the previous duty.
4. Duty of justice – to ensure fair play.
5. Duty of reparation – an obligation to make amends.
6. Duty of gratitude – to repay in some way those who have helped us (owed to special people such as parents), also including loyalty.
7. Duty of self-improvement.

(Jones 2000:22)

As these duties are equal in importance, it is still possible for conflict to arise between them. However, there is a system which can assist in such a conflict – *casuistry*; this system allows for the duties to be prioritized according to the circumstances.

Readers have probably already identified that, although the NHS is generally essentially utilitarian, midwifery, medicine and other similar disciplines tend towards a deontological approach. In fact, the duty with which we are most familiar – the duty of care – would appear to encompass at least the first four of the above duties. This deontological approach is certainly apparent in the text of The Code (NMC 2008).

To assist understanding of the different focus of utilitarianism and deontology when faced with a dilemma, the following non-midwifery story is offered; readers are invited to determine the end:

**Reflective activity 8.2**

Jim is a botanist on expedition in South America. He finds himself in a small town where 20 Indians are lined up ready for execution, following acts of protest against the government. The captain, Pedro, having explained the situation, offers Jim a guest's privilege of killing one of the Indians himself. If he accepts, as a special mark of the occasion, the other Indians will be freed. If he refuses, then there is no special occasion and Pedro will have them all killed as previously planned. (Smart & Williams 1988:98–99)

*You are Jim – what will you do?*

If you are utilitarian, then your decision would be to shoot one (which one is another problem), thus saving the other 19 as a consequence. As a deontologist, however, you would feel a duty 'not to harm' each man; nor would you don a mantle of responsibility and guilt for Pedro's actions.

As midwives, whatever our personal leanings may be, we may be professionally schizophrenic with regard to our ethical actions. Consider the midwife in the next scenario.

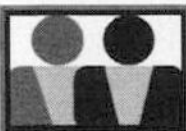

**Case scenario 8.2**

Anita, a midwife, was allocated to a group of women on the ward carrying out her 'duty of care' for each woman in accordance with her 'Responsibility and sphere of practice' (NMC 2004, Rule 6): this approach would be basically deontological, fulfilling duties to each individual.

However, on the next day her remit in managing the overall care of all the women on the ward was to ensure the greatest benefit for the greatest number – both women and staff – by making decisions for the good of the ward as a whole. While clinicians at the bedside, or in people's homes, can be deontological in their approach, the further up the management line that is considered, the more it becomes obvious that a utilitarian approach is essential. It would not be acceptable to society, for instance, if the NHS purse were to be emptied by caring for a few; the limited resources are expected to do as much as possible for as many as possible.

It must be remembered, however, that most people have to deal with conflicts and dilemmas in their lives without knowledge of these theories. However, whether we wish to embrace formal or informal approaches, it is important for healthcare professionals to know something about each of them, if only to understand how and why some decisions are made. It is also useful to have some idea of the approach which managers or clinicians might take when proposals for implementing schemes or changes are being made.

**Reflective activity 8.3**

Consider the tragic situation of the conjoined twins known as Mary and Jodie (Jones & Jenkins 2003); there surely could be no greater professional dilemma for medical and legal practitioners than presented in this case. Analyse the situation through the different philosophical (not legal) viewpoints and determine the decisions which each school might have made.

If you had been a student or qualified midwife assisting in the care of Mary and Jodie, you might have been involved in a case conference. What view would you have put forward and what ethical justification would you have given?

## THE DUTY OF CARE

As health professionals, midwives have a duty of care to those persons who could be affected by their actions or omissions. In midwifery, it is important to note that 'persons' relates directly to the mother and neonate. (Legally, the fetus is not yet a 'person': readers may wish to pursue the subjects of 'personhood' and 'potential', see Harris in 'Further reading'.) This duty of care would include at least the first four deontological duties listed earlier; failure in the duty of care would result in a civil law case for negligence.

### The duty of fidelity

The duty of fidelity requires us to avoid deceiving women and their families, this suggests, therefore, that promises should not be made if they cannot be kept and that truth telling is paramount. An example used earlier, to illustrate a moral conflict, involved a baby with suspected Down syndrome. If the practitioners involved were to withhold the truth from the mother, then they would be failing in their duty of fidelity, however good their motives might be. Anecdotal reports by students and qualified midwives suggest that this deception does occur sometimes, in the paternalistic belief that the mother is being protected.

### The duty of beneficence

The duty of beneficence creates the obligation to help women. This is a positive duty which covers numerous activities, ranging from the various ways of helping to make them comfortable, to the educational aspects of caring for their babies. What this duty does not include is the paternalistic attitude so often experienced within the health service, where practitioners feel that they 'know what is best'. This attitude, although generally well meant, deprives the woman of her right to self-determination (autonomy).

### The duty of non-maleficence

The duty of non-maleficence is a negative duty – to do no harm. On the surface, this would suggest that conducting unpleasant or painful procedures may breach this duty; this would be the case if the intention was to hurt the woman. If the intention is to eventually benefit her and, knowing that she might experience pain or discomfort, she is in agreement, then there is no breach in duty. Administration of analgesic injections, the siting of an epidural analgesic or urinary catheterization would come into this category. This duty, although negative in its statement, can have a positive aspect: that of safety and protection from harm. This includes, among other things, consideration of the environment, observance of drug policies, and adequate education and training of practitioners.

### The duty of justice

The duty of justice requires us to treat women equally, without discrimination. For many people, the word 'discrimination' is immediately associated with terms such as race, skin colour or ethnic origin. While it is essential that we consider these areas, it is also important that we are aware of the other forms of discrimination that can occur, such as between articulate and less articulate women. It is often easier to spend more time with the articulate women, giving as much information and as much choice as possible, than it is with those who require greater explanations or who ask fewer questions. It could be argued that, to consider equality, we should aim to get all women to the same endpoint; this would then necessitate that more time be spent with the less articulate women.

## PRINCIPLES

Knowledge of the underlying moral principles is important, if only to ensure that practitioners are 'talking the same language'. It is not possible, in one short chapter, to consider each of the major principles. However, in the author's opinion, one of the most basic moral principles is that of autonomy, since an understanding and observance of this principle should automatically lead professionals into the understanding and observance of many other principles.

### Autonomy

Autonomy involves self-direction and self-control of one's actions and destiny. It could be argued that it is impossible to be totally autonomous, as society imposes certain rules, often sitting in judgement on the actions of individuals. However, there is a broad band of acceptability in most areas of life, at least in democratic societies, which gives individuals varying degrees of freedom of choice. What is expected of individuals is that their actions and decisions should be rational, i.e. based on sound reasoning. These decisions should then be accepted, whether or not they match the views of others, such as midwives and doctors.

For childbearing women to make rational decisions about their care, the carers must ensure that sufficient information is given at the level and pace required by the individual. Many factors need to be considered. The *environment* should be conducive to the giving and receiving of information. The *language* that is being used should be in the 'mother tongue' of the woman, with the avoidance of jargon and abbreviations. The *circumstances* in which a decision is required may vary – for example, whether there is time for contemplation or whether a fairly urgent situation is faced. Having given the information, it is also important for professionals to assess the woman's understanding of it. These points are of particular importance where midwives are caring for disadvantaged women, such as refugees, asylum seekers and others who enter the country with language or customs incompatibility with British maternity services.

Having determined that a woman has made an informed decision based on what she thinks is sound reasoning, i.e. an autonomous decision, health professionals have no right to overrule that decision (Mental Capacity Act 2005). This principle is inextricably bound to informed consent: if the woman is autonomous, then nothing should be done to her without her prior consent; to do so would be to commit a trespass against the person, i.e. battery (Jones 2000). If her consent is being sought, then she is being considered to be autonomous; therefore, a situation should not arise where, on her refusal to consent to a procedure, professionals attempt to overrule her. There are two groups of people who might be deemed to be not autonomous, therefore unable to give consent. One group includes children, but there is no longer a set age, it depends on the circumstances and degree of rationality of the child (Children Acts 1989 & 2004). The other group includes those who are mentally incapacitated, either by disability or by severe mental illness. With both groups, consent by proxy would be sought. There is also the possibility of temporary mental incompetence, in cases of unconsciousness or possibly the effects of substances. In such cases, the professionals would be expected to act out of necessity, in the best interest of the woman, unless there was sound evidence that the woman would refuse consent if aware of the situation, such as a Jehovah's Witness carrying a card refusing blood products.

The Mental Capacity Act 2005 applies to all healthcare professionals and, from a midwifery perspective, it places into primary law (statute) the position arrived at following decisions made in civil law, in the 1980s/90s, with regard to certain 'enforced caesarean section' cases. Therefore, in both statutory and civil law, it is illegal to enforce any care or treatment on a childbearing woman, even for the sake of the fetus, if she is autonomous and her decision is fully informed. Only diagnosis of mental incapacity, by a psychiatrist, can overrule her decisions and, even then, only treatment that is in her best interests, not those of her fetus or her family, can be undertaken. This principle applies also to young women under 16, except where refusal of treatment could result in her death. Statements in the current edition of The Code (NMC 2008) are in line with this Act. It is important that all midwives familiarize themselves with this Act, particularly the following short sections, the last of which would cover 'living wills' and birth plans:

- The principles
- People who lack capacity
- Inability to make decisions
- Best interests
- Acts in connection with care or treatment
- Acts: limitations
- Advance decisions to refuse treatment: general
- Validity and applicability of advance decisions
- Effect of advance decisions.

It is the author's firm belief that, if women's autonomy were truly considered, then it would be unlikely that the varying aspects of the duty of care would be breached. This would not remove situations of conflict and dilemma, but it would make decision making more straightforward, with all practitioners working to the same ground rules.

The use of reflective practice would assist in this area, by midwives analysing and reflecting upon their actions, particularly with regard to their observance of autonomy, then using this experience to formulate their plans for future decision making.

**Reflective activity 8.4 Client autonomy**

At the end of a shift, consider the clients for whom you cared. In each case consider:

- Which aspects of her care did you discuss with her?
- Which aspects of her care did you not discuss with her?
- What information did you give her?
- What decisions did she make?
- What decisions did you make?
- Did you accept her decisions or did you try to change them?
- What did you write in the records?
- Did you enable her to be autonomous?
- In light of this exercise, what will you do in similar circumstances in future?

Women's autonomy is a relatively new concept. The autonomy of the midwife, however, is not new. Midwives have used the term 'autonomous practitioner' for many years, particularly when trying to explain to the uninitiated the difference between nurses and midwives. Unfortunately, however, this autonomy is not always evident in practice, particularly in the hospital setting. Midwives often plead that they are constrained by the policies within which they are expected to work. This pleading suggests that, either the policies are too constrictive for both the midwife and the woman, and should be addressed, or that some midwives are comfortably hiding behind them. In a survey carried out by the Healthcare Commission in England in 2007, 67% of women said that they were involved in antenatal decision making, with 70% saying that they were involved in decisions during labour and birth. These figures seem very positive, until one considers the plight of the 33% and 30% respectively who felt that they were not always involved.

**Reflective activity 8.5 Midwife autonomy**

Consider your last working week. How many times did you do the following:

- inform a client that the proposed course of action was 'policy'?
- discuss the relevant policy with the client but include the alternatives?
- politely challenge a colleague's (any discipline) decision or course of action because it was not evidence-based?
- notify your manager or supervisor of midwives that a policy needs to be reviewed?
- make a decision based on the circumstances, not on the policy, then **inform** the appropriate person (midwife-in-charge, registrar, consultant) rather than **ask** them?
- assertively justify a decision in relevant documentation, as opposed to wording suggestive of 'covering your back'?

On reflection, given the same circumstances in the future, which of these actions would you change?

## CONCLUSION

This chapter is intended to help readers to accept the need for awareness of moral rights along with the will of individual practitioners to uphold them. An understanding of ethics will help midwives to make decisions in difficult circumstances, even if they do not choose directly to follow the theories outlined. The author firmly believes that observance of ethical principles, especially autonomy, is the most direct route to assisting childbearing women to have the degree of choice and control that each individual feels is right for her. It is possible that the woman who achieves control in childbearing is better placed to do so in the parenting years ahead of her. By practising in this way, the midwife will also be fulfilling personal, professional accountability.

**KEY POINTS**

- Ethics is essential to professional midwifery practice.
- There are numerous ethical principles with which midwives and their students should be familiar.
- Moral conflicts and dilemmas cannot be avoided in some cases; they can be disconcerting but must be resolved. Theories and principles are available to help resolve the dilemmas.
- Professional practice in the NHS requires both deontological and utilitarian consideration.
- The duty of care has an ethical basis and is not only a legal principle.
- Women's autonomy is an essential basis for good midwifery practice – it also enables midwife autonomy.

## REFERENCES


*Children Act 1989*, London, 1989, HMSO.

*Children Act 2004*, London, 2004, HMSO.

Healthcare Commission: *Women's experiences of maternity care in the NHS in England*, London, 2007, Commission for Healthcare Audit and Inspection (CHAI).

Jones SR: *Ethics in midwifery*, ed 2, London, 2000, Mosby.

Jones SR, Jenkins R: *The law and the midwife*, ed 2, Oxford, 2003, Blackwell, pp 123–125.

*Mental Capacity Act 2005*, London, 2005, HMSO.

Smart JJC, Williams B: *Utilitarianism for and against*, Cambridge, 1988, Cambridge University Press.

NMC: *Midwives rules and standards*, London, 2004, NMC.

NMC: *The code: standards of conduct, performance and ethics for nurses and midwives*, London, 2008, NMC.


## FURTHER READING


Beauchamp TL, Childress JF: *Principles of biomedical ethics*, ed 6, Oxford, 2008, Oxford University Press.


This book is a good starting point for gaining depth of understanding of ethical theory beyond the narrow application to midwifery.


Harris J, editor: *Bioethics*, Oxford, 2001, Oxford University Press.


This book has chapters related to beginning-of-life and end-of-life issues, the value and quality of life and professional ethics; all of which are important in midwifery.


Jones SR: *Ethico-legal issues in women's health*. In Andrews G, editor: *Women's sexual health*, ed 3, London, 2005, Baillière Tindall.


Childbearing is just one aspect of women's lives (and not for all women). It is important for midwives to study more broadly into women's health in order to enrich their knowledge of those for whom they provide a service.

Chapter | 9 |

# Law and the midwife

Bridgit Dimond

**LEARNING OUTCOMES**

After reading this chapter, you will be able to:

- understand the language and sources of the law
- have an understanding of the legal framework within which you work in the UK
- make judgements as to when expert help needs to be brought in
- ensure that your practice is within the law
- advise your patients and families.

This chapter includes an introduction to the Courts and how laws are made. It explores the key legislation that affects the practice of midwifery and provision of maternity care services.

## INTRODUCTION TO THE LAW: THE COURTS AND HOW LAWS ARE MADE

### The courts (Fig. 9.1)

The main courts dealing with criminal proceedings are the Crown and Magistrates Courts. Those dealing with civil proceedings are the High Court, the County Courts and the Small Claims Courts. The Court of Appeal and the Supreme Court (which replaced the House of Lords from October 2009) will hear both criminal and civil cases. Where European laws are concerned, there can be an appeal to the European Court of Justice. In the case of issues relating to human rights (see below), appeal is to the European Court of Human Rights in Strasbourg.

In addition to the court system outlined above, there are Coroners Courts and various administrative tribunals that also administer the law, for example, Employment Tribunals.

Since devolution, Northern Ireland, Scotland and Wales are able to enact their own statutes within specified areas.

### Classification of the law

The most common distinction made is between *criminal* and *civil* law. A criminal offence is where the law (statute or common law – see below) forbids a particular activity which can then be followed by criminal proceedings against the accused. The prosecution must establish beyond reasonable doubt the guilt of the accused. In the Crown Courts, if the accused pleads not guilty, a jury will hear the case and determine guilt or innocence.

Civil proceedings take place between individuals and organizations in order that one party can obtain a remedy (for example, an injunction forbidding the other party to act in a particular way) or compensation. In civil courts, the standard of proof is 'on the balance of probabilities'.

Some actions may give rise to both civil **and** criminal proceedings. Thus, touching a person without the person's consent may be both a trespass to the person (which is a civil matter) and also constitute the criminal offence of assault or battery.

Another distinction in law is that between private and public law:

- *Private law* is concerned with matters between private individuals and others or between organizations and individuals. It comes within the ambit of civil law.
- *Public law* is concerned with matters affecting the public. This comprises constitutional law, administrative law and the criminal law.

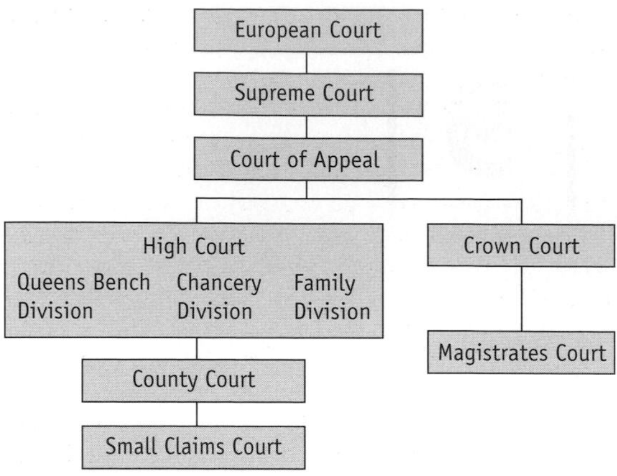


**Figure 9.1** The court hierarchy.

Some statutes may cover both areas: thus, the Children Act 1989 has some sections that deal with matters of a private nature; others deal with public issues, such as the role of local authorities in child protection.

## Sources of the law

The law recognized in this country derives from two main sources:

- legislation – Acts of Parliament, statutory instruments and Regulations and Directives of the European Union
- common law, which is formed from decisions made by courts in particular cases (see below).

### Legislation

Britain is obliged as a member state of the the European Union (EU) to ensure that EU Directives and Regulations are enforced in this country, and appeals can be made to the European Court of Justice.

In the UK, when legislation is proposed, the usual practice is for a consultation paper to be issued (known as a *Green Paper*). Following consideration of the feedback, a *White Paper* is then issued setting out the Government's intentions. The contents of this White Paper are incorporated into a *Bill* which is then passed through the various stages of Parliament and, when agreed by both House of Commons and House of Lords, is signed by the Queen. The Bill then becomes an *Act* and comes into force on a date set either in the Act itself or at a later date set out in a Statutory Instrument. The Act of Parliament may provide for the delegation to Ministers and others of powers enabling detailed rules to supplement the Statute to be enacted. These are known as *Statutory Instruments* or *secondary legislation*. They must be placed before Parliament before coming into effect.

### Common law

Decisions by judges in courts create what is variously known as the *common law, case law* or *judge-made* law. The decisions of the courts create precedents which may be binding on courts below them in the court hierarchy. This is called the doctrine of precedent. Thus, decisions of the Supreme Court (replacing the House of Lords in its judicial format) are binding on those courts below it, but not itself; and decisions of the Court of Appeal are binding on itself and those courts below it.

The doctrine of precedent relies on a recognized system of reporting of judges' decisions, which ensures certainty over what was stated and the facts of the cases. The decisions are recorded in law books such as the *All England Law Reports* or the *Weekly Law Reports*. Every case is identified by the year it was heard, the volume number and page number. For example, the case of *Bolam* v. *Friern Hospital Management Committee* is cited as [1957] 1 WLR 582. This means that it was reported in 1957, in the first volume of the *Weekly Law Reports* at page 582. It is also reported in other series such as the *All England Law Reports*.

The main principles which are set out in a case are known as the *ratio decidendi* (reasons for the decision). Other parts of a judge's speech which are not considered to be part of the *ratio decidendi* are known as *obiter dicta* (things said by the way). Only the *ratio decidendi* are directly binding on lower courts, but the *obiter dicta* are said to be 'persuasive' because they may influence the decision of judges in later court cases. It may be possible for judges to 'distinguish' the current case under consideration from previous cases and not follow them on the grounds that the facts are significantly different.

### The Human Rights Act 1998

The European Convention for the Protection of Human Rights and Fundamental Freedoms (1951) provides protection for the fundamental rights and freedoms of all people. The UK is a signatory, as are many European countries which are not members of the European Union. Thus, Norway is a signatory to the European Convention on Human Rights but not a member of the European Union. The Convention is enforced through the European Court of Human Rights, which meets in Strasbourg. However, following the passing of the Human Rights Act 1998, since 2 October 2000 most of the articles are directly enforceable in the UK courts in relation to public authorities or those exercising functions of a public nature. Of particular significance in healthcare are:

- *Article 2 and the right to life*, which may be used to justify the allocation of more resources, and has already been used (unsuccessfully) to press for the continuation of treatment for a severely disabled baby (*A National Health Service Trust* v. *D Lloyd*, 2000)

- *Article 3 and the right not to be tortured or subjected to inhuman or degrading treatment or punishment* (It has been argued that chaining a pregnant prisoner to a bed during her confinement is a breach of Article 3)
- *Article 5 and the right to liberty and security*
- *Article 6 and the right to a fair trial* (this includes civil hearings and tribunals as well as criminal proceedings)
- *Article 8 and the right to respect of privacy and family life*
- *Article 14 and the right not to be discriminated against* in the recognition of the articles on human rights.

Other articles may also be relevant to the rights of patients and employees.

Under the Human Rights Act 1998, judges have a duty to refer back to Parliament for its consideration, legislation which they consider is incompatible with the rights set out in the European Convention. Parliament can then decide if that Act should be changed. The existence of a right to take a case for violation of rights to the courts of this country does not prevent a person taking a case to the European Court in Strasbourg. Further information including guidance and the latest cases can be obtained from the Ministry of Justice website (www.justice.gov.uk). Organizations exercising functions of a public nature are obliged to recognize and implement rights as set out in the Articles. Section 145 of the Health and Social Care Act 2008 provides for the provision of certain social care to be seen as a public function. Section 145 states that:

> *(1) A person ("P") who provides accommodation, together with nursing or personal care, in a care home for an individual under arrangements made with P under the relevant statutory provisions is to be taken for the purposes of subsection (3)(b) of section 6 of the Human Rights Act 1998 (c. 42) (acts of public authorities) to be exercising a function of a public nature in so doing.*

**Reflective activity 9.1**

Read through and consider Article 3 of the European Convention on Human Rights and analyse the extent to which any woman could claim that her rights under this Article are infringed.

## Midwives rules and the code of professional conduct

The statutory system of the regulation of nursing, midwifery and health visiting set out in the Nurses, Midwives and Health Visitors Act 1979 (as amended by the 1992 Act) went through radical changes following a review of the statutory bodies (JM Consulting 1998) and the revised Health Act (1999) and Orders (2002). In April 2002, the Nursing and Midwifery Council (NMC) was established and has revised much of the guidance originally provided by the UKCC. This includes the Midwives rules and code of practice. Codes of practice are complementary to the rules but, unlike the practice rules, do not have the force of law. Midwives are also expected to comply with the NMC Code of Professional Conduct: standards for performance, conduct and ethics (NMC 2008a) and other guidance from the NMC. Every midwife should ensure that they have copies of all the relevant NMC guidance which is available online from the Nursing and Midwifery Council (www.nmc-uk.org/). Box 9.1 indicates the purpose of the Midwives rules, which are set out under Statutory Instruments, and Box 9.2 sets out the midwife's responsibility and sphere of practice.

**Box 9.1 Aims of the Midwives Rules as set out in Article 42 of the NMC Order 2001**

1. Determine the circumstances in which and the procedure by means of which midwives may be suspended from practice.
2. Require midwives to give notice of their intention to practise to the local supervising authority in the area in which they intend to practise (in addition, if midwives practise in an emergency outside their normal authority they have to notify the new health authority within 48 hours)
3. Require registered midwives to attend courses of instruction in accordance with the rules.

**Box 9.2 Rule 6: Responsibility and sphere of practice**

1. A practising midwife is responsible for providing midwifery care, in accordance with such standards as the Council may specify from time to time, to a woman and baby during the antenatal, intranatal and postnatal periods.
2. Except in an emergency, a practising midwife shall not provide any care, or undertake any treatment, which she has not been trained to give.
3. In an emergency, or where a deviation from the norm which is outside her current sphere of practice becomes apparent in a woman or baby during the antenatal, intranatal or postnatal periods, a practising midwife shall call such qualified health professional as may reasonably be expected to have the necessary skills and experience to assist her in the provision of care.

*(NMC 2004b: 16)*

### Supervision

Midwives are the only group of health professionals to have a statutory system of supervision. Appointed by the local supervising authority, the supervisor of midwives has clear statutory responsibilities in relation to the positive promotion of a high standard of midwifery practice, and the protection of the public. In 2006, the NMC published standards for the preparation and practice of supervisors of midwives and, in 2007, standards for supervised practice of midwives. In 2008, the NMC replaced the ENB publication on midwifery supervision with its own *Modern supervision in action: a practical guide for midwives* (NMC 2009).

## LITIGATION

In 2007–08, 5470 claims of clinical negligence and 3380 claims of non-clinical negligence against NHS bodies were received by the NHS Litigation Authority (which is a Special Health Authority responsible for handling both clinical and non-clinical negligence cases on behalf of the NHS in England). There were 16,959 'live' claims as at 31 March 2008 and it paid out £633,325 million in connection with clinical negligence claims. Of the 45,404 cases dealt with by the NHS Litigation Authority (NHSLA) since its creation in 1995, 9477 (21%) were for obstetrics and gynaecology, but looking at the total value of £6.5 billion, £3.3 billion was spent on obstetrics and gynaecology cases. So, 20% of the cases accounted for 50% of the expenditure, which is explained by the very high cost of obstetric claims (www.nhsla.com/home). The NHSLA estimates that its total liabilities (including claims not yet reported to it) are £21.06 billion. In an effort to reduce the costs of clinical negligence claims, the NHS Redress Act 2006 was passed to establish an alternative route for compensation to be paid without necessitating action in the civil courts. It remains to be seen whether it will become an effective alternative to legal action through the courts.

## NEGLIGENCE

### What is negligence?

Negligence is the most common civil action, brought in situations when the claimant alleges that there has been personal injury, death, or damage or loss of property. Compensation is sought for the loss which has occurred. To succeed in the action, the claimant has to show the following elements:

1. that the defendant owed the person harmed a duty of care
2. that the defendant was in breach of that duty
3. that the breach of duty caused reasonably foreseeable harm
4. that the claimant has suffered harm recognized in law as compensable.

### Duty of care

The law recognizes that a duty of care will exist where one person can reasonably foresee that his or her actions and omissions could cause reasonably foreseeable harm to another person. A duty of care will always exist between the health professional and the patient, but it might not always be easy to identify what this includes. Where there is no pre-existing duty to a person (for example, an existing professional and patient relationship), the usual legal principle is that there is no duty to volunteer services (that is, perform a 'good Samaritan' act). The NMC recognized that there may be a professional duty to volunteer help in certain circumstances in the code published in 2002 (but not included in its revised code of 2008) (NMC 2008a).

In one case, the House of Lords defined the duty of care owed at common law (that is, judge-made law) as being:

> *You must take reasonable care to avoid acts or omissions which you can reasonably foresee would be likely to injure your neighbour. Who then in law is my neighbour? The answer seems to be persons who are so closely and directly affected by my act that I ought reasonably to have them in contemplation as being so affected when I am directing my mind to the acts or omissions which are called in question.*
>
> (*Donoghue* v. *Stevenson*, 1932)

### Breach of duty

#### *Determining the standard of care*

In order to determine whether there has been a breach of the duty of care, it will first be necessary to establish the required standard of care. The courts have used what has become known as the 'Bolam Test' to determine the standard of care required by a professional. In the case from which the test took its name, the court laid down the following principle to determine the standard of care which should be followed:

> *The standard of care expected is 'the standard of the ordinary skilled man exercising and professing to have that special skill'.*
>
> (*Bolam* v. *Friern Hospital Management Committee*, 1957).

The Bolam Test was applied by the House of Lords in a case where negligence by an obstetrician in delivering a child by forceps was alleged:

> *When you get a situation which involves the use of some special skill or competence, then the test as to whether there has been negligence or not … is the standard of the ordinary skilled man exercising and professing to have that special skill. If a surgeon failed to measure up to that in any respect (clinical judgement or otherwise) he had been negligent and should be so adjudged.*
>
> (*Whitehouse* v. *Jordan*, 1981)

In this particular case, the House of Lords found that the surgeon was not liable in negligence and held that an error of judgement may or may not be negligence. It depends upon the circumstances.

This standard of the reasonable professional man following the accepted approved standard of care can be used to apply to any professional person: architect, lawyer, accountant, as well as those working in health. The standard of care which a practitioner should have provided would be judged in this way. Expert witnesses give evidence to the court on the standard of care they would expect to have found in the circumstances before the court. These experts would be respected members of the profession of obstetrics and midwifery, possibly a head of a department or training college, and lawyers would look to the leading organizations of individual professional groups to obtain recommended names.

**Reflective activity 9.2**

Consider any incident of which you are aware, when harm (nearly) occurred to a woman or baby. What potential hearings could take place as a result of this harm and what would have to be shown to secure a conviction/guilt/liability?

In a civil action, the judge would decide in the light of the evidence that has been given to the court, what standard should have been followed.

The standards at the time of the alleged negligence apply; not the standards at the time of the court hearing. This is significant, since many cases take several years to come to court, in which time standards may have changed. Reference is made to literature and procedures which applied at the time of the alleged negligence to establish if a reasonable standard of care was followed.

Experts can of course differ. A case may arise where the expert giving evidence for the claimant states that the accepted approved standard of care was not followed by the defendant or its employees. In contrast, the expert evidence for the defendant might state that the defendant or its employees followed the reasonable standard of care. Where such a conflict arises, the House of Lords has laid down the following principle:

> *It was not sufficient to establish negligence for the plaintiff (that is, claimant) to show that there was a body of competent professional opinion that considered the decision was wrong, if there was also a body of equally competent professional opinion that supported the decision as having been reasonable in the circumstances.*
>
> (*Maynard* v. *W Midlands Regional Health Authority*, 1985)

The determination of the reasonable standard of care was considered by the House of Lords in the case of *Bolitho* v. *City and Hackney Health Authority*, when it was stated that:

> *The court had to be satisfied that the exponents of the body of opinion relied on can demonstrate that such opinion has a logical basis. In particular in cases involving, as they often do, the weighing of risks against benefits, the judge, before accepting a body of opinion as being responsible, reasonable or respectable, will need to be satisfied that, in forming their views, the experts had directed their minds to the question of comparative risks and benefits and had reached a defensible conclusion on the matter.*
>
> *The use of the adjectives 'responsible, reasonable and respectable' (in the Bolam case) all showed that the court had to be satisfied that the exponents of the body of opinion relied upon could demonstrate that such opinion had a logical basis.*
>
> *It would seldom be right for a judge to reach the conclusion that views held by a competent medical expert were unreasonable.*
>
> (*Bolitho* v. *City and Hackney Health Authority*, 1997)

Rule 35 of the new civil court proceedings sets out the duties of experts and assessors. There is a duty to restrict expert evidence to that which is reasonably required to resolve the proceedings. The Rules can be accessed on the website for the Ministry of Justice (http://www.justice.gov.uk/civil/procrules_fin/index.htm).

Government documents (Department of Health 1997, 1998, 1999, 2000) have placed increasing emphasis on standard setting, clinical governance and effective risk management. The National Institute for Health and Clinical Excellence (NICE – www.nice.org.uk), the Care Quality Commission (www.cqc.org.uk – which has replaced the Healthcare Commission) and National Service Frameworks (NSF) are leading to more guidance on standards to be achieved in all departments of a hospital and in community care. They are described in more detail later in this chapter and in Chapters 3 and 7. It is anticipated that these standards will be incorporated into the Bolam Test of reasonable professional practice. Practitioners are expected to follow the results of clinical effectiveness research in their treatment and care of patients. Patients are able to use these national guidelines to argue that inadequate care has been provided in their case, as a result of which they have suffered harm.

In 2008, the four Royal Colleges – Midwives, Obstetricians and Gynaecologists, Anaesthetists, and Paediatrics and Child Health – co-operated in the preparation of a single, comprehensive document setting out 30 standards for maternity care. The document is available on the website of the Royal College of Obstetricians and Gynaecologists (http://www.rcog.org.uk/womens-health/clinical-guidance/standards-maternity-care).

Midwives who decide that, in the light of the specific circumstances of a case, a procedure or protocol or guideline is not entirely appropriate, should ensure that clear documentation is completed including all the circumstances and reasons for the inappropriateness of the guideline, so that their practice can be seen to be justifiable against the standard of the reasonable practitioner.

Communication – between professionals, departments and with patients – is crucial to a reasonable standard of care. This is particularly important where one person is designated as the key worker on behalf of the multidisciplinary team. However, the Court of Appeal has stated that the courts do not recognize a concept of team liability and it is therefore for each individual professional to ensure that his or her practice is in accordance with the approved standard of care (*Wilsher* v. *Essex Area Health Authority*, 1986). Professionals should not take instructions from another professional which they know would be contrary to the standard of care that their profession would require. Failure to follow up a cytology report led to compensation being paid to the dead patient's husband (*Taylor* v. *West Kent Health Authority*, 1997). This is supported by the NMC Code (2008a) which states that:

> *You are personally accountable for actions and omissions in your professional practice and must always be able to justify your decisions. You must always act lawfully, whether those laws relate to your professional practice or personal life.*

### *Has there been a breach of the duty of care?*

Once it has been established in court what the reasonable standard of care should have been, the next stage is to decide whether or not what took place was in accordance with the reasonable standard – that is, whether there has been a breach of the duty of care or not. Evidence will be given by witnesses of fact as to what actually took place. Clear comprehensive documentation will be an important element in determining the facts of what took place. In a case where it was alleged that there had been negligence by a registrar following a forceps delivery, which led to damage to the anal sphincter, the court applied the test of the reasonable standard of care at the time of the birth and found the defendant not to be liable (*Starkey* v. *Rotherham NHS Foundation Trust*, 2007).

## Causation

The claimant must show not only that there was a breach of the duty of care, but that this breach of duty caused actual and reasonably foreseeable harm to the claimant. This requires:

- factual causation to be shown, and also
- evidence that the type of harm that occurred was reasonably foreseeable
- there to have been no intervening cause which breaks the chain of causation.

### *Factual causation*

There may be a breach of the duty of care and harm but no link between them. In the case of *Barnett* v. *Chelsea Hospital Management Committee* (1968), a casualty officer failed to examine patients who came to the A&E department, when they were vomiting very badly. However, the widow of one was unable to obtain compensation, since it was established on the facts that because the man was suffering from arsenic poisoning, he would have died even if reasonable care had been provided. The breach of duty by the doctor therefore did not cause the man's death.

The onus is on the claimant to establish that there is this causative link between the breach of the duty of care and the harm which occurred. In the case of *Wilsher* v. *Essex Area Health Authority* (1988), the claimants failed to establish that excess oxygen (resulting from the placing of a catheter to monitor oxygen in the vein, rather than in the artery) had caused the retrolental fibroplasia suffered by the baby. The House of Lords ordered a new hearing on the issue of causation, because excess oxygen was only one of five factors which might have caused the blindness. The parties then agreed to a settlement.

In a case where a baby suffered brain damage, an allegation that a midwife was negligent in failing to call a registrar an hour earlier to consider a caesarean section succeeded. The court held that this failure had led to the delay in deciding a caesarean delivery was appropriate. The court also held that the registrar was also negligent in failing to recognize the change in contraction patterns (*Khalid* v. *Barnet and Chase Farm Hospitals NHS Trust*, 2007).

### *Reasonably foreseeable harm*

The harm which might arise may not be within the reasonable contemplation of the defendant, so that even though there is a breach of duty and there is harm, the defendant is not liable. This is because a negligent act may set off a 'chain reaction' of consequences and the courts have decided that there should be some limit on the liability of the defendant. For example, a midwife may have delayed in referring a woman for advice from an obstetrician and thus been in breach of her duty of care to the woman, but because of underlying medical problems suffered by the woman, the harm which arose was not reasonably foreseeable by the midwife.

### *No intervening cause which breaks the chain of causation*

It may happen that any causal link between the claimant's breach of duty and the harm suffered by the client is interrupted by an intervening event. For example, an independent midwife contrary to the reasonable accepted practice may have arranged to take a woman in labour in her car, but as a result of a road accident for which the midwife was not responsible, the woman suffered injuries and the baby was stillborn. The road accident would be seen as an intervening event which broke the chain of causation.

## Harm

The final requirement to succeed in an action for negligence is that the claimant or their representatives must establish that the claimant has suffered harm which the court recognizes as being subject to compensation. Personal injury, death, and loss or damage to property are the main areas of recognizable harm. In addition, the courts have ruled that nervous shock where an identifiable medical condition exists (now known as post-traumatic stress syndrome) can be the subject of compensation within strict limits of liability. A test of proximity to the defendant's negligent action or omission has been set by the House of Lords.

## Vicarious and personal liability

It is unlikely that employees will be sued personally, since the employer will usually be vicariously liable for their actions.

To establish the vicarious liability of the employer, the claimant must show the *employee* was *negligent* or was guilty of another wrong whilst acting in the *course of employment.*

Independent practitioners have to accept personal and professional liability for their actions but they may also be vicariously liable for the harm, caused during the course of employment, by anyone they employ. Each of the elements shown above must be established so employers are not liable for the acts of their independent contractors (that is, self-employed persons who are working for them on a contract for services) unless they are at fault in selecting or instructing them.

The employer may challenge whether the actions were performed in the course of employment. For example, a midwife may have undertaken training in a complementary therapy, such as acupuncture. If she used these new skills whilst at work, without the express or implied agreement of the employer, and through use of this therapy caused harm to the client, the employer might refuse to accept vicarious liability on the grounds that the employee was not acting in the course of employment. However, the House of Lords held, in a case involving abuse of pupils at a school boarding house, that the Board of Governors was vicariously liable for the acts of the warden in abusing the claimants: the Home had undertaken the care of the children and entrusted the performance of that duty to the warden and there was therefore sufficiently close connection between his employment and the acts committed by him (*Lister* v. *Helsey Hall*, 2001).

## Liability for student, unqualified assistants: supervision and delegation

Exactly the same principles apply to the delegation and supervision of tasks as to the carrying out of professional activities. Midwives delegating a task should only do so if they are reasonably sure that the person to whom the task is delegated is reasonably competent and experienced to undertake that activity safely. They must also ensure that the person undertaking that activity has a sufficient level of supervision to ensure that the delegated activity can be carried out reasonably safely. Should harm befall a client because an activity was carried out by a junior member of staff, student or assistant, it is **no defence** to the legal action to argue that the harm occurred because that person did not have the ability, competence or experience to carry out that task reasonably safely (*Wilsher* v. *Essex Area Health Authority*, 1986). There will be some midwifery tasks, such as attendance at a birth, which can never be delegated. Other activities may be delegated if the delegatee is assessed as competent and the requisite level of supervision is provided. The NMC has provided guidance on delegation within Midwifery (NMC 2004a) and the Code of Practice issued in 2008 states:

> ***Delegate effectively***
> *You must establish that anyone you delegate to is competent to carry out your instructions*
> *You must confirm that the outcome of any delegated task meets required standards*
> *You must make sure that everyone you are responsible for is properly supervised*

# Defences to an action

The main defences to an action for negligence are listed below:

- Dispute allegations
- Deny that all the elements of negligence are established
- Contributory negligence
- Exemption from liability
- Limitation of time
- Voluntary assumption of risk.

## Dispute allegations

Many cases will be resolved entirely on what facts can be shown to exist. Thus, the effectiveness of the witnesses for both parties in establishing the facts of what did or did not occur will be the determining factor in who wins the case. Clearly, record-keeping and the witnesses in court will play a significant role in determining the facts of what took place. It might appear before the court hearing that one party has a particularly strong case but, unless the facts on which its case rests can be proved in court or are admitted by the other party, the actual outcome of the case might be that the opponent wins.

## Deny that all the elements of negligence are established

The claimant must establish that all elements required to prove negligence are present, that is, duty, breach, causation and harm. If one or more of these cannot be established, then the defendant will win the case. In some situations, the claimant may be able to claim that 'the thing speaks for itself' (i.e. a *res ipsa loquitur* situation). This means that the claimant will say that there is no explanation for the damage other than a negligent act having taken place. If this claim is made, the defendant is then required to explain how what has happened could have occurred without negligence on his or her part.

## Contributory negligence

If the claimant is partly to blame for the harm which has occurred, then there may still be liability on the part of the professional but the compensation payable might be reduced in proportion to the claimant's fault. In extreme cases, if 100% contributory negligence is claimed, such a claim may be a complete defence. In determining the level of contributory negligence, the physical and mental health and the age of the claimant would be taken into account.

The Law Reform (Contributory Negligence) Act 1945 enables an apportionment of responsibility for the harm that has been caused, which may result in a reduction of damages payable. The Court can reduce the damages 'to such extent as it thinks just and equitable having regard to the claimant's share in the responsibility for the damage' (Section 1(1)).

One of the most frequent examples of contributory negligence being taken into account is in road traffic accidents where the injuries sustained by the claimant are greater because the claimant was not wearing a seat belt.

## Exemption from liability

It is possible for people to exempt themselves from liability for harm arising from their negligence, but the effects of the Unfair Contract Terms Act 1977 mean that this exemption only applies to loss or damage to property. A defendant cannot exclude liability from negligence which results in personal damage or death either by contract or by a notice. A midwife could not therefore agree with a woman that she would provide her with a waterbirth on the understanding that the mother would not hold the midwife (or the midwife's employer) liable for any negligence.

Where exemption from liability for loss or damage to property is claimed by the defendant, it must be shown by the defendant that it is reasonable to rely upon the term or notice which purported to exclude liability.

Reasonableness in relation to a notice not having contractual effect means that: 'it should be fair and reasonable to allow reliance on it, having regard to all the circumstances obtaining when the liability arose or (but for the notice) would have arisen' (Unfair Contract Terms Act 1977: S.11 (3)).

Under Section 11(5), it is for those claiming that a contract term or notice satisfies the requirements of reasonableness, to show that it does.

The effect of this legislation is that notices which purport to exempt a department from liability for negligence are invalid if that negligence leads to personal injury or death. However, a notice which excludes liability for loss or damage to property may be valid if it is reasonable for the negligent person or organization to rely upon it.

## Limitation of time

Actions for personal injury or death should normally be commenced within 3 years of the date of the event which gave rise to the harm, or 3 years from the date on which the person had the necessary knowledge of the harm and the fact that it arose from the defendant's actions or omissions. There are, however, some major qualifications to this general principle and these are shown in Box 9.3. As can be seen, in maternity claims, as the action is brought by the baby/child, limitation is potentially 18 years or until death.

The limitation rules are linked to the periods for which records must be retained. The Department of Health has specified minimum retention periods – for maternity records, this is 25 years after last live birth; for other records, this is generally 8 years after treatment concluded or death. The importance of this can be demonstrated by

**Box 9.3 Situations where the limitation of time can be extended**

- Those suffering from a disability:
  - children under 18 years – the time does not start to run until the child is 18 years
  - those suffering from a mental disability – time does not start to run until the disability ends. In the case of those who are suffering from severe learning disabilities or brain damage, this may not be until death.
- Discretion of the judge. The judge has a statutory power to extend the time within which a claimant can bring an action for personal injuries or death, if it is just and equitable to do so.

the case of a woman who had suffered brain damage following heart surgery as a baby at the Bristol hospital, which led to the Kennedy Inquiry (Kennedy Report 2001). She was awarded a seven-figure sum in compensation more than 20 years after the surgery (Rose 2008). Seven further cases were said to be awaiting the outcome and are now likely to be pursued.

The definition of knowledge for the purposes of the limitation of time is that a person must have knowledge of the following facts:

- that the injury in question was significant
- that the injury was attributable in whole or in part to the act or omission which is alleged to constitute the negligence, nuisance or breach of duty
- the identity of the defendant
- if it is alleged that the act or omission was that of a person other than the defendant, the identity of that person and the additional facts supporting the bringing of an action against the defendant.

Knowledge that any acts or omissions did or did not, as a matter of law, involve negligence, nuisance or breach of duty is irrelevant. A person is not fixed with knowledge of a fact ascertainable only with the help of expert advice so long as he has taken all reasonable steps to obtain and, where appropriate, to act on, that advice.

### Voluntary assumption of risk

*Volente non fit injuria* is the Latin term for the defence that a person willingly undertook the risk of being harmed. It is unlikely to succeed as a defence in an action for professional negligence since professionals cannot contract out of liability where harm occurs as a result of their negligence. The defence of *volenti non fit injuria* would not be available to an employer as a defence against a midwife who argued that she had been exposed to HIV/AIDS as a result of negligence by her employer. The employers have a duty to take reasonable care of the health and safety of employees and it cannot be argued successfully that an employee accepts a risk of being harmed as an occupational hazard, where the employer has failed in its duty of care.

### Compensation

The legal term for the amount of compensation to be paid is *quantum* (literally how much). The general rule governing the award of damages is that they should compensate the claimant for the loss s/he has suffered. This means that the claimant should be restored to the position s/he would have been in but for the negligent act.

There are two kinds of damages: *general* and *special* damages. *Special damages* refers to the actual financial losses between the negligent act and the trial (or settlement if there is no trial), for example loss of earnings, purchase of special equipment or adaptations to the home and the costs of medical and nursing care. *General damages* basically reflects compensation for pain and suffering from the injury and loss of amenity (reduced enjoyment of life) plus future financial losses, for example loss of earnings and future expenses.

In some cases of negligence, liability might be accepted by the defendant but there might be disagreement between the parties over the amount of compensation; or there may be agreement over the amount of compensation but liability may be disputed. In others, both liability and quantum might be in dispute.

## CURRENT DEVELOPMENTS IN CIVIL LAW

Significant changes were made to the civil procedures following the Final Report by Lord Woolf (Woolf 1996) which came into force in 1996. He recommended a new system in which the courts would have an active role in case management, including control over the use of expert evidence. He recommended a fast track for cases below a certain financial limit, where experts would normally be jointly appointed by the parties and would not be required to give oral evidence in court. Cases above this limit would be allocated to a multi-track, in which the court would have wide powers to define the scope of expert evidence and prescribe the way in which experts should be used in particular cases. The civil procedures can be accessed on the Ministry of Justice website (http://www.justice.gov.uk/civil/procrules_fin/index.htm).

In spite of these reforms, there are still worries about the delays and cost of litigation and in 2003 the Department of Health published a consultation document *'Making Amends'* (Department of Health 2003) which provided a comprehensive account of the background to the current situation. It looked at the present system of medical negligence litigation and its costs and recommended the introduction of a new scheme for obtaining compensation in clinical negligence cases. The resulting legislation in the NHS Redress Act 2006 is not as radical as proposed in the consultation paper and is still to be implemented. The extent to which the new scheme to recover compensation replaces the use of civil court proceedings remains to be seen.

### Conditional fees

Legal aid is being phased out from personal injury litigation. A system of conditional fees has been introduced whereby the claimant is able to negotiate, with a solicitor, payment on a 'no win – no fees' basis, that is, if the claimant loses, the solicitor does not charge any fees. However, a claimant who does not succeed will have to pay the costs of the successful defendant, and this possibility is covered by taking out insurance to meet these and other costs not covered by the agreement with the solicitor. Recent statutory changes enable a successful party to claim enhanced fees agreed with lawyers under the conditional fee agreement, from the unsuccessful party. In 2008, the NHS Litigation Authority (NHSLA) reported that the annual bill for solicitors representing patients was £90.7 million, double the amount 4 years previously, because of the increase in 'no win – no fee' claims. The bill for NHS lawyers was £43.3 million.

## THE NHS LITIGATION AUTHORITY (NHSLA) AND THE CLINICAL NEGLIGENCE SCHEME FOR TRUSTS (CNST)

In 1995, the NHS Litigation Authority (NHSLA) was established with responsibility for the Clinical Negligence Scheme for Trusts (CNST). This scheme requires member trusts to pay an annual amount into a central pool, from which justified claims over an agreed amount will be paid. This means that NHS trusts do not have to set aside large amounts of money 'just in case' they have to pay out on a major negligence claim. Instead, the risk, and costs, are spread across the NHS and the maximum amount that an NHS trust will have to spend on a single claim is capped.

Great emphasis is placed on the importance of good clinical risk management, as this should reduce the number and cost of legal claims. A system of risk management standards for trusts participating in the scheme has been developed and payments into the pool are based upon assessments of the individual organizations carried out by the CNST. In 2008, the NHSLA piloted through the CNST new clinical risk management standards for maternity. They can be found on the NHSLA website (www.nhsla.com/home). There are three levels of attainment:

**Level 1**: a Trust is required to show that it has the required clinical risk management policies and procedures in place to provide a safe maternity service.
**Level 2**: they must demonstrate that the policies and procedures are being implemented.
**Level 3**: they must show that they are monitoring the implementation proactively to identify problems before they occur.

The identified risk areas are: risk management strategy, emergency caesarean section, pre-eclampsia and eclampsia, clinical risk assessment and postnatal information.

There is a clear financial incentive for NHS trusts to attain the higher levels of participation (as this attracts a discount on their contributions to the central fund) but this also reflects more rigorous practices and thus better care for women and their babies.

The NHSLA oversees the CNST and also administers the scheme for meeting liabilities of health service bodies to third parties for loss, damage or injury arising out of the exercise of their functions. In practice this means claims by employees for accidents at work, or by visitors for accidents taking place in NHS premises.

## CONSENT

It is a general legal and ethical principle that valid consent must be obtained before starting treatment or physical investigation, or providing personal care, to a patient. This principle reflects the right of patients to determine what happens to their own bodies, and is a fundamental tenet of good practice. Health professionals who do not respect this principle may be liable both to legal action by the patient and to action by their professional body or even to criminal prosecution.

There are two distinct aspects of the law relating to consent to treatment. One is the actual giving of consent by the patient, which acts as a defence to an action for trespass to the person. The other is the duty on the practitioner to give information to the patient prior to the giving of consent. The absence of consent could result in the patient suing for trespass to the person. The failure to provide sufficient relevant information could result in an action for negligence. These two different legal actions will be considered separately.

### Trespass to the person

There are two types of trespass to the person. An *assault* is when an individual perceives a threat that she may be touched without her consent. If she is actually touched without her consent, then this is known as *battery*. Thus, threatening behaviour but without any physical contact would be assault, while a vaginal examination carried out without the woman's consent could be battery.

The person who has suffered the trespass can sue for compensation in the civil courts (and in criminal cases a prosecution could also be brought). In the civil cases, the victim has to prove:

- the touching or the apprehension of the touching, and
- that it was a (potentially) direct interference with her person.

The victim does not have to show that harm has occurred. This is in contrast with an action for negligence, in which the victim must show that harm has resulted from the breach of duty of care.

**Reflective activity 9.3**

Analyse the activities which you undertake in relation to women in your care and note the extent to which you obtain consent by word of mouth, consent in writing or consent by non-verbal communication. What changes, if any, do you consider should be made to your practice?

### Defences to an action for trespass to the person

The main defence to an action for trespass to the person is that consent was given by a mentally competent person. In addition, there are two other defences in law, which are:

1. statutory authorization – for example, Mental Health Act 1983 (as amended by the Mental Health Act 2007)
2. the act was performed in the best interests of a mentally incapacitated person under the provisions of the Mental Capacity Act 2005 (see below).

## Consent and negligence

As part of the duty of care owed in the law of negligence the professional has a duty to inform the patient about the significant risks of substantial harm which could occur if treatment were to proceed.

If the harm has not been explained to the patient, and the harm then occurs, the patient can claim that had she known of this possibility she would not have agreed to undergo the treatment. She could then bring an action in negligence. To succeed, the patient would have to show that:

- there was a duty of care to give specific information
- the defendant failed to give this information and in so doing was therefore in breach of the reasonable standard of care which should have been provided
- as a result of this failure to inform, the patient agreed to the treatment, and
- the patient subsequently suffered the harm.

## Elements of consent

For consent to treatment to be valid, it must be given *voluntarily*, by an appropriately *informed* person (the patient or, where relevant, someone with parental responsibility for a patient under the age of 18) who has *capacity* to consent to the intervention in question.

### Voluntarily

To be valid, consent must be given voluntarily and freely, without pressure or undue influence being exerted on the patient by partners, family members or health professionals.

### Informed

To give valid consent, the patient needs to understand in broad terms the nature and purpose of the procedure, together with the risks of the procedure.

The leading case is that of Sidaway where the House of Lords stated that the professional was required in law to provide information to the patient according to the Bolam Test (*Sidaway* v. *Bethlem Royal Hospital Governors*, 1985). It is advisable to advise the patient of any material or significant risks in the proposed treatment and any alternatives to it, and the risks of doing nothing. A Court of Appeal judgement (*Pearce* v. *United Bristol Healthcare NHS Trust*, 1999) stated that it will normally be the responsibility of the doctor to inform a patient of 'a significant risk which would affect the judgement of a reasonable patient'.

To ensure that the patient understands the information which is given, there are considerable advantages in a leaflet being provided (checking, of course, that the patient can understand it). This would also assist if there was any dispute over the information having been given.

### Capacity

The person giving consent must be mentally competent. A child of 16 or 17 has a statutory right to give consent and a child below 16 may, if 'Gillick competent' (or competent according to Lord Fraser's guidelines), also give consent. This means that the child, although below 16, has sufficient understanding and intelligence to enable him or her to understand fully what is involved in a proposed intervention.

The definition of mental capacity is now set out in the Mental Capacity Act (MCA) 2005 and is established in two stages. First, it must be determined if a person has an impairment of, or a disturbance in the functioning of, the mind or brain. Secondly, if so, does this impairment or disturbance cause an inability to make a specific decision? A person is unable to make a decision for himself if he is unable to:

(a) understand the information relevant to the decision
(b) retain that information
(c) use or weigh that information as part of the process of making the decision, or
(d) communicate his decision (whether by talking, using sign language or any other means).

The existence of a mental illness will not automatically mean that a person is incapable of giving a valid refusal of treatment in her or his best interests, as in the case of *Re C*, where a Broadmoor patient was considered to have the capacity to refuse an amputation of the leg which doctors had advised him was indicated as a life-saving measure. An injunction was ordered against any doctors carrying out an amputation on him without his consent (*Re C*, 1994).

### Refusal to consent

The principle of the right of self-determination if the adult is mentally competent has been applied and extended by the Court of Appeal in two cases where a compulsory caesarean section had been carried out. In the first case (*Re MB*, 1997), the pregnant woman suffered from needle phobia and would not agree to an injection preceding the caesarean. The court held that the needle phobia rendered her mentally incapable and therefore it declared that doctors performing a caesarean, acting in her best interests, would not be acting illegally. Under the MCA there is a presumption (which can be rebutted if the evidence exists) that a person over 16 years has the requisite mental capacity to give consent.

The facts of the second case (*St George's Healthcare National Health Service Trust* v. *S*, 1998) are as follows. S was diagnosed with pre-eclampsia and advised that she needed urgent attention, bed rest and admission to hospital for an induced delivery. Without that treatment, the health and life of both herself and the unborn child were in real danger. She fully understood the potential risks but rejected the advice. She wanted her baby to be born naturally.

She was then seen by an approved social worker and two doctors in relation to compulsory admission to hospital under the Mental Health Act 1983 Section 2 for assessment. They repeated the advice which she had been given and she refused to accept it. On the basis of the written medical recommendations of the two doctors, the approved social worker applied for her admission to hospital for assessment under Section 2 of the Mental Health Act 1983. Later that day, again against her will, she was transferred to St George's Hospital. In view of her continuing adamant refusal to consent to treatment, an application was made ex parte on behalf of the hospital authority to Mrs Justice Hogg, who made a declaration that the caesarean section could proceed, dispensing with S's consent to treatment. The operation was carried out and a baby girl delivered. The woman was then returned to Springfield Hospital and 2 days later her detention under Section 2 of the Mental Health Act was ended.

The woman then sought judicial review of her detention, the High Court judgement and the caesarean operation. The Court of Appeal held that the Mental Health Act 1983 could not be deployed to achieve the detention of an individual against her will merely because her thinking process was unusual, even apparently bizarre and irrational, and contrary to the view of the overwhelming majority of the community at large. A woman detained under the Act for mental disorder could not be forced into medical procedures unconnected with her mental condition unless her capacity to consent to such treatment was diminished. The Court of Appeal was not satisfied that she was lawfully detained under Section 2 of the Mental Health Act 1983 because she was not suffering from mental disorder of a nature or degree which warranted her detention in hospital for assessment. Although on the face of the documents her admission would appear to have been legal, her transfer to St George's Hospital was unlawful and at any time she would have been justified in applying for a *habeas corpus* which would have led to her immediate release. The declaration made by the High Court Judge should not have been made on an ex parte basis (that is, without representation of the woman) and was unlawful.

The difference between the two cases is that in the first case the woman was held, as a result of the needle phobia, to be mentally incompetent, and therefore the caesarean section could be carried out in her best interests without her consent. However, in the second case, S was not held to be mentally incompetent and therefore the compulsory caesarean was a trespass to her person. In neither case did the court consider the rights of the fetus to influence the decision-making.

The fetus is not regarded in law as a legal personality until birth. Until then, the wishes of a mentally competent pregnant woman will prevail whatever the effect on the fetus. Since October 2007, the provisions of the Mental Capacity Act 2005 would apply where the woman was assessed as lacking the requisite mental capacity.

## Mental Capacity Act 2005

The Mental Capacity Act 2005 has replaced the common law power to act out of necessity in the best interests of the patient. Where it is established that the patient lacks the capacity to give consent to treatment, treatment can proceed under the Mental Capacity Act 2005 on the basis that it is in the best interests of that individual and is given according to the reasonable standard of the profession. For example, if a woman who had delivered at home, unattended, had a postpartum haemorrhage and was admitted to hospital in a state of collapse, lacking the mental capacity to give consent, with no information available as to her preferences, it would be lawful to examine her and undertake any necessary procedures to preserve her life, including surgery and the administration of blood products, without obtaining prior consent. If time permits, the Act requires steps to be taken to determine what is in the best interests of that person and, in the absence of carers who could be consulted over what was in her best interests, the appointment of an independent mental capacity advocate where serious treatment is being considered.

Action cannot be taken in a person's best interests, unless they lack the mental capacity to give consent. For example, if a mentally competent woman refuses blood or blood products, these cannot be given to save her life should her condition become critical. The Mental Capacity Act enables a mentally capacitated person to draw up an *advance decision*, under which they can refuse treatment at a future time, when they lack capacity. Where life-saving treatment is refused in advance, specific statutory provisions must be satisfied, including a written statement signed by the maker and signed by a witness, making it clear that a life-saving measure is being refused.

## Forms of consent and consent forms

Consent can be given by word of mouth, in writing or can be implied, that is, the non-verbal conduct of the person may indicate that consent is being given, such as offering an arm for an injection. All these ways of giving consent are valid, but where procedures entail risk and/or where there are likely to be disputes over whether consent was given, it is advisable to obtain consent in writing, since it is then easier to establish in a court of law that consent was given.

## What if someone wishes to leave hospital?

It is a principle of consent that a person who has given consent can withdraw it at any time. This means that if people wish to leave hospital contrary to their best interests, unless they lack the capacity to make a valid decision, they are free to go. Clearly, there are advantages in obtaining the patient's signature that the self-discharge or refusal to accept treatment was contrary to clinical advice. If patients refuse to sign a form that they are taking discharge contrary to clinical advice, that refusal must be accepted. It would in such a case be advisable to ensure that there is another professional who is a witness to this and that a careful record is made by both professionals.

Box 9.4 **Abortion Act 1967 Section 1(1) as amended by the Human Fertilisation and Embryology Act 1990**

A person shall not be guilty of an offence under the law relating to abortion when a pregnancy is terminated by a registered medical practitioner if two registered medical practitioners are of the opinion, formed in good faith:

(a) that the pregnancy has not exceeded its 24th week and that the continuance of the pregnancy would involve risk, greater than if the pregnancy were terminated, of injury to the physical or mental health of the pregnant woman or any existing children of her family; or

(b) that the termination is necessary to prevent grave permanent injury to the physical or mental health of the pregnant woman; or

(c) that the continuance of the pregnancy would involve risk to the life of the pregnant woman, greater than if the pregnancy were terminated; or

(d) that there is a substantial risk that if the child were born it would suffer from such physical or mental abnormalities as to be seriously handicapped.

# LAWS REGULATING PREGNANCY, BIRTH AND CHILDREN

## Abortion Act 1967 as amended (Box 9.4)

The provisions set out in Box 9.4, including the requirement to have two registered medical practitioners, do not apply in an emergency when a registered medical practitioner is of the opinion, formed in good faith, that the termination is immediately necessary to save the life, or to prevent grave permanent injury to the physical or mental health, of the pregnant woman.

## Registration of births and stillbirths; births under 24 weeks

The law requires that every birth is registered. When there is a stillbirth, this is registerable if it occurred after 24 weeks or more of gestation. Miscarriages of less than 24 weeks do not have to be registered, but the body must be disposed of with public decency and the wishes and feelings of the parents taken into consideration. Where a live birth is followed by a death (whatever the length of gestation), there must be a registration of both the birth and the death. In other words, if the baby is born alive, even if only for a brief time, and even where the gestation is less than 24 weeks, a birth must be registered, and if the baby subsequently dies, then a death must be registered.

### Human Fertilisation and Embryology Acts 1990, 1992 and 2008

These Acts provide a legal framework within which infertility treatment and embryo growth and implanting can take place. The Human Fertilisation and Embryology Authority is responsible for licensing centres and issuing a code of practice, and has general responsibility for ensuring that the law is followed.

### Criminal law and attendance at birth

A midwife could face criminal proceedings in respect of her work if she offends against the criminal laws, such as health and safety laws or road traffic Acts. If she acts with gross recklessness or negligence in her professional practice, then she could face criminal proceedings. For example, an anaesthetist was held guilty for the death of a patient in theatre where he acted with such gross recklessness as to amount to a criminal offence of manslaughter (*R* v. *Adomako*, 1995).

Section 16 of the 1997 Nurses, Midwives and Health Visitors Act made it a criminal offence for a person other than a registered midwife or a registered medical practitioner (or student of either) to attend a woman in childbirth except in an emergency or undergoing professional training as doctor or midwife. This is re-enacted in Article 45 of the Nursing and Midwifery Order 2001. If the midwife is obstructed by an aggressive partner during a home confinement, she would be able to call upon police powers to assist her.

### Children Acts 1989 and 2004

The Children Act 1989 set up a framework for the protection and care of children and established clear principles to guide decision-making in relation to their care. This is considered in Chapter 15.

## HEALTH AND SAFETY LAWS

The basic health and safety duties are placed upon employers by the Health and Safety at Work Act 1974. This Act has been supplemented by many statutory instruments defining more specific duties in relation to manual handling, protective clothing, and the management of health and safety in the workplace. These statutory duties are enforceable by the Health and Safety Executive in the criminal courts. In addition, they are paralleled by duties placed on the employer under the common law. As a result of an implied term in the employment contract recognized by the courts, every employer must take reasonable care of the physical and mental health and safety of the employee. Therefore, employers may be liable to pay compensation to an employee where:

(a) the employee is known to be suffering from unacceptable stress, *and*
(b) there is reasonable action which the employer could take but fails to take to relieve the situation *and*
(c) as a consequence, the employee suffers from mental harm.

Duties laid down under the manual handling regulations are also paralleled by the employer's responsibility for ensuring that reasonable action (including that of implementing the regulations) is taken to prevent the employee being harmed through manual handling. Every employer has a responsibility to carry out a risk assessment of dangers and hazards in the workplace, including an assessment for substances hazardous to health under the Control of Substances Hazardous to Health Regulations (2002). Regulations also require any incident involving injuries to be reported (RIDDOR; HSE 1995) and further information is available from the HSE website (www.hse.org.uk/riddor). The Medical Devices Regulations (1995) require adverse incidents involving medical devices to be reported to the Medicines and Healthcare Products Regulatory Agency (MHRA) (replacing the Medical Devices Agency [MDA]) in accordance with the notice revised by the MHRA in 2007 and accessible on the MHRA website (www.mhra.gov.uk). Any warnings issued by the Agency must be acted upon. Employees also have a duty to take reasonable care of their own health and safety and those around them.

## LEGAL ASPECTS OF RECORD-KEEPING

Midwives have clear responsibilities under the Midwives' Rules to ensure that their documentation of their midwifery care is kept properly (NMC 2004b, 2008). In addition, if they leave their post, there are specified duties for the transfer of their records. Their supervisor of midwives is also entitled to inspect their records and record-keeping standards. The NMC has updated the guidance on standards in record-keeping (NMC 2009b). It is recommended that records should be kept for at least 25 years. However, where the midwife is aware that a child has been born with serious mental disabilities, it would be wise for those records to be retained until at least 3 years after that person's death, since in the case of those under a mental disability, there is no time limit for bringing a legal action for compensation as long as they are alive.

The Data Protection Act 1998 covers both computerized and manually held records and requires those who deal with personal records to register their storage and use of those records. The duties laid down in the Act are enforced by criminal proceedings. Rights of subject access to personal health records are given by the Act subject to specified exceptions where serious harm would be caused to the physical or mental health of the applicant or another, or where a third party (not being a health professional caring for the patient) who would be identified by the disclosure has requested not to be identified.

## MEDICINES

Midwives have statutory powers in relation to the prescribing of medication. These are set out in the Rules, and guidance is provided in the code of practice (NMC 2008a) and in the standards for medicine management first published by the NMC in 2007. The NMC has also published *Guidance for continuing professional development for nurse and midwife prescribers* (NMC 2009c).

Refer to Chapter 10 for specific laws and rules governing drugs and medicines.

## COMPLAINTS

A new complaints system covering both health and social care was introduced in April 2009. There are two stages within the complaints procedure: local handling and independent review by the Health Service Ombudsman. However, the procedure emphasizes the importance of resolving complaints at local level if at all possible. Further details of the procedure can be obtained from the Department of Health (DH) website (www.dh.gov.uk).

## MISCELLANEOUS LEGAL ISSUES OF RELEVANCE TO THE MIDWIFE

### Care of property

Failure to look after another person's property could lead to criminal prosecution, for example, theft, civil action for trespass to property, or negligence in causing harm to property. In an action for negligence, the person who has suffered the loss or damage of property must establish the same four elements that must be shown in a claim for compensation for personal injury, that is, duty, breach, causation and harm.

Where, however, property is left by a person (known as the bailor) in the care of another person (the bailee), then, should the property be lost or damaged, the burden would be on the bailee to establish how that occurred without fault on his or her part. This is the situation when a client hands over money or valuables for safekeeping in the ward safe. It should be noted that liability for loss or damage to property can be excluded if such an exclusion is reasonable (see the Unfair Contract Terms Act above).

### Vaccine damage

A statutory scheme for compensation was introduced under the Vaccine Damage Payments Act 1979 to compensate those who have suffered harm as a consequence of receiving vaccines. Public health requires a high level of *herd immunity* to ensure that major infectious diseases are eradicated, and, therefore, a high level of vaccination in the community is required. Since it is recognized that there is a tiny risk of harm from these vaccinations, it was accepted that, as a consequence, there should be compensation for those few who suffered such harm as a result of being vaccinated. The amount available has recently been increased from £100,000 to £120,000. Any applicant must establish that he or she has been severely disabled as a result of a vaccination against the specified diseases of diphtheria, tetanus, whooping cough, poliomyelitis, measles, rubella, tuberculosis, smallpox, and any other disease specified by the Secretary of State for Health. The severe disability must be at least 60% (this was formerly 80%). Whether the disability has been caused by the vaccination shall be established on a balance of probabilities. There was a 6-year time limit on making claims but this is being raised to any time up to the age of 18 years. This will enable more persons disabled by vaccines to claim the payment, including those who have already been rejected, who can reapply under the new rules. An applicant under the statutory scheme is not barred from pursuing a claim in negligence, where, if successful, the level of compensation may be far higher. However, an award under the statutory scheme would be taken into account in a negligence payment and vice versa.

### Congenital Disabilities (Civil Liability) Act 1976

This Act enables a child who is born disabled as a result of pre-birth negligence to obtain compensation from the person responsible for the negligent act. The mother can only be sued if she was negligent when driving a motor car (in this case the child would be suing the mother's insurance company). A recent amendment enables those whose children have been disabled during IVF treatment to obtain compensation.

### Negligent advice

There can be liability for negligence in giving advice, but the claimant would have to show that it was clear to the defendant that he or she would rely upon the advice and in so doing had suffered reasonably foreseeable loss or harm. For example, providing a reference for a student or colleague can lead to liability both to the recipient of the reference, if in reliance upon that reference the recipient has suffered harm, and also to the person who is the subject of the reference (*Hedley Byrne & Co Ltd* v. *Heller & Partners Ltd*, 1963). The latter would have to show that the reference was written without reasonable care, and harm occurred to the subject of the reference as a result of potential employers relying upon the reference (*Spring* v. *Guardian Assurance*, 1994). Every care should therefore be taken to ensure that a reference is written accurately in the light of the facts available.

## STATUTORY DUTIES AND THE DUTY OF QUALITY

Statutory duties are placed upon the Secretary of State for Health to provide a comprehensive service to meet all reasonable needs, and these duties are in turn delegated to the NHS organizations. At regional level, there are strategic health authorities (SHAs) which set the overall strategy and monitor the performance of the NHS organizations for which they are responsible. At local level, primary care trusts (PCTs) arrange for the commissioning of health services from NHS trusts and others and provide primary care services through independent contractors such as family practitioners, pharmacists and dentists (in Wales, this is undertaken by local health boards).

### Clinical governance and the duty of quality

Under Section 45 of the Health and Social Care Act 2008, the Secretary of State has the power to prepare and publish statements of standards in relation to the provision of NHS care, which must be implemented by NHS organizations and are monitored by the Care Quality Commission. Failures in fulfilling this statutory duty could result in the removal of a board or the dismissal of its chief executive and chairman.

*The National Institute of Health and Clinical Excellence* (NICE) was established in April 1999 to promote clinical and cost effectiveness across the country. It investigates medicines, and other treatments, and in the light of its research makes recommendations to the Department of Health on the clinical and cost effectiveness of such treatments. In 2008 it issued guidance on induction of labour. This and other guidelines relating to midwifery services are available on the NICE website (www.nice.org.uk). Guidelines and recommendations made by NICE can be used by midwives to press for additional resources if they are aware that the standards of care and services provided in their units are lower than those nationally recommended.

*The Commission for Health Improvement* (CHI) was established under Sections 19 to 24 of the Health Act 1999 as a body corporate (that is, it can sue and be sued on its own account), with significant powers. It was subsequently replaced by the Commission for Health Audit and Inspection (known as the Healthcare Commission) and has since April 2009 been amalgamated with other inspection bodies, including the Commission for Social Care Inspection and the Mental Health Act Commission, into the *Care Quality Commission*. In 2006 the Healthcare Commission published a report on Northwick Park Hospital following the deaths of ten women in childbirth between 2002 and 2005, which is available on its website (www.cqc.org.uk). In January 2008 the Healthcare Commission reported that more than four in ten maternity units offer below average care. Only 64% of hospitals were carrying out the 11 checks on fetal growth as recommended by NICE. In July 2008, in a review on maternity services, the Healthcare Commission concluded that there were significant weaknesses in maternity and neonatal services across England with a shortage of doctors, midwives and basic medical facilities.

### National Service Frameworks (NSFs)

National Service Frameworks are gradually being published in most clinical areas so that there are identifiable quality standards provided across the country. The NSFs are accessible on the DH's specific website (http://www.dh.gov.uk/en/Healthcare/index.htm). The NSF for Children, Young Persons and Maternity was published in 2004. Standard 11 for maternity services sets the following:

> *Women have easy access to supportive, high quality maternity services, designed around their individual needs and those of their babies.*

## FUTURE CHANGES

Since the Cumberlege Report was published in 1993 (Department of Health 1993), there have been many reports recommending the implementation of changes to secure reasonable standards within maternity services in the NHS. The Audit Commission made recommendations in 1997 (Audit Commission 1997) and Reform published a review in 2005 (Bosanquet et al 2005) showing that progress since Cumberlege had been modest. The King's Fund published an independent inquiry into the safety of maternity services in 2008 (King's Fund 2008), making significant recommendations for reform, which is available on its website (www.kingsfund.org.uk/publications). The Healthcare Commission published a major review in 2008 (Healthcare Commission 2008) which raised serious concerns about the standards in maternity services in England, in spite of the nine reports which the Commission had published on maternity services between 2002 and 2008. In 2007 the Department of Health published *Maternity matters* (Department of Health 2007) setting targets to be achieved by 2009 where all women will have choice over the type of care that they receive, together with improved access to services and continuity of care. Raising the standards of maternity services will clearly be a priority of the Care Quality Commission.

## CONCLUSION

This chapter covers a large area of law of considerable importance to midwifery practice. It is suggested that the reader should follow up this chapter by referring to some of the recommended texts to obtain a more detailed knowledge of the law. The current emphasis on human rights, the growth of litigation, the requirement that there must be sound professional practice, all show the importance of midwives having an understanding of the laws which apply to their practice and how essential it is, as in all other areas of their competence, that they keep up to date. In addition, it is clear from the many reports of the Healthcare Commission and other organizations that maternity services are in general failing to comply with the standards set by the CNST, with the guidance published by NICE and with the recommendations of the Healthcare Commission itself. The Care Quality Commission faces a major challenge in ensuring that necessary improvements take place. Midwives are, as a consequence, likely to experience significant changes in future years.

## KEY POINTS

- It is important that the midwife is aware of how laws, statutes and regulations are developed.
- An understanding of the rules and laws governing practice and healthcare can assist the practitioner in developing strategies and approaches which can improve care, and prevent situations which might lead to litigation.
- It is crucial that midwives keep abreast of development and changes within the law.
- The principles of good communication and informed consent are key to quality of care and experience for clients and their relatives.

## REFERENCES


Audit Commission: *First class delivery – Improving maternity services in England and Wales*, London, 1997, The Stationery Office.

Bosanquet N, Ferry J, Lees C et al: *Maternity services in the NHS*, London, 2005, Reform.

Department of Health: *Changing childbirth: report of the expert maternity group*, Chaired by Baroness Cumberlege, London, 1993, HMSO.

Department of Health: *The new NHS – modern – dependable*, London, 1997, The Stationery Office.

Department of Health (DH): *A first class service*, London, 1998, DH.

Department of Health (DH): *Clinical governance*, London, 1999, DH.

Department of Health (DH): *The NHS plan*, London, 2000, DH.

Department of Health (DH): *Making amends: a consultation paper setting out proposals for reforming the approach to clinical negligence in the NHS*, London, 2003, DH.

Department of Health (DH): *Maternity matters: choice, access and continuity of care in a safe service*, London, 2007, DH.

Health and Safety Executive (HSE): *Reporting of Injuries, Diseases and Dangerous Occurrences Regulations (RIDDOR) 1995*. Available online. htttp://www.allriskmgmt.co.uk/hse/accidents/guide.htm# 1 January 2002.

Healthcare Commission: *Towards better births: A review of maternity services in England*, London, 2008, Stationery Office.

JM Consulting: *Independent Review Report of the Nurses, Midwives and Health Visitors Act. Report to the Department of Health*, Bristol, 1998, JM Consulting.

Kennedy Report: *Bristol Royal Infirmary Inquiry, Learning from Bristol: the report of the public inquiry into children's heart surgery at the Bristol Royal Infirmary 1984–1995*, Command paper Cm 5207, London, 2001, The Stationery Office.

King's Fund: *Safe births: everybody's business. An Independent Inquiry into the safety of maternity services in England*, London, 2008, King's Fund.

NHS Litigation Authority. www.nhsla.com/claims/schemes/cnst Accessed August 23, 2010.

Nursing and Midwifery Council (NMC): *Guidance on provision of midwifery care and delegation of midwifery care to others*, NMC Circular 1/2004, London, 2004a, NMC.

Nursing and Midwifery Council (NMC): *Midwives' rules and standards*, London, 2004b, NMC.

Nursing and Midwifery Council (NMC): *Standards for the preparation and practice of supervisors of midwives*, London, 2006, NMC.

Nursing and Midwifery Council (NMC): *Standards for supervised practice of midwives*, NMC Circular 32/2007, London, 2007, NMC.

Nursing and Midwifery Council (NMC): *The code: standards of conduct, performance and ethics for nurses and midwives*, London, 2008, NMC.

Nursing and Midwifery Council (NMC): *Modern supervision in action: a practical guide for midwives*, London, 2009a, NMC.

Nursing and Midwifery Council (NMC): *Record keeping: guidance for nurses and midwives*, London, 2009b, NMC.

Nursing and Midwifery Council (NMC): *Guidance for continuing professional development for nurse and midwife prescribers*, London, 2009c, NMC.

Rose D: Brain damaged woman is first successful case in Bristol baby scandal, *The Times* 14 March 2008, page 11.

Woolf, Lord: *Access to Justice. Final Report by the Right Honourable the Lord Woolf, Master of the Rolls to the Lord Chancellor on the Civil Justice System in England and Wales*, London, 1996, HMSO.

## STATUTES

Children Act (1989) London: HMSO.

Congenital Disabilities (Civil Liability) Act (1976) London: HMSO.

Control of Substances Hazardous to Health Regulations (2002) London: HMSO.

European Convention for the Protection of Human Rights and Fundamental Freedoms (1951) London: HMSO.

Health Act (1999) London: HMSO.

Health and Social Care Act (2008) London: HMSO.

Human Fertilisation and Embryology Act (1990) London: HMSO.

Human Fertilisation and Embryology (Disclosure of Information) Act (1992) London: HMSO.

Human Rights Act (1998) London: HMSO.

Law Reform (Contributory Negligence) Act (1945) London: HMSO.

Mental Capacity Act (2005) London: HMSO.

Mental Health Acts (1983, 2007) London: HMSO.

National Health Service Litigation Authority (Establishment and Constitution) Order (1995) SI No. 2800. London: HMSO.

Nurses, Midwives and Health Visitors Act (1997) London: HMSO.

Nursing and Midwifery Order (2001) London: HMSO.

Primary Care Act (1997) London: HMSO.

Reporting of Injuries, Diseases and Dangerous Occurrences Regulations (RIDDOR) (1995) London: HMSO.

Stillbirth Definition Act (1992) London: HMSO.

Unfair Contract Terms Act (1977) London: HMSO.

Vaccine Damage Payments Act (1979) London: HMSO.

## CASES

*A National Health Service Trust* v. *D Lloyd, Rep Med* [2000] 411

*Barnett* v. *Chelsea Hospital Management Committee* (HMC) [1968] 1 All ER 1068

*Bolam* v. *Friern Hospital Management Committee* (HMC) [1957] 1 WLR 582

*Bolitho* v. *City and Hackney Health Authority* (HA) [1997] 3 WLR 1151

*Bull and Wakeham* v. *Devon Health Authority* [1993] 4 Med LR 117. CA [1989] 2 February 1989 Transcript

*D.* v. *National Society for the Prevention of Cruelty to Children* [1977] 1 All ER 589

*Donoghue* v. *Stevenson* [1932] AC 562

*Hedley Byrne & Co Ltd* v. *Heller & Partners Ltd* House of Lords [1963] 2 All ER 575

*In re MB (Caesarean Section)* [1997] TLR 18 April; *Re MB (Adult Medical Treatment)* [1997] 2 FLR 426

*Khalid v Barnet and Chase Farm Hospital NHS Trust* [2007] EWHC 644 QB, (2007) 97 BMLR 82

*Lister & Others v. Hesley Hall Ltd*, [2001] UKHL 22 [2002] 1 AC 215; The Times Law Report, 10 May 2001; [2001] 2 WLR 1311

*Maynard* v. *W Midlands Regional Health Authority* HL [1985] 1 All ER 635

*Pearce* v. *United Bristol Healthcare NHS Trust* [1999] 48 BMLR 118

*R.* v. *Adomako* House of Lords [1995] 1 AC 171

*Re C (Adult: Refusal of Medical Treatment)* [1994] 1 All ER 819

*Re T (Adult) Refusal of Medical Treatment* [1992] 4 All ER 649

*Starkey v Rotherham NHS Foundation Trust* [2007] LS Law Medical 456

*Secretary of State for the Home Department* v. *Orb* [1995] 1 All ER 677

*Sidaway* v. *Bethlem Royal Hospital Governors* [1985] 1 All ER 643

*Spring* v. *Guardian Assurance plc and others* [1994] TLR 8 July

*St George's Healthcare National Health Service Trust* v. *S* [1998] TLR August 3 CA: 3 All ER 673

*Taylor* v. *West Kent Health Authority* [1997] 8 Med LR 251

*Walker* v. *Northumberland County Council* [1995] 1 All ER 737

*Whitehouse* v. *Jordan* [1981] 1 All ER 267

*Wilsher* v. *Essex Area Health Authority* [1986] 3 All ER 801 CA

*Wilsher* v. *Essex Area Health Authority* [1988] AC 1074 HL

Chapter |10|

# Pharmacology and the midwife

Sue Jordan

## LEARNING OUTCOMES

After reading this chapter, you will be able to:

- appraise the potential benefits and harms of drugs administered in normal labour
- understand the actions of drugs commonly administered in childbirth
- use this knowledge to inform decisions on clinical monitoring, advice and advocacy.

Few women go through pregnancy, childbirth and the puerperium without receiving some form of medication. Ideally, all medication administration, management and monitoring would be based on the results of adequately sized randomized controlled trials with high response rates, supported by large pharmacovigilance follow-up databases and service users' views (Jordan 2008). In practice, this 'gold standard' is rarely achieved in any discipline, and in midwifery there are additional ethical and practical difficulties, which are compounded when investigating the adverse reactions of medication (Jordan 2010, 2007). Therefore, medication administration may be based on biological theories, observations, case reports or even 'custom and practice'.

## THERAPEUTICS IN CHILDBIRTH

Not all treatments are effective, and patients need to be monitored to detect non-response, particularly when antihypertensives, anticoagulants, antiemetics or analgesics are administered. Sometimes, underlying physiological problems may worsen, rendering a previously effective regimen useless; for example, as labour progresses, more analgesia may be required. More predictably, therapeutic failure may be induced by drug interactions – for example, if a patient with hypertension self-medicates with ibuprofen or another non-steroidal anti-inflammatory drug (NSAID). Clinical response shows considerable individual variation, which is not always predictable, and idiosyncratic reactions can occur; for example, some women are unduly sensitive to oxytocin, and therefore infusions are commenced using very low doses.

## ADVERSE REACTIONS

An adverse drug reaction is any untoward and unintended response in a patient or investigational subject to a medicinal product which is related to any dose administered (ICH 1996). Adverse drug reactions can be broadly divided into:

- dose-related and predictable
- neither dose-related nor predictable
- transgenerational effects.

### *Dose-dependent adverse reactions*

These are often the drug's main adverse effects. Since these are often significant and predictable, they are monitored. For example, without adequate monitoring, anticoagulants can cause bleeding, and insulin can cause hypoglycaemia.

Many drugs have more than one action, potentially causing diverse adverse reactions. For example, oxytocin acts on the oxytocic receptors of the uterus, but it also acts on the antidiuretic hormone (ADH) receptors in the nephrons and can cause water retention and fluid overload.

### *Adverse reactions unrelated to dose: hypersensitivity responses*

Some of the most serious adverse events are unpredictable, *idiosyncratic, allergic* or *hypersensitivity* responses, which may occur in any situation with any drug at any dose: common offenders include antimicrobials (particularly intravenous), hormone preparations, dextrans, heparin, vaccines, blood products, iron injections, and local anaesthetics. These adverse events are not related to known physiological actions of the drug, but are initiated when drugs trigger the immune system of susceptible people. They include: *anaphylaxis, drug rashes, bone marrow dysfunction,* and *organ damage*.

A mild hypersensitivity reaction is usually a rash. Once this has occurred, and particularly if any itching was associated, the individual is likely to be sensitized and more likely to have an anaphylactic reaction at the next exposure. Where drugs have similar chemical structures, cross-allergies occur: for example, up to 10% of people allergic to *penicillins* will also be allergic to *cephalosporins*.

### *Transgenerational adverse reactions*

Pregnancy, childbirth, breastfeeding or the developing infant may be affected.

## DRUGS IN PREGNANCY

No drugs have been subjected to randomized controlled clinical trials for teratogenicity in human pregnancy; evidence is largely derived from observational studies, case reports of incidental exposure, and animal studies, and, therefore, no drug has been demonstrated as 'safe'.

Approximately 4.8% of births and 4.0% of live births in Wales in 1998–2003 were associated with a congenital anomaly (CARIS 2007). The causes of about two-thirds of congenital anomalies remain unknown, and fewer than 1% are attributable to prescribed drugs (Ruggiero 2006). Exposure of either parent to a medicinal product at any time during conception or pregnancy should be reported in association with congenital anomalies (ICH 1996).

Relatively few drugs are known to cause fetal malformations, but only drugs that have been used for many years in thousands of women with no evidence of harm can be designated 'generally regarded as safe'. No teratogenic drugs are harmful to the developing fetus in **all** cases. Estimates vary as to the incidence of congenital malformations: up to 30% with *warfarin*, up to 16% with *sodium valproate* (Aronson 2006). However, drugs may affect fetal growth, birthweight, preterm delivery, childbirth, neonatal health and childhood development.

Fetus vulnerability (see website also) is usually considered in stages:

- *Pre-implantation* (0–14 days): may result in death or no effect.
- *Cell division* (14–17 days): medications may cause abortion.
- *Organ differentiation* (18–55 days): a period of vulnerability for several drugs, The central nervous system (CNS), inner ear and palate continue developing after this.
- *During later stages of pregnancy:* the functioning, rather than the structure, of organs may be damaged throughout pregnancy by several drugs, including *alcohol, cocaine, insulin, furosemide,* and *antithyroid agents*. Some can cause neurobehavioural deficits.

Drug administration during pregnancy and breastfeeding is based on assessment of risks and benefits. Prescribing is likely to be restricted if drug exposure is known to result in a consistent pattern of similar anomalies or the incidence of congenital anomalies is above the rate in the population of 4%. The risks of fetal damage depend on several factors as well as the chemical composition of the drug:

- stage of pregnancy
- amount of drug ingested
- number of doses – a single dose may be less damaging than repeated exposure
- other agents to which mother and fetus are exposed
- mother's nutritional status
- genetic makeup of mother and fetus.

This is complicated by epidemiological work linking congenital malformations, particularly cleft lip, cleft palate and congenital heart malformations, with adverse life events associated with severe maternal stress during the first trimester (Hansen et al 2000), and stillbirth with high levels of psychological stress (Wisborg et al 2008).

### Drugs in childbirth

Drugs given during childbirth may have long-term effects. Antibiotics may alter the micro-organisms in the neonate's colon, which, in turn, might affect the regulation of the immune system, allowing development of allergy (Jordan et al 2008, Russell & Murch 2006). Also, drugs administered in labour may reduce the chances of breastfeeding (see opioids, below).

### Pharmacology in pregnancy and lactation

The actions and adverse reactions of any drug depend on the drug and its interactions with the body (*pharmacodynamics*) and on the concentration of the drug in the tissues, which is affected by how the drug is administered, absorbed, distributed and eliminated (*pharmacokinetics*). Following administration, drugs are absorbed, and distributed to their sites of action before being removed from the body: if elimination is compromised, there is a risk of drug accumulation and toxicity in either the woman or the fetus/neonate.

### Breastfed infants

Most drugs pass into breast milk, but the concentrations are often too small to be harmful. Drugs that can be administered to neonates are usually suitable for nursing mothers, for example *paracetamol*. For a few drugs, such as *lithium* or *clozapine*, there are reports of serious adverse reactions in infants (Lawrence & Schaefer 2007).

## DRUG ADMINISTRATION AND ABSORPTION

Absorption makes the drug available for distribution. The extent to which a drug reaches its destination is its 'bioavailability' (Wilkinson 2001:5), and depends on formulation and route of administration.

The formulation of a medicine refers to its physical and chemical composition and includes active ingredients and other chemicals present, the *excipients* or 'packing chemicals'. Excipients:

- stabilize the active ingredient or modify its release
- are listed in the product information
- may be responsible for adverse reactions; for example, sodium can be responsible for fluid retention and sugar for dental caries
- may vary between brands; for example, brands of antiepileptic drugs, mood stabilizers or antipsychotics should not be regarded as interchangeable without advice from a pharmacist or consultant.

### Routes of administration

**Oral:**

- Most convenient drug administration route.
- Presence of food, antacids or bulk laxatives in the stomach can affect drug absorption for up to 2 hours – for example, amoxicillin, iron tablets.
- Administration with food is sometimes advantageous in smoothing the absorption profile – for example, nifedipine, iron.
- Drug molecules from the stomach or small intestine pass to the liver, where they are metabolized and detoxified before entering the systemic circulation. This reduces and delays absorption to a varying, and not always predictable, extent.

**Intravenous administration:**

- Employed when rapid, reliable and complete absorption is required.

**Intramuscular injections:**

- Rapidly deliver drugs to the bloodstream.
- Haemorrhage or shock may delay absorption and adverse reactions.

**Subcutaneous injections:**

- Slower absorption.

**Sublingual or buccal administration:**

- Bypasses the liver.
- Rapid, not necessarily predictable, action.
- Can be useful in emergencies, including recurrent seizures or hypoglycaemia.

**Rectal route:**

- Some cultural considerations and practical difficulties.
- Useful for short-term drug administration, if other routes unavailable.
- Laxatives, antiemetics, analgesics and treatments for ulcerative colitis are sometimes administered this way.
- Drugs absorbed from the upper two-thirds of the rectum pass to the liver.
- Those absorbed from the lower region enter the general circulation – absorption unpredictable.

**Topical applications:**

- Examples, direct application to skin, eyes or ears.
- Systemic effects are reduced, but not abolished.

**Intrathecal (spinal) and epidural administration:**

- Increases the proportion of drug reaching the central nervous system.
- Following intrathecal administration, drug diffuses into the epidural space before circulating (Eltzschig et al 2003). Appreciable quantities are absorbed into the epidural venous plexus and pass to the general circulation, the brain and the fetus.
- Headache, pruritus and fetal bradycardia may occur more commonly with intrathecal than epidural analgesia (Collis et al 2008).
- Technical problems include: failure to flex the spine; kinking of lines; accidental removal of lines; dural puncture; need for re-insertion (Paech 1998).
- Complications include: puncture site tenderness for up to 7 days; dural puncture headache; intravascular injection; infection; epidural haematoma; abscess formation; accidental total spinal anaesthesia. Around 4 per million women suffer persistent neurological complications (Ruppen et al 2006).

### Therapeutic range

Every drug has a therapeutic range for the concentration of drug in plasma and tissues: above this, toxic effects are more likely; below it, the drug is less likely to have the desired effect. For some drugs, the range is narrow, and the therapeutic concentration is close to the concentration at which side-effects appear; for example, antiepileptic drugs, *warfarin, insulin, opioids*. For others, the therapeutic range is wide in most individuals, and there is a larger 'safety margin' between therapeutic and toxic dose. For example, in people not suffering from epilepsy, *penicillins* and *folic acid* are relatively safe, even in overdose.

For a medicine with a narrow therapeutic range, dose administration intervals are calculated to prevent more than twofold fluctuations in plasma concentrations. If strict adherence to dose intervals fails, both toxicity and therapeutic failure are likely. For example, where these drugs require administration twice each day, they should be given 12 hours apart (Wilkinson 2001). Where medicines must be given four times a day – that is, every 6 hours – this may involve disturbing sleep.

## Drug distribution

Movement of drugs around the body is affected by drug properties (lipid solubility and binding), state of the circulation and other organs, pregnancy, breastfeeding, and infancy. Highly lipid-soluble drugs rapidly pass into the brain, fetus and breast milk. For example, *diamorphine* and *fentanyl* are distributed more rapidly than *morphine* – advantageous during emergency caesarean deliveries.

### *Pregnancy*

Most drugs are lipid soluble and cross the placenta during pregnancy, to varying extents, but not all are harmful.

### *Childbirth*

The placenta is an ineffective barrier to the passage of drugs, and the blood–brain barrier is underdeveloped in the fetus. Permeability may be further increased during stress, labour and hypoxia. Drugs administered in labour may enter the fetus, and may cause adverse reactions in the neonate; for example, opioids, local anaesthetics or magnesium can induce respiratory depression.

### *Lactation*

Most drugs pass into breast milk (though concentrations may be too small to be harmful): the amount varies between women, during feeds, with the age of the infant and with use of a breast pump. The relative dose as a proportion of body weight received by the infant depends on the drug administered (for example, the dose of lithium is 80% of maternal dose), and the maturity of the infant's liver and kidneys (Lawrence & Schaefer 2007).

### *Neonates*

The body of the neonate contains a relatively high proportion of water and a low proportion of fat. Any lipid-soluble drugs are therefore distributed into a small volume. Thus, neonates, particularly premature babies, receive different drug doses from adults, even when body weight is taken into consideration.

## Elimination or clearance of drugs

Route of elimination varies with individual drugs, but most are:

- metabolized in the liver
- excreted in the kidneys.

A few drugs (such as magnesium, lithium) are eliminated unchanged, whereas others are extensively metabolized. Some metabolites are active, for example those of *carbamazepine* and *opioids*, while others may cause adverse reactions, such as *pethidine*. Most drugs are excreted via the kidneys, although bile is also an important route of excretion, for example for *oestrogens* and *corticosteroids*.

### Drug metabolism

Most metabolism takes place in the liver, though the gastrointestinal tract and the central nervous system contain enzymes responsible for the metabolism of some drugs. Metabolism deals with and detoxifies foreign substances. Metabolism varies with:

- *genetic makeup/familial tendencies*
- *drug interactions*: rate of metabolism and elimination may be increased or decreased by drugs, foods or herbs.

### Drug excretion

Most drugs depend on the kidneys for excretion. Glomerular filtration rate (GFR), usually considered the best overall measure of the kidneys' ability to eliminate drugs in health and disease (Levey et al 1999), is the volume of fluid filtered into the nephrons every minute, that is, the sum of the volume of filtrate formed each minute in all the functioning nephrons in the kidneys. This represents about 20% of the plasma flowing through the kidneys. In normal pregnancy, the circulating volume expands by some 8 litres, and renal plasma flow and GFR rises by 30–50% in the second trimester and declines towards term. This increases the elimination of certain drugs (Loebstein et al 1997). Therefore, doses of ongoing therapeutic regimens may need to be increased, particularly antiepileptic drugs and low molecular weight heparins. By the fourth week of pregnancy, GFR has risen 20%; therefore, increased drug elimination and decreased drug effects may occur before the woman realizes she is pregnant (Perrone et al 1992).

If GFR falls, elimination of most drugs is impaired, causing accumulation and even toxicity. If GFR is below normal, as occurs in pre-eclampsia, most drugs are administered in reduced doses or at prolonged intervals. In seriously ill women, rapidly changing GFR may complicate administration of *magnesium sulphate*.

The kidneys of the fetus eliminate drugs slowly into the amniotic fluid, which is then ingested through the mouth, further reducing clearance. The GFR of the neonate is only 30–40% of adult values. Therefore, some drugs, such as *magnesium*, may accumulate following maternal administration. These neonates should be observed for signs of muscle weakness, including respiratory depression, for 48 hours after delivery. Some drugs, such as *lithium*, may accumulate during breastfeeding.

## Pharmacodynamics

Most drugs work as a result of the physiochemical interactions between drug molecules and the recipient's molecules: cell receptors, ion channels or enzymes. These chemical reactions may alter the way the cells are functioning, which in turn may lead to changes in the behaviour of tissues, organs and systems.

An agonist will bind to a receptor and alter its functioning. For example *salbutamol*, prescribed for asthma or tocolysis, is a beta$_2$-agonist, *pethidine* is an opioid agonist. Agonists usually augment the normal function of the receptors to which they bind. For example, *pethidine* stimulates the opioid receptors, increasing analgesia, sedation and constipation. Likewise, beta-agonists mimic some of the actions of the sympathetic nervous system, increasing heart rate, dilating bronchioles and relaxing the uterus.

An antagonist will bind to a receptor, blocking it and preventing the agonist reaching its site of action. For example, *naloxone* (*Narcan*) blocks the opioid receptors and reverses the actions of *pethidine*, reducing respiratory depression and sedation, but causing return of pain. Similarly, the beta-blockers (*propranolol, atenolol, labetalol*) block the actions of the sympathetic nervous system, slow and stabilize the heart rate and induce bronchoconstriction: they are contraindicated for people who suffer from asthma, due to the risk of life-threatening narrowing of the airways (BNF 2009:86).

Most drugs act on more than one type of cell, and therefore have multiple effects on the body. For example, nicotine acts on the central nervous system to 'calm the nerves', on the blood vessels to raise blood pressure, and on the respiratory epithelium to cause irritation. Other drugs are relatively specific; for example, penicillins act almost exclusively on bacterial cell walls.

Where drugs act on the same or similar receptors, ion channels or enzymes or have similar actions or adverse reactions, their actions are intensified if they are co-administered. For example, co-administration of two or more sedatives can cause respiratory depression.

The cells' receptors are continually being renewed by their protein-synthesizing machinery. When a drug is administered over a period of time, the cells or their receptors may adapt: the number of receptors available on the cell surface may change in response to the presence of drugs.

### *Tolerance or desensitization*

The continued presence of an agonist may reduce the number of relevant receptors available. This desensitization or downregulation of receptors is believed to be responsible for the loss of response seen with continued use of opiates, oxytocin or beta$_2$-agonists (bronchodilators). For example, prolonged administration of oxytocin may render the uterine muscle unresponsive, leading to the uterus not contracting following delivery, increasing the risk of postpartum haemorrhage. In these circumstances, the uterus will not respond to oxytocin and other agents (for example, prostaglandins, ergometrine) will be needed to combat the haemorrhage (Robinson et al 2003).

### *Supersensitivity*

Conversely, the continued presence of an antagonist or blocking drug may increase the number of receptors. Therefore, if an antagonist is abruptly discontinued, the tissues may be unduly sensitive. For example, abrupt withdrawal of beta-blockers makes the myocardium unduly responsive to stress, which increases the risk of a heart attack.

# DRUGS IN LABOUR

## Analgesics

- Inhalational analgesia
- Opioids
- Local anaesthetics (see website).

Many women request pharmacological pain relief in labour, and all drugs have advantages and disadvantages.

### Inhalational analgesia: nitrous oxide with oxygen (Entonox)

Widespread use of *nitrous oxide* for over a hundred years has established its relative safety. Nevertheless, the administration requires close supervision. There is no indication that *Entonox* affects the progress of labour or breastfeeding. Other methods of analgesia are more effective, but are associated with more adverse reactions, both short and long term.

Inhalation analgesia is achieved by the use of an anaesthetic gas, nitrous oxide, in sub-anaesthetic concentrations. Concentrations of 50% nitrous oxide are needed for effective analgesia. If administered with air, rather than oxygen, hypoxia would ensue. Nitrous oxide is now administered as *Entonox*, using pre-mixed cylinders of 50% nitrous oxide in 50% oxygen as a homogenous gas (BOC 2004).

Nitrous oxide rapidly passes from the lungs to the circulation and brain. Analgesic effects of nitrous oxide are experienced some 25–35 seconds after administration, persisting for about 60 seconds after inhalation ceases. Therefore, women are advised to inhale on palpation of a contraction, rather than wait for the pain to reach a crescendo.

Being lipid soluble, inhalation agents cross the placenta and enter adipose tissue. The concentration of nitrous oxide in the fetus reaches 80% of maternal values within 3 minutes of administration. Like all anaesthetic gases, it is rapidly eliminated through the lungs after delivery. This is an advantage over other analgesics, which depend on the immature liver and kidneys for removal. In both mother and neonate it is estimated that the effects of *Entonox* have worn off after 2 to 3 minutes, although removal from tissues with low blood flow, such as fat, takes longer (Kennedy & Longnecker 1996).

When *Entonox* is inhaled, the women may overbreathe to maximize analgesia, risking the exhalation of too much carbon dioxide, lowering the concentration in the blood, causing:

- vasoconstriction of the placental bed and fetal hypoxia
- maternal hypoventilation between contractions, leading to fetal hypoxia
- cerebral vasoconstriction, causing dizziness
- alkalosis, which may induce tetany.

Therefore, women's respirations are closely supervised during administration of *Entonox*.

### *Actions and adverse reactions*

Anaesthetic gases gradually suppress the reticular activating system in the brainstem, producing four stages, or depths, of anaesthesia:

1. Analgesia
2. Delirium
3. Surgical anaesthesia
4. Depression of the vital centres of the medulla.

When *Entonox* is administered, the aim is to achieve analgesia – excessive administration may give the second stage of anaesthesia, characterized by 'lightheadedness', dizziness, nausea or 'laughing'. Sedation or confusion may occur, though nitrous oxide is insufficiently powerful to produce surgical anaesthesia when used alone. Prolonged exposure to nitrous oxide can inactivate vitamin $B_{12}$ and may also affect pregnancy.

### *Interactions*

The respiratory depressant action of opioids may be compounded by nitrous oxide, causing transient maternal hypoxia (Clyburn & Rosen 1993).

### *Cautions*

Nitrous oxide is contraindicated where abnormal quantities of gas are trapped within the body, for example in women with middle ear occlusion or sinus infections (BOC 2004). Nitrous oxide may also diffuse into air bubbles formed by epidural or intrathecal analgesia, hindering the spread of local anaesthetic (Sweetman et al 2007).

Nitrous oxide should not be administered to women whose level of consciousness is already impaired.

To reduce the risk of cross-infection, including hepatitis C, appropriate microbiological filters should be placed between the patient and the breathing system; supplying clean masks and mouthpieces may not be sufficient (AAGBI 1996, Chilvers & Weisz 2000).

## Opioids

The term 'opioid' is used to describe any preparation acting on the body's opioid receptors, which normally respond to endorphins and enkephalins, the body's natural mood changers and analgesics. Thus, *morphine, diamorphine, pethidine, meptazinol, codeine, buprenorphine (Temgesic), pentazocine (Fortral), fentanyl* and its derivatives, and the 'morphine antagonists' such as *naloxone (Narcan)* are all opioids.

Opioids are used in labour, preoperatively, intraoperatively, postoperatively and in intensive care, for analgesia, sedation and reduction of anxiety. Administration may be intramuscular, intravenous, epidural, intrathecal, oral, transdermal or buccal.

Opioids are rapidly transferred across the blood–brain barrier, the placenta and into colostrum. Transfer is more rapid and complete for the more lipophilic compounds, such as *diamorphine, fentanyl* and *fentanyl derivatives*. The fetus and neonate excrete opioids more slowly than adults, due to the immaturity of their liver enzymes. The concentration of opioids will always be higher in the fetus than in the woman, in proportion to the dose administered. This delayed clearance allows accumulation in the central nervous system, which could be sufficient to produce subtle behavioural changes, such as depression of feeding reflexes (Jordan et al 2005).

Following a single intramuscular dose of *pethidine* to the mother, the fetus receives maximum exposure 2 to 3 hours later; therefore, respiratory depression in the neonate is most likely in babies born at this time. If delivery occurs within 1 hour of pethidine administration, very little drug is transferred to the fetus. Should delivery occur more than 6 hours after administration, much of the pethidine will have been transferred back to the mother, although the active metabolite, normeperidine, will remain in the neonatal tissues, and is gradually excreted over several days. During this time the neonate's behaviour will be suboptimal (irritable and difficult to feed) (Crowell et al 1994). *Pethidine* passes into breast milk, which compounds early difficulties with feeding.

### *Epidural and intrathecal opioids and local anaesthetics*

Epidural administration entails injection into the fat in the narrow space between the dura mater and the bony canal. Intrathecal administration involves placing the drug in the cerebrospinal fluid (CSF) by passing a very thin needle through the dura mater.

Opioids and local anaesthetics may be administered epidurally or intrathecally or in combination as combined spinal-epidural (CSE) analgesia. These are the most effective strategies for pain relief. Epidural or CSE analgesia is usually achieved and maintained with *bupivacaine* and *fentanyl*, with *diamorphine* reserved for urgent situations (NCC 2004).

Following epidural administration, drugs diffuse through the dura, where they act on the receptors in the spinal cord. Absorption is increased at delivery when the mother is spontaneously pushing, and 'top up' injections are usually avoided at this time.

### *Actions*

Opioid receptor binding triggers changes within nerve or smooth muscle cells, usually inhibiting their activity and neurotransmitter release. Several classes of opioid receptors exist and different opioids act selectively.

In general, opioids (endogenous and pharmacological) depress the activity of target tissues and have a calming effect. They inhibit the hypothalamus and 'damp down' the level of activity in the autonomic nervous system, partly by reducing the stress response attributable to noradrenaline (norepinephrine). Sometimes, sedation, mental detachment or euphoria are the predominant effects, and the woman may be able to tolerate pain, while still perceiving sensations.

Opioids regulate endocrine, gastrointestinal, autonomic and immune systems, and may trigger histamine release. They also act directly on the chemoreceptor trigger zone, which activates the vomiting centre, and interact with dopamine in the areas of the brain associated with 'reward'.

### *Adverse reactions*

Opioids produce drowsiness, mental clouding and sometimes euphoria. They inhibit the vital centres in the brainstem of mother and neonate. Sedation is intensified with higher doses and intravenous administration. Epidural administration of >100 micrograms fentanyl or equivalent may sedate and depress the respirations of infants (NCC 2007).

#### ***Respiratory depression***

Opioids act directly on the respiratory centre to depress respiration, reducing the sensitivity of the respiratory centre to carbon dioxide, thereby depressing the normal drive to respiration. Therefore, respiration fails to increase to meet the high metabolic demands of labour. Rate, depth and regularity of respirations are decreased, reducing alveolar ventilation and oxygenation. This effect is intensified if the woman becomes so sedated that she falls asleep. If the circulation is adequate, respiratory depression is maximal within 90 minutes of intramuscular administration. Following administration of normal doses of intrathecal or epidural opioids, maternal respiratory depression, apnoea and sedation may occur 30 minutes later or be delayed up to 16 hours (Clyburn & Rosen 1993).

Respiratory depression during labour may lead to:

- retention of carbon dioxide and respiratory acidosis, in mother and fetus
- hypoxia in mother and fetus, which causes fetal heart rate decelerations
- the fetus developing acidosis – increasing accumulation of pethidine and metabolites.

In the neonate, measurements with fetal scalp electrodes indicate that transcutaneous oxygen tensions fall to 37% of baseline values 7 minutes after the intramuscular administration of 50 mg pethidine but recover within 15 minutes (Clyburn & Rosen 1993). Depression of the central nervous system reduces the neonate's reflexes, including the respiratory reflexes needed to cope with hypoxia and birth (Wagner 1993). Neonatal respiratory depression is occasionally sufficiently severe to warrant rapid reversal with *naloxone*.

#### ***Bradycardia***

Opioids reduce the heart rate, by direct action on the cardiovascular centres in the medulla, by decreasing the activity of the sympathetic nervous system and by reducing anxiety. In labour, this may contribute to a fall in blood pressure and a reduction in placental perfusion. The subsequent depression of the fetal heart rate and loss of fetal heart baseline variability may be interpreted as fetal distress, triggering medical interventions.

Some fetal bradycardia on administration of opioid analgesia by any route is normal, attributed to the transient release of oxytocin, causing a brief tetanic contraction of the uterus (Eberle & Norris 1996). Bradycardia lasting beyond 5 to 8 minutes may be a sign of metabolic stress (Arkoosh 1991).

#### ***Hypotension***

Opioids act on the cardiovascular centres, blood vessels and sympathetic nervous system to produce a fall in blood pressure, exaggerated on standing or sitting up, partly due to inhibition of the baroreceptor reflex. Any hypotension is likely to be exaggerated by the fetus compressing the maternal aorta and vena cava if the mother adopts the supine position.

When opioids are administered epidurally or intrathecally, hypotension is likely to occur within 30 minutes of administration. This may be accompanied by severe fetal bradycardia (Richardson 2000).

### *Thermoregulation*

Opioids impair thermoregulation. Extra care is taken to ensure that the neonate is kept warm.

### *Breastfeeding*

Opioids administered in labour transfer into the fetus, impairing coordination and suckling post birth (Jordan et al 2005). Women who have received high doses of analgesics in labour may need extra support over the first 1–3 days to establish breastfeeding (Jordan 2006).

### *Prolonged labour*

The initial brief tetanic uterine contraction (Eberle & Norris 1996) is superseded by reduced contractility of uterine smooth muscle due to decreased release of oxytocin (Carter 2003). Opioids reduce both the uterine response to oxytocin and the oxytocin release from the posterior pituitary (Thompson & Hillier 1994), diminishing uterine contractions (Carter 2003).

### *Retention of urine and dysuria*

Opioids inhibit the smooth muscle of the bladder and the voiding reflex – a full bladder may inhibit uterine contractions both during labour and post partum.

### *Gastrointestinal effects*

Opioids inhibit the propulsive, peristaltic actions of the gut, while increasing segmental, non-propulsive contractions, particularly in the pyloric region of the stomach, the first part of the duodenum and the colon. Gastric stasis may cause nausea, vomiting, and oesophageal reflux. Opioids contribute to the constipation which commonly follows delivery and decrease gastrointestinal secretions, causing a dry mouth. Spasm of the biliary tract, producing pain on the right side of the abdomen, and gastrointestinal obstruction are rare adverse reactions.

### *Pruritus*

Inhibition of peripheral nerves and histamine release may cause flushing, itching, 'nettle rash' and sweating, particularly following intrathecal administration (Simmons et al 2007).

### *Other potential problems*

These include:

- Myoclonus
- Fluid imbalance
- Suppressed immune responses
- Bronchospasm.

### *Cautions and contraindications*

These include:

- increased intracranial pressure (stroke, head injury): opioids may increase intracranial pressure and obscure vital signs/pupil reflexes
- decreased respiratory reserve, including obesity and kyphosis; contraindicated if carbon dioxide partial pressure is increased
- pregnancy (long-term use) and breastfeeding
- known allergy or dependence on opioids
- renal insufficiency
- neonates and premature babies require proportionately lower doses – fentanyl may cause jaundice.

Conditions that may be worsened include:

- asthma
- convulsive disorders (particularly tramadol, pethidine)
- biliary colic, pancreatitis
- conditions where there is a possibility of paralytic ileus
- pre-existing hypotension – for example, due to haemorrhage
- hypothyroidism or Addison's disease
- acute alcohol intoxication
- liver failure
- phaeochromocytoma
- myasthenia gravis.

### *Interactions*

Hypotension, sedation and respiratory depression may be intensified by: alcohol, antihistamines, barbiturates, anaesthetics (nitrous oxide), benzodiazepines, metoclopramide, phenothiazines, tricyclic antidepressants, and other non-opioid sedatives. Protease inhibitors, cimetidine and, occasionally, ranitidine may have this effect.

Central nervous system toxicity may occur if *pethidine* (possibly also *fentanyl*) is administered within 2 weeks of any *monoamine oxidase inhibitors (MAOIs;* including *moclobemide* and, possibly, *linezolid*) or *selegiline* or *rasagiline* (for Parkinson's).

Myoclonus is more likely with co-administration of: *chlorpromazine, haloperidol, amitriptyline* and some *NSAIDs* (but not *diclofenac*).

Drying of secretions, and therefore need for mouth care, is intensified by co-administration of *hyoscine, cyclizine* or related drugs (see antiemetics).

## **Uterotonics** (for more information, see the website)

Uterotonics or oxytocics are used for induction and augmentation of labour, prevention and treatment of postpartum haemorrhage, and control of bleeding due to incomplete abortion. Uterotonics used in the UK are:

- *prostaglandins*
- *oxytocin*
- *ergometrine*
- *Syntometrine®* – a combination of *oxytocin* and *ergometrine*.

## Prostaglandins

These are 'local hormones' and are commonly used to stimulate uterine contractions.

- *Dinoprostone ($PGE_2$)*, for cervical priming and induction of labour, is administered vaginally.
- *Carboprost (15- methyl-$PGF_{2\alpha}$, synthetic derivative)*, for postpartum haemorrhage, is given by deep intramuscular injection.

### *Actions and adverse reactions*

Prostaglandins act on distinct prostaglandin receptors, affect many systems, and can occasionally cause adverse effects, including hypotension, bronchospasm, pyrexia, sensitization to pain, inflammation, glaucoma, tremor and diuresis. Hypertension may complicate administration of *carboprost*.

Following vaginal administration, the most important adverse reaction is uterine hyperstimulation. Uterine contractions may become abnormal and too intense, leading to pain, fetal compromise or even rupture of the uterus or cervix, with or without previous caesarean delivery. Lower doses and, possibly, gel formulations of *dinoprostone* present less risk (NCC 2008).

## Oxytocin

Oxytocin (Syntocinon®) is manufactured to reproduce the structure and actions of the natural hormone. These actions include:

- uterine contraction at term both by direct action on smooth muscle and by increased prostaglandin production
- constriction of umbilical blood vessels
- contraction of myoepithelial cells (milk ejection reflex)
- bonding (Leng et al 2008)
- attenuation of the stress response (Slattery & Neumann 2008)
- sudden increase or decrease in blood pressure (particularly diastolic)
- water retention.

High-dose oxytocin can shorten prolonged labours (Blanch et al 1998, Sadler et al 2000), while increasing the risk of uterine hyperstimulation (NCC 2007). Failure of induction necessitating emergency caesarean is more likely if the woman has a high body mass index or the baby is heavy (McEwan 2007).

Oxytocin is administered for:

- induction of labour
- augmentation or stimulation of delayed labour by intravenous infusion, to shorten first stage (NCC 2007)
- prevention of postpartum haemorrhage either by:
  - intramuscular injection (alone or combined with ergometrine)
  - slow intravenous injection or intravenous infusion for high-risk women or following caesarean delivery (CEMACH 2005)
- treatment of postpartum haemorrhage by slow intravenous injection or infusion
- incomplete, inevitable or missed abortion (BNF 2009)
- management of retained placenta by injection into umbilical vein (NCC 2007).

Oxytocin acts within 1–4 minutes of intravenous administration; increased uterine contractions begin almost immediately, stabilize within 15–60 minutes of commencing intravenous infusion and last for 20 minutes after discontinuation. Oxytocin is removed by enzymes in the liver, spleen, ovaries and placenta. Estimates of half-life range from 1 to 20 minutes, although pharmacological data indicate a value of 15 minutes (Gonser 1995).

### *Adverse reactions*

#### *Overstimulation of the uterus*

When oxytocin is administered, frequency and force of smooth muscle contractions are increased, intensifying the labour pain, more so than with prostaglandins (NCC 2008). Women report that oxytocin-induced contractions are more painful than those of spontaneous labour. Augmentation of labour with oxytocin carries an inherent risk of uterine hyperstimulation: since some individuals are hypersensitive to oxytocin, infusion always entails risk of tetanic or spasmodic uterine contractions, however low the dose.

During uterine contraction, blood vessels are compressed, impairing delivery of oxygen to the uterus, placenta and fetus. Normally, oxygenation is restored during relaxation, preventing the accumulation of lactic acid. However, if the uterus is overstimulated and relaxation is too brief, fetal hypoxia and acidosis will follow. Uterine tetany or spasm may reduce uterine blood flow to a point where the fetus is asphyxiated.

#### *Fluid retention*

Oxytocin, particularly in high doses, mimics the actions of antidiuretic hormone, and without careful monitoring may produce dangerous fluid retention. Any water retained passes, by osmosis, from plasma into tissue fluids, and thence into the cells, which swell. This causes confusion and disorientation, progressing to convulsions with or without oedema, raised jugular venous pressure and pulmonary oedema, which impairs breathing and oxygenation. The danger is greatest with administration of prolonged high doses of oxytocin, accompanied by infusions of large volumes of electrolyte-free or hypotonic fluids such as 5% glucose (BNF 2009). In reported cases of water intoxication, more than 3.5 litres of fluid had been infused (Sweetman et al 2007).

### *Changes in blood pressure*

In conjunction with its antidiuretic actions, oxytocin may induce vasoconstriction and hypertension, particularly in women with pre-eclampsia. In contrast, administration of large amounts of oxytocin may cause vasodilatation and a sudden profound fall in blood pressure. Vasodilatation complicates haemorrhage.

### *Postpartum haemorrhage*

Protracted administration, particularly at high doses, may exhaust and desensitize the uterine muscle, leaving it unable to contract and respond to oxytocin, increasing postpartum haemorrhage risk. Observational studies have linked induction of labour with increased incidence of postpartum haemorrhage (Magann et al 2005).

Other adverse effects of oxytocin include: nausea, hypersensitivity responses, and, possibly, reduced chances of breastfeeding (Jordan et al 2009, Ounsted et al 1978, Out et al 1988, Rajan 1994, Wiklund et al 2009).

### *Cautions and contraindications*

Oxytocin is contraindicated in the following situations:

- the uterus is already contracting vigorously
- presence of a mechanical obstruction to delivery
- if commenced during the second stage of labour in parous women – associated with a high risk of uterine hyperstimulation (NCC 2007:240)
- risk of uterine rupture
- presence of apparent uterine resistance and/or inertia (BNF 2009).

### *Cautions*

- Oxytocin alone should not be used for induction of labour (NCC 2008).
- Potential disruption to fluid balance and blood pressure makes oxytocin unsuitable for women with pre-eclampsia, cardiovascular disease or those aged over 35 years.
- 'Starved uterus'. Muscle contraction requires both glucose and oxygen. If either of these is not supplied to the contracting muscle, due to starvation or inadequate blood supply (most likely to arise in prolonged labour), the response to oxytocin will be inadequate, and dose increments will be ineffective (Clayworth 2000).

### *Interactions*

- Prostaglandins, oestrogens: if more than one agent promoting uterine contractility is administered, uterine overstimulation is more likely. Six hours should elapse between prostaglandin and oxytocin administration for induction (BNF 2009).
- Vasoconstrictors, such as ephedrine, can induce hypertension (BNF 2009:431).
- Blood, plasma or metabisulphite will inactivate oxytocin if infused in the same intravenous giving set (Alliance Pharmaceuticals, ABPI 2010).

## Ergometrine

*Ergometrine*, used alone, remains important in the management of acute postpartum or post-abortion haemorrhage. With oxytocin in *Syntometrine®*, it is widely used prophylactically for the active management of the third stage of labour.

When *Syntometrine®* is administered:

- The almost immediate effects of oxytocin are followed by the slightly delayed and more sustained contractions induced by ergometrine.
- Ergometrine acts on the inner region of the myometrium, whereas oxytocin and prostaglandins act on the outer myometrium (de Groot et al 1998).

Onset of action is within 1 minute with intravenous administration, and within 3 to 7 minutes with intramuscular administration. Duration of action is 3 to 8 hours. Excretion is via the kidneys.

### *Actions and adverse reactions*

Actions on alpha$_1$ and serotonin receptors underlie the uterine and gut contractility brought about by ergometrine.

### *Contraction of the uterus*

Ergometrine has a rapid stimulant effect on the uterus, particularly at term. There is a danger that the uterus will fail to relax between contractions and ergometrine is never administered before the delivery of all fetuses. Retention of placental fragments may account for the reported association with increased problems with bleeding in the first 6 weeks post partum (Begley 1990).

### *Vomiting and diarrhoea*

Ergometrine mimics the actions of dopamine, and Syntometrine® is more likely to cause nausea or vomiting than is oxytocin alone (McDonald et al 2004). Mild or moderate diarrhoea may result from increased contractility of the gastrointestinal tract.

### *Vasoconstriction*

Ergometrine acts on alpha$_1$ (noradrenergic) receptors in arterioles and veins to bring about vasoconstriction and venoconstriction. This raises total peripheral resistance, and may lead to:

- hypertension
- postpartum eclamptic fits
- reflex bradycardia and reduced cardiac output
- raised central venous pressure
- cold hands and feet
- numbness, paraesthesia, pain, weakness or even gangrene in digits

- cerebral vasoconstriction and sudden severe headache, tinnitus, dizziness, sweating, confusion, retinal detachment, cerebrovascular accident or seizures
- coronary artery spasm and chest pain or palpitations.

### *Breastfeeding*

Ergot alkaloids act on dopamine receptors to suppress prolactin production. One drug in this group, bromocriptine, is prescribed to manage galactorrhoea and, occasionally, to suppress lactation post partum (Jordan et al 2009).

#### *Cautions and contraindications*

The vasoconstrictor properties of ergometrine make it unsuitable for women with pre-existing pulmonary, cardiac or vascular disorders – including pre-eclampsia, eclampsia, migraine and Raynaud's phenomenon – or multiple pregnancy. If sepsis, renal or hepatic failure is present, sensitivity to ergometrine is increased. Ergometrine is contraindicated in the first and second stages of labour (BNF 2009).

**Reflective activity 10.1**

Get access to a computer – either at the university, Trust/hospital library or at home.

Go to the BNF site: http://www.bnf.org/bnf/bnf/current/index.htm.

You will need to register.

Then look up ergometrine.

- Was the information new to you?
- Was the information easily accessible?
- How will you use the site in the future?

## Drugs for third stage

Due to the differences in the side-effect profiles of the drugs, current guidelines (NCC 2007) suggest that oxytocin (10 units) is the prophylactic drug of choice for the prevention of postpartum haemorrhage, and ergometrine should be used only if this is found to be ineffective, or in high-risk cases. Oxytocin is not currently licensed for intramuscular administration (BNF 2009) and intravenous access may be inaccessible. Therefore, the BNF (2009) recommends *Syntometrine®* (comprising ergometrine 500 micrograms plus 5 units oxytocin) by intramuscular injection for the routine management of the third stage. Use of this regimen necessitates the careful exclusion of women who should not receive ergometrine, for example those with pre-eclampsia. In view of the possible disruption to the delicate homeostatic balance at the sensitive transition period of parturition, the impact of exogenous oxytocin needs further research (Jordan et al 2009).

## Drugs for symptom relief

These include:

- antiemetics
  - antihistamines
  - dopamine ($D_2$) antagonists/blockers
- control of gastric acidity
- laxatives
- analgesics
  - non-steroidal anti-inflammatory drugs (NSAIDs)
- heparin
- folic acid
- vitamin K.

For more specific and detailed information on these, see the website.

## Preventive medicines

The midwife should also use every opportunity to emphasize health and wellbeing through advising about healthy diet and exercise, as this may reduce the need for medications such as iron and some vitamins and minerals.

## LEGAL ASPECTS

The principal statute regulating the use of medicines is the Medicines Act 1968, which controls the sale and supply of medicines. Before a drug can be marketed, it must have a Marketing Authorization issued by the Secretary of State for Health. Drugs that have a manufacturing authorization are categorized into three types for the purpose of supply to the general public: *prescription only, pharmacy only* and *general sale*. Controlled drugs are prescription-only medicines that are further regulated by the Misuse of Drugs Act 1971. In health contexts, Misuse of Drugs Regulations 2001 categorizes controlled drugs into five numbered schedules, according to perceived risk of abuse (Griffith & Tengnah 2008).

Registered midwives may supply and administer, on their own initiative, any of the substances that are specified in medicines legislation under midwives exemptions, provided it is in the course of their professional midwifery practice. They may do so without the need for a prescription or patient-specific direction (PSD) from a medical practitioner (NMC 2010).

It is essential that midwives are aware of their statutory obligations around drug administration, and are conversant with legislation governing drugs and medications. In administering medications, midwives must be knowledgeable regarding the storage, use, dosage, effect and methods of administration of any drug used. This includes consideration that any equipment used is correct and properly maintained. Should the midwife be required to administer new drugs or use new equipment to administer medications, this must be under the direction of a medical practitioner (NMC 2004, 2008).

## Midwives and controlled drugs

The legislation governing midwives and controlled drugs includes that the registered midwife can 'possess diamorphine, morphine, pethidine and pentazocine in her own right so far as is necessary for the practice of her profession' (NMC 2008). Supplies of these drugs can be made on the authority of a midwife's supply order signed by the Supervisor of Midwives, or other Appropriate Medical Officer (a doctor authorized in writing by the local supervising authority). The Supervisor of Midwives or other Appropriate Medical Officer should be satisfied that locally agreed procedure is being followed before signing the supply order (that is that the amount being requested is appropriate etc.). Midwife prescribing may be undertaken subject to the requirements set down by the NMC (2006, 2008, 2010).

Once medicines are received – by midwives working in the community or independent midwives – they become the responsibility of the midwife, and should be stored safely and securely, and if no longer required, should be returned to the pharmacy or destroyed following set regulations (NMC 2004, 2008). Where it is necessary for midwives to keep medicines in their homes, the medicines should be placed in a secure, locked receptacle. If necessary, this should be provided by the employing body (NMC 2008).

## CONCLUSION

Drug administration may involve difficult decisions. These problems could be ameliorated by further research into the physiological changes associated with pregnancy, labour and the puerperium that may be responsible for either therapeutic failure or adverse drug reactions, including easily overlooked events, such as failure to breastfeed.

### KEY POINTS

- All drugs taken during pregnancy and childbirth may affect the woman, fetus or newborn.
- The midwife needs to ensure that the woman understands these potential effects.
- Midwives must have contemporary knowledge about drugs, their interactions and possible adverse effects.
- Midwives must follow legal and practice guidelines and procedures for the safe storage, prescription and administration of medications.
- The pharmacist or drugs information department provide useful resources.

Thanks are due to Palgrive/McMillan for permission to adapt from Jordan: Pharmacology for Midwives 2e (Palgrave Macmillan, 2010).

## REFERENCES

Alliance Pharmaceuticals: Summary of product characteristics for Syntocinon®. In ABPI (Association of the British Pharmaceutical Industry) (2010): *Compendium of data sheets and summaries of product characteristics*, London, 2010, Datapharm Publications Ltd (Pharmacy Dept). http://www.medicines.org.uk/

Arkoosh V: *Guidelines for regional anesthesia in obstetrics: viewpoint of an anesthesiologist in a tertiary care center* (website). www.anes.ccf.org:8080/soap/guideline.htm. 1991. Accessed October 2008.

Aronson JK, editor: *Meyler's side effects of drugs: the international encyclopedia of adverse drug reactions and interaction*, London, 2006, Elsevier.

Association of Anaesthetists of Great Britain and Ireland (AAGBI): (1996) *A report received by Council of the Association of Anaesthetists on blood borne viruses and anaesthesia* (website). www.aagbi.org/publications/guidelines/archive/docs/hivinsert96.pdf. 1996. Accessed September 24, 2008.

Begley C: The effect of ergometrine on breast feeding, *Midwifery* 6(2):60–72, 1990.

Blanch G, Lavender T, Walkinshaw S, et al: Dysfunctional labour: a randomised trial, *British Journal of Obstetrics and Gynaecology* 105(1):117–120, 1998.

British Medical Association (BMA) and the Royal Pharmaceutical Society of Great Britain: *British National Formulary* (BNF) (website). www.bnf.org/bnf/. 2009. Accessed April 2009.

BOC: (2004) *Medical Entonox data sheet* (website). www1.boc.com/uk/sds/medical/entonox.pdf. 2004. Accessed September 24, 2008.

CARIS (Congenital Anomaly Register and Information Service for Wales): *CARIS review including 1998–2006 data* (website). www.wales.nhs.uk/sites3/Documents/416/Caris%20Ann%20rep%202006.pdf. 2007. Accessed October 2008.

Carter C: Developmental consequences of oxytocin, *Physiology & Behavior* 79(3):383–397, 2003.

CEMACH (Confidential Enquiries into Maternal and Child Health): *Why mothers die 2000–2002: the sixth report of the Confidential Enquiries into Maternal Deaths in the United Kingdom*, London, 2005, CEMACH.

Chilvers R, Weisz M: Entonox equipment as a potential source of cross-infection, *Anaesthesia* 55(2):176–179, 2000.

Clayworth S: The nurse's role during oxytocin administration, *MCN: American Journal of Maternal and Child Nursing* 25(2):80–85, 2000.

Clyburn P, Rosen M: The effects of opioid and inhalational analgesia on the newborn. In Reynolds F, editor: *Effects on the baby of maternal analgesia and anaesthesia*, London, 1993, Saunders, pp 169–190.

Collis R, Harries S, Lewis E, et al: Regional analgesia for labour. In Clyburn P, Collis R, Harries S, et al, editors: *Obstetric anaesthesia*, Oxford, 2008, Oxford University Press, pp 221–254.

Crowell MK, Hill P, Humenick S: Relationship between obstetric analgesia and time of effective breast feeding, *Journal of Nurse-Midwifery* 39(3):150–156, 1994.

De Groot AN, van Dongen PW, Vree TB, et al: Ergot alkaloids. Current status and review of clinical pharmacology and therapeutic use compared with other oxytocics in obstetrics and gynaecology, *Drugs* 56(4):523–535, 1998.

Eberle R, Norris M: Labour analgesia. A risk-benefit analysis, *Drug Safety* 14(4):239–251, 1996.

Eltzschig H, Lieberman E, Camann P, et al: Regional anesthesia and analgesia for labor and delivery, *New England Journal of Medicine* 348(4):319–332, 2003.

Gonser M: Labor induction and augmentation with oxytocin: pharmacokinetic considerations, *Archives of Gynecology and Obstetrics* 256(2):63–66, 1995.

Griffith RA, Tengnah CA: *Law and professional issues in nursing*, Exeter, 2008, Learning Matters.

Hansen D, Lou H, Olsen J: Serious life events and congenital malformations: a national study with complete follow-up, *The Lancet* 356:875–880, 2000.

International Conference on Harmonisation (ICH): *ICH Harmonised Tripartite Guideline. Guideline for Good Clinical Practice. E6 (R1)*. Marlow, 1996, Institute of Clinical Research.

Jordan S: Infant feeding and analgesia in labour: the evidence is accumulating, *International Breastfeeding Journal* 1:25, 2006.

Jordan S: Adverse drug reactions: reducing the burden of treatment, *Nursing Standard* 21(34):35–41, 2007.

Jordan S: *The prescription drug guide for nurses*, Maidenhead, 2008, Open University Press.

Jordan S: *Pharmacology for midwives: the evidence base for safe practice*, ed 2, Basingstoke, 2010, Palgrave/ Macmillan.

Jordan S, Emery S, Bradshaw C, et al: The impact of intrapartum analgesia on infant feeding, *British Journal of Obstetrics and Gynaecology* 112(7):927–934, 2005.

Jordan S, Storey M, Morgan G: Antibiotics and allergic disorders in childhood, *The Open Nursing Journal* 2:48–57, 2008.

Jordan S, Emery S, Watkins A, et al: Associations of drugs routinely given in labour with breastfeeding at 48 hours: analysis of the Cardiff Births Survey, *BJOG* 116(12):1622–1630, 2009.

Kennedy S, Longnecker D: History and principles of anaesthesiology. In Hardman J, Limbird L, Molinoff P, et al, editors: *The pharmacological basis of therapeutics*, ed 9, New York, 1996, McGraw-Hill, pp 917–936.

Lawrence R, Schaefer C: General commentary on drug therapy and drug risk during lactation. In Schaefer C, Peters PW, Miller RK, editors: *Drugs during pregnancy and lactation: treatment options and risk assessment*, ed 2, Oxford, 2007, Elsevier, pp 609–620.

Leng G, Meddle SL, Douglas AJ: Oxytocin and the maternal brain, *Current Opinion in Pharmacology* 8(6):731–734, 2008.

Levey A, Bosch J, Lewis J, et al: A more accurate method to estimate glomerular filtration rate from serum creatinine: a new prediction equation, *Annals of Internal Medicine* 130(6):461–470, 1999.

Loebstein R, Lalkin A, Koren G: Pharmacokinetic changes during pregnancy and their clinical relevance, *Clinical Pharmacokinetics* 33(5):328–343, 1997.

Magann EF, Evans S, Hutchinson M, et al: Postpartum hemorrhage after vaginal birth: an analysis of risk factors, *Southern Medical Journal* 98(4):419–422, 2005.

McDonald SJ, Abbott JM, Higgins SP: Prophylactic ergometrine-oxytocin versus oxytocin for the third stage of labour, *Cochrane Database of Systematic Reviews* (1):CD000201, 2004.

McEwan A: Induction of labour, *Obstetrics, Gynaecology and Reproductive Medicine* 18(1):1–6, 2007.

National Collaborating Centre for Women's and Children's Health (NCC): *Caesarean section: Clinical Guideline*. London, 2004, RCOG.

National Collaborating Centre for Women's and Children's Health (NCC): (2007) *Intrapartum care: care of healthy women and their babies during childbirth: Clinical Guideline*. London, 2007, RCOG.

National Collaborating Centre for Women's and Children's Health (NCC): (2008) *Induction of labour: Clinical Guideline*. London, 2008, RCOG.

Nursing and Midwifery Council (NMC): *Midwives rules and standards*, London, 2004, NMC.

Nursing and Midwifery Council (NMC): *Standards of proficiency for nurse and midwife prescribers*, London, 2006, NMC.

Nursing and Midwifery Council (NMC): *Standards for medicines management*, London, 2008, NMC.

Nursing and Midwifery Council Circular: *Changes to Midwives Exemptions*, May 2010. www.nmc-uk.org/Documents/circulars. Accessed June 2010.

Ounsted MK, Hendrick M, Mutch, LM, et al: Induction of labour by different methods in primiparous women. Some perinatal and postnatal problems, *Early Human Development* 2(3):227–239, 1978.

Out JJ, Vierhout ME, Wallenburg HC: Breast-feeding following spontaneous and induced labour, *European Journal of Obstetrics, Gynecology and Reproductive Biology* 29(4):275–279, 1988.

Paech M: New epidural techniques for labour analgesia: patient-controlled epidural analgesia and combined spinal-epidural analgesia, *Bailliere's Clinical Obstetrics and Gynaecology* 12(3):377–395, 1998.

Perrone RD, Madias NE, Levey AS: Serum creatinine as an index of renal function: new insights into old concepts, *Clinical Chemistry* 38(10):1933–1953, 1992.

Rajan L: The impact of obstetric procedures and analgesia/anaesthesia during labour and delivery on breast feeding, *Midwifery* 10(2):87–103, 1994.

Richardson M: Regional anesthesia for obstetrics, *Anesthesiology Clinics of North America* 18(2):383–406, 2000.

Robinson C, Schumann R, Zhang P, et al: Oxytocin-induced desensitization of the oxytocin receptor, *American Journal of Obstetrics and Gynecology* 188(2):497–502, 2003.

Ruggiero R: *Visible embryo pharmaceutical guide to drugs in pregnancy* (website). www.visembryo.com/baby/pharmaceuticals.html. 2006. Accessed April 20, 2009.

Ruppen W, Derry S, McQuay H, et al: Incidence of epidural hematoma, infection, and neurologic injury in obstetric patients with epidural analgesia/anesthesia, *Anesthesiology* 105(2):394–399, 2006.

Russell AR, Murch SH: Could peripartum antibiotics have delayed health consequences for the infants? *British Journal of Obstetrics and Gynaecology* 113(7):758–765, 2006.

Sadler L, McCowan L, White H, et al: Pregnancy outcomes and cardiac complications in women with mechanical, bioprosthetic and homograft valves, *British Journal of Obstetrics and Gynaecology* 107(2):245–253, 2000.

Simmons SW, Cyna AM, Dennis AT, et al: Combined spinal-epidural versus epidural analgesia in labour, *Cochrane Database of Systematic Reviews* I(3):CD003401, 2007.

Slattery DA, Neumann ID: No stress please! Mechanisms of stress hyporesponsiveness of the maternal brain, *Journal of Physiology* 586(2):377–385, 2008.

Sweetman SC, Blake P, McGlashan G, et al: *Martindale: the complete drug reference*, London, 2007, The Pharmaceutical Press.

Thompson A, Hillier V: A re-evaluation of the effect of pethidine on the length of labour, *Journal of Advanced Nursing* 19(3):448–456, 1994.

Wagner M: Research shows medication of pain is not safe, *MIDIRS Midwifery Digest* 3(3):307–309, 1993.

Wiklund I, Norman M, Uvnäs-Moberg K, et al: (2009) Epidural analgesia: breast-feeding success and related factors, *Midwifery* 25(2):e31–e38, 2009.

Wilkinson G: Pharmacokinetics. In Hardman J, Limbard L, Molinoff, P, et al, editors: *Goodman & Gilman's: the pharmacological basis of therapeutics*, ed 10, New York, 2001, McGraw-Hill, pp 3–30.

Wisborg K, Barklin A, Hedegaard M, et al: Psychological stress during pregnancy and stillbirth: prospective study, *British Journal of Obstetrics and Gynaecology* 115(7):882–885, 2008.

# Part 2

# Childbirth in context

Chapter 11

# Social, cultural and spiritual context of childbearing

*Tina Heptinstall and Liz Gale*

## LEARNING OUTCOMES

By the end of the chapter, the reader will be able to:

- discuss the construction of social differences between individuals and its influence on midwifery practice
- evaluate the ways in which midwives can develop positive trusting relationships with women and their families.

## INTRODUCTION

The term 'social context' refers to a range of factors that shape and influence our lives, including concepts such as social class, ethnicity, gender, family and faith. Midwives need to understand this wider social context of women's lives in order to appreciate their needs and provide appropriate care, support and guidance. Additionally, in understanding their own social context, including their professional knowledge and power, midwives can develop greater self-awareness and recognize the influence this has on relationships with women and their families. While pregnancy and childbirth are biological processes and universal events, they are also related to specific social settings which are socially created and given meaning. The different meanings and language of pregnancy, childbirth, motherhood and fatherhood have varied over periods of time, across cultures, among women and men and between professional groups (Davis-Floyd 2003, Kent 2000, Squire 2003, Symonds & Hunt 1994).

A society's views encompass a range of differing standpoints and opinions depending upon individual experience. Women's own writing of their experiences of health, children and motherhood are examples from bodies of knowledge through which women understand and explain their lives (Cusk 2008, Douglas 2005, Wolf 2001). Yet this body of knowledge is given scant regard and considered unscientific by the predominantly masculine medical profession. As Kitzinger comments, 'Obstetric language is mechanistic; women's is experiential' (Kitzinger 2005a:60).

In studying western societies, sociologists divide individuals into categories such as race, social class and gender, which tends to imply homogeneity within groups. Such an oversimplification ignores the complexities of these individual lives and often does not account for multiple identities, differences in life events, and an individual's quality of life. As Bilton et al (2002) comment:

> *'... while it may sometimes be legitimate for sociologists to discuss race, class and gender separately, to understand fully the dynamic and complex nature of inequalities in later modernity, we must consider how race, class and gender divisions combine to produce specific effects.'*
>
> (Bilton et al 2002:189)

However, these artificial divisions between individuals is a practical way of examining aspects of society that are of interest and help us understand social organization and social interaction (Bilton et al 2002, Giddens 2006). Social differentiation is important to midwives as it reflects an unequal access to healthcare for certain groups within society. Recognition of this unequal access and the underlying reasons helps midwives to provide appropriate care for the women and their families.

## SOCIAL CLASS AND SOCIAL DISADVANTAGE

Whilst some may argue that differentiation by social class is no longer relevant within society, it continues to be used by statisticians in data gathering. For example, breast-feeding statistics and perinatal mortality rates are both produced using the British Register General classification. Criticized because of its focus on the occupation of the man of the house, consequently excluding the unemployed, retired, lone parents and students, it continues to provide evidence of health inequality gradients; that is, the lower the social class, the greater the incidence of poorer health and social outcomes.

Evidence for this first appeared 30 years ago in the seminal Black Report (DHSS 1980), although at the time the report was suppressed by the Conservative Government. It was brought to a wider audience and discussed further by Peter Townsend et al in their 1988 book *The Black Report and the health divide*. Within it, Townsend et al (1988) focus on those disadvantages that are social or cultural rather than biological differences, such as age or sex. The acknowledgement that health inequalities exist and that it need not be inevitable stems from the Black Report and was followed in 1998 by an independent enqiry into health inequalities led by Sir Donald Acheson (DH 1998). This report recommended that high priority be given to policies that improve health and reduce inequalities for women of childbearing age, expectant mothers and young children.

Health inequalities are clearly linked to income inequality, but income inequality also affects self-esteem and social standing. Access to healthcare is influenced by both economic factors and the motivation to improve one's situation. This may be known as self-efficacy. This concept is linked to the idea of the 'inverse care law' (described in 1971 by Julian Tudor Hart), namely, those in most need of healthcare are least likely to get it. Several factors affect this; local services tend to be of poorer quality – fewer staff caring for sicker people; access tends to be more difficult – restricted appointment times or geographically more difficult to get to; and people are also more likely to suffer multiple external disadvantages – poorer environment, housing and nutrition (Appleby & Deeming 2001). In recent years this multiple disadvantage has come to be known as *social exclusion*, which refers not only to poverty and low income but also to its wider causes and consequences. The Government describes it as:

> *'what can happen when people or areas suffer from a combination of linked problems such as unemployment, poor skills, low incomes, poor housing, high crime, bad health and family breakdown. These problems are linked and mutually reinforcing.'*
>
> (Cabinet Office 2008)

The Acheson report, alongside more recent health policy documents such as the National Service Framework for Children, Young People and Maternity Services (DH 2004), The NHS Plan (DH 2000) and Sure Start local programmes, have all helped to increase the public health profile of midwives. This has been endorsed by the Royal College of Midwives in their position paper The Midwife's Role in Public Health (RCM 2001) and highlighted by both the 2004 and 2007 Confidential Enquiries into Maternal and Child Health (CEMACH 2004, Lewis 2007). While public health has always been part of a midwife's role, more formalized public health midwifery posts are increasingly being developed, at consultant midwife, community-based and management levels.

Addressing health inequalities and poor pregnancy outcomes through service improvements for disadvantaged women is a challenge for midwives (Chapter 23). The National Service Framework, Standard 11 Maternity services (DH 2004) highlighted the need to provide inclusive services, particularly for the most vulnerable who do not acccess maternity services; travellers, homeless women, young pregnant women, young men, those misusing drugs and alcohol, refugees and asylum seekers, women experiencing domestic abuse and women who are HIV positive. Many of these women also experience socio-economic hardship and they have poorer pregnancy outcomes than do women in households with higher incomes. One example of this is poor nutrition among economically disadvantaged women, usually associated with women who are underweight or, increasingly, obese (Guelinckx et al 2008). Inadequate nutrition is linked with low-birthweight babies, who are at increased risk of physical and intellectual disabilites as well as being at greater risk of developing coronary heart disease and diabetes in later life. As Ihunnaya et al (2008:558) commented: 'Birth weight, a leading determinant of infant survival, has implications for public health policy making and practice.' Mcleish (2007) discussed this challenge and identified that while poorer women are aware of the meaning of a healthy diet there are a number of barriers to healthy eating, such as lack of cooking skills, access to affordable quality food, safe storage and putting others first (especially other children). Mcleish (2007) identified that midwives have a key role in providing nutritional advice to pregnant women alongside informing them about the government-funded scheme 'Healthy Start' which gives food vouchers for milk, fresh fruit, fresh vegetables and infant formula milk to women on low incomes and to their young children (DH 2009).

Midwives have a unique opportunity to be welcomed into the homes of such families at a time when the prospect of a new baby provides a motivation to improve their health and lifestyles. Whilst having no financial aid to offer (apart from ensuring that they are claiming their entitled benefits), midwives can, by their recognition of the complexities of some people's lives and by providing the care and respect entitled to these women and their families, help to empower them. Midwives working in these areas of socio-economic deprivation have an important role in building constructive relationships with women and their families as well as with other health professionals and community-based agencies. These may include housing associations, benefit advisors, Connexions (a government-funded support and advice service relating to health, education, work and relationships for 13–19-year-olds), sexual health services, advocacy workers and local voluntary support groups as well as doctors, health visitors and other health professionals; awareness of local services is crucial. Davies (2008) emphasizes how enhanced midwifery care can contribute to improving the lives of women in areas of socio-economic deprivation, particularly in relation to their health, confidence and personal aspirations.

**Reflective activity 11.1**

- Identify three groups of women in your locality who you consider to be socially disadvantaged.
- Outline sources of support available for these women and their families.
- Using one of these groups of women you have identified, how best can midwives work alongside them and guide them in accessing other sources of support?

## ETHNICITY

When considering social disadvantage, it needs to be recognized that amongst those most disadvantaged, certain groups are overrepresented, including black and minority ethnic groups. Britain is increasingly multicultural, particularly in larger cities. Midwives should be aware of different cultural groups and related community support within their localities, but essentially they need to demonstrate a willingness to learn about others and develop relationships that are open and honest.

Differing terminology around race and ethnicity can be confusing. Race is the term often used for the genetic, physical characteristics of individuals, factors that midwives need to be aware of when considering, for example, haemoglobinopathy screening or the significance of pelvic shape for women in labour. However, the biological basis of race does not link it to disadvantage; it is the social construct of ethnicity and its differing perceptions that is important. Phillips & Rathwell (1986) suggest that 'race' is a social construct that has more to do with social structures and power relationships than with biology.

Ethnicity is a difficult concept to define but is generally recognized as 'shared origins' (Sookhoo 2003). This embraces a sense of belonging to a particular community; common geography, beliefs, language and history, but does not imply homogeneity within a group any more than shared views could be expected within the 'white' ethnic group. Within any society, the most dominant ethnic group is likely to be relatively invisible, whilst 'difference' is identified in all other groups. Consequently, it can be hard for those members of the dominant group to recognize racism within their organization and to make the transition to seeing the service as others may see it. Cross-Sudworth (2007) argues that although legislation and policy directives address discrimination and racism, midwives need to actively tackle racism in the workforce as well as in the organization and provision of services. Ethnicity may also be complicated as these 'shared origins' change over generations, between first- and second-generation immigrants and in the meeting and pairing of different cultures and ethnicities. Individuals may describe having a dual heritage, as they recognize the differing cultures and ethnicities of each parent.

For midwives to be able to determine the needs of women, it is clear that generalizations are no more appropriate for women from minority ethnic groups than they are for women from more dominant groups. Effective communication and understanding of the expectations of women from a range of diverse backgrounds is key to what is termed 'cultural competence' (Sookhoo 2003). This does not necessarily require indviduals to be highly competent about all cultures but it is about openness and respect, a willingness to learn and self-awareness.

Without effective communication and unable to establish a relationship with clients, health professionals may fall back on stereotype or making generalized assumptions based on an individual's ethnicity, leading to simple misunderstandings, insensitivity or racist behaviour (Schott & Henley 1996). These tend to be negative and reflect an ethnocentric view that one's own cultural norms are superior to another. Whilst it is important for midwives to try to understand the differences between cultures and cultural practices, some may present ethico-legal challenges at an individual or societal level. Within midwifery, the complex socio-legal arguments around female genital mutilation is one such example, and is discussed in more detail by McCafferty et al (2005). Developing a better understanding of the nature of differences between individuals can result in improved planning and delivery of care. Moreover, cultures are not static and individuals within groups are not all the same.

In the latest Confidential Enquiry into Maternal and Child Health (CEMACH) report, mortality rates were significantly higher for black and Middle Eastern women (Lewis 2007) (see Chapter 16). Black African women, including asylum seekers and newly arrived refugees, were almost six times more likely to die than white women. Refugees and asylum seekers are categories of minority ethnic groups. The care of childbearing refugees and asylum seekers, who have needs unique to their difficult circumstances, is often poorly understood (Mcleish 2002).

An asylum seeker is someone who has fled their country of origin, applied for protection under the Geneva Convention (1951), or Article 3 of the European Convention on Human Rights (torture), with the UK Border Agency at the Home Office, and is awaiting a decision regarding their immigration status. This decision can take many months and in the meantime they are supported financially at levels below income support. They can be detained at any time for indefinite periods, and may be moved at any time (Mcleish et al 2002, Kitzinger 2005b). If an asylum seeker's application has been accepted by the Home Office the applicant is granted refugee status. A refugee is defined under the 1951 United Nations Convention Relating to the Status of Refugees as someone who has a well-founded fear of being persecuted for reasons of race, religion, nationality, membership of a particular social group or political opinion.

Both asylum seekers and refugees are entitled to primary and secondary healthcare without charge (Joels 2008). Despite this entitlement, they can find it difficult to access services (Mcleish 2002). In particular, frequent moves make it difficult for asylum seekers to form relationships with health professionals. They may have considerable health needs, both mental health needs – many will have witnessed or endured violence, rape and torture – and physical health needs – infections such as TB spread rapidly through accommodation and detention centres and many have poor nutrition from earlier deprivations (Kelley & Stevenson 2006). Pregnancy may be a result of rape by oppressors in their country of origin (Dunkley-Bent 2006) or from either consensual or forced intercourse whilst awaiting asylum. The House of Commons Health Committee (2003) concluded that reasons why pregnant asylum seekers may not access care include: their future in the UK was uncertain; isolation from family and friends left them with no support; and an inability to speak English. These same reasons increased their vulnerability and this continues for both mother and child until a final decision is made on their right to remain in the UK.

**Reflective activity 11.2**

- Using local sources (e.g. from library, council and health settings) identify the range of different ethnic groups that live in your locality.
- Talk informally to someone from a different ethnic group to yourself and share your experiences on your upbringing, identifying similarities as well as differences.

## GENDER AND FAMILY PATTERNS

In the same way that different meanings can be attributed to race and ethnicity, so may different meanings be ascribed to the concept of gender. While anatomical and physiological differences between the sexes are biologically determined, gender may be described as the socially or culturally prescribed status of women and men in a society. The associated concepts of femininity and masculinity are similarly socially constructed and, as such, they are not fixed. In common with all social constructs, these expectations will vary between cultures and over time. Although related to it, gender is different from sexuality, which is a social construct of a biological drive. Whilst there are differences between the sexes, of which the ability to have children is a key one, it is the use of those differences as justification for ongoing inequalities between women and men which is challenged by feminist thinking (Squire 2003).

A society's expectation of gender roles reflect ongoing changes in women's lives and family life, yet despite these changes gender inequalities persist and are most visible within career pathways and earning potential. Less visible are inequalities in the division of household chores and the responsibility of childcare. Despite some parents' attempts at avoiding traditional gendered differences in bringing up their children, the influence of society is pervasive. This is reflected in the media representation of appropriate gendered toys and the type of language used to talk to and about small children. Ideas about a person's gender roles and behaviour may be ascribed before birth. Rothman (1994) uses the phrase 'fetal sons and daughters' as she describes how women who know the sex of their child after amniocentesis describe fetal activity in a way that is gender stereotyped. The movements of the males were more often described as 'strong' and 'vigorous' and females were described as 'lively'. Gender stereotyping continues soon after birth as appearance and behaviour are gender related.

The socialization of children is dependent upon more than just gender and is influenced by class, ethnicity, social networks and the interaction with a child's environment. The traditional nuclear family is often portrayed in the media as the norm, yet this image fails to acknowledge the range of different family stuctures. These families include single parents (the majority headed by mothers), parents of children who are adopted or fostered, same-sex parents, those living in extended families, and those within 'blended' or 'reconstituted' families who may have step brothers and sisters on both maternal and paternal sides. The term 'single parent' frequently conjures up images of young mothers and has often been used in a derogatory way within the media, particularly the tabloid press, for many years. Often cited as an indicator for antisocial behaviour amongst children and young people, its links to poverty, aspiration and employment prospects are ignored. Contrary to stereotypes of young women becoming pregnant without thought and young men disappearing early on, 93% of births are registered jointly (soon to become a legal requirement), suggesting that both parents intend to support the child (Department for Work and Pensions 2008).

While midwives need to possess knowledge that family life and structure is not fixed or uniform, their attitudes and actions towards individuals are equally important. One example of this is lesbians and motherhood. Lesbians have some different needs to heterosexual women but many have the same needs during pregnancy, in labour and during early motherhood. The primary tensions for lesbians lie in the values and attitudes of others (Brogan 1997). Much of the literature on lesbians and health focuses on the issue of the power relationship between women and health professionals (Lee 2007, Royal College of Midwives 2000). In their study of lesbian mothers, Wilton & Kaufmann (2001) reported high levels of anxiety among the women about the implications of disclosing their sexual identity as well as an acute awareness of midwives' personal attitudes and prejudices. Overall, the women were satisfied with their care, such as feeling accepted and welcomed, recognition of their partner and a positive attitude towards them as parents. Conversely, some women experienced such 'neutral' attitudes that rendered them almost invisible as lesbians, some were asked unnecessary questions about the biological father of the child and a few experienced hostility arising from moral or religious beliefs of health professionals.

Although family is often assumed to be a place where individuals feel happy and safe, this is not the case for everyone. For example, 30% of abuse towards women starts or worsens in pregnancy (Lewis 2007). Midwives may assume that because a woman is married or lives with a partner or parents she is 'supported'. This may not be the experience for women whose partners are unsupportive because they feel ambivalent or unreceptive towards the woman's pregnancy and forthcoming child. Single mothers living alone may be well supported through family or friendships networks.

Changes in working patterns, for women in particular, have led to many of the changes in family life. Gender equity, for the childless, is closer than it has ever been, with more equitable educational achievements, careers, income and home lives until women have their first child, when, as Gimson (2008:1) comments, 'becoming a mother carries an enormous penalty and the poorer a woman you are, the greater the price you pay.'

For women who have no interruption in their working lives, their overall income remains less than for men, but this discrepancy is exacerbated by the number of children a woman has. More significantly, when considering multiple disadvantage, it is the poorer qualified and lower paid who suffer the largest gap between the income that they would have achieved and that which they earn (Makepeace et al 2004). Over the past two decades there has been a sharp increase in the numbers of mothers who work, although this is disproportionate, with more married women with working partners returning to work than lone mothers, despite both having similar aspirations. Lone mothers cite caring responsibilities and financial concerns as key barriers to work and are frequently amongst those most likely to be in poverty; conversely, married couples are more likely to have a dual income (Millar & Ridge 2001). Despite women being more likely to be employed outside the home, they still undertake the greater share of housework and childcare than men (Crompton & Lyonette 2008, Office for National Statistics 2008), although men are undertaking more childcare responsibilities than they did in the past (Equal Opportunities Commission 2006, O'Brien 2004).

Research from the Economic and Social Research Council (Henwood 2001) found that new fathers were concerned and confused over balancing their roles of provider, nurturer and partner. British fathers are working some of the longest hours in the European Community and these tend to increase in the children's earliest years (Kodz et al 2003). However, it is argued in a more recent study that birth is associated with new fathers reducing the amount of time that they spend at work, although this is not maintained through the child's formative years (Dermott 2006). These long hours can put a strain on both an individual's health and domestic relationships, despite evidence that fathers would rather spend more time with their children (Kodz et al 2003). Several studies from the Equal Opportunities Commission (EOC) suggest that both fathers and mothers would like increased paternal involvement in child care, often to enable the mother to also work, and would welcome policies that allowed for flexible working and parental leave (O'Brien 2004, Thompson et al 2005). Davies (2008) argues strongly for midwives to rethink the way they work and connect with fathers. He suggests that men are eager to get involved but that, 'many maternity services still treat men as an optional extra ... and sometimes even as an unwelcome complication' (Davies 2008:120). Drawing on related evidence, he proposes that midwives should engage more with fathers in addressing smoking, postnatal depression and breastfeeding, in order to meet the needs of mothers and children.

**Reflective activity 11.3**

- Consider how roles of adults within households influence patterns of childrearing.
- Identify the needs of prospective fathers and consider how responsive your services are to them.

## SPIRITUALITY

As midwives have become increasingly aware of the social context of women's and men's lives, an understanding of each woman's inner or spiritual needs is equally important (Davies 2007, Hall & Taylor 2004, Pembroke & Pembroke 2008). Spirituality is often linked to religious faith or belief and sometimes these terms are used interchangeably, but Tanyi (2002) argues that they are different concepts. Broadly, spirituality may be considered to be the search for meaning or purpose in life, whereas faith usually implies a religious belief system with a belief in a higher power or God. Tanyi (2002:500) suggests that 'spirituality is an inherent component of being human, and is subjective, intangible, and multidimensional.'

Jesse et al (2007), in using the terms faith and spirituality interchangeably, describe how for some women spirituality is a significant resource in pregnancy. In their study on the relevance and meaning of spirituality for low-income African-American and Caucasian women in the Midwestern United States, around half of the respondents considered spirituality had an important positive effect on their pregnancy. The women described how they felt guided, supported and protected by their faith; that it gave them strength and confidence; that their faith helped with difficult choices and enabled them to communicate with God.

Hall (2007) provides a more secular approach and she looks at creativity as one expression of spirituality and identifies how creativity is expressed through, for example, poetry, music and story telling. She explores pregnancy and childbirth as intensely creative and life-changing events in a woman's life and how they are marked by 'nesting' (making, purchasing and arranging items in preparation for the for the new baby), the powerful event of birth itself and the experience of breastfeeding. McHugh (2003) argues that not only are the spiritual dimensions of pregnancy and labour neglected, they are difficult to express within a medicalized technological birth environment.

Pembroke & Pembroke (2008) explore the spirituality of midwifery care and consider that the 'capacity to respond loyally and authentically is at the heart of the spirituality of midwifery care' (2008:324). These authors suggest that the midwife is a reassuring calm presence and is available for the woman; not just to do practical things, but to be there, just for her, emotionally. Leap (2000) has also explored this idea of being available for women in her discussions around 'doing less' and 'giving more'.

McHugh (2003) suggests that the 'sense of the spiritual' may be more readily achieved away from large obstetric units; home or birth centres are more appropriate places where the environment and culture embrace a more holistic approach, including a recognition of the spiritual dimensions of labour and birth. Nevertheless, while some physical hospital environments may not appear conducive to the 'sense of the spiritual', midwives can create an appropriate emotional environment in hospital settings through building meaningful, supportive relationships with women during the intense experience of labour and birth.

## CONCLUSION

Midwives need to have an understanding of the social and cultural context of the lives of childbearing women and their families as this impinges on a range of physical and psychological outcomes of pregnancy and early motherhood. Supportive relationships with women and their families and timely interventions and referrals by midwives may mitigate against difficult social circumstances.

**KEY POINTS**

- The construction of motherhood and fatherhood is socially prescribed and socially controlled. Parenting is not a fixed role and changes with societal, moral, political and economic influences.
- Social differences between groups are categorized by social class and gender. This is not a practical way of understanding the norms in the organization of society.
- Midwives should recognize the norms and values of different groups within society in order to provide individualized care to women.

## REFERENCES


Appleby J, Deeming C: *Inverse Care Law, Health Service Journal* 111(5760):37, 2001.

Bilton T, Bonnett K, Jones P, et al: *Introductory sociology*, Basingstoke, 2002, Palgrave.

Brogan M: *Healthcare for lesbians: attitudes and experiences, Nursing Standard* 11(45):39–42, 1997.

Cabinet Office: *What do we mean by social exclusion?* (website). www.cabinetoffice.gov.uk/social_exclusion_task_force/context.aspx. 2008. Accessed February 13, 2009.

Confidential Enquiry into Maternal and Child Health (CEMACH): *Why mothers die 2000–2002*, London, 2004, RCOG Press.

Crompton R, Lyonette C: *Who does the housework? The division of labour in the home*. In Park A, Curtice J, Thomson K, et al, editors: *British social attitudes: the 24th report*, London, 2008, Sage for National Centre for Social Research.

Cross-Sudworth F: *Racism and discrimination in maternity services, British Journal of Midwifery* 15(6):327–331, 2007.

Cusk R: *A life's work*, London, 2008, Faber and Faber.

Davies J: *Completing the maternity jigsaw, The Practising Midwife* 11(11):12–14, 2008.

Davies L, editor: *The art and soul of midwifery: creativity in practice, education and research*, Oxford, 2007, Churchill Livingstone.

Davis-Floyd R: *Birth as an American rite of passage*, ed 2, California, 2003, University of California Press.

Department for Work and Pensions (DWP): *Joint birth registration: recording responsibility* (website). www.dwp.gov.uk/publications/dwp/2008/birth_registration_ia.pdf. 2008. Accessed February 25, 2009.

Department of Health (DH): *Independent Inquiry into Inequalities in Health Report* (Chaired by Sir Donald Acheson), London, 1998, HMSO.

Department of Health: *The NHS plan: a plan for investment, a plan for reform*, London, 2000, The Stationery Office.

Department of Health: *National Service Framework for Children, Young People and Maternity Services*, London, 2004, The Stationery Office.

Department of Health (DH): *Healthy start: a new Welfare Food Scheme* (website). www.dh.gov.uk/en/Healthcare/Maternity/Maternalandinfantnutrition/DH_4112476. 2009. Accessed January 6, 2009.

Department of Health and Social Security (DHSS): *Inequalities in Health; Report of a Research Working Group (The Black Report)*, London, 1980, HMSO.

Dermott E: *The effect of fatherhood on men's employment*, Swindon, 2006, ESRC.

Douglas SJ: *Mommy myth: the idealization of motherhood and how it has undermined all women*, New York, 2005, Simon & Schuster.

Dunkley-Bent J: *Reducing inequalities in childbirth: the midwife's role in public health*. In Page L, McCandlish R, editors: *The new midwifery: science and sensitivity in practice*, ed 2, Philadelphia, 2006, Churchill Livingstone.

Equal Opportunities Commission (EOC): *21st century dad*, Manchester, 2006, EOC.

Giddens A: *Sociology*, ed 5, Cambridge, 2006, Polity Press.

Gimson S: *Listening to mother: making Britain mother-friendly*, London, 2008, Family and Parenting Institute.

Guelinckx I, Devlieger R, Beckers K, et al: *Maternal obesity: pregnancy complications, gestation, weight gain and nutrition, Obesity* 9(2):140–150, 2008.

Hall J: *Creativity, spirituality and birth*. In Davies L, editor: *The art and soul of midwifery: creativity in practice, education and research*, Oxford, 2007, Churchill Livingstone.

Hall J, Taylor M: *Birth and spirituality*. In Downe S, editor: *Normal childhood: debate and the evidence*, Oxford, 2004, Churchill Livingstone.

Henwood K: *Masculinities, identities and transition to fatherhood*, 2001, Economic and Social Research Council (website). www.esrcsocietytoday.ac.uk. Accessed February 24, 2009.

House of Commons Health Committee: *Inequalities in access to maternity services. Eighth report of Session 2002–2003* (website). www.publications.parliament.uk/pa/cm200203/cmselect/cmhealth/696/696.pdf. 2003. Accessed February 25, 2009.

Ihunnaya FO, Williams MA, Sales AE, et al: *Pre-pregnancy body mass index, gestational weight gain, and other maternal characteristics in relation to infant birth weight, Maternal and Child Health Journal* 12(5):557–567, 2008.

Jesse DE, Schoneboom C, Blanchard A: *The effect of faith or spirituality: a content analysis, Journal of Holistic Nursing* 25(3):151–158, 2007.

Joels C: *Impact of national policy on the health of people seeking asylum, Nursing Standard* 22(31):35–40, 2008.

Kelley N, Stevenson J: *First do no harm: denying healthcare to people whose asylum claims have failed*, London, 2006, The Refugee Council.

Kent J: *Social perspectives on pregnancy and childbirth for midwives, nurses and the caring professions*, Buckinghamshire, 2000, Open University Press.

Kitzinger S: *The language of birth*. In Kitzinger S, editor: *The Politics of Birth*, Philadelphia, 2005a, Elsevier.

Kitzinger S *(2005b) Pregnant asylum seekers: the dispossessed*. In Kitzinger S, editor: *The Politics of Birth*, Philadelphia, 2005b, Elsevier.

Kodz J, Davis S, Lain D, et al: *Working long hours: a review of the evidence. Volume 1 – Main report*, London, 2003, Department of Trade and Industry.

Leap N: *The less we do the more we give*. In Kirkham M, editor: *The midwife-woman relationship*, Basingstoke, 2000, Macmillan.

Lee E: *Lesbian users of maternity services: challenges in midwifery care*. In Richens Y, editor: Challenges for midwives, vol 2, London, 2007, Quay Books.

Lewis G, editor: *The Confidential Enquiry into Maternal and Child Health. Saving mothers' lives: reviewing maternal deaths to make motherhood safer 2003–2005. The Seventh Report into Maternal Deaths in the United Kingdom*, London, 2007, CEMACH.

Makepeace G, Dolton P, Joshi H: *Gender earnings differentials over time, across and within cohorts: unequal pay among individuals in British Cohort Studies*

*1991 and 2000, International Journal of Manpower* 25(3–4):251–263, 2004.

McCafferty C, Davis K, Momoh C: *Female genital mutilation*, Oxford, 2005, Radcliffe Publishing.

McHugh N: *Midwives of the soul: the spirituality of births, Midwifery Matters* 97:4–5, 2003.

Mcleish J: *Mothers in exile: maternity experiences of asylum seekers in England*, London, 2002, Maternity Alliance.

Mcleish J: *The challenge of providing dietary advice to disadvantaged pregnant women*. In Richens Y, editor: *Challenges for midwives*, London, 2007, Quay Books.

Mcleish J, Cutler S, Stancer C: *A crying shame: pregnant asylum seekers and their babies in detention*, London, 2002, Maternity Alliance.

Millar J, Ridge T: *Families, poverty, work and care: a review of literature on lone parents and low income couple families*, DWP Research Report No 153, Leeds, 2001, CDS.

O'Brien M: *Shared caring: bringing fathers into the frame*, Working Paper Series No 18, Manchester, 2004, Equal Opportunities Commission.

Office for National Statistics (ONS): *Attitudes to household chores 2000–2001*, London, 2008, 2000 UK Time Use Survey.

Pembroke NF, Pembroke JJ: *The spirituality of presence in midwifery care, Midwifery* 24(3):321–327, 2008.

Phillips T, Rathwell D: *Race and ethnicity*, London, 1986, Croom Helm.

Rothman BK: *The tentative pregnancy: Amniocentesis and the sexual politics of motherhood*, London, 1994, Pandora Press.

Royal College of Midwives (RCM): *Position paper 22: Maternity care for lesbian mothers*, London, 2000, RCM.

Royal College of Midwives (RCM): *The midwives role in public health: Position paper No 24*, London, 2001 (reviewed 2005), RCM.

Schott J, Henley A: *Culture, religion and childbearing in a multiracial society: a handbook for health professionals*, Oxford, 1996, Butterworth Heinemann.

Sookhoo D: *'Race' and ethnicity*. In Squire C, editor: *The social context of birth*, Oxford, 2003, Radcliffe Medical Press.

Squire C, editor: *The social context of birth*, Oxford, 2003, Radcliffe Medical Press.

Symonds A, Hunt S: *The social meaning of midwifery*, Basingstoke, 1994, Macmillan.

Tanyi J: *Towards clarification of the meaning of spirituality, Journal of Advanced Nursing* 39(5):500–509, 2002.

Thompson M, Vinter L, Young V: *Dads and their babies: leave arrangements in the first year*, Working paper 37, London, 2005, Equal Opportunities Commission.

Townsend P, Davidson P, Whitehead M, editors: *Inequalities in health: the Black Report and the health divide*, Harmondsworth, 1988, Penguin.

Wilton T, Kaufmann T: *Lesbian mothers' experiences of maternity care in the UK, Midwifery* 17(3):203–211, 2001.

Wolf N: *Misconceptions: truth, lies and the unexpected on the journey to motherhood*, London, 2001, Chatto & Windus.

Chapter |12|

# Psychological context

Lynne Spencer

## LEARNING OUTCOMES

After reading this chapter, you will:

- appreciate the psychological factors that may affect a woman's experience of pregnancy, childbirth and early motherhood
- appreciate the complexities of communication, and how this affects midwifery practice
- understand the necessity of recognizing each woman and her family as a unique unit.

## INTRODUCTION

Each woman reaches pregnancy by a different road. Some women will have chosen very carefully to have become a mother and be excited by the prospect. Others will have become pregnant earlier than they had wished, whilst some will be unhappy to be pregnant. This last-mentioned group may include those women who have become pregnant by violence or force. It is important therefore that midwives remember that each woman and her family will need care which is planned and organized to support in their individual journey to becoming a family. Midwives need to have great sensitivity and awareness of the processes and dynamics of communication. They may then address the anxieties, fears and worries, often not spoken about by women, but which still need to be made explicit so that appropriate care is offered to women in their individual family units.

In any work on psychological processes or communication, it is important to remember that before we begin to work with others we should examine ourselves, because how we behave and how and when we speak will impact on women, students and other healthcare practitioners with whom we work. In addition, the relationships we develop with a woman and her partner will influence the way a woman experiences her journey to motherhood, and the psychological aspects of her care.

## RELATIONSHIP

It has been recognized for many years that it is the depth and strength of the relationship between client and therapist that makes the difference (P Clarkson, personal communication, 2000) (see website for Case scenario 12.1). This bond or working alliance enables the client to explore their situation and change or remain the same, depending upon their decisions following explorations of their circumstances.

The concept of relationship is so obvious that it is often taken for granted; however, anecdotal evidence and research (Griffith 1990) suggests that it is frequently missing in general practice. Yet, this is an area where clients may have a lifelong provider of care. If this is true in general practice, it could be similar in midwifery.

Women are having fewer babies than formerly. Pregnancy is a time when women may feel vulnerable because so many changes are occurring at such a rapid pace. The meeting with the person who will provide care at this time is important. Some people really enjoy change, it is exciting; others dislike change, as it provokes anxiety, which they try to avoid because they wish for stability or for their life to remain the same.

For some women, the relationship between themselves and the midwives whom they meet may become very important. Women who are without an extended family network or friends are often socially isolated. It is common knowledge that such ordinary human relationships can have a psychotherapeutic value (Clarkson 1996). Women who have a poor relationship with their own mothers and few friends may experience difficulties in pregnancy, childbirth and the first year following the birth of their baby, if they do not receive adequate support from the midwife or a therapist (J Harman, unpublished PhD thesis, 2008). A sound relationship with the midwife will provide stability for the woman and reduce her experiences of anxiety or fear, enabling her to develop confidence in herself.

For a relationship to develop or establish, three components are required:

- trust
- respect
- communication.

## Trust

All adults realize that an individual can betray them; therefore, trust does not exist overnight in any relationship and has to be earned. It has long been recognized that if we have similar traits to another person then we are more likely to like that person, relax in their company and be influenced by them (Cialdini 2001). Women also expect a midwife to 'look after them' or act in their best interest, thus to advocate for them (Fraser 1999). Advocacy goes hand in hand with trust, and this means that midwives need to trust and believe in a woman's ability to be pregnant and give birth so that the woman will believe in her own ability to be pregnant and give birth.

However, in today's maternity services, risk management is an important aspect that influences the ways in which midwives practice. In a hospital setting, midwives respond to the influences of senior practitioners and will change their behaviour to obey or conform to their senior's wishes (Hollins Martin & Bull 2008). If a woman sees this, she may feel differently about her midwife, perceiving that if the midwife conforms, the woman herself may consider the need to conform. If she conforms, she is seen as a 'good' patient. If she does not conform, she may be considered to be a 'problem' patient.

Women may prefer to be seen as the good patient, because the fantasy is that care will be kinder or better. However, the decision to change her behaviour and accept the care offered by a senior practitioner may result in the woman no longer feeling that she has choice, control or a voice to influence what happens to her during her pregnancy or labour. The trust she has in the midwife may be breached and may be irreparable. The woman may also feel angry with herself for not being stronger. She may consider herself weak and if she thinks this about herself, she may also think the same about the midwife.

A second aspect of trust is that if the midwife or student midwife is confident in her own ability to provide care to women and their partners, they, in turn, will have confidence in the midwife. The woman will feel safe. Often women are happy to be cared for by 'brusque' midwives because their behaviour displays confidence, whereas sometimes a very kind midwife can display behaviour which shows a lack of confidence, consequently the woman feels unsafe.

It is important for midwives to develop confidence and competence so that the care they offer to women provides feelings of safety to build trust. However, many students and midwives do not feel confident or competent at the point of registration (Donovan 2008). This perceived lack of confidence and competence will affect the woman/midwife relationship. During her student training, each midwife needs to be nurtured by a mentor who facilitates her practice, providing praise when it is due, encouraging the making of decisions when appropriate and discussing the decisions made (Currie 1999). Consequently, when students qualify and begin to work independently, they do not display or experience anxiety, thus women will feel safe in their care. As a result, an individual woman will be willing to tell the midwife her personal story, which will facilitate accurate history-taking and lead to the appropriate provision of care for the woman and her partner.

A third aspect of trust is compassion, which can also equate to un-possessive love. It is a challenge for midwives to remain compassionate when they are working under pressure. Midwives may work in a delivery ward where there are too few midwives to offer continuous support for women in labour. The pressures may lead to little or no time to comfort a midwife who has attended and been affected by a difficult birth. What happens is that the midwife becomes psychically numb. She switches off her empathy and compassion to protect herself and as a consequence she can be perceived and experienced by women as uncaring and unkind (Kings Fund 2008). The midwife no longer conveys the sense that she understands the experiences of the woman and wants to do something about it (Youngson 2008).

## Respect

Respect for women is the foundation on which all meetings or interventions are built (Egan 2007). It is a way of seeing the woman as a unique individual and is based on maintaining a woman's dignity. The midwife needs to convey in her way of being that she will not cause any harm and that she is skilled, competent and confident in her practice of midwifery. The midwife needs to convey to the woman that she is her advocate and will be with the woman on her journey. This does not mean though that the midwife would collude with the woman. If the woman is drinking more than the recommended amount of alcohol units per week, the midwife will point this out, because this behaviour needs to be challenged. The midwife works on an assumption that women wish to live healthily, so if the woman resists, she will also recognize and respect that it is her right so to do. It is important that midwives are able to suspend judgements; most people are their own worst critics, so women do not need other people to judge them as harshly as they may judge themselves. Respecting women is to keep them as the focus in order to provide woman-centred care.

### Communication

This refers to proficient and appropriate use of specific skills. Many people believe that they are good communicators, yet when asked to identify which communication skills they are using, they are unable to do so. If an individual is unable to identify which skill they are using, they are often not using the skill most appropriate for the situation. Communication skills need to be practised and fine-tuned so that they are used every day. As midwives interact with women each one may require different skills in order for her to feel valued, listened to and understood.

When all three of the above aspects are present, a woman will experience a satisfying relationship that will enable her to cope with the changes which occur during pregnancy, labour and early motherhood.

## THE DYNAMICS OF COMMUNICATION PROCESSES

A simple explanation of communication is that one person speaks to another, who hears and understands what is said and responds to the speaker, as in Figure 12.1.

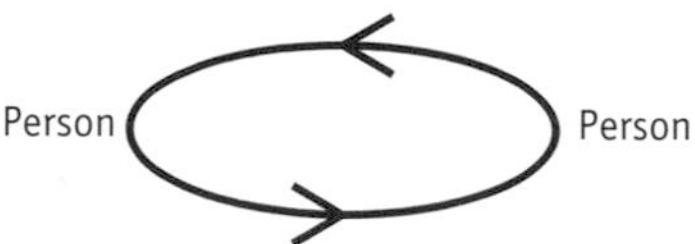


**Figure 12.1** Representation of the communication process.

The diagram shown in Figure 12.1 is very simplistic and does not allow for the complexities surrounding human interaction. What are important to take into consideration are the factors that impede our ability to listen to ourself and others.

Figure 12.2 illustrates some of the factors that midwives, students and women may experience every day which will impede their ability to listen. The factors may be present in one or other or both parties.

Bearing this simple diagram in mind, it is important that each practitioner takes responsibility for themselves to minimize as much as possible the avoidable/preventable factors for both herself and the woman, so that when meeting a woman she can interact with confidence. All of the factors in Figure 12.2 will act as barriers to a relationship developing.

## SPECIFIC COMMUNICATION SKILLS

Communication via body movements and facial expressions take place rapidly and what a person sees may inform a decision-making process more than what is being said or heard. How much we communicate non-verbally continues to be debated. Hargie & Davidson (2004) suggest that what is said contributes a mere 7% of the overall message conveyed. If this is so, then it is important for midwives to become skilled in observing individual women. For example:

- *Body*: her posture; is it upright and relaxed, or crumpled and tense? Does she move with ease, or is her movement restricted? What gestures does she make?
- *Eyes*: are her eyes cast down, or does she look at you with ease? Are her eyes staring or flitting about?
- *Face*: does she look perpetually worried? Or does she bite her lips? Is she frowning or smiling?
- *Voice*: does she speak rapidly or very slowly? Does she seem to struggle to find her words? Is

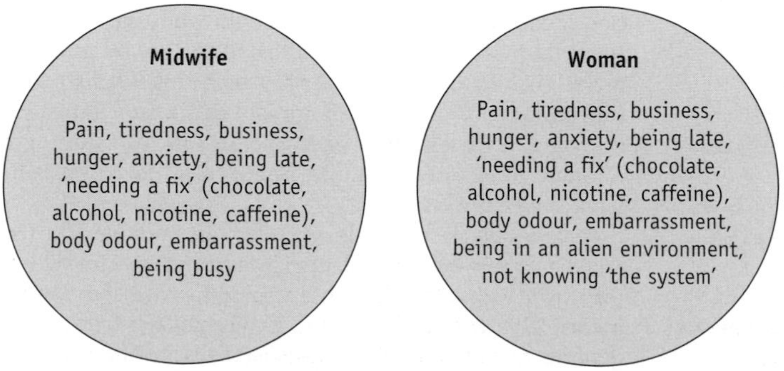

**Midwife**

Pain, tiredness, business, hunger, anxiety, being late, 'needing a fix' (chocolate, alcohol, nicotine, caffeine), body odour, embarrassment, being busy

**Woman**

Pain, tiredness, business, hunger, anxiety, being late, 'needing a fix' (chocolate, alcohol, nicotine, caffeine), body odour, embarrassment, being in an alien environment, not knowing 'the system'

**Figure 12.2** Factors which interfere with listening.

her voice high-pitched? Does she speak loudly or quietly?

- *Personal space*: does she need lots of personal space, or are you able to get physically close to her in your conversations?
- *Physicality*: does she look as if she has prepared herself for her visit, or does she look as if she has not cared for herself? Does she look fit and well or does she look pale and drawn? Does she look physically aroused? Does she seem short of breath? Are her pupils dilated or constricted?

n.b. It is also crucial that the midwife is aware of her own body language, and verbal and non-verbal cues that she might emit, and how these might be translated and understood by the woman and her family.

**Reflective activity 12.1**

It is also useful for midwives to look at themselves in a long mirror and see what the women would see. Not, maybe, a 360-degree mirror, but one in which you see yourself as others might see you. Then ask yourself, do you like what you see? If you do not like what you see, what can you do so that you will like what you see?

This activity may be quite simple: smile so that the smile reaches your eyes; change your hairstyle/colour of your hair; or stand with your head up and your shoulders back, which will immediately make you look 10 lb lighter, and reduce back pain and headaches.

Non-verbal communication such as smiling, nodding your head and beckoning in a welcome expresses warmth and friendliness to the woman. When speaking to a woman it is important to use words that, to her, have a meaning to them and include, with explanation if necessary, professional midwifery terminology so that the midwife does not appear to be condescending. Should the woman see another healthcare practitioner who uses professional terminology, the woman will not feel confused or overwhelmed because she has heard the words previously.

It is important to demonstrate your attention. This is mainly conveyed through body language. Egan (2007) developed the acronym *SOLER*. Prior to meeting a woman for her appointment, it may be useful to repeat the acronym to prime yourself. It is a way of letting go of the previous interaction to focus on the next.

- S *stands for squarely*: it is the positioning of the body to face the woman; it indicates 'I have come to be with you or join you'.
- O *represents open*: crossed arms or holding patient records in front of the body can indicate that you are uncomfortable with the meeting; having your arms by your side indicates a lack of defensiveness, that you feel comfortable meeting the person.
- L *represents an orientation of the body towards the other person*: being able to be flexible to move in to listen if someone speaks quietly; leaning away gives the impression that you are not interested; and a rigid body, that you find being in the person's presence distasteful.
- E *represents eye contact*: the woman may not be looking at you because her culture does not encourage this, but if you look at your client, it demonstrates an interest. It also means that you are able to see when the woman looks towards you for, perhaps, reassurance or acceptance.
- R *represents being relaxed*: a person who fidgets can give the impression that they do not have the time to be with the woman, or they are feeling nervous, which can cause the woman to feel nervous. Being relaxed demonstrates that you are accepting of the woman and of yourself.

Once the woman is sure that she has your attention, it is then important to demonstrate that you are listening to her. At first, passive listening whereby you indicate by para-linguistics, the *'Mm …', 'yes …', 'ok …', 'ahum …', 'right …', using* head nodding and eye contact indicates that you are listening. The same technique can be used whilst speaking to the woman on the telephone to indicate that you are listening and attentive. Be aware that if you are smiling as you talk, this may be transmitted.

What becomes more important is to actively listen, because this will demonstrate not only that you have been listening but also that you have understood. It is this which informs the woman that you do care and that she is an individual.

## Active listening

This involves the use of reflection, paraphrasing, questions and demonstrating the traits of empathy, unconditional positive regard (warmth) and genuineness (see website for Case scenario 12.2).

*Reflection* is the skill whereby the midwife, having listened to the woman, will repeat one or two words back to her to encourage her to continue with what she is saying. If the midwife is not skilled in this, it can sound as if you are mimicking the woman, or just repeating what she has said (Egan 2007). The words are said in the same tone that the woman says them, rather like an echo, so that they resonate in her mind and act as a prompt to go on with what she has been saying.

*Paraphrasing* is the skill whereby the midwife has listened to the woman and then restates in the midwife's own words what the woman has said, the core of the statement (Adler & Rodman 2000). The use of her own words demonstrates that she has absorbed the information, that she understands. Thus, the woman feels understood and supported. If the midwife has incorrectly understood, it gives the woman the opportunity to correct the misunderstanding.

*Questions* can be open, closed, directive and multiple. Many practitioners will ask closed questions, mistakenly thinking that they are open. Too many closed questions can cause women to feel that they have just been interrogated and leave them feeling exposed and vulnerable with, for some, a sense that, 'I don't want to go through that again'.

It is useful for students to practise with each other, taking full records at an initial visit. This can be followed by giving and receiving honest balanced feedback, remembering to give praise so that lessons are learnt. Audio taping or videoing such a session is even more useful because it is then possible to hear and/or see oneself. Many people do not like undertaking such exercises, because they are false; however, if the student performs well in the exercise, then it is likely that the real situation will be even better.

*Empathy* is the ability of the midwife to sense the woman's inner world and communicate that back to the woman. This can be really important when the woman is from a different culture, because she will feel accepted by the midwife.

*Genuineness* is the ability of the midwife to be her real self when working with women and not hide behind a professional façade. Communication from the midwife to the woman should be clear and the midwife clearly hears what the woman has spoken (Egan 2007).

*Unconditional positive regard* is the ability of the midwife to see a woman as a unique person, who is important and whose contribution is valued. If the woman is a drug user, even though the midwife will challenge her in her use of drugs, the midwife still makes clear that she is valued and accepted as a person.

The above skills and traits, used well, will enhance the midwife/woman relationship and enable midwives to perform their functional role, that of midwife; and will assist in identifying whether the woman needs to be referred to a counsellor for ongoing support.

**Reflective activity 12.2**

When you next observe a midwife discussing care with a woman, observe how the above skills are used. How would you use these in the same circumstances?

## THERAPEUTIC COUNSELLING

The midwife is not a therapeutic counsellor; she is a midwife and, as such, needs to learn when to refer women to therapists. Some NHS trusts have specially qualified midwives who can offer ongoing support for women and their partners. Sometimes a midwife may not be able to maintain an emotional distance from a woman and this means the midwife may over-identify with the woman. If this occurs and the NHS trust employs a midwife counsellor who works with women and their families, it would be useful for the midwife to speak to the counsellor to assist the midwife to regain her equilibrium.

## IMPROVING MIDWIFERY CARE

Substandard care caused by poor communication has resulted in the deaths of women (Lewis 2004). This means that every student and midwife must examine communication skills to identify where improvement is necessary. A skills audit and checklist (see website for Tables 12.1a and 12.1b) will assist midwives to identify their own communication skills.

### Interpreters

When a woman is unable to speak English, it is important to offer her the use of an interpreter when she attends for care. However, it is important that interpreters have adequate training so that they ask the questions the healthcare professionals have asked. They need to report back to the midwife exactly what the woman or her partner has said.

It is important that trained or professional interpreters are used so that they do not make assumptions about the woman's answer as this may affect the woman's care adversely. The use of children and family members must be avoided because there may be a lack of understanding of the importance of the questions being asked, or the family member may be reticent to ask the questions owing to feelings of modesty or embarrassment (Bramwell et al 2000) (see Chapter 23). It is important to remember that it takes time to arrange a professional interpreter, which may be impossible during an emergency or during labour (Iqbal 2004). If at all possible, it is important to use the same interpreter at each visit. This will enable the midwife, interpreter and woman to build a trusting respectful tripartite relationship.

## PSYCHOLOGICAL ASPECTS OF PREGNANCY

Each woman will react to the news of being pregnant in a manner relevant to her individual situation. Many changes take place in the childbearing year, physically, emotionally and socially. Physical changes occur whether the woman wants them to or not, although some women will fast to minimize the amount of weight they gain in pregnancy. Some women relish the new identity of mother and adapt without any difficulties; other women do not and find the change of identity difficult, particularly if there has been a difficult relationship with their own mothers, for example, over-controlling or distant. If the woman has many roles to fulfil, she may be torn between the roles she is comfortable with and those which she finds difficult. Equally, a woman's expectations of pregnancy and childbirth will affect how she sees herself in each given situation; does she see herself in control, responding to the changes which happen day by day, or does she see herself out of control, fearful and/or angry? Asking women these questions, and discussing them, may help the midwife see whether a woman has a realistic view of pregnancy and childbirth.

## Family relationships

The woman's relationship with her partner may come under pressure, particularly if the partner feels left out. It is at this time that domestic abuse may present for the first time as the partner becomes insecure and feels jealous (see Chapters 19 and 23). The midwife needs to be observant for signs of such abuse. Finances may become strained as the woman leaves work, even if this is temporary, and this can affect their relationship.

Becoming a parent for the first time challenges a woman's resources:

- Does she have enough basic human support around her?
- Does she have a balanced perception of what is required of the situation?
- Does she have problem-solving skills?

The midwife can help her make an assessment of the above with suggestions regarding how and where further resources may be found.

## Adapting to pregnancy

For some women, this comes naturally; they seem to go with the flow, blooming with health and relishing their pregnancy, not getting upset. Raphael-Leff (1991) referred to these women as facilitators. Others find pregnancy more difficult: the woman feels irked by the fact she is pregnant; it is an inconvenience. These women are referred to as regulators, and may resist the loss of control which pregnancy brings.

# PSYCHOLOGICAL HEALTH DURING PREGNANCY

During the first visit in pregnancy at which a history is taken, midwives should try to identify the woman's perceptions of her mental health. It is also important to identify whether the woman has experienced any previous mental health issue (see Chapter 69). If the midwife has begun to develop a relationship or rapport with the woman, then it is easier to ask this question. If no rapport or relationship exists, then a woman may be loath to disclose this information for fear of stigma or rejection by the midwife.

In the last Confidential Enquiry into Maternal and Child Health (Lewis 2007) the most common cause of indirect deaths and the largest cause of maternal deaths overall was psychiatric illness (for further details, see Chapter 69). It is therefore important to recognize when a woman is mentally ill.

When assessing a woman's psychological health, it is important to establish the following:

- Has the woman experienced any past or present severe mental illness, such as schizophrenia, bipolar disorder (previously known as manic depression), psychosis in an earlier postnatal period or severe depression?
- Has the woman been treated previously by a psychiatrist/specialist mental health team, including care as an inpatient?
- Is the woman already taking drugs for a mental health disorder? If so, is she taking them as prescribed, and if she is, is the practitioner who prescribed the drug aware that she is now pregnant?
- Is there a family history of perinatal mental illness?
- Has the woman experienced in the last month a feeling of being down, depressed or hopeless?
- Has the woman in the last month lost interest or experienced no pleasure in doing things she has always enjoyed doing?

If the woman answers yes to the last two points, it is important to refer her back to her general practitioner for further assessment and support, or to a midwife specialist who will be able to undertake more detailed assessment (see Chapter 69). The general practitioner must be kept informed of any care provided, and the care written in the woman's notes.

**Reflective activity 12.3**

When next taking a history from a woman, reflect whether a comprehensive and detailed history of psychological health was taken, using the above text as a checklist.

Access to counselling in some NHS trusts can be limited. Referral needs to be fast-tracked; or if a woman's mental illness is considered to be mild, such as a mild depression, she can be advised about self-help approaches such as relaxation techniques, or guided imagery to focus on the positive aspects of her life (see Chapter 69 for more serious situations).

Each NHS trust should have a clinical network which provides perinatal mental health services so that women receive the care most appropriate for them (NICE 2007) and midwives must be aware to whom they would refer a woman for the most appropriate care.

## PSYCHOLOGICAL ASPECTS OF CAESAREAN SECTION

The caesarean section rate at an urban hospital known by the author in 1978 was 13%, spontaneous births 80% and instrumental births 7%. In London teaching hospitals at the same time the caesarean section rate was 20%. Birth was no more or no less dangerous than it is today; however, women's belief in their ability to give birth has decreased and the request for elective caesarean sections has increased. Along with this self-doubt is the fear of the pain that is to be experienced or the damage that may be caused by a vaginal birth (see website for Case scenario 12.3).

Women who request birth by caesarean section may be:

- a woman who has heard 'nightmare' stories from friends and families and is just too scared to experience birth, and so is tocophobic: a woman in this situation may have no physical reasons why she cannot give birth spontaneously but is too anxious to do so, and probably experiences anxiety in other aspects of her life
- a woman who has previously experienced a traumatic birth, and does not wish to repeat that experience.

It would be useful for both these women to be referred to a midwife who specializes in counselling and/or be offered psychotherapy with women or encouraged to meet and speak with those who are able to speak of enjoyable birth experiences (see website for Case scenario 12.3). In addition, women who have had a baby born by caesarean section often need the opportunity to reflect upon their labours. If a woman's baby has been born by emergency caesarean section following a few hours in labour with analgesia, she may not be able to remember events clearly. This means she will feel confused and result in her feeling traumatized. She may not have been able to read the non-verbal communication because of her tiredness and the analgesia received; her hearing may have been affected and she may not be able to remember having been told certain information. If this has happened, she may feel very frightened because she felt so out of control and angry as it seemed that no-one spoke to her at the time.

Offering a woman the opportunity to see her notes and discuss this with the midwife who cared for her for the longest period of time so that she may go through the records of her labour will assist in making sense of what has happened. This may decrease her confusion and therefore her anger to help her become calm enough to sleep and also to care for her baby (Smith & Mitchell 1996).

When words such as 'Caesarean section for failure to progress' have been written in the notes (or spoken), a woman is left feeling a failure. She, therefore, begins her parenting/mothering career in a negative mood. This mood can be difficult to shift and self-doubt (which can be confused with depression) can set in, leading to increased anxiety. This will affect the flow of breast milk and thus her ability to feed her baby.

When working through the notes it is important to praise the woman so that she is able to see how well she did and that she did not fail in any way. We need to remember that people require five portions of praise to counterbalance one portion of criticism. This is important not only in our work with women but also with our colleagues. When giving feedback to our students or colleagues we need to remember to balance praise with criticism, because midwives can feel disappointed or a failure when births do not go as expected. Therefore, all women and midwives need appropriate support offered to them by their peers or by supervisors of midwives (Lewis 2004).

## POST BIRTH, THE EARLY DAYS OF MOTHERHOOD

A woman's first experience of contact with her baby will differ according to how she has experienced her pregnancy and her birth and her personal expectations. Some women experience relief, joy, with overwhelming love. Others will experience shock; as the baby will not match the fantasy picture created in their mind:

- The baby may be blonde whereas she was expecting a dark-haired baby.
- She may be expecting a big baby and finds she has a smaller baby.
- She may be filled with loathing because the baby is covered in 'muck'.

All of these experiences are normal, and the way the midwife interacts with the woman will enable expression of these thoughts and feelings so as to adjust to motherhood. It is when a woman is unable to express her thoughts and feelings that she remains anxious and therefore unsettled, unable to enjoy her baby and get to know him or her, and, most importantly, to sleep. Sleep is a great healer and enables the body and mind to recuperate and re-create itself. Sleep deprivation may lead to irritability, tearfulness, tension, anxiety and self-doubt.

At some point in the first 24 hours, the woman and her partner will explore the baby, looking for familial similarities. If a woman is frightened to do this, the midwife needs to assist her in this meeting with her baby. This is usually more successful when the baby is awake and alert, therefore responsive to the parents smiling and crooning. If possible, this meeting is best undertaken within a short period following the birth so that breastfeeding may be initiated. As the midwife is more likely to recognize a baby communicating the desire to feed, she needs, in a warm positive tone of voice, to point out the signs when the baby is looking for mummy to feed him or her, whatever method of feeding has been chosen. The woman can then recognize the signs in the future. In this way, the woman will not feel that she lacks experience. If the woman has chosen to breastfeed, explain to her before she offers the breast to the baby, that she needs to be physically comfortable. Also, demonstrate how to recognize when baby is in the correct feeding position. This will increase a woman's confidence and her ability to breastfeed her baby successfully. Explain that baby will learn along with her, but that all babies have an instinct to suckle.

A quiet period following the birth allows the stress hormones activated in labour to recede and settle, enabling anxiety and fear to decrease so that a woman and her partner may celebrate their success together. This settling often enables the woman to look back on her birth experience with satisfaction as it enables her to regain her control. If this quiet period is missing after a birth, a woman's agitation is likely to increase with the sense of being out of control. This will occur especially when a woman is hurried out of a birthing room because the delivery suite is busy and her bed is needed.

If this does happen, the midwife needs to ensure that wherever the mother is moved, she and her partner are able to have quiet time together. This often means protecting women from initial visits from relatives or friends. This may result in the midwife being unpopular, but the woman, partner and baby come first.

## BABY IN THE NEONATAL UNIT

When a baby is ill and has been removed to a neonatal unit, the woman must be able to see photographs or a digital recording of her baby. A visit, as soon as possible, is also important, by the mother or by her partner, who will report back, or by both together, so that they may see, touch or even hold the baby; as this will reassure parents that the baby is alive and beginning to thrive, which assists in reducing the trauma of the separation (Robinson 2002).

The woman and her partner will need clear explanations of the care and any reasons for plans in caring for the baby. The explanations may have to be repeated or written down so that parents may grasp what has happened. Their anxiety may interfere with their ability to absorb information. If women are separated from their babies, regular updates need to be given for them to understand what is happening and have some control over the situation.

If a woman shows no interest in her baby, this needs to be noted, but not acted upon straight away. The midwife needs to continue offering support to the woman and speaking of the baby as she would with a woman who is besotted with her baby. Most women in this situation adjust and begin to show an interest within 24 to 48 hours of the birth. If the woman continues to express little or no interest in her baby after this period of time, it is important to liaise with the woman's health visitor so that the woman receives extra support on her transfer home.

During the first few weeks following the birth the woman and her family will need to make adjustments to their relationships and the way they live. Most women are surprised by the amount of time it takes to care for a newborn baby. Women may express their dismay when their baby does not feed and sleep for 4 hours, thus allowing them to get on with household chores. The baby may not sleep throughout the night and women will have to get up and feed baby, often three or four times a night, thus they experience sleep deprivation. Resentment is often experienced towards the partner who may have persuaded the woman to artificially feed the baby because, 'Then I will be able to feed baby during the night and take my turn.' Whilst this is often a naïve belief, the partner may have been truthful when expressing this statement, but may not have had any previous experience of life with a baby. If the partner has to return to work immediately following the birth and is expected to be out of the house by early morning and does not return until late evening, it is unlikely that the partner will be able to assist with night feeds. The demands of the daily work routine combined with a disturbed sleep pattern may lead to sleep deprivation causing stress to both parents. It is important for midwives to explore the reality of new parenthood at some point with women and their partners.

## PHYSIOLOGICAL EVENT

Though promotion of birth as a normal physiological event is ideal, it is important to recognize it is a strenuous event. Women used to remain in hospital recuperating from the birth for a period of 10 days, but they now return home within 6 to 48 hours after birth. This is appropriate as the family can begin to make the adjustments required to accept the baby into the home.

Many women have support at home for a week whilst the partner has parental leave. Given that the woman has probably been in hospital for a very limited period of time or had her baby at home, she is likely to be tired from the birth.

In some cultures, women are supported by other female family members for up to 6 weeks. If an aunt or sister is able to move into the house to take over the household chores whilst the woman focuses on mothering her baby and greeting her partner at the end of the day, this is to be welcomed and celebrated. If this is not possible, then encourage the new family to ask friends and family for practical support such as some housework or a cooked meal. A midwife who explains carefully to the woman about increasing her activities slowly, is offering good advice; often women attempt to return to 'normal' too soon and end up being tired or developing mild postnatal depression because they cannot live up to their own high expectations.

## CONCLUSION

The journey from conception through pregnancy, childbirth and early parenting is full of immense change in every aspect of a woman's life. It is a time when a woman is at her most creative and during this creativity she has the right to have midwives who are able to support her to achieve a safe, normal pregnancy and labour that is as happy and enjoyable as possible. The midwife is the health professional who is able to support the woman on her journey and to offer holistic care which takes into account the psychological aspects of the childbearing journey.

### KEY POINTS

- Midwives must learn the skills to develop a working relationship with women and their families.
- Midwives must develop self-awareness so that they understand how they impact on a woman and her decision-making process.
- It is crucial to be aware of the impact of verbal and non-verbal communication.
- Midwives need to recognize that they are role models for women.
- Midwives, rather than medical staff, are more likely to provide emotional support to women and need to refine their communication skills in order to support a woman throughout her journey to becoming a mother.

## REFERENCES


Adler R, Rodman G: *Understanding human communication*, ed 7, Fort Worth, 2000, Harcourt College Publishers.

Bramwell R, Harrington F, Harris J: *Deaf women: informed choice, policy and legislation, British Journal Midwifery* 8(9):545–548, 2000.

Cialdini R: *Influence: science and practice*, Boston, 2001, Allyn and Bacon.

Clarkson P: *The therapeutic relationship*, London, 1996, Whurr Publishers.

Clarkson P: Personal communication. Study Day for Students and Supervisors, MSc Therapeutic Counselling, University of Greenwich, June 2000.

Currie SM: *Aspects of the preparation of student midwives for autonomous practice, Midwifery* 15(4):283–292, 1999.

Donovan P: *Confidence in newly qualified midwives, British Journal of Midwifery* 16(8):510–514, 2008.

Egan G: *The skilled helper*, Belmont, CA, 2007, Brooks/Cole.

Fraser DM: *Women's perceptions of midwifery care: a longitudinal study to shape curriculum development, Birth* 26(2):99–107, 1999.

Griffith S: *A review of the factors associated with patient compliance and the taking of prescribed medicines, British Journal of General Practice* 40(332):114–116, 1990.

Hargie O, Davidson D: *Skilled interpersonal communication: research theory and practice*, ed 4, London, 2004, Routledge.

Hollins Martin CJ, Bull P: *Obedience and conformity in clinical practice, British Journal of Midwifery* 16(8):504–509, 2008.

Iqbal S: *Pregnancy and birth: a guide for deaf women*, London, 2004, Royal National Institute for the Deaf (RNID) and The National Childbirth Trust (NCT).

Kings Fund: *Safe birth: everybody's business*, London, 2008, Kings Fund.

Lewis G: *Why mothers die. 2000–2002 Confidential Enquiry into Maternal and Child Health*, London, 2004, RCOG Press.

Lewis G, editor: *The Confidential Enquiry into Maternal and Child Health (CEMACH). Saving mothers' lives: reviewing maternal deaths to make motherhood safer – 2003–2005. The Seventh Report on Confidential Enquiries into Maternal Deaths in the United Kingdom*, London, 2007, CEMACH.

NICE: *Antenatal and postnatal mental health: clinical management and service guidance*, London, 2007, British Psychological Society and Royal College of Psychiatrists.

Raphael-Leff J: *Psychological processes of childbearing*, London, 1991, Chapman & Hall.

Robinson J: *Separation from the baby – a cause for PTSD? British Journal of Midwifery* 10(9):508, 2002.

Smith J, Mitchell S: *Debriefing after childbirth: a tool for objective risk management, British Journal of Midwifery* 4(11):581–586, 1996.

Youngson R: *Compassion in healthcare: the missing dimension of health reform*, London, 2008, NHS Confederation.

# Chapter 13

# Sexuality

*Karen Jackson*

## LEARNING OUTCOMES

By the end of this chapter, the reader will be able to:

- cite a basic definition of 'sexuality'
- outline the psychological, social and physiological implications of sex and sexuality during pregnancy, childbirth and afterwards
- describe the implications of pregnancy and childbirth for women who are survivors of sexual abuse, women who have undergone female genital mutilation and for women who are lesbians
- list some of the factors that may impact on sex and sexuality for women who are breastfeeding.

### Reflective activity 13.1

Whilst reading this chapter, think of the word 'sexuality'. What does it mean? Write down a simple definition, or words that you would associate with 'sexuality'.

Did you find the task easy? If not, why do you think 'sexuality' is difficult to define?

## SEXUALITY

The word sexuality is scattered liberally throughout contemporary sexual health literature, but the text frequently fails to explore what sexuality actually means. The word itself did not come into being until the modern era, and many authors are reluctant to confine it to a simple definition. This may well be because sexuality is fundamentally dynamic. It has different meanings culturally, its definition changes throughout history, and an individual's feelings and values concerning their sexuality alter as they gain more life experience.

Lion (1982:8) embraces sexuality as a concept that is open to transmutation as 'all those aspects of the human being that relate to being a boy or girl, woman or man, and is an entity subject to lifelong dynamic change. Sexuality reflects our human character not solely our genital nature.' This definition alone demonstrates clearly that sexuality is more than overt sexual behaviour encompassing the complete range of human experience (Pratt 2000). A more recent definition, courtesy of the Royal College of Nursing (RCN 2000, cited on contents page), states that sexuality is: 'an individual's self concept, shaped by their personality and expressed through a heterosexual, homosexual, bisexual or transsexual orientation'. This definition may reflect a more contemporary view of sexuality.

The word 'sex' is usually employed to mean the act of having sex or to distinguish between the 'sexes' – that is, male or female. Gender is the name given to socially and culturally defined characteristics of the sexes – that is, masculinity and femininity.

## PUBERTY AND TEENAGE PREGNANCY

Please see website and Chapters 19, 23 and 32 for more information.

## SEX DURING PREGNANCY

Sex during pregnancy has historically been shrouded in myth, misconceptions and old wives' tales. The advice offered during traditional British antenatal care has been one of abstention, without any evidence to substantiate this stance.

During pregnancy, many couples are fearful of continuing their sexual relationship. They may feel that they may somehow provoke miscarriage, premature labour or damage the fetus; some men have expressed fear of breaking the 'bag of waters' (Kitzinger 1985). Couples can be reassured that this is not the case.

The overriding message from most well-conducted studies is that sex during pregnancy for the vast majority of women is safe and does not lead to any increase in complications (Enkin et al 2000), though male superior position (Ekwo et al 1993) and a vagina colonized with specific micro-organisms, for example *Trichomonas vaginalis* (Read & Klebanoff 1993), have both been associated with preterm birth. More studies are required in this area to provide definitive results. The National Institute for Clinical Excellence (NICE) (2003) antenatal care guidelines stated that health professionals can inform healthy pregnant women that sexual intercourse during pregnancy is not known to be associated with any adverse outcomes.

**Reflective activity 13.2**

A woman who has just had confirmation that she is 8 weeks pregnant asks about sex during pregnancy. Which of the following statements would you agree with:

- Sex is safe for most couples throughout pregnancy.
- Sex should be confined to the second trimester of pregnancy only.
- All forms of sexual activity are safe throughout pregnancy.
- There are certain clinical contraindications to sex in pregnancy.
- Sexual activity generally decreases as pregnancy progresses.
- Some women feel more sexy during pregnancy.

There are a few definite or relative contraindications to different sexual practices or sexual intercourse during pregnancy. Forceful blowing of air into the vagina during oral sex is an absolute contraindication, as this may lead to fatal air embolism (Aston 2005, Lumley & Astbury 1989). The insertion of a foreign body into the vagina may cause damage to the internal structures and introduce infection (Walton 1994). Placenta praevia, vaginal bleeding, history of premature birth and rupture of membranes are often cited as clinical reasons to avoid sex during pregnancy (Aston 2005).

Whilst sex can be enjoyed by couples throughout the whole of pregnancy, other factors may play an important role. Change of body image (see website), tiredness, breast changes, backache and frequency of micturition are some of the things that can affect a pregnant woman's sexuality (Aston 2005). There are many accounts that give a very negative view of sexuality and pregnancy. Kitzinger (1985) states that some women have a distorted view of their bodies during pregnancy, they feel bigger than they really are and think that their partners must find them ugly when in fact the partners often delight in pregnant women and find their physical changes exciting and beautiful.

Conversely, some women have a very positive 'body image' during pregnancy. They feel incredibly attractive and womanly. It is viewed as the ultimate expression of femininity and an eminently powerful symbol of potency and fertility.

Physiological hormonal changes during pregnancy mean that oestrogen and progesterone act together to procure marked pelvic vasocongestion, which occurs as a result of increased vascularity and venous stasis. The results can mean a heightened manifestation of all aspects of sexual intercourse, including orgasm (Aston 2005). For some, this may be the first time that they experience orgasm (Walton 1994). For others, however, vasocongestion may predispose the woman to discomfort during sexual intercourse (Aston 2005).

It is often assumed that there is a linear decrease in sexual activity as pregnancy progresses, but for some women sexual activity may well increase during the second trimester. This may be due to the disorders of pregnancy subsiding and the woman developing a sense of wellbeing. However, it is also well recognized that sex diminishes during the third trimester (Frohlich et al 1990), most probably due to the discomfort and mechanics of having sex with a greatly enlarged abdomen. Alternative positions to the missionary position, such as the man behind the woman or 'spooning', or the woman sitting or kneeling on top of the man, could be explored.. Other non-penetrative options such as self or mutual masturbation, oral sex, fondling or massage or purely kissing and cuddling may also be adopted (Walton 1994).

It is suggested that having sexual intercourse may be an alternative to other methods of induction, the theory being that sperm is rich in prostaglandins, thereby providing a stimulus for ripening the cervix. However, to date, this has been poorly evaluated, and more research is required in this area (Kavanagh et al 2001).

Overall, keeping clear channels of communication open is the most important aspect of maintaining an intimate sexual or non-sexual relationship.

## SEXUALITY AND LABOUR

Labour is usually synonymous with anxiety, discomfort and pain. It is not often viewed as being a 'sexual' experience. It is clear when reading literature in this area that for some women and their partners it can be an intensely pleasurable and sexual experience. The sounds a woman makes during contractions, the organs that are used in the process of childbirth, the overwhelming energies and powers that are at work during labour, are all intimately related to sex and sexuality (Aston 2005, Gaskin 2002, Kitzinger 1985, Williams 1996). Kitzinger (1985:210) describes it thus: 'the most intensely sexual feeling a woman ever experiences, as strong as orgasm, even more compelling than orgasm'. In her book *Spiritual midwifery*, Gaskin (2002) quotes a number of experiences of the sexual nature of childbirth. One woman recounts her birth experience with her husband: 'My rushes (contractions) hardly felt heavy at all, but I knew they must be because I was opening up. We just kept making out and rubbing each other. We got to places that we had forgotten we could get to... going through the birthing I felt his love very strong. It was like getting married all over again' (Gaskin 2002:53). Rabuzzi (1994) cites examples of other couples' erotic experiences of labour. One husband of a woman having a home birth said: 'The birth was not only painless, but very pleasurable. We had never read about this aspect.' He goes on to describe the noises his wife made whilst the baby's head was crowning as being 'orgasmic' and ends with: "what a long way from the pain and agony of conventional myth' (Rabuzzi 1994:120).

If labour can be such a sensual and gratifying experience, it may be a cultural or contextual aspect that makes it generally viewed negatively. It is suggested by some that the scientific and technological procedures have taken childbirth out of the hands of women and set it in the context of the powerful male-dominated institution of the hospital (Cosslett 1994, Williams 1996), where everything is controlled, the medical model's ultimate goal being 'safety' whatever the cost. In contrast, the natural childbirth discourse is focused on the power of the woman, which is more in evidence in home births (Cosslett 1994; Williams 1996). Midwives argue that 'safety' and 'satisfaction' are both achievable.

Nipple stimulation is known to produce oxytocin, and therefore can be performed by the woman or her partner to attempt to initiate or augment labour naturally. Privacy will of course be required if she wishes to try this activity.

## WOMEN REQUIRING SPECIALIZED CARE

There are some groups of women who may need specialized care and attention during pregnancy, labour, childbirth and afterwards. Some are discussed below.

**Reflective activity 13.3**

Listed below is a group of women who you may well care for in clinical practice

- Anne, a woman who is a survivor of sexual abuse
- Lydia, a pregnant lesbian
- Saadah, who underwent female genital mutilation as a child
- Katie, a woman who had chlamydia
- Bernie, a woman who is breastfeeding

What are the issues concerning sexuality for each of these woman?

It is important not to stereotype these women. All will quite probably have similar issues, but in addition: Anne may have to deal with reactivated memories of the abuse; Lydia may have to deal with homophobia and sometimes hostile behaviour; Saadah may be terrified of labour and birth; Katie may face stigma and labelling of being promiscuous; Bernie may have conflict between being a nursing mother and a sexual being.

## SURVIVORS OF SEXUAL ABUSE

The prevalence rate for reported cases of childhood sexual abuse is around 21% for females in the UK. A similar or higher rate is reported in Canada and North America (NSPCC 2007). It is clear, given the high prevalence of childhood sexual abuse, that midwives will, at some point, care for women who have survived sexual abuse. These women may or may not disclose such abuse to their carers.

Memories of abuse, even those that have been partially or wholly repressed, may be triggered by pregnancy and childbirth (Courtois & Riley 1992, Kitzinger 1990). The change in body image, submission to physical contact, and feelings of powerlessness are all factors that are likely to make the survivor regress back to times when she encountered similar susceptibilities.

Women who have been previously sexually abused may display a range of behaviours as follows:

- extreme anxiety over intimate examinations
- needing to be in complete control
- dissociating themselves from the experience or
- being quite uninhibited, engaging freely in sexual banter (Rhodes & Hutchinson 1994).

Some of the styles exhibited by sexual abuse survivors may also be enacted by women who have not been abused; however, in the former group, the behaviour may appear extreme.

Control has been identified as being of grave importance to women who have been sexually abused (Parratt 1994). Therefore, keeping women well informed, ensuring that they are made part of the decision-making process and obtaining informed consent for all procedures are absolute requirements.

### Caring for the lesbian client

It is becoming more common for lesbian couples to fulfil the desire to become parents by using natural or artificial means. These couples will generally enter the maternity services for care and support during pregnancy and childbirth. It is therefore imperative that the needs of these clients are recognized. Many lesbian writers and writers who have explored lesbian issues identify that lesbians as a group are largely ignored and consequently become invisible in texts discussing women's health (Wilton 1996).

Midwives can do much to ensure that a lesbian's experience of pregnancy and childbirth is a positive and empowering one. They can attain this by being knowledgeable about lesbian sexuality, by using non-heterosexist language, by giving appropriate advice, by being non-judgemental and by rejecting socially constructed stereotypes (Hastie 2000).

### Female genital mutilation (FGM)

Please see website and Chapter 58 for further information.

### Sexually transmitted infections (STIs)

Please see website and Chapter 57 for further information.

## PATERNAL PRESENCE AT THE BIRTH

In western societies, there has been a cultural shift from men being virtually excluded from the birthing room, to men being actively encouraged to attend the birth of their child. It is not known what effect paternal presence at birth has on the process of labour or on the subsequent relationship of the couple. It does appear, however, in some studies that the presence of a female companion such as a doula can have numerous positive effects on the outcome of labour (Kennell & Klaus 1991).

One dimension of paternal presence at birth that is rarely discussed is the possible adverse effects on subsequent sexual relationships. Sex therapists working with sexually dysfunctional couples have discovered that the man's experience of what was for him a traumatic labour and delivery has stifled any sexual feelings for his wife/partner (O'Driscoll 1998).

It is the midwife's responsibility to ensure that the couple realize the importance and enormity of the decision for the man 'to be there or not to be there'. They should be encouraged to discuss the issue openly (ideally antenatally) with the pros and cons clearly defined so that they can make an informed choice.

## PERINEAL CARE

See website and Chapter 40 for further information on care of women with perineal problems.

## SEX AFTER CHILDBIRTH

As with sex during pregnancy, many social and cultural taboos surround the issue of sex after childbirth. The main issues appear to be fear of infection and trauma, but there is no evidence to support these possible complications provided that the sexual activity is considerate and gentle (Walton 1994). The woman herself is therefore the best person to regulate when she is ready to resume sexual intercourse. In the past, there appeared to be an unwritten rule that women should abstain from sex until after the 6-week postnatal check, when the GP could give her the 'all clear' to resume sexual relations. It was assumed that all would be well sexually after this period of time. The reality, however, is quite contrary. Limited research in this field demonstrates that childbirth causes high levels of sexual morbidity and states that this is not adequately addressed by health professionals (Barrett et al 2000, Glazener 1997, National Childbirth Trust et al 1994).

There are also a number of areas related to sexuality and childbirth that appear to raise important issues for midwives and the women for whom they care. It is important that family planning is discussed with the woman soon after the birth; one of the reasons for this is that a woman's fertility can return quite soon after giving birth. In addition to this, fear of becoming pregnant can diminish desire for sex.

A reduced libido postnatally may be an indication of underlying problems within the relationship, or could be a symptom of postnatal depression. If this is the case, other professionals will need to be involved in giving specialized care and attention.

However, in the majority of cases, sexual problems following childbirth are directly linked to the pregnancy, the labour and birth, or the baby. This being the case, midwives and other health professionals involved in childbirth are in a prime position to counsel, guide and support parents with sexual anxieties. Some of the more common reasons for breakdown in sexual relations may be related to negative body image, or confusion over adopting the dual roles of mother and lover (see website).

## BREASTFEEDING AND SEXUALITY

The literature surrounding the effect of breastfeeding (Chapter 43) on sexuality and sexual activity is confusing and largely conflicting. Some found a positive effect on sexual activity (Masters & Johnson 1966); some found a negative impact (Alder & Bancroft 1983); and yet others found that there was no effect on sexual interest (Reamy & White 1987).

More up-to-date research further supports the hypothesis that breastfeeding reduces interest in sex (Barrett et al 2000, Glazener 1997). There are two assertions that may be derived from the conflicting evidence: firstly, that further well-conducted, comprehensive research is required in this field; and secondly, that no definitive conclusions **can** be drawn. Therefore, women's sexuality may be affected in any of the ways described and each woman must be cared for, advised and counselled accordingly.

### Breastfeeding, sexuality and sexual difficulties

Alder & Bancroft (1983) found that during the early postnatal period, and particularly if the baby is being breastfed, many women report a significant decrease in libido, or a complete loss of interest in sex.

There may be several reasons why breastfeeding may interfere with sexual relations:

- the mother's requirements for intimacy are being met by the baby
- she feels guilty and thrown into conflict about having sexual feelings whilst breastfeeding
- high prolactin levels and low oestrogen levels may affect libido
- fatigue caused by regular feeding day and night
- the partner's feelings of jealousy towards the baby
- milk ejection during intercourse.

Being sexually stimulated by a suckling baby can provoke feelings of confusion and guilt. The woman may feel that she is somehow perverted (Hulme 1993). It is hardly surprising that breastfeeding as well as sexual intercourse brings about such pleasurable feelings: these basic actions have evolved to secure the survival of the human race (Evans 1992). She should be reassured that breastfeeding is an immensely satisfying experience and one that should be relished.

Milk ejection during intercourse, if this causes a problem to the couple, can be alleviated by breastfeeding the baby or expressing milk prior to coitus. Some couples incorporate this phenomenon into their sexual play (Van Wert 1996); provided that both parties are happy with this, there is no physiological reason to discourage such an activity.

Vaginal dryness has been reported, particularly in breastfeeding mothers, possibly because of low oestrogen levels. An appropriate lubricating gel (water-based if used in conjunction with condoms) may be used to address this problem. This may be discussed in conjunction with family planning advice.

## THE MENOPAUSE

This is a time of immense change when a woman's fertility reduces, though she may continue to be fertile. A reduction in the fertility hormones, in particular oestrogen and progesterone, may cause bodily changes that may also affect a woman's sense of sexuality. Some find this a period of liberation whilst others may experience a sense a loss of opportunities for fertility.

## CONCLUSION

Just because a woman is pregnant, in labour, giving birth, or recovering from birth, she does not cease to be a sexual being. The parameters of 'normality' in terms of sexuality are wide, varied and unique to each woman. As the very essence of sexuality is embodied within childbirth, aspects of sexuality should be considered as an integral part of the care that women receive from midwives. A midwife should have the knowledge and skills to be able to advise, support, educate and counsel women appropriately, which includes acknowledging her limitations and referring to another health professional. For most women, the expert, sensitive care from her midwife will be all that is required.

### KEY POINTS

- Sex during pregnancy is safe for the majority of women.
- Labour for some women can be an immensely satisfying, sensual or sexual experience.
- Sexuality should be an issue considered for all pregnant, labouring and postnatal women, but some women will require special care and attention: survivors of sexual abuse, lesbians, women who have undergone female genital mutilation, breastfeeding mothers.
- Sex following birth should initially be regulated by the woman, i.e. when she feels ready.

## REFERENCES


Alder E, Bancroft J: *Sexual behaviour of lactating women: a preliminary communication, Journal of Reproductive and Infant Psychology* 1(2):47–52, 1983.

Aston G: *Sexuality during and after pregnancy*. In Andrews G, editor: *Women's sexual health*, ed 3, London, 2005, Baillière Tindall.

Barrett G, Pendry E, Peacock J, et al: *Women's sexual health after childbirth. British Journal of Obstetrics and Gynaecology* 107(2):186–195, 2000.

Cosslett T: *Women writing childbirth: modern discourses of motherhood*, Manchester, 1994, Manchester University Press.

Courtois C, Riley C: *Pregnancy and childbirth as triggers for abuse memories: implications for care, Birth* 19(4):222–223, 1992,

Ekwo E, Gosselink C, Woolson R, et al: *Coitus late in pregnancy: risk of preterm rupture of amniotic sac membranes, American Journal of Obstetrics and Gynecology* 1(1):22–31, 1993.

Enkin M, Keirse M, Neilson J, et al: *A guide to effective care in pregnancy and childbirth*, ed 3, Oxford, 2000, Oxford University Press.

Evans K: *Getting back to nature, Modern Midwife* 2(1):14–17, 1992.

Frohlich E, Herz C, van der Merwe F, et al: *Sexuality during pregnancy and early puerperium and its perception by the pregnant and puerperal woman, Journal of Psychosomatic Obstetrics and Gynaecology* 11(1):73–79, 1990.

Gaskin I: *Spiritual midwifery*, ed 4, Summertown, 2002, Book Publishing Company.

Glazener C: *Sexual function after childbirth: women's experiences, persistent morbidity and lack of professional recognition, British Journal of Obstetrics and Gynaecology* 104(3):330–335, 1997.

Hastie N: *Cultural conceptions: lesbian parenting and midwifery practice*. In Fraser D, editor: *Professional studies for midwifery practice*, London, 2000, Churchill Livingstone.

Hulme H: *Grin and bear it, Nursing Times* 89(6):66, 1993.

Kavanagh J, Kelly A, Thomas J: Sexual intercourse for cervical ripening and induction of labour, *Cochrane Database of Systematic Reviews* (2):CD003093, 2001.

Kennell J, Klaus M: *Continuous emotional support during labor in a US hospital. A randomized controlled trial, Journal of the American Medical Association* 265(17):2197–2201, 1991.

Kitzinger S: *Women's experience of sex*, London, 1985, Penguin.

Kitzinger J: *Recalling the pain, Nursing Times* 86(3):39–40, 1990.

Lion E, editor: *Human sexuality in nursing process*, New York, 1982, Wiley.

Lumley J, Astbury J: *Advice for pregnancy*: In Chalmers I, Enkin M, Keirse M, editors: Effective care in pregnancy and childbirth, vol 1, Oxford, 1989, Oxford University Press.

Masters W, Johnson V: *Human sexual response*, Boston, 1966, Little, Brown.

National Childbirth Trust, Victor C, Barrett G: *Is there sex after childbirth? New Generation* 13(2):24–25, 1994.

National Institute for Clinical Excellence (NICE): *Antenatal care: routine care for the healthy pregnant woman*, Clinical guideline 6, London, 2003 (Updated version June 2008), NICE.

National Society for the Prevention of Cruelty to Children (NSPCC): *NSPCC inform. Sexual abuse. Key child protection statistics* (website). www.nspcc.org.uk/inform. 2007. Accessed August 8, 2008.

O'Driscoll M: *Midwives discover sex, The Practising Midwife* 1(4):27–29, 1998.

Parratt J: *The experience of childbirth for survivors of incest, Midwifery* 10:26–39, 1994.

Pratt R: *Sexual health and disease: an international perspective*. In Wilson H, McAndrew S, editors: *Sexual health*, London, 2000, Baillière Tindall.

Rabuzzi K: *Mother with child*, Indiana, 1994, Indiana University Press.

Read J, Klebanoff M: *Sexual intercourse during pregnancy and preterm delivery: effects of vaginal microorganisms, American Journal of Obstetrics and Gynecology* 168(2):514–519, 1993.

Reamy K, White S: *Sexuality in the puerperium: a review, Archives of Sexual Behaviour* 16(2):165–186, 1987.

Rhodes N, Hutchinson S: *Labour experiences of childhood sexual abuse survivors, Birth* 21(4):213–220, 1994.

Royal College of Nursing (RCN): *Sexuality and sexual health in nursing practice*, London, 2000, RCN.

Van Wert W: *When lovers become parents, Mothering* 81(Winter):58–61, 1996.

Walton I: *Sexuality and motherhood*, Cheshire, 1994, Books for Midwives.

Williams C: *Midwives and sexuality: earth mother or coy maiden?* In Frith L, editor: *Ethics and midwifery: issues in contemporary practice*, Oxford, 1996, Butterworth-Heinemann.

Wilton T: *Caring for the lesbian client: homophobia and midwifery, British Journal of Midwifery* 4(2):126–131, 1996.

Chapter |14|

# The health service context and midwifery

*Tara Kaufmann*

## LEARNING OUTCOMES

After reading this chapter, you will be able to:

- identify key developments in National Health Service (NHS) policy and practice
- be aware of how policy developments in the NHS may impact on the role of the midwife and on maternity services
- appreciate the opportunities and threats of NHS change for midwives, mothers, babies and their families.

## INTRODUCTION

Why should midwives concern themselves with change and reform in the wider NHS? Working in the health service can sometimes feel like a constant exercise in rearranging deckchairs, as successive waves of restructuring, targets and priorities lap against the heels of professionals working within the NHS. There are many health professionals who do a very good job of taking care of patients whilst paying little attention to the world outside their own practice or their profession. Getting an understanding of the wider picture of midwifery and the context of the health service makes the midwife more effective and able to work as an advocate for women and families. Without that understanding, it is difficult to respond effectively to change and to proactively use the opportunities that change provides. Recognizing where to obtain funding streams and policy initiatives that can transform the maternity services and the wider services that are associated with maternal, child and family healthcare are frequently lost opportunities, as without a realization of the wider picture midwives may not recognize what could be offered to assist in transforming their service. Importantly, an understanding by midwives of the environment and context of their practice allows more control to be exerted, and helps prevent staff alienation and burnout (Sandall 1999).

It is particularly important for midwives to engage with NHS reform (see Midwifery 2020 website). Too often, midwives feel oppressed rather than supported by the system within which they work. Some see midwives' gradual loss of autonomy – as they came under NHS control, and then into the hospital system over the last few decades – as the loss of a golden age, and believe that the only way to rejuvenate midwifery and improve care for women is to 'liberate' midwives from external control – and, in particular, from control by doctors (Kirkham & Stapleton 2004). Much has been written about the historic battle for control between (male) medicine and (female) midwifery (Donnison 1988) (see Ch. 2), and this polarization is still evident in maternity services today (a battle in which midwives usually fare badly and childbearing women fare worse). While gender is an important factor in this dynamic, there are others: the balance of power and resources between primary and secondary healthcare, between the needs of the ill few and the healthy majority, between regulating quality and allowing local flexibility, between the advancement of knowledge and the strengthening of basic healthcare provision. In other words, midwives are facing similar challenges to those experienced by many others in the NHS, and midwives – as much as anyone else in the health service – can work to influence and benefit from NHS reform.

Midwives are proud to be an 'autonomous' profession, but the reality is that no health worker is truly autonomous in today's NHS. The teams of professionals are all as effective as the partnerships they create, the opportunities seized, and the resources identified and used. That means that engaging with wider NHS reform is of crucial interest to all those concerned about the future of maternity services.

At the time of writing, the UK is undergoing a change of government during the deepest economic crisis that has been known for many years (see website). Years of sustained growth in NHS funding, accompanied by ambitious programmes of service transformation, are on the cusp of plunging into an extended period of austerity and efficiency savings (see website chapter 7). In addition, devolution in the UK has increased the diversity of policy and practice across the UK (DH 2002, Ham 2009). These factors make it increasingly difficult to provide accurate and comprehensive detail on how the NHS is changing. Instead, this chapter will focus on the main policy drivers and trends that are consistent across the UK and across UK governments.

## A LITTLE HISTORY

The creation of the National Health Service, 60 years ago, is rightly remembered as among our nation's finest expressions of collective will. One of the central planks of the post-war reforms that sought to tackle social inequalities, build public health, and create a society that provided its most vulnerable with a safety net 'from the cradle to the grave', the health service still commands great loyalty and affection in the public psyche. Yet preoccupation over the accessibility and effectiveness of the NHS's services is equally a national pastime, and the future of the NHS has become highly contested – between political parties, in the media, and in public discourse.

Before the NHS was established, there was not one single maternity care system: women chose, according to their means, from a plethora of competing providers, including midwives, family doctors, obstetricians and hospitals (private and charitable). The 1946 National Health Service Act, which became operational in 1948, established a comprehensive, if fragmented, model of care, comprising hospital maternity services, community midwifery services (which were under the control of local authorities), and general practitioners. This fragmentation caused duplication and poor continuity, and many midwives were frustrated by what they saw as the encroachment of doctors on the provision of midwifery care. This was exacerbated by the expansion of hospital maternity beds resulting from the 1962 Hospital Plan, and by the Peel Report of 1970 (DHSS 1970), which recommended that all women give birth in hospital, cared for by multidisciplinary teams of midwives, obstetricians, and general practitioners (GPs). In 1973, the National Health Service Reorganisation Act brought all midwives under the responsibility of the NHS.

These reforms, along with the opportunities offered by evolving obstetric expertise, exacerbated the erosion of community-based midwifery. Childbirth became increasingly medicalized, with hospital delivery and many obstetric interventions becoming routine. The development of general management during the early 1980s meant that midwives reported up through general or nursing management, making them feel even more isolated from decision-making power.

Meanwhile, the wider NHS was experiencing repeated restructuring and reform in order to reduce its complex, multi-layered bureaucracy. At the end of the 1980s, it also underwent ideological revolution as the Government aimed to introduce 'market forces' to public services. A competitive internal market was established within the NHS, within which the functions of purchasing and providing were separated. Hospitals, community and ambulance services were encouraged to become self-governing trusts. GPs were encouraged to become fundholders, with power over their own resources and responsibility for purchasing care for their patients. The aim of this was to increase choice and efficiency, but both aims were frustrated: efficiency was undermined by the unavoidable management costs of implementing and running the system, while choice was subverted by the system of block contracts and restrictions on extra-contractual referrals.

## THE NEW NHS

By the time the Labour Party assumed government in 1997, after 18 years of uninterrupted Conservative administration, it appeared that the NHS was feeling sick and tired itself. Those who worked within it were fatigued and demoralized by continued structural reform and the implicit (often explicit) message that they could not run their own affairs efficiently. Conflict over wages, differentials, professional territories and management influence was widespread. Long waiting lists and poor customer care were alienating NHS users and supporters. There was significant public debate about whether the health service had a future, at least in its current form, or whether it should be dismantled and replaced by a system of private insurance funding. The NHS had become a service that was criticized. Each government attempted to make changes but it was an area of political influence as the public wished to retain its service and would not support privatization. Its future management was one of the key reasons why the country felt ready for change. The highlighted areas of deficiency in quality (see Ch. 7) supported an imperative for change.

Then a government was elected that demonstrated ideological commitment to the NHS and increased funding to enable this (see website chapter 7). This led to a Modernisation Agency and agenda (2002) and the revised structure for the NHS (see Fig. 7.1). The record increases in funding provided were matched with a serious commitment to radical reform. As with the previous administration, it was determined to break up the power cabals and vested interests that dominated the NHS, and to harness market forces to drive up quality and secure efficiency. The central strategy of 'the new NHS' was to deliver early performance improvements (in particular, speedier access) and to develop a culture of continuous quality improvement, by:

- setting priority national targets, with penalties for non-compliance
- introducing competition, through patient choice and the opening up of the NHS market to independent providers
- intensive centralized performance management, with earned autonomy for those achieving targets and the introduction of foundation trusts
- strengthening the power of commissioning to lever improved performance from providers, by establishing primary care trusts and developing cross-sectoral commissioning partnerships
- tackling health inequalities
- investing in large-scale development of information technology systems.

Thirteen years on, the impact of these reforms is undoubted but contested. Rising demand has been met by increased resource, with NHS funding more than doubled. Waiting lists fell to their lowest level since records began; a new maximum wait of 18 weeks from GP referral to treatment was secured; nearly all A&E patients were seen, treated, admitted or discharged within 4 hours, new hospitals and health facilities were built; significant progress was made in the management of long-term conditions; there was expansion of staff numbers and staff pay. To a very large extent, the NHS has regained public trust.

Nevertheless, the subsequent relationship between the Government and the NHS has not always been easy. Undoubtedly, many NHS staff welcomed the philosophical underpinning of new policy, and few demurred at the impressive investment produced in 2001 (see website chapter 7). But they became wearied by the relentless cycle of structural reform and centralized micro-management that is implemented by successive governments. Many were deeply alarmed by the Government's commitment to developing a mixed economy of providers, and its efforts to introduce this in a fair and effective way. Many of the professional groups complained about the targets culture, which produced impressive results, and which promoted an inflated sense of its own possibilities, overreached itself and has now been forced into retreat.

At the close of the Labour administration, the NHS was shifting the emphasis of its reform agenda away from speed of access toward quality of care (see Ch. 7), from centrally set targets to local priority setting, from supply-side expansion to demand-side management, and towards the development of a truly primary care-led health service as envisioned by the Darzi Next Stage Review (DH 2008). The scale of change needed in the NHS is clearly evidenced by how much work is still to be done, after a dozen years of full-on modernization (see website).

## THE CHALLENGES OF MODERNIZATION

If there is any unanimity in discussion of the NHS, it is on the necessity of modernization. Calls to abolish or partially dismantle the NHS have quietened down in the face of public hostility, and the focus now is on how the health service can meet the challenges of the future. The concept of 'modernization' has been taken up by all political parties, who have moved away from ideology-driven politics into a focus on effective management – 'what counts is what works'. This helpfully allows all parties to portray their health service plans as common sense and working for and on behalf of 'the people' – and to portray any opposition to new developments and to the increased use of technology to support the health service care and reforms.

There are, undoubtedly, significant and persistent problems in the NHS. Its inflexibility, lack of responsiveness and perceived indifference to patients' wishes, have shown it to be out of step with our modern consumer society. As a monopoly provider of healthcare and thus maternity services, it has been too quick to prioritize its own interests over patients' needs. The services that are provided are not always of high quality: too often, users face excessive delays, fragmentation, poor coordination, and conflicting advice. Maternity care services are not immune to these criticisms. Quality is variable, and clinicians are sometimes slow to adopt best practice or apply research evidence to their practice. Above all, patients often feel that services are not geared to their needs; rather, they are expected to fit into the service's requirements, and sometimes treated with less than full respect.

The causes of these problems are multifactorial. Some are structural; the sheer size of the NHS, and many of its constituent institutions, leads to impersonality and inflexibility. The complexity of the system defies attempts to reform and throws up unexpected effects of the most carefully planned change programme. Persistent over-centralization deadens local initiative and ownership. The barriers between services confuse and alienate patients and disrupt effective, seamless treatment. Hospital and community services are not sufficiently integrated; the gaps between health and social care are even more marked. Links between social care and maternity care are essential as the understanding of birth within its social and environmental context becomes relevant where there is increasing diversity and population movement. Women require a seamless approach in the services offered to them, but increasingly their care is fragmented; for example, a woman and family who require mental health care, maternity services and social support may not have an integrated team to follow her care through.

From the midwifery perspective and the team of care professionals, the volume and pressure of work never seem to allow for adequate communication or relationship-building across these barriers, and the development of information technology and communications systems to help bridge the gap has not been given sufficient priority. Paradoxically, given the problems arising from NHS structures, it is also clear that successive governments' addition to structural change has caused, and is causing, real damage – lowering morale, diverting priorities, consuming resources, and inhibiting the development of expertise and partnerships.

The general public and some clinicians are fond of blaming managers for all the health service's woes, and certainly poor management has played its part in the slow pace of service improvement. Performance management – while necessary and important – has often been badly executed: lack of incentives, targets that are seen as meaningless or perverse, and a culture of blame have all been evident. The very definition of quality is contested between different professions, organizations and sectors.

However, important though it undoubtedly is to ensure that structure serves purpose, and that leadership and management are of the highest quality, culture is the trump card that so often defeats attempts to create change. Ham and Alberti (2002) have written convincingly of the breakdown of the contract between the NHS and its doctors. They point out that the implicit contract, agreed at the founding of the NHS, was based on the government providing resources and the medical profession taking care of clinical standards. Prior to 1948, British doctors were private practitioners and their freedom to practise as they wished was curtailed less by the State than by the strong moral and ethical context in which they worked. Although many were not enthusiastic about the establishment of the NHS, they ceded to government the right to determine the budget and the national policy framework for their work, in return for continued medical control over regulation and clinical decision-making. In these early years of the NHS, managers were administrators and saw their job as facilitating doctors rather than managing them. Patients, too, accepted that 'doctor knows best', and were generally happy to acquiesce to medical authority.

This implicit contract was undermined by the growing consumer movement in the 1960s, the increased publicity given to poor standards, and the medical profession itself becoming more vocal and lobbying for higher budgets to keep pace with growing technological opportunities (see website). Over the next 30 years the implicit contract was further undermined by growing regulation, clinical audit and patient involvement. Public-spending constraints led governments to seek efficiency improvements in the NHS, and increased management power led to strained relationships between managers and doctors. The rise in litigation and challenges to self-regulation further undermined doctors' sense of professionalism (see website chapter 7). Doctors, along with other health professionals and managers, have become increasingly frustrated by their workloads and by the growing gap between what it is possible to do for patients and what can be done with available resources.

### Reflective activity 14.1

*'The values that produce high quality clinicians are not always compatible with either conventional approaches to management or other characteristics of high performance organisations such as team working and effective resource management' (NHS Confederation 2002).*

Do you agree with this? What are the qualities that make a leader in midwifery? (see Ch. 6) What can the profession do to identify, develop and sustain its leaders?

Midwives, meanwhile, have experienced the breaching of their own implicit contract. In the first half of the last century, midwives worked very hard and their pay was poor. Compared with other working women, however, their lot was not so bad. Although their social status never rivalled that of doctors, they worked with a significant degree of autonomy and often enjoyed high status in the communities where they worked. The level of continuity of care they were able to offer provided them with job satisfaction that was some compensation for their long hours. It should also be remembered that they were often unmarried and childless, wedded to the job in a way that today's midwives – many of whom have children, and most of whom believe in a life outside work – could not countenance.

Sixty years of NHS reform have not been altogether negative for midwifery, but they have altered this original agreement out of recognition. NHS midwives generally work shorter hours with lighter caseloads than their predecessors. They have the support of medical back-up, technological and other resources, and employment benefits. Yet the highly risk-averse nature of modern healthcare does not allow for the full flourishing of essential midwifery skills, and as midwives have been drawn into the traditional doctor–nurse dyad that characterizes our system of healthcare, they have lost status and pride. Many midwives would go so far as to argue that the modern hospital environment – fast-moving, technological, strongly directive – is intrinsically oppositional to birthing and to a midwifery philosophy of care.

In addition, the historic drive to professionalize midwifery has had ambivalent results. While it may have saved midwifery from near-extinction, as happened in other countries, it did so at the cost of autonomy from medical direction (and of the livelihoods of many working class midwives). Over 100 years on from the establishment of legal regulation of midwifery in all countries of the UK, midwifery is not fully a profession, and midwives continue to feel devalued by their role and status within the health service. Critically, the status of the midwife – relative to other health professions, and to other working women – has fallen, while consumer expectations have risen.

With the expansion of alternative – and more lucrative – occupations for educated women, this lack of consensus on the relationship between midwifery and its paymaster is finding expression in chronic staff shortages and a growing sense of crisis. The future for midwifery is uncertain, and it is in this area, as much as any other, that the necessity for effective NHS reform is most marked.

**Reflective activity 14.2**

What is happening to improve your service? What plans exist for modernization within your workplace that will affect the service you provide? If you were planning a change programme, what would you put in it?

## LOOKING TO THE FUTURE

The challenges facing the NHS for its next 60 years are not new; they are, rather, persistent and evolving. Our ageing and diversifying society, the growth of long-term health conditions, rising patient and public expectations, the costs and opportunities offered by new technologies, all in the context of a global recession, together demand truly creative solutions, delivering significantly better outcomes for significantly lower costs.

Even without the benefit of a crystal ball, there are some near-certainties about the future:

1. *Efficiencies and economies*: These will not be sufficient to tackle the challenges and pressures facing public services; fundamental change is still necessary, and this change will be contested. Every hospital closure, every move to re-site an A&E service – even in an over-provided area like central London – will attract bitter local opposition and high-profile, politically embarrassing campaigns.
2. *NHS delivery*: The NHS will be expected to deliver more while costing less. The public wants change, but without sacrifice. It expects more than it wants to pay for. Rising expectations are matched by changing demographics: people are living longer, though sometimes with chronic, complex (and expensive) health conditions. More babies with serious disabilities are living into adulthood. The UK society is more diverse, demanding more than a 'one size fits all' approach. There is more geographical mobility and often less community and family support available.
3. *Organizational size and diversity*: The sheer size and complexity of the NHS is a major challenge: most commentators agree that command and control management is doomed in an organization that is so big and diverse, and that employs so many highly educated and professionally autonomous staff. But the NHS is highly politicized, and no government wants to risk too much local autonomy, innovation and risk-taking. How to guarantee national consistency while also developing inspired local leadership, to encourage creativity without taking risks, is a continuing conundrum.
4. *Promotion of health and prevention of disease*: All governments talk about the holy grail of prevention, through better health promotion and better care of people with long-term conditions, delivered more cheaply and more effectively in the community. But although everybody agrees this is necessary, it is not happening fast or effectively. Again, it is simply too high a political risk to divert resources away from treatment.
5. *Health inequalities and diversity of population:* Similarly, all governments recognize the persistence of health inequalities, and there is a growing mountain of evidence on the causes and solutions. But nothing effective happens because many of the causes and solutions lie outside the health arena, in the politically sensitive areas of wealth distribution and tax policy. It is far easier – though ultimately less effective – to focus on lifestyle factors and behaviour change.

The future of the NHS is crucially dependent on its ability to tackle these challenges (see website). The health service is a complex adaptive system – an interconnection of parts sharing an environment, with each part having some freedom to act independently (NHS Confederation 2001). This means that change cannot be delivered by simply issuing instructions and expecting that implementation will just happen; policy pronouncements may have completely unexpected effects when put into practice, and anything that discourages creativity and innovation will slow down the whole system. As the national economy has changed and there will be a period of unprecedented austerity, it will be tempting for the Government to micro-manage the health service towards inflexible, politically driven targets. This will not help to create an environment that encourages innovation, experimentation, partnership and inspirational leadership. Whatever the risks, the government that will truly save the NHS will be the one that can understand and embrace the real drivers of sustainable change, and encourage a more mature public discourse on what can be expected from the nation's health service and how those working within it can achieve it.

## MIDWIFERY IN THE FUTURE NHS

There has probably never been a time that combined the large number of patient satisfaction audits and surveys which express the value of the contribution of midwives with such widespread dissatisfaction within the midwifery workforce. Despite great efforts over the last decade to boost the midwifery workforce, there are still chronic shortages. Despite a national guarantee that women can choose where to give birth, this freedom seems more rhetorical than real. Despite the policy objective of creating a more humane, family-friendly maternity service, there is a trend and a danger that hospital centralization will lead to the creation of huge, impersonal units – what Cathy Warwick, RCM General Secretary, has called 'baby factories' (Campbell 2010).

For the busy midwife in an overstretched maternity unit, national debates about health service policy may seem remote and irrelevant, like the distant buzzing of an irritating fly. But the coming half decade will be tough on everyone in public services; midwives, too, will experience the sharp impact of job losses, centralization and service 'efficiencies', and beyond those immediate challenges, they will need to influence the persisting and critical questions facing the profession.

### What is a midwife?

Midwives have been encouraged to maintain expertise across the breadth of their role, but increasing specialization and role enhancement offers new opportunities and challenges. Can a midwife be an expert community-focused practitioner, working in partnership with a range of partners across health and social care and the primary and secondary sectors, while also providing increasingly technological intrapartum care? Should there be a return to the days when midwives worked either in hospital or the community? Should the profession embrace more specialization – high-dependency care midwives, public health midwives, community support midwives? And what would women want from their future midwife? These are all questions that will need to be addressed in the future context of the health service with diminishing resources.

### Who is in the maternity care team?

Over the last decade, many services have developed health/maternity care assistant roles to support midwives by providing some routine and non-clinical services. How are those roles working in practice? Are we identifying evidence to support their benefits and value for money? How should those roles develop in the future, and is there any scope for developing additional complementary roles? How do these roles impact on the midwife and her role now and in the future? Any future midwifery service will need to identify clarity in roles to provide women with the care they need.

### Redefining partnerships

Who are midwives' natural partners? If the answer is 'women', or 'obstetricians', then extra attention may also be needed for other health and social care partners, whose contribution can be utilized to improve the effectiveness of maternity care. Most midwives are employed by and managed within the acute sector, and this can distort the focus of the partnerships they create and sustain. There is no justification for a claim of providing 'woman-centred' or 'holistic' care if that care is solely framed by acute sector inputs and processes. This does not mean that relationships with obstetricians are obsolete; there is an urgent need to improve them and make them more equal and constructive. But with the transfer of planning and commissioning powers to the primary care sector, midwives should ensure that their communication and influence is appropriately placed and effective.

### Defining priorities, making best use of resources

As more and more tasks and responsibilities are loaded onto an already overburdened workforce, midwives will need to identify and agree the priorities for their working time – the things that must be done and that only midwives can do – and find ways of dropping or reallocating the other tasks. This will involve process mapping, analysis and redesign. In many areas this is long overdue; for example, who can say that if asked to design antenatal and postnatal care from scratch, they would come up with the present structure and content? Similarly, hard choices may need to be made about how best to tailor resources to need in order to produce best outcomes for particular population groups. For example, if continuity of carer or one-to-one care in labour could not be provided to all women, should it be targeted to those who need it most?

## Positioning the profession

In common with some other professional groups within the NHS, midwifery stands at a defining moment in its development. If the profession is serious about achieving full professional status, significantly increasing its remuneration and assuming greater power in decision-making and management, it will need to embrace responsibility (and therefore shoulder blame), develop its own support staff, accept further specialization, actively develop its own evidence-based body of knowledge, develop its management capacity and capability, get slicker at understanding and using the wider NHS agenda, and agree a new contract with its medical colleagues.

The investment needed to do this will be significant and may not be rewarded. It may feel like too high a price to pay to a workforce that is relatively low-paid, has been demoralized by its recent history, is largely female and often has caring responsibilities. There is no right or wrong answer to this question; a number of different pathways are possible and plausible. But midwifery will need to develop greater consensus over its own future, and find the energy and will to drive that consensus forward, if it is to avoid having its fate decided by others.

Whatever the answers to these questions, it is evident that status quo is not an option (see Midwifery 2020). The NHS reform agenda is gathering scope and speed, and the midwifery profession cannot choose to opt out of it (DH 2010). Some midwives may feel that an inordinate amount is being demanded of them in return for their remuneration and reward. Nevertheless, change always creates opportunities, and midwives will want to play their part in ensuring that maternity services – effective, woman-centred, safe and humane maternity services – survive and thrive in the difficult years to come. Midwives will need to discover the work that is being developed through the 'workstream' groups for looking at the vision of the profession for the future (Midwifery 2020). This group, set up by the UK Health Departments, is a collaborative group of professionals and lay groups from governmental and non-governmental bodies and linked to the four countries of the UK. It has set up 'workstreams' comprising core groups of professions and lay persons which are:

- The core role of the midwife
- Workforce and workload
- Education and career progression
- Measuring quality
- Public health.

### Reflective activity 14.3

'In the NHS, everyone thinks power belongs to someone else, that it is somebody else choosing to stop things getting better.' In your experience, is this true? Who do you think are the individuals who exert most influence over what you can and cannot do in your daily work? Are you aware of your own power, and how you exercise it? What are positive and negative uses of power? How can you maximize your own positive use of power?

## CONCLUSION

The NHS will be operating in the context of severe restraint on spending across the public sector in the years ahead. Merely cutting any excesses of time and efficiency will not deliver the scale and scope of change needed. Hospitals will need to find ways to improve demand management, commissioners will need to identify radical new ways of delivering effective care, government will need to resist the temptation to distract these efforts by indulging in any unnecessary organizational restructuring or rebranding.

The health service will continue to struggle with continuing questions over its very existence. There are still many who believe that the dream of a system of universal provision of healthcare, funded by universal taxation, is redundant and doomed to failure, but also many who see the NHS as the foundation block of a society that is committed to fairness and equality.

The future of individual NHS organizations, and indeed of the NHS as a whole, will largely be determined by the ability of health service staff to create innovations and initiatives to demonstrate that, despite chronic shortages, growing pressures, and systemic disincentives, they can deliver a step change in performance capable of transforming the pride of 20$^{th}$ century Britain into the pride of the 21$^{st}$.

The future of health services worldwide is linked to government resources. Maternal and child health are fundamental areas for priorities for health needs. Articulating these needs and raising political awareness of the value of midwifery in promoting health is contingent upon women and midwives working together to have one voice for the future.

### KEY POINTS

- Since its inception in 1948, the NHS has been undergoing a process of constant change.

- Midwives need to be familiar with the structures and systems within the NHS, and their place within this, and be able to visualize opportunities in policy developments, service modernization programmes and changing patterns of care.
- The midwife's focus is on the woman, her baby and family, and any changes to the NHS and its service provision must be seen in this context, and translated to the midwife's practice appropriately.
- Some of the modernization proposals fundamentally change the way acute and primary services will be controlled, and it is crucial that midwives place themselves in a position to influence, contribute and shape services and workforce planning.
- Midwives working within the modern NHS will need to be alert to the changes so that they may innovate and adapt to the changing culture.

## REFERENCES


Campbell D: Midwives' leader warns against 'baby factories', *Guardian society online*, www.guardian.co.uk/society/2010/may/04/maternity-services-nhs-midwives-factory. 4 May 2010.

Department of Health (DH): *The NHS quality, innovation, productivity and prevention challenge: an introduction for clinicians*, London, 2010, TSO.

Department of Health (DH): *High quality care for all: NHS Next Stage Review final report* (The Darzi Report), London, 2008, DH.

Department of Health (DH): *A guide to NHS foundation trusts*, London, 2002, DH.

Department of Health and Social Security (DHSS): *Report of the Sub-Committee on Domiciliary and Maternity Bed Needs* (Chair: Sir John Peel), London, 1970, HMSO.

Donnison J: *Midwives and medical men*, London, 1988, Heinemann.

Ham C: *Health policy in Britain*, ed 6, London, 2009, Macmillan.

Ham C, Alberti KGMM: The medical profession, the public and the government, *British Medical Journal* 324:838–842, 2002.

Kirkham M, Stapleton H: The culture of the maternity services in Wales and England as a barrier to informed choice. In Kirkham M, editor: *Informed choice in maternity care*, Basingstoke, 2004, Palgrave Macmillan.

Midwifery 2020 The Future of the profession website address: www.midwifery2020.org/pages/news.asp. Accessed May 2010.

Modernisation Agency: *Improvement leaders' guide to involving patients and carers*, London, 2002, Modernisation Agency.

NHS Confederation: *Why won't the NHS do as it is told – and what might we do about it?* Leading Edge Briefing No. 1, London, 2001, NHS Confederation.

NHS Confederation: *Creating high performance: why is it so hard?* Leading Edge No. 4, London, 2002, NHS Confederation.

Sandall J: Team midwifery and burnout in midwives in the UK: practical lessons from a national study, *MIDIRS Midwifery Digest* 9(2):147–152, 1999.

# Chapter 15

# Legal frameworks for the care of the child

*Barbara Burden and Michael Preston-Shoot*

## LEARNING OUTCOMES

By the end of this chapter, you will be able to:

- understand the legislative basis and key principles within the Children Act 1989; Children Act 2004 and other relevant legal policies, including the Human Rights Act 1998
- appreciate the range of resources available to support families in caring for their children
- assess the role and responsibilities of local authority and voluntary sector organizations in providing and monitoring services for children and families
- identify the particular needs of children with disability and those from different racial and cultural backgrounds
- evaluate the role and responsibilities of the midwife in assisting councils with social services responsibilities to promote and safeguard the welfare of children in need and at risk
- realize the midwife's contribution to the assessment of children and families.

Note: Please see the website for a list of all the Acts/Statutes referred to in this chapter.

## INTRODUCTION

Safeguarding children and promoting their welfare is the responsibility of every health and social care professional. An increasing emphasis is placed on outcomes, to be delivered through multi-agency working and information-sharing. Repeatedly, government documents continue to highlight the requirement for interagency and interprofessional working to safeguard and promote the wellbeing of children and young people (DCSF 2010, DH 2000a, Laming 2009). Decisions about children's welfare and safety are complex, with high-profile deaths of children, such as Victoria Climbié and Baby P, raising criticisms and anxieties about professional decision-making, leadership and management (DH 2003a, Joint Area Review 2008). Whilst the quality of children's services may be improving, criticisms remain of partnership arrangements, performance management, the involvement of young people in decision-making, the use of assessment to identify need and track progress, and communication to ensure the emergence of a comprehensive picture of a child's needs (Ofsted 2009, Statham & Aldgate 2003). There are also concerns about high thresholds limiting access to services (Corby 2003, Morris 2005) and lack of compliance by local authorities with the legal rules (Preston-Shoot 2010).

This chapter seeks to enable midwives to understand the legislative framework and related policies, procedures and resources, to carry out their role effectively in working together with parents and other professionals to ensure the wellbeing and safety of children. For the definition of the child, please see Box 15.1. Please note that those working outside England and Wales need to access legislation and policy guidelines relevant to that country.

The discussion below may be linked to three scenarios that may be encountered by midwives (see Case scenarios Web 15.1, 15.2 and 15.3 and a range of activities on the website suggested for learning).

## THE CHILDREN ACT 1989

The Children Act 1989, amplified by associated regulations and statutory guidance, covers legislation relating to

**Box 15.1 Legal definition of a child**

The Children Act 1989 defines a child as a person under the age of 18. In current British law, an individual has no legal entity until the moment of birth. Similarly, a person does not become a parent until his or her child is born.

aspects of care, upbringing and protection of children (Braye & Preston-Shoot 2009). This includes the welfare and protection of children in disputed divorce proceedings, children in need, children at risk, children with disabilities or special educational needs, and those who need to live away from home (either short or long term) including children in hospital, boarding schools, residential homes and foster homes. These rules have been amended and supplemented by subsequent legislation, most notably the Family Law Act 1996 (to protect victims of domestic violence), the Children (Leaving Care) Act 2000 (duties regarding young people leaving care), the Adoption and Children Act 2002 (reform of adoption law and changes to the Children Act 1989 provisions, for instance concerning parental responsibility, special guardianship and advocacy), the Children Act 2004 (specifying outcomes for children and requirements for interagency working), the Children and Adoption Act 2006 (sanctions for disrupting contact between children and non-resident parents, and changes to family assistance orders), the Children and Young Persons Act 2008 (amendments to children in need and emergency protection order provisions, and changes concerning accommodated children) and the Apprenticeships, Skills, Children and Learning Act 2009 (creating statutory Children's Trusts and changes to Local Safeguarding Children Boards).

Guidance and regulations produced by central government departments provide detailed information about how legislation should be implemented. When guidance is issued under section 7, Local Authority Social Services Act 1970, it should be followed. Two published examples of these are *Working together to safeguard children* (DCSF 2010) and *Framework for the assessment of children in need and their families* (DH 2000a). These provide blueprints for agencies to work together with children (Fig. 15.1). Guidance has also been issued to clarify how outcomes for children, detailed in the Children Act 2004, should be approached (CWDC 2007, DfES 2005).

The midwife has a universal and accepted role in working with pregnant mothers, newborn babies and their parents, and is in a unique position to comment on all aspects of the health and care of newborn babies (see case scenarios and reflective activities on website). This is in direct contrast to some other professionals, for example, social workers and police, who tend to be involved with families when there is cause for concern. Whilst midwives

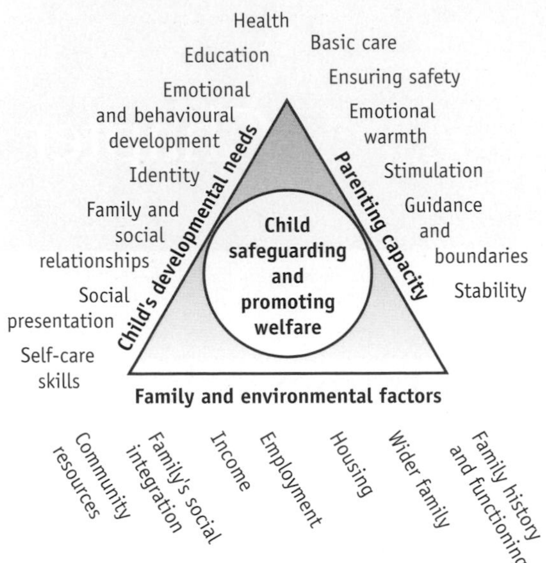


**Figure 15.1** The assessment framework (DH 2000a).

have been involved with all children born in England (approximately 11 million), intervention by councils with social services responsibilities affects only a small proportion of families, estimated to be about 5% (DH 2007). See website and Reflective activity Web 15.2.

## KEY FEATURES OF THE CHILDREN ACT 1989

The Children Act 1989 was formulated on key beliefs about children, young people, parents and the role of the State, which are given statutory recognition in the Act.

These include the following:

- There is a universal duty to promote and safeguard the welfare of the child.
- Children are best brought up within their family, and local authorities have a duty to give support to children and families to facilitate this, when it is safe and appropriate so to do.
- Even where children are separated from their families, they should maintain contact with them, except where this puts them at risk.
- The state should only intervene where it is in the child's best interests and legal measures are only taken as a last resort.
- Professionals should work in partnership with parents, where possible, involving them in the care of, and decisions made about their children.
- The wishes and feelings of children and young people should be sought (depending on their age and level

of understanding), and taken into account when making decisions about their lives.
- The child's welfare should be the paramount consideration in court decisions.
- The race, religion, culture and language of a child should be taken into account in provision of any services.

The Act is clear. The paramount duty for everyone is to *safeguard and promote the welfare of children*. Whilst other objectives, such as working in partnership with parents, are also highlighted, it is important to recognize that these practice principles do not overturn the paramount duty of the local authority to safeguard and promote the welfare of children (Braye & Preston-Shoot 2009, Brayne & Carr 2010, Wilson & James 2007).

## CONTENT AND STRUCTURE OF THE CHILDREN ACT

Of particular interest to midwives are the parts of the 1989 Act that deal with the responsibilities of the local authority (LA) in providing support for children and families (Part III) and the protection of children (Part V).

### Part 1 (section 1): Welfare of the child

The Children Act 1989 begins with a statement that the child's welfare is the paramount issue to be taken into account in decisions made by a court in respect of children and young people (s1:1). The Act advocates avoiding delay in making decisions about a child's upbringing (s1:2) as it can prejudice the welfare of the child. Where the court is required to take action, the Act requires it to take account of the following *'welfare checklist'* (s1:3):

- the ascertainable wishes and feelings of the child concerned (subject to age and understanding)
- the child's physical, emotional and educational needs
- the likely effect on the child of having any changes in their circumstances
- age, sex, background and any characteristics the court considers relevant
- any harm which the child has suffered or is at risk of suffering
- how capable each of the parents and any other person in relation to whom the court considers the question to be relevant, is of meeting the child's needs
- the range of powers available to the court.

Whilst this applies to only parts of the Act and relates specifically to decisions of the court, professionals are expected to take this checklist into account when making decisions about a child.

The Act also states (s1: 5) that courts can only make an order in respect of a child if this would be better for the child than not making an order. This is based on the principle that the state should intervene in private and family life only to the degree necessary. This conforms to Article 8 of the European Convention on Human Rights, with its principle of proportional intervention, incorporated into UK law by the Human Rights Act 1998.

### Part 1 (section 2): Parents and parental responsibility

The concept of *parental responsibility* is described in sections 2, 3, 4 and 5. Parental responsibility is defined as: all the rights, duties, powers, responsibilities and authority, which by law a parent has in relation to the child and his property (Children Act 1989: S.3(1)).

This includes the responsibility to care for, and promote and protect the child's moral, physical and emotional health. Although not specifically defined in the Act, this is generally considered to include decisions in respect of the name, religion and education of the child, the right to consent or not to medical treatment and adoption, to have contact and to arrange for the burial or cremation of a child.

#### Who has parental responsibility?

Having parental responsibility does not automatically equate with being the legal or biological parent of the child. For example, the birth mother automatically acquires parental responsibility at the moment of birth. However, the father does not have parental responsibility automatically unless he has been married to the mother. An unmarried father has parental responsibility if he is registered as the father on the child's birth certificate (an amendment in the Adoption and Children Act 2002), or if the birth mother or a court gives him parental responsibility. Other people may also acquire parental responsibility through decisions of the court, for example grandparents, guardians, foster carers or the local authority. In these circumstances, parental responsibility can be shared amongst several people. The only circumstance in which a birth mother and married father would lose parental responsibility is when their child is adopted or a placement order is made permitting adoption to be planned. If an unmarried birth father has been given parental responsibility, it can in exceptional circumstances be removed by a court. In divorce, both parents retain parental responsibility, even if it is decided that the child should live with one of the parents.

The issue of parenting and parental responsibility is becoming increasingly complicated with the advent of surrogacy and in vitro fertilization. For example, the woman who gives birth is the legal mother and has parental responsibility. Other adults may need to adopt the child in order to become the legal parents.(see website and Reflective activity Web15.3.)

## SUPPORT FOR CHILDREN AND FAMILIES

### The changing nature of family

Practice with children and families needs to take account of the changing nature of family life. The UK has become an increasingly multicultural society, bringing a diversity of ideas in respect of different family structures and ways of life. This diversity has been recognized within the Children Act 1989. Firstly, the Act widened the concept of people who are important to children by allowing absent parents and other relatives to be consulted and involved in decisions about the care of children, and to apply under section 8 for residence and contact orders. Secondly, for the first time in English law, the diversity and multicultural context of families have been recognized and should be taken account of and respected (s1:3). The legal rules have been changed subsequently to recognize civil partnerships, to extend to same-gender couples the right to adopt, to allow step-parents to acquire parental responsibility with the agreement of birth parents, and to create the concept of special guardianship (Adoption and Children Act 2002).

**Reflective activity 15.1**

Find out where your local authority children's services department is. How has it organized its responsibilities to children?

What initiatives do you have in your area for helping vulnerable children and their families?

See if you can obtain a copy of the Children and Young People's Plan for your area? What are the key aims and objectives for your area?

### Poverty and social exclusion

Sources of stress and disadvantage for children and families include poverty and accompanying social exclusion. The Government published *Ending child poverty: everybody's business* (HM Treasury 2008a), its strategy to tackle childhood poverty. In 2009, 2 million children were living in households where there was no adult in paid work, with the impact of poverty on their families being recognized as having a major effect on life chances, health, education and future employment (Hirsch 2009, Platt 2009), especially amongst black and minority ethnic group communities (Butt & Box 1998).

#### Employment rights

Pregnant women and their partners can access a range of benefits to help combat social inequality caused by poverty. Under the Employment Rights Act 1996, women retain employment rights whilst pregnant and should not be discriminated against. This includes paid time off for antenatal appointments, protection from unfair treatment or dismissal, the right to maternity leave, maternity pay, redundancy payment, and return to work following pregnancy (see Reflective activity Web 15.5). The Employment Act 2002 provides that every working father is entitled to paternity leave.

### Family support and the Children Act

Central and local government strategies have been designed to aid vulnerable children. For example, Sure Start programmes have been targeted at children under 4 and their families within some of the most disadvantaged communities, addressing the health and wellbeing of children and families before and after birth. The aim has been to improve the health of children before entry to school to enhance their potential at school. The programmes provide access to family support, advice on nurturing, health services and early learning. Other initiatives include the concept of extended schools and the requirement on local authorities to ensure that they have sufficient children's centres to meet local need (Apprenticeships, Skills, Children & Learning Act 2009).

The Children Act 1989 places a duty on local authorities to target particular services to children defined as being *in need*.

Local authorities have a general duty to:

- safeguard and promote the welfare of children 'in need' and
- promote the upbringing of such children by their families

by providing a range and level of services appropriate to those children's needs (Children Act 1989: s.17(1)).

The definition of a child in need has been extended to include being a victim of, or witness to, domestic violence (Adoption and Children Act 2002, DH 2000b). The requirement that financial support could be given only in exceptional circumstances has been removed by the Children and Young Persons Act 2008. The aim of the duty to children in need within the Children Act is to target services to the most vulnerable, including those at risk, providing support to avoid the need for the state to seek statutory control. Service provision under section 17 may be one means by which a local authority seeks to deliver good outcomes for children and young people as defined in the Children Act 2004. However, financial constraints, reflected in high thresholds and eligibility criteria, have limited this section's effectiveness (Morris 2005).

## FAMILY SUPPORT SERVICES

Part 3 of the Children Act 1989, especially section 17 and Schedule 2, outlines the provision of services for children in need. These services may be provided by the local authority and/or the voluntary and private sector. Such services include family centres, day nurseries, fostering, childminding or playgroups, and support within the home, such as family aides (see website). The local authority may charge for these services, but any person in receipt of income support or family credit is exempt.

### Children living away from home (see website)

The local authority has a duty to provide accommodation in a range of situations, including when children are *in need* and there is no person who has parental responsibility for them, they are lost or abandoned, or the person who has been caring for them is prevented from providing them with suitable accommodation or care. When the local authority accommodates children, they become *looked after* children.

### Accommodation for young babies

Where there are concerns about a young baby, it is likely that the local authority would – unless there is very good reason against such – try to maintain the mother and child in their own home by provision of a family aide and/or home help. If this is not possible, efforts would be made to try to place mother and child together with foster carers who specifically work with mothers. There are still a small number of residential mother and baby homes, predominantly managed by the private and voluntary sector, which provide care, support and training for mothers with specialist needs, such as drug dependency. (For foster care and teenage pregnancy, please see website.)

## ADOPTION (SEE WEBSITE)

Adoption is the dissolution of parental rights and duties, which are subsequently transferred to the new adoptive parent(s).

In some cases, midwives become involved with a mother who has decided to give up her child for adoption. In rare circumstances, the mother may decide that she does not want to care for the baby after birth. If this is the case, then midwives will be involved in planning with councils with social services responsibilities or an adoption agency to manage this process.

## CHILDREN WITH DISABILITIES (SEE WEBSITE)

The Children Act 1989 (section 17) recognizes children with disabilities as children first and includes them in the definition of children *in need*, enabling them to benefit from the same services as other children.

Midwives are at the front line of working with parents who are expecting a child with disability or where a disability is diagnosed at birth. They need to be sensitive to how information is conveyed to parents and ensure openness and honesty. In many cases, this involves referral to paediatric specialists.

An important principle in working with children with disabilities is to ensure that the views and wishes of the child are sought and not to make the assumption that this is not possible.

Disabled children are particularly vulnerable and face an increased risk of abuse in many settings. This may arise in part from social attitudes and special treatment resulting in disabled children being more isolated, more dependent, having less control over their lives and bodies, and being less able to communicate their abuse.

## FEMALE GENITAL MUTILATION

The midwife may also need to be alert to the possibility of some families wishing to have the child 'circumcised'. This might be from an awareness that the mother/family is from a culture where this practice is accepted; and if the mother herself has had this procedure. Occasionally, the mother may ask for information which might alert the midwife. Under the terms of the Female Genital Mutilation Act 2004, it is illegal to have this carried out abroad under the principle of 'extra-territoriality' (see website chapter 58). This is a sensitive and difficult situation, and seeking assistance from the supervisor of midwives and using the guidelines from the Department of Health (DH 2003) can be useful. Midwives must initiate their local child protection process if they feel that a female child is at risk.

## THE PROTECTION OF CHILDREN

The impact of domestic violence on children and adolescents is becoming increasingly recognized and has been well researched (DH 2000b, Hester et al 2006, Humphreys & Stanley 2006). In some circumstances, alcohol and drugs misuse and mental illness may also adversely affect parents' abilities to care for their children (Humphreys & Stanley 2006). Women's refuges have been established to provide a safe haven and advice for women and their children, accessed through the Samaritans, the police or social services. The legal rules have been strengthened to recognize the impact of domestic violence. The Adoption and Children Act 2002 makes a child who is a victim of, or witness to, domestic oppression, a child in need. The Family Law Act 1996 allows a court to add an exclusion order to an interim care order or emergency protection order made under the Children Act 1989, with the objective of removing the perpetrator from the family home rather than the child. If this does not prove possible, then the child may be removed using a granted emergency protection order or interim care order powers.

Along with all other professionals and voluntary sector workers involved with children, midwives have a responsibility to be alert to the possibility of child abuse and to take appropriate action where indicated. Should a midwife have any concerns about a family, she should discuss this with her senior colleagues and others who may be involved in the care of the family. This involves discussion with a supervisor of midwives, senior colleague, or doctor (Box 15.2).

Section 47 of the Children Act 1989 places a duty on any health authority or NHS trust to help a local authority in its inquiries in cases where there is reasonable cause to suspect that a child is suffering or is likely to suffer *significant harm*. It is important for midwives to recognize the roles and responsibilities of other professionals in working with children and access joint multidisciplinary training in respect of assessment and child protection. Where it is agreed, following a *strategy decision*, that a *section 47 enquiry* should be instigated and the child may be at risk of significant harm, the midwife may become involved in a *child protection conference*. If the child is made the subject of a *child protection plan, core group meetings* and *review conferences* will follow.

Box 15.2 **Responsibilities of the senior midwife**

Those who manage midwifery should ensure that:

- There are agreed arrangements to give the name and telephone number of the health visitor to the mother the first week after the birth.
- They provide professional advice and guidance to any midwife who is concerned about a child or who is involved where a child is suspected of being at risk or has been abused or neglected.
- There is an early response to information of a pregnancy in a family where there has been an identified concern. The concern should be shared with other professionals as appropriate.
- Where the mother is known to have abused drugs or alcohol during pregnancy, the risk factors are taken into account for the unborn child and any other children. Where a baby is born with fetal alcohol syndrome or has signs or symptoms of addiction to narcotics, a referral to social services should be made.
- Midwives and nurses in neonatal units are aware that infants separated from their mother at birth may be at greater risk of child abuse later in childhood. Their observations may be the first crucial step in alerting others to an 'at risk' situation.
- Midwives and nurses have an important part to play in promoting parent and child contact to ensure strong parent/child relationships and the development of good parenting skills. This is particularly important where there are problems, e.g. mental or physical illness, physical or learning disability.
- Where the midwife is notified of a child or young person under 18 who is pregnant, she should consider whether there is a child protection concern.
- The special needs of the mother and father are met, e.g. a parent(s) with a disability including a learning disability, referring them to appropriate sources of support.

Adapted from DH 1997: 9–10

## Local Safeguarding Children Boards

Each health authority is required to identify a senior nurse as designated senior professional to the Local Safeguarding Children Board (LSCB). Each NHS trust must also identify a named nurse or midwife to lead on child protection matters (CWDC 2009).

The overall management of the cooperation between various agencies in respect of child protection in any local authority is the responsibility of the Local Safeguarding Children Board (Children Act 2004; Local Safeguarding Children Board Regulations 2006; Apprenticeships, Skills, Children & Learning Act 2009). Each board has a representative at a senior management level from each of the relevant agencies. They have responsibility to develop, audit and challenge local policies and procedures for interagency working and for the safeguarding and promotion of the welfare of children. They must ensure provision is made for training and raising awareness within the wider community, and for monitoring and evaluating the effectiveness of partner agencies, individually and collectively. They will provide regular reports to the Children's Trust, and publish an annual report. They also conduct a serious case review of any particularly difficult cases that arise, or where a child dies as a result of abuse or neglect in their area.

## Significant harm

Important in the assessment of risk is the concept of *significant harm*. If there is reasonable cause to suspect that a child is suffering or is likely to suffer significant harm, the local authority has a duty to make enquiries necessary to enable them to decide whether to take any action to safeguard or promote the child's welfare (Children Act 1989: s.47). This enquiry is commonly known as a *section 47 investigation*.

Harm is defined in section 31(9) and (10) of the Children Act as: *'ill treatment or impairment of health or development'*.

Ill-treatment includes sexual abuse and other forms of ill-treatment that are not necessarily physical (see Box 15.3). The decision as to whether the harm is *significant* is measured on a comparison with the health and development reasonably expected of a similar child. It will be informed by a comprehensive assessment (DH 2000a) and take into account legal advice. Assessments should be child-centred so that the impact of parenting capacity, family and environment on the child can be clearly identified and understood (HM Government 2006).

*Working together to safeguard children* (DCSF 2010) advises that abuse or neglect is caused by inflicting harm. Whilst it is not within the remit of this chapter to provide detail of signs and symptoms of abuse, there are well-documented warning signs that may alert the midwife. Physical abuse includes hitting, shaking, throwing, poisoning, burning, scalding and suffocating. Midwives should be concerned about any bruising on a baby, particularly bruising around the face or on any soft tissues, bruising consistent with an implement being used to hit a child, finger-tip bruising or slap marks, black eyes or ears, bites, scald and burn marks anywhere on the body, or a torn frenulum. Suspicion may be raised if parents delay seeking advice about injuries or if there are discrepancies between the parents' explanation and the actual injuries found.

Emotional abuse may be observed by the midwife in terms of poor emotional bonding and possible rejection of the pregnancy and child, unrealistic expectations and/or demands of the child, constant criticism, unequal treatment, or a child being made to feel worthless and unloved. Failing to meet a child's basic physical or psychological needs in respect of food, clothes and safety, failing to protect the child from harm, and failing to ensure access to appropriate medical care or treatment may be examples of neglect. Failure to follow medical advice through pregnancy and postnatal care, the mental state of the mother, rough handling, and a history of drug or alcohol abuse or domestic violence also give cause for concern.

**Box 15.3 Categories of abuse and neglect**

Abuse and neglect are generally considered under the following categories:

- physical abuse
- emotional abuse
- sexual abuse
- neglect.

These are generally used as the basis for making children the subject of child protection plans.

The time immediately after birth is important in establishing a positive relationship between parent and baby. Prematurity, illness of either mother or child, or other factors, sometimes hinder this relationship. The midwife is a key figure in fostering a positive relationship, recognizing what is likely to support or hinder this.

Whilst stress does not automatically lead to child abuse, it may make it more likely. Sources of stress for families include issues relating to finances, social exclusion (SEU 2001), domestic violence, mental illness of parent, and drug or alcohol abuse (Haggerty et al 2001, Hughes & Owen 2009).

Whilst acknowledging that these factors do not necessarily lead to abuse or neglect, the potential or actual impact of these on a child needs to be assessed and action taken to support the child and family as well as ensuring the child's safety.

A midwife who is involved with a child where there is concern may be involved in a *strategy discussion* with other professionals to share information, determine a plan for *section 47 enquiries*, and consider how to immediately safeguard the child and provide interim services and support. This includes consideration of how to take race and ethnicity into account, including use of interpreters; the needs of other children; decisions about what information should be shared with the family; and the role of the police where an offence may have been committed.

## ASSESSING CHILDREN 'IN NEED' AND THEIR FAMILIES

The *Framework for the assessment of children in need and their families* (DH 2000a) and *Working together to safeguard children* (DCSF 2010) guidelines emphasize that promoting the welfare of children and safeguarding their needs are not separate activities. They aim to refocus attention on preventive work, together with producing a more holistic and interagency assessment focusing on strengths as well as needs (Calder 2000). Assessment begins from the point of referral and emphasizes the corporate responsibility of local authority departments, the NHS and voluntary organizations in contributing to both the assessment and the provision of services to children in need. The assessment seeks to discriminate between different types and levels of need and is crucial to improving the success of services for children. Focus on an interagency approach starts as soon as there are concerns about a child's welfare, not just when there is concern about the child being at risk of significant harm.

The assessment framework takes account of current research to produce an approach that retains the child at the centre of three domains which interact to affect the wellbeing and development of a child within the family (Aldgate & Statham 2001). These are:

(a) the child's developmental needs
(b) parenting capacity
(c) family and environmental factors (see Fig. 15.1).

Where families fail to cooperate with an assessment, and where it remains unclear if criteria are met for application for an emergency protection order, the local authority may apply for a child assessment order which, if granted by the court, requires parents to make the child available for assessment (see Reflective activity Web 15.6).

Midwives are well placed to comment on all three assessment domains, given their close and frequent contact with newborn babies and parents; their skills in assessment, observation and communication; and their knowledge of early childhood development and needs. In visiting the home, midwives may become aware of the care, not only of newborn babies, but also of older children, lifestyles, home conditions, parenting and child abuse. Midwives can identify vulnerable children and refer them to social services for assessment, contributing to the assessment, planning and intervention as required (DH 2003b, Fraser 2003). The most common situations where midwives are involved in working with social workers in respect of children in need or at risk, are pre-birth assessments and post-birth concerns.

## Making a referral

*Working together to safeguard children* states that anyone who believes a child to be suffering, or at risk of suffering, significant harm, should refer their concerns to children's social care departments (DCSF 2010).

Before making a referral, the midwife should discuss concerns with a manager or a supervisor of midwives and, unless this would place the child at increased risk, discuss concerns with the family and gain their agreement for the referral. The GP should also be informed. In making the referral, it is important to be clear about the nature of the concerns and document these, referring only to known facts.

## Consent and confidentiality

Personal information about children and families is subject to a duty of confidence and should not normally be shared without consent. However, the Data Protection Act 1998 permits disclosure of confidential information if it is necessary to safeguard a child. Trusts have local policies regarding this. In circumstances where there are concerns about the child being at risk or suffering significant harm, the overriding duty is to safeguard the child. Information regarding data protection is available in *Information sharing: guidance for practitioners and managers* (HM Treasury 2008b). This is in keeping with the Human Rights Act 1998 and Article 8 of the European Convention because the right to private and family life is a qualified right. Disclosure of otherwise confidential information is permitted providing it is done according to law and is proportional to the need identified to safeguard and promote the child's welfare. When safe to do so, midwives should practise openly and honestly with families about child protection concerns to ensure that this relationship is not compromised and involvement with both parents and child can continue (Calder 2000).

## The midwife's role in assessment

Early identification, assessment and intervention associated with child protection cases are clearly outlined in the *Common Assessment Framework for Children and Young People: a guide for practitioners* (CWDC 2009). This detailed and comprehensive document outlines the role that practitioners play in the multi-agency approach to safeguarding children. The Framework is described as 'a shared assessment and planning framework for use across all children's services and all local areas in England. It aims to help the early identification of children and young people's additional needs and promote coordinated service provision to meet them' (CWDC 2009:8). All children considered at risk of significant harm must be referred directly to children's social services or police, in keeping with Local Safeguarding Children Boards (LSCB) procedures (DCSF 2010).

Where a midwife refers a child, she should confirm this in writing within 48 hours using the *Common Assessment Framework* (see Box 15.4). In turn, the local authority should acknowledge the referral within one working day of receipt. The midwife may be asked to contribute to an assessment of whether a child is in need and, if so, the services which may be appropriate to promote the child's welfare and upbringing within the family (see website). The midwife in respect of women who had been referred (see Case scenarios Web 15.1 and 15.3) would be contacted for information about previous pregnancies, attitudes towards antenatal and self-care, or home conditions, as part of the *initial assessment* phase, which must be concluded within 10 working days (DH 2000a).

In circumstances requiring a more in-depth exploration, a *core assessment* is undertaken, and must be completed within 35 days (DH 2000a). Again, depending on the degree of involvement, the midwife may be invited to provide information, specialist knowledge and advice,

**Box 15.4 Common assessment framework**

'The situations that might lead to a common assessment include where a practitioner has observed a significant change or worrying feature in a child's appearance, demeanour or behaviour; where a practitioner knows of a significant event in the child's life or where there are worries about the parents or carers or home; or where the child, parent or another practitioner has requested an assessment. A common assessment might be indicated if there are parental elements (e.g. parental substance abuse/misuse, domestic violence, or parental physical or mental health issues) that might impact on the child.'

*(HM Government, 2006:4)*

and, in some cases, undertake specific assessments. The midwife is expected to contribute to the *plan* for providing support – *The Child in Need Plan*. However, it is important to note that it is not necessary to wait until the outcome of the assessment to begin to provide services.

## Pre-birth assessment

Pre-birth assessments are undertaken when the local authority is concerned that the baby, when born, will be in need or at risk of significant harm. The safety of the child is paramount, with the pre-birth assessment evaluating the needs of the child and whether support is possible to enable the family to succeed. Assessments include consideration of parenting skills, preparation for the baby, use of medical advice and guidance, and consideration of the family and environment (DH 2000a). In these situations, the identified midwife works with social workers and other professionals in contributing to the assessment.

Particular issues that may trigger a referral to children's social care or a pre-birth assessment are:

- a mother who has a learning disability or physical disability which makes it difficult for her to care for her baby (note that disabled parents are also entitled to assessment and service provision under community care law, the responsibility for which will fall to adult social care departments)
- consistent use of illegal drugs, substances or alcohol by the mother or within the environment
- a mother living with, or having frequent contact with, a violent partner or Schedule 1 offender (a Schedule 1 offender is someone who has been convicted of serious physical or sexual offences, whether or not against children)
- young and vulnerable mothers with no support mechanisms – for example, this may be a girl who is herself 'in need', accommodated by the local authority or subject to a care order
- concerns about the mental health of the mother (or anyone else likely to have care of the child) and the impact of her ill-health on the baby
- extreme poverty or inadequate housing
- families where a child has previously been the subject of a child protection plan or removed from the home
- where pregnancy is the result of rape.

The unborn baby can be made the subject of a child protection plan but no further action can be taken until the child is born.

It has been held that where a local authority wishes to take early action to protect a newly born baby from potentially inadequate parents, they cannot intervene before birth. However, they can intervene immediately after the birth and base this intervention on the mother's behaviour whilst pregnant and the presumption that this would lead to the child being at risk of significant harm (Bainham 2005).

In cases where there is serious concern about the child, they may be made subject to an *emergency protection order* and removed from the mother after birth. This should be planned ahead to enable removal to take place as sensitively as possible. It can be a very traumatic time for all concerned, including professionals, and it is essential that all involved are supported throughout.

## The emergency protection order

Where safe for children to do so, plans to protect a child should proceed in agreement with parents; however, some cases may require emergency action. The Children Act 1989 (section 44) allows for an emergency protection order (EPO) to be made if there is reasonable cause to believe that a child is likely to suffer significant harm if:

- the child is not removed to accommodation; or
- the child does not remain in the place in which he or she is being accommodated.

An EPO can be made if access to a child is being denied as part of a section 47 enquiry. It gives authority to remove a child or cause the child to remain in the protection of the local authority or National Society for the Prevention of Cruelty to Children (NSPCC) for a maximum of 8 days. Police also have powers to remove children to suitable accommodation or to prevent their removal from hospital or safe accommodation (section 46).

In situations where parents are refusing to cooperate with section 47 but there is not sufficient concern to justify an EPO, the local authority can apply for a child assessment order (section 43). This order directs the parents or carer to cooperate with an assessment of the child.

In respect of young babies, an EPO may be applied for at birth if there are concerns that the parent will remove the child. Other examples may include a child who has been seriously injured by a parent who is refusing to allow access to the child or threatening to remove the child from hospital. In line with the best interests of the child, the Family Law Act 1996 allows for a perpetrator to be removed from the home instead of the child, through an *exclusion order* attached to an EPO or interim care order.

## The child protection conference

The child protection conference is the first meeting at which representatives of all the agencies which have dealings with the child or the child's family get together to share and evaluate information and consider the level of risk to a child or children. The conference decides whether the child should be made the subject of a child protection plan and makes plans for the future. Councils with social services responsibilities, or, in some areas, the NSPCC, have responsibility for calling and arranging the conference. Conferences will be led by an independent chair.

The midwife may attend a case conference to present and share information about the child and family, and will be one of many professionals in attendance. Generally, there is a manager representing each agency that attends regularly, including a representative from health, education and the police. Other professionals include social workers and their manager, local authority solicitors, paediatricians, general practitioners, health visitors, housing officers, police, teachers, foster carers, and anyone who may have a significant contribution to make to the assessment. Parents and/or carers are invited to attend but may be excluded if the independent conference chair deems their attendance would potentially jeopardize the welfare of the child (DCSF 2010, HM Government 2006). This sometimes places professionals in a situation where they feel unwilling to speak frankly in front of parents for fear of jeopardizing their relationship with them. However, it is good practice to share child protection concerns openly so parents have an opportunity to respond. (See Reflective activities Web 15.7–15.10 and 15.12.)

All discussions which take place within child protection conferences are confidential. Professionals involved in child protection have their duty of confidentiality to their client overridden by their duty to contribute to the protection of a child at risk. It is important for midwives to be adequately prepared for attendance at a conference. If you are asked to go to a case conference, you are advised to discuss this with your supervisor of midwives. Box 15.5 provides a checklist of things to consider.

### Box 15.5 **Checklist of preparation for a child protection conference**

Who is the health representative attending?
Where and at what time is the meeting to be held?
Will the parents be present?
Do I need a written report?
Am I clear about the information to be presented? – Is my opinion based on facts?
Have I written down notes for myself to assist in my contribution to the conference?
What is my view of the child's developmental needs? – What is my evidence?
What is my view of the parents' capacity to parent? – What is my evidence?
What is my view of family support systems and resources? – What is my evidence?
Have I taken into account the needs of the child as being the primary concern?
What do I think needs to happen to promote the welfare of this child/children?
Is there anything I can contribute to this directly?
Do I know of other resources/aids/assistance, which may be helpful?

### Child protection plan

If a child is made the subject of a plan, a *key worker* is appointed. The key worker is a social worker from either the local authority or NSPCC. They have responsibility for making sure the child protection plan is developed into a more detailed interagency plan, ensuring completion of the core assessment, putting the plan into effect and monitoring it.

A *core group* of professionals, composed of those who have direct contact with the child, is established to develop and implement the child protection plan in conjunction with the family. Members of the core group are jointly responsible for developing, implementing and monitoring the plan. A meeting of the group should take place within 10 working days of the initial conference.

The child protection plan identifies how the child can be protected, including completion of a core assessment, short- and long-term aims to reduce risk to the child and promote the child's welfare, clarity about who will do what and when, and ways of monitoring progress.

If the child is made the subject of a child protection plan, this certainly does not mean that all other work with the child and family ceases. They may also still be eligible to be considered as children 'in need' for whom a range of services may be provided.

### Reflective activity 15.2

Find out who is the designated senior professional and named midwife and doctor in your area.

Obtain a copy of the Local Safeguarding Children Board procedures in your area of practice.

## CONCLUSION

The Children Act 1989, together with subsequent legislation, protects the rights of children, promoting their status within society. Midwives must be aware of the implications of the Act and apply them to their practice. Midwives are uniquely situated to identify risk factors and act as advocates for newborn babies and other children during their professional practice. Detailed and contemporaneous records should be maintained throughout, as these may be required in assessments and child protection conferences (NMC 2008). Key amendments are constantly made to the Children Act and so it is important to keep up to date and access relevant websites and support organizations so that knowledge is current. Using the three case scenarios identified at the beginning of this chapter (available on the website) will have helped you explore aspects of child care law in relation to midwifery practice, through exploration of supporting concepts, on-line materials, and professional and statutory documents. In all cases, it is important that the midwife liaises with the supervisor of midwives and with other professionals, thus perpetuating a multi-agency approach to child support.

## KEY POINTS

- The key features of the Children Act 1989 include paramountcy, parental responsibility, promotion of upbringing within the family where safe to do so, provision of services and support to enable this, and protection of children at risk.
- Midwives need to know the context of working with vulnerable families and how this impacts on their practice.
- The role of the midwife is significant to interagency working, promoting the welfare of children defined by the Children Act as being *in need*, including those at risk of significant harm and requiring protection.
- The midwife plays a vital role in both pre-birth and post-birth assessments.

## REFERENCES


Aldgate J, Statham J: *The Children Act now: messages from research*, London, 2001, The Stationery Office.

Bainham A: *Children: the modern law*, ed 3, Bristol, 2005, Family Law.

Braye S, Preston-Shoot M: *Practising social work law*, ed 3, Basingstoke, 2009, Palgrave Macmillan.

Brayne H, Carr H: *Law for social workers*, ed 11, Oxford, 2010, Oxford University Press.

Butt J, Box C: *Family centred: a study of the use of family centres by black families*, London, 1998, REU.

Calder M: Towards a framework for conducting pre-birth risk assessments, *Child Care in Practice* 6(1):53–72, 2000.

Children's Workforce Development Council (CWDC): *Common Assessment Framework for Children and Young People: practitioners' guide*, Leeds, 2007, CWDC.

Children's Workforce Development Council (CWDC): *The team around the child and the lead professional: a guide for practitioners*, London, 2009, CWDC.

Corby B: Supporting families and protecting children: assisting child care professionals in initial decision-making and review of cases, *Journal of Social Work* 3(2):195–210, 2003.

Department for Children, Schools and Families (DCSF): *Working together to safeguard children: a guide to inter-agency working to safeguard and promote the welfare of children*, London, 2010, HMSO.

Department for Education and Skills (DfES): *Statutory guidance on making arrangements to safeguard and promote the welfare of children under section 11 of the Children Act 2004*, London, 2005, DfES.

Department of Health (DH): *Child protection guidance for senior nurses, health visitors, midwives and their managers*, ed 3, London, 1997, The Stationery Office.

Department of Health (DH): *Framework for the assessment of children in need and their families*, London, 2000a, HMSO.

Department of Health (DH): *Domestic violence: a resource manual for health care professionals*, London, 2000b, DH.

Department of Health (DH): *The Victoria Climbié Inquiry: report of an inquiry by Lord Laming*, London, 2003a, The Stationery Office.

Department of Health (DH): *What to do if you're worried a child is being abused – summary*, London, 2003b, DH.

Department of Health (DH): *Children looked after by local authorities* (website). http://www.dcsf.gov.uk/rsgateway/DB/VOL/v000721/index.shtml. 2007.

Fraser J: *Child protection: a guide for midwives*, ed 2, Cheshire, 2003, Books for Midwives Press.

Haggerty L, Kelly U, Hawkins J, et al: Pregnant women's perceptions of abuse, *Journal of Obstetrics, Gynaecology and Neonatal Nursing* 30(3):283–290, 2001.

Hester M, Pearson C, Harwin N, Abrahams H: *Making an impact: children and domestic violence – a reader*, London, 2006, Jessica Kingsley Publishers.

Hirsch D: *Through thick and thin: tackling child poverty in hard times* (website). www.unicef.org.uk/publications/pdf/ecp_throughthickandthin.pdf. 2009.

HM Government: *The Common Assessment Framework for Children and Young People: supporting tools* (website). www.dcsf.gov.uk/everychildmatters/resources-and-practice/IG00146/. 2006.

HM Treasury: *Ending child poverty: everybody's business* (website). www.hm-treasury.gov.uk/d/bud08_childpoverty_1310.pdf. 2008a.

HM Treasury: *Information sharing: guidance for practitioners and managers* (website). www.dcsf.gov.uk/

everychildmatters/resources-and-practice/IG00340/. 2008b.

Hughes L, Owen H: *Good practice in safeguarding children: working effectively in child protection*, London, 2009, Jessica Kingsley Publishers.

Humphreys C, Stanley N: *Domestic violence and child protection: directions for good practice*, London, 2006, Jessica Kingsley Publishers.

Joint Area Review (Ofsted, Health Commission and HM Inspectorate of Constabulary): *Review of services for children and young people, with particular reference to safeguarding*, London, 2008, JAR.

Laming Report: *The protection of children in England: a progress report*, London, 2009, HMSO.

Morris K: From 'children in need' to 'children at risk' – the changing policy context for prevention and participation, *Practice* 17(2):67–77, 2005.

Nursing and Midwifery Council: *Child protection and the role of the midwife*, London, 2008, NMC.

Ofsted: *The Annual Report of Her Majesty's Chief Inspector of Education, Children's Services and Skills 2008/09*, London, 2009, The Stationery Office.

Platt L: *Ethnicity and child poverty*, Research Report Number 576, London, 2009, Department for Work and Pensions.

Preston-Shoot M: On the evidence for viruses in social work systems: law, ethics and practice, *European Journal of Social Work* 13(4):1–18, 2010.

Social Exclusion Unit (SEU): *Preventing social exclusion* (website). www.socialexclusionunit.gov.uk. 2001.

Statham J, Aldgate J: From legislation to practice: learning from the Children Act 1989 research programme, *Children and Society* 17:149–156, 2003.

Wilson K, James A: *The child protection handbook*, London, 2007, Baillière Tindall.

# Part | 3 |

## Public health, health promotion and childbirth

Chapter |16|

# Epidemiology

Mary Sidebotham and Teresa Walsh

## LEARNING OUTCOMES

After reading this chapter, you will:

- have an understanding of how and why statistical information is collected
- be able to discuss the impact of social and environmental factors upon maternal and neonatal mortality and morbidity
- be critically aware of evidence-based measures which, when implemented, have been shown to reduce maternal and neonatal mortality and morbidity
- appreciate how good midwifery practice can play a positive role in further reducing maternal and neonatal mortality and morbidity.

## INTRODUCTION

Epidemiology is the study of factors affecting the health and illness of populations, and serves as the foundation and logic for interventions made in the interest of public health and preventive medicine. The constantly changing patterns of fertility and childbearing in England and Wales are monitored by the Office for National Statistics (ONS). Information on maternal, neonatal and infant mortality and morbidity is collected and published nationally by the Centre for Maternal and Child Health Enquiries (CMACE) and regionally by regional perinatal health units within the UK. This information plays an important part in future planning for health, education, social welfare and the maternity service needs within the UK.

It is from these data that trends and patterns may be identified and services planned accordingly to meet the needs of current and emerging populations. It is essential that midwives recognize processes for gathering information and utilize these data to inform their day-to-day practice.

## NOTIFICATION AND REGISTRATION OF BIRTHS

Under the National Health Service Act 1977, all births must be notified within 36 hours to the Director of Public Health in the area where the birth occurred. This must be carried out by the midwife or doctor in attendance at the birth, using the local *notification* process that may differ from area to area. Each month a list of births occurring in sub-districts is supplied to the registrar, in order to check whether every birth has been registered.

After the arrival of a new baby, it is a legal requirement to register the birth within 42 days. *Registration* is the responsibility of the child's parents. If the parents fail to register the birth, the duty falls on the occupier of the premises in which the birth took place, usually the midwife or another person of authority, such as a social worker. All midwives must be fully conversant with the legal registration requirements (DPW 2008) (see website).

## FACTS AND FIGURES SURROUNDING FERTILITY AND BIRTH RATES

### General fertility rate

The general fertility rate (GFR) is described as the number of live births per 1000 women aged 15–44. In England

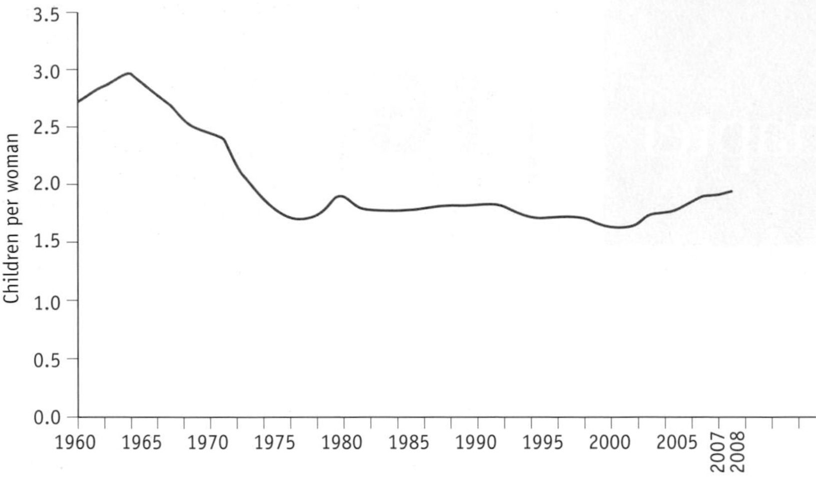


**Figure 16.1** Total fertility rate (TFR) in England and Wales. *(Source: ONS 2008b).*

and Wales, the GFR for 2007 was 62.0, an increase compared with 2006, when the GFR was 60.2 (ONS 2008a).

In 2007, there were increases in fertility rates for all age groups, except for women aged under 20, where the fertility rate fell compared with 2006. The highest percentage increase (6.0%) was observed for women aged 40 and over. For this age group, the fertility rate has risen steadily from 7.3 live births per 1000 women aged 40 and over in 1997 to 12.1 live births per 1000 in 2007. Hence, in the last decade, the number of live births to mothers aged 40 and over has nearly doubled from 12,914 in 1997 to 25,350 in 2007 (ONS 2008a).

## Total fertility rate

The total fertility rate (TFR) is the average number of children a group of women would have if they experienced the age-specific fertility rates of the calendar year in question throughout their childbearing lifespan. The TFR in the UK reached 1.95 children per woman in 2008 (ONS 2008b) (Fig. 16.1). UK fertility has not been this high since 1980.

The UK TFR has increased each year since 2001, when it had dropped to a record low of 1.63. The current level of fertility is relatively high compared with that seen during the 1980s and 1990s. However, the TFR was considerably higher in the 1960s, peaking at 2.95 children per woman in 1964, the height of the 'baby boom' (ONS 2008c). Whereas two children remains the most common family size in England and Wales, an increase in childlessness among women of childbearing age has also been noted in recent years.

## Birth rate

The birth rate is the number of registered live births per 1000 population, and following a decline in the 1990s is now increasing steadily from the rate in 2002 of 11.3 to a rate of 12.8 in 2007 (ONS 2008a).

Because fertility is currently rising faster among women over 30, the average age of childbearing has continued to increase slowly. The mean age for giving birth in the UK was 29.3 years in 2007, compared with 28.6 years in 2001 (ONS 2008a). This could explain, in part, the increasing number of women seeking treatment for infertility, as general fertility decreases with age. Women of 35 are known to be on average half as fertile as those of 31 (Challoner 1999).

## Teenage pregnancy rate

Teenage pregnancy is defined as pregnancy experienced up to and including the age of 19 years, and is frequently further divided into pregnancies up to 15 years of age, and from 15 to 19 years. In 1998, England and Wales were reported to have the highest teenage birth rate in Europe when the birth rate of women aged 15 to 19 years was 30.6 per 1000 women in that age group (UNICEF 2001). Among the developed nations, only the United States had a higher teenage birth rate of 52.1 births per 1000. In response, the British Government introduced a range of measures including the Teenage Pregnancy Strategy in 2000, with the aim of reducing the teenage pregnancy rate by half by 2010, and producing a firm downward trend in the conception rate in the under-16 years age group. Perinatal mortality and morbidity in young mothers is higher than average, so concerted attempts by Government to

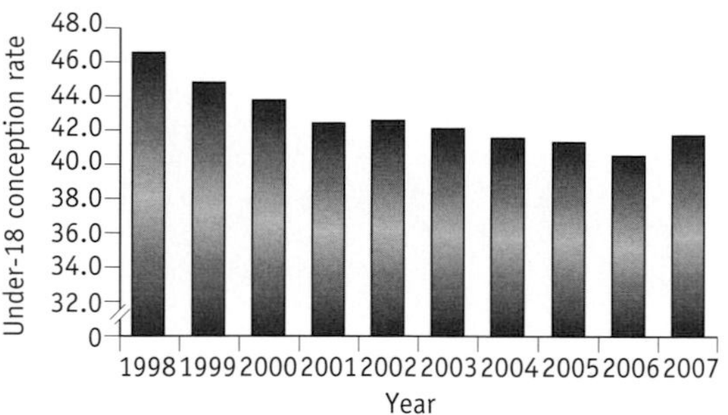


**Figure 16.2** Under-18 conception rate for England: 1998–2007. *(Source: DCSF 2009.)*

improve sex education and make family planning services more accessible to young people have been included in measures to attempt to reduce the teenage conception rate.

Following the introduction of these measures, the ONS figures show teenage pregnancy rates continuing to fall (Fig. 16.2) with a reduction in both the under-18 and the under-16 rates during 2006:

- a 13.3% overall reduction in the under 18 conception rate in England since the 1998 baseline (2% reduction from the 2005 rate)
- a 13% overall reduction in the under-16 conception rate in England since 1998 (1% reduction from 2005)
- between 1998 and 2006, 89% of local authorities have seen an overall reduction in their under-18 conception rate (compared with 83% in 2005)
- the decline in the under-18 conception rate in England contrasts sharply with increases in the conception rate for all other age groups, highlighting the impact of the Teenage Pregnancy Strategy (DCSF 2009).

## FETAL AND INFANT DEATHS

Fetal and infant deaths are divided into defined categories. Whilst there may be similarities between these groups, it is important to look at them individually in order to identify areas for future research, and potential improvement in outcome.

### Stillbirths

*A baby delivered with no signs of life known to have died at 24 completed weeks of pregnancy onwards* (CEMACH 2009).

The stillbirth rate is the number of stillbirths registered during the year per 1000 registered total (live and still) births. In contrast to neonatal mortality, there has been no significant decline in the stillbirth rate since 2000. The stillbirth rate was 5.4 per 1000 total births in 2000 and 5.2 per 1000 in 2007 (Fig. 16.3). The findings from the latest CEMACH report in 2009 suggest that demographic factors known to be associated with stillbirths, such as, obesity, ethnicity, deprivation and maternal age, may be contributing to this lack of progress. In addition, over one-third (40%) of unexplained stillbirths had a birth weight below the 10th centile for gestation and a quarter (26%) of these were below the 3rd centile. This suggests that being small for gestational age may be an important contributor.

### Perinatal deaths

*The perinatal mortality rate comprises all stillbirths and deaths in the first week of life per 1000 registered total births. The group includes all babies who have died 'around' the time of birth.*

The perinatal mortality rate in England and Wales fell from 19.3 per 1000 in 1975 to 7.7 in 2007 (CEMACH 2009) (Fig. 16.3). As with stillbirth, maternal age, obesity, social deprivation and ethnicity remain important risk factors for perinatal mortality.

### Neonatal deaths

*The neonatal mortality rate is the number of deaths of babies within 4 weeks of birth per 1000 registered live births.*

The neonatal mortality rate, like the other mortality rates, is declining in England and Wales and fell from 11.0 per 1000 livebirths in 1975 to 3.3 in 2007 (Fig. 16.4). The majority of neonatal deaths occur in the first day or two after birth, which closely relates the death of the baby to gestational age, labour and delivery.

The causes of perinatal and neonatal deaths occurring in the first week of life are obviously related and may also be responsible for later neonatal deaths; however, other factors, such as infection, may be more strongly implicated in later deaths. The reasons for reduction in the neonatal mortality rate are similar to those responsible for the decline in perinatal mortality (CEMACH 2009).

### Infant mortality

*The infant mortality rate is the number of deaths of infants during the first year of life (including those occurring during the first 4 weeks) per 1000 registered live births in the year.*

There has been a remarkable decline in infant deaths in England and Wales, from 140 per 1000 live births in 1900 to 5.0 per 1000 in 2006 (ONS 2008d) (Fig. 16.4).

The main causes of later infant deaths include:

- infection, mainly acute respiratory and gastrointestinal infection
- congenital malformations
- sudden infant death syndrome (SIDS)

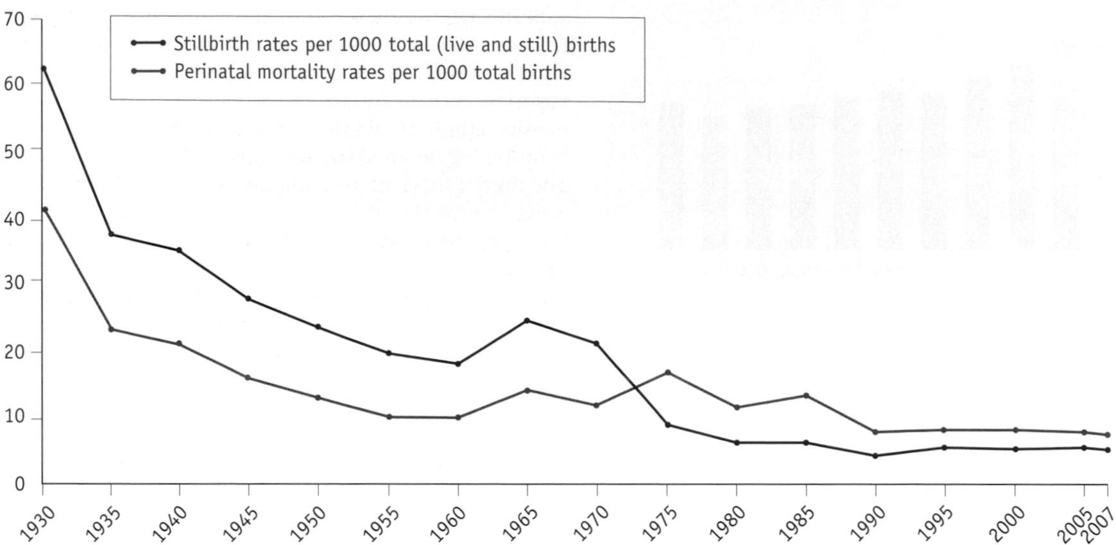


**Figure 16.3** Stillbirth and perinatal death rates in England and Wales. *(Source: ONS 2008d).*

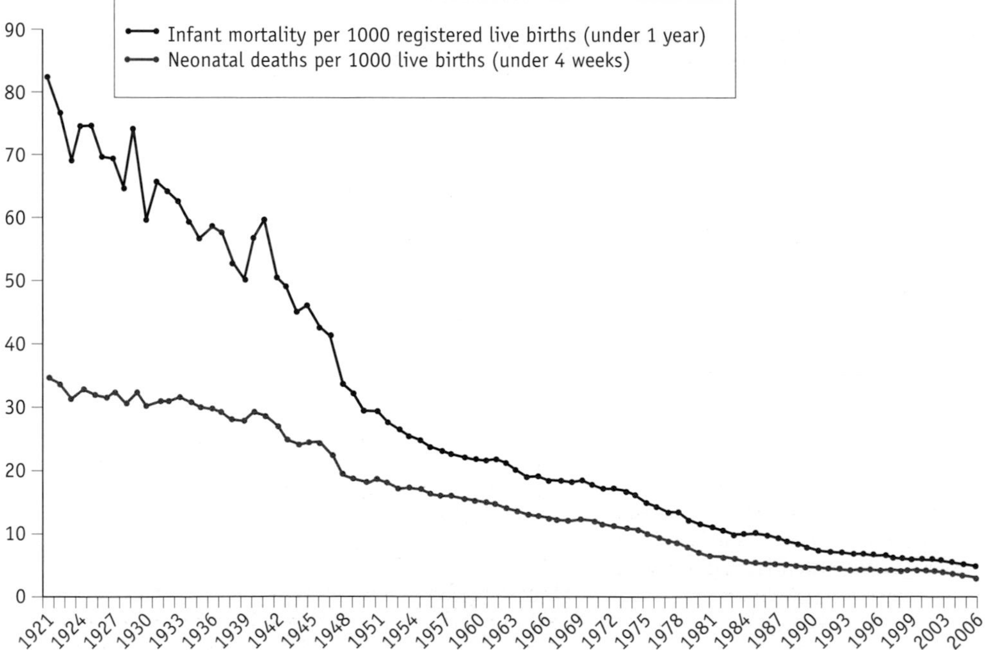


**Figure 16.4** Neonatal and infant death rate in England and Wales. *(Source: ONS 2008d).*

- accidents
- child abuse.

**Reflective activity 16.1**

Review your unit's birth register and other sources of statistical information (as in the reference list).

Note the actual local rate of the following:

- birth rate
- teenage pregnancy rate
- maternal mortality rate
- perinatal mortality rate.

Have these rates changed during the last few years? If so, why do you think this has happened? How has this information been used to design services?

## Predisposing causes and risk factors for fetal, perinatal and infant death

### Social factors

Mortality rates for all categories of death are higher in socioeconomic groups IV and V and the gap between the social classes is widening rather than decreasing (WHO 2005). CEMACH (2009) reported that just over one-third of all stillbirths and neonatal deaths were born to mothers in the most deprived quintiles (compared with the expected 20%). Stillbirth and neonatal mortality rates for mothers resident in the most deprived areas were 1.8 times higher than for those in the least deprived area. Social class differences in access to social and medical care also continue, with women from lower socioeconomic and ethnic minority groups not fully utilizing the services available. This may partly account for the reasons why, when compared with women of white ethnicity, the ethnic-specific mortality rates showed significantly higher stillbirth, perinatal and neonatal death rates for women of black ethnicity (2.7, 2.5 and 2.2 times higher respectively) and Asian ethnicity (2.0, 2.0 and 2.0 times higher respectively) (CEMACH 2009). Low birthweight remains more prevalent in lower socioeconomic and certain ethnic groups. Even if a low birthweight baby survives the perinatal period, recent studies indicate that those who are small or disproportionate at birth, or who have altered placental growth. are at an increased risk of developing coronary heart disease, hypertension and diabetes during adult life (Godrey & Barker 1995). The perinatal mortality rate for babies of unsupported mothers is nearly double that of women who are in a supported relationship.

### Biological and lifestyle factors

Characteristics such as short stature, obesity and maternal age all increase risk. CEMACH (2009) reported that mothers aged less than 20 and above 40 had the highest rates of stillbirth (5.6 and 7.7 per 1000 total births respectively), the highest rates of perinatal deaths (8.9 and 10.3 per 1000 total births respectively) and the highest rates of neonatal deaths (4.4 and 3.4 per 1000 live births respectively).

The impact of obesity on pregnancy outcomes is a growing concern internationally. CEMACH (2009) reported that of the women who had a stillbirth and a recorded body mass index (BMI), 26% (761/2924) were obese (BMI >30), and for neonatal deaths, 22% (356/1609) were obese. Unfortunately, there are no national denominator data available for obese pregnant women in the UK that would provide an estimation of this increased risk.

CEMACH reported that work has commenced on a UK project on obesity in pregnancy which will provide demographic and clinical information on a sample of women with obesity in pregnancy (CEMACH 2008).

The following are all associated with an increase in the overall risk of fetal or maternal mortality.

### Obstetric factors

- Bleeding in pregnancy
- Hypertensive disorders
- Malpresentations
- Malpositions
- Multiple pregnancy
- Cephalopelvic disproportion
- Prolonged labour
- Preterm and postmature labours
- Prolapsed cord
- Rhesus haemolytic disease.

### Medical conditions

- Diabetes mellitus
- Autoimmune disorders
- Haemoglobinopathies
- Renal conditions
- Anaemia
- Respiratory conditions
- Epilepsy
- Infections, such as rubella, cytomegalovirus, toxoplasmosis, listeria, chlamydia, haemolytic group B streptococcus, syphilis and hyperpyrexia.

### Teratogenic factors

Some drugs are known to have a teratogenic effect on the developing fetus, and women should be advised to inform the doctor or pharmacist of their pregnancy. Growing evidence indicates that maternal and passive smoking during pregnancy can have a direct influence on the child in utero, and it has been positively linked with prematurity, low birthweight and stillbirth. The harmful effects remain after birth and links between tobacco exposure and a subsequent increased risk of sudden infant death syndrome, and an increased tendency towards respiratory and infective illness in the child, have been reported. Regular or 'binge' intake of alcohol has been linked to increased risk of miscarriage, growth restriction and fetal alcohol syndrome. Drug abuse is linked to fetal abnormality, growth restriction and an increased risk of sudden infant death (see Chs 23 and 50).

### Dietary deficiencies

Folic acid deficiency preconceptually and in early pregnancy has been shown to be a cause of neural tube defects (MRC Vitamin Study Research Group 1991, Smithels et al 1980, Wald & Bower 1995). Periconceptual vitamin supplementation is therefore advised, especially when there is a history of these malformations. Poor intrauterine nutrition may also affect the long-term health of the individual into adult life (Godrey & Barker 1995).

**Table 16.1 Women's estimated lifetime risk of dying from pregnancy and childbirth**

| Region | Risk of dying |
|---|---|
| Developing countries | 1 in 75 |
| Developed countries | 1 in 7300 |
| Afghanistan | 1 in 7 |
| Sub-Saharan Africa | 1 in 22 |
| Europe | 1 in 1400 |
| UK | 1 in 5100 |
| **All world** | **1 in 92** |

Country-level differences are even more dramatic.

Sources: UNICEF 1996, UNFPA 2007

## MATERNAL DEATHS

The International Classification of Diseases, Injuries and Causes of Death (ICD9/10) defines a maternal death as:

> *the death of a woman while pregnant or within 42 days of termination of pregnancy, irrespective of the duration and the site of the pregnancy, from any cause related to or aggravated by the pregnancy or its management but not from accidental or incidental causes.*
>
> (Lewis 2007)

The maternal mortality rate (MMR) for any year is expressed as the number of deaths attributed to pregnancy and childbearing per 1000 registered total births, or more commonly as the number of deaths per 100,000 maternities. Maternal deaths occurring more than 42 days after pregnancy or childbirth are no longer included in the figures, in line with the international definition of maternal deaths.

The World Health Organization (WHO) Safe Motherhood Initiative was launched in 1987 and maintains its aim to reduce mortality and morbidity significantly among mothers and infants. Most of the annual total of more than 500,000 maternal deaths occur in developing countries, but women still die, albeit in small numbers, in the more affluent nations of the world. There is now a global commitment to find ways to reduce the devastating numbers of maternal deaths. The United Nations Millenium Development Goal 5, *Improve maternal health*, has two targets – to reduce by three-quarters between 1990 and 2015 the maternal mortality ratio, and to achieve universal access to reproductive health by 2015 (UN 2008) (see Ch. 1).

In many countries of the world the maternal mortality rate is difficult to measure owing to the lack of death certificate data (should it exist at all) as well as a lack of basic denominator data, as baseline vital statistics are also not available or unreliable. The recent WHO publication *Beyond the numbers; reviewing maternal deaths and disabilities to make pregnancy safer* (WHO 2004) contains a more detailed examination and evaluation of the problems in both determining a baseline MMR and interpreting what it actually means in helping to address the problems facing pregnant women in most developing countries.

During the triennium 2003–05 there were 295 maternal deaths in the UK, a maternal mortality rate of 13.95 per 100,000 births (Lewis 2007). The slight increase from the maternal mortality rate of 13.07 in the previous triennia is not statistically significant. The UK maternal mortality rate showed steady decline until the mid-1980s but has since remained reasonably static. The maternal mortality rate throughout the world in 2005 is reported as 400 per 100,000 births, which ranges from 8 per 100,000 births in some developed countries to 1400 deaths per 100,000 births in Africa (UNFPA 2007) (Table 16.1).

### Confidential Enquiries into Maternal Deaths

In the UK, a Confidential Enquiry is undertaken into every maternal death to examine factors which may have influenced the outcome, in an attempt to make recommendations and guide future practice. A Confidential Enquiries into Maternal Deaths in England and Wales report was published for each successive 3-year period from the 1952–54 report until the 1982–84 report, and since 1985, reports have included all four countries of the UK. Ascertainment has improved over the last decade as better computer software at ONS is assisting in the recognition of maternal deaths. Reporting has improved owing to the introduction of standards surrounding maternal deaths by

| Table 16.2 Top ten recommendations – Saving Women's Lives report 2003–05 (Lewis 2007) | |
|---|---|
| **1. Pre-conception care** | Pre-conception counselling and support for women of childbearing age with pre-existing serious medical or mental health conditions which could be aggravated by pregnancy. This includes obesity. Especially relevant prior to assisted reproduction |
| **2. Access to care** | Maternity services should be accessible and welcoming to all to promote easier and earlier booking. First appointment should be completed and handheld record given before 12 weeks |
| **3. Access to care** | Pregnant women already 12 weeks at referral should be seen within 2 weeks |
| **4. Migrant women** | Pregnant women from countries where general health may be poorer need full medical assessment and history at booking or as soon as possible. If women are from countries where genital mutilation or cutting is prevalent, this should be sensitively discussed and birth management plans agreed during pregnancy |
| **5. Systolic hypertension requires treatment** | BP 160 mmHg requires antihypertensives. Consider treating at lower recordings if overall clinical picture suggests rapid deterioration is likely |
| **6. Caesarean section** | For some women and babies, caesarean birth is the safest option, but women should be advised that this is not a risk-free procedure and can cause problems in current and future pregnancies. Pregnant women who have previously had caesarean birth must have placental localization in pregnancy to exclude placenta praevia/accreta |
| **7. Clinical skills** | All clinical staff caring for pregnant women must be notified of and have opportunities to learn from critical events and serious untoward incidents in their area of practice |
| **8. Continuing skills training** | All clinical staff must have regular written documented and audited training for:<br>– identification and initial management and referral for serious medical and mental health conditions<br>– early recognition and management of severely ill pregnant women and impending maternal collapse<br>– improvement of basic immediate advanced life support skills |
| **9. Early warning scoring system** | Development and routine use of national obstetric early warning chart for all obstetric women to help with timely recognition of developing critical illness |
| **10. National guidelines** | Urgently require national guidelines for management of<br>– obese pregnant women<br>– sepsis in pregnancy<br>– pain and bleeding in early pregnancy |

local supervising authority (LSA) officers, so what could appear to be an increase in deaths is attributed to improved ascertainment (Lewis 2007).

Information surrounding the care of the woman is gathered by a regional coordinating body, which is then sent to obstetric and, where appropriate, midwifery and/or anaesthetic regional assessors for comment. The assessors send a completed assessment form to the Chief Medical Officer at the Department of Health. In Scotland and Northern Ireland, the system of enquiry is similar but one panel of assessors deals with all cases.

At the Department of Health, only advisors in obstetrics, gynaecology, midwifery and anaesthetics see the forms. An analysis of the cases is undertaken and recommendations are made, highlighting areas of concern and ways of seeking to ensure improvements in future years. The top ten recommendations of the 2003–05 report, which are additional to recommendations made in previous reports, are summarized in Table 16.2.

In the seventh report, *Saving mothers' lives*, for the 3-year period 2003–05, maternal deaths are divided into *direct* deaths, which result from obstetric complications of pregnancy, labour and the puerperium, and *indirect* deaths, which are caused by previously existing diseases or disease that develops during or is worsened by pregnancy (Lewis 2007). Of the 295 maternal deaths assessed for this enquiry, 132 were *direct* deaths (a rate of 6.24 per 100,000 births) and 163 were *indirect* deaths (7.71 per

**Table 16.3 Main causes of maternal death in the UK 2003–2005 (Lewis 2007)**

| Cause | No. of early deaths* | No. of late deaths** |
|---|---|---|
| **Direct** | | |
| Thrombosis and thromboembolism | 41 | 3 |
| Eclampsia and pre-eclampsia | 18 | 0 |
| Early pregnancy deaths (including abortions) | 14 | 0 |
| Haemorrhage (including genital tract trauma) | 17 | 0 |
| Amniotic fluid embolism | 17 | 2 |
| Genital tract sepsis (excluding abortions) | 18 | 3 |
| Anaesthesia | 6 | 0 |
| Other *direct* causes | 1 | 3 |
| **Total *Direct* causes** | **132** | **11** |
| **Indirect** | | |
| Cardiac disease | 48 | 20 |
| Psychiatric, including suicide | 18 | 18 |
| Malignancies | 10 | 27 |
| Other *indirect* causes | 87 | 6 |
| **Total *Indirect* causes** | **163** | **71** |

*Deaths during pregnancy and up to 42 days after end of pregnancy.
**Deaths from 42 days after end of pregnancy, up to 1 year.

100,000 births). Additionally, there were 55 *coincidental deaths* (which are the result of causes not at all related to pregnancy, for example, road traffic accidents) and 82 *late* deaths in the first year after childbirth (Table 16.3).

In keeping with international convention, *coincidental* and *late* deaths are not included in maternal mortality statistics, but are examined in the Confidential Enquiry in case recommendations can be made for service providers.

## Thrombosis and thromboembolism

This remains the commonest cause of direct maternal deaths in the UK, with 41 deaths reported in 2003–05. There were 33 deaths attributed to pulmonary embolism and the remaining 8 were caused by cerebral vein thrombosis. Additionally, three late deaths were due to pulmonary embolism (Table 16.3).

Key recommendations from the Confidential Enquiry report (Lewis 2007) were:

- As obesity is increasing and is a factor in many cases of thromboembolism, all women should have their BMI calculated at the first antenatal visit. Women with a BMI greater than 35 are not suitable for midwife-only care.
- There should be wider use of prophylaxis for women with existing risk factors, and better recognition and investigation of classic symptoms.
- First trimester pregnancy carries a risk and prophylaxis is indicated in situations where there is an increased risk, such as BMI above 40, prolonged bedrest, dehydration, air travel, or familial history.
- Investigations should be carried out on any pregnant or recently pregnant woman with breathlessness, chest pain or leg symptoms to exclude the possibility of deep vein thrombosis and pulmonary embolism.
- All women undergoing caesarean section should be assessed for prophylaxis.
- All women experiencing ovarian hyperstimulation syndrome (OHSS) during assisted conception treatment should be given thromboprophylaxis.

The Royal College of Obstetricians and Gynaecologists has produced guidelines for thromboprophylaxis in pregnancy and the puerperium (RCOG 2004) but the report suggests that further guidelines are needed for women with a BMI greater than 40. There is a need to raise awareness for detection of classic symptoms, especially in women perceived to be at low risk. Deaths occurred where the diagnosis had been delayed or missed, particularly within primary care or accident and emergency settings. There were also a number of women with recognized risk factors who were not offered thromboprophylaxis, emphasizing the continuing need for widespread education in this area.

## Hypertensive disorders of pregnancy

This remains a major cause of maternal death (see Ch. 56), with 18 deaths attributed to this condition during 2003–05; the total number of deaths and mortality rate similar to the previous two triennia. Cerebral complications, mainly intracerebral haemorrhage, were the commonest cause of death. Despite recommendations made in previous reports, there were still substandard aspects of care associated with these deaths. Criticisms were made by panels of failure to react quickly enough to impending signs of eclampsia and lack of seniority and experience within teams caring for these women. There were also examples where healthcare professionals misdiagnosed and failed to make standard routine measurements of blood pressure and urinalysis. Midwives must be vigilant in their approach to early detection and management of any women presenting with risk factors and ensure appropriate management and referral.

The key recommendations (Lewis 2007) for the management of pregnancy-induced hypertension (PIH) include:

- Women with systolic blood pressure of 160 mmHg or above should be treated with antihypertensives. Consideration should be given to commencing treatment at lower systolic pressures if the overall clinical picture suggests likely rapid deterioration with anticipation of severe hypertension.
- Syntometrine should not be administered to hypertensive women for active management of the third stage of labour or when the blood pressure has not been measured.
- Clinicians should anticipate a further rise in blood pressure during intubation and inducing general anaesthesia for emergency caesarean section in women with severe pre-eclampsia, and must take measures to avoid a speed that compromises maternal wellbeing, even when there are concerns about fetal wellbeing.

## Haemorrhage (Chs 54 & 68)

Table 16.3 lists 14 direct deaths due to haemorrhage in 2003–05, in addition, a further 3 deaths from uterine rupture and genital tract trauma are included, which in previous triennia were reported in a separate section (Lewis 2007). The maternal mortality rate remains similar to that for 2000–02 in the UK. Haemorrhage followed caesarean section in 11 of the 14 maternal deaths. Haemorrhage remains a major cause of maternal death through out the world, and it is estimated that a quarter of all maternal deaths are due to haemorrhage (WHO 2005).

The midwife is often the first person to see the woman who may present with acute pain or bleeding. The midwife should always refer a woman who complains of abdominal pain in early pregnancy to a doctor. Similarly, a woman presenting with pain and tender abdomen may have a concealed haemorrhage.

Postpartum haemorrhage will always remain a risk, and midwives must be trained appropriately to manage the situation whilst awaiting medical aid. The woman's haemodynamic status should be checked in pregnancy and when anaemia is detected it should be appropriately treated. Midwives caring for women at home or in birth centres should have access to immediate resuscitation facilities until additional medical assistance can be provided.

The key recommendations made by the CEMACH report 2003–05 encompass many of these points and can be summarized as:

- All staff require specific training to identify and manage maternal collapse, including the identification of hidden bleeding and management of haemorrhage.
- Women should be made aware that caesarean section is not a risk-free procedure and can cause problems for current and future pregnancies.
- All women who have had a previous abdominal delivery should have the placental site identified in the next pregnancy. If in doubt, magnetic resonance scanning as well as ultrasound should be used to exclude placenta accreta or percreta. Pregnancies complicated by placenta percreta require careful multidisciplinary planning.
- Senior clinicians with appropriate surgical experience should be involved in the resuscitation of women with severe haemorrhage from an early stage.
- All maternity staff must have access to the guidelines for management of women who refuse blood products.

## Genital tract sepsis (Ch. 52)

The most recent Confidential Enquiry (Lewis 2007) found there were 18 deaths in 2003–05 attributed directly to genital tract sepsis, and a further 4 deaths in which infection may have played a significant part. This represents an increase from 13 direct deaths in the 2000–02 report. Midwives must be vigilant in the detection and management of any signs of infection. The growing trend towards early discharge from hospital, especially following operative delivery, and reduced postnatal visiting may adversely influence puerperal sepsis rates. The spread of disease can be rapid and devastating; therefore, early detection and treatment are essential. Whilst numbers are small, cases of substandard care are identified throughout the last report, highlighting that care fell short of generally accepted standards.

## Amniotic fluid embolism

There were 19 deaths, including two late deaths, from amniotic embolism in 2003–05 (Lewis 2007), which appears to be an increase from the two previous triennia, but this may be due to increasing efforts in the UK to correctly ascertain this difficult-to-diagnose event. The care of women suffering from this condition is the same as for any maternal collapse before, during or after labour. About 35% of the cases assessed were considered to have received suboptimal obstetric/midwifery care, but this condition carries a high mortality despite prompt treatment and good intensive care. Risk factors include higher maternal age, and, as the average age of childbearing is increasing, this may influence future statistics. Sudden collapse in labour is a common feature in this condition, which should be suspected in any woman regardless of type of labour or delivery. There is little evidence guiding practice towards prevention or treatment and further research would increase understanding and provide information on best practice in its management. A large nationwide prospective study by the United Kingdom Obstetric Surveillance System (UKOSS) to discern the actual incidence of amniotic fluid embolism is currently in progress.

## Indirect causes of maternal death

In 2003–05, the rate for mothers' deaths from *indirect* causes, such as from pre-existing or new medical or mental conditions aggravated by pregnancy (Chs 55 and 69), such as heart disease or puerperal psychosis, had not changed significantly since the previous report (Lewis 2007). Indirect causes outnumber direct causes of death in the UK, whereas worldwide they account for about 20% of maternal deaths (WHO 2005). The commonest cause of maternal death in the 2003–05 triennium was cardiac disease, with 48 deaths attributed to this cause, which has risen clearly since the late 1980s. Although these deaths are classified as indirect maternal deaths, this may change in future reports because lifestyle changes, such as the rising maternal age and obesity in the population, are increasing the incidence of cardiac complaints in the childbearing population generally.

The number of deaths from suicide (Ch. 69), the most common single cause of maternal death in the 2000–02 report (58 deaths), decreased to 37 in 2003–05. This decrease probably indicates that previous recommendations to identify women at risk and offer specialized support services in the antenatal period have been heeded. Most suicides were *late* deaths, occurring more than 42 days but less than one completed year after the end of the pregnancy.

It has been recognized for some time that the underlying root causes of maternal mortality are often social or other non-medical reasons. As with previous UK Confidential Enquiry reports, analysis of the data for 2003–05 reveals that women were more likely to die during pregnancy or childbirth if they were from the most disadvantaged groups in society – socially excluded, lower socioeconomic groups, the very young, and women from certain ethnic communities. It is also clear that vulnerable women with complex social requirements most need care in pregnancy but are least likely to access and maintain contact with maternity services.

Midwives should ensure that services are planned to meet the needs of the most vulnerable women in our society. There should be safeguards built into monitoring systems to ensure that women shown to be at higher risk do not 'slip through the net' (DH 2007).

Midwives should be aware of their professional accountability when caring for women with psychiatric and psychological problems during pregnancy and the puerperium. They should be vigilant in identifying women at risk, and have access to appropriate sources of referral should problems arise. Working within the remit of their professional boundaries, it is essential for midwives to have access to appropriate mental health practitioners at all times.

## STATISTICS INFLUENCING CHANGE: REDUCING MATERNAL, FETAL AND PERINATAL MORTALITY

There are marked geographical differences in mortality rates. Improvements will occur when efforts to improve the whole aspect of the nation's health, through changes in healthcare provision, housing, education, employment prospects and general social welfare, are effective. The detrimental effects of socioeconomic deprivation are recognized universally (DH 2005). Midwives need to influence policy at local, regional and national levels to encourage investment in maternal and child health services.

One of the major influences in the reduction of infant mortality in the last decade has been the reduction in deaths attributed to sudden infant death syndrome (Ch. 50). The 'reducing the risk' information leaflet (DH 2001) is widely distributed to all expectant and new mothers. The Care of the Next Infant (CONI) scheme provides support and resources to families where there is an increased risk of cot death.

Midwives must be aware of their responsibilities in child protection issues, and appropriate training in managing these issues should be widely encouraged. Many families are living in extremely difficult conditions and stress levels are high. There is a growing awareness of the condition 'shaken baby syndrome', illustrated by highly publicized cases where babies, originally thought to have died from cot death syndrome, have been rediagnosed as having been victims of child abuse. Scarce resources should be appropriately targeted to ensure that those families in need of extra support are detected and receive the help that they need. This includes referral to voluntary sector services and agencies, such as the NSPCC, which provide positive parenting support. Parenting skills are highlighted as an important theme within education. Midwives can support this initiative and local schemes by visiting the schools and contributing to the programme. The detrimental effect of domestic violence within families on maternal and infant welfare is also well known. Services must be designed to recognize and support women who are victims of domestic violence (DH 2000, Lewis 2007, RCM 1997).

**Reflective activity 16.2**

What measures are being taken in your area to address the effects of social exclusion and poverty, to ensure that all women have equitable access to care in pregnancy?

There is a growing concern not only about mortality, but also about the quality of life of the survivors. Some babies who survive perinatal complications may be left with a permanent handicap, therefore there is emphasis to measure morbidity, with many regions producing data that relate to outcomes of all babies born below a certain birthweight. The EPICURE study (Wood et al 2000) focuses particularly on the mortality and morbidity of babies born between 24 and 26 weeks' gestation and will provide important information to those planning ongoing services for these children.

Collection of statistics is meaningless unless the information gathered is put to good use.

Being aware of how local, regional and national statistics can be used in the provision and development of services, midwives may contribute to ways of improving clinical practice. They may also contribute to bids for service innovations in all areas, particularly those aimed at reducing inequalities.

## KEY POINTS

- Statistics are an important part of measuring quality and quantity of service, of highlighting shortcomings in practice and supporting the development of appropriate protocols and guidelines to prevent and manage high-risk situations in obstetrics and neonatal care.
- Confidential enquiries into maternal and perinatal mortality are an important strategy towards improving clinical practice and reducing risks for mothers and their babies.
- Midwives play a key role in the gathering of statistical data, and in translating the ensuing reports into practice outcomes. They therefore must be knowledgeable about the whole process and be familiar with the most recently available information.

## REFERENCES


Confidential Enquiry into Maternal and Child Health (CEMACH): *Perinatal mortality 2006: England, Wales and Northern Ireland*, London, 2008, CEMACH.

Confidential Enquiry into Maternal and Child Health (CEMACH): *Perinatal mortality 2007: United Kingdom*, London, 2009, CEMACH.

Challoner J: *The baby makers: the history of artificial conception*, London, 1999, Macmillan.

Department of Children, Schools and Families (DCSF): *Every child matters: teenage pregnancy* (website). www. every childmatters.gov.uk/ teenagepregnancy. 2009. Accessed March 2009.

Department of Health (DH): *Domestic violence: a resource manual for health care professionals*, London, 2000, DH.

Department of Health (DH): *Reduce the risk of cot death: an easy guide*, London, 2001, DH.

Department of Health (DH): *Tackling health inequalities: status report on the programme for action* (website). www.dh.gov.uk/en/ Publicationsandstatistics/ Publications/ PublicationsPolicyAndGuidance/ DH_4117696. 2005. Accessed September 2008.

Department of Health (DH): *Maternity matters: choice, access and continuity of care in a safe service* (website). www.dh.gov.uk. 2007. Accessed December 2008.

Department for Work and Pensions (DPW): *Joint birth registration recording responsibility* (website). www.dwp.gov.uk/publications/ dwp/2008/birth_registration_ia.pdf. 2008. Accessed September 2008.

Godrey KM, Barker DJP: Maternal nutrition in relation to fetal and placental growth, *European Journal of Obstetrics and Gynecology and Reproductive Biology* 61(1):15–22, 1995.

Lewis G, editor: *The Confidential Enquiry into Maternal and Child Health (CEMACH). Saving mothers' lives: reviewing maternal deaths to make motherhood safer – 2003–2005. The seventh report on Confidential Enquiries into Maternal Deaths in the United Kingdom*, London, 2007, CEMACH.

MRC Vitamin Study Research Group: Prevention of neural tube defects: results of the Medical Research Council Vitamin Study, *Lancet* 338(8760):132–137, 1991.

Office for National Statistics (ONS): *Birth statistics: births and patterns of family building England and Wales (FMI) No. 36 – 2007* (website). www.statistics.gov.uk/downloads/ theme_population/FM1_36/ FM1-No36.pdf. 2008a. Accessed July 2009.

Office for National Statistics (ONS): *Births and deaths in England and Wales 2008* (website). www.statistics.gov.uk/pdfdir/ bdths0509.pdf. 2008b. Accessed August 2009.

Office for National Statistics (ONS): *Key population and vital statistics 2006*, Series VS No 33 PPI No 29, Basingstoke, 2008c, Palgrave Macmillan.

Office for National Statistics (ONS): *Mortality statistics: childhood, infant and perinatal: review of the National Statistician on deaths in England and Wales, 2006*, Series DH3 No 39 (website). www.statistics.gov.uk/ downloads/theme_health/ DH3_39_2006/. 2008d. Accessed March 2009.

Royal College of Midwives (RCM): *Domestic abuse in pregnancy*, Position Paper 19, London, 1997, RCM.

Royal College of Obstetricians and Gynaecologists (RCOG): *Thromboprophylaxis during pregnancy, labour and after normal vaginal delivery. Guideline No 37* (website). www.rcog.org.uk. 2004. Accessed November 2008.

Royal College of Obstetricians and Gynaecologists (RCOG): *Registration of stillbirths and certification for pregnancy loss before 24 weeks of gestation (Good Practice No 4)*, RCOG London, 2005, RCOG.

Smithels RW, Sheppard S, Schorah LJ, et al: Possible prevention of neural tube defects by periconceptual vitamin supplementation, *The Lancet* 1(8164):339–340, 1980.

UN: *United Nations Millennium Development Goals* (website). www.un.org/millenniumgoals/. 2008. Accessed January 2009.

UNFPA: *Maternal mortality in 2005. A joint report by UNFPA, WHO, UNICEF and The World Bank* (website). www.unfpa.org/mothers/statistics.htm. 2007. Accessed November 2008.

UNICEF: *Estimates of maternal mortality* (website). www.unicef.org/pon97/p48b.htm. 1996. Accessed November 2008.

UNICEF: *A league table of teenage births in rich nations* (website). www.unicef-irc.org. 2001. Accessed October 2008.

Wald NJ , Bower C: Folic acid and the prevention of neural tube defects, *British Medical Journal* 310(6986):1019–1020, 1995.

World Health Organization (WHO): *Beyond the numbers. Reviewing maternal deaths and complications to make pregnancy safer* (website). www.who.int/reproductive-health/publications/btn/text.pdf. 2004. Accessed March 6, 2009.

World Health Organization (WHO): *The World Health report: make every mother and child count*, Geneva, 2005, WHO.

Wood NS, Marlow N, Costeloe K, et al: Neurologic and developmental disability after extremely preterm birth, *New England Journal of Medicine* 343(6):378–384, 2000.

Chapter |17|

# Nutrition

*Denise Tiran*

## LEARNING OUTCOMES

By the end of this chapter, you will be able to:

- understand the basic principles of good maternal nutrition
- use a knowledge of nutrition to advise women about their diet during pregnancy
- appreciate the value of nutrition as a therapeutic intervention for specific conditions during pregnancy.

Nutrition is the sum of the processes involved in taking in, utilizing and assimilating nutrients. Nutrients such as proteins, carbohydrates, fats, vitamins and minerals are necessary for development, growth, normal functioning and maintenance of life. As the body cannot produce them, they need to be obtained from a variety of food sources. Nutritional status is affected by the amount and quality of food eaten; the digestion, absorption and utilization of food nutrients; and biochemical individuality. In westernized countries, eating enough food is not normally a problem. Many people, however, do not eat the correct balance of nutrients. Malnourishment causes impairment of health. In the United Kingdom it occurs for reasons different to those in developing countries, where food is scarce. Food quality may be affected by nutrient-deficient soil in which crops are grown for human or livestock consumption, or by the use of pesticides. The addition of chemical preservatives, colourings and flavourings to ready-prepared food, and antibiotics to meat, will also adversely influence nutrient absorption and utilization.

Digestion and absorption may be affected by general health or combinations of foods eaten. On the other hand, impaired absorption of certain nutrients may be iatrogenic, as when someone is taking specific drugs. Over-indulgence in some foods can affect absorption of essential nutrients; for example, coffee and tea interfere with absorption of zinc and iron from food. Similarly, alcohol, cigarettes or recreational drug abuse, or environmental factors including lead pollution, may lead to malnourishment through inadequate absorption and utilization of nutrients from food. Each person has unique nutritional requirements which alter according to age, gender, general health, activity level, genetic influences and stressors, including pregnancy. Some people need professional help to direct them towards the most appropriate diet.

## THE IMPORTANCE OF GOOD NUTRITION BEFORE AND DURING PREGNANCY

Midwifery advice about healthy eating during pregnancy can have long-term benefits for the whole family. Inadequate preconceptional and antenatal nutrition may have adverse fetal effects, increasing the risk of perinatal mortality and morbidity, low birthweight or preterm infants, birth defects such as neural tube defects (Carmichael et al 2007, Tamura & Picciano 2006), or maternal complications (Bodnar et al 2006). Impaired maternal nutrition can also adversely affect fetal disease programming, increasing the tendency to hypertension and cardiovascular disease in adult life (Plagemann et al 2008, Woods 2007).

Infertility can be exacerbated by nutritional deficiencies (Chavarro et al 2007, 2008), and dietary advice is a major component of preconceptional care, especially for medical conditons (Tieu et al 2008). Ovulation is dependent on adipose tissue (fat) distribution equal to at least 17% of a woman's total body weight; anorexics are thus less likely to conceive and more likely to miscarry from vitamin and mineral imbalances. Similarly, male infertility due to poor sperm production may be associated with nutritional deficiency exacerbated by contemporary western diets (Eskenazi et al 2005, West et al 2005). A nutritional diet is high in beneficial nutrients such as those that suppress the effects of toxicity caused by environmental pollution, and low in substances such as nicotine, tea, coffee, alcohol and drugs (Vujkovic et al 2007). The contraceptive pill interferes with the absorption of vitamin $B_6$ and zinc and should ideally be discontinued for at least 3 months preconception. Premenstrual syndrome, triggered by magnesium, zinc, vitamin $B_6$ and other vital nutrient deficiency, may impact on conception. Women who are deficient in essential fatty acids, zinc, manganese and vitamin E or who indulge in potentially toxic substances are also more susceptible to recurrent miscarriage (Bailey & Berry 2005, Ronnenberg et al 2007). Controversy continues regarding the amount of caffeine which may provoke miscarriage (George et al 2006). Alcohol has long been recognized as a possible contributor to fetal teratogenicity and morbidity; women are advised to avoid alcohol completely in the first trimester and to limit later consumption to no more than two alcohol units once or twice a week (NICE 2008a). Artificial preservatives can be harmful.

Expectant mothers should be advised to eat as much fresh food as possible, with a minimum of five portions of fruit, vegetables and salad daily. Organically grown food reduces the impact of fertilizer sprays used on crops but it is usually more expensive and the health benefits of organic foods have been questioned recently in the media. Some food-acquired infections may affect fetal wellbeing and women should reduce or eliminate their consumption of foods likely to harbour these pathogens (NICE 2008b). Examples include *Listeria monocytogenes*, found in non-pasteurized milk, soft cheeses such as Brie and Camembert, blue-veined cheeses, meat and vegetable pâtés, and uncooked or undercooked ready-prepared meals, whilst *Salmonella* infection can arise from eating raw or partially cooked meat or eggs or egg products, such as mayonnaise.

## WEIGHT IN PREGNANCY

Most mothers gain between 11 and 15.75 kg (25–35 lb) in weight during pregnancy, but this depends upon maternal diet, activity, food availability, and gestational factors such as sickness or multiple pregnancy. In women of average weight at conception, a balanced diet usually results in full-term babies of adequate birthweight. Preconceptional, gestational and lactational nutrition affect the birthweight, wellbeing and long-term prognosis of infants, with impact on risk of maternal obesity in later life (Uauy et al 2008). Obesity has become a significant issue in the western world, with serious consequences for UK maternity services (Heslehurst et al 2007). The Confidential Enquiry into Maternal and Child Health 2003–2005 found that almost 30% of women who had a stillbirth or neonatal death were clinically obese, while 35% had a body mass index of 30 or above (Lewis 2007). Maternal obesity is associated with an increased risk of gestational diabetes, hypertension, pre-eclampsia, operative delivery and anaesthetic risks, postpartum haemorrhage, infection, thromboembolic disorders and fetal abnormalities (Dixit & Girling 2008), as well as a high risk of long-term weight problems and childhood obesity (Durand et al 2007). Obesity poses a very real risk to the progress and outcome of pregnancy, birth and the puerperium. Steps should be taken to reduce this risk through education, social support, appropriate obstetric care and management.

Women who restrict their energy intake in pregnancy also cause concern. Dieting to lose weight is not recommended antenatally, even for obese women, unless under medical supervision. In societies where lack of food forcibly restricts energy intake, maternal metabolic adaptations enable energy production for fetal growth. However, care must be taken when advising immigrant women in Britain, such as those from the Indian subcontinent. Pregnant Muslim women are required to comply with total fasting during Ramadan; midwives should be aware of current teachings regarding Ramadan, and should ask Muslim women if they are fasting.

Anorexia nervosa and bulimia nervosa are associated with poor pregnancy outcome, including sub-fertility, risk of miscarriage, obstetric complications, intrauterine growth retardation and postnatal depression. Midwives should be alert to signs of possible eating disorders, particularly in women with a very low body mass index, those who appear to have poor body image and those who report prolonged hyperemesis gravidarum.

## ESSENTIAL NUTRIENTS

### Proteins and amino acids

*Required for:*

- development of cells, enzymes, hormones, antibodies, haemoglobin
- buffers, helping to regulate acid–base balance
- controlling osmotic pressure between body fluids
- assisting in the transport of lipids as lipoproteins, and free fatty acids and bilirubin.

*Protein foods:*

- meats, poultry, fish
- cheese, milk, eggs and other dairy produce
- beans, peas and other legumes
- corn, wheat products
- grains, seeds, nuts
- brewer's yeast, soya.

Proteins are digested by being broken down into amino acids and transported to the liver, where amino acid transferase enzymes convert them into a more usable form. Essential amino acids include leucine, lysine, methionine, cystine, phenylalanine and tryptophan; non-essential amino acids include alanine, glutamic acid, glycine and tyrosine. This process requires vitamin $B_6$; consequently, a high protein intake will require an increase in vitamin $B_6$ intake. Pregnant women have higher blood levels of tryptophan, an amino acid converted to serotonin, a calming and antidepressive agent. Certain protein foods are potential infection sources for pregnant women, in particular contaminated meat; advice regarding thorough cooking may prevent gastrointestinal disorders. Raw meat may be contaminated with *Listeria monocytogenes* or *Toxoplasma gondii*, so pregnant women should avoid raw or undercooked meat. *Listeria monocytogenes* may also be present in unpasteurized milk, including in soft cheeses.

## Essential fatty acids

*Required for:*

- energy, heat insulation
- production of active biological substances essential for normal body functioning
- facilitation of absorption of fat-soluble vitamins and calcium
- formation of cell walls throughout the body
- production of prostaglandins.

*Foods containing essential fatty acids:*

- nuts, grains, seeds (omega 6 and 3)
- fruits and vegetables (omega 6)
- sunflower, safflower, soya, evening primrose, wheatgerm oils (omega 6)
- flax/linseeds (omega 3)
- green leafy vegetables (omega 3)
- oily fish, especially salmon, and shellfish (omega 3)
- walnuts (omega 3).

*Foods containing unsaturated fatty acids:*

- vegetable oils: safflower and sunflower, but excluding coconut and palm oil, which are saturated
- oily fish.

*Foods containing saturated fatty acids:*

- animal fats: butter, lard, meat fat
- margarines and vegetable shortening.

Fats are composed of triglycerides, which are broken down during digestion. Most fatty acids are synthesized by the body, with the exception of linoleic acid, linolenic acid and arachidonic acid, which must be obtained from food. Fatty acids are either monounsaturated or polyunsaturated. Unsaturated fatty acids are preferable to saturated ones, and polyunsaturated are the most favourable as they are more readily converted into energy; however, a balance of each type is required for adequate nutrition.

Fatty acids depend on adequate intake of zinc, magnesium, selenium, and vitamins $B_3$, C and E. Fat requirements are slightly increased during pregnancy, for extra energy and to avoid protein calories being misused. Omega-3 fatty acids are essential for the developing fetus, particularly visual and cognitive functioning. They may prevent preterm labour, intrauterine growth retardation, pre-eclampsia and postnatal depression (Cetin & Koletzko 2008, Innis & Friesen 2008).

## Carbohydrates

*Required for:*

- calorie intake: 1 gram of carbohydrate provides 4 calories of energy
- regulation of gastrointestinal function
- balancing the growth of normal bacterial flora against undesirable flora.

*Carbohydrate foods:*

- sugars, fruit sugars and foods containing sugars, including 'hidden' sugars in savoury foods
- breads, pastas, flours, cereals
- potatoes, bananas
- beetroot
- dates, figs
- maple syrup
- sauces, flavourings.

Carbohydrates are classified as sugars (mono- and disaccharides) or starches and fibre (polysaccharides). They are the most easily digested nutrients, which can be stored and released as energy when required, preventing excessive oxidation of fats for energy. All carbohydrates are partly broken down in the mouth but mainly in the small intestine, to the simplest compound, glucose; excess glucose is converted into glycogen and stored by the liver. Carbohydrate intake should equate to approximately half of all food consumed. This may indicate a need to increase starches and fibre and decrease fats and proteins.

## Vitamins and minerals

### Vitamin A

*Required for:*

- growth and repair of cells
- fighting infection
- synthesis of ribonucleic acid (RNA)
- healthy eyes, especially night vision
- protein metabolism
- aids in detoxification processes
- as an antioxidant.

*Foods which contain vitamin A:*

- liver, kidneys
- fish oils
- eggs, dairy produce
- apricots, carrots, other yellow vegetables
- broccoli, parsley, green leafy vegetables.

Deficiency of vitamin A may cause anaemias, blindness, skin disorders, tooth decay, allergies and gastrointestinal disorders. Absorption can be impeded by vitamin D deficiency, alcohol, coffee, mineral oil, nitrate fertilizers and strong glaring sunlight. However, women should be discouraged from taking vitamin A supplements (more than 700 µg) or eating excessive amounts of vitamin A-containing foods, such as liver or liver products, during the first trimester, as birth defects have been reported (NICE 2008b).

### Thiamin (vitamin $B_1$)

*Required for:*

- synthesis of acetylcholine within the cells
- maintenance of healthy nerves, cardiac muscle, digestive tissues
- digestion of carbohydrates.

*Foods which contain thiamin:*

- whole grains
- nuts, seeds, such as sunflower
- brewer's yeast
- fruit, green vegetables
- liver, kidneys
- fish
- eggs, milk.

Thiamin absorption is impaired by stress, food additives, alcohol, coffee, excessive sugar consumption, overcooking vegetables and some antibiotics. Thiamin requirements increase during pregnancy and lactation. Long-term deficiency can lead to irritability, insomnia, weight loss, oedema, poor reflexes and impairment of the cardiovascular, nervous and gastrointestinal systems.

### Riboflavin (vitamin $B_2$)

*Required for:*

- metabolism of fats, proteins, carbohydrates
- wound healing
- regulation of hormones
- growth and development of the fetus.

*Foods which contain vitamin $B_2$:*

- foods which also contain thiamin.

Absorption is adversely affected by antibiotics and the contraceptive pill. Deficiency may cause various external lesions, fatigue, personality disturbance, anaemia, digestive upset and hypertension.

### Niacin (vitamin $B_3$)

*Required for:*

- conversion of food to energy
- metabolism of fats, proteins, carbohydrates
- regulation of hormonal and enzymal actions
- vasodilatation.

*Foods which contain niacin:*

- liver, lean meat
- poultry
- fish
- grains
- yeast
- butter
- nuts.

Absorption of niacin is antagonized by alcohol, stress, coffee, high carbohydrate intake, antibiotics and antitubercular drugs. Various skin and gastrointestinal disturbances may result from inadequate intake, as well as headache, memory loss, insomnia and poor appetite. If a mother is deficient in vitamin $B_6$, her niacin needs will also increase.

### Pyridoxine (vitamin $B_6$)

*Required for:*

- synthesis of proteins
- production of antibodies
- manufacture of erythrocytes
- enzyme reactions
- development of the nervous system
- healthy teeth and gums
- release of stored glycogen.

*Foods which contain pyridoxine:*

- foods which contain other B vitamins
- bananas, grapefruit
- prunes, raisins.

Absorption is affected by some drugs, including the contraceptive pill, cortisone and penicillamine. Pyridoxine requirements increase during pregnancy and lactation; insufficient intake triggers anaemia, neuritis, convulsions, depression, dermatitis and renal calculi.

## Cobalamin (vitamin $B_{12}$)

*Required for:*

- proper functioning of the bone marrow and erythrocytes
- nervous system, including myelin formation
- development of RNA and DNA
- regulation of normal blood ascorbic acid levels
- carbohydrate metabolism.

*Foods which contain cobalamin:*

- liver, kidney
- fish, shellfish.

Absorption may be adversely affected by aspirin, the contraceptive pill, codeine, alcohol and nitrous oxide. Deficiency can result in pernicious anaemia, poor growth, memory loss, nervous disorders and ataxia. Although requirements do not increase significantly during pregnancy, certain women are at risk of deficiency, including vegetarians, epileptics and those with tapeworms. The risk of neural tube defects and that of neurological symptoms, including failure to thrive, irritability and poor milestone development, is increased in the infants of women with vitamin $B_{12}$ deficiency (Dror & Allen 2008, Ray et al 2007).

## Folic acid

*Required for:*

- production of erythrocytes, in conjunction with $B_{12}$
- maintenance of the nervous system
- gastrointestinal tract functioning
- production of leucocytes
- production of choline and methionine
- development of the fetus.

*Foods which contain folic acid:*

- leafy greens
- whole grains, nuts
- oranges
- broccoli
- tuna
- liver, kidney.

The incidence of neural tube defects increases in women deficient in folic acid. The National Institute for Health and Clinical Excellence (NICE) recommends that all women intending to become pregnant should take 400 μg of a folic acid supplement daily before pregnancy and during the first trimester (NICE 2008a). In the mother, folic acid deficiency can lead to some anaemias, depression, nervousness, cell and tissue disruptions, and premature greying or loss of hair and may contribute to placental abruption (Nilsen et al 2008). Impaired absorption and utilization may occur if the woman is stressed, drinks alcohol, has recently discontinued the contraceptive pill, or is taking drugs such as aspirin, sulphonamides or anticonvulsants.

## Vitamin C

*Required for:*

- cell, tissue, nerve, tooth and bone health
- wound healing
- metabolism of amino acids
- facilitation of iron absorption.

*Foods which contain vitamin C:*

- all citrus fruits
- berries
- melons
- tomatoes
- potatoes
- parsley
- green vegetables (cooking destroys it)
- blackcurrants.

Inadequate levels of vitamin C lead to infections, bruising, oedema, haemorrhage, anaemia, poor digestion, tooth and gum disease and scurvy. Some drugs, including aspirin, anticoagulants, antibiotics, diuretics, cortisone, the contraceptive pill and antidepressants, interfere with absorption, as can pollution, industrial toxins, and overcooking or poor storage of food sources. There is some suggestion that daily vitamin C supplementation may reduce the incidence of urinary tract infections in susceptible pregnant women (Ochoa-Brust et al 2007).

## Vitamin D

*Required for:*

- calcium absorption
- healthy bones and teeth
- renal, cardiac, nervous systems
- blood clotting.

*Foods which contain vitamin D:*

- fish liver oils
- liver
- brewer's yeast
- tuna
- avocados
- cereals.

The main source of vitamin D is the sunshine. Drugs such as laxatives and antacids inhibit absorption, therefore women with constipation or heartburn should take care not to overuse them. The mother and fetus both require additional vitamin D to prevent skeletal malformations, rickets, osteoporosis, poor muscle tone, and reduced kidney and parathyroid gland function. Women predisposed to pre-eclampsia should be encouraged to increase their vitamin D intake since vitamin D deficiency may contribute to the disease (Hyppönen et al 2007). Pregnant women who restrict their consumption of milk, a source of vitamin D, protein, calcium and riboflavin, may be at greater risk of having babies of low birthweight (Mannion et al 2006) or who suffer hypocalcaemic convulsions (Camadoo et al 2007). The NICE guidelines advocate vitamin D supplementation for pregnant women with limited exposure to sunlight, such as long-stay antenatal inpatients or those who habitually cover the skin when outdoors. This recommendation also applies to mothers with a body mass index of 30 or above, those who are breastfeeding and those who eat a diet low in foods containing vitamin D (NICE 2008a, 2008b).

## Vitamin E

*Required for:*

- maintenance of erythrocytes
- major bodily functions, including reproduction
- retarding ageing
- helping the body to respond to stress.

*Foods which contain vitamin E:*

- whole grains
- eggs
- leafy greens, broccoli, cabbage
- avocados
- nuts
- liver, kidneys
- cold-pressed vegetable oils.

Vitamin E is destroyed by food processing, rancid fats and oils, and inorganic iron. Absorption is adversely affected by mineral oil, the contraceptive pill, chlorine and thyroid hormone. Requirements for vitamin E increase during pregnancy: indeed, what was originally called vitamin E is now known to be a group of compounds called tocopherols. In humans, deficiency may result in spontaneous abortion, preterm labour, stillbirth, anaemia, and muscular or cardiovascular diseases.

## Calcium

*Required for:*

- formation of bones and teeth
- utilization of iron
- assisting coagulation
- regulation of cardiac rhythm.

*Foods which contain calcium:*

- milk and dairy products: yogurt, egg yolk
- sardines and salmon with bones
- green beans
- bone marrow
- tofu, soya beans.

High-protein or high-phosphorus diets will antagonize calcium absorption, as will either excessive or inadequate physical activity, or stress. Drugs affecting calcium absorption or utilization include antacids, laxatives, diuretics and anticonvulsants. Deficiencies may lead to bone disorders, such as osteoporosis or osteoarthritis, dental problems, palpitations, hypertension, insomnia or muscle cramps. Routine calcium supplementation may be helpful in women at risk of pre-eclampsia or those who have an identified low level of calcium.

## Zinc

*Required for:*

- cell development in the brain, thyroid gland, liver, kidneys, lungs, prostate gland
- skeletal growth, skin, hair, repair of body tissues, wound healing
- metabolism of proteins, carbohydrates and phosphorus
- facilitation of release of stored vitamin A.

*Foods which contain zinc:*

- herrings, oysters, fish bones
- liver, red meat, meat bones
- eggs, milk
- nuts, whole grains
- mushrooms, leafy green vegetables
- paprika.

Zinc requirements rise by approximately 30% during pregnancy to provide for the development of the fetal central nervous system, and 40% in lactating women. Absorption is enhanced by adequate intakes of calcium, copper, vitamins A, $B_6$, $B_{12}$ and C, and certain amino acids. Absorption and utilization are impaired by tea, coffee, alcohol, processed grains, iron tablets, the contraceptive pill, and by excess levels of phytates, found in bran, and calcium. Jewish women may be deficient in zinc, owing to the presence of phytates in unleavened bread. Zinc neutralizes the toxic effects of cadmium, a contributory factor in hypertension; conversely, high levels of cadmium, found in cigarettes, some processed and canned foods, instant coffee and gelatine, inhibit the action of zinc.

Excessive sweating can cause a loss of up to 3 mg of zinc per day. Zinc is lost in the urine at times of stress and during increased diuresis, such as following high alcohol consumption.

Zinc deficiency can lead to retarded growth and mental development, delayed sexual maturity or sterility (semen contains large quantities of zinc). It may exacerbate gestational sickness and worsen the appearance of striae gravidarum. Women who are zinc deficient may have white spots on their fingernails, experience a metallic taste in the mouth and have a poor appetite. Maternal intake of less than 6 mg daily may lead to babies of low birthweight or prematurity and impaired immune systems (Mahomed et al 2007). Zinc antagonizes lead and cadmium, both of which may be found in higher than normal quantities in the bones of stillborn infants; by inference, therefore, adequate zinc levels may decrease the risk of stillbirth caused solely by nutritional deficiencies.

### Iron

*Required for:*

- manufacture of haemoglobin for oxygenation of the blood
- protein metabolism
- bone growth
- resistance to disease.

*Foods which contain iron:*

- red meats, liver
- sardines, pilchards, sprats, whitebait, cockles
- eggs, especially the yolks
- wholemeal bread, chapattis, oatcakes
- cereals
- potatoes, parsley, chives, spinach
- dried fruits, nuts, cherries
- soya beans, red kidney beans, lentils, chickpeas.

An inadequate iron level will lead to anaemia, fatigue, headache, palpitations and heartburn. Supplementation will be required to treat iron-deficiency anaemia. Dietary iron consumption will normally achieve sufficient serum levels, although a high zinc intake, tea, coffee, intestinal parasites, antacids and tetracycline will interfere with absorption. Women who consume adequate amounts of foods containing vitamins C, E, $B_6$, $B_{12}$, folic acid, calcium, copper and other trace elements will normally be able to utilize efficiently the iron from dietary intake. Whilst there is no indication for routine iron supplementation in pregnancy (NICE 2008b), those who require additional iron should be advised to take tablets with orange juice (or other vitamin C-containing drink), which facilitates absorption of the iron, while overconsumption of tea hinders its absorption.

**Reflective activity 17.1**

Make comprehensive lists of foods that contain certain minerals – for example, magnesium, selenium – and identify what might happen if a mother were to be deficient in these elements.

## NUTRITION AS A THERAPEUTIC INTERVENTION

### Nausea and vomiting (Chapter 53)

Many women find that nausea is exacerbated by hypoglycaemia, especially if they are also tired. Advice can be given by the midwife to eat small frequent meals of complex carbohydrate foods, such as bread, cereal or potatoes, but not those that are high in sugar or salt. Bananas are a good source of carbohydrate, and may also help to prevent potassium deficiency. Sickness in pregnancy is worse for women lacking in vitamin $B_6$, magnesium and zinc. Women should be advised to eat foods rich in these substances or to take a good-quality supplement. Reducing the amount of dairy produce may also help, as may increasing the intake of citrus fruits or juices (Tiran 2004, 2006).

### Constipation

The midwife can advise women to increase their intake of high-fibre foods, but more importantly they must increase their fluid intake to at least 2 litres of water daily. Tea consumption should be decreased. Tannin reduces peristalsis and inhibits the absorption of iron, which might result in prescription of iron tablets; these, in turn, exacerbate constipation.

Women should eat plenty of fresh fruits, vegetables, unrefined carbohydrates, seeds, grains and pulses, such as beans (Derbyshire et al 2006). Bran should be *avoided*, unless there is a substantial increase in fluid intake, as it absorbs fluid from the intestines and makes the stool hard, increasing the severity of the constipation. Wheat and wheat products, such as bread and cereals, may increase bloating or abdominal discomfort, particularly if the problem was present before pregnancy, as it may be due to a mild wheat intolerance. Long-term use of laxatives should be discouraged as they will not treat the cause of the problem and can often create other side-effects. Vitamin C supplements may be necessary in some mothers. If iron tablets are prescribed for anaemia and found to exacerbate the problem, other sources of iron-containing foods should be advised. It may be necessary to suggest alternatives to medication, such as herbal liquid preparations, available from healthfood stores.

### Heartburn and indigestion

The mother should be advised to eat small frequent meals and avoid drinking with meals, but maintain a high fluid intake between meals. She should avoid foods which aggravate the condition, such as spicy or greasy foods, as well as coffee, tea, alcohol and cigarettes. Milk and milk products do not always help to relieve the symptoms, and may exacerbate them, as may sugar, sweet foods, wheat and bread. Excessive antacid use should be avoided, especially those containing aluminium, as this may be absorbed and cause mild toxicity. Using large quantities of garlic in cooking can be very helpful. It is best to use whole, peeled but uncut, cloves of garlic which, when cooked, can be squashed and stirred into the food. In this way, adequate quantities of the active ingredients, allicin and other sulphur-containing substances, will be consumed but there will be no excessively strong flavour nor the aftertaste or halitosis, of which many people complain.

## Anaemia

Anaemia may be prevented, or the effects reduced, by encouraging the mother to eat foods rich in iron. Her diet should include plenty of fresh green leafy vegetables, such as cabbage, spinach, watercress, parsley, spring onions, chives, sprouted grains and seeds. Seaweeds, nettle tops and dandelion leaves are also good sources of iron. Dried prunes, raisins, figs and unsulphured apricots are helpful, as are blackcurrants, blackberries, cherries and loganberries. Wholegrain bread, oatcakes and chapattis should be eaten rather than highly refined carbohydrates. Pilchards, salmon, kippers and organic liver also provide iron. Bran should be avoided as it inhibits the absorption of iron from foods. Tea and coffee, particularly when taken with meals, have similar effects. Vitamin C-containing fruits and vegetables that enhance the uptake of iron include kiwi fruits, oranges, rosehips, potatoes, cauliflower, broccoli, brussel sprouts and parsley. If iron supplements are prescribed, the mother should be advised to take them with a glass of orange juice and avoid drinking too much tea or coffee.

**Reflective activity 17.2**

Reflect on some of the women you have cared for during pregnancy and explore how you may have been able to help them to relieve their symptoms by a more efficient management of their diet.

Keep a record during a week of your clinical practice to identify the dietary practices of the women you see: how many of them actively seek advice regarding their nutrition?

## Candida albicans ('Thrush')

*Candida albicans* yeast infection (see Chapter 57) is common in pregnancy and if left untreated can complicate delivery and may develop into a chronic condition. Women on antibiotics, especially those who have had recurrent infections or when antibiotics are required long term, are more susceptible to thrush. Zinc deficiency compromises the immune system, so infection is more likely, and any nutritional deficiencies should be corrected, initially with an increase in foods containing the relevant minerals and vitamins, or with supplements.

Refined carbohydrates and yeast-containing foods exacerbate the condition and facilitate multiplication of the candida, so should be eliminated from the diet, especially white flour, white or brown sugar or any foods containing these. Similarly, foods containing yeast should be avoided, for example, bread, cheese, alcohol, yeast extract, frozen or concentrated orange juice, grapes, grape juice, unpeeled fruits, raisins, sultanas and B vitamin supplements (unless labelled as yeast-free). Food that is not absolutely fresh should not be consumed, whereas foods containing natural antifungal agents, such as garlic, fresh herbs, spices and fresh green leafy vegetables, can be eaten frequently. For vaginal thrush, a whole peeled but *uncut* clove of garlic can be inserted into the vagina to act as a local antifungal agent; daily consumption of garlic in food is also recommended.

# CONCLUSION

Adequate nutrition during pregnancy and lactation is vital for good maternal and fetal health. The midwife is in an invaluable position to educate women, thereby influencing family nutrition and health from the beginning. This chapter has discussed the needs of normal women and no mention has been made of the special nutritional requirements of some mothers, for example, diabetics. Midwives should have a basic knowledge of the main dietary needs of mothers, and be able to advise women accordingly. However, it is also important that midwives are able to identify women more at risk of poor nutrition, so that they can be referred to a specialist nutritional therapist or dietician for appropriate information. It has not been possible here to provide more than a general introduction to the subject of nutrition, but further suggestions are on the website.

**KEY POINTS**

- Good nutrition is essential both before and during pregnancy, for the mother and the fetus. The midwife has a vital role to play in educating parents about good family nutrition.
- There is a correlation between poor nutritional status and physiopathological conditions in pregnancy. Nutrition can be used as a therapeutic tool to correct or treat some of these conditions.
- Midwives require a comprehensive understanding of what constitutes a balanced diet to advise women in their care accordingly.

## REFERENCES


Bailey LB, Berry RJ: Folic acid supplementation and the occurrence of congenital heart defects, orofacial clefts, multiple births, and miscarriage, *American Journal of Clinical Nutrition* 81(5):1213S–1217S, 2005.

Bodnar LM, Tang G, Ness RB, et al: Periconceptional multivitamin use reduces the risk of preeclampsia, *American Journal of Epidemiology* 164(5):470–477, 2006.

Camadoo L, Tibbott R, Isaza F: Maternal vitamin D deficiency associated with neonatal hypocalcaemic convulsions, *Nutrition Journal* 6(9):23, 2007.

Carmichael SL, Yang W, Herring A, et al: Maternal food insecurity is associated with increased risk of certain birth defects, *Journal of Nutrition* 137(9):2087–2092, 2007.

Cetin I, Koletzko B: Long-chain omega-3 fatty acid supply in pregnancy and lactation, *Current Opinion in Clinical Nutrition and Metabolic Care* 11(3):297–302, 2008.

Chavarro JE, Rich-Edwards JW, Rosner BA, et al: Diet and lifestyle in the prevention of ovulatory disorder infertility, *Obstetrics and Gynecology* 110(5):1050–1058, 2007.

Chavarro JE, Rich-Edwards JW, Rosner BA, et al: Use of multivitamins, intake of B vitamins, and risk of ovulatory infertility, *Fertility and Sterility* 89(3):668–676, 2008.

Derbyshire E, Davies J, Costarelli V, et al: Diet, physical inactivity and the prevalence of constipation throughout and after pregnancy, *Maternal & Child Nutrition* 2(3):127–134, 2006.

Dixit A, Girling JC: Obesity and pregnancy, *Journal of Obstetrics and Gynaecology* 28(1):14–23, 2008.

Dror DK, Allen LH: Effect of vitamin B12 deficiency on neurodevelopment in infants: current knowledge and possible mechanisms, *Nutrition Reviews* 66(5):250–255, 2008.

Durand EF, Logan C, Carruth A: Association of maternal obesity and childhood obesity: implications for healthcare providers, *Journal of Community Health Nursing* 24(3):167–176, 2007.

Eskenazi B, Kidd SA, Marks AR, et al: Antioxidant intake is associated with semen quality in healthy men, *Human Reproduction* 20(4):1006–1012, 2005.

George L, Granath F, Johansson AL, et al: Risks of repeated miscarriage, *Paediatric and Perinatal Epidemiology* 20(2):119–126, 2006.

Heslehurst N, Lang R, Rankin J, et al: Obesity in pregnancy: a study of the impact of maternal obesity on NHS maternity services, *British Journal of Obstetrics and Gynaecology* 114(3):334–342, 2007.

Hyppönen E, Hartikainen AL, Sovio U, et al: Does vitamin D supplementation in infancy reduce the risk of pre-eclampsia? *European Journal of Clinical Nutrition* 61(9):1136–1139, 2007.

Innis SM, Friesen RW: Essential n-3 fatty acids in pregnant women and early visual acuity maturation in term infants, *American Journal of Clinical Nutrition*. 87(3):548–557, 2008.

Lewis G, editor: *Saving mothers' lives: reviewing maternal deaths to make motherhood safer – 2003–2005. The Seventh Report on Confidential Enquiries into Maternal Deaths in the United Kingdom*. London, 2007, CEMACH.

Mahomed K, Bhutta Z, Middleton P: Zinc supplementation for improving pregnancy and infant outcome, *Cochrane Database of Systematic Reviews (Online)* (2):CD000230, 2007.

Mannion CA, Gray-Donald K, Koski KG: Association of low intake of milk and vitamin D during pregnancy with decreased birth weight, *Canadian Medical Association Journal* 174(9):1273–1277, 2006.

National Institute for Health and Clinical Excellence (NICE): Quick reference guide: Maternal and child nutrition (website). www.nice.org.uk/nicemedia/pdf/PH011quickrefguide.pdf. 2008a. Accessed January 28, 2009.

National Institute for Health and Clinical Excellence (NICE): Clinical guideline 62: Antenatal care – Routine care for the healthy pregnant woman (website). www.nice.org.uk/nicemedia/pdf/CG062NICEguideline.pdf. 2008b. Accessed January 28, 2009.

Nilsen RM, Vollset SE, Rasmussen SA, et al: Folic acid and multivitamin supplement use and risk of placental abruption: a population-based registry study, *American Journal of Epidemiology* 167(7):867–874, 2008.

Ochoa-Brust GJ, Fernández AR, Villanueva-Ruiz GJ, et al: Daily intake of 100 mg ascorbic acid as urinary tract infection prophylactic agent during pregnancy, *Acta Obstetricia et Gynecologica Scandinavica* 86(7):783–787, 2007.

Plagemann A, Harder T, Dudenhausen JW: The diabetic pregnancy, macrosomia, and perinatal nutritional programming, *Nestle Nutrition Workshop Pediatric Program* 61:91 102, 2008.

Ray JG, Wyatt PR, Thompson MD, et al: Vitamin B12 and the risk of neural tube defects in a folic-acid-fortified population, *Epidemiology* 18(3):362–366, 2007.

Ronnenberg AG, Venners SA, Xu X, et al: Preconception B vitamin and homocysteine status, conception, and early pregnancy loss, *American Journal of Epidemiology* 166(3):304–312, 2007.

Tamura T, Picciano MF: Folate and human reproduction, *American Journal of Clinical Nutrition* 83(5):993–1016, 2006.

Tieu J, Crowther CA, Middleton P: Dietary advice in pregnancy for preventing gestational diabetes mellitus, *Cochrane Database of Systematic Reviews (Online)* (2):CD006674, 2008.

Tiran D: *Nausea and vomiting in pregnancy: an integrated approach to care*, London, 2004, Elsevier.

Tiran D: Nutritional approaches to nausea and vomiting in pregnancy, *RCM Midwives' Journal* 9(9):350–352, 2006/

Uauy R, Kain J, Mericq V, et al: Nutrition, child growth, and chronic disease prevention, *Annals of Medicine* 40(1):11–12, 2008.

Vujkovic M, Ocke MC, van der Spek PJ, et al: Maternal western dietary patterns and the risk of developing a cleft lip with or without a cleft palate, *Obstetrics and Gynecology* 110(2 Pt 1):378–384, 2007.

West MC, Anderson L, McClure N, et al: Dietary oestrogens and male fertility potential, *Human Fertility (Cambridge, England)* 8(3):197–207, 2005.

Woods LL: Maternal nutrition and predisposition to later kidney disease, *Current Drug Targets* 8(8):906–913, 2007.

Chapter 18

# Complementary therapies in maternity care: responsibilities of midwives

*Denise Tiran*

## LEARNING OUTCOMES

By the end of this chapter, you will have an awareness of:

- the responsibilities of midwives when mothers wish to self-administer natural remedies
- the responsibilities of midwives when mothers enquire about consulting independent complementary therapists
- the responsibilities of midwives when caring for mothers who are accompanied in labour by an independent practitioner of complementary therapies, including doulas
- the responsibilities of midwives wishing to use complementary therapies in their own practice.

## INTRODUCTION

There is a huge public interest in complementary therapies (CTs) as an adjunct to conventional healthcare, perhaps due in part to the emphasis on the holistic approach to care in which psychosocial factors are seen to interact with the biological aspects – the body–mind–spirit approach. During pregnancy, women demand more choices and wish to remain in control of their bodies during a period when they can feel very vulnerable. Increasingly, mothers request information and advice on natural remedies since they are often unable to use prescribed drugs to deal with the discomforts of pregnancy, labour and the puerperium. Many women have already consulted independent complementary therapists before conception, either for themselves or for their families, and want to continue to do so once pregnant. Some mothers may wish to seek alternatives to conventional care for the various discomforts of pregnancy, or they may wish to be accompanied in labour by an independent therapist. Enabling women to use CTs empowers them in the childbearing process and provides them with additional resources, which are not only therapeutically effective but also often relaxing and calming. Increasingly, too, midwives wish to incorporate CTs into their own repertoire of tools for assisting mothers during pregnancy, labour and the puerperium.

However, it is essential not to view 'complementary therapies' simply as a single 'add-on' to maternity care, but to appreciate that there are *several hundred* different modalities, each with its own specialist knowledge and skills. There are about 20 therapies commonly in use in the UK today and expectant mothers frequently consult practitioners of massage, reflexology, aromatherapy, acupuncture, shiatsu and hypnosis, or self-administer natural remedies, including herbal, homeopathic and Bach flower remedies. Many midwives now train in specific therapies and are tasked with establishing a complementary therapy service, such as aromatherapy or reflexology, in their maternity unit, especially since the development of low-risk birthing units and efforts to normalize birth and reduce soaring caesarean section rates. There are several examples of maternity CTs services which have been set up by midwives (Burns et al 2000, Dhany 2008, Lythgoe & Metcalfe 2008, Tiran 2001). In Oxford, midwives were trained to use a limited number of essential aromatherapy oils for women in labour and offered the service to over 8000 women over a 9-year period (Burns et al 2000). It was found that mothers greatly enjoyed the aromatherapy for relaxation, pain relief and to facilitate progress, and that maternal satisfaction in their overall labour care was greatly enhanced. It was also shown that essential oils decreased the need for conventional pharmacological analgesics and oxytocics, without compromising safety, as there was less than a 1% incidence of side-effects, all minor, and none affecting fetal wellbeing. Furthermore, an unexpected finding was that midwifery recruitment and retention was improved, as midwives actively chose to work in a unit in which they were encouraged to return to the nurturing of being 'with woman'.

The subject area of complementary therapies in maternity care is a speciality in its own right and is far too complex to cover in a single chapter, especially since many therapies are discrete academic and clinical disciplines, many of which have been covered in depth elsewhere. This chapter therefore explores some of the issues pertinent to the use of CTs in midwifery practice, provides a glossary of terms for the most commonly used therapies, and directs the reader to further sources of information.

## THE NMC POSITION

Midwives are permitted to advise on or to administer CTs and natural remedies if they are adequately and appropriately trained to do so and can justify their actions. The 2008 code specifically identifies that '*the use of complementary and alternative therapies must be safe and in the best interests of those in your care*' (NMC 2008:7). Enthusiasm for integrating CTs into midwifery practice must be balanced by comprehensive contemporary knowledge and understanding, '*based on best available research evidence or best practice*', so that efficacy can be measured and safety can be assured (NMC 2008:7), and any advice on, or suggestions for, healthcare products and services should be evidence-based. Additionally, registrants should work within the limits of their competence and maintain up-to-date practice through '*appropriate learning and practice activities*' (NMC 2008:7). These guidelines can be interpreted according to whether the midwife is caring for women who wish to administer their own natural remedies, women who wish to seek alternative practitioners outside the conventional maternity services, and who are accompanied in labour by a practitioner of CTs, or if the midwife wishes to incorporate CTs into her own practice.

**Reflective activity 18.1**

Brainstorm with a colleague to find out how many different complementary therapies you can name.

### The responsibilities of midwives when mothers wish to self-administer natural remedies

Midwives should recognize that women have the right to self-administer natural remedies. If the midwife is unfamiliar with the effects, indications, contraindications and side-effects, she should discuss this with the mother and, if necessary, consult an appropriately trained practitioner of the relevant therapy for advice, or '*make a referral to another practitioner when it is in the best interests*' of the mother or baby (NMC 2008:5). It would be wise to enquire, when taking the initial booking history, whether the mother uses any natural remedies, such as aromatherapy oils, herbal, homeopathic and Bach flower remedies, in the same way as enquiring about the use of over-the-counter and recreational drugs. Not only does this implicitly give the mother 'permission' to discuss complementary therapies, but it will also alert the midwife to any potential problems which may arise, for example, interactions with drugs or exacerbation of existing medical problems. It is, however, necessary for the midwife to have a basic appreciation of the different therapies in order to assist the mother, for example, understanding the difference between herbal and homeopathic medicines.

It is essential that midwives '*maintain clear and accurate records*' of (any) discussions which they have with the mother about CTs (NMC 2008:8), including recording any questions asked by the mother about CTs or natural remedies. A common subject for discussion is the use of *ginger* for 'morning sickness', with women almost universally (and many midwives) believing, incorrectly, that ginger biscuits offer a suitable remedy to resolve this symptom (personal communications with mothers and midwives). Ginger is not a universal remedy for nausea and vomiting, for whilst it may be effective for some women, it is not safe for those on anticoagulants and other similar medications or for those with blood clotting disorders (Marcus & Snodgrass 2005, Tiran & Budd 2005). In some women the use of ginger will exacerbate their symptoms and may trigger others, such as heartburn. Furthermore, ginger biscuits are not the means by which women should take ginger as there is insufficient real ginger in them to be effective in the long term. Women may obtain temporary relief, but this is mostly as a result of the sugar content of the biscuits increasing blood sugar levels.

Another common question is about the use of the popular herbal remedy *raspberry leaf tea* to tone the uterus in preparation for childbirth, typically asked by the mother as she is leaving the antenatal clinic. Unfortunately, the way in which midwives often tackle this question demonstrates an example of the 'Chinese whispers effect' which pervades midwifery practice, with many midwives having gleaned a little information overheard from colleagues. Some midwives inappropriately interpret this as sufficient 'learning' to permit them to provide women with advice on the subject, which is at best superficial, and sometimes incorrect, potentially even dangerous, particularly as herbal remedies act pharmacologically and can interfere with prescribed medication.

It is essential that midwives understand the contraindications and precautions to raspberry leaf prior to giving specific advice to women, and refer to an expert in the event that their knowledge is incomplete. Many midwives advise women to start taking raspberry leaf after 37 weeks' gestation, a laudable but incorrect precautionary measure to prevent preterm labour. However, if a mother wishes to take raspberry leaf, she should be advised to start taking it earlier, at about 32 weeks' gestation, to allow time for her body to become accustomed to the effects. She should increase the dose gradually from one cup of the tea or one tablet daily to a maximum of four, taking into account any adverse effects on the Braxton Hicks contractions and, if necessary, reducing the dose accordingly.

The use of raspberry leaf as a routine does pose an ethical question about whether or not it is absolutely essential, since any pharmacological agent taken inappropriately can complicate normal physiology, and it may be preferable to advise women with a history of normal eutocic labour to refrain from taking the remedy. Women with any uterine compromise should be advised *not* to take raspberry leaf. This includes those with a previous caesarean section scar, history of preterm or precipitate labour, multiple pregnancy, those due to have an elective caesarean, or mothers with major medical conditions for which they are receiving combined obstetrician/physician care (Parsons et al 1999, Simpson et al 2001).

Some mothers wish to self-administer natural remedies during labour, such as essential oils or homeopathic remedies. They have the right to do so and should be facilitated in this wish where possible, but the midwife should record in the mother's notes and on the partogram when she uses a remedy, even if the midwife is unaware of its action. If the midwife feels, at any time, that using the remedy may be detrimental to maternal or fetal health, the midwife must discuss the situation with the mother, and consult a relevant expert, if possible, to ascertain safety (NMC 2008).

Essential oils, used in aromatherapy, are extremely popular but should be used cautiously since they can affect everyone in the room. Midwives, other staff and the woman's partner and relatives may be adversely affected by inhaling the aromas of the oils, since their chemical constituents can cause drowsiness, nausea or headaches. If it is possible to smell the aromas, the chemicals from the oils are present in the air and will be inhaled. It is not acceptable to use vaporizers with a naked flame in an institutional setting, and if the mother brings an electrical vaporizer into the maternity unit, the wiring will need to be checked by the hospital electrician prior to use. Preplanning is necessary if the mother is to obtain the most effectiveness from the vaporizer, which should be left on for no more than 10–15 minutes at a time. Pregnant midwives should not be exposed to essential oils known to aid uterine contractions, particularly *clary sage* and *jasmine*, as well as large doses of *lavender*, and volatile essential oils should not be used within the anaesthetic room or operating theatre (Tiran 2005).

If the mother wishes to use herbal remedies, which act pharmacologically – and this includes essential oils – care needs to be taken regarding possible interactions with any other drugs the mother may require. For example, pethidine and *nutmeg essential oil* both have a narcotic effect (Grover et al 2002), which may exacerbate any hallucinatory effect and could compromise respiration, especially in the neonate. *Lavender* is known to reduce blood pressure (Hur et al 2007; Kiecolt-Glaser et al 2008), so it may be wise to refrain from using lavender oil once the mother has requested epidural analgesia. *Clary sage* has shown some promising effects on uterine action (Burns et al 2000, Lis-Balchin & Hart 1997), but, by inference, should not be used concomitantly with oxytocics.

Conversely, homeopathic remedies do not act pharmacologically so will not interact with prescribed medications, but need to be used correctly to avoid triggering new symptoms in response to the initial dose (Tiran 2008). Some mothers purchase special 'childbirth homeopathic kits' which include brief instructions on use, but midwives should remember that, as labour progresses, the mother may be less able to make an objective decision regarding the most appropriate remedy, for what is, after all, a very dynamic and rapidly changing clinical situation.

**Reflective activity 18.2**

Keep a record of how often you are asked for information about raspberry leaf tea, arnica for bruising, or the safety of aromatherapy oils in pregnancy and labour, and consider how you respond to these queries.

## The responsibilities of midwives when mothers enquire about consulting independent complementary therapists

Mothers sometimes ask the midwife about visiting an independent therapist, such as an osteopath for backache and sciatica in pregnancy, or a hypnotherapist to prepare for labour. The midwife should record any conversations regarding external therapists and the reasons the mother gives for consulting them.

Practitioners of some therapies can be guaranteed to have received adequate training to treat pregnant women safely. For example, osteopaths and chiropractors, whose professions are statutorily regulated in the same way as midwifery, will have completed a standard nationally regulated pre-registration training which includes reproductive health. However, most therapies are not nationally regulated nor are the training programmes necessarily of the most appropriate academic calibre to prepare practitioners to treat pregnant women at the point of qualification. It is of concern that some therapists presume to treat, even to specialize in treating, expectant mothers without any relevant post-qualifying education (personal communications with therapists). Therefore, midwives should be wary of recommending specific therapies or therapists unless they can vouch for their credentials. It is permissible for midwives to recommend named individuals if they have become acquainted with local reputable and suitably trained therapists, and this may be preferable to leaving a mother to select from advertisements in the local telephone directory. However, if the midwife is not familiar with local practitioners, she should advise the mother to ask about the therapist's training, experience of, and educational preparation for treating pregnant women and to ensure that the therapist is in possession of personal professional indemnity insurance cover. See also 'Additional resources' on website.

A contemporary trend of particular concern is that of mothers nearing term asking therapists to facilitate the onset of labour. This is often before the estimated delivery date and, most commonly, it appears to be reflexologists who are consulted (personal communications with mothers and therapists). Women should be advised that it would be inappropriate to attempt to expedite labour before term and that *any* intervention, even those which are 'natural', could complicate maternal physiology and trigger the cascade of intervention which can occur with a medicalized induction (Tiran 2010). On the other hand, if the mother progresses beyond her expected date and is being 'threatened' with prostin or syntocinon, this may be adequate justification for receiving CTs, such as shiatsu or acupuncture, to facilitate cervical ripening and may make the difference between spontaneous or induced onset of labour (Ingram et al 2005, Lee et al 2004). It is, however, important that midwives and therapists liaise to ensure safe care for the mother.

## The responsibilities of midwives when caring for mothers who are accompanied in labour by an independent practitioner of complementary therapies, including doulas

Some women choose to be accompanied in labour by a lay person who is able to provide complementary therapies. This may be a qualified therapist, or a doula (birth companion) who has acquired some skills in CTs, but who may not always be adequately trained or insured to use them. The midwife remains accountable for the mother's care and has a duty to ensure that intrapartum care is safe and in keeping with normal midwifery care. It is, of course, preferable to encourage the mother to inform her midwife during pregnancy if she thinks she may have a therapist or doula with her during labour. However, occasionally a mother may present in the delivery suite with her supporter, without prior warning.

The midwife should record in the notes and on the partogram when natural remedies or complementary therapies are being used. Some trusts require independent therapists to sign a disclaimer form stating that the therapist acknowledges that the midwife remains responsible for the mother's care, that they have independent insurance cover and that, in the event of an emergency, they agree to discontinue CTs and facilitate the midwife to manage the situation. As with other occasions, if the midwife believes that CTs are inappropriate, she should discuss this with the mother and her lay carer and record the outcome of any discussion.

## Responsibilities of midwives wishing to use complementary therapies in their own practice

If a midwife wishes to use complementary therapies in her own practice, it is not necessary to be a fully qualified practitioner but it is essential to be able to apply principles of the therapy to reproductive physiopathology and to the use of that therapy within an institutional setting. For example, midwives could learn the chemistry, indications, contraindications and precautions, methods of administration and possible side-effects of a selected number of essential oils for use in labour without needing to be fully qualified aromatherapists, but must also relate their use to health and safety issues within the delivery suite, such as not using a vaporizer with a naked flame to dispense aromas into the air because of the fire risks. It would also be acceptable to learn the skill of moxibustion to turn a breech-presenting fetus to cephalic, without becoming a fully qualified practitioner of traditional Chinese medicine (TCM), but midwives would need to fully understand the mechanism of action, indications and contraindications of the technique and have a working knowledge of conventional management of breech presentation.

It is certainly not acceptable for midwives to 'dabble' in complementary therapies, for not only are they jeopardizing the health of women and babies but also they are risking their own professional careers. A genuine desire to act as the mother's advocate by facilitating her use of complementary therapies has, unfortunately, led to numerous examples of midwives who overhear appropriately trained colleagues giving advice on natural remedies but who then take the information they have heard as accurate and proceed to offer this to other women in their care, without adequate training. Common examples are advice about herbal medicines, such as *raspberry leaf* to aid labour or *cabbage leaves* to ease breast engorgement, aromatherapy, including *lavender* and *clary sage* for labour, or

**Box 18.1 Summary of issues for midwives incorporating complementary therapies into their practice**

- Adequate and appropriate education and training in the therapy
- Recognition of professional accountability and service obligations
- Advocacy for and understanding of the rights of the mother
- Communication and collaboration with all colleagues
- Maternal consent; comprehensive and contemporaneous record-keeping
- Policies and protocols
- Evaluation and audit of complementary therapy services and treatments
- Research-based practice where possible

homeopathy, such as *arnica* for post-episiotomy pain. Sadly, in this day of frequent litigation, it is essential for midwives to acknowledge the risks of *any* clinical intervention and be able to justify their actions if they are required to do so in a court of law. It is also vital to recognize that, just because complementary therapies are 'natural', this does not mean that they are always automatically safe.

The issues for midwives incorporating complementary therapies into their practice are summarized in Box 18.1.

Obtaining informed consent and maintaining contemporaneous records is vital, as in all other aspects of care, and midwives must appreciate the limitations of their own professional practice. The NMC regulates the practice of nurses, midwives and health visitors, in order to protect the public, but can only regulate midwives' use of complementary therapies when it relates to their *midwifery* practice. It is not possible for qualifications in different therapies to be added to an individual's entry on the NMC register. It is also important for the midwife to undertake continuing professional development, both of her midwifery practice and the relevant complementary therapy.

When working in an employment situation, rather than as an independent practitioner, midwives wishing to implement CTs within the unit will also need to develop and gain approval for the relevant guidelines and protocols. These should state clearly the rationale for incorporating the specific elements of CTs into midwifery practice, supported by contemporary research or authoritative references. The guidelines should state which midwives are eligible to use the therapy, based on having acquired the relevant initial knowledge and skills and maintaining these via continuing professional development. They may also state which midwives should not use the therapy; for example, it may be advisable to exclude pregnant midwives from using uterotonic essential oils in the labour ward. The guidelines should also identify which mothers may receive the therapy and those for whom it is inappropriate. An example might be the establishment of a reflexology service within the delivery suite, from which mothers with medical or obstetric problems may need to be excluded. Other specific information regarding the use of a particular therapy may be included in a precise protocol, for example moxibustion for breech presentation.

If a midwife is appropriately trained in aspects of complementary therapy and has the permission of her employing authority to incorporate this into her practice, the Royal College of Midwives' and the Royal College of Nursing's personal professional indemnity insurance schemes provide suitable cover. However, the vicarious liability cover of the employing authority will be invalidated unless the midwife has gained permission of the relevant authorities to use complementary therapies in her work. If the midwife also chooses to practise independently as a therapist, she should at present arrange additional insurance cover through one of the complementary therapy organizations; the Royal College of Nursing indemnity insurance covers midwives wishing to use complementary therapies in private practice, but the Royal College of Midwives does not (2010).

**Reflective activity 18.3**

Ask 10 women in your care what they understand by the term 'complementary therapies' and find out whether or not they have used any therapies or natural remedies, either before or during pregnancy, or in a previous labour.

## COMMONLY USED COMPLEMENTARY THERAPIES

**Acupuncture** is based on the principle that the body has energy lines, called meridians, running through it, which link one part of the body to another. There are 365 meridians with over 2000 focus points where energy is concentrated – acupuncture points. When the body, mind and spirit are in optimum health, energy flows along the meridians unimpeded, but disorder or disease causes blockages (stagnation) or over-stimulation (excess) of energy at specific points. Acupuncture needles may be inserted to rebalance the body's internal energy and facilitate a return to homeostasis. *Acupressure* involves the use of thumb pressure to stimulate or sedate the acupuncture points. Acupuncture and acupressure have been effectively used for 'morning sickness' and induction of labour (Can Gürkan & Arslan 2008, Gaudernack et al 2006, Helmreich et al 2006, Selmer-Olsen et al 2007, Shin et al 2007).

**Aromatherapy**, an aspect of *herbal medicine*, involves the use of highly concentrated *essential oils* extracted from plants, the chemical constituents of which have various therapeutic purposes. The therapeutic benefits – or possible risks – of aromatherapy are due to a combination of the chemistry, the effects of the aromas on the limbic system in the brain and the method of administration, most commonly massage, but also added to water, for example in the bath, or used in compresses, suppositories, pessaries, creams, lotions or inhalations. Oral use is not encouraged and, with very few exceptions, oils should not be applied to the skin neat because the chemical constituents may cause skin reactions. Many essential oils are contraindicated during pregnancy, labour and breastfeeding and are contraindicated completely in neonates. Some essential oils are known to raise the blood pressure, others lower it; some potentiate the action of certain drugs or alcohol; all have a range of anti-infective properties. Many oils are relaxing and some contain chemicals that are analgesic. (See Tiran 2000, 2005.)

**Bach flower remedies** (BFRs) are liquid preparations prepared from 38 flowers using minute doses similar to *homeopathy*, but prepared differently. This form of vibrational medicine aims to treat the emotional symptoms associated with disease and disorder. *Rescue Remedy*, the best known, is a combination of five of the 38 remedies and is used for stress, panic and nervous tension, which could be useful for women in the transition stage of labour. There is limited research into BFRs but there is some suggestion that they may have a part to play in relieving pain through psychophysiological effects (Howard 2007), whereas any impact on stress, anxiety and panic is attributed to the placebo effect (Walach 2001).

**Chiropractic** is statutorily regulated by the General Chiropractic Council and is concerned with the relationship of the nervous system to the mechanical structure of the body and places emphasis on spinal joints as well as related muscles and ligaments. It is particularly appropriate for musculoskeletal conditions of pregnancy, especially symphysis pubis diastasis and sacroiliac joint pain (Leboeuf-Yde et al 2002, Lisi 2006).

**Herbal medicine** involves the medicinal use of plants and works pharmacologically in exactly the same way as drugs, which poses the potential problem of interactions with other medication; there is an immense body of research evidence to demonstrate this. Many herbal preparations are contraindicated during pregnancy as they may affect embryonic development, cause miscarriage, or affect the mother's systemic wellbeing, for example raising the blood pressure or interfering with clotting mechanisms (Dugoua et al 2006a, 2006b, 2008).

**Homeopathy** involves the use of minute doses of substances which, if given in their full dose, would actually cause the problems they are attempting to treat. It does *not* work pharmacologically but is a powerful form of energy medicine, and should not be considered harmless. Remedies must be individually prescribed according to the *precise* symptom picture, but also take into account the individual's personality and factors that exacerbate or inhibit symptoms. The popular remedy arnica is used to combat bruising, trauma and shock (Oberbaum et al 2005, Seeley et al 2006).

**Hypnotherapy** is the clinical use of deep relaxation to access the subconscious mind, often likened to daydreaming, and can be used to change behaviour, such as habitual and addictive behaviours. It has been used to good effect to alter women's perceptions of labour pain (Cyna et al 2006, VandeVusse et al 2007).

**Massage** is the applied use of touch and is effective for relieving stress, aiding relaxation, reducing blood pressure and inducing sleep. Touch impulses reach the brain more quickly than pain impulses; therefore massage is effective in easing discomfort in labour (Chang et al 2006, Kimber et al 2008, McNabb et al 2006). Massage can also work to stimulate areas of the body, including excretory processes and the circulation. Baby massage has become increasingly popular and has been found to be of particular benefit for preterm babies (Lahat et al 2007; Mendes & Procianoy 2008).

**Moxibustion** is an element of *TCM* in which sticks of dried compressed mugwort, a herb, are used as a heat source to stimulate acupuncture points where energy is deficient. It is best known in maternity care for effectively turning breech presentations to cephalic (Cardini et al 2005, Neri et al 2007, Tiran 2004, Vas et al 2008).

**Osteopathy** is statutorily regulated by the General Osteopathic Council and aims to restore and maintain balance within the body, particularly in the relationships between the neural, muscular and skeletal systems and by examining and maintaining the biomechanical functioning of the body. It is particularly effective for the treatment of back pain in pregnancy but can be useful for other problems, for example heartburn or carpal tunnel syndrome (Krueger 2006; Tettambel 2007).

**Reflexology** is based on the principle that the feet (and hands) represent a map of the rest of the body, so that by working on specific areas of the feet, other distal parts of the body can be treated, and is thought to be related to acupuncture meridians. Reflexology is *not* simply foot massage, but a very powerful therapy which should be used with caution in pregnancy unless the practitioner has a thorough working knowledge of physiopathology (see Tiran 2002).

**Shiatsu** is a contemporary Japanese form of *acupressure* incorporating the use of simple pressure and holding techniques combined with gentle stretching. Touch is used as a means of adjusting the internal energies of the body, in both treating and preventing energy imbalances (see references for acupressure).

**Traditional Chinese medicine (TCM)** is a complete system of traditional medicine involving *acupuncture*, including cupping (placing special cups over acupuncture points to draw out heat), *moxibustion*, special massage (*tuina*) and Chinese herbs (Dengfeng et al 2007, Li 2007; see also references for acupuncture and moxibustion).

**Yoga** involves learning a series of postures and positions, often in conjunction with meditation and breathing techniques, for relaxation and relief of symptoms. It encourages flexibility, suppleness and strength and is valuable for preparing for labour (Chuntharapat et al 2008, Narendran et al 2005).

## CONCLUSION

Mothers increasingly turn to complementary therapies to expand their options during pregnancy, labour and the puerperium, for relaxation and for specific physiological discomforts. As the general public's use of CTs has risen, so too has the possibility that pregnant women will ask their midwives about the use of CTs. Midwives are in an invaluable position to facilitate women's desires but must balance their enthusiasm for the benefits of CTs with an appreciation of the potential safety issues, and recognize their own professional boundaries when advising mothers. Whilst all midwives should have a basic understanding of the principles, the use of complementary therapies within midwifery is a specialist area of practice. In the same way as some midwives specialize in obstetric ultrasound scanning, parent education, or caring for women with high-risk pregnancies, so too should CTs be seen as a broad subject area which requires in-depth knowledge and skills.

### KEY POINTS

- Midwives have a responsibility to facilitate mothers who wish to self-administer natural remedies or who choose to consult independent therapists during pregnancy and labour, but should work always in the best interests of the mother and baby.
- Midwives wishing to use complementary therapies in their own practice must be adequately and appropriately trained to use them safely and effectively, and able to apply the principles of their chosen therapy to the physiopathology of pregnancy and childbirth.
- Midwives must be able to justify their actions in accordance with NMC regulations and, where possible, use contemporary evidence or best practice to support their use of complementary therapies.

## REFERENCES


Burns E, Blamey C, Errser SJ, et al. The use of aromatherapy in intrapartum midwifery practice: an observational study, *Complementary Therapies in Nursing & Midwifery* 6(1):33–44, 2000.

Can Gürkan O, Arslan H: Effect of acupressure on nausea and vomiting during pregnancy, *Complementary Therapies in Clinical Practice* 14(1):46–52, 2008.

Cardini F, Lombardo P, Regalia AL, et al: A randomised controlled trial of moxibustion for breech presentation, *British Journal of Obstetrics and Gynaecology* 112(6):743–747, 2005.

Chang MY, Chen CH, Huang KF: A comparison of massage effects on labor pain using the McGill Pain Questionnaire, *Journal of Nursing Research* 14(3):190–197, 2006.

Chuntharapat S, Petpichetchian W, Hatthakit U: Yoga during pregnancy: effects on maternal comfort, labor pain and birth outcomes, *Complementary Therapies in Clinical Practice* 14(2):105–115, 2008.

Cyna AM, Andrew MI, McAuliffe GL: Antenatal self-hypnosis for labour and childbirth: a pilot study, *Anaesthesia and Intensive Care* 34(4):464–469, 2006.

Dengfeng W, Taixiang W, Lina H, et al: Chinese herbal medicines in the treatment of ectopic pregnancy, *Cochrane Database of Systematic Reviews (Online)* 17(4):CD006224, 2007.

Dhany A: Essential oils and massage in intrapartum care, *The Practising Midwife* 11(5):34–39, 2008.

Dugoua JJ, Mills E, Perri D, et al: Safety and efficacy of St. John's wort (hypericum) during pregnancy and lactation, *Canadian Journal of Clinical Pharmacology* 13(3):e268–e276, 2006a.

Dugoua JJ, Mills E, Perri D, et al: Safety and efficacy of ginkgo (Ginkgo biloba) during pregnancy and lactation, *Canadian Journal of Clinical Pharmacology* 13(3):e277–e284, 2006b.

Dugoua JJ, Perri D, Seely D, et al: Safety and efficacy of blue cohosh (Caulophyllum thalictroides) during pregnancy and lactation, *Canadian Journal of Clinical Pharmacology* 15(1):e66–e73, 2008.

Gaudernack LC, Forbord S, Hole E: Acupuncture administered after spontaneous rupture of membranes at term significantly reduces the length of birth and use of oxytocin. A randomized controlled trial, *Acta Obstetricia et Gynecologica Scandinavica* 85(11):1348–1353, 2006.

Grover JK, Khandkar S, Vats V, et al: Pharmacological studies on Myristica fragrans – antidiarrheal, hypnotic, analgesic and hemodynamic (blood pressure) parameters, *Methods and Findings in Experimental and Clinical Pharmacology* 24(10):675–680, 2002.

Helmreich RJ, Shiao SY, Dune LS: Meta-analysis of acustimulation effects on nausea and vomiting in pregnant women, *Explore (New York, N.Y.)* 2(5):412–421, 2006.

Howard J: Do Bach flower remedies have a role to play in pain control? A critical analysis investigating therapeutic value beyond the placebo effect, and the potential of Bach flower remedies as a psychological method of pain relief, *Complementary Therapies in Clinical Practice* 13(3):174–183, 2007.

Hur MH, Oh H, Lee MS, et al: Effects of aromatherapy massage on blood pressure and lipid profile in Korean climacteric women, *International Journal of Neuroscience* 117(9):1281–1287, 2007.

Ingram J, Domagala C, Yates S: The effects of shiatsu on post-term pregnancy, *Complementary Therapies in Medicine* 13(1):11–15, 2005.

Kiecolt-Glaser JK, Graham JE, Malarkey WB, et al: Olfactory influences on mood and autonomic, endocrine, and immune function, *Psychoneuroendocrinology* 33(3):328–339, 2008.

Kimber L, McNabb M, McCourt C, et al: Massage or music for pain relief in labour: a pilot randomised placebo controlled trial, *European Journal of Pain (London, England)* 12(8):961–969, 2008.

Krueger PM: Women's reproductive health and neonatal care, *Journal of the American Osteopathic Association* 106(4):181–182, 2006.

Lahat S, Mimouni FB, Ashbel G, et al: Energy expenditure in growing preterm infants receiving massage therapy, *Journal of the American College of Nutrition* 26(4):356–359, 2007.

Leboeuf-Yde C, van Dijk J, Franz C, et al: Motion palpation findings and self-reported low back pain in a population-based study sample, *Journal of Manipulative and Physiological Therapeutics* 25(2):80–87, 2002.

Lee MK, Chang SB, Kang DH: Effects of SP6 acupressure on labor pain and length of delivery time in women during labor, *Journal of Alternative and Complementary Medicine (New York, N.Y.)* 10(6):959–965, 2004.

Li DZ: Use of traditional Chinese herbal medicines during early pregnancy in mainland China, *Pharmacoepidemiology and Drug Safety* 16(8):942–943, 2007.

Lis-Balchin M, Hart S: A preliminary study of the effect of essential oils on skeletal and smooth muscle in vitro, *Journal of Ethnopharmacology* 58(3):183–187, 1997.

Lisi AJ: Chiropractic spinal manipulation for low back pain of pregnancy: a retrospective case series, *Journal of Midwifery and Women's Health* 51(1):e7–e10, 2006.

Lythgoe J, Metcalfe A: Birth of a midwifery acupuncture service, *The Practising Midwife* 11(5):25–29, 2008.

Marcus DM, Snodgrass WR: Do no harm: avoidance of herbal medicines during pregnancy, *Obstetrics and Gynecology* 105(5 Pt 1):1119–1122, 2005.

McNabb MT, Kimber L, Haines A: Does regular massage from late pregnancy to birth decrease maternal pain perception during labour and birth? A feasibility study to investigate a programme of massage, controlled breathing and visualization, from 36 weeks of pregnancy until birth, *Complementary Therapies in Clinical Practice* 12(3):222–231, 2006.

Mendes EW, Procianoy RS: Massage therapy reduces hospital stay and occurrence of late-onset sepsis in very preterm neonates, *Journal of Perinatology* 28(12):815–820, 2008.

Narendran S, Nagarathna R, Gunasheela S, et al: Efficacy of yoga in pregnant women with abnormal Doppler study of umbilical and uterine arteries, *Journal of the Indian Medical Association* 103(1):12–14, 16–17, 2005.

Neri I, De Pace V, Venturini P, et al: Effects of three different stimulations (acupuncture, moxibustion, acupuncture plus moxibustion) of BL.67 acupoint at small toe on fetal behavior of breech presentation, *American Journal of Chinese Medicine* 35(1):27–33, 2007.

Nursing and Midwifery Council (NMC): The code: standards of conduct, performance and ethics for nurses and midwives, London, 2008, NMC.

Oberbaum M, Galoyan N, Lerner-Geva L, et al: The effect of the homeopathic remedies Arnica montana and Bellis perennis on mild postpartum bleeding – a randomized, double-blind, placebo-controlled study–preliminary results, *Complementary Therapies in Medicine* 13(2):87–90, 2005.

Parsons M, Simpson M, Ponton T: Raspberry leaf and its effect on labour: safety and efficacy, *Journal of the Australian College of Midwives* 12(3):20–25, 1999.

Seeley BM, Denton AB, Ahn MS, et al: Effect of homeopathic Arnica montana on bruising in face-lifts: results of a randomized, double-blind, placebo-controlled clinical trial, *Archives of Facial Plastic Surgery* 8(1):54–59, 2006.

Selmer-Olsen T, Lydersen S, Mørkved S: Does acupuncture used in nulliparous women reduce time from prelabour rupture of membranes at term to active phase of labour? A randomised controlled trial, *Acta Obstetricia et Gynecologica Scandinavica* 86(12):1447–1452, 2007.

Shin HS, Song YA, Seo S: Effect of Nei-Guan point (P6) acupressure on ketonuria levels, nausea and vomiting in women with hyperemesis gravidarum, *Journal of Advanced Nursing* 59(5):510–519, 2007.

Simpson M, Parsons M, Greenwood J, et al: Raspberry leaf in pregnancy: its safety and efficacy in labour, *Journal of Midwifery and Women's Health* 46(2):51–59, 2001.

Tettambel MA: Using integrative therapies to treat women with chronic pelvic pain, *Journal of the American Osteopathic Association* 107(10 Suppl 6):ES17–ES20, 2007.

Tiran D: Clinical aromatherapy for pregnancy and childbirth, ed 2, London, 2000, Elsevier.

Tiran D: Complementary strategies in antenatal care, *Complementary Therapies in Nursing and Midwifery* 7(1):19–24, 2001.

Tiran D: Supporting women during pregnancy and childbirth. In Mackereth P, Tiran D, editors: Clinical reflexology: a guide for health professionals, London, 2002, Elsevier.

Tiran D: Breech presentation: increasing maternal choice, *Complementary Therapies in Nursing & Midwifery* 10(4):233–238, 2004.

Tiran D: Implementing aromatherapy in maternity care: a manual for midwives and managers, London, 2005, Expectancy.

Tiran D: Homeopathy in pregnancy: issues for midwives, *The Practising Midwife* 11(5):14–21, 2008.

Tiran D: Complementary therapies in labour and delivery. In Walsh D, Downe S, editors: Essential midwifery practice: intrapartum care, London, 2010, Wiley-Blackwell.

Tiran D, Budd S: Ginger is *not* a universal remedy for nausea and vomiting in pregnancy, *MIDIRS Midwifery Digest* 15(3):335–339, 2005.

VandeVusse L, Irland J, Healthcare WF, et al: Hypnosis for childbirth: a retrospective comparative analysis of outcomes in one obstetrician's practice, *American Journal of Clinical Hypnosis* 50(2):109–119, 2007.

Vas J, Aranda JM, Barón M, et al: Correcting non cephalic presentation with moxibustion: study protocol for a multi-centre randomised controlled trial in general practice, *BMC Complementary and Alternative Medicine* 21(8):22, 2008.

Walach H, Rilling C, Engelke U: Efficacy of Bach-flower remedies in test anxiety: a double-blind, placebo-controlled, randomized trial with partial crossover, *Journal of Anxiety Disorders* 15(4):359–366, 2001.

Chapter |19|

# Health promotion and education

*Jacqueline Dunkley-Bent*

## LEARNING OUTCOMES

After reading this chapter, you will be able to:

- appreciate the scope of health promotion in midwifery practice
- discuss the provision of health promotion within the context of inequalities in health and healthcare provision
- identify the emerging public health role of the midwife in the primary care setting
- apply the principles of health promotion to enhance the health of the woman and her family.

## INTRODUCTION

The importance of the health promotion role of the midwife within the context of health and healthcare provision in the 21st century is crucial in enhancing the health and wellbeing of women and their families. There is potential for developing health gain through utilizing midwifery skills in practice. The notion of health promotion is explored, enabling readers to develop firm foundations for effectively progressing their work in midwifery and their wider public health role.

## THE MEANING OF HEALTH

Health is a state of being to which most people aspire, yet a concept difficult to define, as personal meanings are enshrined in social structure, culture and belief systems. In 1946, the World Health Organization (WHO) described health as a state of complete physical, mental and social wellbeing, not merely the absence of disease or infirmity (WHO 1946). Health is thus seen as an ideal state of being which may be impossible to achieve. In an attempt to clarify the meaning of health, Seedhouse (1997) suggests that health is determined by the individual's socioeconomic and cultural position, the context of which is determined by biological or chosen health potentials that provide an opportunity for the individual to aspire to achieve good health within the context of that health potential.

**Reflective activity 19.1**

What does being healthy mean to you? Jot down your personal definition of 'being healthy'.

Lifestyle behaviours, personal habits and personal constructs of the health of individuals are major contributors to health and illness. These may be affected by the individual's attitudes and beliefs, culture, ethnicity, social class, religion, gender and economic status. It is crucial, therefore, that health professionals are aware of their own attitudes, beliefs and personal constructs of health prior to promoting the health of others.

Health is to be viewed holistically, involving dimensions of health that are inextricably linked and include physical, mental, emotional, societal, sexual and spiritual health. If one dimension is negatively affected, this will have an impact on other dimensions (Ewles & Simnett 2003).

## MODELS OF HEALTH

Health models have been developed to try to explain why some individuals indulge in healthy behaviours and others do not. Well-known models include the *Health Belief Model*, formulated by Rosenstock in the 1960s and developed by Becker in the 1970s (Becker et al 1977), which was specifically designed to explain and predict preventive health behaviours. The *Health Locus of Control*, proposed by Rotter (1966), refers to the personal control over events that people believe they possess and is commonly used to explore how people's beliefs about health and illness affect their behaviour. More information is available in the references and the website.

## REDUCING INEQUALITIES IN HEALTH

Understanding the social, cultural and economic context of health and illness increases the opportunity for health promotion to be meaningful and effective. Poverty and deprivation are linked to poor health outcomes (Lewis 2007). In the UK, the National Health Service (NHS) was set up in 1948 to provide free medical care to the whole population and thereby achieve equality of access to health services for those in need. The hope was this would eliminate or greatly reduce inequalities in health. Perhaps unsurprisingly, this single approach to improving the health of those worst off in society did not succeed. The provision of health services cannot singularly solve inequality in health without addressing factors that influence ill health. Even when health improvements are made for all, inequalities continue to persist. Health inequalities are linked to wider determinants including income, housing, education and other opportunities which must be tackled so that health interventions can be effective (Office for National Statistics 2007).

### A commitment to improve healthcare for all

Over the last three decades, a plethora of policy documents and guidance regarding health inequalities with ways of reducing these in tandem with healthcare provision have been published. The following documents present a useful insight into policy and guidance:

- *The Black Report* (Black et al 1982)
- *Independent inquiry into inequalities in health* (Acheson 1998)
- *Saving lives: our healthier nation* (DH 1999)
- *The NHS plan* (Secretary of State for Health 2000)
- *National Service Framework for Children, Young People and Maternity Services: Core Standards* (DH 2004)
- *Maternity matters: choice, access and continuity of care in a safe service* (DH 2007)
- *Health inequalities: progress and next steps* (DH 2008a).

Some, such as the Black Report, demonstrate substantial differences in mortality and morbidity rates between social class groups and made recommendations to address this (Black et al 1982) though these were not endorsed.

## WHAT IS HEALTH PROMOTION?

WHO defines health promotion as the process of enabling people to increase control over their health, and improve it. Integral to this definition is the notion of empowerment (WHO 1984). An example of empowerment in midwifery practice is the process by which the health professional uses strategies to enable the woman and her partner to lead and take control over their childbirth experience, resulting in development of personal empowerment, skills and control in everyday life.

The midwife's role encompasses a wide range of health promotion initiatives that may not influence immediate behaviour change, including advice and guidance about baby care and parenting. Decision-making, empowerment, debriefing and health education are important for health promotion in midwifery and should be provided throughout the antenatal, labour and postnatal period, as a coherent whole, rather than an activity placed within an antenatal education class.

Health develops by an ongoing relationship between the individual and their environment (Bauer et al 2006). The ultimate aim of health promotion is to provide opportunities for people to move within the context of their biological, intellectual and/or emotional potential (Seedhouse 1997). The momentum of movement, or indeed its maintenance, is likely to be successful only if the most appropriate avenue has been chosen to promote health, that is particular to or within the context of an individual's life. A realistic approach to health promotion would include assessing the context of the woman's living experience and identifying with the woman obstacles that inhibit the fulfilment of health potentials (see website for Case scenario 19.1).

### Mental health promotion

Impaired mental health has a negative impact on emotional and physical health and reduces the individual's capacity to cope with everyday life activities. The process and impact of postnatal depression is one example of how physical, spiritual, emotional and mental health are affected (see Chapter 69).

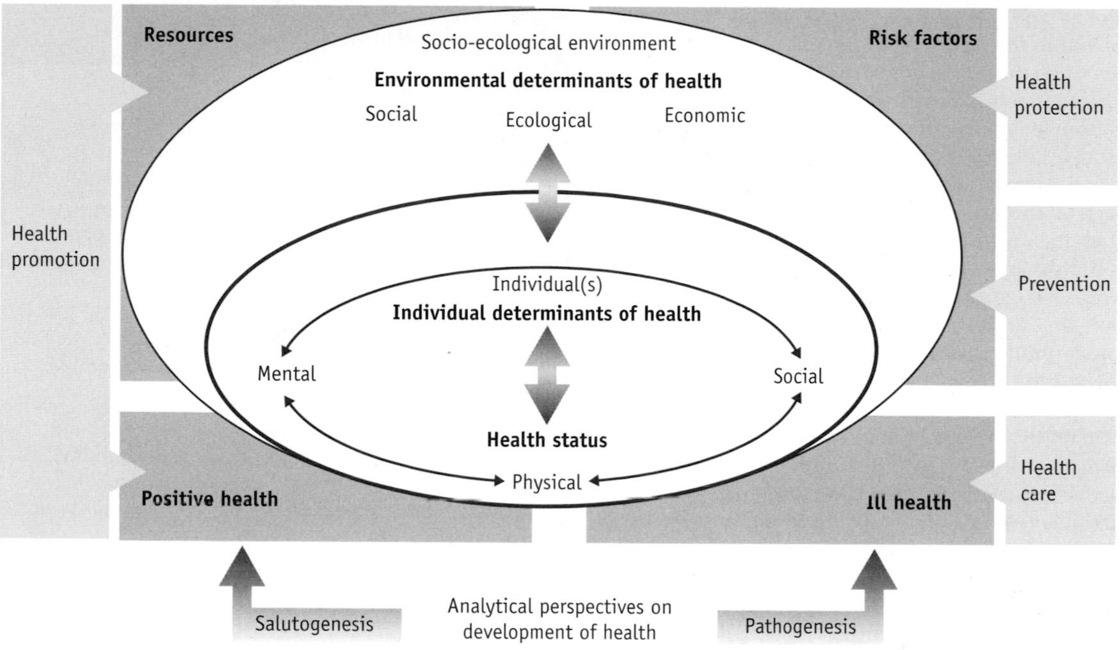


**Figure 19.1** Health Development Model (Bauer et al 2006).

## Sexual health promotion

Addressing sexual health issues may contribute to the overall wellbeing of the woman and family, therefore the midwife has an important role to play in this area of public health (see Chapter 57).

### Sexuality and pregnancy

Sexuality is influenced by health, personal circumstances, self-image and self-esteem. Physical, mental and emotional health influence how individuals view their own sexuality. Pregnancy, childbirth and motherhood challenge personal concepts of sexuality and sexual expression, though the impact of physiological and psychological changes that occur during pregnancy is generally beyond personal control. For example, physiological effects of pregnancy, including pelvic vasocongestion resulting from increasing levels of the hormones oestrogen and progesterone; changes in body image; or 'minor disorders', such as vulval varicosities and haemorrhoids, may change a woman's sexual experiences.

Sexuality in pregnancy is an important aspect of health that is not always addressed appropriately. Some women may feel embarrassed broaching this topic and some midwives, fearing intrusion of privacy, may also be reticent about discussing the issue. There may be religious, cultural and social taboos about having sexual intercourse during pregnancy, but some couples may have anxieties that could be relieved through frank discussion (see Chapter 13).

## A health promotion model

A model may be described as a conceptual framework for organizing and integrating information offering causal links among a set of concepts believed to be related to a particular problem (Seedhouse 1997). There are several health promotion models that assist the practitioner in undertaking health promotion work. Here, only one model will be presented and explored in detail.

The *health development model* (Bauer et al 2006) in Figure 19.1 shows that health development is an ongoing process and health promotion intentional and planned. The model identifies three dimensions of health: physical, mental and social, and shows the interrelationship between health promotion and public health. The arrows pointing between these dimensions show that they are interdependent and interrelated. For example, exercising during pregnancy positively influences mental health and enables interaction and communication with others, thereby supporting social health.

This model shows the central role of *salutogenesis* and *pathogenesis,* which is integral within health and the health promotion process, illustrating that health development is an ongoing process, and health promotion is an intentional and planned approach aiming to sustain change within the health development process.

When using the model it is useful to note that the health of an individual is not created and lived in isolation but results from a dynamic ongoing relationship with the relevant socio-ecological environment, including the cultural dimension (Bauer et al 2006). The health promotion approach taken must therefore reflect this. The model also identifies that an individual's health status determines future health, and can be used as a predictor of health; however, a targeted health promotion approach can improve the health potential of that individual. For example, a mother who smokes may be helped to stop smoking during pregnancy and therefore enhance her life potential and that of her baby.

The majority of studies that set out to establish the determinants of health and ill health are set within the pathogenic paradigm (Tones & Green 2004). Pathogenesis analyses how risk factors of individuals and their environment lead to ill health. Antonovsky (1996) proposed that an additional perspective should be adopted by health promotion practitioners, that of *salutogenesis*, which examines how resources in human life support development towards positive health. Bauer et al (2006) suggest that in real life, *salutogenesis* and *pathogenesis* are simultaneous, complementary and interacting real-life processes.

## Health promotion approaches

A health promotion approach can be described as the vehicle used to achieve the desired aim. An example would be the aim of raising awareness about the efficacy of vitamin K. The ultimate objective may be to enable the woman and her partner to make an informed choice about its use, but the health promotion approach may vary according to the woman, practitioner and context.

Ewles & Simnett (2003) identify five health promotion approaches:

- the medical or preventive
- behavioural change
- educational
- client-centred
- societal change

(see Box 19.1 for practice application).

**Reflective activity 19.2**

Think about your midwifery practice over the past 2 months in terms of public health. How many public health activities have you been involved in?

Reading the next section may increase the number of activities identified.

Box 19.1 **Health promotion in practice**

### Medical approach

Seeks to prevent and/or cure illness through medical intervention.

*Example:* the midwife may offer the woman who is non-immune to rubella the vaccination in the postnatal period and contraceptive advice for a period of 3 months. Education and discussion should form part of this process. Didactic instruction should be avoided.

### Behavioural change approach

Primary focus is on encouraging people to change their behaviour.

*Example:* dietary adjustment to include more fruit and vegetables. This may involve raising awareness through education, empowerment and decision-making. Client-centred work should form part of this strategy to ensure success.

### Educational approach

Provision of information, tailored to meet the individual needs of the client.

*Example:* this approach is generally a precursor for other approaches. Methods that will enhance the educational approach include group work, discussion methods and problem-solving.

### Client-centred approach

This places the client at the centre of an interaction that is based on an equal partnership between the client and the professional. Empowerment is integral to this approach where individuals are encouraged to utilize personal strength toward health gain.

*Example:* making an informed decision about the uptake of antenatal screening tests, and behaviour change including stopping smoking.

### Societal change approach

Health promotion initiatives are focused on societal health and involve, for example, policy planning and political action (Dunkley 2000).

*Example:* political and community action toward the prohibition of smoking in enclosed public spaces and workplaces.

## Health promotion – community action

Health enhancement through community initiatives is well supported (DH 2008b). Health promotion has the potential to influence the health of present and future generations, with scope for a profound impact on reducing inequalities in health. Antenatal and postnatal care is predominantly provided in the community (historically recognized as a key arena to address these issues) where care is accessible with opportunity for flexibility at the point of delivery. Sure Start Children's Centres provide a multi-agency, multidisciplinary focus to healthcare provision, located in the heart of the community, focusing services toward vulnerable women and their families.

The aim of Children's Centres is to improve the health and wellbeing of children and their families through achieving health and reducing inequalities.

They bring together childcare, health, family support and early education to improve access to services. It is commonplace to have midwives based in Children's Centres providing maternity care within a multi-agency family-focused setting. With additional support from maternity services, midwives have the potential to develop services in areas where they have the greatest reach, including supermarkets, community centres and mobile bus services. Healthcare provision in an environment outside of the hospital setting increases opportunities for developing equal partnerships between midwives and women – reducing the potential for medical dominance and power.

Although traditionally midwives have provided postnatal care up until 28 days postpartum, the National Childbirth Trust found that women reported they had insufficient help and information between 11 to 30 days after birth, compared with the first 10 days (DH 2004). The *National Service Framework for Children, Young People and Maternity Services*, Standard 11 (DH 2004) suggests that midwifery-led services should be provided for the mother and her baby for at least a month after birth or discharge from hospital, and up to three months or longer depending on individual need.

This is a time when most families may be more receptive to health promotion, particularly with a new baby at home. The Royal College of Midwives (RCM) emphasizes the strength of midwifery within the community setting, encouraging the development of the midwife's public health role (RCM 2000, 2001).

Provision of maternity care to members of the travelling community and immigrant families presents challenges to the midwife's role in relation to equality and access to healthcare provision and services. Eviction orders, commonly associated with the travelling community owing to unlawful caravan parking, cause disruption in midwifery care provision. Local authorities proceeding with eviction orders are required to liaise with the relevant statutory agencies, to enable practitioners to fulfil statutory obligations, particularly where pregnant women and neonates are involved.

In 2007, asylum seeker applications in the UK totalled 23,430 (including dependants) (Home Office 2007). The Reproductive Health for Refugees Consortium made recommendations which included the need for culturally sensitive reproductive health, and appropriate referral systems, should obstetric emergencies arise. The health of pregnant asylum seekers is frequently compromised by lack of antenatal care, stressful, tortuous journeys from countries of origin, turmoil caused by war, oppression and poor nutrition. Their health disadvantage increases the risk of perinatal mortality and morbidity (Lewis 2007) and renders them ill-prepared for childbirth and parenting, particularly if antenatal care has been sparse (see Chapter 23).

It is for this reason that all pregnant mothers from countries where women may experience poorer overall general health, and who have not previously had a full medical examination in the UK, should have a medical history taken and clinical assessment made of their overall health by their obstetrician or GP (Lewis 2007). In particular, female asylum seekers arriving in the UK from certain countries in Africa and the Middle East may have undergone female genital mutilation (FGM) and as such require sensitive history-taking to ensure that an appropriate care plan is developed for pregnancy, labour and the postnatal period (see Chapter 58).

### Preconception care

Preconception care is described as the 'passport' to positive health during pregnancy. The aim of care is to optimize the chances of conception, ensure maintenance of a healthy pregnancy, and promote a healthy outcome for mother and baby (see Chapter 20).

## HEALTH PROMOTION IN MIDWIFERY

### Diet and nutrition

The midwife can provide effective health education in the area of diet and nutrition and may contribute to long-term healthy lifestyle changes (see Chapter 17). The health promotion approach chosen must be client-centred and include health education and empowerment. Behaviour change may also be necessary to promote immediate and long-term health. In an ever-changing healthcare climate where facts and knowledge change as new research emerges, the midwife must maintain current knowledge regarding diet and nutrition as the woman and her family naturally look to the midwife for advice.

New recommendations issued by the Food Standards Agency (FSA) on caffeine, for example, call for a reduction in caffeine consumption during pregnancy from no more than 300 mg to less than 200 mg (FSA 2008). This recommendation is based on two linked studies which showed that babies of pregnant women who consumed between 200 and 299 mg of caffeine per day were at an increased risk of fetal growth restriction which could result in low birthweight and/or miscarriage (CARE Study Group 2008).

## Exercise during pregnancy

Most people are well aware of the benefits of exercise and sport, and many women are fitness conscious. Knowledge and understanding regarding exercise during pregnancy will assist the midwife in supporting women who wish to exercise during pregnancy (see Chapter 22).

Exercise has many positive benefits for the individual, including:

- mental wellbeing, improvement in stamina and posture, and maintenance of good muscle tone
- during pregnancy, an improvement in cardiovascular function and reduction in excess weight gain, and has been found to have a protective effect on coronary heart disease, osteoporosis and hypertension (Paisley et al 2003)
- may reduce symptoms of fatigue, varicosities and swelling of extremities (RCOG 2006a, ACOG 1994)
- a primary role in preventing the development of gestational diabetes mellitus and helps to improve glycaemic control in women with the condition (Bung & Artal 1996).

It is important to adhere to safety principles during exercise, to enable physiological adjustment to take place, and midwives can use these to advise women (see website for Web Box 19.1). Women should avoid strenuous exercise to exhaustion (may cause blood flow diversion from the uterus, with resultant acute fetal hypoxia) (RCOG 2006a) and 'jumpy jerky' movements (NICE 2008).

Just as the maternal system copes with gradual respiratory and cardiac adjustment during pregnancy, the body also adjusts during exercise in a pregnancy identified as low risk. The woman who leads a sedentary lifestyle before pregnancy should be encouraged to undertake gentle exercise during pregnancy (NICE 2010); for example, aquanatal exercise may be a preferred option because of the benefits of non-weight-bearing activity, hydrostatic pressure, buoyancy and upthrust. Additionally, the increased mobility experienced reduces strain on joints and may relieve backache (Dunkley 2000). Walking and swimming may also be useful.

## Smoking in pregnancy

Smoking is the largest single preventable cause of mortality and is responsible for reducing the female advantage in life expectancy (ASH 2008). It is a major cause of coronary heart disease, stroke, chronic bronchitis, and lung and other cancers, and is also associated with reduced fertility and early menopause in women (BMA 2004). In pregnancy, smoking is related to spontaneous abortion, placenta praevia, placental abruption, low birthweight and preterm labour (Dewan et al 2003, George et al 2006, Kyrklund-Blomberg et al 2005). Other reports show an association between maternal smoking and wheeze during early childhood (Lux et al 2000).

Women from lower socioeconomic groups are more likely to smoke during pregnancy, which significantly increases the risk of perinatal and infant mortality. Children who are exposed in the home to cigarette smoke are more likely to develop otitis media and asthma and have higher hospitalization rates for severe respiratory illness. *Smoking kills* (Secretary of State for Health 1998) detailed the Government's commitment towards helping people quit smoking and reducing the prevalence of those who start. The report identified the provision of funding toward delivering expert help to those most in need and the phasing out of tobacco advertising by 2006. The smoke-free legislation in the UK in 2007 (2004 in Ireland) saw the prohibition of smoking in enclosed public places and workplaces from 1 July 2007 in England.

A report published by ASH (2008) presented a review of progress since 1998 and an agenda for a comprehensive tobacco control strategy. Nationally, smoking in pregnancy fell from 23% in 1995 to 19% in 2000 and then to 17% in 2005, indicating that the *Smoking kills* target for 2005 was met and the 2010 target is achievable. As there is significant underreporting of smoking during pregnancy, however, the current data are unreliable (ASH 2008).

### Smoking cessation: the midwife's role

The midwife's role facilitates women's reception of the support, guidance and advice that is offered, which is generally well received and acted upon (Lumley et al 2004). This unique relationship provides a window of opportunity for health education, which, if delivered appropriately, will not negatively alter the dynamics of the midwife–woman relationship but form an integral part of clinical practice. A client-centred approach and empowerment are more likely to secure and strengthen the midwife's relationship with the woman and ultimately achieve the health promotion goal than are persuasion, cajoling and scaremongering.

At the first antenatal visit, the midwife establishes the smoking status of the woman, her partner and other members of her household. Specialist smoking cessation counselling should be offered to all pregnant women who smoke (ASH 2008). Midwives may also choose to identify the woman's readiness to change her smoking behaviour and include her partner, if present, in the discussion. Prochaska et al (1993) developed the behaviour change cycle to assist health professionals in identifying the readiness of clients to change their smoking behaviour (see Box 19.2).

The midwife must increase her understanding of the complex nature of nicotine addiction experienced by smokers and view the process of cessation as more than cutting down or stopping. Women who are highly dependent on tobacco may feel guilty and inadequate at not being able to give it up. The midwife must be encouraging and

Box 19.2 **The model of behaviour change in practice**

**Precontemplator**

Not interested in stopping, has no intentions of stopping

What can I do?

- Present the risk factors and offer damage-limitation advice
- Refer for smoking cessation counselling

**Contemplator**

Is thinking about stopping, may have been thinking about stopping for several years

What can I do?

Encourage the woman to:

- Attend smoking cessation counselling services
- Explore reasons for wanting to stop; explore barriers to stopping
- Discuss preparation needed in order to stop – this may involve removing all ashtrays and similar appliances
- Consider triggers to smoking, e.g. telephone, coffee, after a meal, and think of an alternative strategy
- Consider substitutes for habitual feelings, e.g. something in the mouth or hand
- Consider substitutes if smoking is regularly used as a relaxer, or ice melter
- Consider strategies which may help to overcome the nicotine craving; think of times when the craving is strongest and consider strategies which may help to overcome this

**Ready for action**

Ready to stop – may need help and support in doing so

What can I do?

Encourage the woman to:

- Attend smoking cessation counselling services
- Choose a time to give up when there are fewer triggers to smoke (e.g. stress)
- Set a date to stop and stick to it (make plans for stopping as detailed in the contemplator section)

**Relapse**

Stopped smoking but has restarted

What can I do?

- Unsuccessful attempts to quit work toward successful quitting; the smoker may learn valuable lessons after each relapse episode, which may increase the chances of future success
- Encourage the woman to make a list of everything that went wrong, think of strategies which may reduce the likelihood of relapse
- Encourage her to attend smoking cessation counselling services

NB. Strategies must be client led and not prescribed by the midwife, whose role is primarily facilitating the discussion and offering support and guidance.

supportive and ready to offer help to women who express the desire to stop smoking, particularly if they are reluctant to attend smoking cessation counselling. Ten minutes of counselling interaction may be sufficient as an effective intervention for smoking cessation (Lancaster et al 2000).

Reducing the number of cigarettes smoked should generally be discouraged, but praised if this action is taken prior to contact with the midwife. Whilst cutting down, people tend to drag on the cigarette more frequently than usual, inhale more deeply and smoke the cigarette as far to the end as is physically possible (Dunkley 2000). The amount of noxious chemicals inhaled may therefore be the same as the dose inhaled prior to cutting down, when the nature of the smoking behaviour was casual.

Together with current knowledge of specialist support services available in the local area, the midwife can also offer health education leaflets, 'quit line' numbers and information about self-help groups, but leaflets should not be used as a replacement for discussion, personal support, sign-posting to other services and advice. Nicotine replacement therapy is considered an option for some women and may be prescribed by their GP after consultation and counselling (NICE 2008).

## Damage limitation

Overwhelming evidence shows the association between secondhand smoke and sudden infant death syndrome (SIDS) – 86% of cot deaths occur in families where the mother smokes (ASH 2008). Further evidence points toward the long-term effects of postnatal neonatal exposure, with associations made between secondhand smoke and heart disease, and increased risk of asthma attacks among those already affected. An association has also been made between secondhand smoke breathed by the pregnant non-smoker and increased maternal circulating absolute nucleated red blood cell counts, which suggests there may be subtle negative effects on fetal oxygenation (Dollberg et al 2000).

The midwife has a responsibility to provide health information and education to women and their families to reduce the damage to the fetus/infant, without making the parents feel guilty. Through two-way communication with the woman and her partner, the midwife should establish the nature of the smoking behaviour and establish their readiness to change. If the woman is ready to stop smoking, the midwife should refer her for specialist support. However, if the woman is not ready to stop, damage limitation advice should be offered. This can involve exploring strategies for reducing the tobacco exposure to the neonate by suggesting that a smoke-free environment is created for the baby; that parents use another room to smoke – outside or near a window. Parents must be actively encouraged to explore strategies that best work for them rather than those prescribed by the midwife. This encourages ownership of plans made and ultimately ensures effectiveness.

## Alcohol intake during pregnancy

Alcohol ingestion is a socially accepted behaviour that forms part of everyday social interaction in the western world. Over the past 30 years, the number of women drinkers has increased more than that of men. Excessive alcohol intake is potentially lethal, affecting virtually every organ and system in the body, including the liver, gastrointestinal tract, and cardiovascular and neurological systems. It affects nutrition by suppressing the appetite and by altering the metabolism, mobilization and storage of nutrients (Wardlow 2000). Excessive or chronic alcohol abuse is associated with several vitamin and mineral deficiencies, including folic acid, vitamin B, magnesium and iron. Learning difficulties, loss of memory and other mental problems are associated with infants born to parents who have abused alcohol (Chang et al 1998). Women's tolerance of alcohol is lower than that of men because of differences in body size, absorption and metabolism. They have a higher proportion of fat to water; therefore alcohol becomes more concentrated in body fluids and damaging effects such as gastritis, pancreatitis, peptic ulcers and malnutrition are more likely to develop.

Drinking alcohol during pregnancy is both teratogenic and fetotoxic (NICE 2008) and excessive intake during pregnancy is associated with fetal alcohol syndrome and fetal alcohol spectrum disorder (see Chapter 48).

### Safe measures of alcohol during pregnancy

Despite numerous research studies, to date there is no universally acceptable safe measure of alcohol consumption during pregnancy. In the USA, alcohol consumption of any amount during pregnancy or for women considering a pregnancy is not recommended – advice consistently given since 1981 by the US Surgeon General's Office. Alcohol-containing products also carry a health warning.

In the UK this advice is not endorsed and a range of options are available that allow some drinking during pregnancy. For example, the Department of Health report *Sensible drinking* (DH 1995) initially suggested that to minimize the risk to the developing fetus or women trying to get pregnant, no more than one or two units of alcohol per week should be ingested, and this slightly altered on the DH website in 2008 to they 'should not drink more than 1–2 units of alcohol once or twice a week and should not get drunk'. This view was endorsed by the National Institute for Health and Clinical Excellence (NICE) antenatal care guidelines stating that women should avoid alcohol during the first trimester and then limit their intake to one to two units once or twice a week for the remainder of their pregnancy (NICE 2008). Whilst there is no evidence of harm from low levels of alcohol intake, there is uncertainty regarding a safe level of alcohol consumption during pregnancy and, as such, complete abstinence of alcohol ingestion during pregnancy should be considered in line with the US Surgeon General's advice (Mukherjee et al 2005).

### Antenatal screening

During the antenatal period, starting at the booking visit, questions relating to alcohol intake should be specific and focused enough to identify women who have a drinking problem. At the first antenatal visit, the midwife should ask the woman if she drinks alcohol. Common responses include, 'no', 'yes', 'not really', or 'just socially'. Further enquiry must follow to establish clear meaning and specific information to ensure the appropriate health promotion approach is taken. There is a general trend toward underreporting, which will inhibit the identification of high-risk drinkers (RCOG 2006b, Stoler & Holmes 1999). Heavy drinkers may book late for maternity care and require intensive counselling with referral to specialist agencies to help them reduce alcohol consumption. Highlighting teratogenic effects on the fetus forms part of health education, but midwives should be sensitive in ensuring that the information they provide is balanced and informed, and does not result in fear or guilt, as this may impede the woman's ability to reduce drinking levels.

A useful way of taking a drinking history is to ask specifically about the preceding 7 days. If alcohol has been consumed, the amount in units should be recorded. If intake is higher than RCOG guidelines, the midwife should discuss this with the woman and explore ways of reducing the amount and nature of alcohol intake. While ingesting two units of alcohol over a week may be considered safe (RCOG 2006b), this amount in one evening may not be. A screening tool to detect alcohol abuse recommended by the RCOG is the T-ACE questionnaire (Sokol et al 1989) (see website).

## Drugs in pregnancy

Pregnant women should be advised to take only those drugs that are prescribed by a doctor. The *British National*

*Formulary* (BMA & RPSGB 2008), also available online, offers an excellent guide on drugs contraindicated in pregnancy (see Chapters 10 and 23 and the recommended reading list for further information about drugs in pregnancy and drug misuse).

## Domestic violence

Domestic violence (formerly referred to as domestic abuse) poses a serious threat to women's health and may be emotional, sexual, physical or financial abuse and can result in homicide. It is well established that violence towards women increases during pregnancy (DH 2007, Mezey 1997). The perpetrator is usually the male partner or ex-partner but domestic violence may occur in same-sex relationships, or from other family members.

Abused women and abusers come from all cultural, educational, racial, religious and socioeconomic backgrounds. Midwives must be able to recognize women at risk of violence and provide information and support, acting as a conduit to local resources, support networks and services available (Box 19.3).

### Prevalence

Research indicates that domestic violence is widespread in the UK, but it is difficult to obtain reliable statistics as it is generally underreported and therefore a hidden crime. It occurs in all parts of society and is reported to account for 25% of violent crime in the UK (DH 2007). One in three women will experience domestic violence at some time in their lives. It is estimated that 30% of domestic violence starts in pregnancy (Home Office 2004). Reasons for this are numerous and may include feelings of overpossessiveness, jealousy and denial of the women having any other role than spouse. The perpetrator may feel jealous of the woman's ability to produce a child, or see the fetus as an intruder. He may also become violent because of strained finances or reduced sexual activity (DH 2005).

### Risk to the woman and fetus

Domestic violence during pregnancy has been associated with adverse pregnancy outcomes, including low birthweight (Kaye et al 2006). The physical and psychological risks to the woman and fetus are overwhelmingly high, and the fetus may be injured or may die during the pregnancy. During 2003–05, the deaths of 19 pregnant or recently delivered women who were murdered were reported to the Confidential Enquiries into Maternal Deaths in the UK (Lewis 2007). The ages of these women ranged from 16 to 45. Five could not speak English and, alarmingly, in all cases the husbands acted as interpreters. It is suggested that many more such deaths are unreported and that this number of 19 should be treated as a

**Box 19.3 Domestic abuse: new and existing recommendations**

Once multi-agency support services are in place this Enquiry [CEMACH] continues to recommend that routine enquiries should be made about domestic abuse, either when taking a social history at booking, or at another opportune point during a woman's antenatal period.

Whenever possible, all women should be seen alone at least once during the antenatal period to enable disclosure more easily if they wish.

When routine questioning is introduced, this must be accompanied by the development of local strategies for referral to a local multidisciplinary support network to whom the woman can be referred if necessary.

Local trusts and community teams should develop guidelines for the identification of, and provision for further support for, these women, including developing multi-agency working to enable appropriate referrals or provision of information on sources of further help.

Information about local sources of help and emergency helplines such as those provided by Women's Aid should be displayed in suitable places in antenatal clinics, for example in the women's toilets or printed as a routine at the bottom of hand-held maternity notes or cooperation cards.

Clear, relevant and complete information must be passed from the GP to the antenatal care team, at booking, which accurately details any past current or past medical, psychiatric, social or family history.

It must be remembered that health professionals, too, are victims of abuse.

Women with known significant features of domestic abuse should not be regarded as 'low risk' and should be offered multidisciplinary care in a supportive environment. If they choose midwifery led care the midwife should receive support and advice from an experienced superior.

All health professionals should make themselves aware of the importance of domestic abuse in their practice. They should adopt a non-judgemental and supportive response to women who have experienced physical, psychological or sexual abuse and must be able to give basic information to women about where to get help. They should also provide continuing support, whatever decision the woman makes concerning her future.

(Lewis 2007:173)

**Box 19.4 Possible signs of domestic abuse in women**

| | |
|---|---|
| Frequent appointments for vague symptoms | Frequent missed appointments |
| Injuries inconsistent with explanation of cause | Multiple injuries at different stages of healing |
| Woman tries to hide injuries or minimise their extent | Patient appears frightened, overly anxious or depressed |
| Partner always attends unnecessarily | Woman is submissive or afraid to speak in front of her partner |
| Woman is reluctant to speak in front of partner | Partner is aggressive or dominant, talks for a woman or refuses to leave the room |
| Suicide attempts – particularly with Asian women | Poor or non-attendance at antenatal clinics |
| History of repeated miscarriages, terminations, stillbirths or pre-term labour | Injuries to the breasts or abdomen |
| Repeat presentation with depression, anxiety, self-harm or psychosomatic symptoms | Recurring sexually transmitted infections or urinary tract infections |
| Non-compliance with treatment | Early self discharge from hospital |

None of the above signs automatically indicates domestic abuse. But they should raise suspicion and prompt you to make every attempt to see the woman alone and in private to ask her if she is being abused. Even if she chooses not to disclose at this time, she will know you are aware of the issues, and she might choose to approach you at a later time. If you are going to ask a woman about domestic violence, always follow your Trust's or Health Authority's guidance. Or follow the guidance in Section 3.3 of the *Responding to Domestic Abuse* handbook.

(DH 2005:48)

minimum. Seventy women reported to the enquiry had features of domestic violence. Most women proactively self-reported domestic abuse to a health professional before or during pregnancy (Lewis 2007). All women were reported to have at least two identifiable risk factors of domestic violence detailed in Box 19.4. None were referred for help or advice. It is important to note that more than 80% of women who died from direct or indirect causes of domestic violence booked late for maternity care (after 24 weeks) or received minimal or no antenatal care (Lewis 2007).

## Risks to other family members

In households where there is domestic violence, the children within that household may be affected. They may observe the abuse or be injured directly or indirectly as a result of the abuse (Home Office 2004). The fear experienced and the psychological consequences are immeasurable and may well influence the child's emotional development. The child may also try to protect younger siblings or take on the role of prime carer. It is reported that 52% of child protection cases involve domestic abuse (Home Office 2004).

## The midwife's role

Due to the number of domestic violence cases that commence in pregnancy, the Department of Health set up the Domestic Abuse and Pregnancy Advisory Group in 2005. This group recommends how health services can meet the needs of pregnant women who are experiencing abuse. It contributed to the development of a handbook for health professionals offering a practical guide on domestic abuse, routine enquiry and training (DH 2005). Routine enquiry for domestic violence during pregnancy has been found to increase the rate of detection, enabling women who disclose domestic violence to seek help early (Bacchus et al 2004).

Routine enquiry about domestic violence should only be carried out if appropriate education and training has been provided, guidelines developed to support staff, and support/referral systems are current and reliable.

When violence is suspected, the best way to confirm suspicion is by direct questioning, which may include the following questions:

- Has somebody been hurting you?
- Did somebody cause these injuries?
- Do you ever feel frightened of your partner, or other people at home?
- Have you ever been slapped, kicked or punched by your partner?

The woman may choose to deny being abused, but awareness that help is available is useful. For some women, however, pregnancy provides a unique opportunity for change and disclosure of violence may therefore be likely (Bacchus et al 2004). Routine enquiry of all women antenatally reduces the chances of targeting certain female and male groups that conform to personal stereotypes of those who are likely to be abused and those who may be abusers. Common difficulties for routine enquiry include:

- finding an appropriate time to ask the question, particularly when the woman is accompanied by her partner
- denial of abuse and subsequent non-attendance for antenatal care
- lack of supervision services for midwives who receive disclosure. (Without supportive structures in

place, direct questioning must be approached with caution.)

In anticipation of some of these difficulties, several maternity services inform the woman via the booking appointment letter that she will be required to see the midwife alone on at least one occasion during the pregnancy.

Fostering a safe, nurturing and private environment during antenatal visits, with the midwife expressing genuineness, positive regard, empathy and honesty, may provide the woman with an opportunity to seek help should she feel the need. Survivors of domestic violence often feel ashamed about being abused by their partner, have low self-esteem and have conflicting feelings about disclosure, including the repercussions of their actions. Very often, leaving the abuser is not considered a favourable option. Some women are financially and emotionally dependent on their abusers, who often have control over all domestic arrangements. Religious and cultural influences often encourage people to stay in abusive marriages where separation or divorce is considered unacceptable.

The midwife should understand the nature of domestic violence, be sensitive to clues that may suggest abuse (see Box 19.4) and be aware of the impact of abuse on everyday life. When the woman and the midwife are not in the company of the partner – for example, when showing the woman where the toilet is – this may provide an opportunity for the woman to disclose something about how she is feeling that may be indirectly related to the abuse.

Although considered a viable approach, direct questioning is not the *only* option for obtaining information. Some midwives may be reluctant to acknowledge domestic violence or ask questions about it because of:

- their fear of offending
- fear of disclosure
- lack of knowledge of what action to take if this occurs
- feeling that it is a private matter and belief that it is not a part of their role.

Staff should be trained in conflict avoidance to ameliorate the course of violence (DH 2005) and this often increases their confidence.

Each maternity unit and midwifery group practice should have current details about domestic violence units and the Women's Aid Federation, who provide a safe refuge for those who need it (see details on the website). The Samaritans, Relate and Victim Support all offer support services to survivors of domestic violence. The midwife should be able to supply the woman with relevant local telephone numbers and addresses.

## Teenage pregnancy

A teenager is described in different contexts to be a young person under the age of 18, 19 or 20 years of age. The Teenage Pregnancy Strategy considers the key teenage pregnancy group to be those who are under 18 years of age (Department for Children, Schools and Families [DCSF) et al 2008); the Every Child Matters programme (The Treasury 2003) focuses on those between birth and 19 years of age; and the Infant Feeding Survey define their youngest group to be the under-20s for the measurement of national breastfeeding and smoking rates (refer to the website and see Chapters 16 and 23).

## Employment and health

For the majority of women, work during pregnancy does not pose a threat to their health or that of their babies (NICE 2008). For some, it may be necessary to modify working practices to promote safety and comfort.

The pregnant woman should avoid heavy lifting. Seating for sedentary workers should be supportive to the back because of increased lumbar lordosis. Standing for long periods should be avoided and rest periods instituted because of the risk of development of varicosities. Smoky environments should be avoided because of the risks associated with passive smoking.

Some occupations may be hazardous to the health of the fetus and expectant mother, including exposure to toxic chemicals (such as lead, pesticides, anaesthetic gases and radiation). Utilization of protective clothing in the home and the workplace, where appropriate, and adhering to safety parameters and work codes will minimize exposure to teratogenic hazards. This makes it important for the midwife to establish the woman's normal working environment, identify any potential hazards, and provide a conduit for further information should this be required (see website).

## Travel

The midwife has a responsibility to raise awareness about travel and health. The most basic but essential information can reduce the risk of harm to the woman, fetus and infant. The UK Government made a commitment to reducing the number of road traffic accidents by one-tenth by 2010 among children and young people in England. Health education during the antenatal period should include issues relating to car seats and the correct application of seatbelts during pregnancy. Pregnant women must be informed about the correct use of seatbelts, including the correct positioning of the seatbelt above and below the uterus (NICE 2008).

Other travel advice given to pregnant women may need to include information about airline travel, particularly 'long haul' flights, when the risk of venous thrombosis is increased. Most airlines will not carry pregnant women after 32 weeks' gestation.

## EVALUATION

Evaluation is the process by which criteria to determine the value of an idea or method are formulated. The aim of this is to demonstrate the success of the method based on designated aims and learning outcomes.

Without the use of appropriate evaluation tools, the potential to challenge the efficacy of midwifery health promotion is reduced. Evaluation is a worthwhile process and should be used to demonstrate the impact and outcome of interventions deemed to enhance health. Knowledge about the most suitable methods of evaluation is essential not only to highlight the most effective health interventions but also to demonstrate their efficacy to key stakeholders who influence resource allocation. Midwives may use qualitative or quantitative methods of data collection to formulate evaluation results (see Chapters 5 and 7).

Health promotion evaluation can be extremely difficult for the midwife, particularly when assessing long-term success of a health intervention or behaviour change. Other areas that present challenges in terms of evaluation include awareness raising and empowerment.

### Reflective activity 19.3

Consider the content of this chapter, and draw up a list of referral agencies for the issues mentioned: Women's Refuge; alcohol support; local exercise classes; and contacts such as local nutritionist, social worker and health visitors. You can add to this list as you seek out more information for women and families in your area, and you can use this as a reference resource.

## CONCLUSION

Health promotion is an integral part of the midwife's role, with many potential health-gain benefits for the childbearing population. Understanding the context of health and illness is a key factor in promoting health, and choosing the appropriate health promotion approach to achieve the desired aim is essential if the health promotion approach is to be effective. The midwife's scope of practice provides room for the public health role to be enhanced and community initiatives to be embraced. The midwife is a vital resource in terms of advice and information on diet, smoking and exercise, and may be a useful means of promoting a healthy lifestyle. The woman may look at her midwife as a role model, and her attitudes and activities may carry as much weight as her words.

The current UK political health agenda recognizes the valuable contribution midwives make to the health of the nation. Rigorous robust evaluation of all health promotion activities will provide evidence of the impact of the midwife's work in terms of health gain.

### KEY POINTS

- The concept of health and the meaning of health promotion are fundamental to the role of the midwife.
- The midwife needs to be aware of her own attitudes, behaviours and understanding of health in order to develop an effective health promotion approach to apply to midwifery practice.
- The midwife should expand her knowledge of women's health and screening to enable her to meet the public health agenda.
- It is important to provide realistic and appropriate health promotion strategies, and develop a mechanism for evaluation of their effectiveness.

## REFERENCES

Acheson D (Chair): *Independent inquiry into inequalities in health*, London, 1998, The Stationery Office (TSO).

Action on Smoking and Health (ASH): *Beyond smoking kills: protecting children reducing inequalities*, London, 2008, ASH.

American College of Obstetricians and Gynecologists (ACOG): *Exercise during pregnancy and the postpartum period*, Technical Bulletin No. 189, Washington DC, 1994, ACOG.

Antonovsky A: The salutogenic model as a theory to guide health promotion, *Health Promotion International* 11(1):11–18, 1996.

Bacchus L, Mezey G, Bewley S, et al: Prevalence of domestic violence when midwives routinely enquire in pregnancy, *British Journal of Obstetrics and Gynaecology* 111(5):441–445, 2004.

Bauer G, Davies J, Pelikan J: The EUHPID Health Development Model for the classification of public health indicators, *Health Promotion International* 21(2):457–462, 2006.

Becker MH, Haefner DP, Kasl SV, et al: Selected psycho-social models and correlates of individual heath-related behaviours, *Medical Care* 15(5):27–46, 1977.

Black D, Morris JN, Smith C, et al: *Inequalities in health: the Black Report*, Harmondsworth, 1982, Penguin.

British Medical Association (BMA): *Smoking and reproductive life* (website). www.bma.org.uk/images/smoking_tcm41-21289.pdf. Accessed August 2010.

British Medical Association (BMA), Royal Pharmaceutical Society of Great Britain (RPSGB): *British National Formulary*, ed 56, London, 2008, BMA.

Bung P, Artal R: Gestational diabetes and exercise: a survey, *Seminars in Perinatology* 20(4):328–333, 1996.

CARE Study Group: Maternal caffeine intake during pregnancy and risk of fetal growth restriction: a large prospective observational study, *British Medical Journal* 337:a2332, 2008.

Chang G, Wilkins-Haug L, Berman S, et al: Alcohol use and pregnancy: improving identification, *Obstetrics and Gynecology* 91(6):892–898, 1998.

Department for Children, Schools and Families (DCSF), Department of Health and Royal College of Midwives (RCM): *Teenage Pregnancy. Who cares? A guide to commissioning and delivering maternity services for young parents*, ed 2, London, 2008, DCSF/DH/RCM.

Department of Health: *Sensible drinking: report of an Interdepartmental Working Group*, London, 1995, DH.

Department of Health (DH): *Saving lives: our healthier nation; a contract for health*, London, 1999, The Stationery Office (TSO).

Department of Health (DH): *National Service Framework for Children, Young People and Maternity Services: core standards*, London, 2004, DH.

Department of Health: *Responding to domestic abuse: a handbook for health professionals*, London, 2005, DH.

Department of Health (DH): *Maternity matters: choice, access and continuity of care in a safe service*, London, 2007, DH.

Department of Health (DH): *Health inequalities: progress and the next steps*, London, 2008a, DH.

Department of Health: *The Health and Personal Social Services Programmes. Departmental Report*. Presented to Parliament by the Secretary of State for Health by Command of Her Majesty, 2008b.

Dewan N, Brabin B, Wood L, et al: The effects of smoking on birthweight for gestational age curves in teenage and adult primigravidae, *Public Health* 117:31–35, 2003.

Dollberg S, Fainaru O, Mimouni FB, et al: The effect of passive smoking in pregnancy on neonatal nucleated red blood cells, *Paediatrics* 106(3):E34, 2000.

Dunkley J: *Health promotion in midwifery practice: a resource for health professionals*, Edinburgh, 2000, Baillière Tindall.

Ewles L, Simnett I: *Promoting health, a practical guide*, 5 ed, London, 2003, Baillière Tindall.

Food Standards Agency (FSA): *Caffeine consumption during pregnancy* (website). www.food.gov.uk/news/newsarchive/2008/nov/caffeinenov08. 2008. Accessed November, 2008.

Foresight: *Preconception care services* (website). www.foresight-preconception.org.uk/aboutus.aspx. Accessed August, 2010.

George L, Granath F, Johansson AL, et al: Environmental tobacco smoke and risk of spontaneous abortion, *Epidemiology* 17(5):500–505, 2006.

Home Office (HO): *Safety and justice: sharing personal information in the context of domestic violence*, London, 2004, HO.

Home Office (HO): *Asylum seeker applications in the UK* (website). www.ukba.homeoffice.gov.uk/asylum. 2007. Accessed March 6, 2009.

Kaye D, Mirembe F, Bantebya G, et al: Domestic violence during pregnancy and risk of low birthweight and maternal complications: a prospective cohort study at Mulago Hospital, Uganda, *Tropical Medicine and International Health* 11(10):1576–1584, 2006.

Kyrklund-Blomberg NB, Granath F, Cnattingius S: Maternal smoking and causes of very preterm birth, *Acta Obstetricia et Gynecologica Scandinavica* 84(6):572–577, 2005.

Lancaster T, Fowler G: Training health professionals in smoking cessation, *Cochrane Database of Systematic Reviews*, (2):CD000214, 2000.

Lewis G, editor: The Confidential Enquiries into Maternal and Child Health (CEMACH). Saving mothers lives: reviewing maternal deaths to make motherhood safer 2003–2005. The Seventh Report on Confidential Enquiries into Maternal Deaths in the United Kingdom, London, 2007, CEMACH.

Lumley J, Oliver SS, Chamberlain C, et al: Interventions for promoting smoking cessation during pregnancy, *Cochrane Database of Systematic Reviews* (4):CD001055, 2004.

Lux AL, Henderson AJ, Pocock SJ: Wheeze associated with prenatal tobacco smoke exposure: a prospective, longitudinal study. ALSPAC Study Team, *Archives of Disease in Childhood* 83(4):307–312, 2000.

Mezey GC: Domestic violence in pregnancy. In Bewley S, Friend J, Mezey G, editors: *Violence against women*, London, 1997, RCOG Press, pp 77–85.

Mukherjee RAS, Hollins S, Abou-Saleh MT, et al: Low level alcohol consumption and the fetus, *British Medical Journal* 19(330):375–376, 2005.

National Institute for Clinical Excellence (NICE): *Antenatal care: routine antenatal care for the healthy pregnant woman*, NICE clinical guideline 62, London, 2008, NICE.

National Institute for Health and Clinical Excellence: *Weight management before, during and after pregnancy*, NICE Public Health Guidance PH27, London, 2010, NICE.

Office for National Statistics (ONS): *Health inequalities in the 21st century* (website). www.statistics.gov.uk. 2007. Accessed March 6, 2009.

Paisley TS, Joy EA, Price RJ: Exercise during pregnancy: a practical approach, *Current Sports Medicine Reports* 2(6):325–330, 2003.

Prochaska J, Diclemente C, Norcross C: In search of how people change: applications to addictive behaviours, *Addictions Nursing Network* 5(1):3–16, 1993.

Rotter JB: Generalized expectancies for internal versus external control of re-enforcement, *Psychological Monographs* 80(1):1–28, 1966.

Royal College of Midwives (RCM): *Vision 2000*, London, 2000, RCM.

Royal College of Midwives (RCM): *Position Paper: The midwife's role in public health*, London, 2001, RCM.

Royal College of Obstetrics and Gynaecology (RCOG): *Exercise in pregnancy, Statement number 4*, London, 2006a, RCOG.

Royal College of Obstetricians and Gynaecologists (RCOG): *Alcohol consumption and the outcomes of pregnancy, Pregnancy Guideline Statement No. 5*, London, 2006b, RCOG.

Secretary of State for Health: *Smoking kills*, London, 1998, The Stationery Office (TSO).

Secretary of State for Health: *The NHS plan: a plan for investments. A plan for reform*, Cm4818-1, London, 2000, The Stationery Office (TSO).

Seedhouse D: *Health promotion philosophy, prejudice and practice*, Chichester, 1997, John Wiley.

Sokol RJ, Martier SS, Ager JW: The T-ACE questions: practical prenatal detection of risk-drinking, *American Journal Obstetrics and Gynecology* 160(4):863–870, 1989.

Stoler J, Holmes L: Under-recognition of prenatal alcohol effects in infants of known alcohol abusing women, *Journal of Paediatrics* 135(4):405–406, 1999.

The Treasury: *Every child matters*, London 2003, The Stationery Office (TSO).

Tones K, Green J: *Health promotion: planning and strategies*, London, 2004, Sage.

Wardlow G: *Contemporary nutrition: issues and insights*, ed 4, USA, 2000, McGraw Hill Higher Education.

World Health Organization (WHO): *Constitution*, New York, 1946, WHO.

World Health Organization (WHO): Health promotion: a discussion document on concepts and principle, Geneva, 1984, WHO.

Chapter |20|

# Preconception care

Barbara Burden and Trish Jones

## LEARNING OUTCOMES

After reading this chapter, you will:

- appreciate the concepts involved in undertaking a preconception history and screening tests
- be able to evaluate preconception care advice for parents.

## INTRODUCTION

The aim of preconception care is to maximize the health of prospective parents prior to conception. This ensures they are at the peak of their health potential at the point of conception and organogenesis (17–56 days following conception) when the potential for fetal abnormality is highest, thus attempting to achieve maximum health potential of the developing baby. In an ideal world, prospective parents would present themselves to an appropriately trained healthcare professional for health screening at least 6 months prior to a planned conception. In reality, this is not usually perceived as essential by prospective parents and health professionals and it is only in retrospect when pregnancy outcome is compromised that parents seek to identify what could have prevented or reduced this outcome. Preconception care, therefore, needs to be aimed at any individual, male or female, with the potential for conception.

With the developing public health role of the midwife in providing total care for the family, every health promotion activity undertaken must include elements of preconception advice. Preconception care must be included in routine health screening activities offered by a variety of healthcare professionals, in health promotion literature and classes, in schools, during family planning or cervical screening sessions (Kierman 2006), in pregnancy testing kits, at post-abortion counselling and in any potential health education experience. Reproductive sexual health is already discussed in schools, with the aim of reducing teenage pregnancy, and this example could be applied to components of preconception care, to inform adolescents of the importance of planning and preparing for pregnancy. Women who have negative pregnancy tests should be targeted for preconception information in readiness for subsequent pregnancy. Preconception advice should be offered to women during the antenatal and postnatal periods.

Preconception care varies considerably internationally, nationally and locally, reaching a small segment of the community, usually clients who are motivated, articulate and aware of their needs, or clients who have had a compromised pregnancy and are preparing for future pregnancy. The type of screening available to women and their partners varies; thus, advising women on preconception care is often confusing. The difficulty with preconception care is that it is not perceived as a priority by healthcare professionals and is not readily available to women. Only in retrospect when pregnancy outcome is compromised do women and their partners seek information or advice on care for subsequent pregnancy. With appropriate preconception care, the care and treatment required during pregnancy is significantly reduced. For example, providing preconception care to women with diabetes reduces hospital admissions, length of stay in hospital, intensity of care of newborn infants and subsequently shortens the infant's period of hospitalization (Kendrick 2004).

This chapter outlines some of the areas of interest to women and their partners attempting to conceive. Each area of interest is subdivided into advice a midwife could offer to women and partners and further reading or Internet addresses for additional information. It is important to remember that patterns of treatment are continually changing as new ideas and research results emerge and, therefore, midwives need to monitor changes and implement them into their care provision.

**Reflective activity 20.1**

Determine what preconception care is available to you locally. For example:

- Are preconception care clinics offered at your local health centre or hospital?
- Are there healthcare professionals willing to offer advice in areas such as HIV, genetic counselling or health promotion?

## AIM OF PRECONCEPTION CARE

The aim of preconception care is to increase the health of prospective parents, ensuring they are at the peak of their health potential at the point where conception occurs and throughout the period of organogenesis, enhancing the health of the developing baby.

**Organogenesis** This is the period of early fetal development (17–56 days following conception) where the early cell mass of conception becomes organized into three layers: ectoderm, mesoderm and endoderm; each responsible for development of different organs or body parts in the developing baby (see Ch. 29).

## OBJECTIVES OF PRECONCEPTION CARE

The objectives of preconception care are to:

- maximize the health of prospective parents and hence the health of the baby, creating a constructive environment in which conception and fetal development occur
- reduce perinatal and maternal mortality and morbidity
- provide information to prospective parents, enabling them to make informed choices about the care they receive and their readiness to be parents
- evaluate the genetic potential of women and their partners and the need for genetic counselling
- advise on discontinuation of contraception, enabling planning of conception and reduction of unplanned pregnancies
- inform prospective parents of elements of maternity services, enabling informed choice on the type of care required and where that care takes place.

## TAKING A PRECONCEPTION HISTORY

When a woman and her partner present for preconception care, the supporting practitioner records a personal history. The most important aspect of preconception care is the need for a full and detailed health history from both partners and others identified as being significant, such as where genetic screening is required. The aim of the session is to assess, educate and counsel prospective parents on optimum health in preparation for pregnancy. The information obtained at this interview guides the care process, providing a baseline for subsequent comparative tests.

The interview must be undertaken in an environment where clients feel at ease, with confidentiality and privacy ensured. Appropriate allocation of time for appointments should be available, enabling time to listen and advise and undertake necessary screening tests. All tests are explained in detail, information sheets are provided and informed consent obtained. At some point it is recommended that each partner be interviewed privately so that they may disclose personal information which they do not wish their partner to know.

### The preconception care assessment

The process of risk assessment in preconception care presumes the potential for adverse outcome in pregnancy (see website). The assessment focuses on identification of conditions relating to risk, assessing prospective parents' risk of complications in pregnancy and interventions required to reduce severity of those complications. It should contain a detailed medical, psychological and social history, physical examination and health screening of both prospective parents. The need to link risk assessment to health promotion activities ensures preconception care focuses not only on diagnosis and treatment but also on creating a healthy environment for the proposed conception through advice and guidance.

Both the woman and her partner should be involved in the discussion to provide the following information:

- health status – that is, rubella immunity, hepatitis B status, body mass index (BMI)
- sexual history – such as contraceptives, sexually transmitted disease, infertility
- family history, to include genetic history, even if sperm or egg donors are used
- medical/surgical history
- psychological history
- substance use – for example, drugs, smoking, alcohol
- history of infections

- obstetric and gynaecological history
- contact with environmental hazards
- nutritional history
- occupational history.

Once a detailed history has been taken, areas of health promotion or risk are identified and screening tests performed. Not all of the following tests may be offered or deemed necessary, as they will depend on individual needs and services available. However, specialist support services are available through organizations such as Foresight.

### Screening tests

- Physical examination to identify any medical or surgical conditions requiring referral to members of the multi-professional team
- Blood pressure measurement
- Cardiac function
- Thyroid function
- Respiratory function
- Review of gastrointestinal activity
- Weight
- Sexual health status, such as vaginal, urethral or anal swabs
- Cervical smear
- Serum screening:
  - for haemoglobinopathies
  - full blood count
  - rubella status
  - tuberculosis status
- Assessment of vitamin, zinc and lead levels
- Hair analysis:
  - nutritional state
  - exposure to toxic metals
- Karyotyping/genomics (Dolan et al 2007)
- Urinalysis for protein, ketones, glucose and bacteriuria.

## Providing information to prospective parents

Results of screening tests are given to clients as the information becomes available, taking care not to overload the couple with details. Verbal information is supported by documents, information via the Internet, and referral to other multi-professional teams. It is important not to assume a prior level of knowledge, particularly in relation to issues such as basic anatomy, sexual health or knowledge of support services.

## NUTRITION

The importance of an adequate diet at conception and during pregnancy is identified as a key factor in adult health, with associated links to illness such as coronary heart disease (DH 2000). There is a direct relationship between nutritional intake, malnutrition and suboptimal nutrition in pregnancy and maternal and child health (Reifsnider & Gill 2000). Women with conditions requiring specific diets or nutritional requirements are referred or advised to seek specialist advice from a dietician. The aim is to ensure that women have a healthy body weight, sensible eating habits and suitable nutritional stores at the point of conception (Cuco et al 2006). Diet in pregnancy is influenced by morning sickness, hyperemesis, pica (food cravings) and dislike of certain foods. Nutritional assessment is important because of the increase in malnutrition and the recognition that someone who is obese can also be malnourished.

The body mass index (BMI) is still the recognized method of estimating nutritional status. A BMI of 20 or less indicates that the individual is underweight, whereas a BMI of 30 or over is indicative of obesity. Energy intake should be increased by approximately 200 calories per day during pregnancy, but no change is required while preparing to conceive.

Table 20.1 outlines the information, advice and further reading on nutrition that a midwife may find helpful when offering preconception advice on nutritional intake.

## INFECTION

Infection in the mother, and in some cases the father, may affect the developmental phases of the fetus. Infections should be diagnosed and treated prior to conception and advice given on prevention of reinfection (Table 20.2). Routine serum screening can assess immunity to infections such as rubella, and where immunity is not detected, vaccination must be offered prior to conception. Infection that causes a significant rise in body temperature may result in spontaneous abortion in early pregnancy. The impact of mumps should be considered when exploring a medical history from prospective fathers, because of associated infertility in men.

## SEXUALLY TRANSMITTED DISEASE

A full and detailed sexual history must be obtained before conception to assess potential risk. This area of health is often the most difficult to discuss but must be explored during the interview to determine associated risk factors. Sexually transmitted diseases, infections and infestations are on the increase and individuals need to be routinely screened. Where infections are indicated, barrier methods of contraception should be used until treatment is completed. Suspected cases are referred to genitourinary

**Table 20.1 Nutrition: preconception care, advice and further reading**

| | Information and advice | Further information |
|---|---|---|
| Obesity | Lack of essential nutrients in the first trimester influences organogenesis and fetal formation<br>Advise women to achieve a BMI of 21–29 prior to conception<br>Unsupervised dieting is not advised during pregnancy although a healthy low-fat diet may help regulate weight gain<br>Refer to dietician | Galtier-Dereure et al 2000 |
| Eating disorders<br>– Anorexia<br>– Bulimia | Discussion of eating habits, although women may be reluctant to disclose information<br>Advise women to achieve a BMI of 21–29 prior to conception<br>Refer to general practitioner for referral to dietician, psychologist or psychiatrist<br>Bulimia often improves during pregnancy, with 34% no longer suffering after pregnancy | Siega-Riz et al 2008 |
| Vitamin deficiency and supplements | If following a healthy diet, vitamin supplements are unnecessary unless medically indicated<br>Advise women that some medications contain vitamin A, which can be teratogenic, for example, treatment for acne<br>Avoid foods high in retinoids, such as liver and fish liver oil, as they contain high levels of vitamin A | http://www.nutrition.org.uk/ |
| Folic acid deficiency | Advise to take folic acid, remembering to take higher dose if epileptic<br>Alcoholics, smokers and lactating women are at increased risk of folic acid deficiency. 4 mg of folic acid is taken daily 2–3 months prior to conception to the end of the first trimester following a previous neural tube defect or if epileptic. 0.4 mg of folic acid is taken daily 2–3 months prior to conception to the end of the first trimester in a first or subsequent pregnancy where there is no history of neural tube defects<br>Increase consumption of leafy vegetables and wholemeal products | Lumley et al 2000 |
| Calcium deficiency<br>– Osteoporosis<br>– Rickets<br>– Osteomalacia | Many women do not meet the recommended daily intake of 700 mg of calcium even when not pregnant<br>Advise on daily intake of calcium, milk, cheese, fish and yogurt<br>Refer to dietician | |
| Caffeine | Reduces implantation; two cups per day reduces the rate of conception by 27%<br>Advise to lower caffeine intake or cease | http://www.eatwell.gov.uk/agesandstages/pregnancy/trybaby/ |
| Anaemia | Anaemia should be diagnosed before pregnancy and the cause found and treated<br>Advise on diet, such as bread, pulses, red meat and spinach | |

**Table 20.2 Infections: preconception care, advice and further reading**

| | Information and advice | Further information |
|---|---|---|
| Rubella virus (German measles) | Avoid contact with infected persons for 7 days before and 5 days after rash appears<br>Ask the GP to check immunity status and vaccinate prior to conception<br>Avoid pregnancy for 3 months following vaccination<br>Higher fetal risk in the first trimester<br>Advise mothers on vaccinating children | http://www.nhs.uk/Conditions/Rubella/Pages/Prevention.aspx |
| Erythema infectiosum (slapped cheek disease) | Avoid children with the disease. It is thought to be communicable 1 week before symptoms appear to 1 week after onset of symptoms | Morgan-Capner & Crowcroft 2000 |
| Listeriosis (*Listeria monocytogenes*) | A food-borne pathogen found in soil, water and some vegetation<br>Wash hands when dealing with food<br>May be present in ready-to-eat food, meat pies, pâtés, unpasteurized milk or goat's milk, soft cheeses, such as Feta, Camembert, Brie and Stilton, and can survive and multiply in refrigerators at temperatures of 6°C or above<br>Re-heat all food to steaming point, as this kills the pathogen<br>Avoid contact with sheep during lambing and avoid handling silage<br>Treated with antibiotics<br>Takes up to 8 weeks for illness to emerge, so advise against pregnancy during that time | http://www.nhs.uk/Conditions/Listeriosis/ |
| Toxoplasmosis | Caused by the parasite *Toxoplasma gondii*<br>If tested prior to pregnancy and shown to carry the infection, then women are not at risk during pregnancy<br>No risk to healthy women unless they have a compromised immune system<br>Wear gloves when dealing with cat litter boxes<br>Wash hands thoroughly following gardening or contact with soil<br>Thoroughly cook meat<br>Avoid raw or cured meat<br>Wash hands after handling meat, fruit and vegetables (because of soil contamination) | Turner 2000 |
| Tuberculosis | Treat prior to conception<br>Vaccinate prior to travelling to areas where TB is prevalent<br>Seek advice from GP if in contact with infected persons | Bothamley 2006 |
| HIV/AIDS | Steady maintenance of low viral load and high CD4 count prior to conception reduces risks to the baby<br>Continued unprotected sex results in an increased viral load<br>Sperm washing and artificial insemination is available but not on the NHS<br>Treatment with AZT<br>Referral to sexual health team | http://www.bhiva.org/files/file1030325.pdf |

Table 20.2 Continued

| | Information and advice | Further information |
|---|---|---|
| Chickenpox virus (varicella zoster [VZ]) | The majority of mothers who have had chickenpox develop lifelong immunity which protects their baby during pregnancy<br>Test for VZ antibody; if not present, can receive varicella zoster immune globulin<br>1 in 3 women suffer spontaneous abortion following infection<br>Avoid pregnancy for 3 months following vaccination<br>At-risk groups include schoolteachers, childcare workers and nursery nurses<br>Avoid infected individuals. If in contact and not immune, advise to use contraception until end of incubation period | http://www.nhs.uk/conditions/Chickenpox/ |
| Hepatitis B | Assess hepatitis status<br>Vaccinate before conception if in at-risk category – for example, body piercing, tattoos<br>May recommend liver function tests to assess severity of disease | http://www.nhs.uk/Conditions/Hepatitis-B/ |
| Group B streptococcus (GBS) | May have no effect. 25% of women of childbearing age have GBS in their vaginas with no apparent symptoms<br>Advise women they require intravenous antibiotic therapy in labour or following rupture of membranes, to reduce the incidence of transmission to their baby | www.gbss.org.uk |
| Cytomegalovirus | May be asymptomatic as the virus lives within the salivary glands in 'healthy' adults<br>Wash hands before preparing meals | Azam et al 2001<br>http://www.nhs.uk/Conditions/Cytomegalovirus/ |
| Tetanus | *Clostridium tetani* spores are found in soil, dust and gut of animals<br>Wash hands following gardening or dusting | http://www.nhs.uk/Conditions/Tetanus/Pages/Introduction.aspx |

medicine clinics. Further information on sexual health is included in Chapter 57.

**Reflective activity 20.2**

Access the Health Protection Agency website at http://www.hpa.org.uk/. Review the various types of sexually transmitted diseases, evaluating them in relation to preconception care and the information required during discussion on a sexual history.

## MEDICAL CONDITIONS

Women and their partners who have a medical condition must attend for preconception care within a multi-professional team, consisting of specialist practitioners, obstetricians, physician and midwives. Most medical conditions, if managed effectively throughout organogenesis and the first trimester, result in sucessful outcome for mother and baby at birth (Table 20.3). In each case, early referral to the medical team is paramount.

## GENETICS

One of the most important activities in preconception screening is assessment of risk of genetic anomalies in prospective children (Table 20.4). The level of risk is linked to the chance of a baby inheriting an abnormality from its family. A family pedigree is constructed as part of the preconception interview or with a geneticist. Pregnancy is not the time for genetic screening, as this should be completed before conception. Historically, genetic anomalies were linked to a given population, but now with a migratory world population it is difficult to label specific groups as being more at risk than others. At present, genetic counselling is only provided to a small sample of the community and in most cases does not reach those who are most at risk. The emphasis is currently

**Table 20.3 Medical conditions: preconception care, advice and further reading**

| | Information and advice | Further information |
|---|---|---|
| Diabetes | Involve specialist practitioners, such as diabetic liaison midwife, dieticians, physician<br>Aim to control preconception glycaemia, reducing the incidence of fetal malformations at conception and organogenesis<br>Measure glycosylated haemoglobin (HbA1) as this gives information of blood glucose levels over previous 4–6 weeks | Kendrick 2004<br>McElvy et al 2000 |
| Epilepsy | Seek advice on anticonvulsant therapy prior to conception as this may help reduce the incidence of fetal malformations<br>Medication levels may be reduced<br>Anticonvulsant drugs are teratogenic<br>Take folic acid daily. The dose should be discussed with and prescribed by a GP or physician | British Epilepsy Association<br>http://www.epilepsy.org.uk<br>Helpline: 0808 800 5050 |
| Phenylketonuria | Is monogenic, autosomal recessive and affects phenylalanine metabolism<br>Phenylalanine is present in milk, meat, fish, cheese and eggs<br>Refer to dietician<br>Advise woman to maintain blood phenylalanine levels between 120 and 360 mmol/L through a low-phenylalanine diet before conception occurs and during first trimester | http://www.nhs.uk/conditions/Phenylketonuria/ |
| Hypertension | Review hypertensive medication as it may influence fetal development<br>Refer to medical team | Robson & Waugh 2008 |
| Systemic lupus erythematosus (SLE) | Pregnancy is not advised in women with active nervous system involvement<br>Control associated kidney disease for 6 months prior to conception<br>Use barrier contraceptive methods during these 6 months<br>Refer to physician and specialist clinics | http://www.nhs.uk/conditions/Lupus/Pages/Introduction.aspx |
| Thyroid conditions | Surveillance of thyroid function required<br>Refer to medical team | Robson & Waugh 2008 |
| Multiple sclerosis | Does not appear to increase obstetric complications<br>Refer to support organizations for specialist needs and advice | http://www.nhs.uk/conditions/Multiple-sclerosis/Pages/Introduction.aspx<br>http://www.mssociety.org.uk/ |
| Cancer | Clients or partners receiving chemotherapy or treatments affecting spermatogenesis or oogenesis should seek advice on storing sperm and ova<br>Should have a cervical smear prior to conception<br>Cancer has different outcomes in pregnancy, so it is important to seek early advice prior to conception<br>In some instances, delay of conception may be advised to enable treatment of cancer to commence | Grady 2006<br>Sood et al 2000 |

**Table 20.4 Genetics: preconception care, advice and further reading**

| | Information and advice | Further information |
|---|---|---|
| Cystic fibrosis | Lung function determines severity of maternal outcome during pregnancy<br>Refer to dedicated cystic fibrosis team including obstetricians | Edenborough et al 2000<br>http://www.cysticfibrosis.co.uk |
| Sickle cell anaemia | Refer to specialist team | http://www.sicklecellsociety.org<br>Villers et al 2008 |
| Thalassaemia | Detection of carrier status<br>Genetic counselling<br>Referral into the healthcare system early in pregnancy | Sickle cell and thalassaemia support project |
| Tay–Sachs disease | A fatal genetic disorder that destroys the central nervous system<br>Autosomal recessive disorder<br>Send woman and partner for genetic screening prior to conception<br>Referral to genetic counsellor | http://www.ntsad.org/ |

on diagnosis and treatment during pregnancy rather than prevention before pregnancy (Harper 2004).

## ENVIRONMENT AND LIFESTYLE

The environment and individual lifestyles influence development of our children, not only during childhood but also during the period of organogenesis (Table 20.5). Stereotypical ideas of social class are now merging, making it difficult to determine the lifestyle of specific groups, as drinking, smoking and drug addiction cross all social barriers. The effect of some drugs on conception and organogenesis was first identified following the administration of thalidomide in the 1960s as a treatment for morning sickness, and as new drugs appear on the market the impact on the next generation of children has yet to be recognized.

The preconception history must include an assessment of risks associated with employment, exercise, drug consumption and smoking, plus questions on physical abuse, use of alternative therapies and exposure to toxic substances. It is important not to make assumptions about individuals but to ask detailed questions to secure a full and detailed history.

## REPRODUCTIVE SEXUAL HEALTH

Barrier methods of contraception are recommended during the preparation phase for pregnancy. These are non-invasive methods with no direct influence on the body or conception. The morning-after pill is not discussed here as its function is to terminate pregnancy rather than promote it (see Ch. 27). However, preconception care advice should be included in the packaging for distribution to women (Table 20.6).

## DISABILITY

The term disability covers an extensive range of physical and mental conditions and abilities. Because the variety and scope of clients' ability is so varied, it is necessary to refer women to appropriate specialists as early as possible prior to pregnancy, so that effective screening and care management can occur (see Table 20.7).

## MIDWIFERY AND OBSTETRIC ASPECTS

A poor obstetric or midwifery history alerts the midwife to potential problems in a subsequent pregnancy; therefore, it is essential to obtain a full obstetric and midwifery history when discussing preconception care (Table 20.8).

## CONCLUSION

The relevance of preconception care to the health of future generations still remains a minor component of health promotion, even though the impact could increase the health potential of children, both in the short and long term. Improving the health of prospective parents in turn,

**Table 20.5 Environment and lifestyle: preconception care, advice and further reading**

| | Information and advice | Further information |
|---|---|---|
| Employment | Advice varies with type of employment<br>Risk assessment to protect from occupational hazards<br>Access health and safety policies at work for information on preconception and pregnancy-related issues<br>Should avoid jobs which involve:<br>– vibrating machines<br>– toxic substances<br>– excessive cold or heat<br>– heavy lifting<br>– long travelling times<br>Advise to discuss any concerns with employer<br>Remember to enquire about partner's employment | |
| Stress | Avoidance of severe stress during the period of organogenesis<br>Refer to psychologist, GP, employer's occupational health department or other relevant organizations | |
| Exercise | Do not take up new exercise when pregnant; take it up before pregnancy and maintain<br>Avoid contact sports, such as kickboxing, and sports that increase core body temperature, as these are associated with spontaneous abortion<br>Avoid hot saunas, steam rooms and spas that increase core body temperature | Heffernan 2000 |
| Smoking | Reduces sperm count in men<br>Both partners should stop smoking 4 months prior to conception as cigarettes produce carbon monoxide and nicotine, reducing oxygen supply to the fetus, causing vasoconstriction of spiral arterioles in the placenta<br>Refer to support groups<br>Advise to keep away from smoky environments | NHS Smoking Helpline: 0800 169 0169<br>http://smokefree.nhs.uk/smoking-and-pregnancy/ |
| Alcohol | Alcohol crosses the placenta, being metabolized by the fetus once liver enzymes mature in the second half of pregnancy; is toxic in early pregnancy<br>Decreases sperm count, motility of sperm and causes sperm malformations<br>Is a testicular toxin resulting in poor sperm production, abnormal sperm cells, sterility and impotence<br>Abstain from consumption of alcohol for at least 4 months prior to conception<br>Discourage 'binge' drinking particularly during organogenesis | Krulewitch 2005 |
| Drugs (social and prescribed) | Increased risk of structural anomalies during organogenesis, such as in the heart and great vessels, digestive system and musculoskeletal system<br>Parents may not wish to disclose information<br>May need to cease administration, reduce intake or supplement with less hazardous substitutes<br>Refer to specialist practitioners | Floyd et al 2008 |
| Alternative therapies | Therapies that include administration of herbal remedies require careful monitoring of type and quantity. Treatment should be prescribed by a registered therapist, and therefore care should be taken when self-prescribing (see Ch. 18) | http://www.grcct.org/ |

**Table 20.5 Continued**

| | Information and advice | Further information |
|---|---|---|
| Violence against women | Advise women on support services<br>Refer parents to support organizations such as Relate | Saunders 2000 |
| Pets | Special precautions should be taken when handling pets, their feeding bowls or excrement. Direct contact is not necessary as cross-infection can occur from the handler to another person or through pet equipment<br>Toxoplasmosis is transmitted through cat faeces<br>Advise to avoid contact with reptiles as 9 out of 10 carry *Salmonella*<br>Salmonella from birds, insects, mammals and reptiles can result in meningitis or septicaemia<br>*Escherichia coli* may result in food poisoning and fetal death | |
| Hazardous substances | Recommend organically grown foods<br>All foods should be thoroughly washed<br>Farmers should reduce contact with pesticides or insecticides<br>Avoid using garden insecticides, touching pet flea collars, and anti-lice shampoos | (for all entries in this section) http://www.foresight-preconception.org.uk/books_literaturesummaries.htm |
| Solvents | Found in a variety of occupations, such as printing, dry cleaning, painting, leather industries, anaesthetics, gardening, pharmaceutics and housework<br>Limit work with solvents | |
| Lead | Comes from exhaust fumes, soil, food, drinking water, lead cooking utensils<br>Wearing of protective clothing at work if in contact<br>Mineral analysis prior to conception<br>Filter water and avoid lead cooking equipment<br>High levels of lead in men linked to infertility<br>Lead moves from maternal bones to the fetus during pregnancy | |
| Cadmium | Reduce contact with cigarette smoke, plumbing alloys, paint, batteries, fertilizers<br>Filter water<br>High levels of cadmium in men are linked to infertility<br>Reduce smoking and alcohol intake as both activities increase cadmium levels<br>Mineral analysis prior to conception | |
| Zinc | Found in red meat, cereals, cheese and nuts<br>Levels reduced in alcohol drinkers<br>Low levels related to infertility in men<br>Mineral analysis prior to conception | |
| Aluminium | Derives from kitchen utensils, some foods cooked in aluminium pans, particularly apple and rhubarb, antacids and kitchen foil<br>Filter water<br>Replace kitchenware with stainless steel, enamel or glass<br>Advise mineral analysis prior to conception | |
| Mercury | Derives from tinned tuna, weed killers and dental amalgam; therefore dental treatment should be undertaken prior to conception or involve non-mercury-based amalgam<br>Filter water<br>Advise mineral analysis prior to conception | |

**Table 20.6 Reproductive sexual health: preconception care, advice and further reading**

| | Information and advice | Further information |
|---|---|---|
| Oral contraception | (see Ch. 27)<br>Cease administration 3 months before conception. Use alternative barrier methods, enabling the body to regulate hormones prior to conception and increase mineral stores such as copper and zinc<br>Reduces zinc, manganese and vitamins A and B | |

**Table 20.7 Disability: preconception care, advice and further reading**

| | Information and advice | Further information |
|---|---|---|
| Disability | Refer to specialist organizations<br>Refer to members of the multi-professional team<br>Vary depending on the type of disability | http://www.disabledparentsnetwork.org.uk/ |
| Mental health | Some drugs lead to birth defects; for example, diazepam causes congenital malformations if taken during first trimester<br>Refer to psychiatrist/GP | Frieder et al 2008 |

**Table 20.8 Midwifery and obstetric aspects: preconception care, advice and further reading**

| | Information and advice | Further information |
|---|---|---|
| Poor obstetric history | Need to know what occurred previously to manage preconception care appropriately<br>This depends on the type of obstetric incident<br>Refer to midwife or specialist obstetrician to review previous case(s) or advise on care in pregnancy | See relevant chapters within this book |

influences the health of their children and grandchildren. What appears insignificant information in one generation may have a compounding impact in the next. By informing prospective parents of their health status, information such as sickle cell status can be documented and used to inform other family members or partners. Any healthcare activity should involve aspects of preconception care and include both partners, taking account of the diverse nature of society, human actions and the environment. Preconception care involves a team approach including any health professional offering specialist advice. As preconception care involves such diverse issues it is impossible to include detailed information within this chapter. You are, therefore, reminded to access other relevant sources, review new evidence as it is published, and access your local preconception facilities, so that you can actively inform women of the local services available.

## KEY POINTS

- Preconception care enhances and informs the health of prospective parents, creating the best possible environment at the point of conception.
- Opportunities exist in any healthcare encounter for healthcare professionals to offer preconception advice.
- Midwives need to have access to information on preconception care to be able to offer advice to parents, evaluate the potential outcome of pregnancy and refer to other specialists, such as medical practitioners, diabetic liaison, psychologists, sexual health practitioners or physiotherapists.

## REFERENCES


Azam A, Vial Y, Fowler C, et al: Prenatal diagnosis of congenital cytomegalovirus infection, *Obstetrics and Gynecology* 97(3):443–448, 2001.

Bothamley D: Tuberculosis in pregnancy: the role for midwives in diagnosis and treatment, *British Journal of Midwifery* 10(4):182–185, 2006.

Cuco G, Fernandez-Ballart J, Sala J, et al: Dietary patterns and associated lifestyles in preconception, pregnancy and postpartum, *European Journal of Clinical Nutrition* 60(3):364–371, 2006.

Department of Health (DH): *Coronary heart disease: national service framework for coronary heart disease: modern standards and service models*, London, 2000, DH.

Dolan S, Biermann J, Damus K: Genomics for health in preconception and prenatal periods, *Journal of Nursing Scholarship* 39(1):4–9, 2007.

Edenborough F, Mackenzie W, Stableforth D: The outcome of 72 pregnancies in 55 women with cystic fibrosis in the United Kingdom 1977–1996, *British Journal of Obstetrics and Gynaecology* 107(2):254–261, 2000.

Floyd L, Jack B, Cefalo R, et al: The clinical content of preconception care: alcohol, tobacco, and illicit drug exposures, *American Journal of Obstetrics and Gynecology* 199(6 Suppl 2):S333–S339, 2008.

Frieder A, Dunlop A, Culpepper L, et al: The clinical content of preconception care: women with psychiatric conditions, *American Journal of Obstetrics and Gynecology* 199(6 Suppl 2):S328–S332, 2008.

Galtier-Dereure F, Boegner C, Bringer J: Obesity and pregnancy: complications and cost, *American Journal of Clinical Nutrition* 71(5 Suppl):1242S–1248S, 2000.

Grady M: Preconception and the young cancer survivor, *Maternal and Child Health Journal* 10(5):s165–s168, 2006.

Harper PS: *Practical genetic counselling*, ed 6, London, 2004, Arnold Publications.

Heffernan A: Exercise and pregnancy in primary care, *Nurse Practitioner* 25(3):42–56, 2000.

Kendrick J: Preconception care of women with diabetes, *Journal of Perinatal and Neonatal Nursing* 18(1):10–27, 2004.

Kierman L: Family planning services: an essential component of preconception care, *Maternal and Child Health Journal* 10(5):s157–s160, 2006.

Krulewitch C: Alcohol consumption during pregnancy, *Annual Review of Nursing Research* 23:101–134, 2005.

Lumley J, Watson L, Watson M, et al: *Periconceptional supplementation with folate and/or multivitamins to prevent neural tube defects, The Cochrane Library*, Issue 1, Oxford, 2000, Update Software.

McElvy S, Miodovnik M, Rosenn B, et al: A focused preconceptional and early pregnancy programme in women with type 1 diabetes reduces perinatal mortality and malformation rates to general population levels, *Journal of Maternal–Fetal Medicine* 9(1):10–13, 2000.

Morgan-Capner P, Crowcroft N: Guidance on the management of, and exposure to, rash illness in pregnancy. Report of the Public Health Laboratory Services Working Group (website). www.hpa.org.uk/HPA/Topics/InfectiousDiseases/InfectionsAZ/1200577813065. 2000. Accessed December 8, 2009.

Reifsnider E, Gill S: Nutrition for the childbearing years, *Journal of Obstetric, Gynecologic and Neonatal Nursing* 29(1):43–55, 2000.

Robson S, Waugh J: *Medical disorders in pregnancy: a manual for midwives*, London, 2008, Wiley Blackwell.

Saunders E: Screening for domestic violence during pregnancy, *International Journal of Trauma Nursing* 6(2):44–47, 2000.

Siega-Riz A, Haugen M, Meitzer H, et al: Nutrient and food group intakes of women with and without bulimia nervosa and binge eating disorders during pregnancy, *American Journal of Clinical Nutrition* 87(5):1346–1355, 2008.

Sood A, Sorosky J, Mayr N, et al: Cervical cancer diagnosed shortly after pregnancy: prognostic variables and delivery routes, *Obstetrics and Gynecology* 95(6 Pt 1):832–838, 2000.

Turner A: Causes, prevention and treatment of toxoplasmosis, *British Journal of Midwifery* 8(11):722, 2000.

Villers M, Jamison M, De Castro L, et al: Morbidity associated with sickle cell disease in pregnancy, *American Journal of Obstetrics and Gynecology* 199(2):125e1–125e5, 2008.

Chapter |21|

# Education for parenthood

Tandy Deane-Gray

## LEARNING OUTCOMES

After reading this chapter, you will be able to:

- analyse the significant needs of parents in their transition to parenthood, so that classes and activities can be focused to enable them to feel more prepared
- explore methods of integrating and facilitating parenting skills into programmes and other activities delivered to parents, so that they may be more prepared for the emotional impact of having a baby
- outline the current government initiatives that influence the provision of parent education
- practise appropriately in the delivery of parent education and leading of groups.

*'Pregnancy and the first years of life are one of the most important stages in the life cycle. This is when the foundations of future health and wellbeing are laid down, and is a time when parents are particularly receptive to learning and making changes. There is good evidence that the outcomes for both children and adults are strongly influenced by the factors that operate during pregnancy and the first years of life. We have always known this, but new information about neurological development and the impact of stress in pregnancy, and further recognition of the importance of attachment, all make early intervention and prevention an imperative.'*

(DH 2008a:6)

## WHAT COULD THE FOCUS BE FOR PARENTHOOD EDUCATION?

Education for parenthood should be seen as part of a lifelong journey, and as a means of helping parents acquire understanding of their own social, emotional and psychological needs and those of their infants (Smith 1997). Parenting programmes form part of the early intervention services that promote positive perinatal outcomes (DH 2008a). These support the transition to parenthood particularly for new parents, in preparing them for their new roles and responsibilities. Specifically, they include enhancement of the parent–infant relationship and relationships within the family, as well as problem-solving skills, and encourage families to identify and take advantage of supportive networks within local communities (DH 2008a, Smith 1997).

'Traditional' parenthood education classes can and do help parents to form social networks, as they may meet others in similar circumstances. However, the focus for healthcare providers and voluntary organizations is often, in general, preparation for birth; concentrating on the physical aspects of pregnancy and possible care of the baby (Crisp 1994). Classes are often provided for women only, yet Lloyd (1999) suggests it is more effective to work with both parents. Unfortunately, as Nolan's (2005) critical review of the literature points out, it is difficult to draw any conclusions as to the effectiveness of classes, as the quality of the research is flawed, although parents do seem to enjoy them.

Parents-to-be themselves concentrate on the physical aspects of pregnancy and managing practical aspects, such as work and childcare. The psychological impact of impending parenthood is given little or no attention (Barnes & Balber 2007). Consequently, parents complain that they are unprepared for the emotional impact of having a baby (Woollett & Parr 1997). The Child Health Promotion Programme (CHPP) (DH 2008a) is urging progression in education for parenthood to services which are evidence based and promote the health and wellbeing of children. This chapter will help practitioners to refocus their programmes to provide education for parenthood, promoting some features that will form a successful programme.

## WHAT ARE PARENTS' NEEDS?

Often, formal parenting sessions have been designed around what professionals **think** women and their partners need to know (Nolan 2005). When parents are asked where they obtained their information, it is either by reading, watching television or talking to friends and family. Antenatal classes are often viewed as inaccessible (particularly for fathers or other partners), or do not include parenting. When it is addressed, it is viewed as impractical or unrealistic by parents (Coombes & Schonveld 1992, Deave & Johnson 2008, Wilkins 2006). In some areas, access to antenatal/parenting courses has been reduced or even made unavailable.

Studies investigating the needs of new parents postnatally suggest they would have liked to have been more prepared for the changing relationship between their partner and themselves (Deave & Johnson 2007) (Box 21.1, Fig. 21.1).

Parents find that their established routines are thrown into confusion, so there is a need to develop coping skills (Wilkins 2006). Fathers have great difficulty in finding a

**Box 21.1 What do parents need to address in education for parenthood groups?**

- The psychological, social and emotional changes for themselves and their infants
- The changing relationship between the couple and incorporating their baby
- Self-knowledge and problem-solving skills
- Developing attachment and sensitive responsiveness to infants
- Practical aspects of baby care
- Postnatal issues

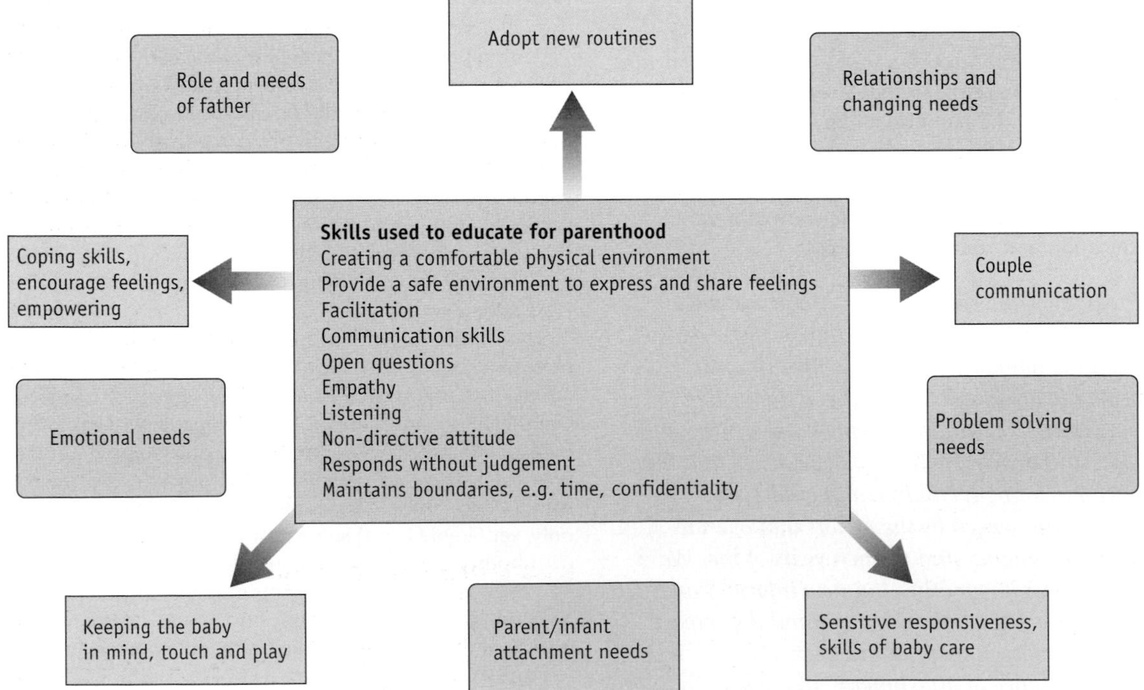


**Figure 21.1** Supporting the transition to parenthood: skills used to facilitate development in the tasks of parenthood, so parents can meet their own needs.

role, and classes do not always focus on their perspective, resulting in feelings of helplessness and isolation (Deave & Johnson 2007, World Health Organization 2007). Additionally, it is more effective to work with both parents, not just mothers (Lloyd 1999). Nolan (1997) also found antenatal classes were often deficient in covering postnatal issues and parents also wanted practical aspects of baby care included. It is also important to be aware of different family patterns, and their particular needs, such as lesbian mothers and their partners (RCM 2000).

In addition to the needs of parents, the Child Health Promotion Programme (CHPP) (DH 2008a) report asks that professionals empower parents through a focus on their strengths and promotion of self-knowledge. This recognizes their expertise in personal self-knowledge and knowledge of their new infant, with finally promotion of their attachment, which encourages empathy and sensitive responsiveness towards their infant. This attunement to infants and development of attachment leads to loved and loving individuals, who do not become antisocial individuals. The Worldwide Alternatives to Violence (WAVE) Trust report (WAVE Trust 2005) summarizes the importance of this intervention and outlines the brain development that can be impaired when parenting is not good enough. As such, this also promotes the mental wellbeing of future generations, one of the goals of the Darzi report (DH 2008b).

The CHPP (DH 2008a) cites several programmes that seem to meet both the needs of parents and the government recommendations in promoting attachment, the only one in the antenatal period being *First steps in parenting* (Parr 1996, 1998, Parr & Joyce 2009). Probably the most important determinant of programmes such as this, is the quality and skills of the practitioners who deliver them. It is imperative that midwives learn group work skills, how to facilitate rather than teach, and develop the ability to communicate with sensitive responsiveness (Deane-Gray 2008). This investment in practitioners has been demonstrated as making a considerable difference when working with new parents (Douglas & Brennan 2004).

## PARENT EDUCATION AND GROUP WORK

Group facilitation is not generally part of pre-registration midwifery programmes, though some students learn presentation and seminar skills. Consequently, the style often adopted in classes can be directive, with a high level of 'teacher' input and a low level of acceptance of ideas, behaviours and feelings. Closed questions are often used, which do not invite discussion or sharing of feelings, and so parents' responses become restricted (Underdown 1998). This suggests that assessment of the amount the 'leader' speaks in relation to the group members is a useful indicator as to how successful the leader is in facilitating and encouraging group interaction when delivering parent education.

### Effective facilitation

Ockenden (2002) suggest that facilitators listen first and then consider informing. Listening involves noticing and reflecting on the message underlying the question asked (Deane-Gray 2008). What are the parents really asking? For example, 'What would you suggest for backache?', may really be a concern that the pregnancy is normal, or they want someone to hear how uncomfortable they are feeling and are looking for some sympathy. On the other hand, they may be seeking coping strategies as sleep is disturbed and additional work pressures are causing anxiety (Ockenden 2002). Giving an anatomical explanation or stating that back pain is normal would be a reply that missed the interpersonal cues of parents, and thus the answer provided would be one-dimensional. Part of facilitation is effective communication. In observing a group, the skill of the facilitator in listening can be ascertained by how questions are answered – sometimes by another question. An example might be managed further, by the facilitator responding to the question about backache, through asking another question, such as: 'What is it that worries you about your backache?' or a statement that invites the parents to talk, such as: 'Tell me more', or one that opens it to the group: 'Is this a concern for others here?' Indeed, effective communication and supporting transitions are two of the basic areas of expertise required for those working with children and their families as outlined in *Every child matters* (DfES 2005). The skills of group facilitation and the factors that contribute to successful groups cannot be addressed in detail in such a short chapter. Please look at the resources and recommended reading on the website for more on groups and skills to encourage interactive learning.

Group-based parenting programmes that are interactive in learning have been suggested to be most effective in supporting parents (Lloyd 1999). Parents value the interaction of sharing the recent experiences of other expectant and new parents (Wilkins 2006). Group discussions enable parents to understand that their feelings are normal and an effective group can be a strong source of non-stigmatizing support which increases parents' confidence in their own ideas and abilities.

### Learning environment

In order for parents to approach a task with confidence, it is essential that the physical and psychological climate be comfortable, so they feel enabled to direct their own learning, which is one of Knowles' (1990) assumptions of adult learners (Box 21.2). The midwife needs to create and control the environment that assists prospective parents to

**Box 21.2 Assumptions of adult learners**

- Adults are self-directed in their learning and need to be responsible for their own decisions
- Adults have experiences of life which represent the richest resource for learning. They build on personal experience
- Adults are problem-centred rather than topic-centred in the acquisition of knowledge, they need to know why they need to learn
- Adults have a readiness to learn things that help them cope effectively with life situations and the developmental tasks of their social roles
- Adults are motivated to learn when they perceive that it will help them perform tasks they confront in their life situations

(Based on Knowles 1990:57)

direct their learning by negotiating and agree the aims and agenda of the course together with the group. Knowles (1990) also suggests as adult learners their learning is grounded in personal experience. They can build on their experiences as they orientate their learning towards the development of new tasks in their adaptation to new social roles of being parents. To facilitate this learning, it is useful to note that adults are self-motivated and have a problem-centred approach as opposed to a subject-centred approach to the acquisition of information (Knowles 1990). Using this model, the midwife (facilitator) cannot claim full control but is a joint 'shareholder' with the learner. The facilitator needs to adopt a non-directive role that aims to 'make it possible (through an enabling process) for another person to achieve goals' (Craddock 1993). This is what is truly meant by facilitation.

Empowering is enabling parents such that they feel they lead the discussion; this gives a sense of ownership that usually leaves them feeling better equipped to make the many decisions new parenthood brings (Fig. 21.2). Wickham & Davis (2005) suggest that a more empowering approach to education for parenthood can be achieved through empowering midwives. In particular, they give examples of experiential exercises to help student midwives realize how they can manage groups. They argue that practitioners prepared in this way, are able to empower parents to feel central and in control of their own experience.

The skill in preparing a session is providing experiences that engage parents, building on their experiences. However, before undertaking any form of facilitation, the facilitator must have a depth and breadth of understanding of the subject. In planning and preparing a session, the information needs to be current. This requires a literature search prior to teaching, and perhaps discussion with colleagues. The skill then is in the presentation, trusting that the method chosen will engage the parents, cover the key issues and empower them. It is also important to reflect on the session, incorporating an evaluation of both the 'performance' and the achievement of the group outcomes, in order to validate what has worked well and what requires further development for the future (Nolan 2002). Using practical activities, such as group work, discussion and experiential activities, keeps the group active and assists in meaningful learning. It is well known that adults learn most effectively by experience, perhaps best summed up by Confucius:

*I hear I forget*
*I see I remember*
*I do I understand*

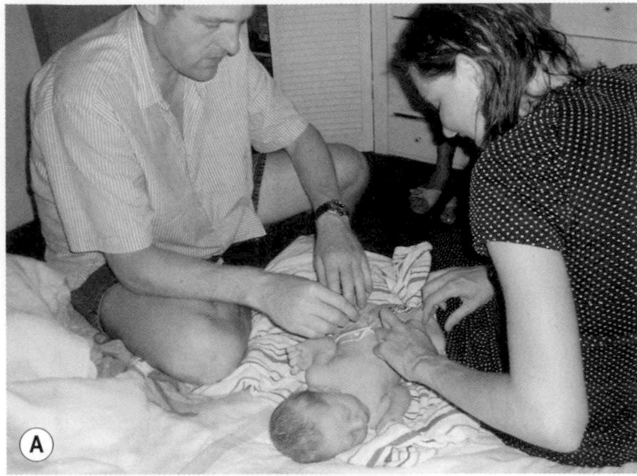


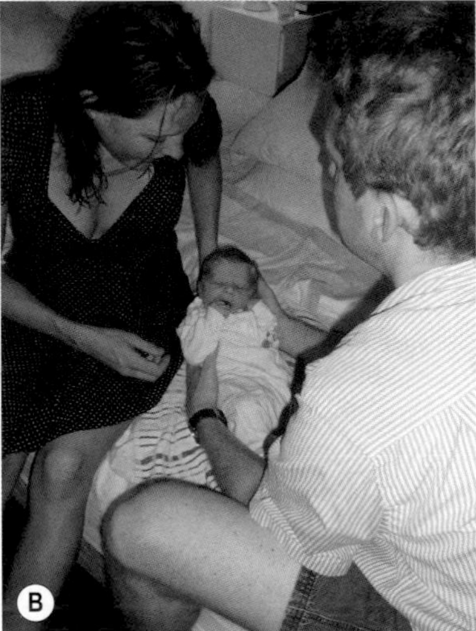


**Figure 21.2** An example of empowerment – parents dress their newly born infant themselves.

**Box 21.3 Session plan: aims and objectives**

**Session A**

Aim

To instil confidence in couples in their ability to cope with the pain of labour

Objectives

- To explore the parents' past experience and knowledge of pain and pain management
- To help couples communicate their different needs and emotions, and develop coping and problem-solving skills together
- To enable partners to participate in effective support for labour

**Session B**

Aim

To provide information about the methods of pain relief

Objectives

- The parents will know the advantages and disadvantages of the various methods of pain relief, both pharmacological and physiological
- The parents will practise alternative positions for back pain
- Parents will have explored/discussed the various ways they can cope with pain by using such strategies as water or massage

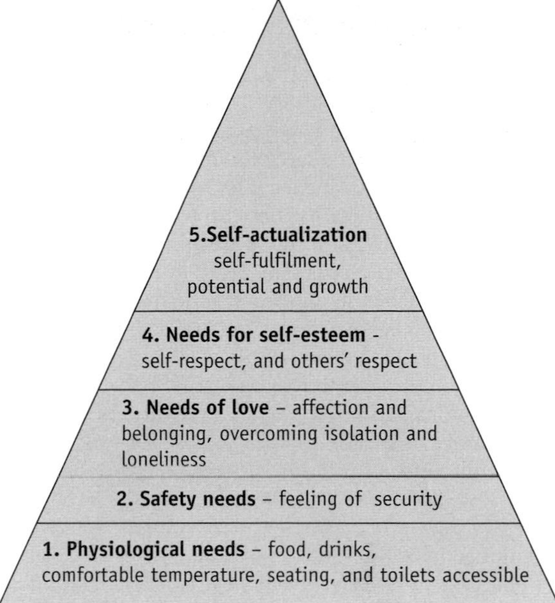


**Figure 21.3** Maslow's (1943) hierarchy of needs.

**Reflective activity 21.1**

Consider a topic that parents are likely to want to discuss, such as pain relief. Outline for yourself what content you would want to include and what you think parents might need. Compare your thoughts with the session suggested in Box 21.3, including your aims, objectives, content, and adult learning methods.

As there is limited time and resources to provide parenting as well as childbirth preparation (which parents expect when they attend classes), it is proposed that childbirth topics are used as a 'hanger' onto which parenting is included. The session outlined in the website (see website for Web Figure 21.2) is an example of how the aspects discussed thus far in the chapter (see Figure 21.1) might be included in a session on pain relief. The comments are expansions on the content and process, based on the experience of several groups.

Planning is crucial to providing a successful session. It is useful to develop a session plan, including aims (that is, what the general purpose of the session is) and objectives (what the participants will be able to do/understand after the session) (Priest & Schott 1991). Compare the two sessions of aims and objectives in Box 21.3 with your session plan. (See website for session plan template.)

In Box 21.3, Session B is a more traditional session, whereas Session A has more potential to empower and help couples make decisions together; more likely to explore ideas, behaviours and feelings; and help fathers explore their role. However, fathers are more likely to be able to do this if the session encourages the same gender talking to each other, as their needs differ (Parr 1996).

In order to structure your session so that it is interactive and participative, it is useful to draw upon the theories of group 'life'. Groups need nurturing, as all individuals need to feel safe before they can expose themselves and be open to participating in a group.

**Reflective activity 21.2**

Personally reflect on a time when you felt comfortable in new group and a time when you felt uncomfortable in a group. What makes a group safe to participate and engage in?

## GROUP DYNAMICS AND THE LIFE CYCLE OF GROUPS

Feelings of warmth and welcoming, respect and trust for each other, not being judged, finding a friend, knowing the environment, knowing the rules, and refreshments; are the answers other students come up with from Reflective activity 21.2. All of these answers are mirrored in Maslow's (1943) hierarchy of needs (Fig. 21.3), as people yearn for order and predictability in their world. The physiological needs are the strongest needs because if a person were deprived of all needs, these must come first; as each level is satisfied, then they can move potentially to the next level.

The Stanford and Roark model of the process of groups may be a useful structure for you to use for your classes, as it begins with a warm-up, proceeds to a middle work phase and ends with integration (Edwards & Nichols 2000). In the warm-up phase the parents disengage from previous activities and tune in to the new situation. There are many warm-up exercises that can be used (Brandes & Norris 1998) to help the group to get to know each other in a non-threatening way. Fundamentally every session should embrace the concept of Maslow's (1943) hierarchy of needs. So things that instil safety and trust in a group, such as the forming of ground rules, are useful here. These can be formed initially by asking the parents to state what they need to feel safe in this group.

Earlier it was suggested that parenting programmes need to embrace the promotion of attachment theory. The beginning of a group is an ideal time to use parents' experiences, to draw out the needs of babies. Compare for yourself Figure 21.3 and Box 21.4. The feelings that a parent instils in their baby for emotional development are similar to those they themselves want from a group to feel safe. It is possible to discuss this with the group and so highlight that a baby as a person has needs of safety in their family group.

### Box 21.4 **Emotional regulation and needs of infants**

- Observer who *listens* and sees their strengths and helps them with their difficulties
- Warm and responsive interactions with caretakers. The mothers' task is to respond *empathetically* – to mind read. Baby has no control or bad intent, they learn they can self regulate through maternal containment. They then learn to soothe the self, for example, by sucking.
- Structure and routine, but flexible, that give boundaries. Providing psychological and physical holding, holding also relieves anxiety – they feel held together.
- Maintains interest by providing things to look at and do through play and touch, but in tune e.g. recognise a yawn means 'leave me to sleep'.
- Vocalisation reinforced by response-dialogue. Hearing and being heard – respond to parent voice, familiar gives sense of security, and babies need to hear talking to develop speech.

(Drawn from Paavola 2006, DfES 2005, Wave Trust 2005)

### Reflective activity 21.3

Observe the facilitation of three different groups of Parent Education.

Note how the facilitators encourage group participation, and measure the ratio of time parents and facilitators speak. Did the parents get to say how they feel? Was everyone included? Were the worries and concerns elicited?

Reflect on the skills of the facilitator, and the factors that could impact on running a successful group.

## Groups

The age, gender, economic circumstances and ethnicity of individuals who comprise the group need to be considered, and it can be useful to encourage the same gender to talk to each other, as their needs differ (Parr 1996).

Setting priorities without being biased about what you think they need to know (and feeling you must tell them all of it) is often difficult, but the learning is ultimately the responsibility of the parents, which is in line with Knowles' (1990) assumptions of adult learners. The *warm-up phase* can include finding out what the group want to cover and what their expectations and fears might be. The group can be set 'homework' with activities such as watching a video in advance of the group to help direct the parents' learning.

The *work phase* is where learning takes place and the parents focus on the task. During this phase, the topics to be covered during a session need to be structured by the leader, but agreed with the group. Group size may influence the choice of activity, but dividing the group into pairs enables parents to work with different people. This allows them to explore other views and work with all the members of the group (Rolls 1992).

The last phase, the *integration phase*, requires reflection on personal meaning, integrating the understanding, significance and usefulness of the session for the future. This phase is more than the end of the session. It is the achievement phase for the parents. The facilitator encourages and validates learning by giving feedback on aspects of performance and correction of misconceptions.

## Facilitation of the group

Your facilitation and structure will help promote the non-threatening atmosphere and comfort of the group. When you consider what helps or hinders the contribution of individuals in learning groups, the environment, as discussed, needs to be warm and receptive. But also when 'warming up' to a topic, it takes time to let go of the cares of the day. So give time for the topic to sink in by repeating instructions several times and allow the individual silence with space for their own thoughts first. Remember when you ask a small child a complex question they often will take quite some time before they respond.

Returning to the original topic of a session on pain relief, a possible warm-up exercise could be a discussion or a quiz. This can be assisted by a self-reflection exercise of asking individuals to think about the most painful experiences they have had.

### Discussion groups

To help people begin a discussion, it is always helpful to get them to share initially with the person next to them. To build on experience and encourage discussion on pain relief, ask same-sex pairs (not couples) to talk about pain they have experienced in their lives. This helps focus on the purpose of pain, their normal reaction and beliefs about pain, and how they cope with pain. After they have discussed with one person, you can invite a group discussion by possibly using some of the questions below to raise more issues for the group. But remember to facilitate, by summarizing and moving the topic on by asking others if their experience is similar or different.

- What did you notice about your discussion together?
- What is your reaction to another's pain, such as headache?
- What do you want to do if someone is crying?
- What does pain mean to you?
- What makes it easier or seem more painful?
- What do you imagine labour is like for the baby?

Printing some pictures from the internet on pain and labour and asking the parents to pick one up and then discuss the picture with a same-sex person is an alternative way of engaging interest.

This approach may suggest that the session leader is not providing information, which parents may want, and it is useful to reflect on the following:

- Can you ask parents to come prepared to discuss pain relief?
- How do people who never attend a class cope?
- Do you discuss a birth plan with women?
- Where do parents get information?

As discussed earlier, midwives are not the sole source of information for parents. Giving information in advance of the group session, by offering the loan of a book or video, or asking parents to do 'homework' of reading about a topic will often be a good way of directing the parents' learning and may save some time. Setting priorities without being biased about what **you** think they need to know (and feeling you must tell them all of it) is often difficult, but learning is ultimately the responsibility of the parents, which is in line with Knowles' (1990) assumptions of adult learners.

### Quiz

A fun set of questions can act as an icebreaker. Stocktaking worksheets can provide a starter for discussion. For example, to begin a discussion on pain relief, a list of questions on the facts, feelings and myths can be posed, then responses shared with other members of the group.

## Work phase of group 'life'

Using the phases of groups can help structure the sessions and aid your management as a facilitator. For the parents it forms a 'holding' which leads to greater cooperation of groups. This work phase focuses attention on the group, providing a bridge between 'job' and group. This is where learning takes place and the parents focus on the task. During this phase, topics to be covered during a session need to be structured by the leader, but agreed with the group. This work phase of the session incorporates the teaching plan, which includes a good structure and examination of the events occurring during learning (Frederick 2000). Group size may influence the choice of activity, but dividing the group into smaller groups enables parents to work with different people. This allows them to explore other views and work with all the members of the group (Rolls 1992). Instructions may need repeating two or three times as it helps people to internalize what is asked of them. Parents should be organized as required for the exercise chosen and understanding checked before they begin the exercise. Before moving on, the facilitator should ensure that individuals in the group have completed the exercise to their satisfaction. This will provide a link to the next piece of work, or to an evaluation.

Following Knowles' (1990) assumptions for adult learners, the methods chosen to facilitate learning in this phase could use problem solving and focus on decision making. This will also help the couple's relationship. Two suggested approaches are detailed below.

### Stories and scenarios

These are used as case studies and the facilitator can build up a fictitious 'library'. Parts of the story are distributed and the parents are asked to discuss the circumstances – for example, early labour beginning while out shopping together. When they have discussed the situation fully, the next part of the story is given. Here you can have fun and give different outcomes to different groups, so one progresses quickly and finds themselves going to the nearest hospital, while another goes home to feed the dog. This helps parents to consider realistic situations, test ideas and explore attitudes as to when and if they require pain relief.

### Problem solving

Realistic problems are posed for small groups of parents to solve. Examples of topics are:

- 'You arrive at the delivery suite after labouring at home for 12 hours, and are told you are in early labour. What do you do?'
- 'You enter the pool and find you do not like it. What do you do?'
- 'Your mother comes with you in labour and says this is just the beginning and you should have an epidural. What will you do?'

This approach challenges and encourages self-direction and self-investigation of resources available.

## Integration phase of group 'life'

The last phase, integration, requires reflection on personal meaning, integrating the understanding, significance and usefulness of the session for the future. This phase is more than the end of the session. It is the achievement phase for the parents. The facilitator encourages and validates learning by giving feedback on aspects of performance and correction of misconceptions.

Couples can engage in a wind-down of the session, giving them time together to discuss what they will take away from the session (Box 21.5). The facilitator can ask for feedback, or simply ask couples to state a word that encompasses the session for them.

### Evaluating effectiveness

Writing the aims and objectives in a session plan will clarify the bigger picture of what might be achieved, however, it also important to ensure that the environment is prepared by being warm and inviting, seats placed in a circle rather than classroom style, and that there is a good range of equipment and resources to assist in the session. More information is available on the website.

Box 21.5 **What parents find helpful**

- Awareness of their attitude to pain
- Strategies to cope
  - Mental
  - Physical
- Partner role
- Help in decision making
- Sharing their feelings, fears

It is important to evaluate both individual sessions and the whole programme. The midwife can evaluate from her perspective, matching the group learning with the planned aims and objectives, but it is also important that the parents can express their views. This will enable a process of continual improvement.

## CONCLUSION

This chapter suggests that midwives should deliver parenting programmes that support the government agenda (DH 2008a). In order to meet this agenda and the needs of parents, these groups need focusing to promote parents' own understanding of their emotional, social and psychological transition to parenthood. The content of sessions needs to include changes in relationships, attachment and sensitive responsiveness towards infants as well as practical baby care. Promotion of problem-solving and decision-making skills prepares parents to manage and develop their coping skills in this major life transition, which in turn promotes self-knowledge and empowerment.

The skills midwives need to develop in order to enable and prepare parents and families are those of group work skills, facilitation, communication and empowerment. The determinants of success and quality in education for parenthood lie in midwives developing these skills. The midwife must also ensure that programmes integrate evidence-based knowledge, focus on parent needs and are delivered with an empowering philosophy enabling parents to feel more prepared for their new role.

### KEY POINTS

- Midwives are in a privileged position to support parents in their transition to early parenthood, providing education that can facilitate this more fully, particularly including needs of parents and promoting attachment through the parent/infant relationship.
- The Government has given parenting a high priority and this is congruent with the changing role of midwives in developing their public health role.
- Midwives need to fully develop their facilitation and group management skills to promote interaction and learning in groups.
- Groups require the leader to manage the balance between the building of the group and achievement of the task and this must be supported by the use of evidence-based practice and reflective skills.
- Good facilitation and group work will usually promote effective and meaningful learning and enable parents to access information, learn from a wide range of sources with other parents and develop their repertoire of life skills.

## REFERENCES


Barnes DL, Balber L: *The journey to parenthood: myths, reality and what really matters*, Oxford, 2007, Radcliffe Publishing.

Brandes D, Norris J: *The gamesters' handbook (1, 2 & 3)*, London, 1998, Nelson Thorn.

Coombes G, Schonveld D: *Life will never be the same again: a review of antenatal and postnatal education*, London, 1992, Health Education Authority.

Craddock E: Developing the facilitator role in the clinical areas, *Nurse Education Today* 13(3):217–224, 1993.

Crisp S: *Counting on families: social audit report on the provision of family support services*, London, 1994, Exploring Parenthood.

Deane-Gray T: Effective communication. In Peate I, Hamilton C, editors: *Becoming a midwife in the 21st century*, Sussex, 2008, John Wiley

Deave T, Johnson D: *The needs of parents in pregnancy and early parenthood, final report*, Bristol, 2007, Centre for Child and Adolescent Health and University of Bristol.

Deave T, Johnson D: *Transition to parenthood: the needs of parents in pregnancy and early parenthood*, Glasgow, 2008, International Confederation of Midwives 28th Triennial Congress.

Department for Education and Skills (DfES): *Common core of skills and knowledge for the children's workforce. Every child matters. Change for children*, London, 2005, HMSO.

Department of Health (DH): *The child health promotion programme, pregnancy and the first five years of life*, London, 2008a, HMSO.

Department of Health (DH): *High quality care for all, NHS next stage review final report (Prof Lord Darzi report)*, London, 2008b, HMSO.

Douglas H, Brennan A: Containment, reciprocity and behaviour management: preliminary evaluation of a brief early intervention (the Solihull approach) for families with infants and young children, *International Journal of Infant Observation* 7(1):89–107, 2004.

Edwards M, Nichols F: Group process. In Nichols F, Smith-Humenick S, editors: *Childbirth education: practice, research, and theory*, Philadephia, 2000, WB Saunders.

Frederick A: The teaching–learning process. In Nichols F, Smith-Humenick S, editors: *Childbirth education: practice, research, and theory*, Philadelphia, 2000, WB Saunders.

Knowles M: *The adult learner: a neglected species*, ed 4, Houston, 1990, Gulf Publications.

Lloyd E: *What works in parenting education?* London, 1999, Policy & Research Unit Barnardos.

Maslow AH: A theory of human motivation, *Psychological Review* 50(4):370–396, 1943.

Nolan M: Antenatal education: failing to educate for parenthood, *British Journal of Midwifery* 5(1):21–26, 1997.

Nolan M: Evaluating parent education. In Nolan M, editor: *Education and support for parenting: a guide for professionals*, London, 2002, Baillière Tindall.

Nolan M: Childbirth and parenting education: what the research says and why we may ignore it. In Nolan M, Foster J, editors: *Birth and parenting skills: new directions in antenatal education*, Edinburgh, 2005, Elsevier.

Ockenden J: Antenatal education for parenting. In Nolan M, editor: *Education and support for parenting: a guide for professionals*, London, 2002, Baillière Tindall.

Paavola L: *Maternal sensitive responsiveness characteristics and relations to child early communicative and linguistic development*, Oulu, 2006, Oulu University Press.

Parr M: *PIPPIN: Support for couples in the transition to parenthood*, PhD dissertation, London, 1996, University of East London.

Parr M: A new approach to parent education, *British Journal of Midwifery* 6(3):160–165, 1998.

Parr M, Joyce C: 'First steps in parenting': developing nurturing parenting skills in mothers and fathers in the pregnancy and postnatal period. In Barlow J, Svanberg P, editors: *Keeping the baby in mind. Infant mental health in practice*, London, 2009, Routledge.

Priest J, Schott J: *Leading antenatal classes: a practical guide*, Oxford, 1991, Butterworth Heinemann.

Rolls L: *Team development, a manual of facilitation for health educators and health promoters*, London, 1992, Health Education Authority.

Royal College of Midwives (RCM): *Position paper 22. Maternity care for lesbian mothers*, London, 2000 (reviewed 2005), RCM.

Smith C: *Developing parenting programmes*, London, 1997, National Children's Bureau.

Underdown A: Investigating techniques used in parenting classes, *Health Visitor* 7(2):65–68, 1998.

Wickham S, Davis L: Are midwives empowered enough to offer empowering education? In Nolan M, Foster J, editors: *Birth and parenting skills: new directions in antenatal education*, Edinburgh, 2005, Elsevier.

Wilkins C: A qualitative study exploring the support needs of first time mothers on their journey towards intuitive parenting, *Midwifery* 22(2):169–180, 2006.

Woollett A, Parr M: Psychological tasks for women and men in the transition to parenthood, *Journal of Reproductive and Infant Psychology* 15(2):159–183, 1997.

World Health Organization (WHO): *Fatherhood and health outcomes in Europe*, Copenhagen, 2007, WHO Regional Office for Europe.

Worldwide Alternatives to *Violence (WAVE) Trust: Violence and what to do about it*, Surrey, 2005, Wave Trust.

Chapter 22

# Physical preparation for childbirth and beyond, and the role of physiotherapy

*Gill Brook*

## LEARNING OUTCOMES

After reading this chapter and practising the suggested activities, you will:

- have increased your awareness of the effects of pregnancy, labour and the postnatal period on the musculoskeletal system
- understand the benefits of exercise during pregnancy and postnatally
- feel competent to advise women in your care on appropriate exercise and strategies to minimize the symptoms of any musculoskeletal dysfunctions they are experiencing
- have an understanding of the role of physiotherapy in relation to women during the childbearing year and history of the specialty
- know when and how to refer women in your care to a women's health physiotherapist, where available.

## INTRODUCTION

This chapter aims to equip midwifery students and midwives with the knowledge and skills required to understand issues such as exercise, good posture, relaxation techniques and effective physical preparation for pregnancy and childbirth, plus common musculoskeletal dysfunctions in pregnancy and childbirth. This will enable them to advise and support women in their care and recognize situations when referral to another professional is indicated. The author is a women's health physiotherapist and will refer to the role throughout, with further information on the specialty towards the end of the chapter.

## EXERCISE AND SPORT DURING PREGNANCY

Pregnancy is a time when women are often receptive to health education messages. This can include the introduction of exercise as not just having short-term benefits during the pregnancy and childbirth period, but also holding long-term health gains. There is evidence that exercise during pregnancy can benefit both the woman and fetus (RCOG 2006a) and is harmful to neither, provided the pregnant woman is progressing normally and healthily (Artal et al 2003). Therefore it is suggested that women should be encouraged to start, or continue with, appropriate exercise to derive the associated health benefits (NICE 2008, NICE 2010, RCOG 2006a). These include a reduction in fatigue, varicosities and peripheral swelling; a lower incidence of insomnia, stress, anxiety and depression; and, possibly, weight-bearing exercise in pregnancy may result in a shorter labour and a decrease in delivery-related complications (RCOG 2006a). In addition, a randomized study of women with gestational diabetes (Bung et al 1991) found that more than three-quarters of those following an exercise programme demonstrated improved glucose tolerance, so exercise is recommended for this group (RCOG 2006b). There is no robust evidence that exercise will prevent the onset of gestational diabetes in women (Artal & Sherman 1999).

It has been suggested that babies born to exercising women may tolerate labour better and be less likely to demonstrate signs of stress, such as meconium (RCOG 2006a).

There appears to be some variation between what are considered absolute or relative contraindications to (aerobic) exercise in pregnancy (ACOG 2002) and conditions requiring medical supervision while undertaking exercise in pregnancy (RCOG 2006a). Guidance produced by physiotherapists (ACPWH 2004) suggests the contraindications and precautions indicated in Table 22.1.

The aim of exercise during pregnancy should be to maintain or moderately improve fitness levels (ACPWH 2004) without trying to reach peak fitness or train for competition (RCOG 2006a). It is impossible to go into any detail of different regimens within the constraints of this chapter, but the needs of different women will vary, based on whether they were a complete non-exerciser, non-regular exerciser, regular exerciser or elite athlete before conception (ACPWH 2004). Women should be advised to monitor their level of effort during exercise, to ensure that they are not overexerting themselves, and if using a gym, should seek advice from professional staff.

Commonly described tools are the talk test, Borg's scale of perceived exertion, and heart rate (RCOG 2006a):

- During exercise, the woman should be able to hold a conversation, and not become too breathless to talk
- On a scale of 'very, very light' through to 'very, very hard' exertion, she should aim for 'somewhat hard'; around the middle of the Borg scale
- The suggested maximum heart rate during exercise varies, depending on a woman's exercise habit pre-conception and her age, and she should ensure that she knows how to take her own pulse, and her optimum heart rate before starting exercise.

Women should avoid overheating during exercise, as a maternal core temperature over 39.2°C might be teratogenic in the first trimester (RCOG 2006a). They can minimize this risk by drinking sufficient fluids during exercise, and avoiding exercise in very hot conditions. Women must also know when to stop exercising, and seek a medical opinion. This includes onset of symptoms such as dizziness, faintness or headache; shortness of breath before exertion or breathlessness during exercise; any pain, e.g. abdomen, pelvic girdle; painful uterine contractions; decreased fetal movements; vaginal loss, urinary incontinence, ruptured membranes; swollen leg(s); muscle weakness (RCOG 2006b).

Regular exercisers familiar with a particular activity or sport, such as walking, aerobics, swimming or dancing, can usually continue with it.

Those unaccustomed to exercise should be advised to start with 15 minutes of continuous exercise three times a week, gradually increasing to 30-minute sessions four times a week or daily (RCOG 2006a). Exercise in water, often referred to as *aquanatal exercise*, may offer a feeling of weightlessness, and reduced jarring of the joints, possibly offering some relief from aches and pains, an increase in energy and better sleeping (Brook et al 2008).

**Table 22.1 Absolute contraindications and precautions to exercise in pregnancy***

| Absolute contraindication | Precaution |
|---|---|
| Serious cardiovascular, respiratory, renal or thyroid disease | Asthma |
| Poorly controlled type 1 diabetes | Diabetes type 1 if insulin regimens are well controlled and exercise is moderate – discuss with diabetic consultant, nurse or GP |
| Risk of, or current, premature labour | History of miscarriage |
| Cervical incompetence | Vaginal bleeding |
| History or risk of intrauterine growth retardation and premature labour – reduce activity after 12 weeks | Reduced fetal movement |
| Hypertension – should be discussed with the woman's doctor | Pre-pregnancy hypertension |
| Placenta praevia after 26 weeks' gestation – should be discussed with the woman's doctor | Placenta praevia |
| | Vaginal bleeding |
| Hypertension – should be discussed with the woman's doctor | Pre-pregnancy hypertension |
| Severe rhesus isoimmunisation | |
| Sudden swelling of ankles, hands or face | Anaemia |
| Acute infectious disease | |
| | Extreme obesity |
| | Breech presentation |
| | Extreme underweight (BMI <12) |
| | Heavy smoking |
| | Thyroid disease |

*Adapted from ACPWH 2004.

Scuba diving is contraindicated during pregnancy as the fetus is not protected against decompression sickness and gas embolism, and women should be warned that contact sports and pursuits which might result in a fall, such as horse riding, could result in fetal trauma (ACPWH 2004, RCOG 2006a).

Readers are advised to access appropriate sources – for example, ACPWH 2004, RCOG 2006a and 2006b – for further and updated evidence-based information, before discussing recreational exercise with pregnant women in their care.

**Reflective activity 22.1**

What exercise groups are available specifically for pregnant or postnatal women in your area? If possible, ask to attend one, or check whether any women you know have attended them, and assess their value. Record this information for future reference.

## Muscle groups

Two muscle groups that are affected more than others by pregnancy and childbirth because of their position, structure and function are those of the pelvic floor and abdominal wall. The pelvic floor is described and illustrated elsewhere within this book, but it is also useful to understand the structure and function of the abdominal muscles (Fig. 22.1).

The abdominal muscles have various roles, including protection and support for the abdominal contents. More specifically, their main functions are flexion of the lumbar spine (*recti abdominis*), side flexion and rotation of the spine (external and internal obliques) and postural support (*transversus abdominis*, working with the pelvic floor muscles) (Brook et al 2008). As pregnancy progresses, the abdominal muscles are stretched considerably by the gravid uterus, causing recti abdominis to become longer, wider and thinner (Y Coldron, unpublished PhD thesis, 2006). In addition, the linea alba (an area of connective tissue in the midline) may become wider and thinner (*divarication*) or even split (*diastasis*). Although there is little information on the effect of pregnancy on transversus abdominis (Brook et al 2008), its role along with the pelvic floor muscles – that is, support for the intra-abdominal organs, lower spine and pelvic girdle joints – is significant.

Many women's health physiotherapists will include pelvic floor muscle and transversus abdominis exercises in any advice they give to pregnant women, whether it is in a parent education session, exercise class, or during

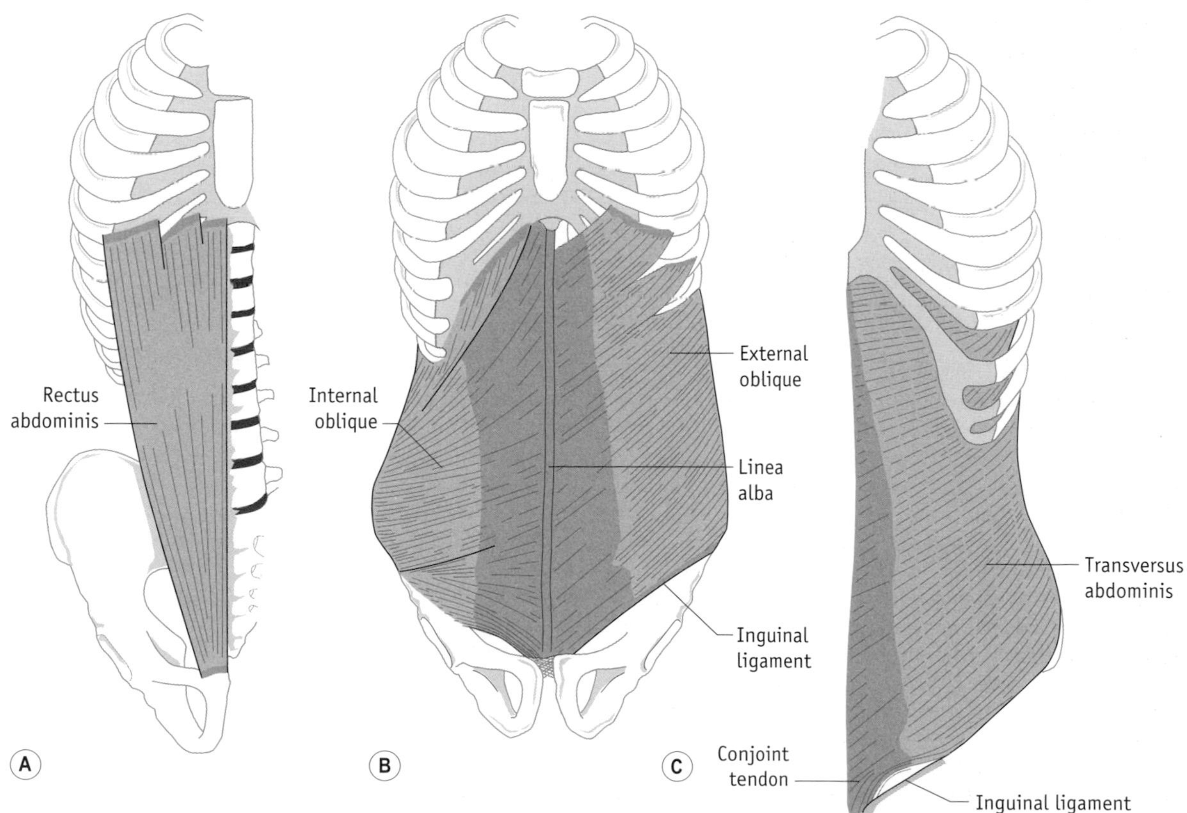


**Figure 22.1** Muscles of the abdominal wall. **A.** Right rectus abdominis. **B.** Right internal oblique and left external oblique muscles. **C.** Left transversus abdominis. *(Palastanga et al 2006, reproduced with permission)*

individual assessment of a musculoskeletal problem. Midwives may wish to do the same.

## Pelvic floor muscle exercises

There is evidence that pelvic floor muscle exercises during pregnancy can prevent urinary incontinence (Mørkved et al 2003) and reduce the likelihood of prolonged second stage labour (Salvesen & Mørkved 2004). The National Institute for Health and Clinical Excellence (NICE) has suggested that pelvic floor muscle training should be offered to women in their first pregnancy as a preventive strategy for urinary incontinence (NICE 2006a).

In non-pregnant women, research has suggested that a sizeable minority of women given verbal instructions on pelvic floor muscle exercises will not perform an optimum contraction (Bump et al 1991) and recent advice on the management of urinary incontinence suggests that a digital assessment of the muscles should be undertaken prior to commencing a course of exercises (NICE 2006a). Physiotherapists have been advised against such examination on pregnant women if there is a history of miscarriage or the woman has been advised to avoid sexual intercourse whilst pregnant (CSP 2003). Also, vaginal examination would not be practical in many situations when a pregnant woman is being advised on pelvic floor muscle exercises, e.g. parent education session, or exercise classes. Therefore, it is important that physiotherapists, midwives and any other health professionals teaching pelvic floor muscle exercises give clear instructions. There are many different ways to do this, including:

> *'Imagine you are trying to stop yourself breaking wind, and at the same time trying to stop your flow of urine midstream' (Brook et al 2008); the 'lift' analogy, i.e. closing the doors (a squeeze) and moving upstairs (a lift); the action of a vacuum cleaner (Bø & Mørkved 2007).*

If women are not sure that they are contracting correctly, they could look at the perineum using a hand mirror, and see if the area lifts away from the mirror as they squeeze. Alternatively, they could try to stop the dribble at the end of voiding but should not stop midstream as this may disturb normal neurological activity (Bø & Mørkved 2007) and affect emptying.

Advice on how often to exercise and how many squeezes to undertake varies from author to author but a recent review of evidence suggests building up to 8–12 near-maximum contractions three times a day. In addition, any women experiencing stress or urge urinary incontinence should also squeeze before and during those activities which make them leak, e.g. cough, sneeze, on their way to the toilet (Bø 2007). A study of 23 pregnant women complaining of stress urinary incontinence (Miller et al 2008) showed they could reduce leakage by undertaking this anticipatory contraction, often referred to as 'the Knack'.

**Reflective activity 22.2**

Try a series of pelvic floor contractions yourself. How can you best describe this to someone else? Try teaching this to a family member or friend who does not know anything about the pelvic floor.

## Transversus abdominis exercises

Although many women have heard of pelvic floor muscles, far fewer will be aware of *transversus abdominis*, although this may change owing to recent interest in gym ball exercise and Pilates, which focus on core stability. Professionals may prefer to use a lay term such as 'deep' or 'support' muscle.

As the muscle lies under other layers, it is difficult to feel or see, so, as with pelvic floor muscle exercises, clear instructions are necessary. One description is:

> *'Place your hand on the lower part of your tummy under your bump. Breathe in through your nose. As you breathe out, gently draw in your lower tummy away from your hand towards your back, then relax' (ACPWH 2001).*

As with pelvic floor muscle exercises, a review of the literature regarding exercise and pregnancy-related pelvic girdle pain (Vleeming et al 2008) suggests that researchers use a range of exercise regimens, but the Association of Chartered Physiotherapists in Women's Health (ACPWH) suggests a contraction lasting up to 10 seconds, with up to 10 repetitions, repeated six to eight times per day (ACPWH 2001).

## Low back and pelvic girdle pain

Many women experience lower back or pelvic girdle pain during pregnancy. Low back pain normally refers to pain of (lumbar) spinal origin, while pelvic girdle pain (PGP) originates in the symphysis pubis or sacroiliac joints (Brook et al 2008). Different authors report great variations in incidence, from 4% to 76.4%, largely due to wide methodological differences, but there is strong evidence to suggest 20% is accurate for PGP (Vleeming et al 2008). There are many factors that make pregnant women prone to low back pain or PGP, including fatigue, increased joint mobility related to hormonally induced changes in collagen, pressure on pain-sensitive structures by remodelled collagen, weight gain with an associated change in posture, and pressure from the growing fetus (Barton 2004a). Specific risk factors are probably a history of previous low back pain or trauma to the pelvis (Vleeming et al 2008) but in many cases no reason is identified (ACPWH 2007a). Common signs and symptoms include pain, difficulty walking (a waddling gait), clicking or grinding in the anterior or posterior pelvic joints, and difficulty with activities such as housework and sexual intercourse (ACPWH 2007a). Pain may occur in one or more of a variety of sites around the lower back, posterior or anterior pelvis, hips and groins, and common triggers include standing on one leg (e.g. climbing stairs, dressing) and straddling movements (e.g. getting in and out of the bath, turning in bed) (ACPWH 2007a). Evidence-based guidance for the management of pregnancy-related PGP recommends exercise in pregnancy, specific stabilizing exercises postnatally, physiotherapy, a pelvic belt for short periods, acupuncture, and appropriate analgesia (Vleeming et al 2008). Current guidance on the management of backache during pregnancy (NICE 2008) suggests women should be advised that exercising in water, massage therapy, and group or individual back care classes might help to ease their symptoms.

Midwives are often the first health professional with whom pregnant women will discuss any PGP, and having excluded any other possible cause of the symptoms, such as urinary tract infection, Braxton Hicks contractions, or labour, the midwife needs to explain the condition, advise on analgesia and offer general advice such as that in Table 22.2 (ACPWH 2007a).

Although rare, osteoporosis can occur during pregnancy, most commonly affecting the vertebrae, ribs and pubis (Barton 2004a). Symptoms such as backache and groin pain may make it difficult to differentiate it from other musculoskeletal dysfunctions. It should be considered, particularly if women are subject to other risk factors, such as long-term use of corticosteroids, thyroid problems, malabsorption disorders (e.g. coeliac disease), smoking, poor diet or low bodyweight (Carne 2008).

## Posture and moving and handling

As every pregnant woman is affected by hormonal changes and, to varying degrees, postural adaptations to accommodate the developing fetus, then all are at risk of the various musculoskeletal dysfunctions discussed. Consequently, every pregnant woman should be offered appropriate advice to minimize the chance of such problems developing. Although such advice might not be as specific as that shown in Table 22.2, it could include advice on posture in standing (Fig. 22.2A), sitting (Fig. 22.2B) and lying (Fig. 22.2C), movement on and off a bed (Fig. 22.2D) and lifting (Fig. 22.2E) (Barton 2004a).

The midwife can assist women in understanding the importance of posture, and clarifying good back care. This includes getting up from the examination couch, which, if the woman sits up from a lying position, imitates performing a sit-up and puts great strain on the abdominals as well as the back. Encouraging the woman to move to a side-lying position and then swing her legs down whilst pushing herself up with her arm, and suggesting that she

**Table 22.2 General advice for women experiencing pregnancy-related pelvic girdle pain***

| Advice | It can help to: |
|---|---|
| Remain active within the limits of pain | Avoid activities which she knows make the pain worse |
| Accept offers of help and involve partner, family and friends in daily chores | Ask for other help if needed |
| Rest is important | Rest more frequently, or sit down for activities that normally involve standing, e.g. ironing |
| Avoid standing on one leg | Dress sitting down |
| Consider alternative sleeping position | Lie on her side with pillows between legs for comfort. Turn 'under' when turning in bed, or turn over with knees together and squeeze buttocks |
| Explore alternative ways to climb stairs | Go upstairs one leg at a time with the more pain-free leg first and the other leg joining it on the step |
| Plan the day | Bring everything needed downstairs in the morning and set up changing stations both up and downstairs. Have drinks on hand, e.g. thermos flasks. A rucksack may be helpful to carry things around the house, especially if crutches have to be used |
| Avoid activities that involve asymmetrical positions of the pelvis | Avoid sitting cross-legged. Avoid reaching, pushing or pulling to one side. Avoid bending and twisting to lift or carrying anything on one hip, e.g. toddlers |
| Consider alternative positions for sexual intercourse | Try lying on the side or kneeling on all fours |
| Organize hospital appointments for the same day if possible | Combine appointments for antenatal care and physiotherapy |

*ACPWH 2007a, reproduced with permission.

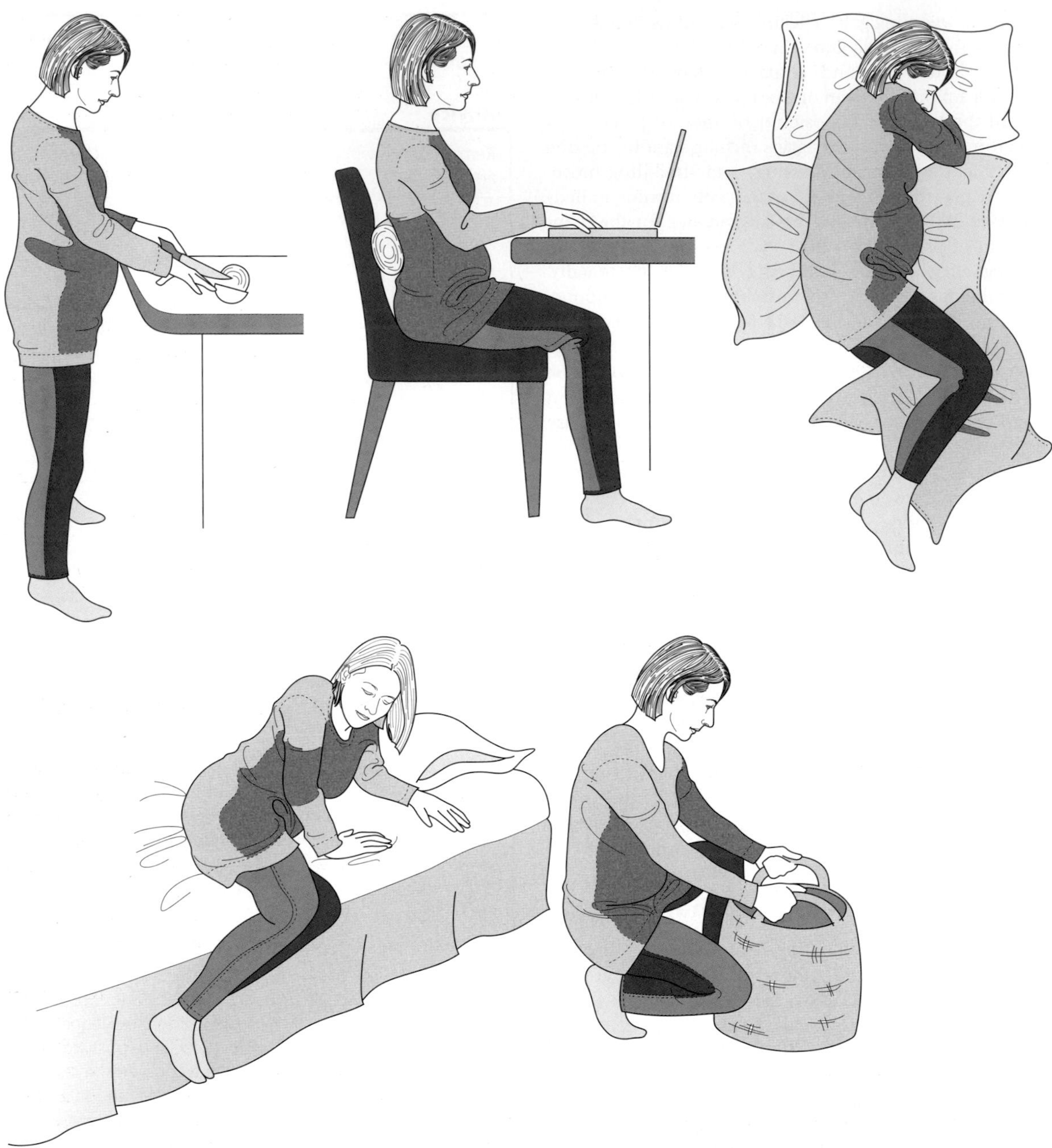

Figure 22.2 **A.** Good posture in standing. **B.** Good sitting posture. **C.** Example of a comfortable sleeping position. **D.** How to get on and off the bed. **E.** Good lifting technique. *(ACPWH 2001, reproduced with permission.)*

does this at home when getting in and out of bed, can be of great help.

## Referral to physiotherapy

If there is a women's health physiotherapy service available locally, the midwife, obstetrician or general practitioner should be able to request assessment and treatment. In some places, pregnant women may be able to self-refer. When and to whom to refer may also depend on local protocol, the confidence and experience of the midwife concerned, and the physiotherapy service available (see later section on women's health physiotherapy). For example, some physiotherapists might offer advice or exercise groups for pregnant women, whilst others may only accept referrals for women with a specific musculoskeletal dysfunction that has not responded to advice from the midwife or doctor.

**Reflective activity 22.3**

Are there women's health physiotherapists working in your area? What services do they offer? How can you access them? Record this information for future reference. Could you spend some time with them, to discuss your respective work?

## RELAXATION

The use of relaxation in pregnancy and labour goes back to the mid-20[th] century, if not before. Grantly Dick-Read referred to relaxation as 'a condition in which the muscle tone throughout the body is reduced to a minimum' (Dick-Read 1954), while physiotherapist Helen Heardman preferred 'reduction to a minimum of mental and muscular energy conducive with life' (Heardman 1959). It has been suggested that relaxation and breathing awareness during labour may help address the *pain–anxiety–tension cycle,* act as a distraction technique, increase tolerance of pain, and offer a coping strategy (Schott & Priest 2002). Studies of parent education sessions indicate that some women might be made more aware of pain relief techniques rather than improving their own ability to cope with pain (Fabian et al 2005). Simple 'sighing-out-slowly breathing' is more likely to be used than a relaxation technique taught in classes (Spiby et al 1999). A systematic review of randomized controlled studies of complementary and alternative therapies for labour pain, including breathing (respiratory autogenic training), hypnosis and massage, found no proof of efficacy (Huntley et al 2004).

However, despite the lack of evidence to support their effectiveness, midwives are still advised to support women's use of breathing and relaxation techniques and massage they have chosen to use in labour (NICE 2007). In addition, relaxation may be considered a useful 'life skill' for dealing with stress caused by changes in lifestyle (Fordyce 2004) and – of particular relevance to expectant and new mothers – coping with the stresses of pregnancy (Brayshaw 2003), a crying baby or rebellious toddler (Schott & Priest 2002).

Health professionals teaching relaxation should ideally understand and believe in what they are teaching, and have practised the techniques before introducing them into their practice (Schott & Priest 2002). There are many different techniques, but physiological relaxation devised by Laura Mitchell is taught widely by physiotherapists and midwives (Brayshaw 2003). The method is based on the physiological concept of reciprocal relaxation – i.e. if one group of muscles is tightened, then the opposite group will relax. People who are stressed or tense adopt a typical posture, e.g. fists clenched, shoulders hunched. The Mitchell technique addresses tension in different parts of the body with a set of instructions for each joint:

- Move (out of the position of stress, by tightening the opposite muscle group)
- Stop
- Feel the new position (ACPWH 2007b, Brayshaw 2003).

Physiological relaxation can be practised in any suitable, comfortable position, using the instructions in Box 22.1. Eventually, the participant should be able to memorize the instructions in bold, and use the technique whenever required, and for a range of life situations that might cause stress.

**Reflective activity 22.4**

Practise the relaxation technique in Box 22.1 yourself a few times. When you are familiar with it, try it out when you feel tense or stressed. This will help with your teaching of the technique, and how you explain the effect.

## POSTNATAL EXERCISE AND ADVICE

Postnatal exercises target the abdominal and pelvic floor muscles as the groups most affected by pregnancy and birth, and are designed to aid a return to previous fitness levels (ACPWH 2010). *Transversus abdominis* and pelvic floor muscle exercises may be taught as they were during pregnancy (see above) and women reminded that these exercises can be practised in a variety of positions, so can be undertaken whenever and wherever they are remembered.

Whereas previous generations of new mothers might rest at home or in hospital for a period of days or even weeks before expecting to return to 'normal' activities, current expectations are for a much speedier recovery (Barton 2004b). It is, therefore, pertinent to encourage appropriate, safe exercises as soon as possible to help return the soft tissues to their pre-pregnancy condition and minimize the risk of musculoskeletal problems. Current guidance (ACPWH 2010) gives no specific time at which to start, just suggesting as soon as possible, but a woman's choice may be influenced by any pre-existing or de novo musculoskeletal dysfunction, labour, or delivery. In a study of 1193 women Thompson et al (2002) found that primiparous women and those who had undergone an assisted vaginal delivery reported more perineal pain than others, whilst those who had undergone caesarean section reported a higher incidence of exhaustion and

Box 22.1 **Physiological relaxation***

**Pull your shoulders towards your feet** away from your ears, making the neck longer. Stop. Feel your shoulders are lower and neck feels longer.

**Elbows out and open**. Keep your arms supported, on the bed or chair, then push them slightly away from your sides, opening out the elbow joints. Stop. Feel your elbows are open and slightly away from your side.

**Fingers and thumbs long and supported**. Open out your fingers and thumbs, keeping your wrists resting on their support. Stop. Feel your fingers and thumbs fall back onto their support

**Turn your hips outwards**. Feel your thighs and lower legs roll outwards. Stop. Be aware that your legs are slightly apart and turned outwards.

**Move your knees gently until comfortable**. Stop. Feel the resulting comfort in your knees.

**Push your feet away from your body**. Bend at the ankles gently pointing your toes. Stop. Feel your feet hanging loosely from the ankle joints.

**Press your body into the support** using the floor, bed or back of the chair. Stop. Feel the pressure of your body on the support.

**Press your head into the pillow or chair**. Feel the movement in your neck as you do this. Stop. Feel your head lying in the hollow you have made for it.

**Drag the jaw down** keeping your lips closed. Stop. Feel your teeth are no longer touching and your lips are gently touching.

If it is stuck against the roof of your mouth **bring your tongue down and let it lie in the middle of your mouth**. Stop. Feel your tongue resting on the floor of your mouth, the tip touching your lower teeth.

If they are not already closed, **close your eyes**. Do not screw them up. Stop. Be aware of the darkness.

Make the space between your eyebrows and hairline as wide and wrinkle-free as possible. Try not to frown – **smoothe the skin over your forehead from your eyebrows into your hair, continuing the movement over the top of your head and down the back of your neck**. Stop. Feel the smoothing of the skin.

**Take a deep breath,** expanding forward slightly above the waist and around the lower ribs, **then breathe out easily,** at your own rate.

*Adapted from ACPWH 2007b, Brayshaw 2003.

bowel problems. In the absence of evidence that early, appropriate exercise is detrimental to such women, midwives can encourage it. It is suggested (Barton 2004b) that the pumping action of pelvic floor exercises assists venous and lymphatic drainage, removing traumatic exudate, so reducing symptoms.

If a woman has experienced a stillbirth or neonatal death, exercise and a return to normal physical activity may be a low personal priority. However, written advice, which can be consulted when the time is right, is a useful resource (ACPWH 2007c).

Women are advised to avoid stronger abdominal exercises until they have good *transversus abdominis* control, especially if a significant divarication or diastasis – over three fingers' width – persists (Brook et al 2008). This can be checked by a physiotherapist or midwife by asking the woman to lie flat on her back (one or no pillows), with her knees bent and feet flat on the bed. The fingers of one hand are placed widthways on her abdomen, just above or below the umbilicus. As the woman is asked to lift her head and shoulders and reach down towards her feet, it is possible to feel the *recti abdominis* muscle bellies pressing against the fingers, and you can then gauge the gap in finger widths (Barton 2004b).

**Reflective activity 22.5**

Check *recti abdominis* on a friend, family member or colleague who has had children. Compare to a nulliparous woman. Are you confident in what you are doing and feeling? Could you ask a more experienced midwife or women's health physiotherapist for guidance?

There are no published studies which suggest that a rapid return to exercise or sport would, in the absence of medical complications, prove detrimental, but advice is that exercise regimens should be resumed gradually, be individualized (Artal et al 2003), not resuming high impact activity too soon (RCOG 2006a). Advice from a midwife or physiotherapist can include brisk walking, or swimming when there has been no vaginal bleeding or discharge for 7 consecutive days (ACPWH 2010).

Some maternity units will have no or limited inpatient postnatal physiotherapy input. In the latter case, physiotherapists may restrict their service to women with postnatal complications, such as ongoing or delivery-related musculoskeletal dysfunctions, third or fourth degree tears, postnatal urinary retention, or rectus abdominis divarication or diastasis. Although guidance on postnatal care (NICE 2006b) suggests that backache should be managed as in the general population, European guidelines on the management of pelvic girdle pain (Vleeming et al 2008) recommend specific stabilizing exercises postnatally.

## WOMEN'S HEALTH PHYSIOTHERAPY

Physiotherapists in the UK have a long history of advising and treating women during pregnancy and the postnatal period (see website). The ACPWH promotes the role of the physiotherapist in women's health; improvement of knowledge and skills and informing members of relevant professional and political developments. It fosters mutual understanding and provides opportunities for inter-professional learning in order to facilitate good working relationships between members of the healthcare team and their professional bodies, and to promote all relevant aspects of health education and patient care (ACPWH 2008).

The role of women's health physiotherapists in the UK is diverse, usually including the care of women antenatally and postnatally, and often involvement in parent education sessions. Clinicians may be specialists in the treatment of pregnancy-related musculoskeletal dysfunctions (ACPWH 2008). Many treat incontinence (both female and male) and other pelvic floor muscle dysfunctions, and may care for women undergoing gynaecological surgery. In addition, other areas of practice might include neonatal paediatrics, osteoporosis, menopause, breast care, and lymphoedema management (Brook 2007).

The Department of Health has proposed that there is a place for physiotherapy in the multi-professional team offering antenatal care (DH 2004), and that care from a range of maternity professionals including midwives, obstetricians and other specialists should be available (DH 2007). Physiotherapists are the experts in musculoskeletal assessment (Barton 2004a), and current evidence-based guidance on the management of pregnancy-related pelvic girdle pain (Vleeming et al 2008) recommends exercises in pregnancy; an individualized treatment programme focusing on specific stabilizing exercises as part of a multifactorial treatment for the condition postnatally; individualized physical therapy; manipulation or joint mobilization as a possible test for symptomatic relief; acupuncture; and possibly the trial of a pelvic belt for symptomatic relief. Most, if not all, of the above are within the scope of practice of many physiotherapists working within women's health and are not commonly practised by other professionals working within maternity services.

Unfortunately, there appears to be little or no consistency of provision of women's health physiotherapy around the UK (Brook 2007). This is a disadvantage to other professionals, such as midwives, who may or may not have access to such specialist services. It is reported (Brook 2007) that a unit handling 6000 deliveries a year might have anything between the equivalent of one and four full-time physiotherapists offering a range of women's health services. The last 20 years has seen a large increase in their role within continence services with a decrease in obstetric work, possibly related to a lack of appropriate research in the specialty (Mantle 2004).

## CONCLUSION

Midwives are the prime care providers and advisors for women during their childbearing year. As continuity of care is recommended (NICE 2008) it is ideal if midwives are knowledgeable and competent to offer advice on posture and exercise in pregnancy and the management of musculoskeletal dysfunctions, as well as a return to normal activities postnatally. They must also know what additional services are available locally, including those offered by women's health physiotherapists, so that safe, high-quality maternity care is available for all women and their partners (DH 2007). This period is an ideal time to provide advice on posture, exercise and moving and handling that women can go on to use during their early parenthood and beyond.

### KEY POINTS

- A clear understanding of the normal and altered anatomy and physiology enables the midwife to identify deviations from normal, and consult and refer appropriately.
- Appropriate exercise and the development of relaxation techniques during pregnancy and the postnatal period can have short-term and long-term health benefits for the woman.
- The midwife should provide individualized advice and information regarding exercise and posture.

## REFERENCES

American College of Obstetricians and Gynecologists (ACOG): Exercise during pregnancy and the postpartum period. ACOG Committee Opinion No 267, *Obstetrics and Gynecology* 99(1):171–173, 2002.

Artal R, Sherman C: Exercise during pregnancy: safe and beneficial for most, *The Physician and Sportsmedicine* 27(8):1–9, 1999.

Artal R, O'Toole M, White S: Guidelines of the American College of Obstetricians and Gynecologists for exercises during pregnancy and the postpartum period, *British Journal of Sports Medicine* 37(1):6–12, 2003.

Association of Chartered Physiotherapists in Women's Health (ACPWH): *Fit for pregnancy. Essential exercises and helpful advice to get you into shape for the birth of your baby* (website). www.acpwh.org.uk/docs/FitforPregnancy.pdf. 2001. Accessed July 3, 2010.

Association of Chartered Physiotherapists in Women's Health (ACPWH): *Fit and safe to exercise in the childbearing year. Advice for chartered physiotherapists and other health professionals* (website). www.acpwh.org.uk/docs/Fit_and_Safe_(physio).pdf. 2004. Accessed July 3, 2010.

Association of Chartered Physiotherapists in Women's Health (ACPWH): *Pregnancy-related pelvic girdle pain. Guidance for health professionals* (website). www.acpwh.org.uk/docs/ACPWH-PGP_HP.pdf. 2007a. Accessed July 3, 2010.

Association of Chartered Physiotherapists in Women's Health (ACPWH): *The Mitchell method of simple relaxation* (website). www.acpwh.org.uk/docs/ACPWH-Mitchell.pdf. 2007b. Accessed July 3, 2010.

Association of Chartered Physiotherapists in Women's Health (ACPWH): *Exercises and advice after the stillbirth or death of your baby* (website). www.acpwh.org.uk/docs/ACPWH-PostNatal.pdf. 2007c. Accessed July 3, 2010.

Association of Chartered Physiotherapists in Women's Health. (ACPWH): *About us* (website) http://www.acpwh.org.uk. 2008.

Association of Chartered Physiotherapists in Women's Health (ACPWH): *Fit for the future: essential exercises and advice after childbirth (website)* www.acpwh.org.uk/docs/leaflets/ACPWH-FFFuture.pdf. Accessed July 3, 2010.

Barton S: Relieving the discomforts of pregnancy. In Mantle J, Haslam J, Barton S, editors: *Physiotherapy in obstetrics and gynaecology,* ed 2, London, 2004a, Butterworth-Heinemann, pp 141–164.

Barton S: The postnatal period. In Mantle J, Haslam J, Barton S, editors: *Physiotherapy in obstetrics and gynaecology,* ed 2, London, 2004b, Butterworth-Heinemann, pp 205–247.

Bø K: Female stress urinary incontinence. Pelvic floor muscle training for stress urinary incontinence. In Bø K, Berghmans B, Mørkved S, et al, editors: *Evidence-based physical therapy for the pelvic floor,* Edinburgh, 2007, Churchill Livingstone, pp 171–187.

Bø K, Mørkved S: Pelvic floor and exercise science. Motor learning. In Bø K, Berghmans B, Mørkved S, et al, editors: *Evidence-based physical therapy for the pelvic floor,* Edinburgh, 2007, Churchill Livingstone, pp 113–119.

Brayshaw E: *Exercises for pregnancy and childbirth. A practical guide for educators, Edinburgh,* 2003, Books for Midwives.

Brook G: *Women's health physiotherapy service, National Association of Primary Care Review* summer edition:163–165, 2007.

Brook G, Coldron Y, Evans G, et al: Physiotherapy in women's health. In Porter S, editor: *Tidy's physiotherapy,* ed 14, Edinburgh, 2008, Churchill Livingstone, pp 113–144.

Bump R, Hurt WG, Fantl JA, et al: Assessment of Kegel pelvic muscle exercise performance after brief verbal instruction, *American Journal of Obstetrics and Gynecology* 165:(2) 322–329, 1991.

Bung P, Artal R, Khodiguian N, et al: Exercise in gestational diabetes: an optional therapeutic approach? *Diabetes* 40(Suppl 2):182–185, 1991.

Carne K: Osteoporosis. In Porter S, editor: *Tidy's physiotherapy*, ed 14, Edinburgh, 2008, Churchill Livingstone, pp 182–198, 2008.

Chartered Society of Physiotherapy (CSP): *Clinical guidelines for the physiotherapy management of females aged 16-65 with stress urinary incontinence,* ed 2 (website). www.csp.org.uk/uploads/documents/csp_guideline_sui.pdf. 2003. Accessed July 20, 2008.

Department of Health (DH): *National service framework for children and maternity services. Standard 11,* London, 2004, DH.

Department of Health (DH): *Maternity matters: choice, access and continuity of care in a safe service,* London, 2007, DH.

Dick-Read G: *Childbirth without fear. The principles and practice of natural childbirth,* London, 1954, William Heinemann.

Fabian HM, Radestad IJ, Waldenström U: Childbirth and parenthood education classes in Sweden. Women's opinion and possible outcomes, *Acta Obstetricia et Gynecologica Scandinavica* 84(5):436–443, 2005.

Fordyce J: The antenatal period. In Mantle J, Haslam J, Barton S, editors: *Physiotherapy in obstetrics and gynaecology,* ed 2, London, 2004, Butterworth-Heinemann, pp 93–139.

Heardman H: *Physiotherapy in obstetrics and gynaecology*, Edinburgh, 1959, Livingstone.

Huntley AL, Thompson Coon J, Ernst E: Complementary and alternative medicine for labor pain: a systematic review, *American Journal of Obstetrics and Gynecology* 191(1):36–44, 2004.

Mantle J: Editorial, *Journal of the Association of Chartered Physiotherapists in Women's Health* 94:3, 2004.

Miller JM, Sampselle C, Ashton-Miller J, et al: Clarification and confirmation of the Knack maneuver: the effect of volitional pelvic floor muscle contraction to preempt expected stress urinary incontinence, *International Urogynecology Journal* 19(6):773–782, 2008.

Mørkved S, Bø K, Schei B, et al: Pelvic floor muscle training during pregnancy to prevent urinary incontinence: a single-blind randomized controlled trial, *Obstetrics and Gynecology* 101(2):313–319, 2003.

National Institute for Health and Clinical Excellence (NICE): *Urinary incontinence. The management of urinary incontinence in women* (website). www.nice.org.uk. 2006a. Accessed July 20, 2008.

National Institute for Health and Clinical Excellence(NICE): *Postnatal care. Routine postnatal care for women and their babies* (website). www.nice.org.uk. 2006b. Accessed August 17, 2008.

National Institute for Health and Clinical Excellence (NICE): *Intrapartum care. Care of healthy women and their babies during childbirth* (website). www.nice.org.uk. 2007. Accessed August 10, 2008.

National Institute for Health and Clinical Excellence (NICE): *Antenatal care. Routine care for the healthy pregnant woman* (website). www.nice.org.uk. 2008. Accessed July 20, 2008.

National Institute for Health and Clinical Excellence (NICE): Weight management before, during and after pregnancy, P427 Public Health Guidance, July 2010. London, 2010, NICE.

Palastanga N, Field D, Soames R: *Anatomy and human movement,* ed 5, Oxford, 2006, Butterworth-Heinemann.

Royal College of Obstetricians and Gynaecologists (RCOG): *Statement No. 4. Exercise in Pregnancy*, London, 2006a, RCOG.

Royal College of Obstetricians and Gynaecologists (RCOG): *Recreational exercise and pregnancy: information for you,* London, 2006b, RCOG.

Salvesen KÅ, Mørkved S: Randomised controlled trial of pelvic floor muscle training during pregnancy, *British Medical Journal* 329(7462):378–380, 2004.

Schott J, Priest J: *Leading antenatal classes. A practical guide*, 2 ed, Oxford, 2002, Books for Midwives.

Spiby H, Henderson B, Slade P, et al: Strategies for coping with labour: does antenatal education translate into practice? *Journal of Advanced Nursing* 29(2):388–394, 1999.

Thompson JF, Roberts CL, Currie M, et al: Prevalence and persistence of health problems after childbirth: association with parity and method of birth, *Birth* 29(2):83–94, 2002.

Vleeming A, Albert H, Östgaard HC, et al: European guidelines for the diagnosis and treatment of pelvic girdle pain, *European Spine Journal* 17(6):794–819, 2008.

Chapter |23|

# Vulnerable women

Claire Homeyard and Anna Gaudion

## LEARNING OUTCOMES

After reading this chapter, you will:

- understand the importance of the mother–midwife relationship and what midwives can do to support vulnerable women
- realize how the wider determinants of health may affect pregnant women and their babies
- appreciate the effects of being a pregnant teenager
- be aware of the effects of drug and alcohol misuse in pregnancy, signs of domestic abuse and the type of questions to ask
- realize the importance of signposting women to appropriate agencies and services for further information and advice.

## INTRODUCTION

Women who find themselves disadvantaged may have multiple social needs that affect their uptake and use of maternity services (DH 2007a). This chapter will provide an overview of the particular needs of these women and some introductory pointers to raise awareness and ensure that the most vulnerable women and those with chaotic lifestyles receive appropriate maternity care. The UK National Service Framework for Children, Young People and Maternity Services, Standard 11 champions the importance of inclusive maternity services (DH 2004a).

## DOMESTIC ABUSE

Domestic abuse can be defined as:

> *'Any incident of threatening behaviour, violence or abuse (psychological, physical, sexual, financial or emotional) between adults who are or have been intimate partners, or family members; regardless of gender, sexuality, disability, race or religion.'*
>
> (BMA 2007:1)

The term domestic abuse also includes a number of issues more prevalent in minority ethnic groups, such as forced marriage, female genital mutilation/cutting and 'honour crimes'.

### *Key facts*

- Domestic abuse forms a quarter of all violent crimes in the UK.
- 14% of maternal deaths occurred in women who had told a health professional they were in an abusive relationship.
- 20% of women in England and Wales assert that their partner has physically assaulted them.
- In 2003–2004 nearly all the female homicide victims were killed by their partner or ex-partner.
- At least 30% of cases first start in pregnancy.
- 40–60% of women are abused during pregnancy.
- Domestic abuse is a child protection issue (Lewis 2007).

Domestic abuse is underreported, mostly due to fear of reprisal, stigma and a continued relationship with the perpetrator, therefore any statistical data need to be interpreted with caution.

Domestic abuse is a major public health issue as during pregnancy it may result in direct harm to the pregnancy, such as preterm birth (Newberger et al 1992) antepartum haemorrhage and perinatal death (Janssen et al 2003), and also indirect harm through a woman's inability to access antenatal care (NICE 2008). Domestic abuse has long-term consequences upon a woman's mental health, with increased likelihood of the victim suffering from anxiety, depression and psychosomatic symptoms (BMA 2007).

A number of professional and governmental bodies, including the Royal College of Midwives (RCM 1999), the British Medical Association (BMA 2007), the Royal College of Obstetricians and Gynaecologists (RCOG 1997) and the Royal College of Psychiatrists (RCPsych 2002), advocate that all pregnant women should be asked about domestic abuse. This should form part of the needs, risk and choice assessment at the booking visit. Suggested questions include:

- 'Are you afraid at home?'
- 'Has your partner ever hit you?'
- 'As an adult have you ever been emotionally or physically hurt by your partner or someone important to you?' (DH 2005).

The process of routine enquiry for domestic abuse has been shown to be acceptable to women (Ramsay et al 2002). By asking all women and explaining it is a routine question, it helps to destigmatize domestic abuse and it also gives 'permission' for the woman to disclose at this time or at a later date.

All women, regardless of disclosure, should be provided with information and contact helplines for support and advice. Where a partner or other person is present, the question should be asked at a later date or an excuse found for the midwife to talk to the woman alone. In situations where a woman does not speak English, the question should be asked through an interpreter and not a family friend or relative. Where possible, the interpreter should be female and have received some instruction on domestic abuse.

A midwife's role is to let the woman know that she can disclose if and when she is ready. The midwife should refer on and not act as a caseworker for the woman.

It is important that a woman reaches her own decision about what to do. It may be that the woman:

- calls a helpline
- contacts the police
- gets legal advice
- seeks emergency accommodation
- returns temporarily to her abusive partner after making a safety plan.

Midwives need to be vigilant and sensitive to possible indicators of domestic abuse, including:

- late booking or poor engagement with antenatal care
- repeated presentation to services or frequent unexplained admissions
- depression, anxiety and self-harm
- injuries of different ages, especially to the neck, breasts, head, abdomen and genital areas
- pelvic pain, frequent urinary tract infections, vaginal infections and sexually transmitted diseases
- partner always present during appointments and dominates the questions
- woman appears evasive or reluctant to talk
- poor obstetric history – repeated miscarriages, terminations, preterm labour, stillbirths or low birthweight babies; the pregnancy may also be unplanned or unwanted (DH 2005).

Documentation of the issues or concerns is imperative, but this should not be in the handheld notes. Confidentiality is important, but, where there is multi-professional working, it is important that information is shared. There are limits to confidentiality. If there are reasons to suspect children are at risk, safeguarding and protection takes precedence. This needs to be explained to the woman.

The Home Office guidance (Taket 2004) recommends the following mnemonic to aid the approach:

**R** Routine enquiry
**A** Ask direct questions
**D** Document findings safely
**A** Assess women's safety
**R** Resources – give women information and respect their choices.

**Reflective activity 23.1**

What ethical dilemmas can arise for the midwife when a pregnant woman with two other young children refuses to discuss the domestic abuse she is experiencing?

## DRUG AND ALCOHOL MISUSE

The risks of physical, psychological and social harm for women who have significant problems related to alcohol and drug use during pregnancy are well documented (DH 2007b). It is also potentially harmful for the baby. Whilst the risks associated with smoking during pregnancy are also recognized, they are not covered in this chapter (see Chapter 19). There are a number of illicit substances used by women in pregnancy, including cocaine, heroin, cannabis and benzodiazepines. Poly-substance misuse – for example, opiates and alcohol – is not uncommon (Lewis 2007).

Substance misuse is often compounded by other factors, such as poverty, social exclusion and homelessness (Kaltenbach & Finnegan 1997). Pregnant drug-using women are therefore at increased risk of poorer general health and other health-related problems, including bloodborne viruses, such as hepatitis B and C. They should be cared for as part of a wider integrated multiprofessional team which includes addiction, neonatal and social services.

Substance misuse during pregnancy increases the risk of poor pregnancy and newborn outcomes (DoH 2007b), including:

- placental abruption (Hulse et al 1998)
- stillbirth and neonatal death
- preterm delivery and intrauterine growth retardation (Gillogley et al 1990)
- low birthweight and sudden infant death syndrome (Hepburn 2005)
- neonatal abstinence syndrome (Shaw & McIvor 1995)
- physical and neurological damage
- fetal alcohol syndrome (DH 2007b).

Midwives should be alert to the fact that substance misuse may be associated with past or current experiences of abuse and with psychiatric or psychological problems (Klee 1997).

## Antenatal care

Substance misuse makes a significant contribution to maternal mortality, with 11% of all pregnant women who died between 2003 and 2005 having alcohol or drug problems (Lewis 2007). Women often book late. This may be owing to a number of issues, including chaotic lifestyles, poor service accessibility, fear of being judged, and avoidance of social services (Lewis 2007). The booking history should include sensitive routine enquiry about all substance misuse; this includes the use of alcohol, tobacco, prescribed or non-prescribed and legal and illegal drugs. However, for some women, pregnancy may act as a positive incentive to change substance-misusing behaviour.

If it emerges that a woman has a problem with drug or alcohol misuse, she should be encouraged to attend addiction services, or specialist maternity services where available. Antenatal services should arrange a multi-professional assessment of the extent of the woman's substance use, including type of drugs, level, frequency, pattern, and method of administration, and consider any potential risks to her unborn child from current or previous drug use.

## Intrapartum care

Routine care during labour should be provided, with careful observation of mother and fetus for signs of withdrawal. Commonly seen symptoms in the mother include restlessness, tremors, sweating, abdominal pain, cramps, anxiety and vomiting. In addition, the fetus is at increased risk of hypoxia and fetal distress, as the effects of drug misuse can cause placental insufficiency (DH 2007b).

## Postnatal care

All mothers and babies should be transferred to the postnatal ward unless there is a medical reason for admission to the special care baby unit. Breastfeeding should be promoted where possible; however, this is contraindicated if the woman is:

- injecting
- using poly substances
- using crack, cocaine or large doses of amphetamines
- HIV positive (Day & George 2005).

Neonatal abstinence syndrome (withdrawal symptoms) occurs in 55–94% of neonates exposed to opiates in utero (American Academy of Pediatrics Committee on Drugs 1998). Commonly seen symptoms include sneezing, poor feeding, irritability, high-pitched cry and tremors (Shaw & McIvor 1995). Hyperphagia can also occur, usually associated with weight loss, but occasionally with excessive weight gain (Shephard et al 2002).

Close follow-up and multi-agency support to keep women in treatment programmes is essential; this is particularly significant if the baby is removed from the woman. Relapse can be a problem and the latest Confidential Enquiry into Maternal and Child Health (CEMACH) report highlighted that a majority of women who died with known alcohol or drug misuse problems did so after 42 days postnatally (Lewis 2007).

## Safeguarding children

It is estimated that there are between 250,000 and 350,000 children of problem drug users in the UK (Home Office 2003), representing 2–3% of children under the age of 16 in England and Wales (Lewis 2007). Midwives and addiction services need to be aware of the laws and issues that relate to child protection. If they have any concerns, they must contact their designated named lead for child protection, supervisor of midwives or social services for advice.

**Reflective activity 23.2**

At the booking visit, a woman who works as a barrister tells the midwife that she used to smoke cannabis but stopped when she discovered she was pregnant. She subsequently misses two antenatal appointments. When you ring her to find out why, she states that she has been extremely busy at work. She is quite dominant in her personality and promises you that she will attend the next appointment. She doesn't. What action would you take?

# TEENAGE PREGNANCY

In June 1999 the Social Exclusion Unit produced a report on teenage pregnancy and parenthood (see Ch. 13). The report highlighted two main goals:

**Table 23.1 Under-18 conceptions for England: 1998–2006**

| Year | Under-18 conceptions | Under-18 conception rate* | Percent leading to legal abortion |
|---|---|---|---|
| 1998 | 41,089 | 46.6 | 42.4 |
| 1999 | 39,247 | 44.8 | 43.5 |
| 2000 | 38,699 | 43.6 | 44.8 |
| 2001 | 38,461 | 42.5 | 46.1 |
| 2002 | 39,350 | 42.7 | 45.8 |
| 2003 | 39,553 | 42.2 | 46.1 |
| 2004 | 39,593 | 41.6 | 46.0 |
| 2005 | 39,804 | 41.3 | 46.8 |
| 2006† | 39,003 | 40.4 | 48.9 |

*Per thousand females aged 15–17.
†2006 data are provisional.
Source: Office for National Statistics and Teenage Pregnancy Unit, 2008.

- to reduce the rate of teenage conceptions, with the specific aim of halving the rate of conceptions among under 18s by 2010
- to get more teenage mothers into education, training or employment, to reduce the risk of long-term social exclusion.

The provisional 2006 under-18 conception rate for England of 40.4 per 1000 girls aged 15–17 represents an overall decline of 13.3% since 1998, the baseline year for the Teenage Pregnancy Strategy (ONS 2008; see Table 23.1). The under-18 conception rate is now at its lowest level for over 20 years; however, it is still one of the highest in Western Europe, with approximately 90,000 teenagers becoming pregnant annually (DCSF 2008). Poorest areas of the country are most affected.

It is recognized that becoming a teenage mother can have negative consequences on a woman's physical and mental health and limits social and educational opportunities, which may impact on future economic wellbeing (DfES 2006). Children born to teenagers are more likely to have poorer health and social outcomes in later life (Swann et al 2003) and daughters are more likely to become teenage mothers themselves (Berrington et al 2005).

### *Effects on child health*

- Rates of infant mortality are 60% higher than rates for infants of mothers aged 20–39
- Affected by late antenatal booking, increased rates of smoking and poor diet
- Babies born with low birthweight (see Ch. 44), linked to higher rates of smoking throughout pregnancy, compared with babies of older mothers (DfES 2006)
- Increased likelihood that babies are bottle-fed (Botting et al 1998)
- Children have an increased risk of accidents resulting in admission to A&E (Peckham 1993).

### *Effects on mental and emotional health*

- Higher rate of postnatal depression than older mothers
- Increased risk of relationship breakdown and therefore living alone, often in poor conditions
- Children are more likely to experience behavioural problems, including hyperactivity (DfES 2006).

### *Effects on economic wellbeing*

- Young mothers' attendance in education, employment or training (EET) beyond the compulsory school-leaving age is low, with approximately 30% of them aged 16–19 being in EET, compared with about 90% of all 16–19-year-olds. This can have a negative impact on their job prospects in later life.
- Children of teenage mothers are therefore at increased risk of living in poverty, compared with those born to mothers in their twenties. They also have lower academic attainment and a higher risk of being unemployed in later life (DfES 2006).

A number of key areas have been identified which can make a difference in reducing teenage pregnancy rates and therefore limit the negative health impact that is associated with it:

- 'Joined up working' – the solution rests with a number of services, including health, youth support, education and social care
- Shared data – to assist with strategic development of services
- Promotion of contraception, including community contraception services
- Sex and relationship education (DCSF 2008).

## BLACK, MINORITY AND ETHNIC WOMEN

Population movements worldwide have resulted in changes to the profile of women using NHS maternity services. The number of people from black and minority ethnic (BME) communities in Great Britain is increasing (CHAI 2008).

There is a strong association between ethnicity, deprivation and poor outcomes in maternity care (Lewis 2007). There is a higher risk of infant death for babies born to mothers from East or West Africa and the Caribbean (London Health Observatory 2007). The Bangladeshi and Pakistani groups make up a four-times larger proportion of the population in the most deprived areas and for black Caribbean and black African groups the proportion is two-and-a-half times higher (DH 2007c).

The arrival of new communities, primarily from the enlarged European Union, has also increased demand on maternity services (Darzi 2007, 2008). These groups share some common characteristics:

- lack of awareness of the maternity services
- poor access and engagement
- language and literacy difficulties
- poor general health
- prejudice
- poverty.

Migrants are not a homogenous group and can be divided into the following:

- asylum seekers and refugees
- 'refused' asylum seekers
- 'illegal' immigrants
- individuals who enter the UK with visa clearance (visas are issued for reasons such as tourism, marriage, study, employment or visiting family).

Recently arrived asylum seekers and women with no recourse to public funds are likely to be more vulnerable than people who have come for employment (Taylor & Newall 2008).

**Reflective activity 23.3**

A 17-year-old Chinese woman, Chew Yeen, attends your booking clinic. She is an hour late for the appointment and tells you in broken English that she walked to the appointment but got lost. She is accompanied by a friend who only speaks Cantonese. From your assessment, you think she is about 28 weeks pregnant. She repeatedly tells you, 'Everything is fine, no problem'. How would you meet the needs of this woman?

### Asylum seekers and refugees

#### Background and definitions

The 1951 Refugee Convention (UNHCR 1951) defines a refugee as:

> *'any person who ... owing to a well-founded fear of being persecuted for reasons of race, religion, nationality, membership of a particular social group or political opinion, is outside the country of his (or her) nationality and is unable or, owing to such fear, is unwilling to avail himself (or herself) of the protection of that country'.*

An asylum seeker is defined as:

> *'a person who has left their country of origin and has applied for refugee status in another country and is waiting for the decision' (UNHCR 1951).*

The term 'failed' asylum seeker is used to describe people who have had their asylum claims refused, who have lost their appeals and who have reached the end of the process (Bennett et al 2007).

Pregnant women who have been displaced from their country of origin may have a number of key issues in common:

- severe loss through the death, often traumatic and witnessed, of loved ones
- physical assault, sexual harassment, rape
- poor general health
- depression
- loneliness
- domestic abuse
- stress of overwhelming domestic responsibilities (Burnett & Peel 2001).

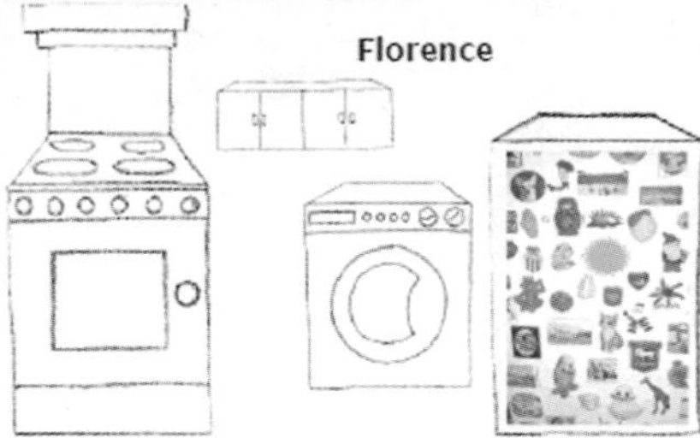

"It's easier to find out about getting
a new kitchen................ for the issue
that is likely to involve many women,
most women, there is nothing. What
you need is advertisments telling
you what to do and where to go and
then of course people would "
Florence


**Figure 23.1** Florence. (Artist Heidi Cutts, The Polyanna Project. All Rights Reserved 2007©)

Asylum seekers from some countries may have additional health needs; for example, women born in sub-Saharan Africa are disproportionately affected by HIV (Health Protection Agency 2008). Women from some countries, for example Somalia and Sudan, may have undergone female genital cutting (Powell et al 2002).

Although there are some examples of good practice in designing maternity services to meet asylum seekers' needs, many asylum seekers find it difficult to access care (Gaudion & Allotey 2008; Harris et al 2006; Project London 2007, 2008). Access to services is made more difficult because of transience of residence, relative poverty and uncertainty within a complicated asylum process (see website for video: Florence ... the experience of becoming a mother in exile).

Evidence in the latest CEMACH report demonstrates that the care provided for women who are seeking asylum in the UK does not always provide for their needs; for example, black African women, including asylum seekers and newly arrived refugees, have a mortality rate nearly six times higher than their white counterparts (Lewis 2007). The report highlights that this may reflect not only cultural factors implied in ethnicity but also social circumstance. Significantly, the report recognized that for this group of women there may be additional risk factors, including poor overall health status and underlying and possible unrecognized medical conditions, such as cardiac disease.

Teenagers who are seeking asylum are particularly vulnerable because of their situation; living in poverty with uncertainty and because of a lack of familial support and a lack of experience inherent in their youth (Gaudion & Allotey 2008).

### Access to maternity services

Accessing services by women who are not well integrated into a community is challenging simply because of the principle 'you do not know what you do not know' (Gaudion et al 2007a; Homeyard & Gaudion 2008). There is little information in the public domain about how to access services (Fig. 23.1; Gaudion et al 2007b) (see website). Current and changing entitlement to NHS maternity care has led to another potential barrier to accessing antenatal care. The Department of Health guidance states that women should be given access to care (DH 2004a); however, the way this is implemented varies between hospitals. The request for payment for care from newly arrived migrants may not come as a surprise for them as they may have arrived from countries where antenatal and intrapartum care is routinely purchased.

Confusion over the 2004 regulations regarding entitlement to NHS care has impacted on access to care for some women (Kelly & Stevenson 2006). The guidelines for Entitlement to Health Care are under review but they currently state that maternity care is classed as immediately necessary care. This means that all antenatal, birth and postnatal care should be provided irrespective of ability to pay (DH 2004b).

## Language

Caring for women whose main language is not English can present problems for staff (CHAI 2008). It is of particular concern as it may lead to women receiving suboptimal care because:

- the woman may not be able to talk about intimate issues or discuss her past history adequately
- the correct information may not be conveyed where a person 'acting' as an interpreter does not have the level of language proficiency needed
- the person translating may be a perpetrator of domestic abuse.

It is important to remember that women may have a basic working knowledge of the English language that enables them to go shopping or catch a bus but this does not mean that they will have the vocabulary to fully understand issues around antenatal screening or understand the relevance of their past medical and obstetric history on their current pregnancy. In the latest CEMACH report, 48 of the women who died spoke little or no English (Lewis 2007).

The National Service Framework stipulates that all NHS maternity providers should have an interpreting and advocacy service (DH 2004a). Additional solutions may include having staff who speak commonly used languages, access to a language line and translation of commonly used maternity information publications (CHAI 2008). A recent needs assessment conducted at Brunel University on asylum seekers in maternity services found:

- a lack of interpreting services
- women did not understand the antenatal screening choices
- women were unaware of domestic abuse services
- women were frightened and ill-prepared for the birth of their baby because they were unable to communicate their concerns
- misinterpretation of the health professional's body language, leaving women frightened that something must be wrong (Gaudion & Allotey 2008).

### Gypsy, Roma and Traveller women

Gypsy, Roma and Traveller communities are the largest ethnic minority group in Europe. The Commission for Racial Equality (2006) estimated that there were approximately 200,000 to 300,000 people in the UK. They are also the most marginalized and comprise a number of different ethnic groups. Sensitive targeted outreach services to enable women to access and use maternity services is important. A study at Sheffield University found that these women have a higher rate of miscarriage, stillbirth and infant death (Parry et al 2004).

Travellers and Gypsy women may have difficulty accessing maternity services for a number of reasons:

- They may not be registered with a general practitioner and therefore unable to access care through this route.
- Although many Traveller and Gypsy women live in houses, many also live in caravans or trailers. Either through choice or because they are evicted from land, they move around the country, often visiting relatives and friends. This means that continuity with a midwife or even a service is disrupted.
- They may have poor literacy skills and therefore not understand information about booking times and procedures that are sent to them.
- They may have encountered hostility and discriminatory attitudes within the health service previously.
- Traveller sites are often in marginalized parts of town not well served by public transport, therefore making attendance more difficult (Parry et al 2004).

Within the Traveller and Gypsy community, women marry young and having children is an important part of their cultural identity. 'Mochadi', a term used to describe cultural issues of cleanliness and modesty, are important. The functions of cleanliness include all activities from washing, food preparation, and relationships. Washing hands is particularly important, especially before handling food and in the morning after getting dressed.

Women's issues are not discussed when men are present, including pregnancy. Although women should be offered the option of their husbands accompanying them at the birth, it should be recognized that this is not the norm for them. Childbirth is 'understood' as polluting and therefore best away from the home and in a hospital. This is a way of limiting the effects of the contamination of the process (Okley 1983). Privacy and modesty also affects uptake of breastfeeding, as women do not like to 'expose' their breasts in public or even on-site where their husbands or other men might see them. Some Traveller and Gypsy women may prefer not to be cared for by a male health professional.

Improving service provision for Gypsy, Roma and Traveller women needs to include designing a flexible service near the site, if not on-site; a system so that women can directly access a midwife and that when they move, the midwife can ring ahead and arrange ongoing care.

## POVERTY AND DESTITUTION

Research has shown that as poverty increases there is a corresponding increase in infant deaths (DH 2007a). Reducing infant mortality and increasing life expectancy are a Government priority. The infant mortality part of the Public Service Agreement states that 'starting with children under one year, by 2010 to reduce by at least 10% the gap in mortality between the routine and manual group and the population as a whole' (DH 2007d).

The 'routine and manual group' includes people working in lower supervisory or technical jobs, semi-routine and routine occupations, for example, cleaners, bar staff/waitress, shop assistants, train or bus drivers, sewing machinists, plumbers and people working in call centres (DoH 2007d).

A third of all the women whose deaths were investigated in the last CEMACH report were either single or unemployed or in a relationship where both partners were not employed. In England, women who lived in the most deprived areas were five times more likely to die than women living in the least deprived areas (Lewis 2007).

In the UK there are a number of factors that can make a woman destitute, including:

- ill health or pregnancy, especially for economic, illegal or irregular migrants
- domestic abuse for migrants where the woman's visa is spousal and she has no recourse to public funds
- becoming 18 or 21 for former unaccompanied asylum-seeking children
- women whose asylum claim has been rejected (Taylor & Newall 2008).

Women who have no recourse to public funds are particularly vulnerable, not just in terms of healthcare but the whole remit of social provision for themselves and their children. They have limited options; although some basic support (Section 4 support) may be possible, it is often linked, for 'failed' asylum seekers, to being returned to their country of origin (Home Office 2007). Other options include voluntary return, support from local authorities under Section 21 of the National Assistance Act 1948, Section 17 of the Children Act 1989 or Section 117 of the Mental Health Act 1995 (Taylor & Newall 2008).

## CONCLUSION

Meeting the challenges of maternity service provision for women who are, because of age, ethnicity, immigration status or social situation, more vulnerable, is not easy. None of the groups discussed are homogenous; every woman is an individual and may 'fall' into more than one of the above categories. Each individual woman presents from a different culture, ethnicity, religion, identity, family structure and educational background; each with unique life experiences that inform their interpretation of and uptake of maternity services. Their needs are correspondingly diverse.

The central most important issue is communication; no midwife or other health professional should work in a silo, and information sharing is crucial. It is not necessarily about specialist services but treating women as individuals and being able to signpost to services that are specialized in order to maximize outcomes for mother and baby. Good practice in maternity care can help build the necessary early links with women and families and ensure that agencies are in place so that they all work together to provide a coherent and responsive service. With complex cases, it is important to consult with the supervisor of midwives, who can offer advice and support.

## KEY POINTS

- All midwives must be sensitive to the issues of vulnerable populations and carefully discern situations where pregnant women require multi-professional services.
- Information sharing and communication in language that women can understand is essential to promote safe and effective care.
- Women and their babies in vulnerable groups are more likely to suffer morbidity and mortality.
- All pregnant women should have a needs, risk and choice assessment by 12+6 weeks of pregnancy.
- Midwives need to be vigilant and sensitive to the individual needs of vulnerable women.
- There is a strong association between ethnicity, deprivation and poor outcomes in maternity care.
- Women who have no recourse to public funds are particularly vulnerable.

## REFERENCES


American Academy of Pediatrics Committee on Drugs: Neonatal drug withdrawal, *Pediatrics* 101(6):1079–1088, 1998.

Bennett K, Heath T, Jeffries R: *Asylum statistics. United Kingdom 2006. Home Office Statistical Bulletin* (website). www.ukba.homeoffice.gov.uk/sitecontent/documents/residency/publicfunds.pdf. 2007. Accessed August 16, 2008.

Berrington A, Diamond I, Ingham R, et al: *Consequences of teenage motherhood: pathways which minimise the long-term negative impacts of teenage childbearing*, Southampton, 2005, University of Southampton.

Botting B, Rosato M, Wood R: Teenage mothers and the health of their children, *Population Trends* 93:19–28, 1998.

British Medical Association (BMA): *Domestic abuse: a report from the BMA Board of Science*, London, 2007, BMA.

Burnett A, Peel M: Health needs of asylum-seekers and refugees, *British Medical Journal* 322(7285):544–547, 2001.

Commission for Healthcare Audit and Inspection (CHAI): *Towards better births; a review of maternity services in England*, London, 2008, CHAI.

Commission for Racial Equality (CRE): *Good practice: Gypsies and Irish Travellers: the facts* (website). http://83.137.212.42/sitearchive/cre/gdpract/g_and_t_facts.html#one. 2006. Accessed August 16, 2008.

Darzi A: *NHS next stage review, interim report. Our NHS, our future*, London, 2007, Department of Health.

Darzi A: *A framework for action. Healthcare for London*, London, 2008, NHS.

Day E, George S: Management of drug misuse in pregnancy, *Advances in*

*Psychiatric Treatment* 11:253–261, 2005.

Department for Children, Schools and Families (DCSF): *Teenage Pregnancy Independent Advisory Group Annual Report 2007/8*, London, 2008, HMSO.

Department for Education and Skills (DfES): *Teenage pregnancy next steps: guidance for Local Authorities and Primary Care Trusts on effective delivery of local strategies*, London, 2006, DfES.

Department of Health (DH): *Maternity Standard, National Service Framework for Children, Young People and Maternity Services*, London, 2004a, DH.

Department of Health (DH): *Implementing the overseas visitors' hospital charging regulations: guidance for NHS Trust hospitals in England*, London, 2004b, HMSO.

Department of Health (DH): *Responding to domestic abuse: a handbook for health professionals*, London, 2005, DH.

Department of Health (DH): *Implementation plan for reducing health inequalities in infant mortality: a good practice guide*, London 2007a, DH.

Department of Health (DH): *Drug misuse and dependence: UK guidelines on clinical management*, London, 2007b, DH.

Department of Health (DH): *Tackling health inequalities. Status report on the programme for action*, London, 2007c, DH.

Department of Health: *Review of the Health Inequalities Infant Mortality PSA Target*, London, 2007d, HMSO.

Gaudion A, Allotey P: *Maternity care for refugees and asylum seekers in Hillingdon. A needs assessment*, Uxbridge, 2008, Brunel University.

Gaudion A, Godfrey C, Homeyard C, et al: *The Hackney women's wheel report*, London, 2007a, The Polyanna Project.

Gaudion A, Godfrey C, Homeyard C, et al: *The Hackney women's wheel visual diary*, London, 2007b, The Polyanna Project.

Gillogley KM, Evans AT, Hansen RL, et al: The perinatal impact of cocaine, amphetamine, and opiate use detected by universal intrapartum screening, *American Journal of Obstetrics and Gynaecology* 163(5 Pt1):1535–1542, 1990.

Harris M, Humphries K, Nabb J: Delivering care for women seeking refuge, *RCM Midwives Journal* 9(5):190–192, 2006.

Health Protection Agency: *Pregnant women* (website). http://www.hpa.org.uk/web/HPAweb&HPAwebStandard/HPAweb_C/1203084355122#f4. 2008. Accessed August 16, 2008.

Hepburn M: Social problems in pregnancy, *Anaesthesia and Intensive Care Medicine* 6(4):125–126, 2005.

Home Office: *Hidden harm: responding to the needs of children of problem drug users*, London, 2003, Home Office.

Home Office: *UK Border Agency. Section 4 Support* (website). www.ukba.homeoffice.gov.uk/asylum/support/apply/section4. 2007. Accessed February 1, 2009.

Homeyard C, Gaudion A: Safety in maternity services: women's perspectives, *Practising Midwife* 11(7):20–23, 2008.

Hulse GK, Milne E, English DR, et al: Assessing the relationship between maternal opiate use and antepartum haemorrhage, *Addiction* 93(10):1553–1558, 1998.

Janssen PA, Holt VL, Sugg NK, et al: Intimate partner violence and adverse pregnancy outcomes: a population-based study, *American Journal of Obstetrics and Gynecology* 188(5):1341–1347, 2003.

Kaltenbach K, Finnegan L: Children of maternal substance misusers, *Current Opinion in Psychiatry* 10(3):220–224, 1997.

Kelly N, Stevenson J: *First do no harm: denying health care to people whose asylum claims have failed*, London, 2006, Refugee Council.

Klee H: *Illicit drug use, pregnancy and early motherhood: an analysis of impediments to effective service delivery*, Manchester, 1997, Manchester Metropolitan University.

Lewis G, editor: *The Confidential Enquiry into Maternal and Child Health (CEMACH). Saving mothers' lives: reviewing maternal deaths to make motherhood safer 2003-2007: The Seventh Report on Confidential Enquiries into Maternal Deaths in the United Kingdom*, London, 2007, CEMACH.

London Health Observatory: *Born equal? A briefing on inequalities in infant mortality in London. Executive summary* (website). www.lho.org.uk/Download/Public/12371/1/Infant_Mortality_ExecutiveSummary.pdf. 2007. Accessed August 16, 2008.

National Institute for Health and Clinical Excellence (NICE): *Antenatal care: routine care for healthy pregnant women. Clinical Guideline Number 6*, London, 2008, NICE.

Newberger EH, Barkan SE, Lieberman ES, et al: Abuse of pregnant women and adverse birth outcome: current knowledge and implications for practice, *Journal of the American Medical Association* 267b):2370–2372, 1992.

Office for National Statistics and Teenage Pregnancy Unit (ONS): *Under 18 conceptions for England: 1998-2006* (website). www.everychildmatters.gov.uk/_files/6D17854AF93522B6D2C32EE0A954ADA8.doc. 2008. Accessed August 24, 2008.

Okley J: *The Traveller-Gypsies*, Cambridge, 1983, Cambridge University Press.

Parry G, Van Cleemput P, Peters J, et al: *Health status of Gypsies and Travellers in England*, Sheffield, 2004, University of Sheffield.

Peckham S: Preventing unplanned teenage pregnancies, *Public Health* 107(2):125–133, 1993.

Powell R, Lawrence A, Mwangi-Powell F, et al: Female genital mutilation, asylum-seekers and refugees: the need for an integrated UK policy agenda, *Forced Migration Review* 14:35, 2002.

Project London: *Report and recommendations. Improving access to healthcare for the communities most vulnerable* (website). www.medecinsdumonde.org.uk/doclib/104524-report2007light.pdf. 2007. Accessed August 16, 2008.

Project London: *Report and recommendations. Improving Access to Healthcare for the Communities most Vulnerable 2006* (website). www.medecinsdumonde.org.uk/doclib/155511-plartwork.pdf. 2008. Accessed August 16, 2008.

Ramsay J, Richardson J, Carter YH, et al: Should health professionals screen women for domestic violence? Systematic review, *British Medical Journal* 325(7359):314–318, 2002.

Royal College of Midwives (RCM): *Domestic abuse in pregnancy*, London, 1999, RCM.

Royal College of Obstetricians and Gynaecologists (RCOG): *Violence against women*, London, 1997, RCOG Press.

Royal College of Psychiatrists (RCPsych): *Domestic violence CR102*, London, 2002, Royal College of Psychiatrists.

Shaw NJ, McIvor L: Neonatal abstinence syndrome after maternal methadone treatment, *Obstetrical and Gynecological Survey* 50(7):511–513, 1995.

Shephard R, Greenough A, Johnson K, et al: Hyperphagia, weight gain and neonatal drug withdrawal, *Acta Paediatrica* 91(9):951–953, 2002.

Social Exclusion Unit: *Teenage pregnancy: report by the Social Exclusion Unit*, London, 1999, The Stationery Office.

Swann C, Bowe K, McCormick G, et al: *Teenage pregnancy and parenthood: a review of reviews. Evidence briefing*, London, 2003, Health Development Agency.

Taket A: *Tackling domestic violence: the role of health professionals*, London, 2004, Home Office.

Taylor B, Newall N: *Maternity, mortality and migration: the impact of new communities*, Birmingham, 2008, Heart of Birmingham Teaching NHS Primary Care Trust.

United Nations High Commissioner for Refugees (UNHCR): *Definitions and obligations* (website). www.unhcr.org.au/basicdef.shtml. 1951. Accessed August 16, 2008.

# Part 4

# The anatomy and physiology of fertility, conception and pregnancy

# Chapter 24

# Anatomy of male and female reproduction

*Barbara Burden and Maria Simons*

## LEARNING OUTCOMES

After reading this chapter, you will have:

- explored the anatomical structures of the pelvis, its corresponding joints and ligaments, and their significance for midwifery practice
- considered the dimensions, angles and axes of the pelvis and how these may influence birth outcomes
- examined the anatomical structures of the female reproductive system and their significance to midwifery practice
- explored how the uterus changes during pregnancy, how it functions during labour, birth and the third stage of labour, and the normal processes of involution in the postpartum period
- reviewed the structures of the male reproductive system and their significance for fertility and conception.

## INTRODUCTION

An understanding of the anatomy of human reproduction enables the translation of abstract concepts of anatomy to normal physiology, function and processes of conception, pregnancy, labour, birth, postpartum and related disorders. This chapter provides a reference point for application to midwifery practice, increasing understanding of the physiological aspects of the birthing process. This brings together theory and practice, enabling knowledge and understanding to be applied in the midwife's practice and in health promotion. Greater understanding of the structure of the human body increases knowledge of how it functions and why it sometimes deviates from the norm.

The chapter, with its supportive literature, links with other chapters demonstrating how anatomy and physiology may be applied to midwifery practice.

## THE PELVIS

The human pelvis supports the upper body and transmits its weight to the lower limbs, enabling movement in an upright posture. In the female, the pelvis serves as a protective bony ring encircling the reproductive organs, bladder and rectum. In pregnancy, physiological processes effect subtle changes in the composition, shape, plane of inclination and internal dimensions of the true pelvis. These changes enable the female skeleton to support the gravid uterus and are essential to the mechanisms involved in the process of childbirth.

The pelvis consists of four pelvic bones (see Fig. 24.1):

- two innominate
- one sacrum
- one coccyx.

The innominate bones are each divided into three regions:

- ilium
- ischium
- pubis.

### Joints and ligaments of the pelvis

The joints of the pelvis connect the innominate bones at the pubis anteriorly and to the sacrum posteriorly, and the

*Sacral foramina*
Four pairs of foramina (or holes) are present in the sacrum, through which the four sacral nerves pass.

*Ala*
An ala projects laterally on each side of the sacral promontory and the superior surface of the first sacral vertebra. The alae extend to articulate with the ilium on both sides.

The anterior surfaces of the alae form part of the landmarks of the pelvic brim.

*Acetabulum*
A round cup-shaped socket on the external surface of the innominate bone with which the head of the femur articulates to form the hip joint. Two-fifths of the acetabulum is formed by the ilium, two-fifths by the ischium and one-fifth by the pubis.

Malformation, disease or injury of the hip joint can result in a reduction in abduction of the legs. This may result in hip and back pain in pregnancy, inability to abduct the hips during vaginal examination and delivery, and inability to adopt certain positions in labour such as the lithotomy or squatting position.

*Symphysis pubis*
A cartilaginous joint between the anterior portions of the two pubic bones. There is increased mobility and size in this cartilage during the last months of pregnancy.

*Ischial tuberosity*
The thickened portion of the body of the ischium providing attachment points for the sacrotuberous ligament. This is the section of the pelvis that takes the full weight of the body when sitting. Women with painful perineums can be advised to sit with their knees apart and the pelvis tilted, allowing the tuberosities to take the weight of the body, so the mother is sitting on a triangular-shaped base, relieving pressure in the perineum.

The distance between the tuberosities is estimated to be 10 cm. A reduction in this dimension may indicate a reduced pelvic outlet. Although this dimension is difficult to measure, a midwife may assess the distance by placing a closed fist on the perineum between the tuberosities. The knuckles of the fist should fit comfortably between the tuberosities in a normal gynaecoid pelvis.

*Sacral promontory*
The prominent upper margin of the first sacral vertebra.

The measurement between the sacral promontory and the anterior surface of the pubis is the anteroposterior diameter of the pelvic brim. A reduction in this diameter can influence the descent and engagement of the presenting part of the fetus into the pelvis.

*Lumbar vertebra (5th)*
Articulates with the first sacral vertebra. The position of the lumbar vertebrae influences the angle of pelvic inclination.

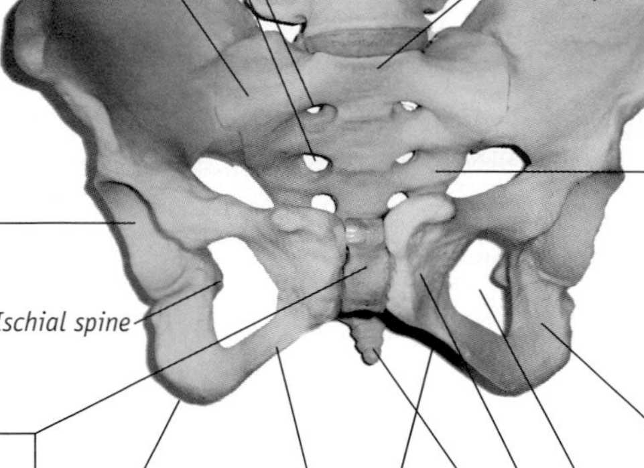


*Pubic arch*
The arch created by the inferior rami of the pubes. The angle of the pubic arch is significant to the dimensions of the pelvic outlet. The optimal angle should be 90°, which is a feature of the gynaecoid pelvis.

Reduction in the pelvic outlet may result in obstructed labour, prolonged labour, persistent occipitoposterior positions and excessive fetal skull moulding.

*Coccyx*
A small triangular-shaped bone that articulates with the lower end of the sacrum. It is composed of four fused rudimentary vertebrae and provides attachment points for ligaments, muscle fibres of the anal sphincter and the ischiococcygeus muscle of the pelvic floor.

During the birth of the baby, the coccyx moves backwards to enlarge the pelvic outlet

*Ilium*
Forms the upper expanded part of the innominate bone. It gives rise to the female shape of the hips.

*Anterior superior iliac spine*
A prominent anterior protrusion of the ilium that can be palpated through the lateral abdominal wall. The distance between the left and right anterior superior iliac spines does not necessarily indicate the capacity of the true pelvis.

*Iliac crest*
The curved upper border of the ilium. Women refer to this part of the pelvis as their hips.

*Sacrum*
Lies between the ilia, forming the rear of the pelvis. It consists of five fused vertebrae forming a wedge shape perforated by four sets of foramina through which the sacral nerves pass.

In a gynaecoid pelvis the sacrum's anterior surface is concave and a feature of the rounded cavity, allowing room for the fetal head to descend. It also plays a part in directing the baby through the pelvis around the curve of Carus (see Fig. 24.3).

*Ischium*
A thickened L-shaped bone that connects to the ilium posteriorly and to the pubis anteriorly.
The medial surface has attachment points for the ischiococcygeus muscle of the pelvic floor.

*Obturator foramen*
A triangular hole created by the borders of the ischium and the pubis. It is covered by the obturator membrane, through which pass the obturator nerve and blood vessels leading to the thigh.

*Pubis*
Forms the anterior portion of the pelvis and has two arms called rami. The inferior ramus attaches to the ischium, and the superior ramus to the ilium at the iliopectineal eminence. It forms one-fifth of the acetabulum. The inferior ramus forms the boundary for the obturator foramen and the pubic arch, under which the baby must pass during birth.

**Figure 24.1** The female pelvis. **A.** Anterior view of pelvis.

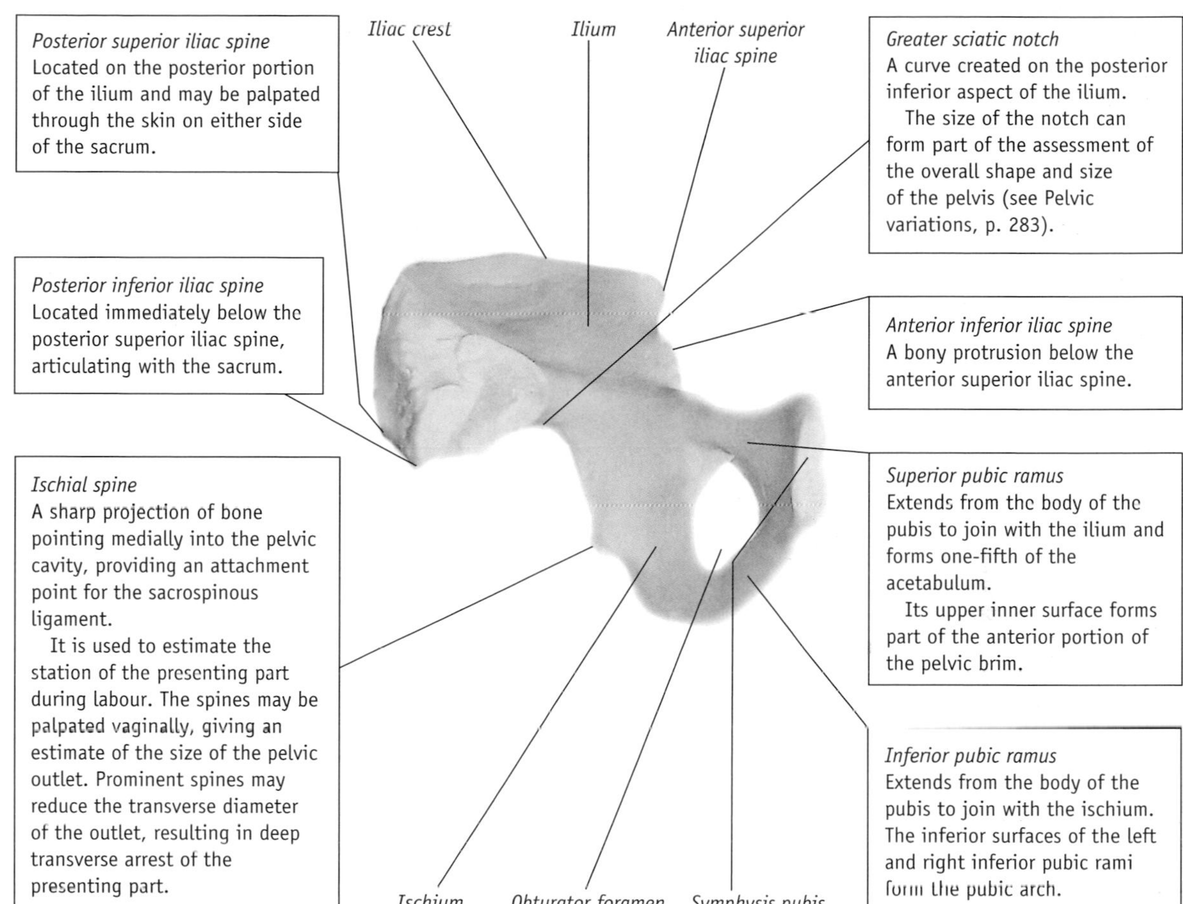

Posterior superior iliac spine
Located on the posterior portion of the ilium and may be palpated through the skin on either side of the sacrum.
Iliac crest
Ilium
Anterior superior iliac spine
Greater sciatic notch
A curve created on the posterior inferior aspect of the ilium.
The size of the notch can form part of the assessment of the overall shape and size of the pelvis (see Pelvic variations, p. 283).
Posterior inferior iliac spine
Located immediately below the posterior superior iliac spine, articulating with the sacrum.
Anterior inferior iliac spine
A bony protrusion below the anterior superior iliac spine.
Ischial spine
A sharp projection of bone pointing medially into the pelvic cavity, providing an attachment point for the sacrospinous ligament.
It is used to estimate the station of the presenting part during labour. The spines may be palpated vaginally, giving an estimate of the size of the pelvic outlet. Prominent spines may reduce the transverse diameter of the outlet, resulting in deep transverse arrest of the presenting part.
Superior pubic ramus
Extends from the body of the pubis to join with the ilium and forms one-fifth of the acetabulum.
Its upper inner surface forms part of the anterior portion of the pelvic brim.
Inferior pubic ramus
Extends from the body of the pubis to join with the ischium. The inferior surfaces of the left and right inferior pubic rami form the pubic arch.
Ischium
Obturator foramen
Symphysis pubis


**Figure 24.1 Continued B.** Inner surface of left innominate bone.

sacrum to the coccyx (see Fig. 24.2). These joints are cartilaginous in type, consisting of plates of fibrocartilage. The pelvis also provides attachment points for ligaments, which are bands of tissue connecting two structures. In normal circumstances, ligaments do not possess the ability to stretch, and therefore prevent excessive movements within the joints, enhancing stability.

In pregnancy, the hormones *relaxin, progesterone* and *oestrogen* affect the joints and ligaments, enabling some movement of the joints to facilitate birth. Pelvic pain sometimes occurs during pregnancy, birth or post partum and is thought to be linked to overstretching of ligaments in the pelvis and lower spine (Rost et al 2004).

## The true pelvis

The *true pelvis,* through which a baby negotiates passage during labour and birth, is the most significant part of the pelvis. This is divided into three regions, known as the *brim, cavity* and *outlet* (see Fig. 24.3). As the presenting part descends into the pelvis, the baby negotiates each aspect of the true pelvis simultaneously. For example, in a cephalic presentation, as the baby's head crowns, the presenting part negotiates the outlet, most of the baby's head is in the cavity and the shoulders are at the brim.

It is important to appreciate that the pelvis is three-dimensional. The pelvic measurements of the brim, cavity and outlet are viewed through a cross-section, whereas measurements incorporated in the pelvic conjugates are viewed through a sagittal section. These two measurements inform a *pelvic assessment.*

## Pelvic measurements (Fig. 24.4)

**The pelvic brim** is the inlet to the *true pelvis* and is almost circular, except posteriorly, where the sacral promontory juts into the brim (see Fig. 24.5).

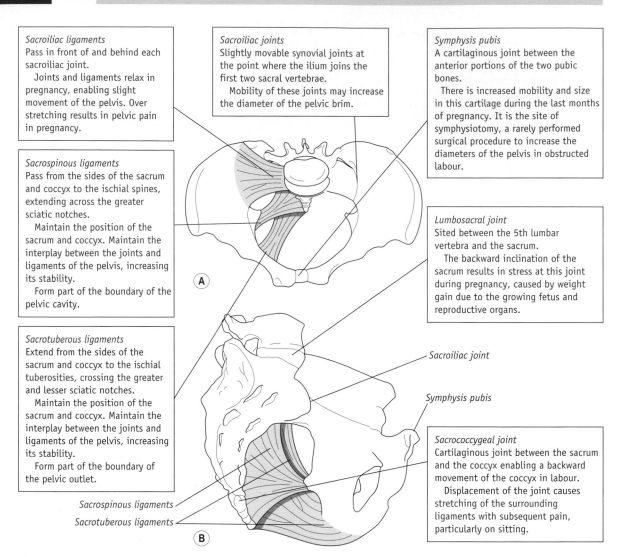

*Sacroiliac ligaments*
Pass in front of and behind each sacroiliac joint.
Joints and ligaments relax in pregnancy, enabling slight movement of the pelvis. Over stretching results in pelvic pain in pregnancy.

*Sacroiliac joints*
Slightly movable synovial joints at the point where the ilium joins the first two sacral vertebrae.
Mobility of these joints may increase the diameter of the pelvic brim.

*Symphysis pubis*
A cartilaginous joint between the anterior portions of the two pubic bones.
There is increased mobility and size in this cartilage during the last months of pregnancy. It is the site of symphysiotomy, a rarely performed surgical procedure to increase the diameters of the pelvis in obstructed labour.

*Sacrospinous ligaments*
Pass from the sides of the sacrum and coccyx to the ischial spines, extending across the greater sciatic notches.
Maintain the position of the sacrum and coccyx. Maintain the interplay between the joints and ligaments of the pelvis, increasing its stability.
Form part of the boundary of the pelvic cavity.

*Lumbosacral joint*
Sited between the 5th lumbar vertebra and the sacrum.
The backward inclination of the sacrum results in stress at this joint during pregnancy, caused by weight gain due to the growing fetus and reproductive organs.

A

*Sacrotuberous ligaments*
Extend from the sides of the sacrum and coccyx to the ischial tuberosities, crossing the greater and lesser sciatic notches.
Maintain the position of the sacrum and coccyx. Maintain the interplay between the joints and ligaments of the pelvis, increasing its stability.
Form part of the boundary of the pelvic outlet.

*Sacroiliac joint*

*Symphysis pubis*

*Sacrococcygeal joint*
Cartilaginous joint between the sacrum and the coccyx enabling a backward movement of the coccyx in labour.
Displacement of the joint causes stretching of the surrounding ligaments with subsequent pain, particularly on sitting.

*Sacrospinous ligaments*

*Sacrotuberous ligaments*

B

**Figure 24.2** The ligaments and joints of the pelvis. **A.** Superior view. **B.** Sagittal section.

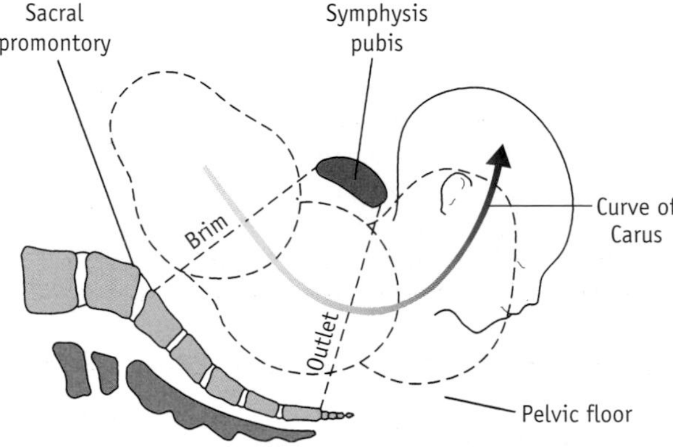


**Figure 24.3** The axis of the true pelvis.

The landmarks of the pelvic brim describe the interplay between the fetus and the pelvis as the presenting part descends, and are a fundamental part of the assessment of descent and engagement of the presenting part. It is not the components of the brim that are important, it is the part that the brim plays as a whole in the assessment of progress during pregnancy and labour. This is the first test that the fetus has to pass as it descends through the pelvis. The midwife assesses engagement of the presenting part during abdominal and vaginal examinations (see Chs 35–37).

**The pelvic cavity** extends from the brim to the outlet of the pelvis. In the anteroposterior view the cavity is wedge shaped: shallow at the front and deep at the back. Viewed from above it is circular in shape in a gynaecoid pelvis and

| | Anteroposterior | Right and left oblique | Transverse |
|---|---|---|---|
| **Brim** | From upper inner border of the symphysis pubis to sacral promontory<br>**11 cm** | From the sacroiliac joint to the iliopectineal eminence<br>**12 cm** | Between widest points on the iliopectineal lines<br>**13 cm** |
| **Cavity** | From inner border of the symphysis pubis to the curve of the sacrum<br>**12 cm** | Right and left from the sacroiliac joint, fanning out to measure a point between the upper and lower pubic rami<br>**12 cm** | From right inner surface of the ischium to left inner surface of the ischium<br>**12 cm** |
| **Outlet** | From lower border of the symphysis pubis to sacrococcygeal joint<br>**13 cm** | From the sacrospinous ligament to the obturator foramen<br>**12 cm** | Transverse from the right to the left ischial spines<br>**11 cm** |

**Other measurements:** Sacrocotyloid diameter from sacral promontory to iliopectineal eminence – 9 cm

**Figure 24.4** Pelvic measurements.

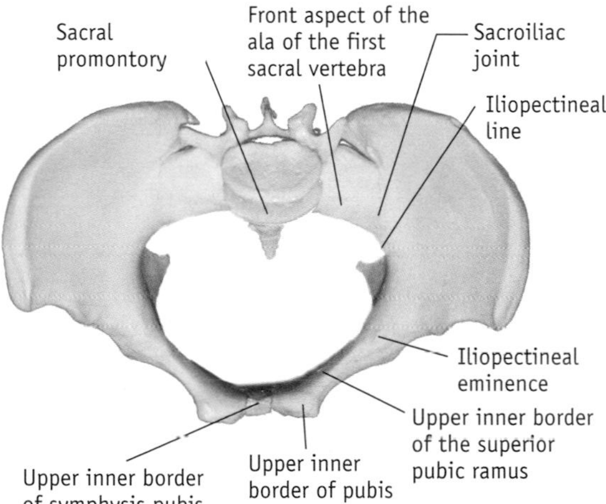


**Figure 24.5** Superior view of the pelvis to show the landmarks of the pelvic brim.

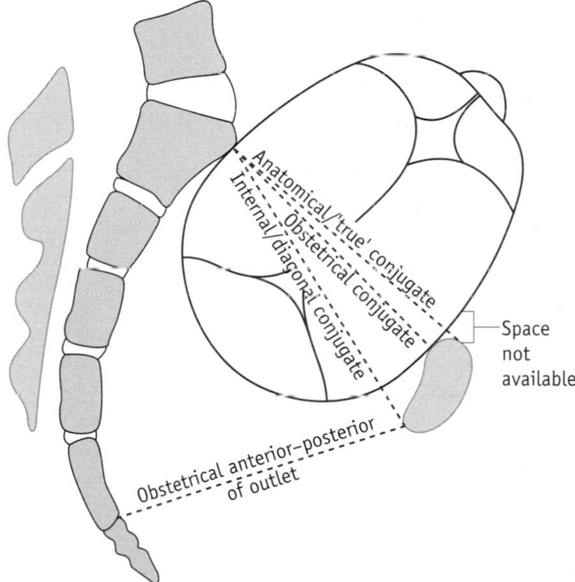


**Figure 24.6** The relationship of the pelvic conjugates and the fetal negotiation of the conjugates.

designed to facilitate the descent and rotation of the presenting part. The boundaries of the cavity are:

- curve of the sacrum
- sacroiliac joints
- sacrospinous ligaments
- ischia
- superior pubic ramus
- inferior pubic ramus
- bodies of the pubes
- symphysis pubis.

**The pelvic outlet** is diamond shaped and partly bound by ligaments. It can be described in two ways:

- by anatomical structure
- by obstetric dimension – that is, the space available through which the baby must pass during birth (see Fig. 24.6).

The anatomical boundaries for the outlet of the pelvis are:

- tip of the coccyx
- sacrotuberous ligaments

- ischial tuberosities
- pubic arch.

The obstetric outlet is bounded by:

- inner border of the base of the sacrum
- sacrospinous ligaments
- ischial spines
- lower inner border of the symphysis pubis.

## Pelvic conjugates

A *conjugate* is a measurement taken from one point in the pelvis to another. In midwifery there are the *anatomical, obstetrical* and *internal (diagonal) conjugates* (Fig. 24.6).

### Anatomical conjugate

- Measured from upper outer border of symphysis pubis, measuring across the pubic bone
- Adds approximately 1.25 cm to all measurements
- Includes space **not available** to the fetus as it enters the pelvic brim.

### Obstetric conjugate

- Measured from sacral promontory to upper inner border of symphysis pubis
- The fetus negotiates this smaller dimension.

### Internal or diagonal conjugate

- Estimated at vaginal examination as part of a pelvic assessment
- Measured from posterior inferior surface of the symphysis pubis to the sacral promontory
- Measurement varies in individual women
- Unusual to identify the sacral promontory on vaginal examination (conjugate measures between 12 and 13 cm, longer than the length of most practitioners' fingers)
- If detected, it indicates that the diameters of the pelvis are reduced and referral for obstetric consultation should be sought.

**Reflective activity 24.1**

To appreciate the interplay between the regions of the pelvis you need to consider the three-dimensional structures of the regions of the brim, cavity and outlet and how they interrelate to form the anatomical dimensions.

Use a model of the pelvis to locate the structures identified in the text relating to the brim, cavity and outlet.

## Angles and planes

These are mathematical concepts applied to the pelvis. When standing, the pelvis slopes into a position where the pubis is lower than the sacral promontory – described as an angle of 55° to the horizontal or to the floor. This slope continues through the cavity, reducing its angle to 15° at the outlet. The fetal head must negotiate the curve created by the changing angles within the pelvis as it enters the pelvic brim in a downward and backward direction. It emerges from the outlet in a downward and forward direction as the presenting part reaches the pelvic floor. The curve created in the pelvis is known as the *curve of Carus*.

The term *plane* describes the relationship between the pelvis and a flat surface, such as the floor, highlighting the tilt of the pelvis in a normal female skeleton. Hypothetical angles are then created in relation to the degree of tilt of a particular individual (see Figs 24.7 and 24.8), which provide a representation of the angles in relation to the planes of the pelvis. Figure 24.8 shows the axis (curve of Carus), an imaginary line through which a fetus rotates as it passes through the pelvis.

In an abnormal pelvis, the plane of the pelvis may be significantly altered, affecting the axis of the birth canal and consequently the direction of the fetus through the

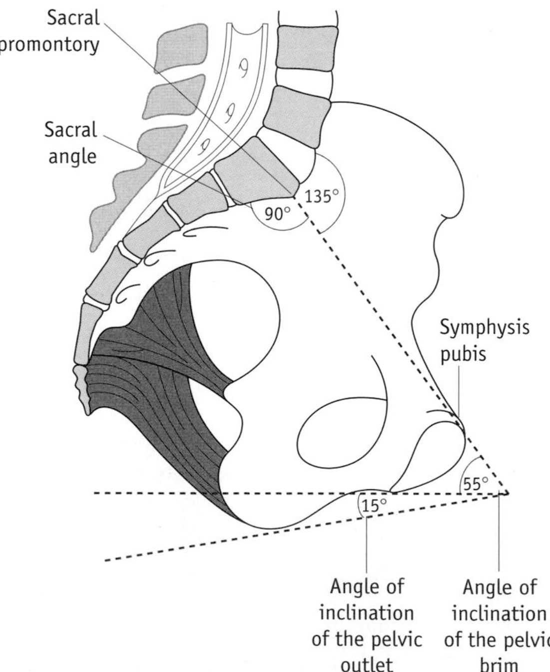


**Figure 24.7** The pelvis, showing the degrees of inclination: inclination of the pelvic brim to the horizontal, 55°; inclination of pelvic outlet to the horizontal, 15°; angle of pelvic inclination, 135°; inclination of the sacrum, 90°.

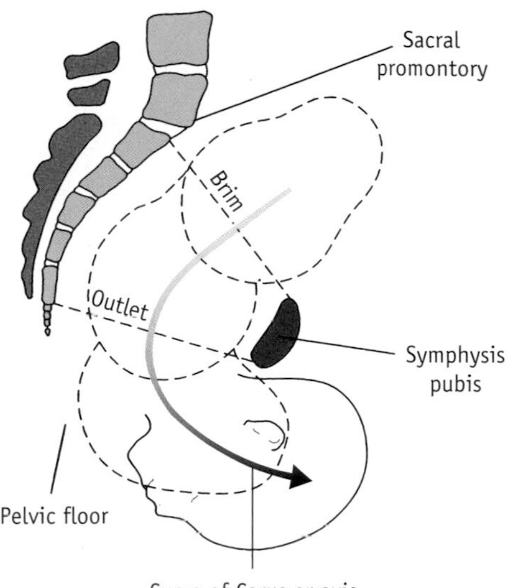


**Figure 24.8** The axis of the birth canal in upright position.

pelvis. The midwife needs to consider the axis of the birth canal when women adopt alternative positions for childbirth during labour and delivery.

1. *Sacral angle.* The angle between the plane of the brim and the anterior surface of the first sacral vertebra. Usual measurement of 90°. (Measurements of less than 90° suggest a cavity smaller than the brim: more than 90°, larger than the brim.)
2. *Angle of inclination of the pelvic brim.* The angle that the plane achieves with the horizontal when a woman is standing is approximately 55°. If greater than 55°, there may be delay in engagement of the presenting part in the pelvis.
3. *Angle of inclination of the pelvic outlet.* This is the 15° angle the upper inner border of the obstetric outlet makes with the horizontal when the woman is in a standing position.

**Reflective activity 24.2**

Rotate Figure 24.2 to represent the woman in a variety of positions, i.e. standing, 'all fours' and squatting. Note the direction of the presenting part of the fetus during descent in all positions. What is the impact of these positions on labour?

The *subpubic angle* is between the two inferior pubic rami forming the pubic arch (Fig. 24.1). In a gynaecoid pelvis, this should be approximately 90°, enabling two finger widths to sit in the apex of the pubic arch during vaginal pelvic assessment.

## Pelvic variations

Although there are four recognized pelvic categories (Caldwell et al 1940) (Table 24.1), variations within these categories can occur. Some women may have mixed features, such as a gynaecoid posterior pelvis and android forepelvis. The most important factor is the *true* pelvic space available for the fetus to descend and emerge from the pelvis. The pelvic size and shape cannot be viewed in isolation from other factors, such as position and size of fetus and processes of labour.

Other factors that may influence the size and shape of the pelvis include:

- injury and disease (Phillips et al 2000)
- dietary deficiencies – in young women these can have a direct influence on the growth and shape of the pelvis (Carruth & Skinner 2000).

## Other pelvic types identified

Any injury or disease of pelvic bones may significantly affect the dimensions of the pelvis, impacting on the outcome of labour and birth. Table 24.2 outlines the classification and characteristics of *unusual pelves*, each of which may have a mixture of characteristics, with the shape depending upon the degree and timing of damage. It is important that the midwife assesses women at risk of pelvic dysfunction as early as possible antenatally.

## Pelvic assessment

Pelvic assessment enables estimation of whether the fetus will successfully pass through the pelvis during labour and delivery, by assessing the pelvic size and outlet. Although this can be undertaken at any time before or during pregnancy, the relationship of the pelvis to the fetal skull can only be assessed from 37 weeks' gestation (antenatally or during labour). Pelvic assessment is no determinant of outcome but contributes to the overall assessment of pelvic adequacy.

The assessment must include:

- abdominal examination – assessing engagement and descent of the presenting part
- vaginal examination – determining the size and shape of the pelvis by assessing the following:
  - prominence of sacral promontory (usually cannot be palpated on vaginal examination)
  - prominence of ischial spines and, if identified, the distance between them
  - angle of pubic arch (usually accommodates two finger widths at the apex of the arch)
  - prominence of ischial tuberosities (usually accommodates four knuckle widths when measured externally at the level of the perineum).

**Table 24.1 Pelvic categories**

| Characteristics | Gynaecoid/ female type | Justo minor pelvis | Android/male type | Anthropoid | Platypelloid |
|---|---|---|---|---|---|
| **Shape of brim** | Round | Round – but small | Triangular – 'heart shaped' | Oval (widest in the anteroposterior diameter) | Bean shaped – flattened |
| | | | | | |
| **Depth of pelvis** | Shallow – straight walls | Shallow | Deep – convergent walls | Deep – straight | Shallow – divergent walls |
| **Subpubic arch** | 85–90° | 90° | 60–75° (narrow) | More than 90° | More than 90° |
| **Sciatic notch** | Wide | Wide – but small | Narrow | Wide | Narrow |
| **Ischial spines** | Not prominent, blunt | Not prominent | Prominent and narrow interspinous diameter | Not prominent but may have narrowed interspinous diameter | Blunted, usually widely separated – not prominent |
| **Sacrum** | Deep &curved | Straight – flattened | Straight – flattened and long | Long and narrow – may be slightly curved | Broad, flat and concave |
| **Transverse diameter of outlet** | 10 cm | Usually less than 10 cm<br>May be android characteristics present – may reduce outlet | Less than 10 cm | More than 10 cm | More than 10 cm |
| **Implications for midwifery** | Most favourable design for positive outcomes of childbirth | Miniature Gynaecoid pelvis<br>Outcomes depend on relationship between degree of size of pelvis and size of fetus | Fetal head may attempt to engage in the occipitoposterior position.<br>Deep transverse arrest may result (See Ch. 64 Excessive moulding and caput of fetal skull) | Women with this pelvis are said to be tall and 'well-built'.<br>Pelvis is large and should accommodate the fetus as it descends during labour.<br>Diameters may result in persistent occipitoposterior position leading to a 'face-to pubes' delivery | Fetal head engages in the transverse diameter. This shape of pelvis may require the fetal head to negotiate the brim using a movement called asynclitism (see Fig. 24.9 and website). This movement occurs where the baby's head tilts in one direction and then the other to enable the biparietal diameter of the fetal skull to engage in the pelvic brim and for descent to occur. Deep transverse arrest may result, as the fetal head may be unable to rotate in the pelvic cavity |
| **Estimated incidence** | 50% | | 20% | 25% | <5% |

**Table 24.2 Classified unusual pelves**

| Characteristics | Rachitic pelvis | Asymmetrical pelvis (Naegele's type) | Robert's pelvis | Osteomalacic pelvis | Spondylolisthetic pelvis |
|---|---|---|---|---|---|
| Shape of brim | Bean shaped<br>Reduced anteroposterior diameter | Asymmetrical – may be absence of one sacral ala | Inlet narrow and significantly contracted | Usually grossly altered | |
| Depth of pelvis | Flattened | May be normal | | Convergent walls | |
| Ischial spines | | One may be prominent | Likely to be reduced interspinous diameter | | |
| Sacrum | Lower end swings back to increase size of cavity<br>May be bent at the middle | | | | |
| Transverse diameter of outlet | Increased in size | May be altered | May be altered | Reduced bituberous diameter is less than 8 cm | May be altered – usually drastically contracted |
| Causes | May result following childhood rickets.<br>The soft bones are distorted by body weight. Can be caused by inadequate diet and vitamin D deficiency | Deficient development of one side of the pelvis often with bony fusion of the sacroiliac joint on the affected side.<br>Sometimes known as Naegele's pelvis. May be caused by congenital dislocation of one hip, poliomyelitis or an accident | Deficient development on both sides of pelvis with fusion of the sacroiliac joints.<br>Rare form of extreme pelvic contraction | A severe pelvis deformity occurring in adults as a result of vitamin D deficiency.<br>Distortion is different from that of childhood rickets as the condition occurs while walking and standing. Upward pressure on the legs and pelvis forces the sides of the pelvis inwards and the weight of the body on the spine forces the sacral promontory forwards | The fifth lumbar vertebra slips forward over the sacrum. The sacral promontory is pushed backwards and the tip of the sacrum pushed forward |
| Implications for midwifery | May lead to obstructed labour.<br>Fetal head may be deflexed, and usually enters the pelvis with the sagittal suture in transverse.<br>Head – asynclitism (see Fig. 24.9) | May result in a reduced incidence of vaginal delivery | May result in a reduced incidence of vaginal delivery | In parts of the world where osteomalacia is endemic, a woman may develop the condition between pregnancies, resulting in a normal vaginal delivery followed by a complicated labour or delivery. | Results in an extreme contraction of the true conjugate |

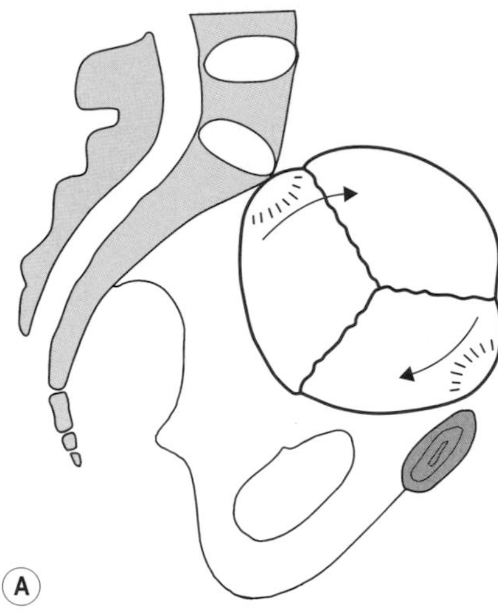


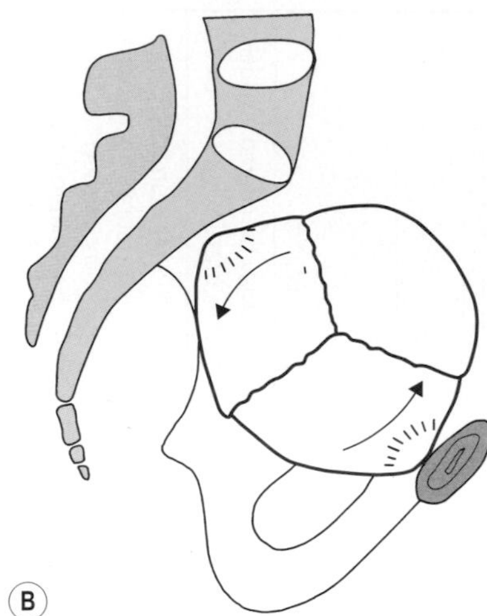


**Figure 24.9** Posterior asynclitism.

It may also include:

- X-ray examination (Sibony et al 2006)
- ultrasound scans
- computed tomography and magnetic resonance imaging (Chen et al 2008, Huerta-Enochian et al 2006).

Other factors must also be considered to enable a complete assessment to be made of the overall capacity of the woman's true pelvis:

- assessment of normality of her gait
- height
- shoe size less than 4
- previous successful vaginal delivery
- non-engagement of fetal head at 38 weeks (primigravida)
- history of rickets
- previous pelvic injury
- previous trial of labour or prolonged labour
- malpresentation, such as a breech
- extent of caput or moulding of the fetal skull during labour.

**Table 24.3 Anatomical relations to the vagina**

| View | Section of the vagina | Associated structures |
|---|---|---|
| Anteriorly | Upper half<br>Lower half | Bladder<br>Urethra |
| Posteriorly | Upper third<br>Middle third<br>Lower third | Pouch of Douglas<br>Rectum<br>Perineal body |
| Superiorly | Centrally<br>Above lateral | Cervix<br>Fornices<br>Ureters and uterine arteries |
| Inferiorly | Vaginal orifices and vestibule | |
| Laterally | Upper<br>Middle<br>Lower | Parametrium<br>Pubococcygeus muscles<br>Perineal muscle<br>Bulbocavernosus muscles |

## FEMALE REPRODUCTIVE ANATOMY

The primary function of the female reproductive system is production and transmission of ova and provision of a nurturing environment for the fertilized ovum and developing fetus. It has the ability to accommodate the developing fetus, expel the baby and placenta at birth, and return to its near pre-pregnant state during the puerperium. The study of the female reproductive system is fundamental to the midwife's understanding of gynaecology, pregnancy, birth and the impact birth has on the female reproductive anatomy. The structures identified with the female reproductive system include internal and external genitalia and the pelvis organs and structures (Table 24.3), particularly the bladder, urethra and rectum. In addition, uterine muscular support, blood supply, nerve supply and lymphatics are identified. This knowledge needs to be studied in conjunction with the pelvic floor muscle structure (see Ch. 40).

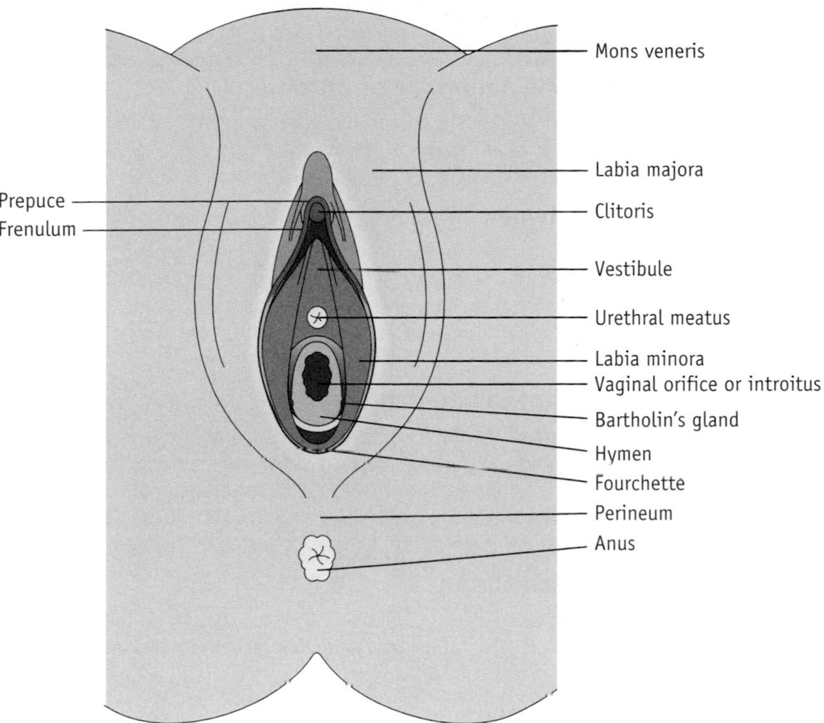


**Figure 24.10** Female external genitalia. (See Box 24.1 for further information.)

## Fetal development

During the first 6 weeks following fertilization, male and female gonads undergo identical forms of development. In female fetuses the ovaries descend a short distance from their position below the kidneys to sit in the pelvic cavity closely alongside the fallopian tubes. Their primary function of ovum production commences under the influence of female hormones during puberty (see Ch. 31).

## External genitalia

Knowledge of the anatomy of the female external genitalia (Fig. 24.10 and Box 24.1) provides a foundation for application to midwifery practice during the process of labour and birth, in relation to labial and perineal tears; episiotomy; tears to the urethral meatus or clitoris; fistulae and female genital mutilation.

Any of the following structures may be damaged during the birthing process and must be assessed following birth:

- labia majora
- labia minora
- clitoris
- vestibule
- urethral meatus
- vaginal orifice
- Bartholin's glands.

**Blood supply** is via the pudendal arteries and drainage is through corresponding veins. The external genitalia are vascular structures that facilitate healing and which bleed heavily when traumatized.

**Lymphatic drainage** occurs via the inguinal glands.

**Nerve supply** is from branches of the pudendal nerve.

## Internal genitalia

Knowledge of female internal reproductive anatomy (Fig. 24.11) enables the understanding of:

- pregnancy, birth and postpartum processes, including growth and development of the uterus in pregnancy
- uterine function in labour, birth and delivery of the placenta
- function of the muscle structures of the uterus in haemostasis and postpartum haemorrhage
- involution of the uterus and return of the anatomical structures to the pre-pregnant state
- influence of breastfeeding on involution

Box 24.1 **Female external genitalia**

### Mons veneris

Pad of fat over the pubic bone, covered by skin and, after puberty, hair.

### Labia majora

One of two thick folds of fatty tissue (labia majora) covered with skin, extending from the mons to the perineum. The inner surface contains sebaceous glands.

### Labia minora

One of two small, smooth folds of skin (labia minora) between the labia majora, containing sweat and sebaceous glands. Anteriorly, the labia minora encircle the clitoris, forming the prepuce and a smaller, lower fold called the frenulum. They meet posteriorly to form the fourchette.

### Clitoris

Highly sensitive erectile tissue about 2.5 cm long. Consists of two erectile bodies called the corpora cavernosa and a glans clitoris of spongy erectile tissue.

### Vestibule

Extends from clitoris to the fourchette and contains urethral and vaginal orifices. Contains the vestibular glands known as Skene's and Bartholin's glands.

### Urethral meatus

Situated between the clitoris anteriorly and vaginal orifice posteriorly and is the external opening of the urethra, connecting superiorly to the bladder.

### Vaginal orifice or introitus

Located posteriorly to the urethral meatus, opening into the vagina above, with the ability to stretch to accommodate the emerging baby at birth.

### Hymen

A thin membrane partially occluding the vaginal introitus – easily ruptured with the use of internal tampons, physical exercise and intercourse. Further rupture occurs during vaginal delivery, resulting in the remaining tissue forming tags – *carunculae myrtiformes*.

### Bartholin's glands

The ducts of the glands emerge on either side of the vaginal orifice on the inner surface of the labia minora. They secrete mucus to lubricate the vulva, and production increases during sexual arousal. They should not be palpable during vaginal examination unless obstructed or infected.

### Fourchette

Created as the labia minora join posteriorly to the vaginal orifice, and used as a landmark for correct alignment during perineal suturing.

### Perineum

Extends from the fourchette to the anal margin, covering the pelvic floor muscles.

### Prepuce

A loose fold of skin covering the clitoris.

### Frenulum

A small ligament maintaining the position of the clitoris.

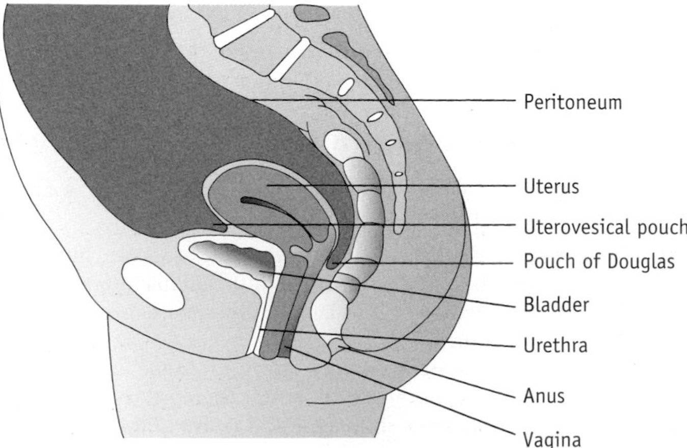


**Figure 24.11** Female pelvic organs in sagittal section.

- genital tract infection
- gynaecological conditions such as:
  - infection (Bartholin's abscess, postpartum infection)
  - infertility and fertility
  - fibroids, ectopic pregnancy, uterine prolapse, carcinoma, ovarian cysts, and cervical screening.

## Vagina

The vagina is a fibromuscular tube directed upward and backward approximately parallel to the pelvic brim. It is important to note the angle of the vagina when conducting vaginal examinations and teaching women the correct insertion of pessaries, tampons and contraceptive diaphragms.

The vagina extends from the vulva to the cervix; the anterior wall is approximately 7.5 cm long and the posterior wall 10 cm. The walls of the vagina lie in apposition until it widens at the upper portion where the cervix projects into the vagina at right angles, forming four recesses (*fornices*). The anterior fornix is shallow and the lateral fornices are deeper. The posterior fornix is deepest, which facilitates pooling of semen during intercourse, increasing the opportunities for sperm to swim through the cervix.

There are no glands in the vagina: moisture is provided by secretions from the cervical glands and transudation of serous fluid from blood vessels. Vaginal secretions are acid (pH 4.5); providing an unfavourable environment for spermatozoa, and counteracted by the alkaline reaction of semen and cervical mucus. The vagina contains lactic acid produced by the action of lactobacilli (Döderlein's bacilli) on glycogen in the squamous cells of the vaginal lining, causing vaginal acidity. Lactobacilli normally inhabit the vagina without pathology. The lactic acid produced helps destroy pathogenic bacteria that may enter the vagina. In prepubescent girls and postmenopausal women, the vagina acidity is around pH 7, creating a favourable environment for the growth of vaginal infections, such as *Candida albicans*.

**Structure** The walls of the vagina have four layers:

- interior layer of squamous epithelium arranged in transverse folds called rugae, enabling vaginal expansion and stretching during childbirth
- vascular layer of elastic connective tissue
- involuntary muscle layer with outer longitudinal fibres and inner circular fibres
- outer layer of connective tissue – part of the pelvic fascia containing blood vessels, lymphatics and nerves.

Following childbirth, the vaginal walls must be examined for damage, and assessment made to establish a plan of care.

**Function** The vagina is able to distend to facilitate the passage of the penis during intercourse, and the baby during childbirth.

**Blood supply** is via the middle haemorrhoidal arteries, arising from a branch of the internal iliac arteries; drainage is through corresponding veins.

**Nerve supply** is via sympathetic and parasympathetic nerves from the plexus of Lee–Frankenhäuser (situated in the floor of the pouch of Douglas in the region of the uterosacral ligaments) originating from branches of the second, third and fourth sacral nerves.

**Lymphatic drainage** The lower third of the vagina drains into the inguinal glands and the upper two-thirds into the internal iliac glands.

## Uterus

The uterus is a muscular, vascular, pelvic organ, often described as shaped like an upturned pear. It is situated with the bladder anteriorly and the rectum posteriorly, and normally is in a position of anteversion (leaning forward towards the bladder) and anteflexion (curved forward on itself).

The uterus is divided into the body and the cervix. The narrow end of the uterus is inserted into the vagina and the upper body communicates with the fallopian tubes at the upper lateral surfaces (Fig. 24.12 and Box 24.2).

**Structure**

*Endometrium* is the lining of the uterus which constantly changes throughout the woman's reproductive lifecycle. It has the ability to shed during the menstrual cycle and be maintained and thickened during pregnancy.

The endometrium is composed of:

- vascular connective tissue, called stroma, containing tubular glands
- a layer of ciliated columnar epithelium covering the stroma
- where the stroma dips to the level of the myometrium it is covered with non-ciliated cells.

*Myometrium* consists of plain muscle fibres and constitutes seven-eighths of the thickness of the uterine wall. In the non-pregnant state, the muscle layers are not clearly defined (Fig. 24.13).

In pregnancy, they become thicker and more defined as three layers of muscle:

1. *Inner circular*:
   - sited mainly in the cornua and around the cervix
   - assists cervical dilatation during labour.
2. *Middle oblique or spiral*:
   - thickest in the upper body of the uterus, where the placenta is normally situated
   - have the ability to contract powerfully to act as natural ligatures to blood vessels following placental separation during the third stage of labour.

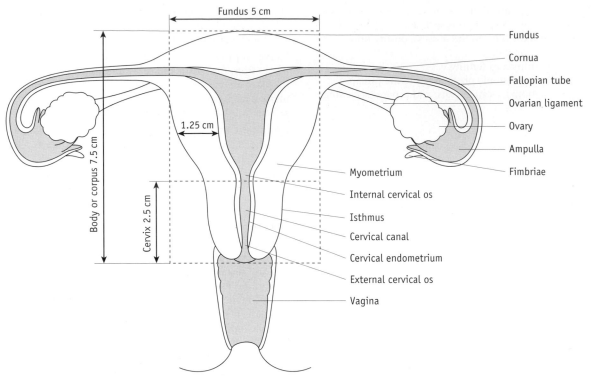

Figure 24.12 The non-pregnant uterus, fallopian tubes and ovaries. (See Box 24.2 for further information.)

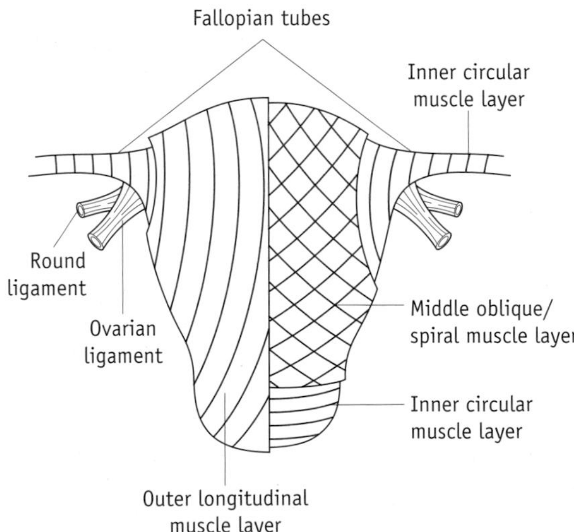


Figure 24.13 The three layers of uterine muscle.

3. *Outer longitudinal*:
   - extend from the cervix anteriorly over the uterus to the cervix posteriorly
   - have the ability to shorten in labour as the uterus contracts and retracts – facilitating descent and expulsion of the fetus, placenta and membranes.

*Perimetrium* is a layer of peritoneum draped over the uterus and fallopian tubes, continuous with the peritoneum covering the bladder, extending to the lateral walls of the pelvis (see Fig. 24.11). Folds in the peritoneum form:

- between the bladder and the uterus – the uterovesical pouch
- between the uterus and the rectum – the pouch of Douglas (this is a recognized site for infection if the membrane is breached during surgery or trauma).

### Functions

- Provision of an environment conducive to the implantation of a fertilized ovum
- Nurture of the developing fetus
- Growth and expansion to accommodate the growing fetus and placenta
- Contraction, retraction and expulsion of the fetus, placenta and membranes during birth and maintainenance of haemostasis following birth

Box 24.2 **The non-pregnant uterus, fallopian tubes and ovaries**

### Body or corpus

The upper two-thirds of the uterus. The cavity of the body is triangular in shape. The structure is made up of the fundus, cornua (singular cornu) and the isthmus.

### Cervix

The lowest third of the uterus – cylindrical in shape with its lower half projecting into the vagina at right angles.

### Internal cervical os

At the top of the cervical canal, its walls are in close apposition in the newly parous woman. It dilates and thins, becoming part of the lower uterine segment during the first stage of labour.

### External cervical os

Situated at the bottom of the cervical canal, its walls are in close apposition in the pre-pregnant state, remaining partially dilated in parous women.

Examination of the external os forms part of the assessment of progress during labour.

### Cervical endometrium or *arbor vitae*

The cervical endometrium is arranged in deep folds to facilitate the passage of spermatozoa through the cervical canal. The upper two-thirds is made up of columnar epithelium containing compound racemose glands secreting alkaline mucus. The cervical mucus is thin at the time of ovulation to facilitate spermatozoa. At other times it is thick in consistency, acting as a plug that assists in the prevention of infection in the uterus. The lower third is composed of stratified squamous epithelium continuous with that of the vagina.

### Fundus

The upper rounded part of the body of the uterus above the insertion of the two fallopian tubes. It may be palpated:

Antenatally:

- to assess fetal growth (weeks of gestation)
- to determine fetal lie and presentation

In labour:

- to assess uterine contractions
- to establish descent of the fetus
- to assess contractility of the uterus following expulsion of the placenta and membranes as an assessment of potential homeostasis

Postnatally:

- to determine involution.

### Fallopian tubes

Two tubes extending laterally from the uterus and opening into the peritoneal cavity. Each tube is approximately 10 cm long and 1 cm in diameter varying along its length. Hairs on the inner surface guide the ova towards the uterine cavity.

Scarring or obstruction caused by infection or trauma may lead to ectopic pregnancy and infertility. Tubes may be surgically ligated for sterilization purposes.

### Cornu

Formed at the junction of the uterine body and fallopian tube.

### Ovarian ligament

This ligament suspends the ovary in a position close to the fimbriae of the fallopian tube to increase the probability of the ovum entering the fallopian tube.

### Ovary

The female gonad that produces predetermined cells destined to become ova. Ovaries are endocrine organs producing oestrogen and progesterone and small amounts of the male hormone, androgen.

### Fimbriae

Finger-like projections on the end of the fallopian tube that help to waft the ovum from the ovary to the fallopian tube.

### Ampulla

Dilated distal portion of the fallopian tube where fertilization of the ovum usually occurs.

### Isthmus

The junction between the body of the uterus and the cervix. During pregnancy there is growth and development of this junction, creating the lower uterine segment.

### Cervical canal

This is a potential tube connecting the external os and the internal os. A plug of mucus (the operculum) forms here during pregnancy and is expelled when cervical activity and dilatation commence.

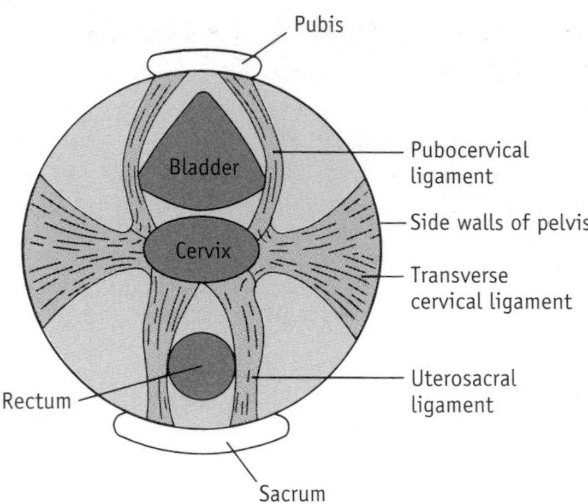


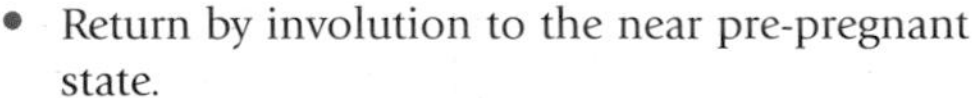
**Figure 24.14** Superior view of uterine ligaments and supports.

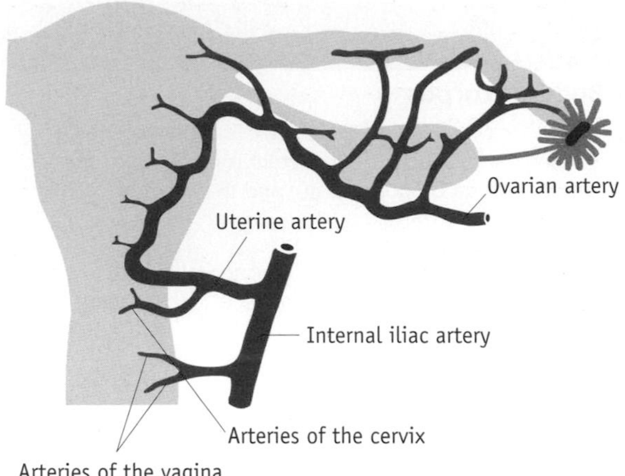


**Figure 24.15** Blood supply to the uterus and its appendages.

- Return by involution to the near pre-pregnant state.

**Uterine ligaments** maintain the normal anteverted, anteflexed position of the uterus. Damage to these ligaments may occur as a direct result of childbirth, especially prolonged labour; chronic constipation and straining; poor lifting techniques; poor posture and obesity. The effect may not be seen until later in life at the menopause, where declining levels of oestrogen cause muscle and ligament atrophy and loss of function. The result of this may be uterine prolapse and associated stress incontinence and defecation difficulties (Fritel et al 2005).

The uterine ligaments (Fig. 24.14) are:

- *Transverse cervical ligaments* (2): extend from the cervix laterally to the side walls of the pelvis.
- *Uterosacral ligaments* (2): pass back from the cervix to the sacrum, encircling the rectum, and maintain the position of anteversion.
- *Pubocervical ligaments* (2): pass forwards from the cervix to the pubic bones, offering limited support to the uterus.
- *Round ligaments* (2): arise at the cornua of the uterus, descending through the broad ligament and the inguinal canals to the labia majora. They help to maintain the uterus in a position of anteversion.
- *Broad ligament*: a double fold of peritoneum extending from the lateral borders of the uterus to the side walls of the pelvis.

**Blood supply** is via uterine and ovarian arteries; drainage is by corresponding veins (Figs 24.15 and 24.16). This provides a rich supply of blood vessels to facilitate growth of the uterus and placenta during pregnancy and supports the growth and development of the fetus. Blood vessels

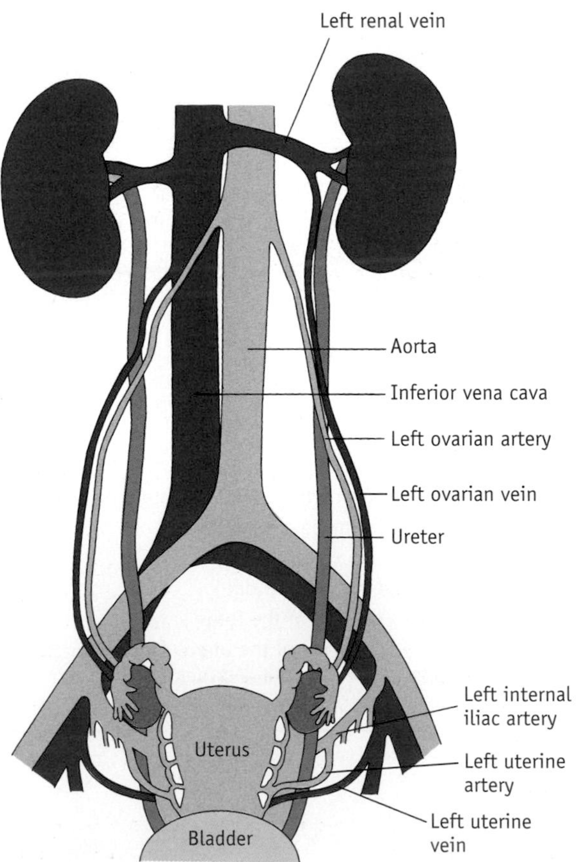


**Figure 24.16** Blood supply to the uterus. Note where the ovarian vein terminates.

to the uterus are twisted in the non-pregnant state and have the ability to uncoil as the uterus expands during pregnancy.

Breaches of this system can occur during pregnancy, labour and through trauma to the genital tract. This may cause severe haemorrhage, increasing the incidence of mortality and morbidity for both mother and baby (Lewis 2007, MCHRC 2001).

*Uterine arteries and veins* The uterine artery arises from a branch of the internal iliac artery and enters the uterus at the level of the internal cervical os, turning at right angles following a spiral course along the lateral border of the uterus, joining with the ovarian artery, with a branch to the cervix and vagina. Uterine veins follow the arteries and drain into the corresponding internal iliac veins.

*Ovarian arteries and veins* The ovarian arteries arise from the descending aorta and cross the urethra and internal iliac arteries before passing over the pelvic brim to enter the broad ligament just below the ovary. Branches of the ovarian artery supply the fallopian tubes and connect with the uterine artery. The right ovarian vein connects with the inferior vena cava and the left ovarian vein connects with the left renal vein.

**Nerve supply** is both sympathetic and parasympathetic. The sympathetic nervous system to the pelvis is a continuation of the aortic plexus (sometimes called the presacral nerve), and lies in front of the fifth lumbar vertebra and the sacral promontory. It passes downwards, joining branches of the lumbar sympathetic chain lying on the floor of the pouch of Douglas. The parasympathetic nervous supply emerges from the sacral foramina to join the Lee–Frankenhäuser plexus. The nerves then pass to the uterus and other pelvic viscera (Waugh & Grant 2006).

**Lymphatic drainage** The lymphatic vessels and nodes draining lymph away from the pelvic organs accompany the main arteries and veins, with nodes sited along the iliac vessels and the aorta. Drainage from the upper portion of the uterus is to the lumbar and hypogastric nodes, and from the lower portion to the hypogastric nodes.

**Cervix** In women who have never been pregnant the cervix can be palpated as a firm structure similar in consistency to the tip of the nose and the cervical os is closed, whereas in a multigravid woman who is not pregnant the cervical os may remain partially dilated.

During pregnancy the cervix may appear to be blue owing to the abundant blood supply, and towards the end of pregnancy it becomes softer as it 'ripens' in preparation for labour.

*Squamocolumnar junction* Carcinoma of the cervix is most likely to occur at the junction between the upper columnar epithelium and the lower stratified squamous epithelium.

## MALE REPRODUCTIVE ANATOMY (Fig. 24.17)

The function of the male reproductive system is the production of spermatozoa and their transfer to the female during sexual intercourse for the creation of new human life. It could be argued that once successful fertilization of the ovum has occurred, the need for knowledge of the male reproductive system is of little importance to the midwife. However, there are a number of issues that could be considered, such as sexual intercourse in pregnancy, transmission of sexually transmitted diseases (see Ch. 57) and understanding of some of the causes of infertility (see Ch. 28).

### Fetal development

In the fetus the male testes are located in the abdomen just below the kidneys, similar to the female. The gonads form distinct structures under genetic and hormonal influences (Johnson 2007). In the seventh or eighth month of pregnancy, male testes descend with the spermatic cord through the right and left inguinal canals and at birth should be located in the scrotum of the term infant (Snell 2000).

For more information on the male reproductive system, see the website.

## MIDWIFERY IMPLICATIONS

Knowledge of anatomy of human reproduction can help identify women who might require different care, treatment and advice, enabling the midwife to plan the most appropriate care during pregnancy, labour and puerperium, and also identify problems which may occur in the fetus and neonate. Early contact with women can identify those who may require further investigations, or referral to the obstetrician for specialist care.

At the booking visit, the woman's medical and family history must be explored, identifying potential problems which may have been caused by nutritional issues, such as rickets, osteomalacia or anorexia nervosa (Dimitri & Bishop 2007, Ekeus et al 2006). The midwife can identify whether the pelvis may have changed from its original shape through trauma, surgery or oesteoporosis (Leggon et al 2002, Phillips et al 2000) and identify normal changes in gait and in posture, as well as pelvic arthropathy, pelvic pain and symphysis pubis diastasis (Divekar & Keith 2004).

During labour, the midwife uses her understanding of pelvic anatomy to assess pelvic shape and size, using the woman's history, clinical examination, abdominal

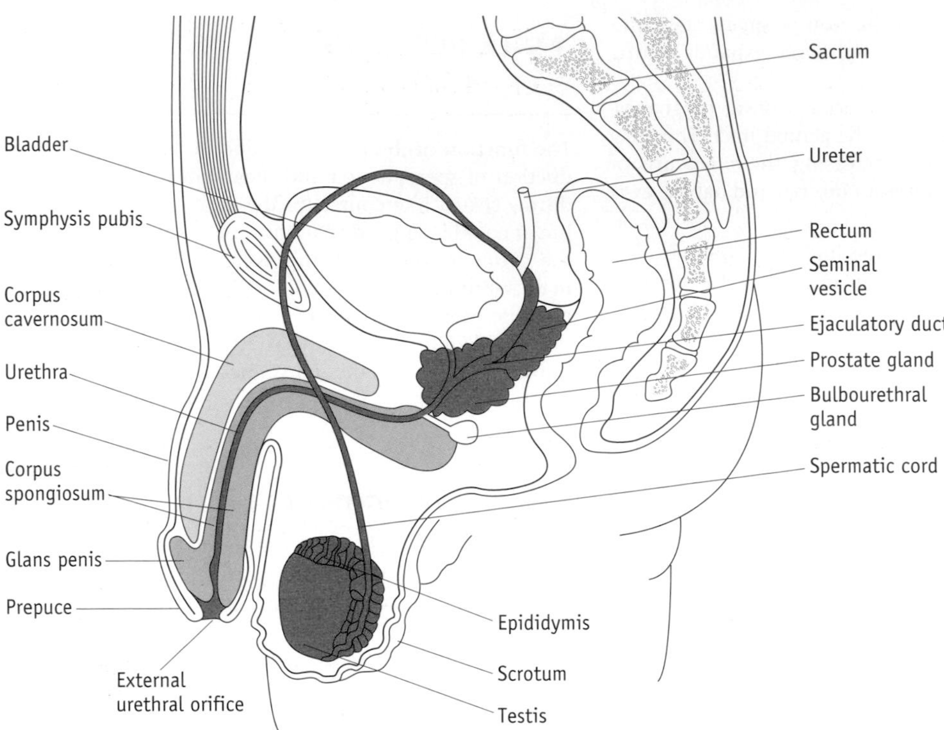


**Figure 24.17** Sagittal section of the male reproductive system.

palpation and vaginal examination, to provide information to help formulate a dynamic and appropriate plan of care for labour and birth. At this point, the midwife may be able to reduce the rate of prolonged labour, or identify dystocia early, and thus have a significant effect on morbidity.

During the postnatal period, the midwife assesses uterine involution and return to its pre-pregnant state. Any deviations from normal must be swiftly identified and appropriately referred. This includes problems caused by birth trauma, male and female circumcision, stress incontinence, contraceptive methods, sexually transmitted diseases (Ch. 57), and sexual function and dysfunction. During neonatal examination (Ch. 41) the midwife establishes the normality of neonate genitalia and educates the mother accordingly.

## CONCLUSION

Knowledge of human reproduction provides the foundation on which to place everyday practice. This understanding of how human reproductive anatomy is constructed and functions enables a midwife to apply the concepts to both the normal physiological process of childbirth and the concepts of obstetrics. It enables midwifery practitioners to utilize a common language to discuss midwifery and obstetric practice issues with other healthcare professionals. This supports and enhances the midwife's role as a health promoter and practitioner, interpreting complex health issues and relating them accurately and in appropriate terminology to women and their families.

## KEY POINTS

- A sound comprehension of the reproductive system provides a basis for an understanding of physiological and pathological conditions related to midwifery practice.
- Detailed anatomical information can be related to how the pelvis impacts on the normal and abnormal mechanisms of labour.
- Knowledge of anatomy provides a foundation for understanding how pregnancy impacts on the health of the pelvis; and how pathological conditions and extrinsic factors impact on the pelvis during parturition.

- Knowledge of anatomy of human reproduction can be applied to the study of obstetrics, gynaecological and urogenital health and pathology to enable practitioners to offer care, treatment and advice.
- An understanding of pelvic anatomy enables a midwife to assess pelvic shape and size, providing information to help formulate a plan of care for labour and birth.

## REFERENCES


Caldwell W, Moloy H, D'Espop A: The more recent conceptions of pelvic architecture, *American Journal of Obstetrics and Gynecology* 40(4): 558–565, 1940.

Carruth BR, Skinner JD: Bone mineral status in adolescent girls: effects of eating disorders and exercise, *Journal of Adolescent Health* 26(5):322–329, 2000.

Chen M, Coackley F, Kaimal A, et al: Guidelines for computed tomography and magnetic resonance imaging use during pregnancy and lactation, *Obstetrics and Gynecology* 112(2):333–340, 2008.

Dimitri P, Bishop N: Rickets: new insights into a re emerging problem, *Current Opinion in Orthopedics* 18(5):486–493, 2007.

Divekar P, Keith L: Pubic symphysis diastasis during pregnancy, *Female Patient: Obstetrics and Gynaecology Edition* 29(9):24–34, 2004.

Ekeus C, Lindberg L, Lindblad F, et al: Birth outcomes and pregnancy complications in women with a history of anorexia nervosa, *British Journal of Obstetrics and Gynaecology* 113(8):925–929, 2006.

Fritel X, Ringa V, Varnoux N, et al: Mode of delivery and severe stress incontinence: a cross sectional study among 2625 perimenopausal women, *British Journal of Obstetrics and Gynaecology* 112(12):1646–1651, 2005.

Huerta-Enochian GS, Katz VL, Fox LK, et al: Magnetic resonance-based serial pelvimetry: do maternal pelvic dimensions change during pregnancy? *American Journal of Obstetrics and Gynecology* 194(6):1689–1694, 2006.

Johnson MH: *Essential reproduction*, ed 6, Oxford, 2007, Blackwell.

Leggon R, Wood G, Indeck M: Pelvic fractures in pregnancy: factors influencing maternal and fetal outcomes, *Journal of Trauma* 53(4):796–804, 2002.

Lewis G, editor: *The Confidential Enquiry into Maternal and Child Health (CEMACH). Saving mothers' lives: reviewing maternal deaths to make motherhood safer 2003–2005. The Seventh Report on Confidential Enquiries into Maternal Deaths in the United Kingdom*, London, 2007, CEMACH.

Maternal and Child Health Research Consortium (MCHRC): *Confidential Enquiry into Stillbirths and Deaths in Infancy, 8th Annual Report*, London, 2001, MCHRC.

Phillips A, Ostlere S, Smith R: Pregnancy-associated osteoporosis: does the skeleton recover? *Osteoporosis International* 11(5): 449–454, 2000.

Rost C, Jacqueline J, Kaiser A, et al: Pelvic pain during pregnancy: a descriptive study of signs and symptoms of 870 patients in primary care, *Spine* 29(22):2567–2572, 2004.

Sibony O, Alran S, Oury J: Vaginal birth after cesarean section: X-ray pelvimetry at term is informative, *Journal of Perinatal Medicine* 34(3):212–215, 2006.

Snell RS: *Clinical anatomy for medical students*, ed 6, London, 2000, Lippincott Williams & Wilkins.

Waugh A, Grant A: Ross and Wilson anatomy and physiology in health and illness, ed 10, London, 2006, Churchill Livingstone.

Chapter |25|

# Female reproductive physiology

*Mary McNabb*

## LEARNING OUTCOMES

After reading this chapter, you will be able to:

- understand the underpinning physiology of the neurohormonal aspects of reproduction, including formation and development of ovarian follicles; the role of external–internal ovarian innervation in follicular development, and the bi-directional communication axis between the oocyte and its surrounding somatic cells
- appreciate the critical role of ovarian steroid hormones in regulating key markers of female reproductive health
- describe the menstrual and ovarian cycles in relation to female health, preparation for conception, and childbearing.

## INTRODUCTION

Knowledge of the complexities underpinning reproductive physiology enables the midwife to assess the woman's general and sexual health and apply this to the individual's menstrual and ovarian cycles, and conception.

This chapter includes a detailed account of the sequence of events within the ovaries, before, during and after ovulation, and ovarian neuroendocrine regulation of hypothalamic–pituitary gonadotrophin responsiveness, across the infertile cycle. The chapter concludes with ovarian steroid regulation of the uterine and mammary cycles and recent markers of female reproductive health. More in-depth information on the underpinning physiology is available on the website.

From puberty to menopause, ovarian activity is characterized by cyclic development of several follicles; maturation and ovulation of a selected follicle, and subsequent formation and regression of the corpus luteum. This episodic pattern of ovulation requires cyclical release of steroid and peptide hormones that imposes a corresponding cyclicity on many organ systems; levels of sexual arousability; and differing behaviours (Chapman et al 1998, Chidambaram et al 2002, Haselton et al 2007, Salonia et al 2005, Tarin et al 2002, Webb 1986).

Evidence of increased sexual motivation during the periovulatory phase of the cycle has been found in humans and other primates, but these behaviours are far less evident and reliable than the monthly shedding of bloody endometrial tissue at the end of the luteal phase. Consequently, the term *menstrual cycle* is used as an indirect measure of the *ovarian cycle*. Both cycles are driven by the dynamic pattern of negative and positive feedback between ovarian steroids and peptide hormones, and gonadotrophins from the anterior pituitary gland and hypothalamus.

## THE OVARIAN CYCLE

The ovarian cycle has three distinct phases:

1. The *follicular* phase prepares the female reproductive system to receive spermatozoa.
2. *Ovulation* of a fertilizable oocyte.
3. The *luteal* phase prepares the female to receive and nurture the conceptus.

In humans, the first and third phases take approximately 14 days each, while the second takes about 15 minutes (Lousse & Donnez 2008) (Fig. 25.1).

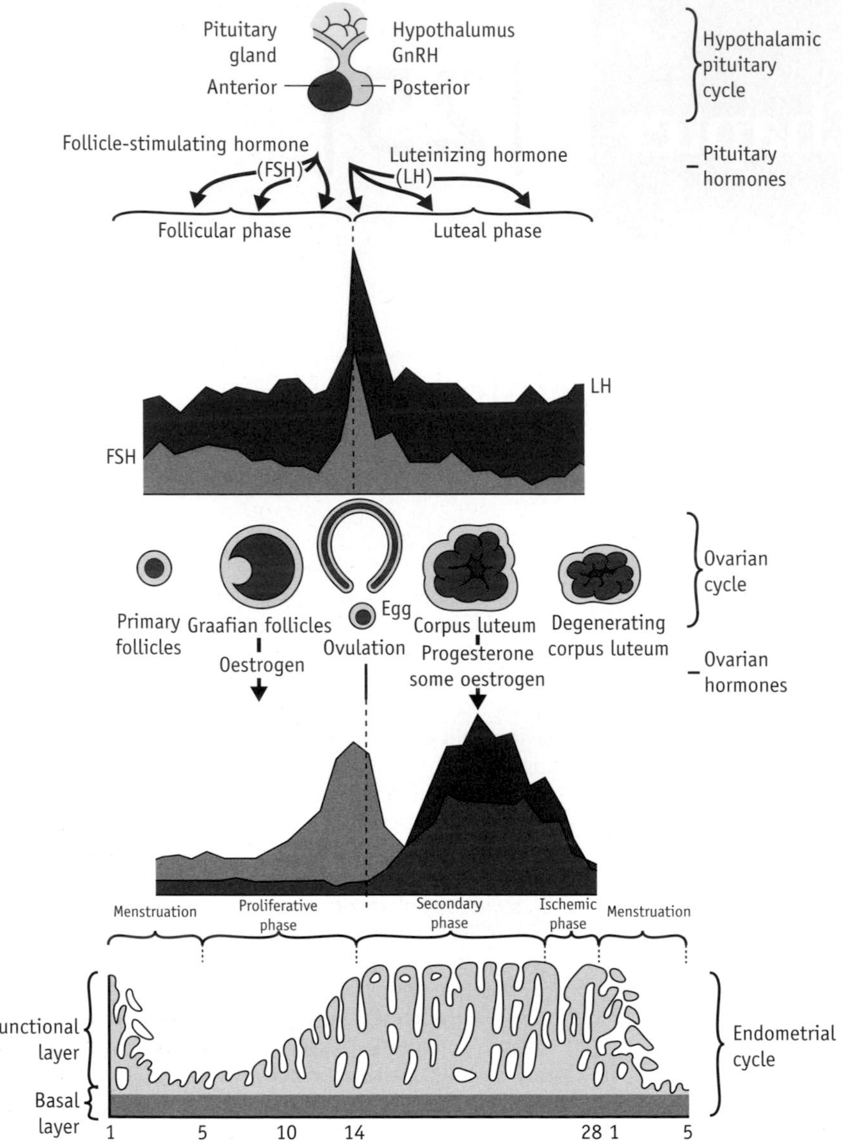


**Figure 25.1** Hypothalamic–pituitary–ovarian–endometrial changes during an ovulatory cycle. *(Reproduced with permission from Blackburn 2007:36.)*

Fertility depends on ovarian production of one *dominant follicle* per cycle, with the capacity to *ovulate* a fertilizable oocyte. From puberty to menopause, a few primary follicles are recruited every day into a pool of growing follicles, producing a continuous trickle of developing follicles.

Of the 15–20 follicles recruited, one *selected follicle* demonstrates increased cell proliferation and differentiation; expansion of thecal vascularity; rapid accumulation of antral fluid; and rising capacity for steroid and peptide hormone secretion (Geva & Jaffe 2000, Gougeon 1996, Seifer et al 2002). Following selection, this growing follicle regulates changes in hypothalamic–pituitary gonadotrophin activity during oocyte maturation and ovulation, and following the mid-cycle LH/FSH surge, when it differentiates into a functional *corpus luteum* or *postovulatory follicle* (Baker & Spears 1999, Hodgen 1982, Kunz et al 1998, Nakao et al 2007) (Fig. 25.2).

At mid-cycle, the *dominant follicle* becomes visible to the naked eye as a large bulge under the surface epithelium of the ovary. The enclosed oocyte acquires meitotic and developmental competence and subsequently undergoes

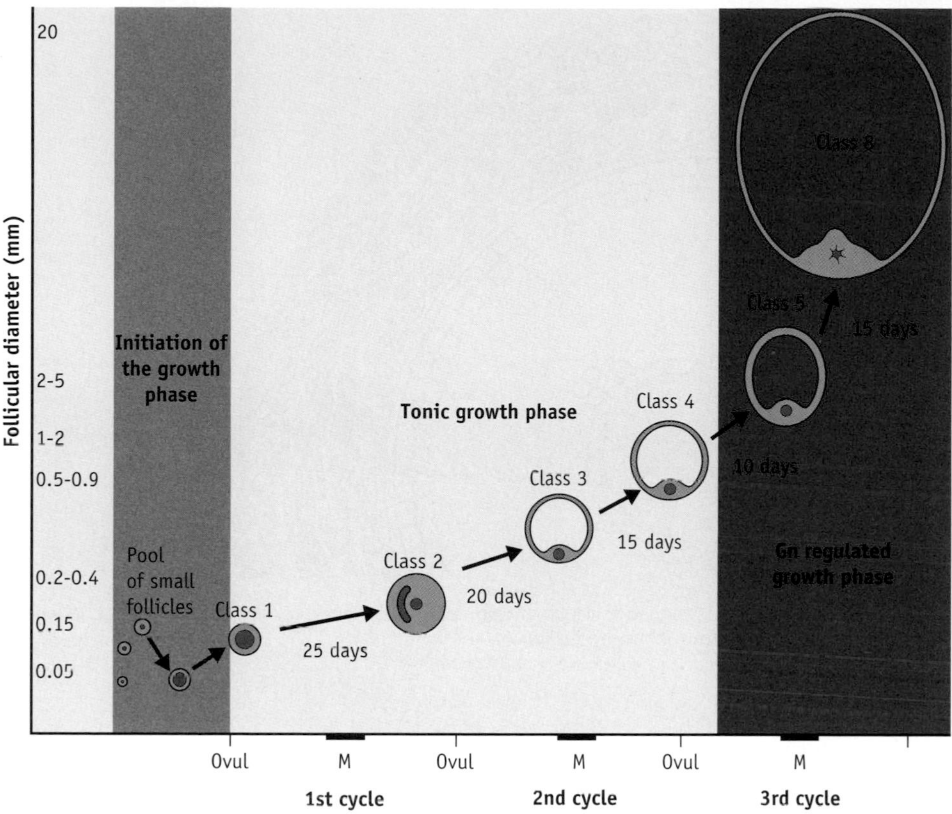


**Figure 25.2** Complete follicular growth trajectory across three successive cycles. Progression through stages 1–4 relies to some extent on pituitary gonadotrophins while stages 5–8 occur during the follicular phase following the third menses from initiation of the growth phase. Exponential growth, selection and dominance are regulated by rising levels of FSH and by varying sensitivity to FSH within the selected cohort. Key: M, Menses; Ovul, ovulation; Gn, gonadotrophin. *(Reproduced with permission from Blackburn, 2007:55.)*

a profound reorganization of the nucleus and cytoplasm, in preparation for fertilization and blastocyst formation (Canipari 2000, Gilchrist et al 2008).

## Ovarian regulation of gonadotrophins

The ovary contains thousands of highly differentiated cells and functions as a complex neuroendocrine–autocrine–paracrine gland, synchronizing hypothalamic, pituitary, ovarian, uterine and mammary activities, throughout the cycle (Behrens et al 1995, Hirshfield 1991, Kunz et al 1998, Nakao et al 2007, Armstrong & Webb 1997).

The ovarian cycle temporarily modulates the secretory patterns of pituitary and hypothalamic gonadotrophins, through a changing balance of hormonal secretions, in successive cohorts of antral follicles, the dominant follicle and its successor, the postovulatory follicle or corpus luteum (Baker & Spears 1999, Hodgen 1982). Across the cycle, ovarian steroid and peptide hormones act through negative and positive feedback mechanisms on the synthesis and pattern of release of hypothalamic gonadotrophin-releasing hormone (GnRH); pituitary gonadotrophins FSH and LH and their responsiveness to GnRH, in conjunction with other modulatory hormones and neurotransmitters operating on pituitary and hypothalamic gonadotrophin cells (Ball 2007, Nakao et al 2007, Smith & Jennes 2001).

Antral fluid has a key role in follicular growth, oocyte maturation, ovulation and fertilization (Tse et al 2002).

As the dominant follicle increases in size (Fig. 25.3), rising synthesis of oestrogens and progesterone lead to a parallel rise in circulating concentrations.

### Mid-cycle LH/FSH surge

The LH/FSH surge is temporally associated with attainment of peak secretion of oestrogens following a rapid rise in progesterone 12 hours earlier (Micevych & Sinchak

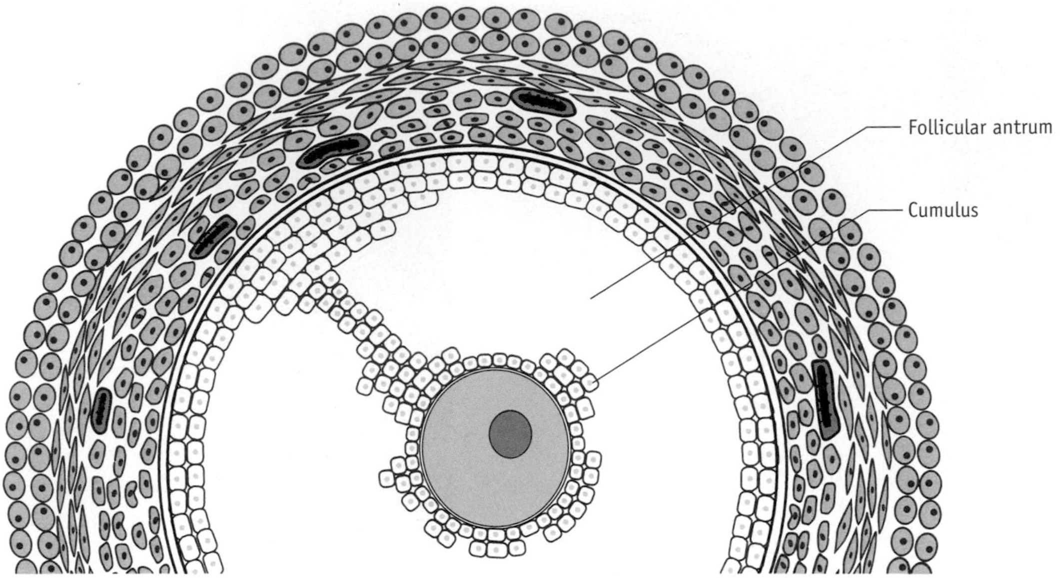

**Figure 25.3** Expanded antral follicle with a fully developed follicular antrum leaving the oocyte surrounded by a distinct layer of granulosa cells. *(Reproduced with permission from Johnson 2007:84.)*

2008, Stouffer 2003). In the hypothalamus, oestrogens induce a rise in synthesis of neuroprogesterone and neuroprogesterone receptors, and these events initiate the pulsatile release of GnRH, which then stimulates the surge release of LH needed for ovulation (Micevych & Sinchak 2008, Smith & Jennes 2001) (Fig. 25.4).

A wide variety of peptides have also been shown to interact with steroids, ions and other paracrine factors, as well as GnRH, in regulating LH and FSH secretion, particularly around ovulation (see website).

During the ovulatory cycle, oxytocin levels vary in the hypothalamo-hypophysial complex, medulla and cerebrospinal fluid (Evans 1996, Salonia et al 2005). In the peripheral circulation, higher levels of oxytocin coincide with the mid-cycle LH surge – variations have been found in oxytocin and oxytocin receptors in granulosa and stromal cells, as well as in uterine and cervical tissue across the ovarian cycle (Behrens et al 1995, Kunz et al 1998). Evidence suggests that central oxytocin plays a key role in regulating the LH surge, by acting directly on GnRH neurons and stimulating sexual behaviour around ovulation.

Uterine and cervical oxytocin cooperate in conjunction with prostaglandin $E_2$ ($PGE_2$)and the preovulatory surge in oestrogens from the dominant follicle. These interactions promote fertilization, by softening cervical tissue and stimulating cervico-fundal contractions, to rapidly transport waves of spermatozoa from the posterior vaginal fornix to the isthmic portion of the fallopian tube (Behrens et al 1995, Drobnis & Overstreet 1992, Kunz et al 1998).

## The preovulatory follicle

Following the LH/FSH surge, fibroblasts within the *theca externa* lay down connective tissue and *theca interna* and mural granulosa cells begin to differentiate from a predominantly oestrogen-secreting tissue into a highly vascularized corpus luteum with progesterone as its major steroid hormone and a rapid rise in progesterone receptors (Stouffer 2003).

During the critical preovulatory period, the oocyte also secretes molecules that enhance oestrogens and inhibit progesterone secretion by *cumulus granulosa cells* (Gilchrist et al 2008, Sutton et al 2003) which also express oxytocin receptors. Oxytocin appears to modulate progesterone secretion while stimulating progesterone receptors on granulosa cells and a variety of regulatory molecules, including growth factors, integrins, prostaglandins and intracellular messengers involved in the process of ovulation.

## Oocyte maturation

Throughout the growth phase of the oocyte, progression of *meiosis* is arrested at the diplotene or germinal vesicle stage of prophase 1. Within 12 hours of the LH/FSH surge, the fully grown oocyte is reactivated to briefly resume meiosis, while complex maturational changes occur in the cytoplasm to support fetilization and the surrounding cumulus cells expand (Sutton-McDowall et al 2010). FSH receptors are present on the entire surface of human

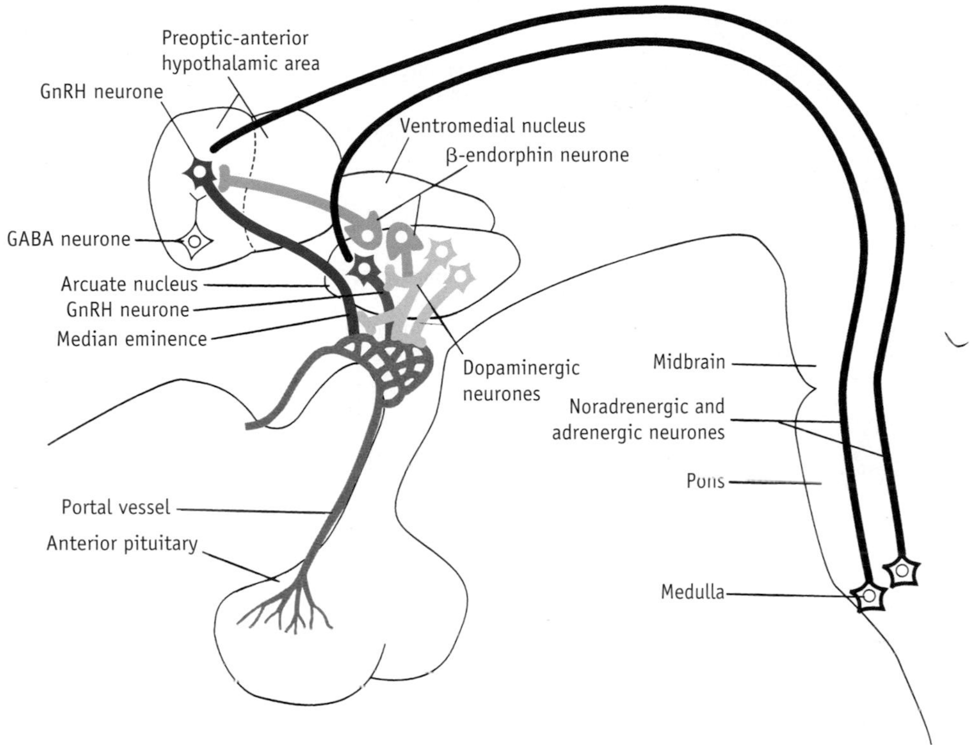


**Figure 25.4** Some of the postulated neurochemical reactions that may control GnRH secretion. *(Reproduced with permission from Johnson 2007:116.)*

oocytes, suggesting that FSH has direct control of oocyte maturation (Meduri et al 2002).

## Preparation for the corpus luteum

Prior to ovulation, mural granulosa and theca interna cells differentiate predominantly into progesterone-secreting theca-lutein and granulosa-lutein cells that remain in the ovary following ovulation, and rapidly expand to form the highly vascularized corpus luteum (Niswender et al 2000, Stouffer 2003) (see website).

## Ovulation

The LH/FSH surge dramatically increases blood flow and vascular permeability in thecal capillary networks that descend to the basal lamina. The rapid increase in size and vascularization of the follicle is accompanied by the local release of the prostaglandin $PGE_2$ and of vasodilatory substances like histamine and bradykinin. $PGE_2$ initiates the breakdown of collagen fibres within the thecal compartment, and other molecules cause an inflammatory reaction from within. FSH and progesterone also initiate proteolytic enzyme activity that loosens, distends and finally erodes the follicle wall at its weakest point (Brannstrom et al 1996).

Within 12 hours of the LH/FSH surge, progesterone replaces oestrogens as the *dominant steroid hormone* synthesized by theca and mural granulosa cells. This shift in steroid hormone production is accompanied by a rise in prostaglandin output which activates enzymes that weaken and distend the follicle wall.

Between 36 and 42 hours following the surges, the apex of the follicle begins to bulge below the surface of the ovary, rupturing at its weakest point, allowing antral fluid to flow into the peritoneal cavity, carrying the expanded *oocyte–cumulus* complex into the fallopian tube (Brannstrom et al 1996).

At ovulation, the dominant follicle releases the hugely expanded oocyte–cumulus complex from the surface of the ovary (Fig. 25.5). Immediately afterwards, the cumulus cell mass regulates acceptance of the oocyte by the fimbriae of the fallopian tube and subsequently functions as a hormonal and metabolic unit in the lumen of the uterine cavity, optimizing conditions for the enclosed oocyte and zona pellucida to undergo final maturational changes in preparation for fertilization, implantation, and embryo formation (Talbot et al 2003).

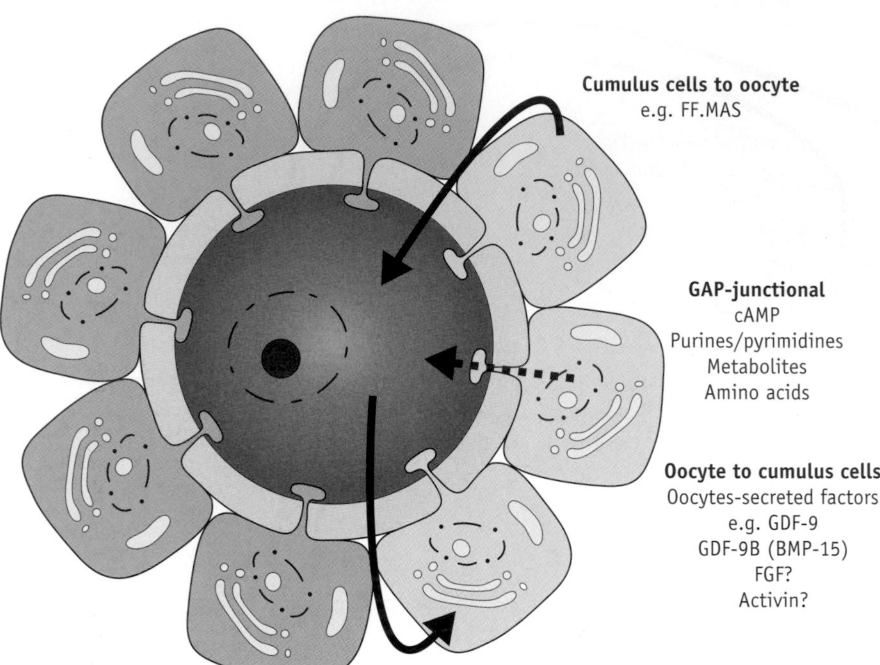


**Figure 25.5** Bi-directional oocyte–cumulus cell communication: paracrine (bold arrow) and gap-junctional (dashed arrow) communication between oocyte and cumulus cells. Factors transmitted include follicular-fluid meiosis-activating sterol (FF-MAS); growth differentiation factor-9 (GDF-9), fibroblast growth factor (FGF) and activin. *(Reproduced with permission from Sutton et al 2003:37.)*

## The corpus luteum – reprogramming the postovulatory follicle

When the cumulus–oocyte complex leaves the ovary, residual cells of the dominant follicle undergo rapid remodelling, including cell growth, proliferation and final differentiation, accompanied by a rapid increase in blood flow and lymphatic drainage (Alexander et al 1998, Redmer & Reynolds 1996, Stocco et al 2007). These changes allow the corpus luteum to expand rapidly to become the most active and highly vascularized autocrine–paracrine–endocrine gland in the body, with a lifespan of approximately 14 days (Duncan 2000, Stocco et al 2007).

At the peak of its activity, in the mid-luteal phase of the cycle, the corpus luteum measures up to 2 cm in diameter and produces up to 25 mg progesterone per day, although the majority of its cells are non-luteal in origin (Duncan 2000, Niswender et al 2000, Redmer & Reynolds 1996).

The convoluted ovarian arterial branches are enmeshed by a responsive venous network surrounding the ovary, providing an effective means of adapting local blood flow to the dynamic state of the enclosed follicles across successive cycles (Alexander et al 1998) (see website).

## Luteinization

The preovulatory LH surge triggers luteinization or terminal differentiation of theca and granulosa cells within a few hours of ovulation (Stocco et al 2007). Both cells synthesize progesterone as the primary steroid hormone. This acts locally to sustain luteal cell function and stimulate its own secretion (Stocco et al 2007). Androgens and oestradiol are also synthesized (Niswender et al 2000).

# CYCLICAL CHANGES IN REPRODUCTIVE ORGANS

Ovarian regulation of gonadotrophs before, during and after ovulation imposes a corresponding cycle on the functional layer of the endometrium and fallopian tubes, mucosal secretions of the cervix, and the structure and secretions of vaginal tissue (Gipson et al 2001). The functional zone of the endometrium undergoes successive phases of proliferation, secretion and regression, while mammary epithelial cells undergo proliferation and involution across the ovarian cycle (Herbison & Pape 2001, Russo & Russo 1987, Smith 2001, Smith & Jennes 2001).

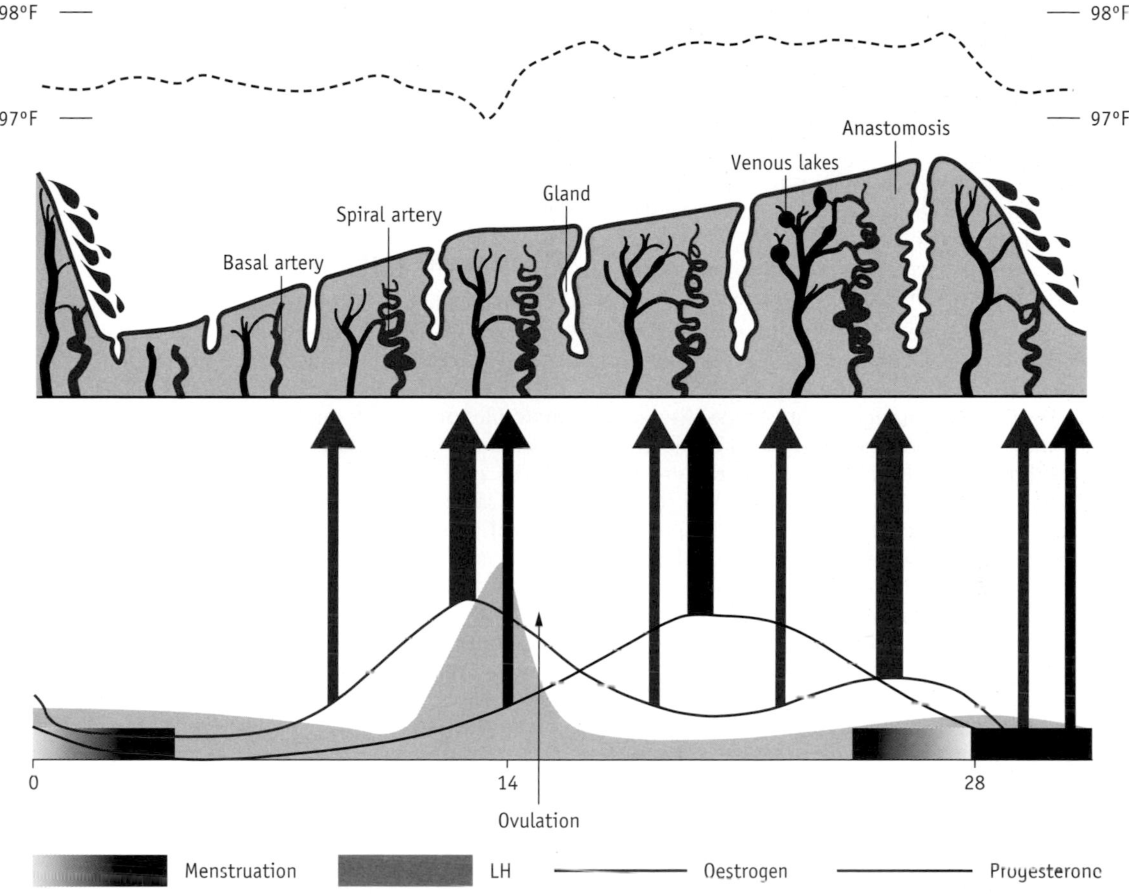


**Figure 25.6** Changes in human endometrium during the menstrual cycle. Underlying ovarian steroid hormone changes are indicated below and basal temperature is indicated above. Thickness of arrows indicates strength of action. *(Reproduced with permission from Johnson 2007:151.)*

## The endometrial cycle

The endometrial cycle (Fig. 25.6) is divided into three phases, which normally take place over 28–30 days:

1. *Proliferative phase* follows menses and may last from 9 to 23 days. Under the influence of oestrogens and local growth factors, blood vessels begin to proliferate; the endometrium grows thicker and softer, and the tubular glands lengthen and become tortuous towards the end of this phase.
2. *Secretory phase* lasts between 8 and 17 days following ovulation. Under the influence of progesterone and oestrogens, the endometrial layer becomes even thicker; spiral arteries lengthen and become more coiled; the endometrial glands become tortuous as they expand with secretions until about 25% of the endometrium is occupied by glands (see website).
3. *Menses* lasts about 4–6 days. Rapidly falling levels of progesterone and oestrogens induce episodes of spasm and relaxation of the spiral arteries in the functional layer of the endometrium. Loss of integrity of vascular tissue leads to dissolution of the endometrium down to its basal layer. The lining is expelled aided by uterine contractions and the total volume shed is around 50–100 mL.

### Cyclical endometrial activity

Cyclical regeneration of the functional layer of the endometrium that culminates with pre-decidualization at around 8–9 days after ovulation, begins towards the end of menses. During the follicular phase, rising concentrations of oestrogens stimulate an intense proliferation of epithelial and stromal cells. This is followed by differentiation of glandular and stromal cells, and continued growth and tubal formation of endometrial vascular cells, which is largely regulated by rising levels of progesterone, following ovulation. During the luteal phase, the functional zone is characterized by changes in cell morphology and extracellular matrix composition that transform it into a secretory, paracrine/autocrine gland. Throughout the secretory phase, the endometrium clearly differentiates into three layers, with numerous gap junctions:

- a superficial compact zone contains decidualized stroma with attenuated non-secretory glands
- a middle spongy zone consists of distended glands with abundant secretions
- a basal zone with extensive development of protein synthesis and secretion (Irwin & Giudice 1998).

As illustrated in Figure 25.6, from the mid-secretory phase to the end of menstruation, thickness of the functional layer declines from 5–8 mm to 1–3 mm, as the functional layer is shed along with its connective tissue matrix and the highly specialized arterioles are reduced to around one-third of the length reached by the onset of menses (Bakos et al 1993, Dockery et al 1990, Rogers 1996, Smith 2000, Starkey 1993). During the premenstrual phase, endometrial cells release increasing levels of proteolytic enzymes that degrade the extracellular matrix, and highly potent and long-lasting vasoconstrictors called endothelins that act on the spiral arterioles (Ohbuchi et al 1995). From the second day after bleeding commences, remaining stromal cells respond to the reduced oxygen tension by synthesizing *vascular endothelial growth factor* (VEGF), which stimulates repair of the vascular bed and elongation of the remaining blood vessels, by the fifth day of the cycle (Maas et al 2001). These blood vessels have an essential role in tissue reconstruction during the proliferative phase of the cycle (Rogers 1996, Smith 2001).

## The proliferative phase

By around day 5 of the endometrial cycle, cell proliferation commences when endometrial and myometrial oestrogen receptors are stimulated by increased secretion of oestrogens from the cohort of developing follicles. During this phase, oestrogens stimulate a rise in the number of ciliated cells in the luminal epithelium and expression of a variety of mitogenic factors, including VEGF, that stimulate a marked proliferation of luminal epithelial, glandular and vascular endothelial cells (Ferrara & Davis-Smith 1997). At the same time, oestrogens directly inhibit endometrial angiogenesis, while vascular permeability rises and endometrial blood flow increases, to peak just before ovulation (Ma et al 2001).

Stromal fibroblasts enlarge and show signs of increased protein synthesis and association with microfibrils of collagen that become denser and thicker just before ovulation. An insoluble pericellular matrix of collagen and fibronectin forms a tight meshwork primarily around glandular and basement membranes of the luminal epithelium (Dockery et al 1990, Fraser & Peek 1992, Shiokawa et al 1996, Starkey 1993). With the surge in oestrogens that follows selection of the dominant follicle, a three- to fivefold increase occurs in endometrial thickness, and oestrogen-dependent intracellular receptors for progesterone are synthesized. During the late proliferative phase, secretory glands enlarge and become thicker and more convoluted, while proliferation in epithelial and stromal cells continues until 3 days following ovulation (Irwin & Giudice 1998, Strauss & Coutifaris 1999).

## The secretory phase

Within the uterus, endometrial glandular cells accumulate glycogen, regulatory proteins, sugars and lipid droplets, and their secretory activity reaches a maximum around 6 days after ovulation. In anticipation of fertilization, these molecules prepare for implantation and provide essential nutritional and regulatory secretions for the conceptus (Budak et al 2006, Burton et al 2007, Cheon et al 2001). At the same time, progesterone stimulates glandular and stromal cells to release human chorionic gonadotrophin (hCG) and increase expression of two potent angiogenic factors: angiogenin in stromal cells and VEGF in stromal cells and neutrophils associated with microvessel walls (Alexander et al 1998, Gargett et al 2001, Ma et al 2001). As illustrated in Figure 25.7, a subepithelial capillary plexus has formed into a complex network of vessels by the mid-secretory phase and newly regrown arterioles become increasingly more spiral as they lengthen more rapidly than the endometrium thickens (Gargett et al 2001, Strauss & Coutifaris 1999).

## Pre-decidualization

During the secretory phase, stromal cells synthesize and release a growing number of new matrix proteins together with surface expression of their receptors, including laminin, fibronectin and integrins, while the earlier cross-linking collagen fibrils are degraded. This process of matrix remodelling creates a looser and more soluble structure and, from the mid-secretory phase onwards, stromal cells also express a variety of regulatory peptides involved in cell replication and haemostasis. Stromal tissue undergoes further differentiation, and individual cells become larger and oedematous, which contributes to the overall thickening of the endometrium.

From the late secretory phase, further changes occur within the endometrium which are regulated by relaxin, progesterone, prolactin and leptin (Budak et al 2006, Gubbay et al 2002, Haig 2008). The endometrial stroma immediately surrounding the arterioles undergoes *decidualization* as it synthesizes a number of hormones and other molecules and is infiltrated by lymphoid cells.

In the event of fertilization, these changes provide an appropriate nutritive, regulatory and immunoprotective environment for the emerging embryo until 9–10 weeks' gestation (Alexander et al 1998, Gonzalez et al 2003, Gubbay et al 2002, Lane et al 1994, Starkey 1993).

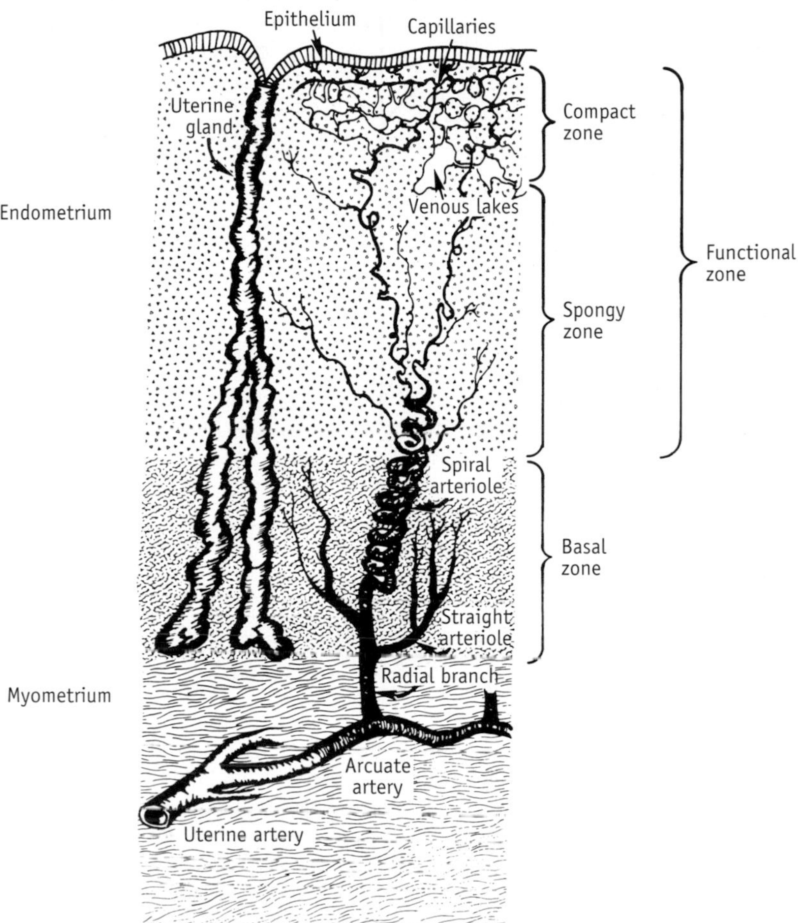


**Figure 25.7** The arterial supply to the uterine endometrium. These specialized endometrial blood vessels arise within the myometrium, as the arcuate arteries. Small straight arterioles supply the basal unchanging layer of the endometrium. As they leave the basal portion and enter the spongy and compact tissue that underlies the luminal epithelium, their thick smooth muscle coat formed by circular and longitudinal layers becomes progressively thinner, and by the time these blood vessels reach the subepithelial surface of the endometrium, they consist only of endothelial cells (Abberton et al 1999). *(Reproduced with permission from Strauss & Coutifaris 1999:219.)*

## Cyclical changes in the cervix and vagina

Significant changes occur in the cervix and vagina throughout the cycle, which facilitate the passage of spermatozoa. During the follicular phase, the muscles of the cervix relax, causing the cervical os to dilate slightly (to around 3–4 mm) at the time of ovulation. The epithelial cells begin to secrete clear watery and 'stretchable' mucus mid-cycle.

Under the influence of rising levels of progesterone following the mid-cycle LH/FSH surge, the cervix becomes firmer and more tightly closed and cervical secretions become scant, viscous and cellular, making it more difficult for spermatozoa to enter the uterus. In addition, relaxin and progesterone relax muscle layers in the isthmic portion of the tube, which assists movement of the conceptus towards the uterine cavity (Downing & Hollingsworth 1993, Johnson 2007).

Lined with stratified squamous epithelium, the vagina is also responsive to oestrogens and progesterone. During the follicular phase, vaginal cells proliferate and begin to accumulate glycogen, which is fermented to lactic acid by the normal bacterial flora. This provides a slightly acid environment, which acts as an anti-infective agent. During sexual excitation, the acidity of vaginal fluid is partly neutralized by the increased blood flow to the pelvic region,

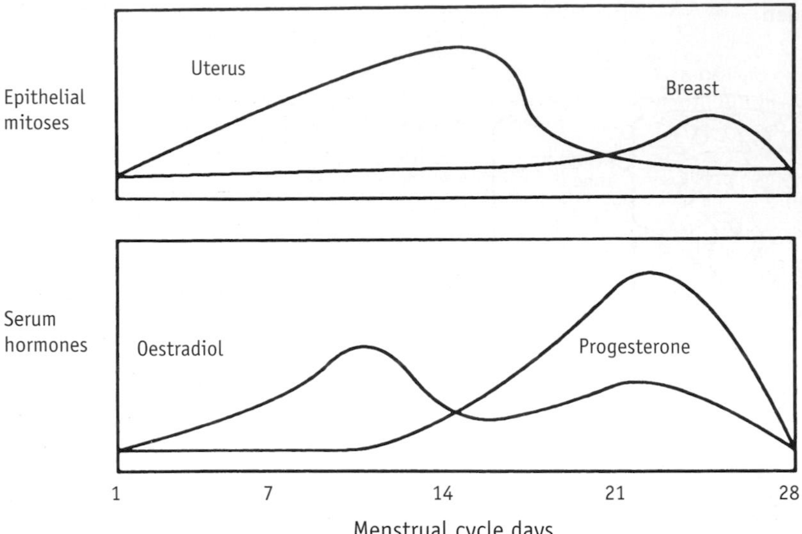


**Figure 25.8** Changes in epithelial mitosis of breast and endometrium, and serum oestradiol and progesterone levels during the menstrual cycle. *(From Yen, 1999:210.)*

and this alters the pH, making it more receptive for the ejaculated sperm.

## The mammary cycle

The female mammary gland undergoes a surge of cell division during puberty and a cyclical pattern of proliferation and involution until approximately 35 years. During this period, hormonally induced increases in cell proliferation and *apoptosis* (programmed cell death) do not return the gland to the starting point of the previous cycle but provide for a cumulative budding of new lobules (Vorherr 1974).

During each cycle, episodes of increased mitosis and apoptosis follow a contrasting pattern to that of the endometrium (Fig. 25.8). Mammary epithelium shows decreased DNA synthesis and mitotic divisions during the first half of the cycle and maximal proliferation that peaks during the luteal phase of the cycle and is followed by a shorter period of increased apoptosis (Russo & Russo 1987). A contrasting pattern of cellular activity in uterine and mammary epithelium is reflected in cyclical differences in steroid hormone receptor concentrations in the two organs of reproduction. Mammary tissue receptors for oestrogen (as in the endometrium) decline during the second half of the cycle; those for progesterone remain fairly constant throughout both phases of the cycle (Soderqvist et al 1993). During the second half of the cycle, secretory activity may also occur together with increases in breast volume, because of the significant rise in extracellular levels of VEGF that stimulates angiogenesis and increases vascular permeability (Dabrosin 2003).

## CONCLUSION

It is important to understand the complex mechanisms and neurohormonal influences that synchronize the ovarian, menstrual and mammary cycles, and how these impact on the woman's body. This ensures that the midwife can accurately calculate the expected date of delivery; help the woman to understand how the calculation is made; and enable her to see how these cycles begin the physiological preparation for pregnancy, childbirth and lactation.

### KEY POINTS

- The normal menstrual cycle can indicate general health, wellbeing and nutritional status of the woman.
- During each cycle, the uterus facilitates reception, maturation and transport of spermatozoa from the vagina to the fallopian tube, while the inner layers of the uterus prepare to receive and directly nourish the blastocyst.
- The ovarian, menstrual and mammary cycles are driven by dynamic patterns of negative and positive feedback between ovarian steroids and peptide hormones, and gonadotrophins from the anterior pituitary gland and hypothalamus.
- An understanding of the complex neurohormonal relationships during the cycle will assist in recognizing the normal cycle and in appreciating the simultaneous changes in other organ systems.

## REFERENCES


Abberton KM, Taylor NH, Healy DL, et al: Vascular smooth muscle cell proliferation in arterioles of the human endometrium, *Human Reproduction* 14:1072–1079, 1999.

Alexander H, Zimmermann G, Wolkersdorfer GW, et al: Utero-ovarian interaction in the regulation of reproductive function, *Human Reproduction Update* 4(5):550–559, 1998.

Armstrong DG, Webb R: Ovarian follicular dominance: the role of intraovarian growth factors and novel proteins, *Reviews of Reproduction* 2:139–146, 1997.

Baker SJ, Spears N: The role of intra-ovarian interactions in the regulation of follicle dominance, *Human Reproduction Update* 5(2):153–165, 1999.

Bakos O, Lundkvist O, Bergh T: Transvaginal sonographic evaluation of endometrial growth and texture in spontaneous ovulatory cycles – a descriptive study, *Human Reproduction* 142:142–157, 1993.

Ball GF: The ovary knows more than you think! New views on clock genes and the positive feedback control of luteinizing hormone, *Endocrinology* 148(7):3029–3030, 2007.

Behrens O, Mascheko H, Kupsch E, et al: Oxytocin receptors in human ovaries during the menstrual cycle. In Ivell R, Russell J, editors: *Oxytocin*, New York, 1995, Plenum Press, pp 485–486.

Blackburn ST: *Maternal, fetal & neonatal physiology: a clinical perspective*, ed 3, Philadelphia, 2007, Saunders.

Brannstrom M, Mikuni M, Peterson CM: Ovulation-associated intraovarian events. In Filicori M, Flamigni C, editors: *The ovary: regulation, dysfunction and treatment*, Amsterdam, 1996, Elsevier Science, pp 113–123.

Budak E, Sanchez MF, Bellver J, et al: Interactions of the hormones leptin, ghrelin, adiponectin, resistin, and PYY3-36 with the reproductive system, *Fertility and Sterility* 85(6):1563–1581, 2006.

Burton GJ, Jauniaux E, Charnock-Jones DS: Human early placental development: potential roles of the endometrial glands, *Placenta* 28(suppl A):S64–S69, 2007.

Canipari R: Oocyte–granulosa cell interactions, *Human Reproduction Update* 6(3):279–289, 2000.

Chapman AB, Abraham WT, Zamudio S, et al: Temporal relationships between hormonal and hemodynamic changes in early pregnancy, *Kidney International* 54:2056–2063, 1998.

Cheon KW, Lee H-S, Parhar IS, et al: Expression of the second isoform of gonadotrophin releasing hormone (GnRH-II) in human endometrium throughout the menstrual cycle, *Molecular Human Reproduction* 7(5):447–452, 2001.

Chidambaram M, Duncan JA, Lai VS, et al: Variation in the renin angiotensin system throughout the normal menstrual cycle, *Journal of the American Society of Nephrology* 13:446–452, 2002.

Dabrosin C: Variability of vascular endothelial growth factor in normal human breast tissue in vivo during the menstrual cycle, *Journal of Clinical Endocrinology and Metabolism* 88(6):2695–2698, 2003.

Dockery P, Warren MA, Li TC, et al: A morphometric study of the human endometrial stroma during the peri-implantation period, *Human Reproduction* 5(5):494–498, 1990.

Downing SJ, Hollingsworth M: Action of relaxin on uterine contractions – a review, *Journal of Reproduction and Fertility* 99:275–282, 1993.

Drobnis EZ, Overstreet JW: Natural history of mammalian spermatozoa in the female reproductive tract, *Oxford Reviews of Reproductive Biology* 14:1–45, 1992.

Duncan WC: The human corpus luteum: remodelling during luteolysis and maternal recognition of pregnancy, *Reviews of Reproduction* 5:12–17, 2000.

Evans JJ: Oxytocin and the control of LH, *Journal of Endocrinology* 151:169–174, 1996.

Ferrara N, Davis-Smith T: The biology of vascular endothelial growth factor, *Endocrine Reviews* 18:4–25, 1997.

Fraser IS, Peek MJ: Effects of exogenous hormones on endometrial capillaries. In Alexander NJ, d'Arcangues C, editors: *Steroid hormones and uterine bleeding*, Washington, 1992, AAAS Press, pp 67–79.

Gargett CE, Lederman F, Heryonto B, et al: Focal vascular endothelial growth factor correlates with angiogenesis in human endometrium. Role of intravascular neutrophils, *Human Reproduction* 16(6):1065–1075, 2001.

Geva E, Jaffe RB: Role of vascular endothelial growth factor in ovarian physiology and pathology, *Fertility and Sterility* 74(3):429–438, 2000.

Gilchrist RB, Lane M, Thompson JG: Oocyte-secreted factors: regulators of cumulus cell function and oocyte quality, *Human Reproduction Update* 14(2):159–177, 2008.

Gipson IK, Moccia R, Spurr-Michaud S, et al: The amount of MUC5B in cervical mucus peaks at midcycle, *Journal of Clinical Endocrinology and Metabolism* 86(2):594–600, 2001.

Gonzalez RR, Leary K, Petrozza JC, et al: Leptin regulation of interleukin-1 system in human endometrial cells, *Molecular Human Reproduction* 9(3):151–158, 2003.

Gougeon A: Regulation of ovarian follicular development in primates: facts and hypotheses, *Endocrine Reviews* 17(2):121–155, 1996.

Gubbay O, Critchley HOD, Bowen JM, et al: Prolactin induces ERK phosphorylation in epithelial and CD56 + natural killer cells of the human endometrium, *Journal of Clinical Endocrinology and Metabolism* 87(5):2329–2335, 2002.

Haig D: Placental growth hormone-related proteins and prolactin-related proteins, *Placenta* 29(suppl A):S36–S41, 2008.

Haselton MG, Mortezaie M, Pillsworth EG, et al: Ovulatory shifts in human female ornamentation near ovulation, women dress to impress, *Hormones and Behavior* 51:40–45, 2007.

Herbison AE, Pape J-R: New evidence for estrogen receptors in gonadotrophin-releasing hormone neurons, *Frontiers in Neuroendocrinology* 22:292–308, 2001.

Hirshfield AN: Development of follicles in the mammalian ovary, *International Reviews of Cytology* 124:43–101, 1991.

Hodgen GD: The dominant ovarian follicle, *Fertility and Sterility* 38(3):281–300, 1982.

Irwin JC, Giudice LC: Decidua. In Knobin E, Neill JD, editors: *Encyclopedia of reproduction*, Vol 1, San Diego, 1998, Academic Press, pp 823–835.

*Nature* 428:145–150, 2004.

Johnson MH: *Essential Reproduction*, ed 6, Oxford, 2007, Blackwell Scientific.

Kunz G, Noe M, Herbertz M, et al: Uterine peristalsis during the follicular phase of the menstrual cycle: effects of oestrogen, antioestrogen and oxytocin, *Human Reproduction Update* 4(5):647–654, 1998.

Lane B, Oxberry W, Mazella J, et al: Decidualization of human endometrial stromal cells in vitro: effects of progestin and relaxin on the ultrastructure and production of decidual secretory proteins, *Human Reproduction* 9(2):259–266, 1994.

Lousse J-C, Donnez J: Laparoscopic observation of spontaneous ovulation, *Fertility and Sterility* 9(3):833–834, 2008.

Ma W, Tan J, Matsumoto H, et al: Adult tissue angiogenesis: evidence for negative regulation by estrogen in the uterus, *Molecular Endocrinology* 15(11):1983–1992, 2001.

Maas JW, Groothuis PG, Dunselman GA, et al: Endometrial angiogenesis throughout the human menstrual cycle, *Human Reproduction* 16(8):1557–1561, 2001.

Meduri G, Charnaux N, Driancourt M-A, et al: Follicle-stimulating hormone receptors in oocytes? *Journal of Clinical Endocrinology and Metabolism* 87(5):2266–2276, 2002.

Micevych P, Sinchak K: Minireview: Synthesis and function of hypothalamic neuroprogesterone in reproduction, *Endocrinology* 149(6):2739–2742, 2008.

Nakao N, Yasuo S, Nishimura A, et al: Circadian clock gene regulation of steroidogenic acute regulatory protein gene expression in preovulatory ovarian follicles, *Endocrinology* 148(7):3031–3038, 2007.

Niswender GD, Juengel JL, Silva PJ, et al: Mechanisms controlling the function and life span of the corpus luteum, *Physiological Reviews* 80(1):1–29, 2000.

Ohbuchi H, Nagai K, Amaguchi M, et al: Endothelin-1 and big endothelin-1 increase in human endometrium during menstruation, *American Journal of Obstetrics and Gynecology* 173(5):1483–1490, 1995.

Redmer DA, Reynolds LP: Angiogenesis in the ovary, *Reviews of Reproduction* 1:182–192, 1996.

Rogers PA: Structure and function of endometrial blood vessels, *Human Reproduction Update* 2(1):57–62, 1996.

Russo J, Russo IH: Development of the human mammary gland. In Neville MC, Daniel CW, editors: *The mammary gland*, New York, 1987, Plenum Press, pp 67–93.

Salonia A, Nappi RE, Pontillo M, et al: Menstrual cycle-related changes in plasma oxytocin are relevant to normal sexual function in healthy women, *Hormones and Behavior* 47:164–169, 2005.

Seifer DB, Feng B, Shelden RM, et al: Brain-derived neurotrophic factor: a novel human ovarian follicular protein, *Journal of Clinical Endocrinology and Metabolism* 87(2):655–659, 2002.

Shiokawa S, Yoshimura Y, Nagamatsu S, et al: Expression of B1 integrins in human endometrial stromal and decidual cells, *Journal of Clinical Endocrinology and Metabolism* 81(4):1533–1540, 1996.

Smith SK: Angiogenesis and implantation, *Human Reproduction* 15(suppl 6):59–66, 2000.

Smith SK: Angiogenesis and reproduction, *British Journal of Obstetrics and Gynaecology* 108(8):777–783, 2001.

Smith MJ, Jennes L: Neural signals that regulate GnRH neurones directly during the oestrus cycle, *Reproduction* 122:1–10, 2001.

Soderqvist G, von Schoultz B, Tani E, et al: Estrogen and progesterone receptor content in the breast epithelial cells from healthy women during the menstrual cycle, *American Journal of Obstetrics and Gynecology* 168(3):874–879, 1993.

Starkey PM: The decidua and factors controlling placentation. In Redman C, Sargent I, Starkey P, editors: *The human placenta*, Oxford, 1993, Blackwell Scientific, pp 362–413.

Stocco C, Telleria C, Gibori G: The molecular control of corpus luteum formation, function, and regulation, *Endocrine Reviews* 28(1):117–149, 2007.

Stouffer RL: Progesterone as a mediator of gonadotrophin action in the corpus luteum: beyond steroidogenesis, *Human Reproduction Update* 9(2):99–117, 2003.

Strauss J, Coutifaris C: The endometrium and myometrium: regulation and dysfunction. In Yen SSC, Jaffe RB, Barbieri RL, editors: *Reproductive endocrinology*, Philadelphia, 1999, Saunders, pp 218–256.

Sutton ML, Gilchrist RB, Thompson JG: Effects of in-vivo and in-vitro environments on the metabolism of the cumulus-oocyte complex and its influence on oocyte developmental capacity, *Human Reproduction Update* 9(1):35–48, 2003.

Sutton-McDowall ML, Gilchrist RB, Thompson JG: The pivotal role of glucose metabolism in determining oocyte developmental competence, *Reproduction* 139:685–695, 2010.

Talbot P, Shur BD, Myles DG: Cell adhesion and fertilization: steps in oocyte transport, sperm–zona pellucida interactions, and sperm–egg fusion, *Biology of Reproduction* 68:1–9, 2003.

Tarin JJ, Gomez-Piquer V: Do women have a hidden heat period? *Human Reproduction* 17(9):2243–2248, 2002.

Tse JYM, Chiu PCN, Lee KF, et al: The synthesis and fate of glycodelin in human ovary during folliculogenesis, *Molecular Human Reproduction* 8(2):142–148, 2002.

Vorherr H: Development of the female breast. In Vorherr H, editor: *The breast*, New York, 1974, Academic Press, pp 1–18.

Webb P: 24-hour energy expenditure and the menstrual cycle, *American Journal of Clinical Nutrition* 44:614–619, 1986.

Yen SSC: The human menstrual cycle: neuroendocrine regulation. In Yen SSC, Jaffe RB, Barbieri RL, editors: *Reproductive endocrinology*, Philadelphia, 1999, Saunders, pp 191–217.

Chapter |26|

# Genetics

*Simon Hettle and Jean Rankin*

## LEARNING OUTCOMES

At the end of the chapter, you will:

- have a basic understanding of genetics, including cell division, modes of inheritance and the chromosomal influences on reproduction
- be aware of methods used in diagnosing fetal genetic abnormalities
- appreciate the significance of genetics and its applications for midwifery practice.

## INTRODUCTION

Genetics is the study of inheritance and variation in both individuals and populations and has its origins in man's curiosity about reproduction and inheritance, including inquisitiveness about both normal and abnormal developments – for example, why do certain diseases 'run in families', whilst others do not?

Virtually all pregnant women will want to know if their baby is within the spectrum of that which is regarded as 'normal', and advances in genetics can both help to answer this question and have other great practical benefits in the field of human reproduction: for example, the probability that a child will suffer from a particular genetic disease can be calculated, allowing parents to make informed choices in planning their families; it may be possible, in a few cases, to replace or supplement defective genes so that the diseases they cause can be cured ('gene therapy'); the potential of stem cells is also on the horizon. Hence, it is important that practitioners in this area are aware of both fundamental principles and relevant applications of genetics. There are many ethical questions associated with genetics and it is also important that these are fully addressed.

## GENES, CHROMOSOMES AND DNA

A gene is typically defined as a unit of inheritance. Genes are found on chromosomes, which are long, thread-like structures in the nucleus of the cell; each chromosome is made up of one DNA (deoxyribonucleic acid) molecule with many different proteins associated with it. Many genes are arranged throughout its length in a fixed manner, one after the other (Fig. 26.1).

DNA is the major single component of each chromosome and it acts as an information store: all the information necessary for the structure, function, reproduction and development of an organism is stored in a stable and coded form.

The DNA molecule is a long, thin molecule and consists of two strands wound around each other to form a double helix (Fig. 26.2): it is like a ladder in which the two uprights, whilst still remaining joined together by the rungs, are twisted round each other to form two interweaving spirals. In the DNA molecule, the 'uprights' are made of alternating sugar residues and phosphate groups ('sugar–phosphate backbones') and the 'rungs' are composed of organic bases, each rung consisting of two bases. There are four different bases: two purine bases – *adenine (A)* and *guanine (G)*; and two pyrimidine bases – *cytosine (C)* and *thymine (T)*. Each 'rung' is made up of a pair of bases, one purine and one pyrimidine, and the pairing arrangements in these 'rungs' are very specific:

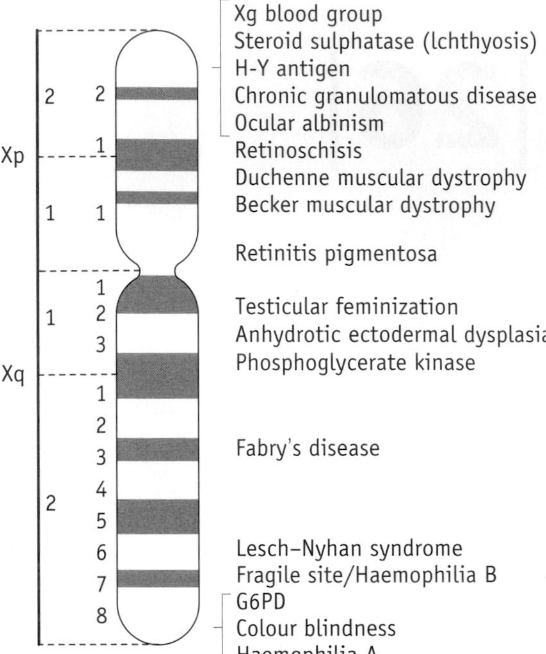


**Figure 26.1** Diagrammatic representation of the human X-chromosome showing some of the inherited characteristics carried.

- adenine *always* pairs with thymine
- guanine *always* pairs with cytosine.

The information stored in DNA needs to be decoded and used to make cellular and organismal components (a process known as 'gene expression'); most commonly, the stored information in DNA is used to direct the production of proteins. There are thousands of different proteins in the body (for example, collagen in tendons, haemoglobin in red blood cells), each with its own specific metabolic role to play. Any protein is made up of amino acids joined together in a chain. Each protein has its own specific amino acid sequence determining its function.

The encoding of information on a DNA molecule is achieved by specifying the precise order (sequence) of the bases along the molecule's length. Information is stored in the form of three-base units (*codons*). Each codon specifies a particular amino acid in a protein. Hence, the sequence of bases in a DNA molecule directly determines the sequence of amino acids in a protein and thus the function of that protein. (Another definition of a gene is, 'that part of a DNA molecule which contains the series of codons necessary to encode a particular protein'.)

The information stored in DNA is decoded using two processes: *transcription* and *translation*. In transcription (which takes place in the nucleus), part of the DNA molecule is used as a template to produce a molecule of

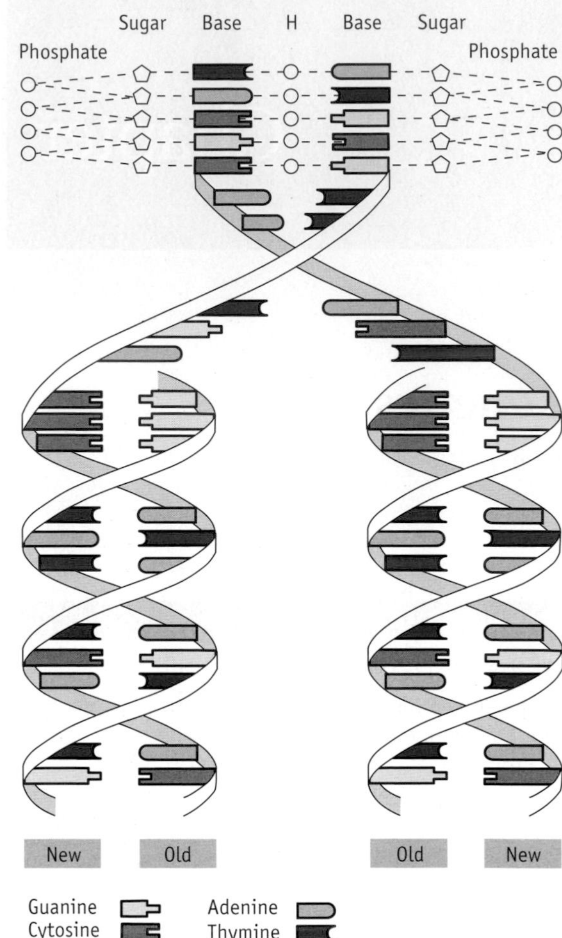


**Figure 26.2** Diagram of a DNA double helix, including the process of replication.

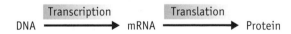


**Figure 26.3** Processes involved in the expression of a gene.

messenger RNA (mRNA) and this mRNA then undergoes translation (on the ribosomes in the cytoplasm of the cell) to produce the protein specified ultimately by the DNA (Fig. 26.3).

Ribonucleic acid (RNA) is the other kind of nucleic acid found in the cell. Unlike DNA, it is single-stranded and it also contains the pyrimidine base uracil (U) instead of thymine. There are three different forms of RNA found in the cell, and all of these are involved in the decoding of information from DNA. These forms are: mRNA; rRNA (ribosomal RNA – a major component of the ribosome) and tRNA (transfer RNA – crucial in translation as an 'adaptor' molecule between mRNA and protein).

**Reflective activity 26.1**

Briefly review the processes involved in the expression of a gene.

## THE HUMAN GENOME

The entire genetic complement of a cell or organism is referred to as its genome. Within the nucleus of all nucleated human cells (apart from the gametes – sex cells – ova and spermatozoa), there are 46 chromosomes: thus, the human genome comprises 46 chromosomes. These chromosomes are arranged in 23 (homologous) pairs, and within each of these pairs, one member is derived from the father, the other from the mother. One of these pairs is the sex chromosomes: in the female, this pair consists of two X chromosomes; in the male, it consists of one X and one Y chromosome. The remaining pairs are collectively known as autosomes and the chromosomes in this group are numbered by length, No. 1 being the longest and No. 22 the shortest (see Fig. 26.7).

Each chromosome carries a specific and particular set of genes and thus each individual carries two copies of any one gene, one copy derived from each parent. Any gene has different forms (or *alleles*). Classically, a gene has two different alleles. Different alleles produce differences in the appearance (or *phenotype*) of the individual. For example, the colour of the iris in the eye is controlled by a single gene which has two alleles – one allele causes the iris to be pale (blue or grey), the other allele causes it to be dark (brown, green or black).

With respect to any one gene, therefore, an individual can have two copies of one allele, two copies of the other allele (arrangements known as *homozygous*) or one copy of each (*heterozygous*). (Thus, for the hypothetical gene A with two alleles – A and a – the combinations AA, aa and Aa are possible.) Clearly, an individual who is homozygous for one allele would have the phenotype associated with that particular allele, but what of heterozygous individuals? In this case, one allele typically 'overrides' the other, an effect described as *dominance* of one allele over the other allele (which is known as the *recessive* allele).

One outcome from the Human Genome Project is that it is now known that the human genome contains a total of some 20,000 genes (Klug et al 2009).

## CELL DIVISION

There are two different types of cell division:

- mitosis, which leads to the production of two daughter cells identical in chromosome number to the parent cell (46 in humans; Fig. 26.4)

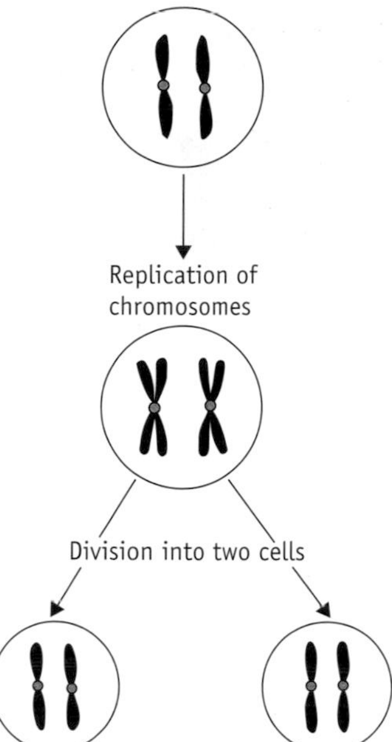


**Figure 26.4** Mitosis.

- meiosis, which leads to the production of four daughter cells, but each containing only half the number of chromosomes of the parent cell (23 in humans; Fig. 26.5).

Mitosis occurs extensively during prenatal development to increase cell numbers, in the adult in tissues where cells are routinely lost (such as skin) and in some of the repair processes that occur following tissue damage. Meiosis only occurs during the production of gametes in the gonads. The reduction in chromosome number is essential if sexual reproduction is to take place without doubling the amount of genetic material in each generation. Note that some rearrangement of genetic material can occur during meiosis; this is an important part of the genetic variation that is an essential feature of sexual reproduction (Fig. 26.6).

Copying (replication) of DNA occurs during both mitosis and meiosis and it is very important that this occurs accurately, so that errors are not introduced into the DNA, with possible consequent changes in the structure and function of encoded proteins. One very important way in which this is ensured is by the 'semi-conservative' mechanism of DNA replication: a parental DNA molecule separates into its two component strands and each of these is then used as a template for the assembly of a new strand. The strict rules of base pairing (A always pairing with T, G with C) ensure that each new double-stranded molecule is an exact copy of the parent molecule (See Fig. 26.2; Russell 2006).

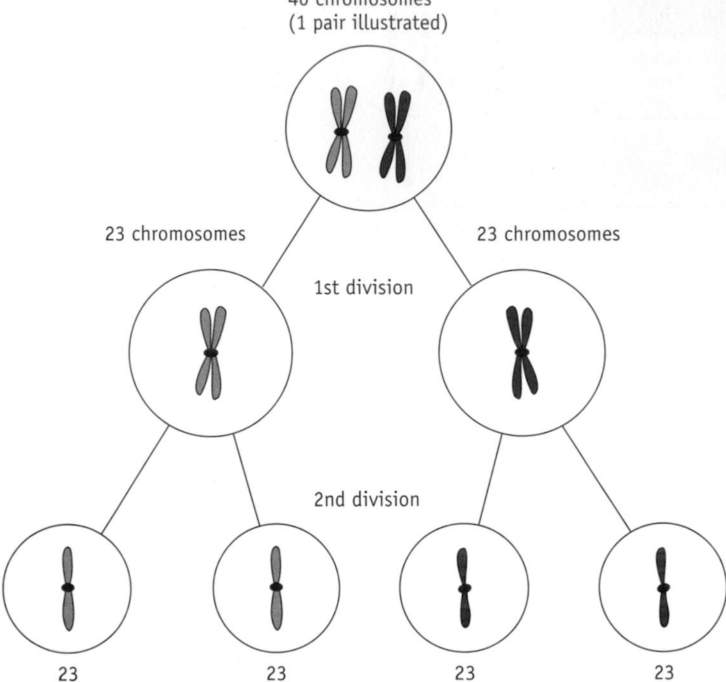


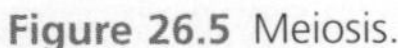
**Figure 26.5** Meiosis.

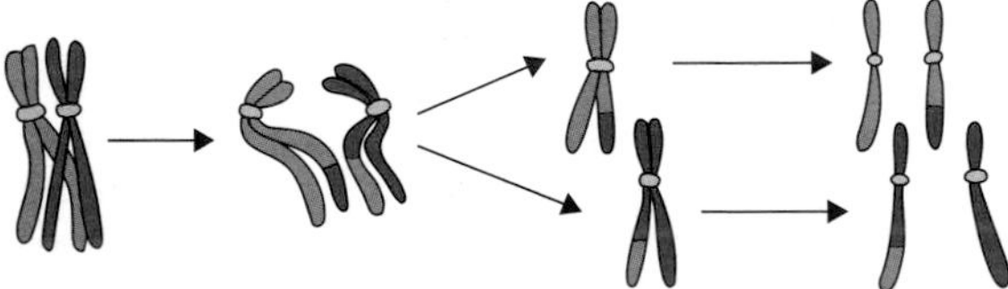

**Figure 26.6** Crossover of genetic material in meiosis.

## CHROMOSOMAL ANALYSIS AND ANOMALIES

The study of chromosomes is called cytogenetics. Chromosomes can be isolated from accessible adult tissues (such as lymphocytes from the blood) or from amniotic fluid or chorionic villi when information about the embryo/fetus is required. The process of examining the chromosomes is referred to as *karyotyping* and it can provide very valuable information about the genome of the cell (Fig. 26.7A,B).

If there is an abnormal number of chromosomes present after fertilization (often due to abnormal events during meiosis), or if there is some alteration in structure, the pregnancy may result in miscarriage or an abnormal fetus. Generally, very major abnormalities (for example, involving whole or large pieces of chromosomes) are likely to have very serious effects. It has been shown that the majority of severe chromosomal abnormalities are not compatible with normal development. Embryos with such defects die at an early stage of development – for example, approximately 15% of pregnancies terminate in spontaneous abortion, with about 50% of these being chromosomally abnormal (Lockwood 2000).

Several different types of chromosomal abnormality are known:

- the presence of three chromosomes of one type is called *trisomy*
- the presence of only one member of a pair is called *monosomy*
- a structural change arising from the loss of a chromosome fragment is known as a *deletion*
- a *translocation* occurs when a chromosome fragment breaks off and is added to another chromosome
- a *reciprocal translocation* occurs if two chromosomes exchange fragments with each other.

The commonest chromosomal birth anomaly is Down syndrome, where there are 47 chromosomes instead of 46 (termed trisomy 21 – three copies of chromosome 21) (Fig. 26.8A). The incidence is 1.5 per 1000 live births and this figure rises with maternal age (Cummings 2003). There are only two other examples of trisomies that are consistent with life – trisomy 13 and trisomy 18 – and

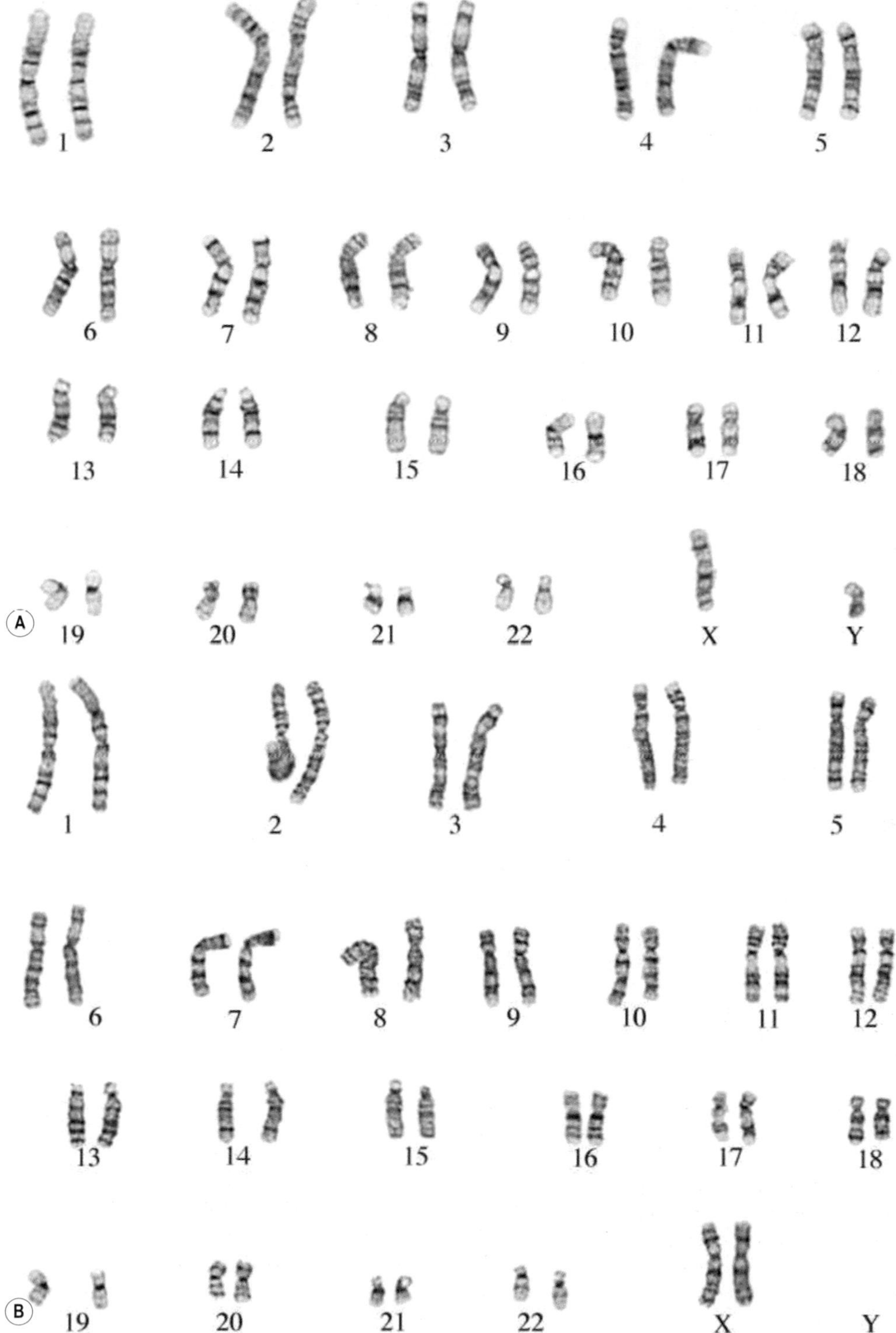


**Figure 26.7 A.** A normal human male karyotype. **B.** A normal human female karyotype.

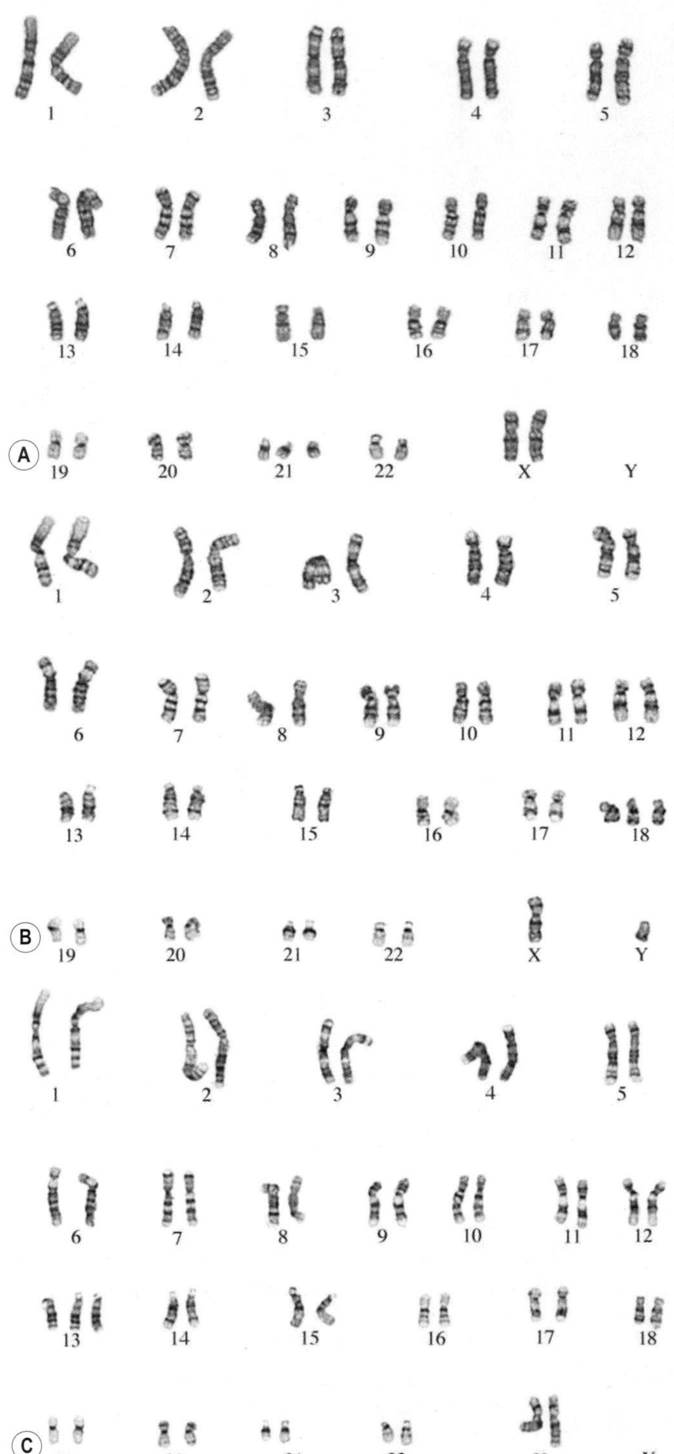


**Figure 26.8** **A.** Karyotype of a female patient with Down syndrome (trisomy 21). **B.** Karyotype of a male patient with Edward syndrome (trisomy 18). **C.** Karyotype of a female patient with Patau syndrome (trisomy 13).

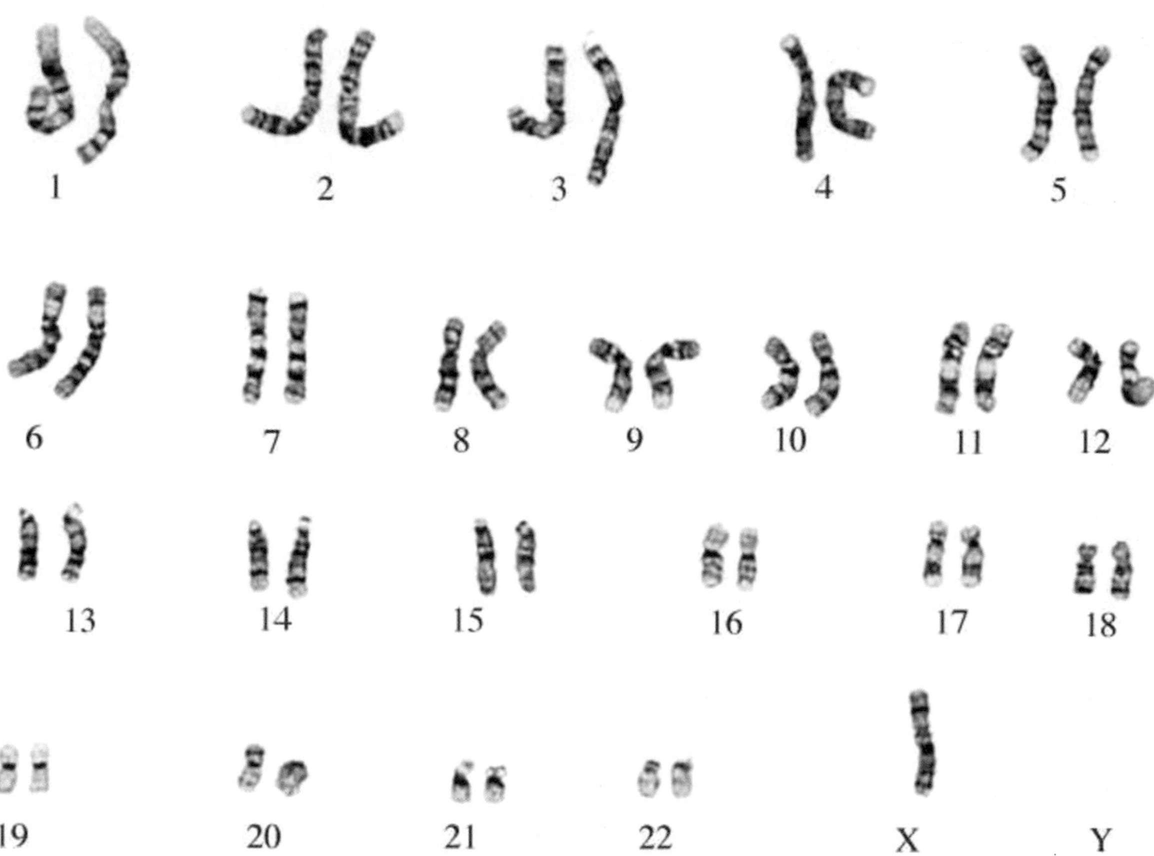


**Figure 26.9** Karyotype of a patient with Turner syndrome (monosomy X).

even in these cases, the defects are many and severe, and affected individuals typically survive for only a short time after birth (Fig. 26.8B,C).

Other common chromosomal anomalies occur among the sex chromosomes; for example, 1.3% of implanted conceptions may carry one X-chromosome without a Y or second X (monosomy X, Turner syndrome – the only viable human monosomy) (Fig. 26.9). Very few of these fetuses survive – about 0.4 per 1000 live-born girls. More common at birth are other anomalies such as XXX (0.65 per 1000 girls), XYY, and XXY or XXXY (1.5 per 1000 boys – Klinefelter syndrome; Cummings 2003) (Fig. 26.10). These sex chromosome anomalies, however, generally produce fewer ill effects than the autosomal anomalies, though these effects can still be serious for the affected individual.

**Reflective activity 26.2**

Visit a cytogenetics laboratory to observe karyotyping.

## MODES OF INHERITANCE

Genetic characteristics (including genetically determined diseases) can be inherited in one of four principal ways:

- autosomal dominant inheritance
- autosomal recessive inheritance
- X-linked dominant inheritance
- X-linked recessive inheritance.

Note that the usual patterns of dominance and recessiveness do not apply in the cases of genes carried on the sex chromosomes – see below.

Common types of genetic disease include:

- enzyme deficiency states ('inborn errors of metabolism'): typically recessive in terms of inheritance, because many metabolic processes can proceed at an adequate rate with reduced levels of enzymes
- defects in structural proteins (such as in connective tissue): typically dominant in terms of inheritance; reduced levels of these proteins and/or the presence

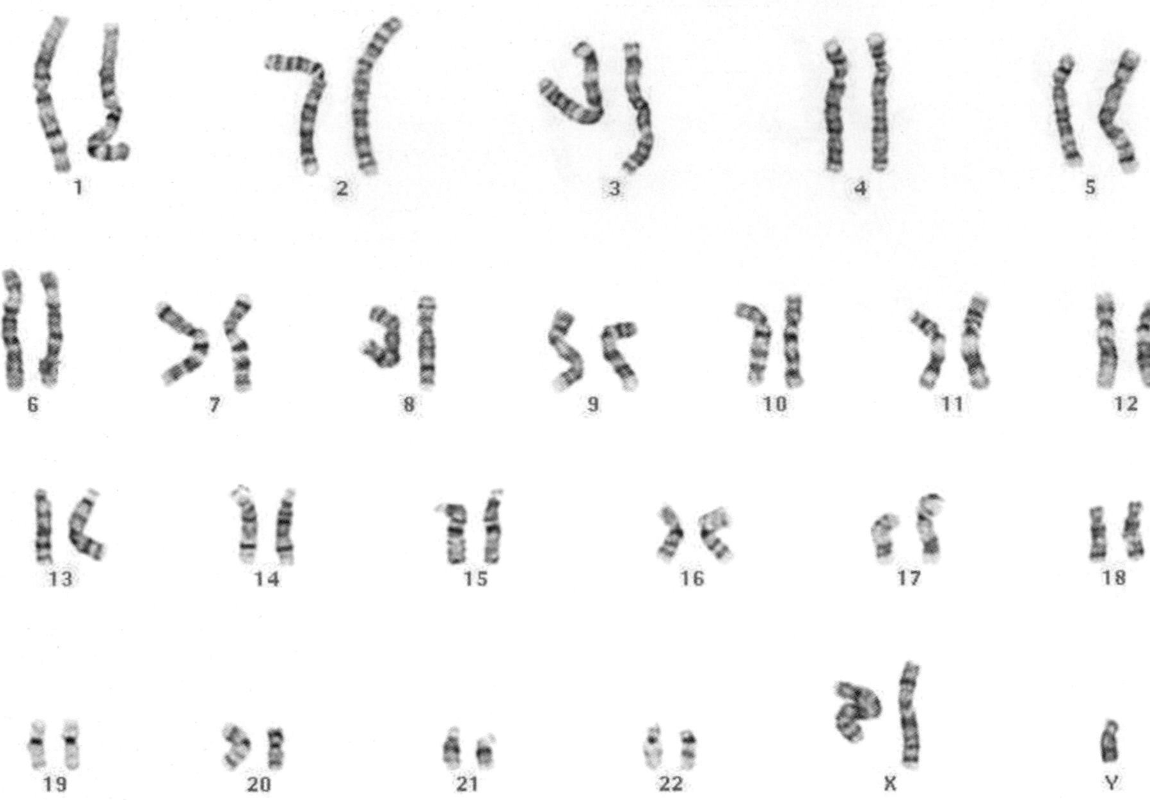


**Figure 26.10** Karyotype of a patient with Klinefelter syndrome (XXY).

of abnormal protein molecules will often cause pathological effects.

## Autosomal characteristics/diseases

Most human genetic diseases are due to mutations in autosomal genes, simply because there is much more genetic material in total in the 22 pairs of autosomes than in the single pair of sex chromosomes.

A homozygous person can only transmit one type of allele to any child they have, whilst a heterozygous person ('carrier') can transmit either of their two alleles to a child. Which allele a heterozygous parent transmits in any particular case is a random event, so there is a 1 in 2 (50%) chance of the child inheriting either allele. Thus, the following situations can arise:

- If both parents are homozygous for the same allele (dominant or recessive), then all their children will also inevitably be homozygous for that allele (Fig. 26.11).
- If one parent is homozygous for one allele and the other parent homozygous for the other allele, then all their children will inevitably be heterozygous (Fig. 26.12).

| | Paternal alleles | |
|---|---|---|
| Maternal alleles | A | A |
| A | AA | AA |
| A | AA | AA |

**Figure 26.11** Inheritance pattern – two homozygous parents, each carrying the same allele.

| | Paternal alleles | |
|---|---|---|
| Maternal alleles | A | A |
| a | Aa | Aa |
| a | Aa | Aa |

**Figure 26.12** Inheritance pattern – two homozygous parents, each carrying a different allele.

- If both parents are heterozygous, then there is a 1 in 4 (25%) chance of them producing a homozygous recessive child, a 1 in 4 (25%) chance of them producing a homozygous dominant child, and a 2 in 4 (50%) chance of them producing a heterozygous child. Note that in terms of phenotypes, the chance

| | Paternal alleles | |
|---|---|---|
| Maternal alleles | A | a |
| A | AA | aA |
| a | Aa | aa |

**Figure 26.13** Inheritance pattern – two heterozygous parents.

of producing a child of the dominant phenotype is 3 in 4 (75%) and of producing a child of the recessive phenotype is 1 in 4 (25%) (Fig. 26.13).

Thus, whilst both autosomal dominant and recessive characteristics/diseases occur in both males and females, dominant characteristics tend to be present in each generation, whilst recessive ones do not. This difference arises because a recessive characteristic can only be seen in the children of a heterozygous parent and either an affected parent or another heterozygous parent. If the particular recessive allele is rare, the probability of this happening is low. In practice, it is often found that parents of an individual affected by a rare recessive characteristic are related to each other (such as first cousins); thus, so-called 'consanguineous unions' are more likely to bring together two heterozygous parents.

If two parents are themselves unaffected and have a child with a recessive characteristic/disorder, it indicates that both of them must be heterozygous. There may then be concern about whether any subsequent child they may have will also be affected. In such a case, it is important to appreciate that the risk of any one particular child suffering from the recessive condition is always 1 in 4 or 25% (Fig. 26.13).

Further problems arise with diseases in which the disease process is either very variable in its severity (for example, myotonic dystrophy) or does not become apparent until later in life (such as Huntington's disease). In the first case, it is possible for people to have and transmit the disease without suffering any serious ill effects themselves (although subtle signs of such diseases can often be detected); in the second, many sufferers have had their families before they realize they carry a mutant allele. In either case, parents may unknowingly pass on mutant alleles to their children and thus have several affected children.

Examples of recessively inherited autosomal conditions include phenylketonuria, galactosaemia and cystic fibrosis; examples of dominantly inherited autosomal conditions include achondroplasia, Marfan syndrome and Huntington's disease.

## Sex-linked characteristics/diseases

Sex-linked conditions are those for which the relevant genes are carried on the sex chromosomes. They are more complex in their inheritance patterns than are autosomal characteristics because of the genetic difference between men and women.

Obviously, there are genes on both the X chromosome and the Y chromosome and hence both X-linked and Y-linked characteristics are known. There are very few genes on the Y chromosome (which is very small) and there are thus very few Y-linked characteristics. As a result of this, Y-linked characteristics are seldom considered and the terms 'X-linked' and 'sex-linked' are often used interchangeably. Note that the genes carried on the two sex chromosomes are quite different.

Only one of the two X chromosomes is active in any cell in a woman's body, the other is inactive (a 'Barr body'). Which X is inactive in any one cell is random and differs throughout the cells of the woman's body.

A very important consequence of the difference in sex chromosome complement between men and women is that men will always exhibit a characteristic resulting from the allele that they carry on their X chromosome since they do not have a second X chromosome. With respect to women, the situation for X-linked characteristics is very similar to that for autosomally determined characteristics: any one woman can be homozygous dominant, homozygous recessive or heterozygous for any gene on the X chromosome. Thus, a woman will only exhibit a recessive X-linked characteristic if she is homozygous recessive. This means that such a woman must be the child of a father who exhibits that characteristic and either a 'carrier' mother or a mother who also exhibits that characteristic, and, since these combinations of parents are very rare, such women, too, are very rare.

Both X-linked dominant and recessive characteristics/diseases are known and their patterns of inheritance can be summarized as follows:

- In X-linked recessive inheritance, there is never male-to-male transmission of the characteristic (since a father must pass on his Y chromosome if the child is to be male) (Fig. 26.14A). Also, as explained above, it is most usual to see only males affected by the condition. Thus, this type of disease is most typically carried by women of normal phenotype and affects mostly their sons. A woman who carries such a disease will transmit it (on average) to 1 in 2 of her children – thus, half her sons will be affected and half her daughters will be carriers (Fig. 26.14B). A man who has such a condition will pass on the disease allele whenever he passes on his X chromosome; all his daughters therefore must be carriers (assuming the mother is homozygous for the normal allele), while his sons cannot be affected (Fig 26.14C).
- In X-linked dominant inheritance, because the mutant allele is carried on the X chromosome, an affected male cannot pass it on to his sons, but must

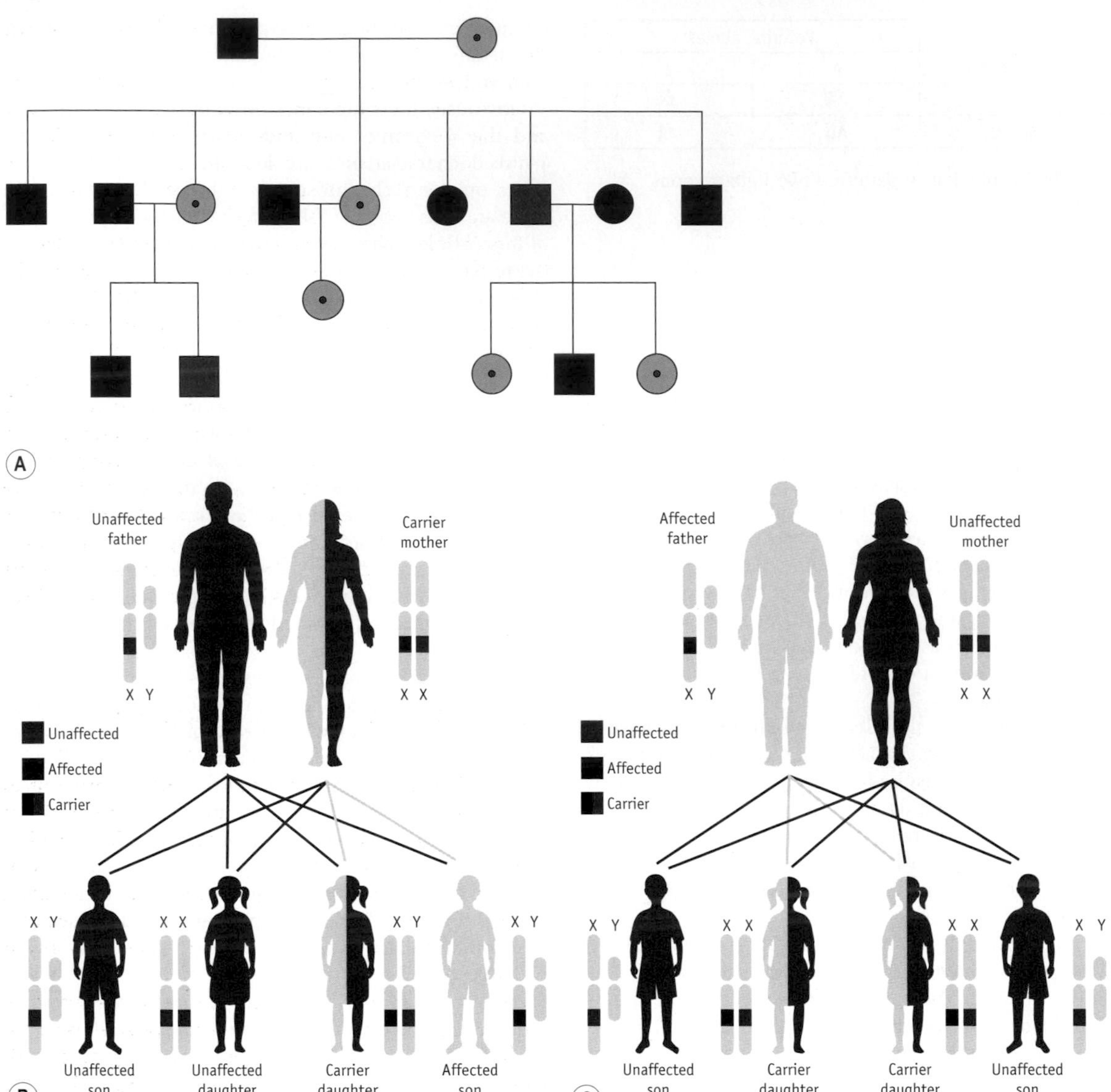


**Figure 26.14 A.** Pedigree diagram of X-linked recessive inheritance. **B.** Diagram of X-linked recessive inheritance with carrier mother. **C.** Diagram of X-linked recessive inheritance with affected father.

pass it on to all of his daughters, while an affected female will pass the mutant allele on to half her sons and half her daughters. Thus, if a father is affected with the disease, only his daughters will be affected (Fig 26.15A); if a mother is affected, then half of all her children (sons and daughters equally) will be affected (Fig 26.15B).

Among the best-known examples of X-linked recessive diseases are Duchenne muscular dystrophy, red/green colour-blindness, and the haemophilias. There are only a few X-linked dominant diseases, one example being hypophosphataemic (vitamin D-resistant) rickets.

It is important to note that, in any generation, new mutations can arise during meiosis and, clearly, the above inheritance patterns will then not be applicable.

## Polygenic and multifactorial characteristics

Many inherited characteristics/diseases are influenced by several genes rather than just one or two. Such characteristics are said to be polygenic ('many genes'), and the details of their inheritance patterns are often difficult to define precisely owing to the interplay between the

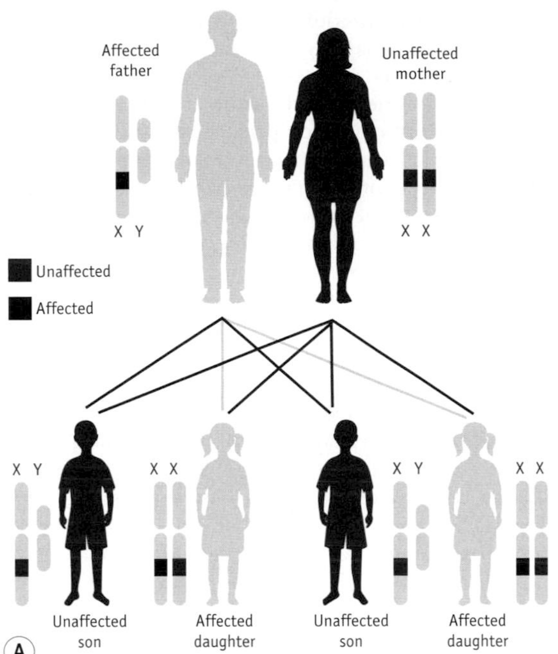


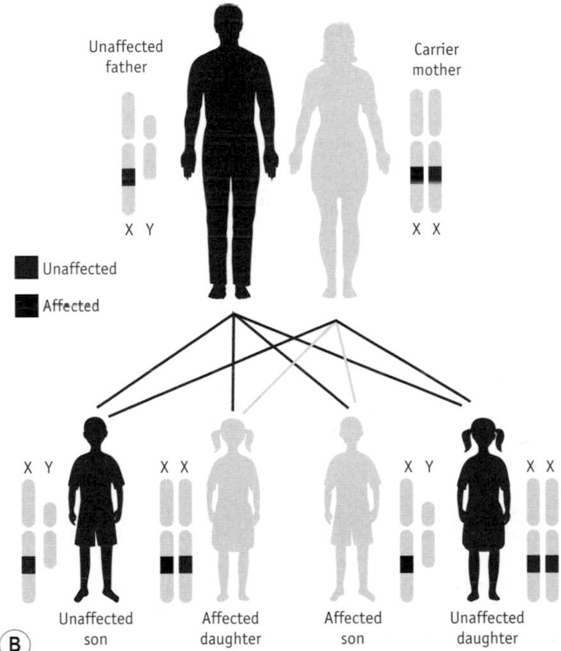


**Figure 26.15 A.** Diagram of X-linked dominant inheritance with affected father. **B.** Diagram of X-linked dominant inheritance with affected mother.

different alleles of the various genes involved (Cummings 2003).

Polygenic inheritance should not be confused with situations where several genetic disorders can cause the same effect, for example, blindness. There are many different inherited conditions that cause blindness, but most of them are simple autosomal recessive or X-linked conditions with only one mechanism operating.

If environmental factors, such as diet, as well as genetic ones are important in determining the precise nature of a physical characteristic or disease process, the characteristic/disorder is said to be *multifactorial* in origin – examples of such disorders include neural tube defects and many cases of cleft lip and/or palate. Most characteristics (for example, height) and diseases (such as atherosclerosis – a very common and serious disease of larger arteries) are, in fact, multifactorial in origin, often involving several genes and several environmental factors. It can prove very difficult to determine the precise risk status of any one individual for any particular condition in such cases owing to the large number of different contributory factors involved and the great range of ways in which these can vary.

## ORIGIN OF GENETIC DISEASES

In considering inherited disease, the problem arises as to why such conditions exist. New mutational events occur frequently – for example, because of errors in DNA replication during cell division, or exposure to mutagenic environmental agents, such as various forms of ionizing radiation (e.g. X-rays, ultraviolet light) or mutagenic chemicals (e.g. complex organic molecules in tobacco smoke).

Single new mutations can produce a dominant autosomal disease or a sex-linked disorder. Recessive disorders, however, cannot be explained so simply because both parents must carry the same mutation for the condition to occur. Rare recessive diseases may be explained by the lack of natural selection against a mutation that causes the heterozygous individual no ill effects, thus allowing the mutation to remain until, eventually, two people carrying the same mutation meet and produce a child who then suffers from the particular disease. There are, however, a number of relatively common recessive autosomal diseases (for example, sickle cell anaemia, cystic fibrosis) for which explanations of their high frequency of occurrence must be found. In general terms, such high frequencies are thought to be explained by the existence of some selective advantage that is peculiar to the 'carrier' (heterozygous individual). In some cases, the precise nature of this advantage has been determined. For example, in the case of sickle cell anaemia (in which the mutation occurs in the gene for one of the components of the gas transport protein haemoglobin), whilst those people who suffer from this disease (homozygous mutants) often die prematurely, those who carry one normal allele and one mutant ('sickle cell') allele show an increased resistance to malaria compared with people carrying two copies of the normal allele. Thus, in malarial areas, as the heterozygous person enjoys a selective survival advantage, the mutant allele is selected for and achieves a high frequency (Cummings 2003). In other cases, the precise nature of the advantage remains to be elucidated – it could be that carriers have some advantage in sexual competition, or that gametes carrying such alleles are somehow preferred, but evidence to support these hypotheses has yet to be produced.

Cummings (2003), Russell (2006) and Klug et al (2009) provide excellent, more detailed coverage of all the above material. Also, see the website for further reference to diagrams, animations and other supporting material.

## ASSESSMENT OF EMBRYO AND FETUS

Our ability to usefully assess the genetic make-up of the embryo and fetus has increased with further understanding of genetic influences on disease. Parental and social expectations of normal/perfect babies appear greater than ever before. Those involved in providing care now need to be aware of developments in this field to enable them to provide appropriate up-to-date information to women and their partners.

The process of screening and diagnosing genetic disorders has advanced significantly in recent years, making it seem easier to assess fetal normality earlier in pregnancy. Prenatal screening and diagnosis need to be differentiated. The Department of Health (2007) and NICE (2008) have laid down national standards for prenatal screening tests that should be offered to all pregnant women. Screening tests usually identify particular individuals or specific populations at increased risk and may just show the probability of a problem with the fetus. In most cases, further specific diagnostic tests are required to give a more definitive diagnosis of fetal abnormality.

## GENETIC COUNSELLING/ADVICE

Women and their partners in a higher-risk category are faced with some challenging decisions early in pregnancy, or before conception. These individuals will need opportunities to seek accurate, relevant, up-to-date information and time to consider the options available. Specialists trained in genetic counselling may be involved in the process, with the midwife having input in a facilitative and supportive role.

The role of genetic counselling is to facilitate effective decision-making, enabling deliberation on the internal and external factors that need to be considered for individuals to make the right choice for them. Examples of internal factors may include personal values and beliefs, previous experiences, and expectations of the present pregnancy or subsequent pregnancies, whilst external factors may relate to cultural values, religious beliefs, family and friend influences, economics, education, and social circumstances. It cannot be assumed when partners are involved that both parties will hold similar views and beliefs about the situation which may threaten their expectations of the baby.

Pre-conception counselling may be conducted in cases of a known or suspected family history of genetic disorders, or a previous pregnancy affected by a genetic disorder (such as cystic fibrosis [CF]). This will allow informed decisions to be made regarding family planning. (It is important to note, however, that this pre-conception approach cannot provide absolute certainty that any child will be disease-free. This is because, firstly, many diseases – such as CF – can be caused by a large number of different mutations and it is both technically demanding and very resource-intensive to screen for all of these. Secondly, even if the parents' somatic DNA is shown to be free of mutations, there is always the possibility that a new mutation could arise during gamete formation in one or both parents.) However, even with this caveat, this application of molecular genetic research has proved to be of great benefit to families with a history of genetic disease.

In the majority of cases, midwives become involved when meeting pregnant women. In providing advice to facilitate informed choices, there should be adequate explanations of the processes, risks, benefits, accuracy of the tests (including information on false positives/negatives), outcomes and alternatives for any assessments offered. This should include a focus on how far advanced the pregnancy will be before the test can be completed and how long the results may take to become available (Chapple 2006).

**Reflective activity 26.3**

Arrange a visit to an ultrasound department, and consider both the information requested by women and their partners, and the information given to them.

What impact did this experience have on your information-giving to women?

The key to successfully supporting women and their partners through this process lies in an awareness of the influence of effective communication skills, acknowledging their values and beliefs. The midwife can facilitate the woman/couple making an autonomous decision by building a trusting relationship and knowing the woman and partner's expectations and beliefs.

Effective counselling enables couples to believe that they have made the right decisions for them, which includes accepting the consequences. All circumstances need to be handled with sensitivity because some individuals may not have previously considered the possibility of fetal abnormality. Unfortunately, one of the difficulties with effective decision-making in pregnancy is the lack of time available to make significant decisions as gestation continues – especially for women who book late in pregnancy.

Owing to a variety of reasons, such as limited family histories and variations observed in severity of a disease process, it can sometimes be difficult to provide clear guidelines as to inheritance, significance of outcomes and the effect(s) on individuals in any one particular counselling situation. With this in mind, any information offered needs to clarify the gaps in knowledge as well as the advances made in the related field.

Once risk factors have been established, information should be provided on their potential impact on the fetus and baby, including options for treatment, if any, and the nature and course of any possible resultant illnesses. Whilst advances in medicine have considerably altered the outlook for many conditions (for example, persons with cystic fibrosis now have a greatly improved life and health expectancy), it is obviously important that advice is realistic, both highlighting the advances made and stressing the drawbacks currently experienced. Often, referral to specialist support groups may be useful at this time.

Equally, it is essential to discuss the impact of tests on the woman with any significant other people in her life, as influences might be consequential to the responsibility and acceptance of any decisions made.

Once counselled, women (and their partners) will have decisions to make. The choices open to them may include:

- not becoming pregnant and opting for fostering or adoption
- utilizing the facilities available for infertility treatments – that is, opting for artificial insemination by donor
- continuing with the pregnancy and 'hoping for the best'
- undergoing prenatal diagnostic tests, with the option to:
  - continue with the pregnancy regardless of outcome
  - terminate the pregnancy if a positive diagnosis is made
- using other available alternatives where possible, e.g. gene therapy.

The choices are nearly always complex, and consequently it is crucial that accurate knowledge is available to facilitate the best personal decisions. Case scenarios 26.1 and 26.2 on the website illustrate situations that may arise.

## SCREENING FOR RISK INDICATORS

The primary aim of screening for risk indicators/markers is to provide accurate information to facilitate fully informed decisions about proceeding with diagnostic tests to confirm or exclude a genetic disorder. There are various indicators and the utility of these in individual cases may depend on available information, previous history, the duration of gestation, and parental expectations of normality. Midwives have a major role to play in prenatal screening programmes (Chapple 2006).

### History taking

History taking has a key role in planning care for the pregnant woman (and partner). It provides detailed information and an opportunity for relationship-building between the woman and the midwife, which, although always important, may be particularly relevant for further decision-making. An accurate, detailed personal, family, medical and obstetric history is essential in identifying risk factors that expose the pregnancy to genetic disorders, which should ideally include relevant details of the biological father of the fetus. Sensitivity to the fact that information is not always available is important, especially where there is no contact with the father or where infertility treatment has been used to achieve the pregnancy.

Consideration of racial and/or geographical origins may also be appropriate (such as with Tay–Sachs disease in Ashkenazi Jews, or haemoglobinopathies in women of Mediterranean, African or Asiatic origin). Situations such as consanguinity should also be examined.

Following the history taking, the midwife and woman/couple should consider the need for further screening. Prior to any decisions, it is essential that the woman is aware that further screening may ultimately lead to a decision about keeping or terminating the pregnancy. For some women, this may be unthinkable and they should be clearly aware of this scenario, whereas for others, having this choice would be essential. Some women may choose to continue with screening anyway, with the view that they would like to know details and prepare for the birth accordingly.

### Ultrasound scanning (USS)

NICE (2008) recommends that routine USS is ideally carried out at 10 weeks' and before 14 weeks' gestation. For more details about USS, see Chapter 33. In the UK, routine USS in early pregnancy has been used for detection of clinically unsuspected fetal malformations (Neilson

2001). Many units now offer USS at 11–14 weeks' gestation, which may predict a risk of chromosomal abnormality by measuring the amount of fluid behind the neck of the fetus, specifically the nuchal fold thickness. It is measured in millimetres, computer recorded in conjunction with maternal age, and used to determine a predictive risk rate. Second trimester USS is usually offered to women between 18 and 20 weeks' gestation for structural anomalies. Diagnostic USS may be carried out in a variety of specific circumstances during pregnancy, such as when the fetus is perceived to be at particularly high risk of malformation.

### Biochemical/maternal serum screening

- Alpha-fetoprotein (AFP) serum screening should ideally be carried out around 13–14 weeks' gestation (see Chapter 33). AFPs are fetal proteins present in maternal serum and amniotic fluid. A raised level of AFPs may indicate intrauterine death, multiple pregnancies, or, most commonly, an open neural tube defect. A lower than expected reading may imply a chromosomal abnormality, for example, Down syndrome.
- Enzyme levels can be assayed to detect inborn errors of metabolism. Alpha-fetoprotein and acetylcholinesterase levels can be measured to help identify and distinguish between neural tube defects, anencephaly, and ventral wall defects such as gastroschisis and omphalocele that may have been suspected during anomaly scanning. Hormone levels can be assessed to diagnose adrenogenital syndrome.

Biochemical screening tests can utilize combination tests to determine risk factors. They can incorporate serum AFPs, unconjugated oestriol and human chorionic gonadatrophin, measured with maternal age and weight in relation to gestational age.

### Integrated (combined) testing

NICE (2008) has recently recommended that all women are offered a combination of tests in the first trimester to determine the risk of the unborn baby having Down syndrome. These tests may not yet be available through all NHS services. The tests comprise nuchal translucency ultrasound scan plus blood tests to measure levels of beta-human chorionic gonadotrophin (β-hCG) and pregnancy-associated plasma protein-A (PAPP-A). These tests should be performed between 11 and 13 weeks and are the most efficient method of detecting Down syndrome (90% as compared to 65% with second trimester serum screening). When necessary, the tests may be repeated between 15 and 20 weeks. The benefit of the 'combined test' is that it would reduce the number of women proceeding to invasive tests. Screening by combining maternal age, nuchal scan and blood biochemistry (for maternal serum free β-hCG and PAPP-A) gives a pick-up rate of over 90%. Recent audit figures (NICE 2008) are an impressive 95% with a false positive.

## DIAGNOSTIC TESTS

Diagnostic tests are carried out to give definitive results for abnormalities and genetic conditions when required. The procedures usually carry risk factors and it is important that women/partners are fully informed of these and the potential outcomes before making a decision to proceed with the test. Risks include compromising the ongoing pregnancy, pregnancy loss, getting false-positive or false-negative results, and having to face the dilemma of deciding whether to proceed with the pregnancy or choose termination. These choices may be more difficult for some women than for others, depending on their expectations, beliefs and needs for their pregnancy, as well as multiple psychosocial influences.

The purpose of testing is to assess the status of the genome of an individual embryo/fetus. Each individual's genome is unique (with the exception of that of identical twins). In order to be able to recognize individual sequences of DNA, techniques have been developed to provide methods of analysis for the DNA of an individual. These techniques use genetic probes (which are labelled fragments of DNA) to determine whether a particular DNA sequence is present or absent. Embryonic/fetal genome analysis is only one application of this technology: others include forensic science and paternity disputes.

DNA can be isolated easily from any human cell that is alive and has a nucleus, including buccal cells and skin fibroblasts. The DNA probe is a copy of a relevant sequence that is identifiable and can be used as a 'probe' to hybridize a corresponding copy of the sample.

### Preimplantation genetic diagnosis (PGD)

Preimplantation genetic screening (PGS) (also known as embryo screening) remains an experimental intervention and comprises procedures that do not look for a specific disease but are used to identify embryos at risk. The technique has to be considered before conception and involves extrauterine assessment of the embryo itself; it can thus provide certainty that the embryo is free of the genetic defects that the particular identification/screening procedure used is able to detect. It has two stages: firstly, in-vitro fertilization techniques are used to create embryos, which are then tested for particular genetic disorders and/or to establish their sex (where the disorder is sex linked). The two major technologies used for single gene cell analysis involve the polymerase chain reaction (PCR – a technique to increase the amount of DNA available for analysis) and fluorescence in-situ hybridization (FISH – the use of fluorescently labelled DNA probes for the detection of single gene defects). It is not feasible to screen for all possible genetic defects and each embryo is screened only for those particular genetic defects likely to occur. After these tests, healthy embryos are implanted into the mother's uterus using techniques developed for infertility treatments. However, many women fail to achieve a pregnancy after the transfer of good-quality embryos. Following a systematic review of literature to date, there are insufficient data to determine whether PGS is an effective intervention in IVF/ICSI for improving live-birth rates (Twisk et al 2006).

This intervention is fraught with ethical issues, especially from those who believe in the sanctity of human life, and about the numbers of embryos that may perish or become damaged during the process. Currently, PGD appears to be only used for severe/life-threatening disorders and ongoing work is regulated through the independent body HFEA (Human Fertilisation and Embryology Authority) overseeing the use of gametes and embryos in fertility and research (www.hfea.gov.uk).

## Chorionic villus sampling (CVS)

CVS is performed to obtain a biopsy of chorionic tissue from the developing embryo (see Ch. 33). The procedure involves placing a fine catheter/forceps by the transcervical or transabdominal route in conjunction with USS. DNA/cytogenetic analysis for chromosomal studies and some biochemical studies can be performed on the tissue biopsy. CVS should not be carried out before 11 weeks' gestation as a precaution to prevent damage to the fetus.

## Amniocentesis

Amniocentesis is performed to obtain a sample of amniotic fluid, which contains cells shed from the surface of the fetus and membranes (see Ch. 33). It can be performed at various stages of gestation but is traditionally undertaken between 16 and 18 weeks' gestation when maternal age, history or screening indicates a high risk of abnormality. The cells are usually first cultured to determine the fetal karyotype and for detailed DNA analyses (including fetal sexing). The biochemical constituents of the fluid may be tested for non-specific indicators of abnormality (for example, AFPs), for the accumulation of specific metabolites in suspected inborn errors of metabolism, or, in later pregnancy, for fetal assessment. The main limitation of the test at this relatively advanced gestational age is the time taken to culture the cells, with results not being available until around 20 weeks' gestation (see Ch. 33).

In a systematic review of 14 randomized controlled trials, Alfirevic et al (2003) compared safety and accuracy of transcervical and transabdominal CVS with early and second trimester amniocentesis. They concluded that second trimester amniocentesis is safer than transcervical CVS and early amniocentesis, with transabdominal CVS being preferred when an early diagnosis is required. There appeared to be increased risks of spontaneous miscarriage, pregnancy loss and neonatal talipes associated with earlier amniocentesis. Regarding second trimester amniocentesis, there was a non-significant increase in pregnancy loss of 1% compared with a control group (3% versus 2%), with a significant increase noted in spontaneous miscarriages (2.1% versus 1.3%). Results may occasionally be ambiguous, and there is also a small risk of cells failing to grow or contamination by maternal cells.

## Fetoscopy

In this technique, the fetus is observed through a fine fibreoptic telescope, during which samples of tissue may be removed under direct vision, for analysis. It may be used to diagnose skin disease, such as epidermolysis bullosa lethalis, by skin biopsy. The technique may be used to perform therapeutic interventions, such as blood transfusion in rhesus incompatibility.

## Cordocentesis

This technique is used to obtain a sample of fetal blood to screen for chromosomal abnormalities, haemophilia and haemoglobinopathies (see Ch. 33). It is carried out using USS to guide a fine needle to the base of the umbilical cord, where a sample of fetal blood is extracted for analysis and/or karyotyping.

All screening and diagnostic tests carry some risks, psychological and/or physical; consequently, the decision to proceed or not needs to be carefully measured. The role of the midwife is, therefore, to ensure that couples are given the opportunity to make fully informed autonomous decisions.

# APPLICATIONS OF GENETICS

The development of molecular genetic techniques in the medical field has already yielded many benefits, for example, production of human insulin by genetically modified bacteria for use in diabetes (Russell 2006).

It is important to note that there are potential problems associated with genetic modification and activities are thus closely regulated by statutory bodies (for example, the UK Advisory Committee on Genetic Modification, the Health

& Safety Executive). Of particular relevance to midwifery is the fact that the manipulation of human gametes is internationally prohibited. This is to avoid deliberately and directly changing the overall genetic constitution (the 'gene pool') of the human species, the consequences of such changes being both unpredictable and irreversible. The only human cells permitted to be genetically modified are the somatic cells (that is, all cells other than the gametes) and modifications to these cells are tightly regulated.

One of the most obvious applications of genetics in midwifery practice is genetic screening of parents and/or embryo (discussed above), but there is also much recent research in genetics from which developments that decrease the morbidity and mortality currently associated with many diseases may arise. In applying this research to clinical situations, the emphasis is on both prevention and cure.

Another obvious potential application of molecular genetic research in medicine is to replace or repair missing or defective alleles with normal ones – 'gene therapy'. This process involves the insertion of genetic material directly into cells to alter the functioning of those cells (thus, to allow them to produce the normal, functional version of a protein). Success has been achieved in the treatment of some diseases (such as adenosine deaminase deficiency – Klug et al 2009), but there have also been some serious adverse consequences (that is, one fatality during gene therapy treatment – Klug et al 2009). Thus, both technical and safety-related problems remain regarding gene therapy, but this is still an active area of research with some promise.

Another possibility is the range of therapeutic options potentially available based on the use of stem cells – 'cell-based regenerative therapies' (National Institutes of Health Stem Cell Information website – http://stemcells.nih.gov), which involves not only complex scientific issues but also complex ethical ones too. The use of stem cells opens up a wide range of novel therapeutic options, but much work remains to be done, with respect to both the scientific and ethical issues, if these too are to be safely and reliably available in the clinical situation.

Media reports about advances in genetic technologies and their applications are both frequent and often dramatic. Consequently, parents/prospective parents may have unrealistic expectations in this area, beyond the current limits of these technologies. These approaches may well prove to be of great benefit in due course, but until both the relevant complex scientific and/or ethical issues are resolved, they remain potential therapeutic options only. It is, therefore, important to be aware of what these technologies both can and cannot achieve when dealing with parents/prospective parents.

Finally, there are resource issues to be considered in relation to these technologies, all of which are resource-intensive. Even when technology is available, consideration will have to be given to the already limited healthcare resources. It may be possible to argue in this context that the potential financial benefits of having children born free from genetic disease outweigh the cost of providing effective life care for a child/adult suffering from the condition. Nonetheless, this will inevitably have to be balanced with the needs of the general population in allocation of funds.

## CONCLUSION

The possibilities for the future are potentially very great and the midwife will need to be aware of these technologies, as parents frequently request information following media coverage. For the midwife, this will include understanding the basis of genetics and the reality of current success in genetic engineering, including the risk:benefit ratios. The message for healthcare professionals is the need to provide appropriate and effective information to enable women and their partners to make informed decisions about the best course of action for them at present.

### KEY POINTS

- A good understanding of cell division, chromosomes and diagnostic testing is important when talking to parents whose baby has an abnormality or to potential parents in whose families there is history of genetic disease.
- Midwives require a sound knowledge of genetics and modes of inheritance to identify women and babies who might be at risk and to select the appropriate screening method and recognize when referral is necessary.
- Genetic engineering may have only a limited impact on the role of the midwife at present, but knowledge of the processes and possibilities in this field is (and will increasingly be) important in terms of effective communication with parents.

## REFERENCES


Alfirevic Z, Sundberg K, Brigham S: Amniocentesis and chorionic villus sampling for prenatal diagnosis, *Cochrane Database of Systematic Reviews* 2003(3):CD003252, 2003.

Chapple J: Simplifying antenatal screening: what midwives need to know, *British Journal of Midwifery* 14(4):193–196, 2006.

Cummings MR: *Human heredity – principles & issues*, ed 6, Pacific Grove, 2003, Thomson/Brooks-Cole, 2003.

Department of Health (DH): *Collaborative commissioning of national screening programmes*, London, 2007, DH.

Klug WS, Cummings MR, Spencer CA et al: *Concepts of genetics*, ed 9, New Jersey, 2009, Pearson Benjamin Cummings.

Lockwood CJ: Prediction of pregnancy loss, *Lancet* 355(9212):1292–1293, 2000.

National Institute for health and Clinical Excellence (NICE): *Antenatal care – routine care for the healthy pregnant woman*, NICE clinical guideline 62, London, 2008, NICE.

Neilson JP: Ultrasound for fetal assessment in early pregnancy, *Cochrane Database of Systematic Reviews* (2):CD000182, 2001.

Russell PJ: *Genetics – a molecular approach*, ed 2, San Francisco, 2006, Pearson Benjamin Cummings.

Twisk M, Mastenbroek S, van Wely M, et al: Preimplantation genetic screening for abnormal number of chromosomes (aneuploidies) in in vitro fertilization or intracystoplasmic sperm injection, *Cochrane Database of Systematic Reviews* (1):CD005291, 2006.

Chapter |27|

# Fertility and its control

*Rosemary Towse*

## LEARNING OUTCOMES

After reading this chapter, you will be able to:

- understand the influence of the psychological effects of childbearing upon the reactions of the woman and her partner in resuming sexual intercourse and the use of contraception
- understand the importance of individual history taking from the woman prior to giving information and advice
- understand the physiological principles of each method of family planning
- evaluate the differing methods of contraception available to women and their partners, including: the advantages and disadvantages of the different methods available; the importance of accurate advice concerning the timing of resumption of the use of contraception
- know the agencies available for the woman and her partner to seek further information and advice.

The control of fertility does not just involve the use of contraceptive techniques but is also a political issue with governments worldwide regulating access to various forms of contraception and abortion. The health of women and their families is linked to being able to control their fertility and, therefore, midwives and other health professionals have an important contribution to make toward the reproductive and sexual health of women.

Worldwide, 1 in 5 pregnancies end in abortion. In England and Wales in 2006 the abortion rate rose to 18.3 per 1000 women aged 15 to 44, with rates varying from 3.9 for the under 16 years to 35 for 19-year-olds (DH 2007). Britain has one of the highest rates for teenage pregnancies in Europe, with 90,000 teenagers becoming pregnant every year, 8000 being under 16 years old. The Government teenage pregnancy strategy has aimed to halve this number by 2010 (Social Exclusion Unit 1999), though indications suggest that this target will not be achieved.

Having an unplanned pregnancy can be a traumatic experience for the woman and her partner and it is therefore important that both have access to information about contraception and the services available to them. This chapter will cover details of the different contraceptive methods and also the midwife's contribution to the contraceptive and sexual care of the mother.

Family planning services and contraceptives are provided free under the UK National Health Service. A couple or an individual requiring family planning advice and supplies may go either to their general practitioner or to a community family planning clinic. In some areas there is also a domiciliary service for selected clients who, for some reason, do not attend the clinics. A variety of clinics may be provided including 'drop-in' clinics for young people as well as the more traditional sessions. Some clinics also specialize in specific areas such as psychosexual counselling.

## RESUMING RELATIONSHIPS FOLLOWING CHILDBEARING

Women vary in their approach to resuming marital relations after childbirth and it is common for newly delivered mothers to feel extremely tired and also guilty about their reluctance to have sexual intercourse. For the man, the effects of witnessing a delivery can be a highly emotional experience and may result in tension or guilt (Clement 1998), but problems of changed sexual relationships are often regarded as the fault of the woman. The man may feel rejected when the baby is establishing a relationship with its mother, and mothers experiencing postnatal depression may find their satisfaction with the relationship with their partner is reduced. This, in turn, may increase the man's guilt and frustration. Women have far better opportunities than men for obtaining advice on these intimate matters, so it is important that the midwife takes the time to provide opportunities for counselling or, where necessary, referral to specialist counsellors.

## METHODS OF CONTRACEPTION

### The ideal method

The ideal method should be an effective, acceptable, simple, painless method or procedure which does not rely on the user's memory:

- 100% safe and free from side-effects
- 100% effective
- 100% reversible
- easy to use
- independent of sexual intercourse
- used by or obviously visible to the woman
- independent of the medical profession
- protective against sexually transmitted diseases
- acceptable to both partners, all cultures and religions
- cheap and easy to distribute.

**Reflective activity 27.1**

Using the ideals stated above, consider each of the methods of contraception. Give a rating out of 10 for each method.

Think of situations where some criteria may be considered more important to the woman/couple than others.

### Male contraception

#### *Coitus interruptus (withdrawal method)*

This is a method which is used by a large number of couples at some stage in their relationship. It depends on the man withdrawing his penis from the vagina before ejaculation takes place and thus requires control. This may be acceptable to some couples but may cause considerable frustration and stress in others.

Because of the risk of leakage of seminal fluid before withdrawal, coitus interruptus is not considered a very safe method. If no other alternative is acceptable, the use of a spermicide pessary or foam would reduce the risk of conception by helping to destroy any sperm released into the vagina before withdrawal.

#### *Condom or sheath*

The condom or sheath is probably the most widely used contraception in the first few months after childbirth. As a barrier method, it not only provides protection against conception but also is effective in preventing the transmission of sexually transmitted diseases, including HIV (Everett 2004). For this reason, many couples use this in addition to other methods and the regular use of condoms should be encouraged as part of the promotion of safer sex. Condoms, however, cannot protect against local infestations such as scabies and lice. Because of the strong links between specific types of the human papillomavirus (HPV) and cervical cancer (Guillebaud 2007), it is reasonable to assume that condoms may reduce the risk of cervical neoplasm.

In the UK, condoms can be obtained free from family planning clinics and Department of Sexual Health clinics, or purchased at chemists or other retail outlets, with a wide variety of sizes, textures and flavours being available. Condoms should no longer be used if lubricated with spermicide, as this is thought to increase the risk of HIV transmission (Guillebaud 2007). Most condoms are made from latex. Occasionally, men and women report sensitivity to the latex, and condoms made from a hypoallergenic latex can be tried. Rarely, an allergy to the latex occurs; the Avanti condom, which is made from polyurethane, can be used in these situations. A new condom, called *Ez.on*, is also made from polyurethane and is slightly different in shape to conventional ones, with a tight base but a looser-fitting shaft, thus theoretically making it less likely to break and allowing more sensation for the man.

The midwife should never assume that either partner knows how to use condoms correctly and safely, and if necessary she should be prepared to explain the correct method for using a condom. The golden rules for safe use of condoms include:

- Only use condoms with the BSI or CE kitemark.
- Never use after the use-by date.
- Never use if the inner packaging around the condom is damaged.
- Condoms should only be used once.
- Take care with fingernails or rings that might snag the rubber.
- Never use with oil-based products, as these weaken the rubber and may cause it to break (these include baby or bath oil, cold cream, suntan oil, Vaseline; lipstick, aromatherapy oils and massage lotions).
- Medicines such as Nystatin or other antifungal creams and pessaries and some oestrogen creams may have the same effect as above.

Following use, in the event of damage or spilling of seminal fluid, unless another contraceptive is already being used, the woman should seek advice from her GP or family planning clinic regarding the need for emergency contraception. The condom has a failure rate of 2–12%.

### *Future developments*

Male hormonal contraception is presently under research. Current trials are mainly using progestogens that inhibit production of follicle-stimulating hormone (FSH) and luteinizing hormone (LH), thus reducing sperm production, with testosterone replacement needed to prevent side-effects. Other trials are using androgen, which induces sperm suppression (Herdiman et al 2006). The aim is to prevent sperm production whilst having no effect on ejaculation. Apart from the effectiveness of this type of contraception, there is the issue of whether women would be happy to rely on their male partner for contraception of this type.

## Female contraception

### Physiological methods (Fig. 27.1)

For some people, this is the only acceptable method of contraception. The 'safe period' refers to the time during the menstrual cycle when conception is less likely to take place. It is known that ovulation occurs approximately 14 days before the onset of the next menstrual period and that fertilization is possible up to 5 days before and 2 days afterwards. Allowing an extra day either end, intercourse should be avoided for these 10 or 11 days during the cycle.

Theoretically, this is very easy; however, in practice, to determine the exact time of ovulation takes time and patience. It will also depend upon the regularity of the woman's menstrual cycle. The physiological return of ovulation following childbirth is variable and difficult to assess, making this method very unreliable in the first few months after childbirth. Various methods have been developed to allow the 'safe period' to be worked out.

### *The standard days method (SDM)*

This is based on the abstinence from unprotected sexual intercourse on days 8–19 of every cycle, assuming the woman has a regular cycle of 26–32 days.

### *The 2 day method*

This is based on the presence of cervical secretions seen by the woman. Fertility is assumed when any secretions are present and also the following day.

Both the SDM and the 2 day method have the advantage of being simpler than the traditional calendar, temperature and *Billings* methods. However, any woman wanting to use these must be advised to seek expert help in order to determine their suitability and ensure correct explanation of the techniques. Both methods have shown good efficacy in women with regular cycles.

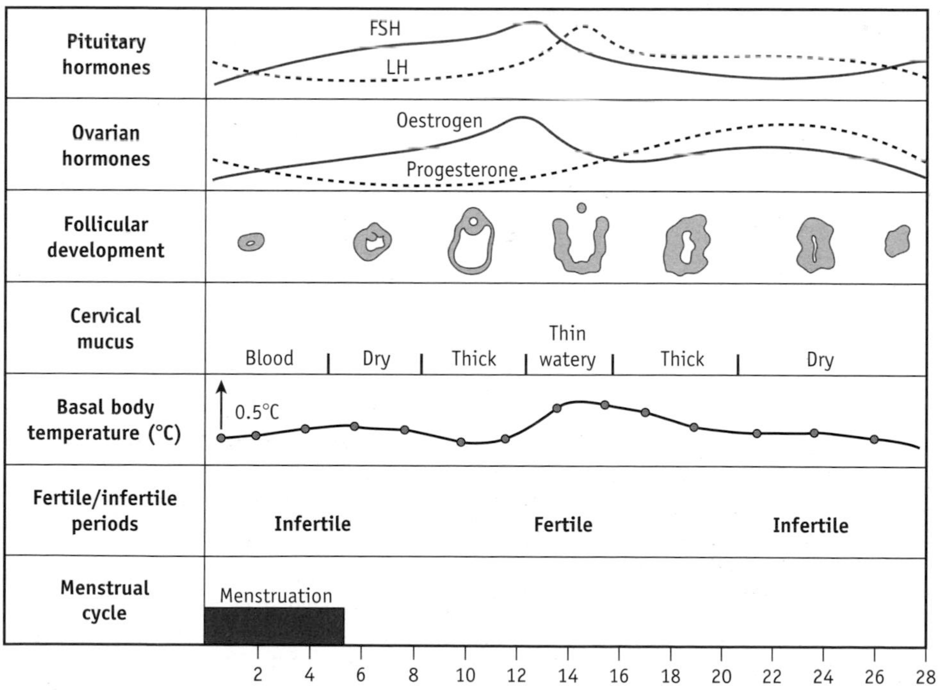


**Figure 27.1** Physiological changes within the reproductive system during the menstrual cycle.

### *Lactational amenorrhoea method (LAM)*

This is a fairly efficient method which can be used in the fully breast feeding mother in the first 6 months postpartum, providing certain criteria are met:

- The mother must be fully breastfeeding, day and night.
- The baby should not be receiving any feed supplements.
- The mother should be under 6 months postpartum.
- The mother should be totally amenorrhoeic. Bleeding in the first 6 weeks postpartum is not included.

If any of the criteria change, the mother is potentially fertile. It is estimated that this method has a failure rate of 2% (Guillebaud 2007).

### *Persona*

Persona combines the features of a micro-laboratory and a microcomputer and is designed to enable calculation of the potentially fertile and unfertile parts of the cycle. The device measures levels of LH and oestrogen breakdown products (E-3-G), by testing the urine with a dipstick that inserts into the machine. The device calculates the likely date of ovulation well in advance, and allowing for sperm survival time, the woman is then shown 'green' days when conception is unlikely and 'red' days when conception could occur. To provide the machine with sufficient information for these calculations, a minimum of 16 tests in the woman's first cycle and eight in subsequent cycles are required. Persona can only be used if the cycles are within 23–35 days in length.

Persona may be of limited value following childbirth, as it requires the woman to have two successive cycles of 23–35 days and this makes it inappropriate for use in breastfeeding mothers. With perfect use, the failure rate of Persona as a contraceptive tool is 6 per 100 woman years; however, for the typical user the rate is higher (Guillebaud 2007). Persona can be used for planning a pregnancy but there are few references to the efficacy of Persona used for this purpose.

## Barrier methods

### *Occlusive caps*

These devices cover the cervix and mechanically obstruct the entrance of spermatozoa.

They are made in a variety of sizes and must be fitted individually. Caps are checked for fit at regular intervals, especially after childbirth or loss or gain of weight. With correct and conscientious use, the rate of pregnancy can be as low as 2 per 100 woman years, but a more typical rate would be 5–10 per 100 women years (Guillebaud 2007). Cervical caps are less effective as a contraceptive in multiparous women.

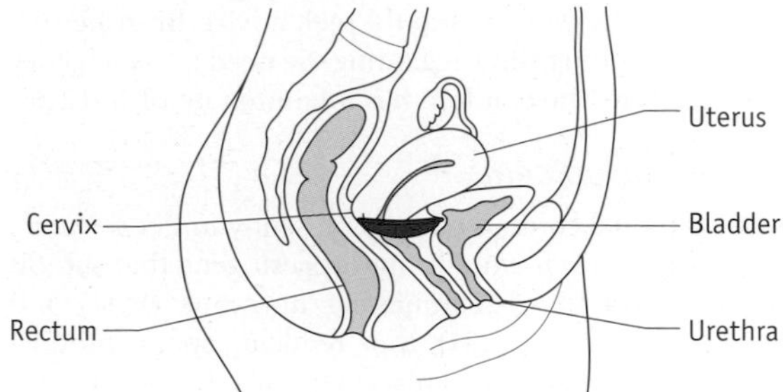


**Figure 27.2** Sagittal section of the pelvis showing a diaphragm in position.

### *The diaphragm or Dutch cap*

This is one of the oldest methods of female contraception and has changed very little in design. A postnatal mother who wishes to use a diaphragm should not be fitted until 6–8 weeks postnatally, to allow the uterus and cervix to return to a non-pregnant size and the vaginal muscles to regain their tone. The shallow rubber diaphragm has a circular spring around the perimeter, allowing it to be compressed and inserted into the vagina rather like a tampon, with the diaphragm lying between the posterior fornix of the vagina posteriorly and the suprapubic ridge anteriorly (Fig. 27.2). The diaphragms come in graduated sizes and must be fitted individually.

A woman who has used a diaphragm before may require a larger size after childbirth and this may need adjustment as the vaginal muscle tone improves. A diaphragm that is too large protrudes and causes discomfort, or may produce extra pressure, giving rise to urethritis-type discomfort; however, if too small, it will move around and will not provide protection. A well-fitting diaphragm is unobtrusive and will not be noticed during intercourse. It should remain in situ for 6 hours after intercourse and is then removed at a convenient time. Failure rates vary from 4% to 18%, depending on the care and consistency of the woman.

### *Other caps* (Fig. 27.3)

Other types of cap less commonly used may be very useful in particular cases. They all rely on suction to remain in place. The use of lubricants on both surfaces and the removal after 6 hours remain a consistent feature of use.

*Vault caps* sit in the fornices of the vagina covering the cervix and have no spring rim and are useful when vaginal tone is poor.

The *cervical cap* is designed to fit over the cervix and it may be useful for women who have a straight-sided cervix. A disposable silicone rubber cap called the Oves cap is now available. Once the woman has been fitted for size, she can buy these herself from a chemist. The Oves cap can be kept in place for up to 48 hours.

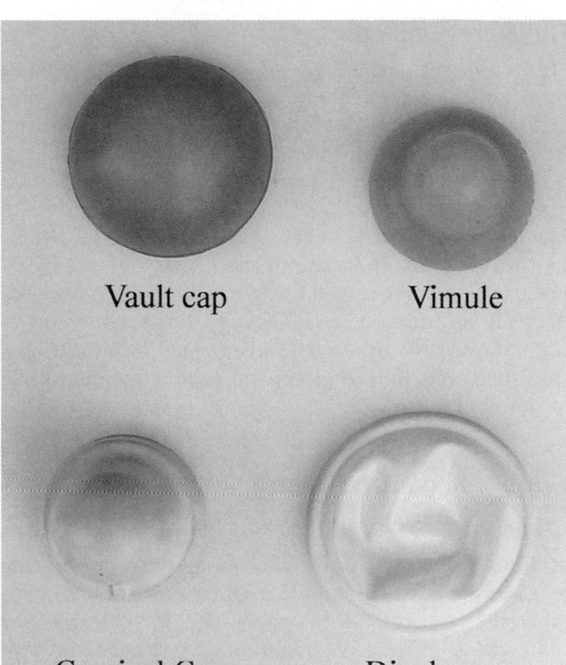


**Figure 27.3** Occlusive caps.

The *vimule* is a combination of vault and cervical cap and has a powerful suction capability and is used to cover the cervix that is small, irregular or partially amputated.

Other varieties of caps are being evaluated at present. The Lea's shield and the FemCap are both made of silicone rubber and can be left in for up to 48 hours. One study found a failure rate of 10.5–14.4 per 100 woman years (Guillebaud 2007).

### *Female condoms*

The Femidom is a polyurethane tubular condom consisting of a loose-fitting polyurethane sheath with a flexible ring at either end. It is inserted so that the condom lines the vagina. A soft but firm plastic ring at the entrance covers the genitalia and needs to be steadied in position during intercourse. This condom provides protection both from pregnancy and from sexually transmitted diseases. It has a failure rate of 5% (Guillebaud 2007). Like caps, these can be fitted prior to sexual intercourse. The female condom contains a spermicide-free lubricant. Being made from polyurethane, avoidance of oil-based products is not necessary.

### *The contraceptive sponge – Today Sponge®*

The contraceptive sponge is a small, one-size, soft, doughnut-shaped foam device made from polyurethane, with a loop at one end for easy removal. It contains spermicide, and is normally placed internally into the vagina to act as a contraception method. The sponge prevents pregnancy in two ways:

- It has a contour that, when correctly placed, covers the cervix. This works to block sperm from entering the uterus.
- If sperm do get past, the sponge absorbs such and kills off the rogue sperm with the spermicide contained within the device.

It can be inserted in advance of intercourse, and has an effectiveness rate of 83–87%.

## Long-acting reversible contraception (LARC)

This term refers to four specific contraceptive methods: intrauterine contraceptive devices (IUCDs), the intrauterine system (IUS or Mirena), progesterone injections and implants. These methods are particularly important as they are highly effective and do not affect fertility long term. In addition, they are useful for those who have compliance problems with other methods. NICE recommends that these methods should be discussed with all women who ask for information about contraception (NICE 2005).

## Intrauterine contraceptive devices and intrauterine systems

Intrauterine contraceptive devices (IUCDs) have been used all over the world since Biblical times. Nowadays, IUCDs are small plastic devices that are placed in the uterine cavity by means of a special introducer. All have copper or copper and silver stems that increase the efficiency of the device. The mode of action of IUCDs is complex and multifactorial. They act as a sterile foreign body in the uterine cavity and the resultant physiological action is potentiated by the addition of copper. The copper has a toxic effect on sperm and ova, preventing fertilization. It is rare to find viable sperm in the uterine cavity, making it very unlikely that IUCDs ever act as an abortive agent. It is also thought that the device causes some reduction in tubular contraction, thereby reducing the speed of the ovum along the fallopian tube, and there is some evidence of infrequent ovulation while the device is in situ. There may also be an increased production of prostaglandins in the uterus, which increases uterine activity and causes the expulsion of a fertilized ovum. A secondary action of inhibiting implantation is relevant when used as part of emergency contraception. The IUCD inhibits implantation and there is also a direct blastocystotoxic effect. There is no evidence that copper IUCDs increase the risk of ectopic pregnancies which are related to the risk of pelvic inflammatory disease (Guillebaud 2007).

The introduction of an IUCD following delivery is generally delayed until 6 to 8 weeks postpartum, when

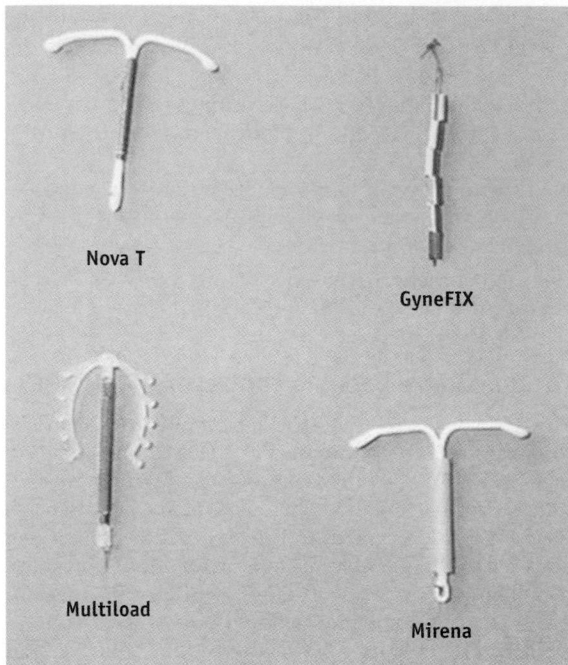


**Figure 27.4** Examples of intrauterine contraceptive devices.

involution of the uterus is likely to be complete. If it is inserted earlier, it may not remain in the optimum position and is more likely to be expelled. Particular care is required after caesarean section, to ensure that the wound has fully healed. In some cases, an IUCD is inserted at the time of termination of pregnancy, if requested by the woman.

A number of types are now available (Fig. 27.4). The GyneFIX, unlike the others, is frameless, consisting of six copper bands threaded onto a length of suture material. One end is provided with a knot, which is inserted into the fundus and acts as an anchor.

An increase in the length and heaviness of menstruation with an IUCD may make this an unsuitable method for women who already have menorrhagia. Women with dysmenorrhoea may find the pain is worsened by the introduction of a device. Women with recurrent infection in the reproductive tract may be advised to use another method. While the device does not introduce infection, any infection, particularly sexually transmitted infection, that may occur is likely to be more difficult to treat.

The devices remain in situ for 5–8 years, depending on type, and require only minimal supervision following insertion. They have an excellent record in preventing pregnancy, with a failure rate ranging from 0.3 to 3 per 100 woman years (Everett 2004). If pregnancy does occur when the device is in situ, removal is advised as soon as possible as there is an increased risk of mid-trimester abortion.

### *The Mirena intrauterine system (IUS)*

This is a newer type of coil, the stem of which contains a progestogen reservoir that allows a slow release of progestogen. The effects are mostly local, so that ovulation frequently continues to occur. The proximity of the progestogen to the endometrium reduces its thickness, so that after an initial few weeks of erratic bleeding episodes the blood loss diminishes, and amenorrhoea is common (Szarewski 2006). The progestogen also causes a physiological mucus plug to form in the cervix, which safeguards the uterus from infection as well as impeding sperm penetration. Statistically, it is as effective as sterilization. It lasts for 5 years, and, following removal, fertility returns rapidly to normal.

## Hormonal contraception

### *Oral contraception*

Millions of women take oral contraceptives worldwide and it is the most commonly used form of contraception especially amongst young people. The oral contraceptive pill contains either a combination of oestrogen and progestogen (the combined pill or COC), or progestogen on its own (the progestogen-only pill or POP). The main controversies have concerned the risk of venous thromboembolism (VTE) in pill takers. The background risk for VTE in women not taking hormones is 5 per 100,000, compared with 60 per 100,000 during pregnancy. In women taking the COC, the risk varies from 15 to 25 per 100,000, depending on the type of pill. Midwives should always advise any women taking the pill to seek professional advice if they have any concerns, before stopping taking the pill.

### *Combined pill*

This pill acts by suppressing the production of gonadotrophins from the anterior pituitary gland and thus inhibiting ovulation. It also alters the consistency of the cervical mucus, making it impenetrable to sperm; reduces the motility of the uterine tubes so that the sperm have difficulty in passing along the tube; and causes a change in the endometrium, making it unsuitable for implantation. The latter three back-up mechanisms are due to the action of progesterone.

The timing of administration of the combined pill is important, to prevent ovulation from occurring. For complete efficiency, the course should begin on the first day of the menstrual period and continue for 21 days. This is followed by 7 days without tablets (or, in some cases, 'dummy' pills), during which time withdrawal bleeding occurs. When taken correctly, the combined oral contraceptive pill is virtually 100% reliable (Guillebaud 2007). In cases of antibiotics being prescribed or the woman developing diarrhoea and vomiting, the COC will no longer provide reliable contraception. Other precautions such as condoms should be used during this time and for a further 7 days afterwards.

There are a number of contraindications to its use, so any woman who has a personal or family history of medical problems should seek advice. For women over 35 years, the COC is contraindicated if the woman either smokes or is significantly overweight with a BMI above 40, as there is an increased risk of thromboembolic disease, myocardial infarction and cerebral vascular accident. Other methods of contraception that do not contain oestrogen should then be employed.

After childbirth, the mother who is not breastfeeding may start the combined pill 21 days postpartum. The regimen of 21 days of pills followed by 7 pill-free days is followed. The oestrogen content of the pill is inclined to reduce lactation by suppressing prolactin and is also passed to the baby, albeit in small quantities, in the breast milk, so the combined contraceptive pill is not recommended for breastfeeding mothers. If started on day 21, it is effective immediately.

### *Progestogen-only pill*

The POP is an effective method of contraception postpartum and is ideal for breastfeeding mothers. The progestogen does not affect lactation and any small quantity passing through the milk is not a problem for babies. The mother commences at 21 days after delivery and takes the tablets continuously from packet to packet without a break. Mothers should be advised that progestogen may cause erratic bleeding patterns, but this usually settles after a few months and the periods may gradually disappear. Breastfeeding mothers are unlikely to see any bleeding until breastfeeding is stopped.

Progestogen acts by causing cervical mucus to form a natural plug in the cervix which prevents the sperm entering the uterus, and also reduces the motility of the fallopian tubes. In some cases, the progestogen also causes suppression of ovulation.

The reported pregnancy rate with the progestogen-only pill is 0.3–3.1 per 100 woman years, with the rates reducing with age (Guillebaud 2007). The POP has to be taken within 3 hours of the same time each day, making this an unsuitable method if the woman has a bad memory or an erratic lifestyle. A newer POP, called *Cerazette*, has a 12-hour leeway for missed pills, similar to the COC. In addition to the normal mode of action, it will in many cases prevent ovulation and in many cases cause amenorrhoea, making it a highly effective pill.

#### *Hormonal patch*

The patch is the equivalent of the combined pill, containing oestrogen and progestogen. The patch is applied to a clean dry area of skin such as on the abdomen or upper arm. Each patch lasts for 7 days, when it is replaced, for a total of 3 weeks, followed by a patch-free week. The patch is resistant to normal bathing but some women find detachment of the patch a problem. There is some evidence that there is an increased cumulative effect of oestrogen using this method, with an increased risk of thromboembolic problems (Weisberg 2006).

#### *NuvaRing*

Similarly to the Evra patch, this ring contains oestrogen and progestogen, and is placed in the vagina for 3 weeks and then removed for 1 week. During this latter time, a withdrawal bleed will occur, and at the end of the 7 days, a new ring is inserted. It has a failure rate of 1–2 per 100 woman years.

#### *Injectable contraceptives*

These consist of a progestogen given as a deep intramuscular injection. The method has a low failure rate of about 0–1 per 100 woman years for *Depo-Provera®* and 0.4–2 per 100 woman years for *Noristerat®*. There is no evidence that it has any detrimental long-term effect on fertility; however, by nature of its mode of action, a return to fertility may be delayed. The average time from the last injection to conception is 9 months (Guillebaud 2007).

### *Depo-Provera (DMPA)*

Depo-Provera 150 mg is most commonly used and is repeated at 3-monthly intervals. It acts by suppressing ovulation and making the cervical mucus impenetrable to sperm, causing changes in the endometrium which may lead to irregular bleeding or amenorrhoea. It is ideal for those with a poor memory and is often used by women who are unable to take the COC, e.g. smokers over 35 years who prefer the injection to the time limitations of the POP.

Depo-Provera can usually be commenced at 6 weeks postpartum provided that the woman has not had unprotected intercourse. If given before 6 weeks, it may provoke bleeding and, at a time when secondary postpartum haemorrhage may occur, could make diagnosis of pathology difficult. It does not affect lactation. There is some evidence that Depo-Provera reduces the risk of pelvic inflammatory disease, endometriosis and endometrial carcinoma (Bigrigg et al 1999).

Recent research suggests that Depo-Provera may adversely affect bone density, particularly if the woman is already at risk for developing osteoporosis in later life. Despite the lack of evidence from controlled trials, the recommendation is that it should not be used as a first-line contraceptive unless no other method is suitable. When Depo-Provera is used, ideally it should not be used for more than 2 years (Guillebaud 2007).

### *Noristerat*

Norethisterone enanthate 200 mg may be given intramuscularly every 8 weeks; however, it is not licensed for long-term use and is used less often than Depo-Provera. It has a similar action to Depo-Provera but is less likely to cause irregular bleeding.

#### *Future developments*

Two once-a-month combined injectables, Cyclofem and Mesigyna, are being used in some countries but are not yet licensed in the UK (IPPF 2002). These cause a monthly bleed similar to the COC.

### *Implants*

Implanon is a contraceptive implant currently used in the UK. It consists of a single rod containing a progestogen on a slow-release carrier. It is the size of a hair grip and is inserted superficially under the skin of the upper arm using a minor surgical technique and local anaesthetic. The implant lasts for 3 years before needing to be replaced. This regimen produces highly effective care-free protection with a failure rate of 0–0.07 per 100 woman years. Like other progesterone methods, it can cause irregular bleeding, although this often reduces with time. About 25% become amenorrhoeic (Reynolds 1999/2000). The mode of action is by inhibiting ovulation, preventing thickening of the endometrium and increasing the viscosity of the cervical mucus. The implant can be inserted from day 21 postpartum. When removed, fertility returns rapidly.

## Emergency contraception

There are various reasons why women may need emergency contraception. These may include unprotected sexual intercourse (no contraception used, rape, failed coitus interruptus), failure of a barrier method (split condoms, dislodged caps), missed pills or injection, or expulsion of an IUCD. Whilst some parts of the menstrual cycle may be regarded as low risk for conception, if the woman has irregular periods or is unsure of her dates, no time can be regarded as safe. In practice, therefore, most women who present with such situations will be prescribed emergency contraception. There are currently two forms of emergency contraception available.

### *Emergency contraception (oral)*

The most widely used form is an oral progestogen preparation called Levonelle 1500, which contains levonorgestrel (a synthetic derivative of progesterone). This is taken as soon as possible after the unprotected sexual intercourse and always within 72 hours. If taken within 24 hours, the percentage of pregnancies prevented is about 95%, whereas this drops to 58% if not started until 49 to 72 hours afterwards (RCOG 2000). The pills will only affect the reported episode of unprotected sexual intercourse and cannot protect the rest of the cycle. A new preparation called ellaOne, which can be used up to 5 days after unprotected sexual intercourse, is available on prescription. It is an important part of health education in the community, especially in schools and colleges. Oral emergency contraception can be obtained free from family planning clinics, GPs, or A&E departments. It can also be bought without prescription at pharmacies.

### *Emergency IUCD contraception*

In the event of unprotected intercourse having occurred, a copper intrauterine contraceptive device may be fitted up to 5 days after the probable day of ovulation in that cycle. It can also be used later in the cycle if within 5 days of a single episode of unprotected intercourse (Guillebaud 2007). If used before ovulation, the IUCD interferes with the development of the follicle and thus prevents or delays ovulation. If used later in the cycle, its action is thought to inhibit implantation (Guillebaud 2007). Although less often used, it is a highly effective method of emergency contraception, with a failure rate of no more than 0.1% (RCOG 2000).

## Sterilization

Tubal ligation or the application of potentially removable clips to the uterine tubes in women and ligation of the vas deferens in men are considered permanent methods of sterilization.

Before these procedures are carried out, it is essential that the couple is carefully counselled, with consideration being given to the psychosocial aspects of the decision as well as to the physical factors concerned with the procedure. Most couples accept sterilization without regret, but unless all eventualities have been carefully thought through, later events may lead to regret and some may use the operation to rationalize disturbances that arise later in life (IMAP 1999). A percentage of those who are sterilized request reversal at a later date, although the success rate is low. The advent of contraceptive methods such as the Mirena IUS, which is as reliable as sterilization, causes amenorrhoea in many cases and yet is removable, is an option for couples who are not totally sure about future plans.

Female sterilization, unless performed at the same time as a caesarean section, is seldom carried out earlier than 6 to 8 weeks after delivery and by that time any problems affecting the baby which could influence the couple's decision are usually evident. The failure rate for female sterilization after 10 years is 1 in 200 and failure may occur several years after the procedure. The rate is slightly lower for older women (Everett 2004). It is worth noting that the effectiveness is less than that of the COC for women under 27 years.

### *Vasectomy*

This involves ligation of both deferent ducts (vas deferens) (Fig. 27.5). It is an easier and safer procedure than tubal ligation and can be done as an outpatient procedure under local anaesthetic. Ligation of the deferent ducts prevents the sperm reaching the seminal vesicle and ejaculatory duct. As spermatozoa may survive in the ducts for some time, the couple should continue to take contraceptive precautions until two sperm-free specimens of seminal

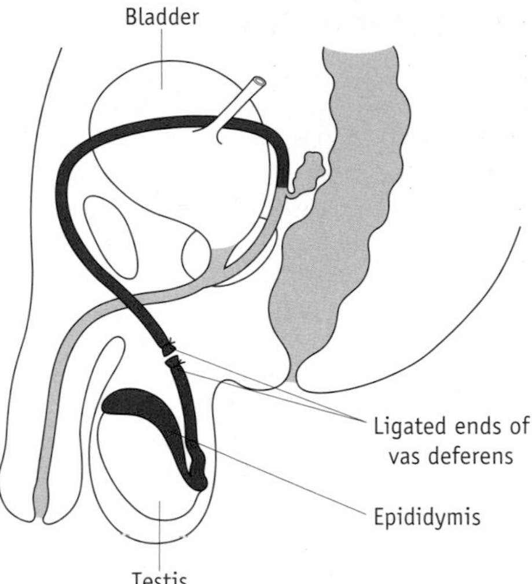

**Figure 27.5** Ligation of the vas deferens.

fluid have been produced. This will take a minimum of 3 months. Again, skilled counselling is essential before a final decision is made. The man should understand that sexual desire and activity are not affected by the operation. Despite concerns about an increased risk of testicular cancer after vasectomy, recent studies have found no evidence to support this (Pryor 1999). The failure rate is 1 in 2000.

## THE ROLE OF THE MIDWIFE IN THE PROVISION OF CONTRACEPTIVE ADVICE

Many women conceive their first child unintentionally, and although this may result in a wanted child, it is not always possible to adapt well to unplanned parenthood.

Family planning is a specialist area, and midwives, whilst knowing the principles involved, also need to be aware of their limitations and when to refer the woman to a family planning clinic or domiciliary service. During discussions, the midwife may also detect cues which could highlight the need for specialist referral, help and advice, for example, in cases of medical disorders or where there are signs of psychosexual problems.

### Factors to be considered

When the midwife discusses contraception with a mother and her partner, a variety of issues that may influence the woman's choice need to be considered (Box 27.1). By discussing these factors, the midwife will be able to give more accurate advice to the woman about choices available, as well as advising her about the best place to obtain the contraception she wants or where to get further information. It is important that the mother does not assume she carries on with her pre-pregnancy contraception without advice. The midwife should not assume that the parents have a reliable knowledge of contraception, and confirming the knowledge before offering advice will quickly indicate if there are misunderstandings to be addressed. The midwife should appreciate that no prior contraception may have been used.

Box 27.1 **Factors that need to be considered when choosing contraception**

- Age
- General health
- Smoking
- Obesity
- Lifestyle/employment
- Experiences of family and friends
- General views on contraception
- Cultural or religious constraints
- Previous methods used which failed
- Partner's views
- Obstetric history, e.g. parity or hypertension
- Level of intelligence/memory
- Ability or willingness to go to a family planning clinic
- Long-term plans for future pregnancies
- Stability of the relationship
- Level of efficacy demanded by the couple from their contraceptive
- Couple's feelings about each type of contraceptive
- What is available
- Any disability that could affect either partner's ability to use a particular method
- Method of infant feeding
- History of menstrual problems, e.g. PMS
- Views about menstruation
- Characteristics of menstrual periods – i.e. normally 'heavy' or 'light'
- Drugs being taken
- Risk from sexually transmitted diseases

**Reflective activity 27.2**

Consider situations you have met where some of these factors were significant for the woman in deciding on her choice of contraception.

## Timing to start contraception

The return of ovulation following delivery varies individually, but research suggests that the earliest possible ovulation occurs 30–35 days postpartum. It is therefore advisable to commence protection before this time. Mothers who breastfeed their babies on demand are likely to suppress ovulation for a long time. Exactly how long will depend on the suckling of the baby at frequent intervals and include at least two full feeds during the night. Babies who vary in their feeding requirement and occasionally sleep through the night will not stimulate enough prolactin to provide control of ovulation. The return of menstruation, when it occurs, indicates retrospective return of ovulation 14 days before. It is therefore important that the mother understands that printed information on packets of hormonal contraceptives does not relate to postpartum situations, and that such contraception needs to be commenced independently of menstruation.

When oral contraception is started on day 21 postpartum, it provides full protection from the first day. If commenced later, other precautions such as condoms should be used for the first 7 days. For any sexual intercourse after day 21, some form of contraception should be used. Following a termination or spontaneous abortion, contraception can be started with immediate effect.

## Special groups

### Teenagers

Young people remain one of the biggest challenges for the family planning services. Sexual activity can start early, sometimes as young as 10–12 years of age, usually unbeknown to the parents. Many have unprotected sexual intercourse partly due to their attitude towards risk taking and partly due to either ignorance about contraception and conception or fear of seeking advice (Andrews 2004). Many young people assume that approaching their GP or attending a family planning clinic will automatically involve information being passed to their parents and some youngsters will risk a pregnancy rather than seek contraceptive advice.

There is often a difference in attitude between girls and boys regarding sexual activity and contraception, with girls more likely to seek help than boys. Despite sex education at school, many young people are ignorant about basic issues such as contraception, conception and safer sex (Andrews 2004).

For young persons under 16 years of age, no contraception can be given, even condoms, unless they are shown to be Fraser competent. Following the Gillick ruling in 1985, the present legal situation is that under 16-year-olds can independently seek medical advice and receive treatment providing they can show that they are competent to do so. In contraceptive terms, provided that the doctor is assured that the young person understands the potential risks and benefits of the treatment/advice being given and the doctor believes that the person is likely to have sexual intercourse without contraception, the doctor is not breaking the law by providing contraception if it is believed that it is in the person's best interest. The value of parental support is always emphasized and the youngsters are encouraged to talk to their parents about the consultation. All consultations are confidential regardless of age.

### Older mothers

With an increasing number of women having babies in their 30s and 40s, contraception for this age group is an important issue. With increasing age, fertility is reduced, with fertility levels at 40 years being half those at 25 years (Guillebaud 2007). This suggests that some of the methods unsuitable for the highly fertile woman may be acceptable in the older woman. The COC pill can be continued until the menopause in the older woman provided that she is not overweight, does not smoke and does not suffer from migraine. For women with these problems, the POP is the oral contraceptive recommended for those aged over 35 years. The IUCD is another good method for the older woman and the Mirena IUS in particular is useful as it prevents menorrhagia, which is common in older women, and provides protection from endometrial hyperplasia and carcinoma. Barrier methods are also popular, and for those around the menopause, the Today sponge® may provide sufficient contraception. Many women request sterilization and the midwife should be able to refer the woman for counselling.

### Medical disorders

Any woman with a long-standing or newly acquired medical disorder needs expert advice in relation to contraception. Some drugs can interfere with the effectiveness of hormonal contraception and some conditions require specialist knowledge. Some women with conditions that make childbearing particularly hazardous, such as severe heart disease, may request sterilization or at least a highly effective method. Cardiovascular disorders, haematological disorders, hypertension, diabetes, migraine and liver diseases all require individualized advice (Guillebaud

2007). Midwives should ensure that the woman knows where to seek help before deciding on any particular method of contraception.

Through continuity of care, the midwife can provide advice and support to women regarding the choices that are available to control their fertility and plan their family appropriately.

## KEY POINTS

- Resuming relationships following childbirth can be difficult for some couples.
- A variety of contraceptive methods are available, including physiological, barrier, hormonal and intrauterine devices.
- Methods vary in their suitability for the individual, therefore the role of the midwife is to give information allowing the woman and her partner to make an informed choice.
- The midwife must appreciate the individuality of each woman and her partner, taking account of age, family spacing, culture, religion and health backgrounds.

## REFERENCES


Andrews G: *Women's sexual health*, ed 2, London, 2004, Ballière Tindall.

Bigrigg A, Evans M, Gbolade B, et al: Depo provera. Position paper on clinical use, effectiveness and side effects, *British Journal of Family Planning* 25(2):69–76, 1999.

Clement S: *Psychological perspectives on pregnancy and childbirth*, London, 1998, Churchill Livingstone, pp 227–241.

Department of Health (DH): *Statistical bulletin. Abortion statistics, England and Wales: 2006*, London, 2007, DH.

Everett S: *Handbook of contraception and reproductive and sexual health*, Edinburgh, 2004, Ballière Tindall.

Guillebaud J: *Contraception today*, ed 6, London, 2007, Informa Healthcare.

Herdiman J, Nakash A, Beedham T: Male contraception: past, present and future, *Journal of Obstetrics and Gynaecology* 26(8):721–727, 2006.

International Medical Advisory Panel (IMAP): IMAP statement on voluntary surgical contraception, *IPPF Medical Bulletin* 33(4):1–4, 1999.

International Planned Parenthood Federation (IPPF): (2002) IMAP statement on hormonal methods of contraception, *IPPF Medical Bulletin* 36(5):1–8, 2002.

NICE: *Long-acting reversible contraception* (website). <www.nice.org.uk/guidance/CG30>. 2005. Accessed September 2010.

Pryor JP: Screening issues in male genital tract cancer. In Kubba A, Sanfilippo J, Hampton N, editors: *Contraception and office gynecology*, London, 1999, WB Saunders, pp 415–425.

Reynolds A: Implanon – a new contraceptive implant, *Primary Health Care* 9(10):14–15, 1999/2000.

Royal College of Obstetricians and Gynaecologists (RCOG), Faculty of Family Planning and Reproductive Health Care: Guidance April 2000. Emergency contraception: recommendations for clinical practice, *British Journal of Family Planning* 26(2):93–96, 2000.

Social Exclusion Unit: *Teenage pregnancy*, London, 1999, Department of Health.

Szarewski A: Choice of contraception, *Current Obstetrics and Gynaecology* 16(6):361–365, 2006.

Weisberg E: Ortho Evra contraceptive patch, *IPPF Medical Bulletin* 40(1):3–4, 2006.

Chapter 28

# Infertility and assisted conception

Debbie Barber

## LEARNING OUTCOMES

After reading this chapter, you will be able to:

- understand the causes of female and male infertility
- be aware of the investigations and treatment options, including drug regimens and side-effects of treatments
- apply understanding of biological functions of fertilization and embryology
- explore the social, physical and emotional impact of infertility and impact on pregnancy and childbirth
- examine the legal, ethical, socioeconomic and psychological implications both for health professionals and for individuals with fertility issues.

## INTRODUCTION

Midwives will frequently care for couples that have received assistance in achieving their pregnancy. It is important to understand the processes they have to go through to become pregnant, which can contribute to the attitudes and anxieties demonstrated by individuals and create greater challenges for the midwifery team. Most couples will have received their fertility treatment in the private sector and occasionally the transition into normal NHS care may itself be stressful. This chapter provides a background on the issues related to infertility and the factors contributing to the patients' approach to their pregnancy. It is useful for midwives to establish links with their local fertility services to provide support and information on patients to ease the transition into their care. Improved networking between fertility nurses and midwives would complement care provided in both areas. Awareness of the range of treatment options and the side-effects from treatment provides insight into both the physical and emotional condition of couples requiring midwifery care.

Multiple births are a key issue of concern in both areas of practice and it is essential that couples understand the risks and the care required when pregnant. Singleton pregnancies with the prevention of twin and triplet pregnancies are the ultimate goal of all fertility clinics, requiring appropriate management and monitoring of treatment. Many nurses and midwives have specialized in fertility, providing care and extending their role to perform ultrasound scanning, intrauterine insemination, embryo transfer and implications counselling (Barber 2002). Where possible, it is important for midwives and nurses to normalize pregnancies for couples, enabling them to enjoy their much-desired pregnancy.

Technological advances within the field of reproduction have increased public awareness of infertility and demand for related services. Approximately one in six couples will experience problems conceiving a child (Hull et al 1985, Templeton et al 1990) and will seek assistance to achieve a pregnancy. Since the birth of the world's first 'test-tube baby' over 30 years ago, over one million babies have been born in the UK from in vitro fertilization (IVF). Research has highlighted the stigma, psychological morbidity and long-term implications caused by the experience of infertility on couples (Kerr et al 1999), and these factors impact on successful and unsuccessful couples. Over 95% of service provision exists within the private sector, thus providing a financial hurdle that couples must overcome prior to commencing their treatment.

## HUMAN FERTILISATION AND EMBRYOLOGY AUTHORITY (HFEA)

The HFEA was created by the 1990 Act to license and monitor clinics performing various fertility treatments (including IVF, donated egg/sperm/embryo procedures, or research on embryos). All licensed clinics must have a delegated 'person responsible' who ensures that the conditions of the licence are carried out. Several forms of treatment are not controlled by the HFEA but may still potentially create similar problems to licensed treatments, including funding, ovarian hyperstimulation and multiple births. The HFEA carries out annual inspections to enable clinics to renew their licences, which include reviewing the welfare of any potential child, clinical and laboratory standards, protocols for practice in all areas and the safety of patients and their families.

As well as a *Code of Practice* and information to staff and patients, the HFEA maintains a formal register of information regarding specific donors, donor treatments and children born from these treatments (HFEA 2009). (For more information, see the website).

**Reflective activity 28.1**

How does regulation impact on the delivery and management of care of couples undergoing infertility treatments?

## CAUSES OF INFERTILITY

See Table 28.1.

### Anovulation

Anovulation may be diagnosed by the GP and may be corrected by drug therapy to initiate ovulation with an anti-oestrogen, such as *clomifene* – a common treatment for polycystic ovary syndrome (PCOS). Anovulation must be investigated as it may be caused by pathology such as hyperprolactinaemia, which could be corrected and prevent the woman undergoing fertility treatments.

Elevated levels of prolactin inhibit the normal hormonal feedback loop that initiates ovulation. If serum prolactin is elevated to 1000 mU/L, the test should be repeated. This could be caused by stress or from a prolactin-secreting pituitary adenoma or macroadenomas diagnosed with MRI. Treatment includes *bromocriptine* or *cabergoline*, which reduce the elevated levels of prolactin and restore normal endocrine activity and facilitate ovulation.

Anovulation can be divided into primary and secondary amenorrhoea – these are primarily caused by pituitary tumours, pituitary ablation, Kallmann syndrome and cancer treatments (see Box 28.1).

**Table 28.1 Main causes of infertility**

| | Incidence |
|---|---|
| Anovulation | 26% |
| Endometriosis | 3% |
| Tubal damage | 13% |
| Unexplained | 30% |
| Male factor | 30% |

(Snick et al 1997)

### Polycystic ovary syndrome (PCOS)

This syndrome is frequently detected in women undergoing investigations for anovulation (Kousta et al 1999). It is characterized by cystic ovaries with more than 10 cysts, 2–8 mm in diameter, distributed around and through an echodense, thickened stroma (Fig. 28.1).

Endocrine features include a raised serum level of luteinizing hormone (LH) and/or testosterone, causing symptoms of acne, hirsutism (hyperandrogenism), oligoamenorrhoea and obesity (Box 28.2). The hypersecretion of LH is associated with menstrual irregularity and infertility. Obesity leads to hypersecretion of insulin, stimulating ovarian secretion of androgens with increased risk of the development of type 2 diabetes (Kousta et al 2000). Anovulation is also associated with endometrial hyperplasia due to increased oestrogen production unopposed by

Box 28.1 **Primary and secondary amenorrhoea**

**Primary**

Congenital abnormalities
Hyperprolactinaemia
Hypogonadotrophic hypogonadism
Hypopituitarism
Polycystic ovary syndrome
Premature ovarian failure

**Secondary**

Exercise-related
Hyperprolactinaemia
Hypogonadotrophic hypogonadism
Hypopituitarism
Polycystic ovary syndrome
Premature ovarian failure

Source: Balen & Jacobs 1997

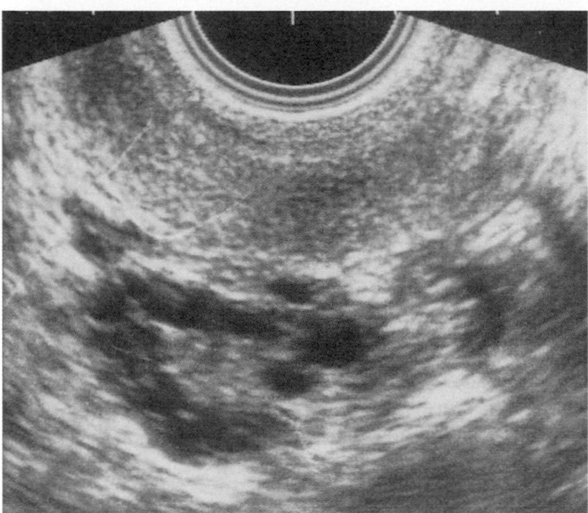

**Figure 28.1** Ultrasound scan illustrating a polycystic ovary.

**Box 28.2 Signs and symptoms of polycystic ovary syndrome**

- Obesity
- Menstrual disturbance
  - Amenorrhoea
  - Oligomenorrhoea
- Hyperandrogenism
  - Acne
  - Hisutism
  - Alopecia
- Acanthosis nigricans
- Endocrine disturbances
  - Insulin
  - Testosterone
  - Androstenedione
  - Sex-hormone-binding globulin (SHBG)
  - LH
  - Prolactin

progesterone (Balen & Jacobs 1997). Women with a body mass index (BMI) >28 kg/m$^2$ and <20 kg/m$^2$ will have decreased fertility. There is an associated deficiency in gonadotrophin production with excessive weight loss, due to diminished production of gonadotrophin-releasing hormone (GnRH).

### Ovarian failure

Ovarian failure can happen at any age. If prior to puberty, it is commonly associated with chromosomal abnormality, such as Turner syndrome (45X) (see Ch. 26), or sterility resulting from radiotherapy or chemotherapy for childhood malignancy. Ovarian failure linked with raised gonadotrophins and cessation of periods prior to the age of 40 is associated with autoimmune failure, infection, previous surgery and cancer treatments. There is also a suggested link with familial forms of fragile X (Balen & Jacobs 1997).

## Endometriosis

This is caused when endometrial tissue is located outside the uterus, around the pelvis. This may be noted at laparoscopy as blue/black pigmentation (old lesions), red vasculated lesions (active lesions) and white non-pigmented papules (just activating) (Gould 2003). Retrograde menstruation is thought to be the most common cause of endometriosis but altered immune function is also thought to be associated with the condition. It causes pelvic pain, dyspareunia, dysmenorrhea and infertility. Pelvic adhesions, especially around the ovaries and tubes, with cystic lesions on the ovaries, called *endometriomas*, are common. Symptoms are linked with the menstrual cycle, age and hormonal therapy; treatments include drugs that interfere with the cycle. One group are *GnRH agonists*, which cause pituitary desensitization, inducing amenorrhoea; another are inhibitors of gonadotrophin secretion, such as *danazol*, which also have androgenic effects that cause unpleasant side-effects, including hot flushes, acne, oily skin, hirsutism, reduced libido, weight gain, nausea and headaches. Both groups of drug temporarily stop menses and reduce levels of antiendometrial autoantibodies (Balen & Jacobs 1997).

## Tubal factors

Tubal damage is commonly associated with pelvic inflammatory disease (PID), ectopic pregnancy, sterilization and adhesions. Increases in sexually transmitted diseases increase the risk of PID and tubal damage. Chlamydia is the most frequently reported infection and is often asymptomatic, which increases the risk of cross-contamination and failure to treat (Byrd 1993). Adhesions commonly result following pelvic infection and subsequently create further problems, including distortion and/or blockage of the fallopian tubes; development of hydrosalpinx; impaired tubal motility and movement of the oocyte; and ovarian adhesion against the pelvic sidewall, which may interfere with the movement of the oocyte into the fimbria of the fallopian tube (Dechaud & Hedon 2000), increasing the risk of ectopic pregnancy (see Ch. 54 and website).

## Unexplained infertility

Unexplained infertility is the inability to conceive after 1 year without any identified causative factors. Approximately 40–65% of couples in this category will conceive spontaneously within 3 years (Balen & Jacobs

**Table 28.2 WHO criteria for a normal sperm count**

| | |
|---|---|
| Volume | 2 mL or more |
| pH | 7.2 or more |
| Count | ≥20 × $10^6$/mL (azoospermia is diagnosed when no sperm is found in the ejaculate and oligospermia is diagnosed when the concentration of sperm is vastly reduced) |
| Motility | 50% or more with forward progression, or 25% or more with rapid progression (within 60 minutes of ejaculation) (abnormal = asthenozoospermia) |
| Morphology | The 1999 edition of the WHO manual does not define normal ranges for morphology but notes that data from IVF programmes suggest that as sperm morphology falls below 15% normal forms (teratozoospermia), the fertilization rate decreases |
| MAR test (Antisperm antibodies) | <50% of motile sperm with adherent particles |
| Immunobead test (Antisperm antibodies) | <50% of motile sperm with adherent beads |
| Source: WHO 1999 | |

1997). Age has a direct effect on the duration of time to try to conceive naturally prior to commencing fertility treatment.

Treatment options consist of improving fertility initially for the woman with drugs to enhance ovulation. Also it is possible to improve sperm function by inseminating prepared sperm into the uterus (intrauterine insemination [IUI]).

## Male infertility

Male factor infertility contributes to 30% of couples seeking treatment. A decline in semen quality over the last few decades has been suggested, though the evidence remains inconclusive with little scientific knowledge of the aetiology (Shakkebaek & Keiding 1994). A full and comprehensive history of each case is an essential element in the assessment of male fertility and should include:

- assessment of previous fertility
- frequency of intercourse
- coital difficulties
- past history of sexually transmitted disease
- history of mumps orchitis
- history of cryptorchidism
- history of scrotal, inguinal, prostatic or bladder neck surgery
- testicular injury
- testicular cancer – exposure to gonadotoxic agents, e.g. chemo/radiotherapy
- vasectomy
  (Thornton 2000).

**Causes of infertility include:**

- undescended testes – most common congenital abnormality, also linked with abnormal spermatogenesis
- hypogonadotrophic hypogonadism – associated with low levels of follicle-stimulating hormone (FSH) and testosterone and is sometimes linked with Kallmann syndrome
- cystic fibrosis – gene mutations are strongly related to congenital bilateral absence of the vas deferens (CBAVD), a defect associated with the bilateral regression of the mesonephric duct
- testicular failure (increased FSH levels)
- cryptorchidism – sevenfold increased risk of testicular cancer (Thornton 2000)
- retrograde ejaculation – congenital or following surgery to either prostate or bladder neck
- antisperm antibodies – anything that disrupts the normal blood–testes barrier can result in the formation of antisperm antibodies, including:
  - vasectomy and vasectomy reversal
  - testicular torsion
  - testicular biopsy
  - varicocele
  - inflammatory reactions in the genital tract
  - infections (orchitis, prostatitis)
  - congenital absence of the vas deferens (seen in the majority of cystic fibrosis patients).

Tests should include the following:

- Sperm count and analysis (see Table 28.2).
- Endocrine assessment – serum measurements of:
  - FSH
  - LH
  - testosterone
  - prolactin.
- Karyotyping.
- Thyroid function screening.
- Genetic analysis and cystic fibrosis screening in cases of azoospermia and oligozoospermia (<5 × $10^6$/mL):
  - chromosomal microdeletions – may lead to suboptimal spermatogenesis
  - chromosomal abnormalities responsible for suboptimal semen parameters, including Klinefelter syndrome (XXY)
  - Down syndrome – may cause hypogonadism in males, resulting in azoospermia or subfertility.

Various solutions to these problems are available and micromanipulation techniques, such as intracytoplasmic sperm injection (ICSI), have helped to overcome many male infertility problems (see website). Previously, steroids were administered to decrease the male immune response and thus improve chances of fertilization, but now are rarely used. Environmental factors such as pesticides, alcohol, cigarettes and drug abuse can reduce male fertility and a decrease in consumption of recreational toxins may sometimes improve semen parameters.

## FEMALE INFERTILITY – TREATMENT AND MANAGEMENT

### Ovulation induction

There are two types of drug regimen for ovulation induction – the most basic of fertility treatments.

- *Clomifene citrate* – an anti-oestrogen used to treat PCOS. Dosage is from 50 mg up to 100 mg to induce ovulation. It is taken from day 2 to day 6 of the cycle and should only be prescribed for up to six cycles where the woman has ovulated (RCOG 2003). The drug can cause cervical mucus thickening, headaches and visual disturbances.
- *Gonadotrophin*, commonly subcutaneous *FSH* to stimulate ovulation. Close monitoring is essential for these women as they are at risk of high-order multiple pregnancy and ovarian hyperstimulation syndrome (OHSS).

OHSS occurs if too many follicles are stimulated during a treatment cycle of ovulation induction (OI), intrauterine insemination (IUI) and in vitro fertilization (IVF). As many follicles are stimulated, especially in the case of PCO and PCOS, this causes abdominal ascites, pleural and pericardial effusions, discomfort, nausea, vomiting, difficulty breathing, electrolyte imbalance leading to dehydration, and an increased risk of deep vein thrombosis. Ultrasound examination reveals enlargement of the ovaries to a diameter greater than 5 cm (Fig. 28.2).

### Donor insemination (DI)

This treatment is appropriate for couples with azoospermia, paternal genetic abnormalities or those unable to afford IVF and ICSI, with national success rates of 9.6% per cycle (Thornton 2000). DI is carried out during the woman's own natural cycle or with superovulation. Monitoring with transvaginal ultrasound is undertaken to identify one leading follicle prior to ovulation and insemination. When more than two leading follicles are stimulated with superovulation, the cycle should be cancelled due to the risk of multiple pregnancy.

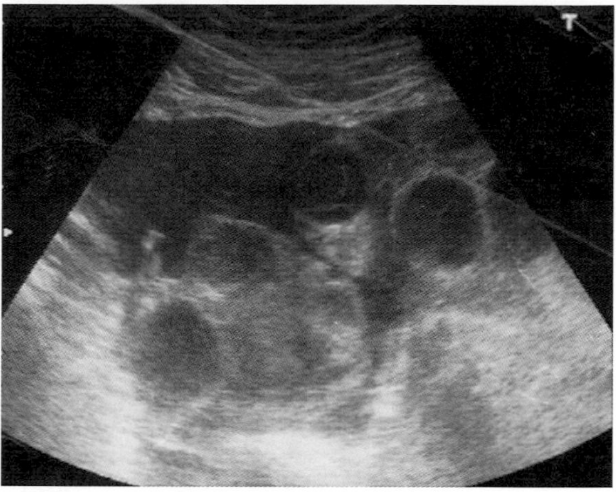

**Figure 28.2** Ovarian hyperstimulation syndrome (OHSS).

### Intrauterine insemination (IUI)

IUI involves monitored superovulation and insemination of prepared sperm 35 hours post administration of human chorionic gonadotrophin (hCG) to initiate ovulation. The semen may be prepared for insemination using one of a variety of techniques, including sperm *swim up* and *gradient density* procedures (see website). This treatment is appropriate for slightly suboptimal sperm parameters, unexplained infertility with normal semen parameters and factors such as female age. It does not provide information on potential problems associated with fertilization and has lower success rates than does IVF.

### Gamete intrafallopian tube transfer (GIFT)

GIFT has generally been superseded by IVF, though is still offered by some clinics. GIFT involves superovulation, following which the oocytes are removed via laparoscopy and a prepared sperm sample is deposited into the fallopian tube to facilitate fertilization. Consequently, this is not suitable for women with tubal damage and it yields no information on the possible fertilization problems.

### IVF

Louise Brown was born in 1978 following pioneering work by Steptoe and Edwards, and since that time IVF has enabled many thousands of couples to achieve a much-desired child. The technique combines superovulation, transvaginal ultrasound-guided oocyte retrieval, insemination of oocyte with sperm in the laboratory, fertilization and replacement of embryos.

Debate surrounds the number of embryos to be replaced in the uterus but many clinics in the UK routinely replace

**Table 28.3 Drug treatments for infertility**

| | Short protocol | Long protocol | GnRH antagonists |
|---|---|---|---|
| Flexibility | Less flexible | Flexible regimen – can be scheduled during working week | Shorter treatment with fewer injections for the woman<br>Currently less favoured drug choice for treatment |
| Success rates | Lower pregnancy rates | Better pregnancy rates | GnRH prevents LH surge |
| Timing for commencement | First half of the cycle designed to use stored FSH | Luteal phase | Within the first half of the cycle |
| GnRH agonist | Commenced on day 2 | (Inhaled or injected) from day 21 of cycle | |
| | Exogenous *FSH* on day 3 | Pituitary suppression is achieved with 14 days | Several days of *FSH* administration precede GnRH |
| Monitoring | Transvaginal ultrasound to measure the size of the follicles (should be approximately 18 mm) prior to administration of hCG and then oocyte retrieval | Hormone levels are checked for desensitization | Once a woman has a leading follicle of approximately 14 mm the drug is injected daily along with the gonadotrophin |
| | Generally lower doses of gonadotrophins are used and the time period is more patient-friendly | Once the woman is downregulated: daily injections of *FSH* to initiate superovulation are commenced | |
| | | Once there are three follicles of approximately 18 mm, *hCG* is administrated 35 hours prior to oocyte retrieval | |

two embryos, achieving similar pregnancy rates to three-embryo replacements.

Current IVF treatments use daily injections of drugs (gonadotrophins) to induce the development of multiple follicles in the ovaries. The oocytes mature within these follicles, are collected and are fertilized in the laboratory.

Immature eggs from unstimulated ovaries can also be collected, matured in the laboratory for 24–48 hours and, once mature, fertilized prior to embryo transfer. Hence, oocyte maturation happens in the laboratory rather than the body.

## Drug management (Table 28.3)

Superovulation is achieved with the administration of *FSH* injections – a purified preparation delivered subcutaneously via autoinjector (dosage from 50 to 350 IU), which recruits a cohort of follicles and promotes development and maturation (Fig. 28.3). To ensure

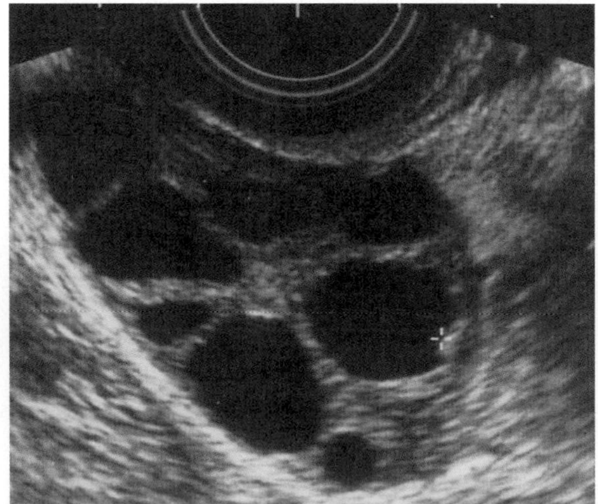

**Figure 28.3** Ultrasound scan of a stimulated ovary.

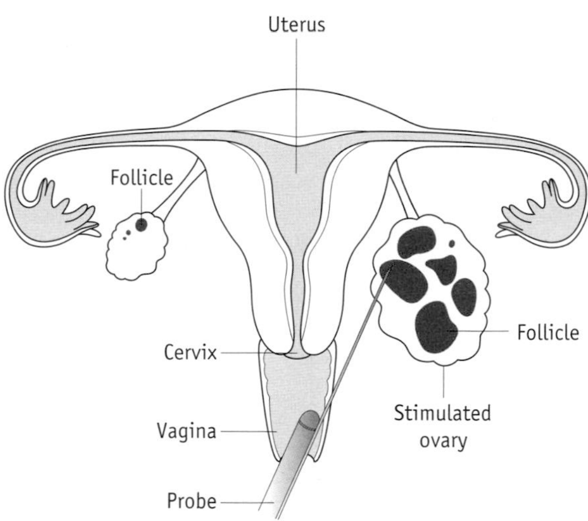


**Figure 28.4** Oocyte recovery. *(Courtesy of Janet Currie, Sister, Oxford Fertility Unit, Level 4, Women's Centre, Headington, Oxford.)*

maturation of the follicles and oocytes, administration of *hCG* is required 35 hours prior to oocyte retrieval.

To establish appropriate management of superovulation and avoid premature ovulation due to the LH surge, many units incorporate *GnRH agonists* or antagonists to prevent ovulation (administered either subcutaneously or nasally). These bind to GnRH receptors on the pituitary gonadotrophins and desensitize the pituitary. The antagonists lead to immediate suppression and are used for a much shorter time, and initiate a flare response which causes a withdrawal bleed in the woman.

## Oocyte collection

This is undertaken as an outpatient procedure using transvaginal ultrasound (Fig. 28.4). Intravenous sedation reduces levels of pain and anxiety and partners can accompany the women through the procedure. Follicles are aspirated using gentle suction via a preset vacuum pump into small tubes, which are identified by the embryologist. A microscope is required to identify the cumulus/oocyte mass. Follicles are frequently reinflated with culture medium to encourage recovery of oocytes. Retrieved oocytes are placed in the incubator with appropriate labelling of the dishes and compartment in the incubator and are double witnessed to ensure correct safety procedures.

## Sperm preparation

Sperm samples may be collected either prior to oocyte retrieval or following the procedure, but should be prepared within 30 minutes of production. Sperm preparation follows the same procedure as described in the IUI treatment. Semen samples may be frozen and

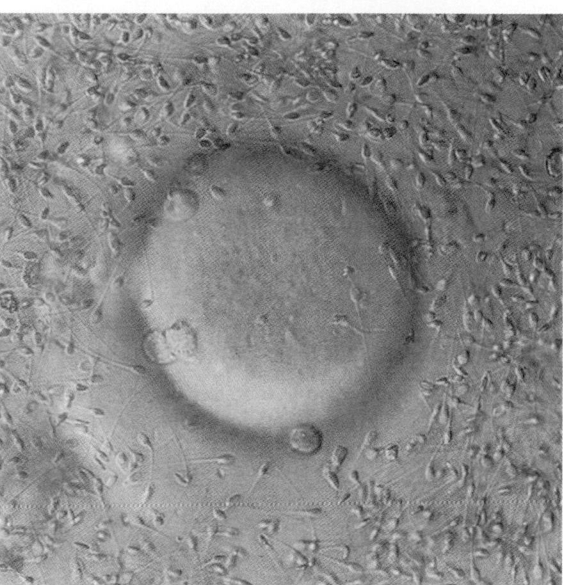

**Figure 28.5** Egg and sperm. *(Courtesy of Dr Susan Pickering, Senior Lecturer, Division of Women's Health, Kings College, London.)*

subsequently defrosted for preparation prior to insemination. After insemination, the spermatozoa and oocytes (Fig. 28.5) are cultured overnight, then, approximately 16–18 hours later, are assessed for signs of fertilization, and the number and grade of polar bodies extruded from the oocyte. These criteria can also aid in the detection of abnormal fertilization. The appearance of two pronuclei – one each from the sperm and oocyte – signifies normal fertilization. Occasionally, more than two pronuclei are detected, indicating abnormal fertilization, and these embryos should not be transferred.

## Fertilization

Fertilization commences when the sperm binds to the zona pellucida of the oocyte (for more information, see website and Ch. 29).

## Embryo grading

Embryos are closely monitored for quality and potential ability to implant and create a pregnancy. Embryo grading is based on visual morphological criteria; it cannot rule out the possibility of a genetic abnormality within the embryo and therefore does not guarantee the selection of a viable embryo for replacement. Preimplantation genetic diagnosis (PGD) is the only way to identify a potential genetic anomaly, including: chromosomal, X-linked, autosomal recessive and dominant, and mitochondrial abnormalities (ESHRE PGD Consortium Steering Committee 2000).

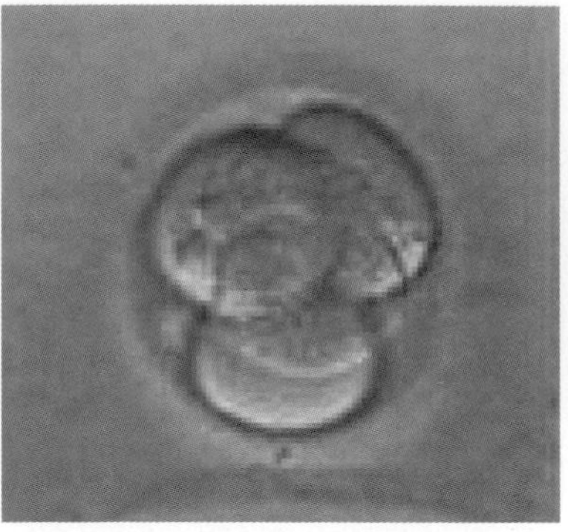

**Figure 28.6** Four-cell embryo. *(Courtesy of Dr Susan Pickering, Senior Lecturer, Division of Women's Health, Kings College, London.)*

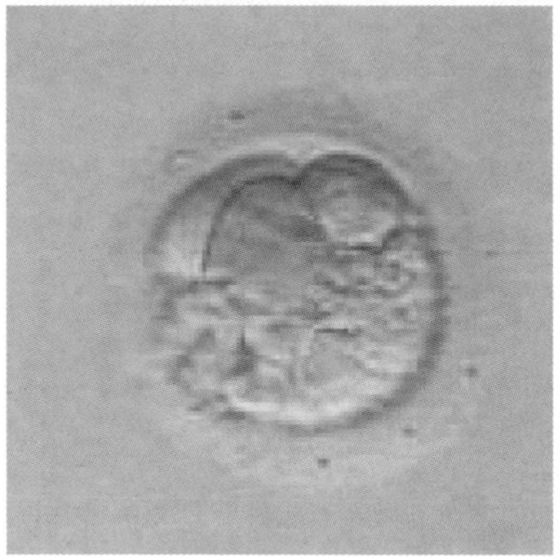

**Figure 28.7** Fragmentation. *(Courtesy of Dr Susan Pickering, Senior Lecturer, Division of Women's Health, Kings College, London.)*

For more information on embryo grading, see website.

### *Fragmentation*

The causes of fragmentation within the embryo (Fig. 28.7) are unknown and have been linked with poor culture conditions and blastomere loss through apoptosis, possibly from chromosomal abnormalities. Whatever the underlying pathology, fragmentation is clearly associated with decreased implantation (Scott 2002). The process of fragmentation has been identified as early as the two-cell stage and continues to develop throughout cleavage.

## Embryo transfer

Embryo transfer takes place approximately 48 hours after oocyte recovery. The embryo normally contains several blastomeres at this stage, ranging from two to six in number (Fig. 28.6). Embryos may be cultured for 5 days until they have reached blastocyst stage before returning

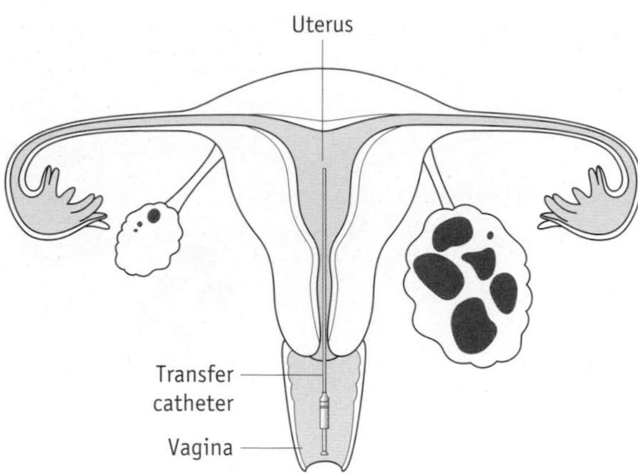


**Figure 28.8** Embryo transfer. *(Courtesy of Janet Currie, Sister, Oxford Fertility Unit, Level 4, Women's Centre, Headington, Oxford.)*

them into the uterus, but there is no evidence to prove that blastocyst replacement provides better pregnancy rates than do the day-2 transfers.

A speculum is inserted into the vagina, and the cervix is wiped with a dry swab to remove excess mucus. The embryos are placed into a fine plastic catheter and passed, sometimes by ultrasound guidance, through the cervix into the endometrium (Fig. 28.8). If the cervix is convoluted or a tight internal os is encountered, the malleable outer sheath of the catheter is adapted to pass through the obstruction. After embryo replacement, the woman is placed on luteal support to prevent a fall in progesterone levels, which could directly affect the function of the endometrium at this crucial time during potential implantation. Commonly, progesterone pessaries are administered twice daily until the pregnancy test is performed 14 days post embryo transfer. After IVF treatment, the ovaries contain multiple corpora lutea, which remain enlarged for the subsequent few weeks; these may contribute to symptoms of bloating and discomfort and the woman should be advised of the symptoms.

**Blastocyst transfer** is another treatment option for couples undergoing IVF treatment. During normal physiological fertilization the sperm fertilizes the oocyte in the fallopian tube, which moves down the tract until it reaches the endometrium around day 5 post fertilization. Blastocyst development has been difficult to achieve in vitro due to inadequate culture media. As technology has developed, improved sequential media have resulted in higher rates of blastocyst development. Embryos are usually replaced on day 2 or 3, which does not correlate with implantation *in vivo*. As some embryos will not reach blastocyst stage but look completely normal at the day 2–3 stage, it has been suggested that blastocyst transfer enables the embryologist to assess the quality of the embryo for longer and in greater detail, allowing a better choice of

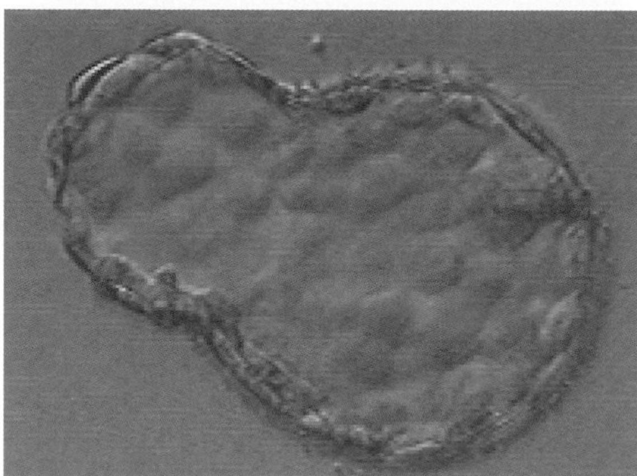

**Figure 28.9** Hatching blastocyst. *(Courtesy of Dr Susan Pickering, Senior Lecturer, Division of Women's Health, Kings College, London.)*

embryos with increased implantation potential (Fig. 28.9). New technology associated with blastocyst transfer has improved success rates and centres are beginning to replace single blastocysts to maintain good pregnancy rates and decrease the multiple pregnancy rate. Blastocysts can be frozen to ensure patients can maximize their potential chance of success from a fresh cycle. *Vitrification – a* new technique of ultra-rapid freezing – allows the embryo to be chilled to liquid nitrogen temperatures (−196 °C) in a fraction of a second (Mukaida et al 2006).

**Table 28.4 Comparison of IVF and IVM**

| | IVM | IVF |
|---|---|---|
| | New | Well established |
| Fertilization rate* | 77% | 78% |
| Cleavage rate* | 95% | 94% |
| Risk of ovarian hyperstimulation syndrome (OHSS) | Reduced | High risk |
| OHSS rate* | 0% | 12.1% |
| Treatment cycles | Shorter | |
| Treatment | hCG injection only | Daily injections required to stimulate ovaries |
| Oocytes | Fewer collected and fertilized | |
| Implantation, clinical pregnancy and live birth rates | Reduced rate – not significant | |
| Pregnancy rate | Difficult to predict at present | Good success rate |

*Data from a case–control study

## In vitro maturation (IVM)

Women who have polycystic ovaries are most at risk of developing OHSS when undergoing fertility treatment, and *in vitro maturation (IVM)*, which does not require fertility drugs, has been licensed in the UK. Without the superovulation of the ovaries there is no risk of the syndrome developing. This technique is established internationally and in 2007 the first babies (twins) were born in the UK.

IVM is appropriate in women with infertility requiring assisted conception and the success rate is known to be significantly related to the number of immature oocytes retrieved, and can be predicted by the antral follicle count (AFC). IVM may be particularly beneficial to women who have an AFC of more than 20. Women with PCOS or with ultrasonographic evidence of polycystic ovaries who are ovulating may be particularly amenable to IVM.

Standard IVF involves a lengthy process of pituitary downregulation with GnRH analogues followed by stimulation by gonadotrophins. This process is time consuming, the drugs involved are known to have side-effects, and the typical cost of drug treatment per cycle is currently around £600–1200. The only drug used in a cycle of IVM is a single injection of hCG 35 hours prior to oocyte collection. IVM has been demonstrated to be an effective treatment for infertile women with polycystic ovaries, although IVF is currently the gold standard treatment for infertility. Approximately 25–50% of women attending IVF clinics have PCO or PCOS (Jurema & Nogueira 2006).

There are many women presenting for fertility treatment for whom both treatments may be appropriate. It is essential they have reliable information on which to base their choice of treatment. No randomized controlled trials currently exist that compare IVF and IVM, although there has been a case-control study comparing such (see Table 28.4).

There were no cases of OHSS in the IVM group. Severe OHSS occurs in around 1 in a 100 standard IVF cycles and usually requires admission to hospital for a few days. Severe OHSS is even more common in women who have polycystic ovaries on ultrasound scan or who have PCOS.

### Advantages of IVM treatment compared with IVF

Studies from Scandinavian IVM programmes, in which only one or two embryos are transferred, report pregnancy rates in the region of 15–25% per cycle, though this is higher (≈30%) for women less than 36 years of age. In the region of 400 babies have been born worldwide from IVM treatment. Recent studies examining the health of these children have been reassuring, showing no increase in rates of abnormality. However, it must be recognized that the number of babies born is still relatively limited (Jurema & Nogueira 2006).

### Factors affecting success in IVM treatment

One of the main factors affecting the success rate of IVF treatment, and possibly IVM, is the age of the woman.

The more eggs collected, the more embryos are produced, and greater the choice of embryos for transfer. The total number of resting follicles measured during a routine ultrasound scan is known as the antral follicle count (AFC) (see website) – shown to be an important predictor of success with IVM. On average, immature eggs are retrieved from half of the antral follicles present. However, as with IVF, there is always the risk that no eggs will be retrieved even when follicles are present or that those that are will not mature, fertilize or produce transfer embryos.

## Cryopreservation

The cryostorage of semen, an essential service provided by most assisted conception units, is offered to patients who are or have:

- undergoing IVF treatment
- been diagnosed with malignant disease (prior to chemotherapy and radiotherapy)
- prior to potentially damaging pelvic surgery
- prior to vasectomy procedure
- poor-quality semen after vasectomy reversal
- a declining sperm count
- production difficulties
- geographical separation of the couple at the time of oocyte retrieval
- when a clean, tested sample is required.

The freezing/thaw procedure, however, will damage the cells and may reduce pre-freeze motility.

*Embryo freezing* can be performed provided that enough suitable spare embryos are available post embryo transfer. Embryos may be frozen at the pronuclear or the cleavage stage (two to eight cells); and must be good quality (grades 1, 2 and 3 or A, B and C) with less than 20% cytoplasmic fragmentation (Dale & Elder 1997) for the best chance of survival following the freeze/thaw procedure. It has been suggested that uneven blastomeres and large amounts of fragmentation could inhibit survival potential.

*Cryopreservation of oocytes* provides a treatment option for women prior to cancer treatment that may cause temporary or permanent sterility. Unfortunately, success rates from the use of frozen eggs is very low and only one baby has been successfully born from this technique in the UK.

## Egg donation

In the UK, egg donation is maintained altruistically, primarily by anonymous donors, though occasionally donation from a family member or friend may be offered. This treatment can be used by women following the onset of premature menopause; genetic abnormality; or multiple failed IVF attempts.

Due to the national shortage of donated eggs, the National Gamete Donation Trust was established to promote altruistic donation. Many fertility units have long waiting lists for donors and have introduced alternative options, such as egg sharing. This treatment provides reduced-cost IVF treatment to couples willing to donate half of their eggs to another recipient couple. This creates ethical debate and the HFEA have produced guidelines for good practice and further review the appropriateness of the treatment for couples (HFEA 2009). Any couple who donate eggs have to undergo thorough counselling, detailed history taking, and investigations including karyotyping, blood grouping, screening for infections such as hepatitis A, B and C, HIV and syphilis, and cystic fibrosis screening. To donate eggs, the donor undergoes a full IVF cycle, which is time consuming and risky. Those with pre-existing disease and familial cancers are normally dissuaded from donation. Contraindications would include any uncertainty from partners.

Some patients travel overseas to obtain donated eggs, creating further problems for UK professionals as other countries do not have regulatory bodies, such as the HFEA, so there are no restrictions on the number of embryos that can be replaced. This has led to an increase in multiple births in the UK, which has serious consequences for all involved.

## Surrogacy

Surrogacy involves a couple commissioning a woman to act as a host for their own genetic embryo and is a solution for women without a uterus or for whom a pregnancy may be contraindicated. It is illegal in the UK to pay a surrogate, but they may have their expenses paid. In English law, the woman who gives birth to the baby is the legal mother of the child, irrespective of the genetic origin of the child. The genetic parents therefore have to apply to adopt the child from the birth mother and this may be problematic should she change her mind about giving up her baby.

# OUTCOME FROM IVF TREATMENTS

Outcome studies have closely monitored the births and development of children conceived from the techniques. Factors contributing to adverse outcome associated with assisted reproductive technology (ART) include maternal age, medical indications for infertility, paternal age and multiple pregnancies. The ICSI procedure has raised several issues as the process can potentially use sperm carrying genetic abnormalities, structural defects introduced by mechanical or biochemical damage when introducing foreign material into the oocyte and bypassing the natural selection process of fertilization (Kurinczuk 2003). Genetic screening is offered to couples requiring ICSI with poor sperm parameters (see website).

Multiple births create further problems with morbidity and mortality of children conceived from ART (Koivurova et al 2002). Women who have IVF are 20 times more likely to have a multiple pregnancy. Approximately 24% of all IVF births are multiple, which means that 40% of IVF babies are twins or triplets (One at a Time 2009). Twins and triplets have increased risks of cerebral palsy:

twins – 13.2 per 1000 confinements – 8 times higher than singletons
triplets – 75.9 per 1000 – 47 times higher than singletons (Petterson et al 1993).

Petterson et al (1993) suggested that 1 in 10 pregnant women with twins and 1 in 5 pregnant women with triplets, whatever the mode of conception, who reach 20 weeks' gestation, will experience at least one of the following: a child with cerebral palsy, an infant death , stillbirth.

One of the treatment options now offered to couples to alleviate the situation is *multifetal pregnancy reduction* – frequently performed in the United States. Data suggest that surviving twins from the procedure have an eightfold increase of cerebral palsy and an eightfold increased risk of periventricular leukomalacia (Geva et al 1998). The preferred option in the UK is to replace fewer embryos (either two or one) to reduce the incidence of multiple births (Hazekamp et al 2000) (Fig. 28.10).

The health of the mother may also be affected. Of mothers pregnant with twins, 20% experience hypertension, 30% will develop pre-eclampsia, and there is a 12% risk of developing gestational diabetes, and this increases the likelihood of longer periods of hospitalization during pregnancy together with a negative impact upon the family (see Ch. 59).

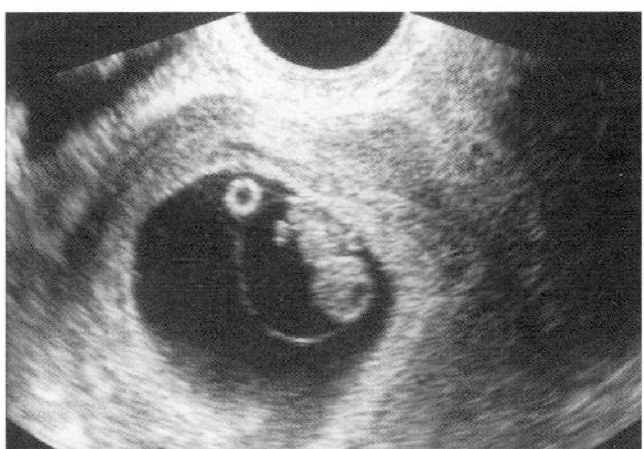

**Figure 28.10** Eight-week pregnancy.

## STRESS AND INFERTILITY

Infertility may have a great impact on an individual's physical and psychological wellbeing (Hammarberg 2003, Kerr et al 1999, Pfeffer & Woollett 1983). The process of IVF is invasive, time consuming, and involves intimate procedures including vaginal ultrasound scanning, transvaginal ultrasound oocyte recovery, embryo transfer, administering injections and producing a sperm sample. Couples frequently feel stigmatized and embarrassed by their infertility, and can experience a growing sense of isolation, creating stress and anxiety in their daily lives. Success rates are low, so many couples experience multiple episodes of grief and loss leading to depression. Emotions described by couples include loss of self-esteem, mourning, threat, guilt, marital problems and also health problems (Guerra et al 1998).

The costs incurred by IVF treatment are a major stress factor for couples undergoing treatment. The government has initiated a review of fertility treatments by the National Institute of Clinical Excellence (NICE) that will establish national standards for fertility treatment and end the 'postcode lottery' that currently exists. According to the latest draft, three attempts with fresh embryos and three attempts with frozen provide the best chance of achieving a pregnancy. One in six couples experience problems with fertility in Britain, and there are approximately 27,000 IVF attempts every year; 80% of cycles take place in private practice. If the cycles were provided by the NHS, it would cost an estimated £400m and there are concerns how the income would be generated (BBC News 2003).

**Reflective activity 28.2**

How would you, as a midwife, help a couple normalize their pregnancy and childbirth experience after fertility treatment?

Counselling is an integral part of the process of fertility treatment, whatever stage a couple may be undergoing, and this is provided throughout the programme independently by licensed units. Mothers who conceive by IVF have higher anxiety levels related to the survival and normality of the unborn babies, damage caused by childbirth and separation from babies after birth, compared with matched controls (McMahon et al 1997). Midwife support during pregnancy is crucial to these couples, who may feel more vulnerable than parents who have conceived naturally. It is important for couples to normalize the pregnancy after the intensity of the fertility treatment, and this may be challenging for the team caring for the couples in primary, secondary and tertiary care.

Understanding the causes of infertility and the treatment processes are important so the midwife can perceive the degree of stress and the financial burden of assisted conception. Couples who experience difficulty with conception have to deal with the stress, frustration and stigma associated with being infertile. Many undergo treatments that have a low level of success that are not available on the NHS. The whole experience may damage them and their relationships and many will not achieve a long-desired pregnancy. It is important for midwives to understand the processes couples have undergone to achieve their pregnancy.

### KEY POINTS

- The midwife needs to be aware of the causes of infertility in men and women, and all treatment options, including drug regimens and potential side-effects.
- Infertility and its treatment can have major long-lasting social, physical and emotional effects on the women and family and their adaptation to pregnancy and childbirth.
- Infertility and its management are carefully regulated in the UK, and the midwife needs to understand current regulations, and legislation.

## REFERENCES


Balen A, Jacobs H: *Infertility in practice*, New York, 1997, Churchill Livingstone.

Barber D: The extended role of the fertility nurse – practical realities, *Human Fertility* 5(1):13–16, 2002.

BBC News: *'More IVF' on the NHS* (website). http://news.bbc.co.uk. 2003.

Byrd C: Chlamydia trachomatis genital infections, *The West Virginia Medical Journal* 89(8):331–333, 1993.

Child T, Adul-Juli A, Huleki B, Tan SL: In vitro maturation of oocytes from unstimulated ovaries, normal ovaries, polycystic ovaries and women with polycystic ovarian syndrome, *Fertility & Sterility* 76:936–942, 2001.

Dale B, Elder K: *In vitro fertilization*, Cambridge, 1997, Cambridge University Press.

Dechaud H, Hedon B: What effect does hydrosalpinx have on assisted reproduction? The role of salpingectomy remains controversial, *Human Reproduction* 15(2):234–235, 2000.

ESHRE PGD Consortium Steering Committee: ESHRE Preimplantation Genetic Diagnosis (PGD) Consortium: data collection II (May 2000), *Human Reproduction* 15(12):2673–2683, 2000.

Geva E, Lerner-Geva L, Stavorosky Z, et al: Multifetal pregnancy reduction: a possible risk factor for periventricular leukomalacia in premature newborns, *Fertility and Sterility* 69(5):845–850, 1998.

Gould D: Women's health – endometriosis, *Nursing Standard* 17(27):47–53, 2003.

Guerra D, Llobera A, Veiga A, et al: Psychiatric morbidity in couples attending a fertility service, *Human Reproduction* 13(6):1733–1736, 1998.

Hammarberg K: Stress in assisted reproductive technology: implications for nursing practice, *Human Fertility* 6(1):30–33, 2003.

Hazekamp J, Bergh C, Wennerholm U, et al: Avoiding multiple pregnancies in ART, *Human Reproduction* 15(6):1217–1219, 2000.

Human Fertilisation and Embryology Authority (HFEA): *Human Fertilisation and Embryology Authority Code of Practice*, ed 5, London, 2001, HFEA.

Human Fertilisation and Embryology Authority (HFEA): *Code of Practice and Guidelines* (website). http://guide.hfea.gov.uk/guide/. 2009.

Hull M, Glazener C, Kelly N, et al: Population study of causes, treatment and outcome of infertility, *British Medical Journal* 291(6510):1693–1697, 1985.

Jurema M, Nogueira D: In vitro maturation of human oocytes for assisted reproduction, *Fertility and Sterility* 86(5):1277–1289, 2006.

Kerr J, Brown C, Balen A: The experience of couples who have infertility treatment in the United Kingdom; results of a survey performed in 1997, *Human Reproduction* 14(4):934–938, 1999.

Koivurova S, Hartikainen A, Gissler M, et al: Neonatal outcome and congenital malformations in children born after in-vitro fertilization, *Human Reproduction* 17(5):1391–1398, 2002.

Kousta E, White D, Cela E, et al: The prevalence of polycystic ovaries in women with infertility, *Human Reproduction* 14(11):2720–2723, 1999.

Kousta E, Cela E, Lawrence N, et al: The prevalence of polycystic ovaries in women with a history of gestational diabetes mellitus, *Clinical Endocrinology* 53(4):501–507, 2000.

Kurinczuk J: From theory to reality – just what are the data telling us about ICSI offspring health and future fertility and should we be concerned, *Human Reproduction* 18(5):925–931, 2003.

McMahon C, Ungerer J, Beaurepaire J, et al: Anxiety during pregnancy and fetal attachment after in-vitro fertilization, *Human Reproduction* 12(1):176–182, 1997.

Mukaida T, Oka T, Goto K, et al: Artificial shrinkage of blastocoels using either a micro needle or a laser pulse prior to the cooling steps of vitrification improves survival rate and pregnancy outcome of vitrified human blastocysts, *Human Reproduction* 21(12):3246–3252, 2006.

One at a Time: www.oneatatime.org.uk/126.htm. 2009.

Petterson B, Nelson K, Watson L, et al: Twins, triplets, and cerebral palsy in births in Western Australia in the 1980's, *British Medical Journal* 307(6914):1239–1243, 1993.

Pfeffer N, Woollet A: *The experience of infertility*, London, 1983, Virago.

Royal College of Obstetricians and Gynaecologists (RCOG): *Long-term consequences of polycystic ovary syndrome – Guideline No. 33*, London, 2003, RCOG.

Scott L: Embryological strategies for overcoming recurrent assisted reproductive technology treatment failure, *Human Fertility* 5(4):206–214, 2002.

Shakkebaek K, Keiding N: Changes in semen in the testis, *British Medical Journal* 309(6965):1316–1317, 1994.

Snick H, Snick T, Evers J, et al: The spontaneous pregnancy prognosis in untreated subfertile couples: the Walcheren primary care study, *Human Reproduction* 12(7):1582–1588, 1997.

Templeton A, Fraser C, Thompson B: The epidemiology of infertility in Aberdeen, *British Medical Journal* 301(6744):148–152, 1990.

Thornton S: *Infertility in men. Update Postgraduate Centre Series – Infertility*, Amsterdam, 2000, Excerpta Medica.

World Health Organization: *WHO laboratory manual for the examination of human semen and sperm-cervical mucus interaction*, ed 4, Cambridge, 1999, Cambridge University Press.

Chapter |29|

# Fertilization, embryonic, fetal and placental development

Mary McNabb

## LEARNING OUTCOMES

After reading this chapter, you will be able to:

- understand critical events in the process of fertilization, transport of spermatozoa, cumulus–oocyte complex, sperm–oocyte interactions and progressive formation of the blastocyst following fertilization
- explore interactive signals between blastocyst, endometrium and ovary that regulate attachment and implantation
- understand the brief period of 'endometrial receptivity' required for successful attachment, implantation and placental formation
- appreciate the distinct environmental conditions for embryonic and fetal phases of gestation and key features of embryonic and fetal life.

## INTRODUCTION

This chapter will build on Chapters 24, 25 and 27. The *luteal* phase of the fertile cycle initiates very distinct trajectories for mother and *conceptus* (see website). Following the luteinizing hormone/follicle-stimulating hormone (LH/FSH) surge, hormonal signals from the corpus luteum induce extensive adaptations in maternal renal, cardiovascular, respiratory, immunological, metabolic, endometrial and mammary systems. When fertilization occurs, these accelerate in response to signals from the conceptus and the endometrium. Before and after implantation, paracrine 'cross-talk' between conceptus and the endometrium prepares for attachment, implantation, differentiation of the trophoblast and development of the conceptus. At the same time, neuroendocrine signals are relayed from conceptus to the pituitary–ovarian and pituitary–thyroid regulatory axes; the peripheral immune system and maternal brain. These extend the functional lifespan of the corpus luteum; induce adaptations in maternal thyroid, stress and immune systems; and alter maternal sleep–wake cycles and food preferences, to accommodate the fertile cycle.

Following successful *maternal recognition* of the presence of the conceptus, adaptations that began following ovulation are enhanced and others specific to the fertile cycle are initiated. Maternal adaptations meet the distinct requirements of the conceptus during the first trimester and prepare for very different conditions needed to sustain fetal and neonatal life. Beginning with fertilization, this chapter focuses on the *regulation of implantation, trophoblast infiltration,* unique features of the *gestational sac* and *formation of key organ systems* during the first trimester. It will then examine fetoplacental interactions, including the fetoplacental circulation and endocrine unit; functional dynamics of amniotic fluid, lung formation and development in preparation for extrauterine life.

## FERTILIZATION

Spontaneous fertilization requires synchronized maturation and transport of the cumulus–oocyte complex (COC) and thousands of spermatozoa, within a tight timeframe. Once the COC is picked up by fimbriae of the fallopian tube, the oocyte has an estimated lifespan of 6–24 hours and spermatozoa 24–48 hours following arrival in the vaginal cavity (Johnson 2007:176). Both cells rapidly undergo a series of developmental and maturational processes, ensuring that only one of the 2–4 million spermatozoa that arrive in the vagina during sexual intercourse acquires the capacity to fuse with the oocyte membrane and release the sperm nucleus into the oocyte cytoplasm (Evans 2002, Kaji & Kudo 2004, Talbot et al 2003).

Following ovulation, the *cumulus cell mass* remains metabolically coupled to the oocyte through gap junctions. These somatic cells undertake a number of complex activities, including secretion of growth factors and antioxidants for the enclosed oocyte, facilitate oocyte travel and pickup and activate the capitation processes, all of which enable effective and successful fertilization (see website).

## The fallopian tubes

The fallopian tubes have critical functions following ovulation. The inner linings and secretions facilitate bi-directional transport of oocyte and spermatozoa; create favourable conditions for oocyte maturation, sperm storage, capacitation, fertilization and successive cleavage of the fertilized egg; and aid its transport towards the designated implantation site in the uterus (Leese et al 2001, Shafik et al 2005) (Fig. 29.1).

Anatomically part of the uterus, inner layers of the fallopian tubes are continuous with those in the cavity. They are composed of an internal mucosa of ciliated and secretory epithelium sensitive to changes in pituitary gonadotrophins and ovarian steroids, across the cycle (Casan et al 2000, Lei et al 1993). Intermediate layers of smooth muscle contain blood, lymph vessels, and steroid-sensitive adrenergic neurons that enable coordinated tubular motility, for the journey of the blastocyst to the uterus (Habayeb et al 2008; Wang et al 2004, 2006).

Around ovulation, smooth muscles display characteristic movements that bring the *infundibulum*, or distal portion of the tube, into apposition with the ovary containing the dominant follicle, by a change in orientation of muscles surrounding the ovarian fimbriae (Hunter 1988, Zervomanolakis et al 2009). One fimbria – slightly longer than the rest – reaches out to the tubal pole of the ovary and involutes, in synchrony with ovulation, to pick up the COC from the peritoneal cavity, into the enlarged trumpet-shaped *infundibulum*, lined with a very dense layer of ciliated secretory epithelium.

Oocyte and blastocyst transport within the tube is facilitated by:

- presence of cumulus cells around the oocyte
- sweeping movements of cilia towards the uterine cavity
- presence of 'pacemaker cells' that induce smooth muscle contractions (Shafik et al 2005)
- oestrogen-induced acceleration of oocyte movement within the tube
- LH- and progesterone-induced relaxation of the isthmic–ampullary junction, where fertilization takes place (Johnson 2007:176–177)
- relaxation of circular muscles of the isthmus by coupling of adrenergic and endocannabinoid signalling to regulate blastocyst transport through the isthmus–uterine junction (Wang et al 2004).

Following fertilization, the blastocyst enters the *isthmus*, which has thick mucosal folds and the greatest concentration of muscle fibres. The diameter increases from 1–2 mm at the uterotubal junction, to more than 1 cm at its distal end, with a lumen ranging from 1 to 100 mm.

The *interstitial portion* is continuous with the uterine cavity and characterized by a marked increase in ciliated cells, and alterations in the shape of secretory cells. Muscles at the uterotubal junction are formed from four

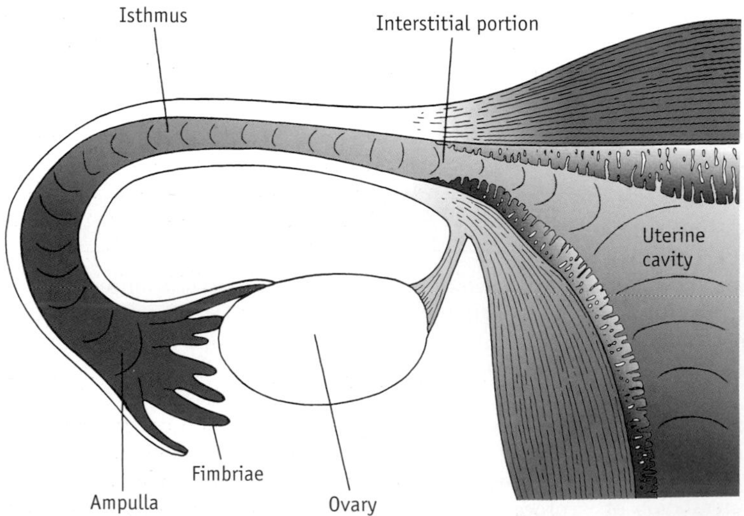


**Figure 29.1** Female reproductive tract. *(Reproduced with permission from Carlson 1994:15; Fig. 1-13.)*

bundles. These hormonally sensitive interlacing spiral fibres allow strong constriction and relaxation of the interstitial portion of the tube. This regulates sperm transport and storage, and movement of the blastocyst towards the uterine cavity (Hunter 1988, Wildt et al 1998).

## Cyclical changes

Across the ovarian cycle, the tubular mucosa undergoes cyclical alterations similar to the endometrial lining of the uterus. In the first half of the cycle, secretory and ciliated cells become larger under the influence of oestrogens. Around ovulation, ciliated cells become broader and lower while secretory cells become more distended with fluid. Following ovulation, microscopic holes appear in secretory cell membranes, which coalesce to release secretions accumulated during the first half of the cycle (Hunter 1988).

Higher rates of ciliary movements within the tube ipsilateral to the dominant follicle are regulated by increased blood flow, higher temperature and higher concentrations of ovarian steroids, compared to the contralateral tube (Zervomanola et al 2009). Around ovulation, beating of the dense concentration of cilia in the fimbriated portion is closely synchronized, propelling the COC into the ampulla. During this period, cilia in the ampulla also beat in the direction of the isthmus, suggesting that they further propel the COC towards the site of fertilization, taking the newly fertilized egg and surrounding cells from the ampulla and aiding subsequent movements of the *zygote* towards endometrial implantation (Hunter 1988).

The tubular environment is highly responsive to changing metabolic needs of the oocyte and blastocyst, through rhythms in secretion of growth factors, antioxidant enzymes and other regulatory molecules, and the supply of chemical and nutritive factors within the fallopian tubes following ovulation (Lapointe et al 2005). The oocyte and blastocyst are exposed to rhythmic secretion of growth regulatory molecules, and precisely timed modulations occur in oxygen tension, glucose concentrations, electrolytes and macromolecules, in different parts of the tube. The composition of tubular fluid complements the low rate of metabolite consumption in the oocyte and newly fertilized egg (Fleming et al 2004, Leese 1995, 2002, Leese et al 2001).

During their journey through the fallopian tube, the oocyte and blastocyst are composed of avascularized cells that undergo maturational changes and a highly regulated series of cleavage divisions, while utilizing exogenous sources of nutrients and growth factors.

Both demonstrate optimal functioning in an alkaline environment, with low concentrations of glucose and oxygen and plentiful supplies of albumin and growth factors (Leese 1995). The nutritive environment of the tubular lumen is regulated by hormonally induced secretions of the tubular mucosa and metabolic activities of the cumulus cell mass which surrounds the oocyte and blastocyst until implantation (Leese et al 2001) (Fig. 29.2).

## Sperm transport

Spermatozoa enter the genital tract in approximately 3–4 mL of seminal fluid which buffers the acidity of vaginal secretions. Over 99% are immediately lost by leakage from the vagina. Those remaining spend variable times in the cervix, showing differential states of motility and rates of transport through the uterus which may increase the chances of fertilization. This reservoir of spermatozoa in the cervix are actively transported in successive waves of peristalsis to a second sperm reservoir site in the isthmus, and finally to the fertilization site, at the isthmic–ampullary junction (Bahat et al 2003, Kunz et al 1998, Wildt et al 1998, Zervomanolakis et al 2009).

Cyclical changes in the vaginal canal around ovulation provide a protected environment for ejaculated sperm. This is mirrored by cyclical changes in cervical and vaginal tissues, including relaxation and widening of the cervix, and an increase in the quantity of cervical mucus, which demonstrates a characteristic 'stretchiness' that facilitates sperm transport (Drobnis & Overstreet 1992).

## Sperm capacitation

During their active transport through the genital tract, spermatozoa undergo a final series of maturational changes before a small number are ready for fertilization. The first of these is *capacitation,* caused by interactions between spermatozoa and secretions of the cervix, uterus and fallopian tube during their journey to the site of fertilization. Capacitation is when the composition of the cell membrane undergoes removal of most glycoprotein molecules added during ejaculation. Capitation seems to induce hyperactive motility, providing increased thrusting power and alterations in cell surface properties enabling entry to the zona pellucida surrounding the oocyte cell membrane (Alberts et al 2002, Drobnis & Overstreet 1992). Sperm also acquire:

- *thermotactic responsiveness* enabling navigation from the storage site in the *isthmus* to the warmer fertilization site at the isthmic–ampullary junction
- *short-lived chemotactic receptors* – these are activated in sperm reaching the isthmic storage site and precisely guide the sperm towards the oocyte in the isthmic–ampullary junction (Bahat et al 2003).

## Fusion of oocyte and spermatozoon

The final set of morphological transformations in spermatozoa are stimulated by binding to the zona pellucida. During this critical process, the acrosome swells and its membranes fuse with the overlying plasma membrane

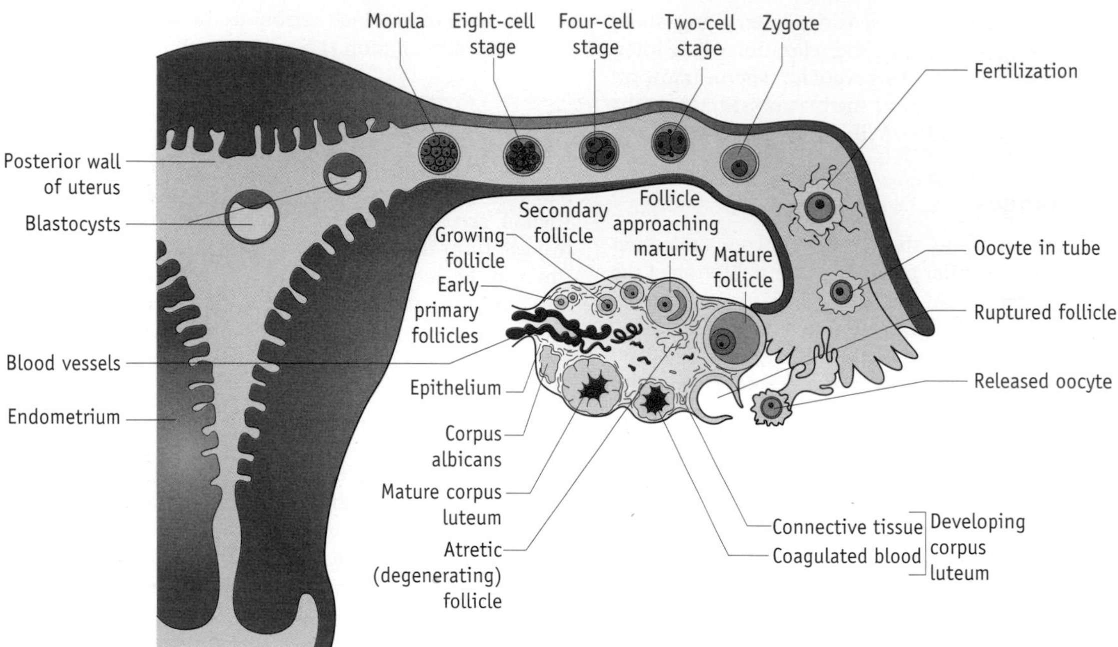


**Figure 29.2** The cumulus–oocyte complex and the corpus luteum following ovulation. *(Reproduced with permission from Blackburn 2007:74.)*

(see Fig. 29.3). Initially, attachment is very loose, involving a number of spermatozoa. Firmer binding follows as an oocyte-binding protein on the sperm head region is recognized by sperm receptors on the zona pellucida. The inner plasma membrane at the apical end of the spermatozoa fuses with the outer membrane of the acrosome and forms a series of membrane-bound vesicles. Proteolytic enzymes released by the *acrosome reaction* digest sections of the zona pellucida surrounding the sperm head. Subsequent movement through the zona occurs very rapidly, creating immediate access to the oocyte membrane. Only spermatozoa that have undergone this *acrosomal exocytosis* can fuse with the oocyte. Usually, the spermatozoon that makes first contact with the oocyte proceeds to fertilization. In the process of fusion, the plasma membrane of the sperm head is enveloped by microvilli on the oocyte surface (Johnson 2007, Tosti & Boni 2004).

Immediately after oocyte and spermatozoon fusion, the *cortical reaction* occurs. This is a series of ionic changes occurring in the oocyte cytoplasm, and cortical granules formed following ovulation bind to the oocyte membrane, thus releasing their content into the space between the surface of the oocyte and the surrounding zona pellucida. The vesicles contain enzymes that modify the structure of the plasma membrane blocking the entry of further spermatozoa.

## From zygote to ...

The *zygote* is the newly formed cell containing maternal and paternal chromosomes and measures about 0.15 mm in diameter (FitzGerald & FitzGerald 1994:12). Within 2–3 hours of fertilization, the zygote proceeds with the final phase of meiosis that was halted immediately following fertilization, transmitting one set of chromosomes to the next generation. The remaining set is discarded to a second *polar body*, on the periphery, which later undergoes apoptosis, along with the first one formed at ovulation (Fig. 29.3). Female chromosomes then divide mitotically, yielding one haploid set within the main body of the cytoplasm.

The cytoplasmic content of the sperm cell membrane combines with that of the oocyte and over the next 2–3 hours the sperm nuclear membrane gradually breaks down. Between 4 and 7 hours after cell fusion, two sets of haploid chromosomes are formed into male and female pronuclei, as each becomes surrounded by distinct membranes, in opposite poles of the cell. During this period, chromosomes synthesize DNA in preparation for the first mitotic division. As chromosomal content increases, the pronuclear membranes break down, bringing together two sets of male and female chromosomes. These events form the diploid complement of a new individual and the cell

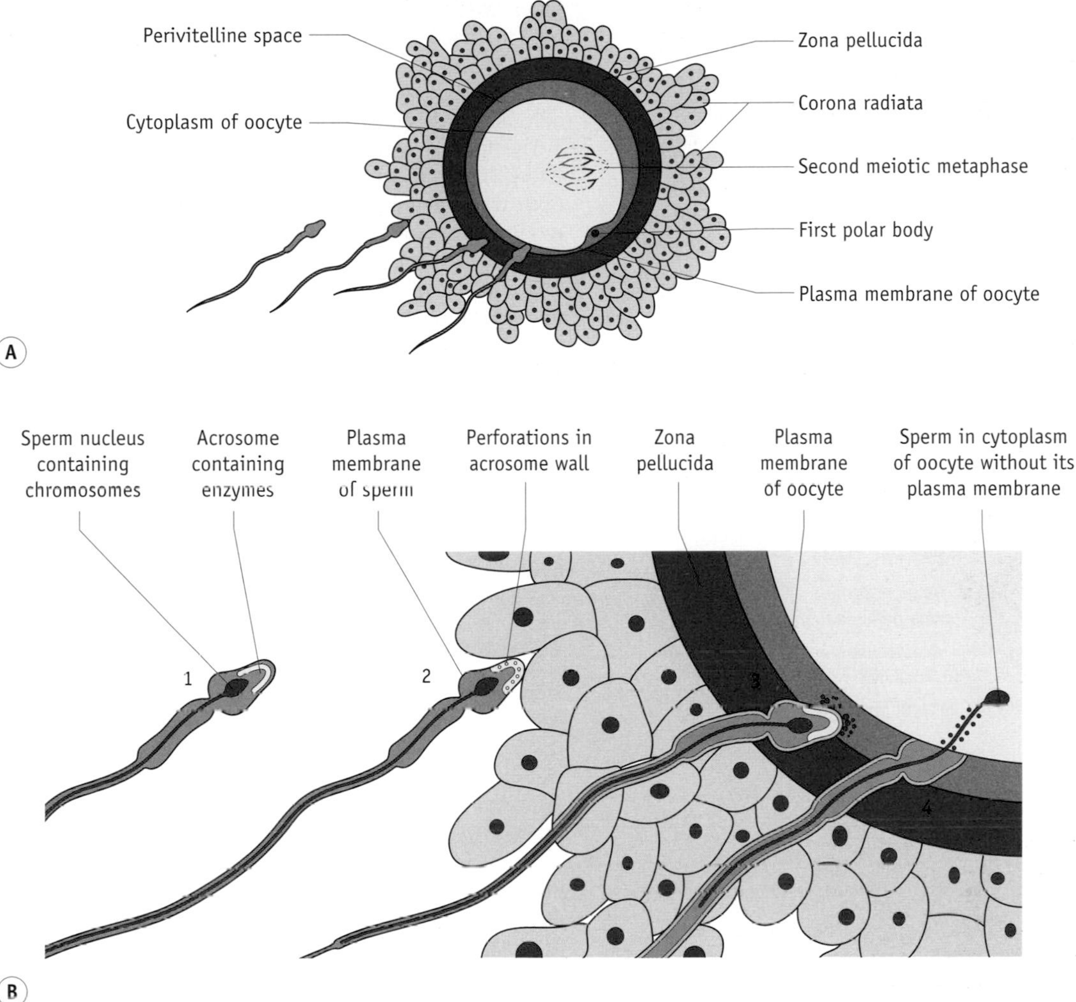


**Figure 29.3** Fertilization and cortical reaction. After capacitation, the plasma membrane of the sperm and the outer membrane of the acrosome fuse and the membranes break down, releasing enzymes that allow the sperm to penetrate the corona radiata. Sperm digest their way through the zona pellucida via enzymes associated with the inner acrosomal membrane. Sperm are engulfed by the oocyte plasma membrane. Cortical granules are released when the sperm cell contacts the membrane. These granules cause other sperm in contact with the membrane to detach. *(Reproduced with permission from Moore & Persaud 2008:30; Fig. 2-14A,B.)*

immediately proceeds with a first mitotic division, passing its genetic material to two daughter cells and forming the two-cell conceptus (Downs 2008) (Fig. 29.4).

## ... morula

Successive rounds of cleavages occur at approximately 12-hour intervals until 8–16 increasingly smaller cells are formed within the zona pellucida and remaining fragments of the cumulus cell mass. When cell cleavage has produced 8–16 cells, the conceptus changes its morphology and undergoes compaction to become a *morula* (resembling a mulberry) (Fig. 29.4). This process maximizes contiguity between adjacent cell membranes (see website).

Glucose is consumed in increasing quantities and the morula utilizes a large number of growth factors for replication (Leppens-Luisier et al 2001), including epidermal growth factor (EGF), insulin-like growth factors (IGFs), and hypoxia-inducible factors (HIFs) (Leese 1995). All blastomeres show intense staining for gonadotrophin-releasing hormone (GnRH), in possible readiness to

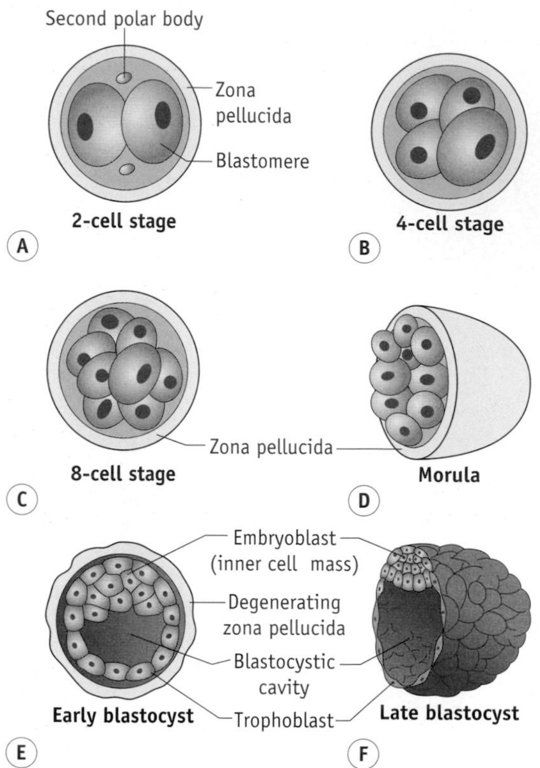


**Figure 29.4** Various stages of cleavage and formation of the blastocyst. *(Reproduced with permission from Moore & Persaud 2008: 36; Fig. 2-18A–F.)*

stimulate human chorionic gonadotrophin (hCG) release just before implantation (Casan et al 1999, Kikkawa et al 2002). During this phase of formation, the morula remains within the zona pellucida. This smooth outer covering provides an overall structure preventing premature adhesion of the blastomeres to the wall of the fallopian tube and providing an immunological barrier between maternal tissue and the genetically distinct cells of the morula (Johnson 2007).

## ... to blastocyst

Over 24 hours, the morula continues cell cleavage to 16–32 cells. Between these two points, outer cells commit to trophoblast lineage, while the inner cell mass (ICM) retains the capacity for pluripotency. Expression of critical genes for blastocyst formation commences in the 16-cell morula (Armant 2005). Outer cells begin to pump fluid internally to form a fluid-filled cavity called the *blastocoele*. Nudged to one side by this fluid, the ICM expresses gap junctions, allowing transfer of ions and small molecules from one cell to the next (Downs 2008). Meanwhile, the outer layer underlying the zona pellucida differentiates into flattened *trophectoderm* cells that combine with the zona to protect the ICM from destruction by maternal immune cells and signals the endometrium to initiate adhesion (Schultz 1998).

The fertilized egg has now become a *blastocyst* (Fig. 29.4). The trophoectoderm expresses mRNA for leptin and both outer and inner cells express mRNA, protein and receptors for GnRH, and the cannabinoid receptor ($CB_1$) (Battista et al 2008, Casan et al 1999).

Composed of 34–64 cells, the blastocyst is programmed to prepare for the embryonic phase of formation, beginning as a free-living organism immersed in uterine secretions actively accumulated by the trophoblasts and utilized as metabolic substrates, while exchange of oxygen and carbon dioxide occurs by diffusion (Burton et al 2002, Leese 1995). Over the next 3 days, *paracrine cross-talk* between the blastocyst and endometrium coordinates blastocyst activation with differentiation of the endometrium to a receptive state, from 7–9 days following ovulation (Fitzgerald et al 2008, Simon et al 1997).

## The corpus luteum

During the fertile cycle, the functional lifespan of the corpus luteum extends from 14 to around 280 days, but the endocrine–paracrine regulation is not well understood, particularly after the first 6 weeks of pregnancy (Handschuh et al 2007, Muyan & Boime 1997, Oon & Johnson 2000).

Research suggests that the close connections between uterine and ovarian arteriovenous systems deliver hCG and other regulatory factors from the endometrium and blastocyst, to the corpus luteum, from the early luteal phase of fertile cycles (see website).

## Relaxin

Following the LH/FSH surges, large luteal cells (LLCs) and small luteal cells (SLCs) develop the capacity to secrete peptide and steroid hormones, in equal amounts. *Relaxin*, a peptide hormone of the insulin-like growth factor family, is a major hormone of the corpus luteum of pregnancy. Beginning during the luteal phase, under the stimulatory influence of LH/hCG, relaxin secretion peaks at 10 weeks' gestation, decreases by around 20% and is present in maternal plasma, at stable concentrations, for the remainder of pregnancy (Bell et al 1987). Ovarian relaxin:

- induces endometrial stromal differentiation during the luteal phase and stimulates decidual prolactin – initiating and maintaining endometrial decidualization (Jabbour & Critchley 2001)
- operates with hCG and progesterone to activate transcription of glycodelin A, a major glycoprotein from the endometrial glands with nutritive and

immunomodulatory functions (Burton et al 2002, 2007, Glock et al 1995, Telgmann & Gellersen 1998, Tseng et al 1999)
- regulates changes in maternal thirst and osmoregulation
- central and peripheral relaxin induces renal and systemic vasodilatation, pituitary GH secretion, plasma volume expansion and increased adipose tissue sensitivity to insulin during the first half of pregnancy (Chapman et al 1997, Davison et al 1990, Kristiansson & Wang 2001, Santoro et al 1994, Vokes et al 1988).

## Hormonal signals

Within a week of fertilization, intact hCG (see website) appears in the maternal circulation and rapidly increases in the first 4 weeks after implantation, reaching peak levels of more than 100,000 mIU/mL around 9–10 weeks' gestation, before falling rapidly to levels under 50,000 mIU/mL from around 18–20 weeks, until the end of pregnancy (Chard et al 1995, Kosaka et al 2002). In contrast, α-hCG levels increase progressively until term (Nagy et al 1994). At present, the exact mechanisms regulating intact hCG secretion are not well understood. Placental GnRH and leptin regulate secretion for the first 8 weeks of pregnancy (Islami et al 2003). Thereafter, hCG secretion as well as uterine and placental expression of LH/hCG receptors seem to be maintained by an autoregulatory mechanism (Cameo et al 2004, Kikkawa et al 2002). As pregnancy progresses, rising levels of fetal adrenal steroids seem to inhibit placental hCG (Tsakiri et al 2002).

hCG appears to have a fundamental role in regulating the establishment, development and maintenance of human pregnancy and the onset of labour (Ambrus & Rao 1994, Handschuh et al 2007, Ticconi et al 2007). Before attachment, trophectoderm cells of the blastocyst secrete hCG (Lopata et al 1997). Following attachment, hCG is released from mitotically active mononuclear cytotrophoblast cells, multinuclear syncytiotrophoblasts and extravillous cytotrophoblasts that differentiate from the trophoblast following implantation (Handschuh et al 2007, Muyan & Boime 1997). This early pregnancy rise in hCG secretion by the syncytiotrophoblast, extraplacental chorion and endometrial lining of the uterus and fallopian tubes constitutes the first neuroendocrine signal that induces *maternal recognition* of the fertile cycle (Handschuh et al 2007).

# PREPARATION FOR IMPLANTATION

In readiness for implantation, endometrial glands accumulate glycogen, proteins, a variety of growth factors, sugars and lipid droplets, and secretory activity peaks at around 6 days after ovulation (Burton et al 2002, 2007). Some secretions supply the conceptus with essential nutritional and regulatory molecules until around 9 weeks' gestation, while growth factors stimulate proliferation of cytotrophoblast cells following implantation and secretion of hCG and human placental lactogen (hPL) by the syncytiotrophoblast from 6 to 12 weeks (Burton et al 2007, Hustin & Franchimont 1992, Jauniaux et al 2003).

Ovarian progesterone stimulates increased expression of two potent angiogenic factors: angiogenin in stromal cells and *vascular endothelial growth factor* (VEGF) in stromal cells and neutrophils associated with microvessel walls (Gargett et al 2001, Ma et al 2001). By the mid-secretory phase, a subepithelial capillary plexus has formed into a complex network of vessels (see Web Fig. 29.1) and newly regrown arterioles become increasingly spiral as they lengthen more rapidly than the endometrium thickens (Gargett et al 2001, Starkey 1993, Strauss & Coutifaris 1999).

## Pre-decidualization

During the secretory phase, stromal cells release a growing number of new matrix proteins together with surface expression of their receptors, including laminin, fibronectin, collagen and integrins, while the earlier cross-linking collagen fibrils are degraded. This process of matrix remodelling creates a thicker, looser and more soluble structure for trophoblast infiltration (see website).

## Blastocyst–endometrial communication

When fertilization occurs, the designated attachment site undergoes extensive synchronized changes transforming it from a usual state of active rejection of blastocyst attachment, to a brief state of receptivity, forming a 'window of implantation' commencing 7 days after ovulation (Fitzgerald et al 2008, Hustin 1992, Hustin & Franchimont 1992, Lessey 2000). Some changes are regulated by paracrine cross-talk with the free floating blastocyst, while others are activated by attachment.

As the blastocyst hatches from the zona pellucida, around 6 days after fertilization, trophoblast cells surrounding the ICM make initial contact with the endometrium, by close apposition of trophoblast plasma membranes with the apical membranes of surface epithelial cells, followed by rapid proliferation and formation of junctional complexes with the surface epithelium. Apical membranes of epithelial cells display a variety of progesterone- and oestrogen-induced changes that facilitate cell recognition and interaction with the trophectoderm. These include a progressive shortening of the microvilli, creating a flatter surface, reduced thickness of the normally dense coating of glycoproteins, and inhibition of gap junctions, facilitating adhesion (Fride 2008, Hustin & Franchimont 1992, Johnson 2007, Lessey 2000).

(For more information, see website.)

## Adhesion and attachment

Around the designated site of implantation, the luminal epithelium expresses calcitonin and the blastocyst-dependent heparin-binding epidermal growth factor (HB-EGF). As the zona pellucida is shed, direct communication between cell adhesion molecules and their receptors on trophoblast and surface epithelium begins the dynamically balanced processes of attachment, implantation and trophoblast replication (Fitzgerald et al 2008) (see website).

## IMPLANTATION – ENDOMETRIAL RESPONSE

The surface epithelium, uterine glands and decidua show distinct responses to implantation. As the tiny blastocyst lodges in the crypt of the endometrial folds and localized oedema moulds a chamber around the trophoblast surface, epithelial cells above the newly created site multiply rapidly to form a complete cover for the embedded blastocyst enveloped in a growing mantle of differentiating trophoblast cells, by approximately 9 days following fertilization (Armant 2005). More extensive hormone-induced changes occur within the underlying decidua, producing a range of matrix proteins to form a loose lattice-type network allowing free passage of water, ions and large molecules to the trophoblast cells.

Like epithelial glands, decidual cells synthesize and release specific glycoproteins. One of these has been identified as a growth factor-binding protein that may participate in regulating the pace and extent of trophoblast implantation (Hustin & Franchimont 1992). Decidual cells that release relaxin have also been found to contain prolactin, which is regulated by a number of factors from adjoining cells in the decidua, placenta and membranes. Activities of decidual prolactin include regulation of glandular secretions, expression of adhesion and proteolytic molecules, and modulation of specific aspects of the immune response (Gubbay et al 2002, Jabbour & Critchley 2001) (see website).

## IMPLANTATION – MYOMETRIUM

Within the myometrium, hCG and progesterone induce cellular enlargement and depress the excitability of uterine muscle by decreasing the uptake of cellular free calcium, blocking the ability of oestrogens to stimulate α-adrenergic receptors and downregulating myometrial gap junctions (Ambrus & Rao 1994, Phillips et al 2005, Ticconi et al 2007). Rising levels of progesterone act centrally to depress oxytocin neuronal activity, which is likely to cause a decline in uterine peristalsis during implantation (Rodway & Rao 1995).

## FORMATION OF THE CYTOTROPHOBLAST SHELL AND GESTATIONAL SAC

Once the blastocyst has embedded in the decidua, rapidly proliferating trophoblast cells follow three distinct pathways, dividing into weakly proliferating *villous cytotrophoblasts* (vCTBs) that subsequently fuse to form a syncytium of terminally differentiated *multinucleated syncytiotrophoblasts* (STs) while the stem cell population of vCTBs form a monolayer directly beneath the STs to renew them. Some of these responses include processes that reduce rejection of the growing embryo (see website).

During the first trimester, STs actively take up secretions from the surrounding endometrial glands and contribute to gaseous and waste exchange (Ellery et al 2009). Throughout pregnancy, they are the major source of hormones, receptors, growth factors and regulatory enzymes (Burton et al 2007, Ferretti et al 2007, Habayeb et al 2008, Islami et al 2003, Jauniaux & Gulbis 2000, Tarrade et al 2001). These include hCG, human placental growth hormone (hPGH), prolactin, atrial natriuretic peptide (ANP), leptin, oestrogens, progesterone, and a growing list of regulatory glycoproteins including GnRH, corticotrophin-releasing hormone (CRH) and thyrotrophin-releasing hormone (TRH) (Cootauco et al 2008, Douglas 2010, Ferretti et al 2007, Pasqualini 2005).

As trophoblast differentiation proceeds, the ICM first subdivides into primary *endoderm* and *ectoderm* cell groups, both of which contribute to embryonic and extra-embryonic tissues (see Fig. 29.5). During the second week of life, regulatory cells within the ectoderm establish a defining organizational structure called the *primitive streak*, which establishes polarity of the body axis and consequently positions all embryonic organs and extra-embryonic compartments, while the endoderm group form a major part of the yolk sac, which performs the functions of a mature placenta, during the first trimester (Downs 2008, Jones 1997).

Over the last 10 years, major advances have been made in identifying the unique biology of this period of gestation (see website).

While the cytotrophoblast shell acts as an effective barrier to maternal concentrations of oxygen, the

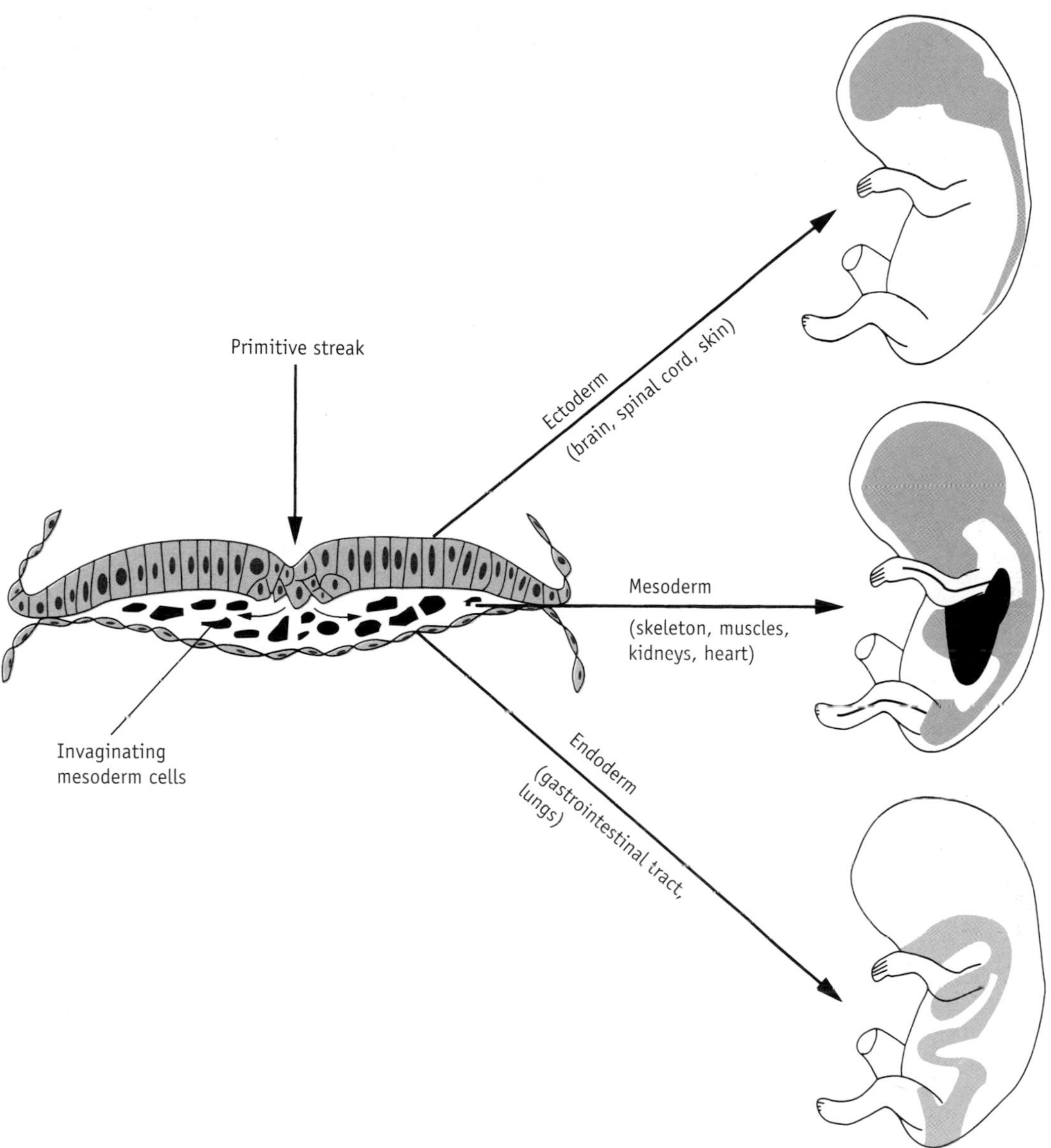


**Figure 29.5** The trilaminar disc illustrating endoderm, ectoderm and mesoderm. *(Reproduced with permission from Dunstan 1990:214.)*

expanding syncytiotrophoblastic mantle erodes the epithelium of surrounding endometrial glands, releasing their secretions into the extracellular matrix (Burton et al 2007). Glandular secretions enter channels forming around the cytotrophoblast shell. This activity is evident from 17 days post conception and only begins to decline when embryonic formation is complete, at the end of the first trimester (Burton et al 2007, Jauniaux & Gulbis 2000).

## HISTIOTROPHIC NUTRITION

During the first 8–10 weeks of pregnancy, the secretory pattern of epithelial glandular cells extends that of the *luteal phase,* with continued glycogen secretion and a rapid rise in a number of glycoproteins (Burton et al 2001, 2007; Muller-Schottle et al 1999). These include glycodelin A, relaxin, hCG, α-tocopherol transfer protein,

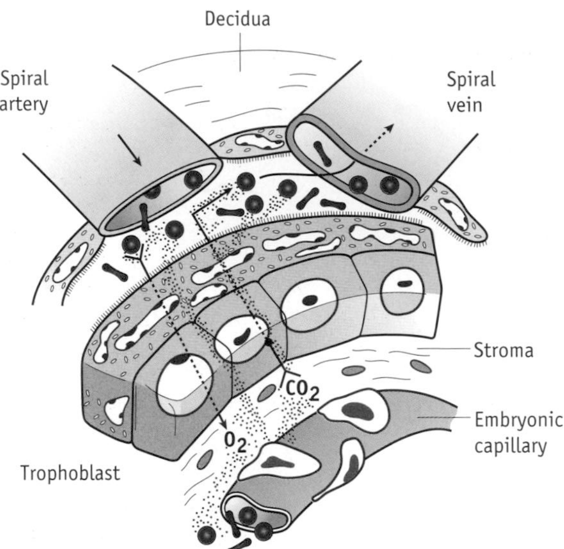


**Figure 29.6** Diagram showing uteroplacental circulation and the trophoblast barrier. *(Reproduced from Jauniaux & Gulbis 1997: 229; Fig. 13.3, with kind permission of OUP. www.oup.com)*

a powerful antioxidant, and MUC-1, a large progesterone-dependent glycoprotein (Burton et al 2002, 2007, Jauniaux et al 2004). Synthesis of glycodelin A parallels the profile of hCG in the maternal circulation during the first trimester. This glycoprotein regulates endometrial receptivity, has potent immunosuppressive activity, and is phagocytosed by the ST for recycling in anabolic pathways within the extra-embryonic compartment. MUC-1 is also taken up by the syncytiotrophoblast membrane and provides a rich and energy-free source of amino acids for its synthetic requirements (Burton et al 2002, Seppala et al 2002, Tseng et al 1999). The transfer pathway for these molecules is histiotrophic (extracellular) rather than haemotrophic (vascular) which characterizes the fetal phase of gestation (Burton et al 2002) (Fig. 29.6).

## CONDITIONS FOR EMBRYOGENESIS AND EARLY PLACENTAL FORMATION

Recent studies suggest that the optimal environment for embryonic and early placental formation includes a reduced oxygen tension of between 2.5% and 5% (see website). Embryonic haemoglobin, which lasts for the first 8 weeks of gestation, combines with oxygen at very low tension found in interstitial fluids. Until the middle of the second month of gestation, all embryonic erythrocytes are nucleated; hence, blood viscosity remains very high and the mean radius of the emerging villous vascular system is very low (Jauniaux et al 2003). The conceptus therefore derives external nutritional support histiotrophically, from secretory products of the decidua and uterine glands. These secretory products are initially phagocytosed by the trophectoderm of the blastocyst, then by vCTBs and the endoderm of the yolk sac (Burton et al 2001, 2002).

Developments within the endometrium fully complement this activity (see Web Fig. 29.1). From the luteal phase of the cycle, glandular cells secrete rapidly increasing amounts of glycoproteins promoting cell growth and organ differentiation. The underlying decidua undergoes considerable biochemical and structural adaptations, forming an array of matrix proteins and differentiated secretory cells that provide:

- growth-promoting factors for the emerging embryo
- immunoprotection for trophoblast infiltration
- a variety of regulatory hormones, including: prolactin, relaxin, renin, retinol-binding protein and prostaglandins (Burton et al 2002, Hustin & Franchimont 1992, King et al 2001, Starkey 1993).

## FORMATION OF EXTRA-EMBRYONIC FLUID COMPARTMENTS

As implantation of the blastocyst proceeds during the first 2 weeks after ovulation, the extra-embryonic mesoderm lining the cytotrophoblast shell progressively increases, and contains isolated spaces by 12 days after fertilization. At the same time, the ICM becomes a bilaminar disk, composed of high columnar cells (*primary ectoderm*) on the dorsal surface and a layer of differentiated cuboidal cells on the ventral surface, adjacent to the blastocyst cavity (*primary endoderm*). Over the next few days, a wave of new endodermal cells migrate from the primary endoderm, to line the blastocyst cavity and form the *primary yolk sac* or *exocoelomic cavity* during the fourth week of gestation. The complex fluid is derived from an ultrafiltration of maternal serum through villous stromal channels and from the secondary yolk sac, which forms at the beginning of the fourth week of gestation. Containing high concentrations of amino acids, regulatory proteins, vitamins and hormones, this fluid acts as a reservoir of molecules, prior to their use by the yolk sac during the first 8–10 weeks of pregnancy (Jauniaux & Gulbis 2000, Jauniaux et al 1994).

Once the primary yolk sac forms, a thick acellular material called the extra-embryonic mesoderm is secreted between the exocoelomic membrane and the cytotrophoblast. Over the next couple of days, this tissue divides to form a second chorionic cavity, between the primary yolk sac and the cytotrophoblast. An inner layer of cytotrophoblast cells delaminate to form amniogenic cells. Some differentiate into amnioblasts and organize into a specialized, semi-permeable membrane composed of a single layer of cuboidal epithelial cells on a loose connective tissue matrix (Jauniaux & Gulbis 2000). Formation of the primordial amniotic cavity seems to arise by cavitation of the primary ectoderm, which opens and then reforms to create a complete membrane around the amniotic cavity containing the emerging embryo.

Fluid formed within the amniotic cavity is largely secreted by the emerging embryo, containing much lower concentrations of all molecules and trace elements than fluid in the exocoelomic cavity (Jauniaux & Gulbis 2000). This indicates that the amniotic membrane separating the two compartments is *not permeable* to large molecules, and most glandular and trophoblast proteins are probably absorbed by the embryo through the secondary yolk sac (Jauniaux & Gulbis 2000, Jauniaux et al 1993, 1994). As illustrated in Figure 29.7, during the first 8 weeks of embryonic formation, the amniotic cavity is dwarfed by the larger and highly dynamic exocoelomic cavity containing the free-floating yolk sac, which directly nourishes and regulates the emerging embryo until around 10 weeks' gestation (Jauniaux & Gulbis 1997, Jones 1997).

## THE SECONDARY YOLK SAC

Around 12 days following fertilization, the primary yolk sac breaks up into a number of smaller vesicles while the endoderm beneath the embryonic disk grows out to form the *secondary yolk sac*. The secondary yolk sac grows rapidly, becoming larger than the amniotic cavity by the fifth week of gestation (Jones 1997). With successive foldings of the emerging embryo during the dynamic process of gastrulation, between 3 and 6 weeks' gestation, the neck of the secondary yolk sac is constricted to form the yolk stalk, which connects the definitive yolk sac to the primitive gut.

Until it begins to degenerate at around 9 weeks' gestation, the secondary yolk sac consists of three distinct layers:

- An outer layer of *extra-embryonic mesoderm* that completely lines the chorionic or exocoelomic cavity: this has a well-developed microvillous brush border and numerous pinocytotic vesicles within the cytoplasm which enhances its capacity for absorption of molecules from the surrounding exocoelomic fluid.
- A middle *splanchnic mesoderm* containing blood islands: this contains free collagen fibrils and sinusoidal blood vessels induced by the innermost

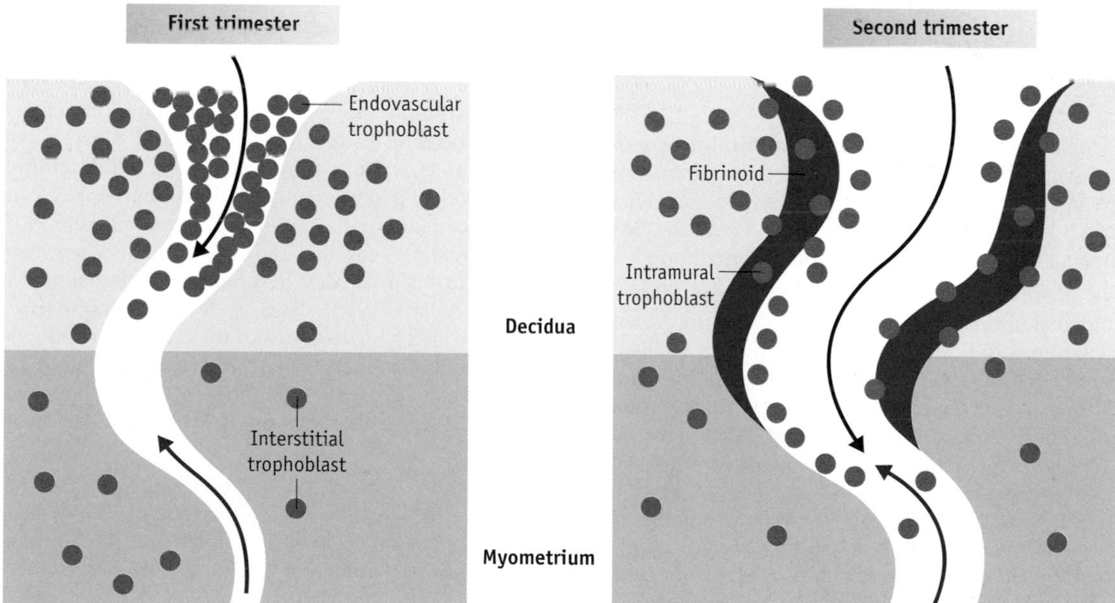


**Figure 29.7** Diagram illustrating endovascular trophoblast migration into decidual segments of spiral arteries during the first trimester (left) and interstitial migration into the myometrial segments from 12-14 weeks. Red arrow: direction of maternal blood flow; black arrow: direction of endovascular trophoblast migration. *(Reproduced with permission form Pijnenborg et al 2006:948: Fig. 7.)*

endodermal layer of the yolk sac. Central cells of the blood islands fuse to form primitive vascular channels within the mesodermal connecting stalk, extending towards the emerging embryo where they make connections with the endothelial tubes associated with the tubular heart and major vessels (Jauniaux et al 2003, Jones 1997).

- An endodermal layer facing the yolk sac lumen (Jauniaux & Moscoso 1992, Jones 1997) is made up of large columnar cells with glycogen deposits and a well-developed capacity for protein biosynthesis. These cells are interspersed with large microvillous-lined channels that open out into the cavity of the yolk sac and seem to be involved in secretion of waste products. Many proteins and enzymes involved in energy metabolism and digestion are synthesized by the endodermal layer, including alpha-fetoprotein, antitrypsin, albumin and transferrin, before the embryonic liver takes over at around 9–10 weeks' gestation (Jones 1997).

Blood cells and capillaries develop within the centre of the chorionic villi. At approximately 19 days, the two sets of vessels establish contact, creating the beginnings of a vascular connection between the embryonic compartment and the early placenta (Carlson 1994:72). Blood cell formation in the secondary yolk sac continues until haematopoiesis begins in the embryonic liver and spleen at around 8 weeks' gestation (Jauniaux & Moscoso 1992).

## FORMATION OF KEY ORGAN SYSTEMS

At present, there are well-characterized anatomical descriptions of sequential periods of human embryo formation and fragmentary findings on regulators of individual systems (Calvo et al 2002, Moore & Persaud 2008, Williams 2008). (See website for more information.)

**At 2–4 weeks' gestation:** precursors of the thyroid, renal, adrenal and gonadal organs begin to form. Experimental findings indicate that distinct progenitor cells of the anterior pituitary gland appear well before the gland takes shape, around 7 weeks' gestation (Moore & Persaud 2008, Simmons et al 1990, Tsakiri et al 2002). Five distinct cell types are defined by the trophic hormones produced; prolactin and growth hormone (GH) from lactotrophs and somatotrophs; thyroid-stimulating hormone (TSH) from thyrotrophs; luteinizing hormone (LH) and follicle stimulating hormone (FSH) from gonadotrophs; and proopiomelanocortin (POMC), which gives rise to adrenocorticotrophic hormone (ACTH), from corticotrophs.

**At 7.5 weeks' gestation:** prolactin receptors are present in a wide variety of emerging organs, notably mesenchymal cells surrounding the developing adrenal cortex, kidneys, lungs, pancreas, duodenum, as well as cardiac and skeletal myocytes (Freemark et al 1997). These and other findings indicate that prolactin released from the pituitary has a key role in cell proliferation and differentiation that begins from the end of the first trimester. Cellular distribution of expression of prolactin receptors alters as its functions change from inducing cell proliferation, to hormone synthesis and organ maturation, as pregnancy advances (Freemark 1999, Symonds et al 1998).

**At 8 weeks' gestation:** thyroid hormone receptor proteins are present in the brain, and thyroxine ($T_4$) of maternal origin is present in coelomic fluid 2 weeks earlier (Iskaros et al 2000). Current evidence on the relative concentrations of maternal thyroid hormone in maternal serum and embryonic fluid compartments shows that transfer during early pregnancy is tightly regulated by a significant rise in the presence of enzymes in the decidua and gestational sac that metabolize $T_4$ and $T_3$ to inactive compounds (Calvo et al 2002, Liggins 1994). The emerging embryo is exposed to rigidly regulated levels of maternal thyroid hormones to regulate neuronal proliferation and migration of neurons in different parts of the brain (Williams 2008).

The urogenital systems and adrenal cortex are formed from mesoderm, one of three definitive germ layers derived from the primary ectoderm (Downs 2008, Kempna & Fluck 2008). A longitudinal elevation of mesoderm – the *urogenital ridge* – forms on either side of the dorsal aorta. The part giving rise to the renal system is the *nephrogenic cord*, while the adrenal cortex and bipotential gonads are initially part of the adrenogonadal primordium, between the urogenital ridge and dorsal mesentery, until they become distinct organs at around **4 weeks'** gestation (Goto et al 2006, Moore & Persaud 2008). During the fifth week of gestation, precursors of adrenal cells form cords that migrate and accumulate at the cranial end of the *mesonephros* – the first set of kidneys – where they condense to form the first outline of the adrenal glands (Mesiano & Jaffe 1999). Large spherical primordial sex cells appear in a restricted area of the endoderm and yolk sac stalk and are subsequently carried along the hind gut to the *gonadal ridge* where they become incorporated in the primary sex cords (Jauniaux & Moscoso 1992, Jones 1997).

**By 6–7 weeks:** adrenal and renal systems begin to function before the genital system. Two distinct zones have differentiated, a small outer definitive zone and an inner temporary or fetal zone that forms 80–90% of the cortex (Goto et al 2006, Tsakiri et al 2002).

**From 7 to 12 weeks' gestation:** cortisol is synthesized in the transitional zone, which is located at the interface between the definitive and fetal zones. Cortisol exerts negative feedback regulation on ACTH release from the emerging anterior pituitary gland, which is critical to prevent excess ACTH from stimulating adrenal hyperplasia, resulting in increased synthesis of precursors for androgen synthesis (Goto et al 2006, Kempna & Fluck 2008). This early release of cortisol protects the emerging female embryo from the virilizing effects of androgens and facilitates normal female sexual differentiation of the external genitalia at **7–12 weeks'** gestation (Goto et al 2006; Mesiano & Jaffe 1997, 1999).

**By 9 weeks' gestation:** the definitive kidneys have begun to excrete urine into the surrounding fluid and the onset of glomerular filtration is reflected in the marked rise in protein composition of amniotic fluid between the first and second trimester (Calvo et al 2002, Moore & Persaud 2008). Throughout fetal life, waste products are not processed by the kidneys but are transferred from amniotic fluid into maternal blood for elimination by the maternal kidneys (Moore & Persaud 2008).

While these and other organ systems unfold during the first **9–10 weeks** of gestation, placental formation remains within the boundaries of the decidua.

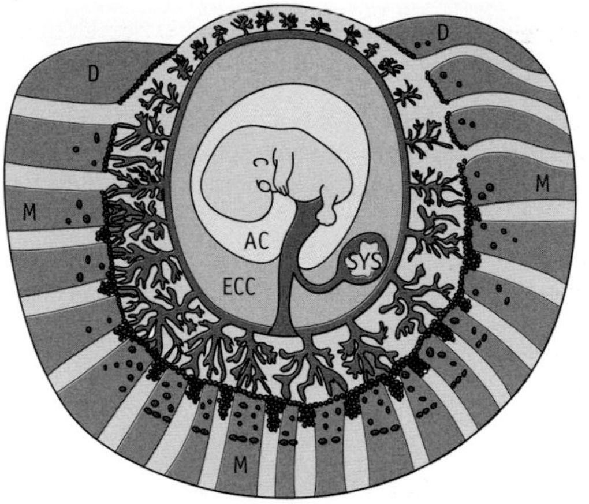

**Figure 29.8** Diagram of a gestational sac at 8–9 weeks' gestation, showing the myometrium (M), decidua (D), placenta (P), and exocoelomic cavity (EEC), the largest space inside the gestational sac from 5–9 weeks' gestation. Arrows indicate uteroplacental blood circulation beginning in the periphery of the placenta. *(Reproduced with permission from Burton et al 2006:203; Fig. 8.)*

## THE DECIDUOCHORIAL PLACENTA

During formation of anchoring villi, proliferating extravillous cytotrophoblasts (evCTBs) extend from the syncytium, forming columns of cells that enter decidual blood vessels. As this process continues, the intervillous space begins to open, exposing the migratory extravillous trophoblast cells to a physiological increase in oxygen tension, from 9 weeks' gestation. This environment alters the expression of specific transcription factors that triggers the expression of an invasive population of migratory evCTBs (Caniggia et al 2000). In addition, evCTBs also express receptors for hPGH which has recently been found to increase the invasive potential of evCTBs in culture (Lacroix et al 2005). Further differentiation of the extravillous cells to a more invasive phenotype allows them to enter and remodel the spiral arteries, to create the low-resistance vascular system that is essential for fetal growth (Caniggia & Winter 2002, Caniggia et al 2000, Hustin 1992).

During the first 12 weeks, extravillous trophoblast migration into the spiral arteries occurs primarily within the decidual segments. First the distal tips of these blood vessels are plugged with evCTBs that extend from the trophoblastic shell or the proliferating tips of the emerging villi. Sheets of these endovascular trophoblasts migrate along the capillary walls, against maternal blood flow, and accumulate within the lumen of the spiral arteries (see Fig. 29.8). During the subsequent process of vascular infiltration, cells strip away sections of the endothelium and burrow beneath this layer, to replace elastic tissue and smooth muscle with cytotrophoblast cells that appear to surround themselves with large quantities of fibrinoid material. Later, surface endothelial cells grow over the new underlying tissues. Throughout, the convoluted walls of the spiral arteries are converted into tubes of fibrinoid material with no elastic tissue or smooth muscle fibres. This results in terminal coils of the spiral arteries reaching 2–3 mm in diameter and underlying segments undergo a generalized non-uniform dilation as pregnancy advances and lose the capacity to respond to the vasomotor influences of continued autonomic innervation (Burton et al 2009, Douglas 2010, Hustin et al 1988, Pijnenborg et al 2006).

During the first **10 weeks of pregnancy**, ultrasound studies suggest that decidual blood vessels do not reach the intervillous space. While small amounts of plasma percolate through the plugs from these low-pressure vessels, chorionic villous sampling has rarely demonstrated the presence of maternal blood. As illustrated in Figure 29.6, current evidence suggests that during the first 9–10 weeks, the intervillous space is not immediately connected with the maternal circulation and is not yet bathed by maternal blood (Hustin & Schaaps 1987). As illustrated in Figure 29.9, estimates of uterine blood flow also support this evidence. In non-pregnant women, uterine blood flow is approximately 45 mL/min, rising by around 10 mL/min during the first trimester. In contrast, much larger increases occur during the second and third trimesters, to reach over 750 mL/min by the end of pregnancy (Burton et al 2009, de Swiet 1991:51).

## FROM EMBRYO TO FETUS

From 12 weeks onwards, trophoblast infiltration extends into myometrial segments of many spiral arteries (Pijnenborg et al 2006). Evidence suggests that this infiltration largely occurs through the endometrial stroma to enter the vessel walls from the outside (Burton et al 2009). As in decidual segments, this activity replaces muscular and elastic tissue with fibrinoid material that converts them into widened, funnel-like tubes with no capacity to respond to the vasomotor influences of continued autonomic innervation (Caniggia et al 2000). At the same time, the trophoblast shell becomes thinner and more irregular as fetal growth enlarges its internal volume (Jauniaux et al 2003). An increasing number of extravillous cells become distinct from the shell surface and these gradually open up low-pressure flow of maternal blood within the intervillous space. Experimental evidence suggests that the velocity of blood flow from the spiral arterioles to the intervillous space is similar to an actively flowing brook entering a reed-filled marsh (Burton et al 2009, Ramsey et al 1976) (Fig. 29.10).

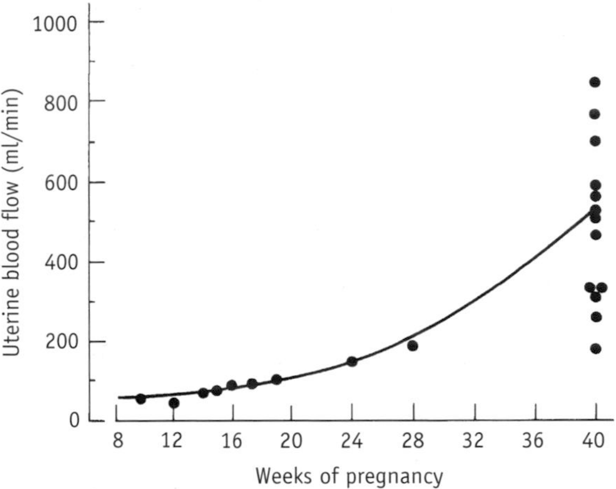


**Figure 29.9** Uterine blood flow in pregnancy. *(Reproduced with permission from Chamberlain and Broughton Pipkin 1998:51.)*

This direct communication between maternal blood and placental villi coincides with the onset of rapid growth of the fetus and placenta. During this phase, the roughly formed organ systems undergo progressive differentiation and rapid growth that requires large increases in uteroplacental size and blood volume (Mark et al 2006). Structural alterations to all segments of uterine blood vessels create conditions for the emergence of an expanding low-pressure system that optimizes gas and nutritional exchange across the placental interface (Burton et al 2009).

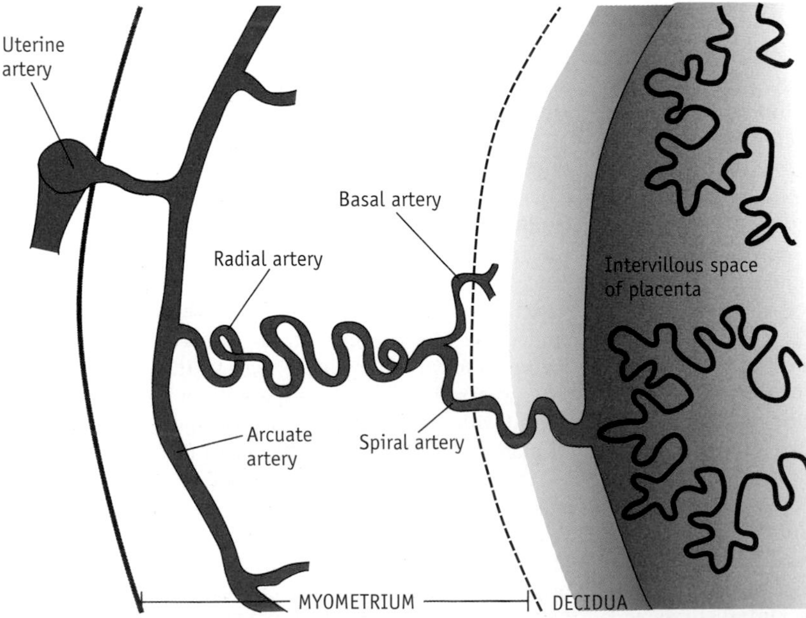


**Figure 29.10** The arterial supply to the placenta.

## GROWTH OF THE AMNIOTIC COMPARTMENT

Between 7 and 12 weeks' gestation, the production of amniotic fluid increases from 3 to 30 mL (Jauniaux & Gulbis 2000). This causes the amnion to swell, until it takes over the chorionic space, bringing amnion and chorion in contact for the first time and enclosing the embryo, except for the umbilical area, within a single cavity. As the sac subsequently grows into the endometrial cavity, this portion of the chorion is gradually compressed against the decidua capsularis – the area of decidual lining surrounding the site of implantation. With continued growth, blood supply is reduced and these villi slowly degenerate, although trophoblast cells between them remain viable for the remainder of the pregnancy. This portion of the chorion (*chorion laeve*) forms an interface between the amnion and areas of decidua not occupied by the definitive placenta (Fig. 29.11).

The *chorion laeve* has the following features:

- Diverse layers of metabolically active tissue (in spite of absence of a direct blood supply).
- Composed of a layer of fibroblast cells that are contiguous with the amnion, a reticular layer, a type of basement membrane and 2–10 layers of trophoblast cells that are closely applied to the decidua capsularis.

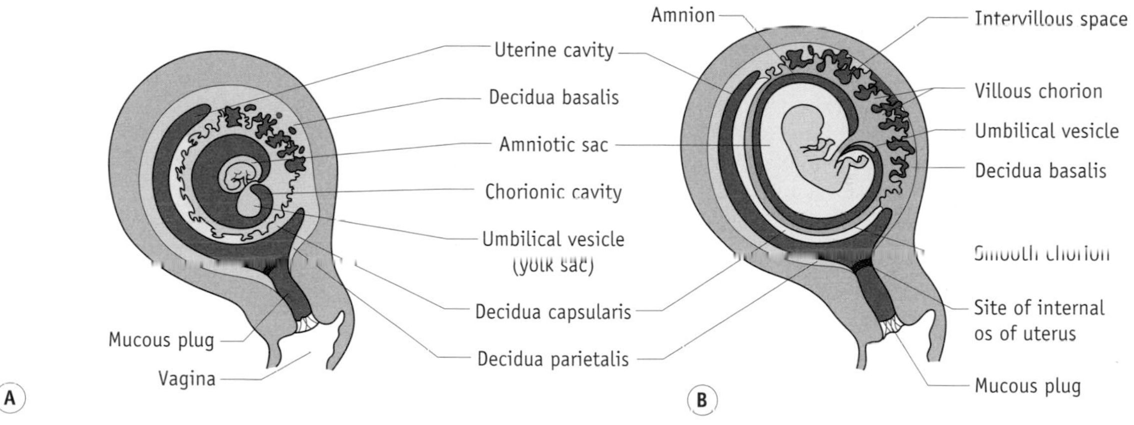


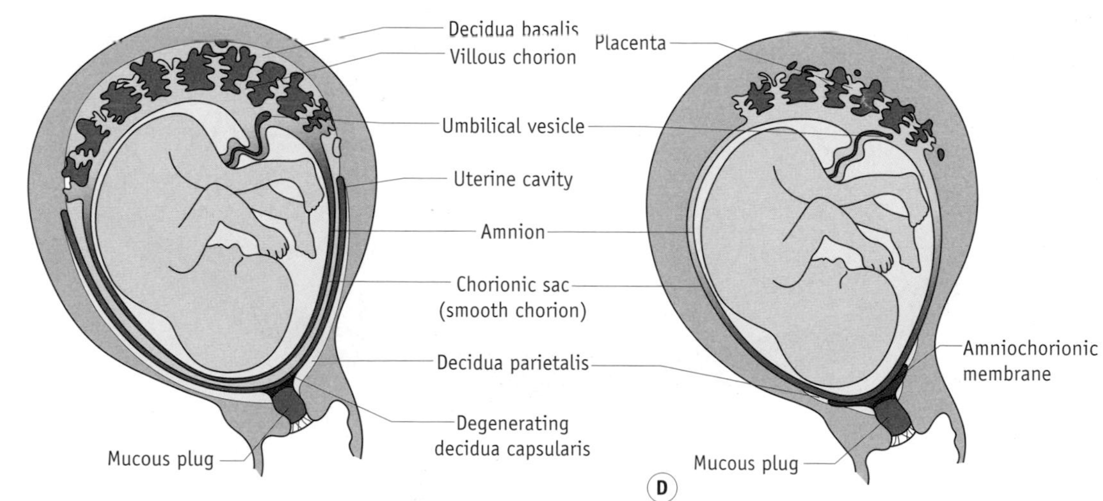


**Figure 29.11** Diagram illustrating changes within compartments of the gestational sac and the changing relations of membranes to the decidua from 12 to 22 weeks' gestation. *(Reproduced with permission from Moore and Persaud 2008:112; Fig. 7-1D–F.)*

- Produces a number of enzymes that degrade locally synthesized molecules including prostaglandins, oxytocin and platelet-activating factor, and brain natriuretic peptide (BNP) which inhibits oxytocin-induced contractility (Carvajal et al 2009). In this way, the chorion protects the myometrium from direct exposure to contractile forces during pregnancy (Erwich & Keirse 1992).

## THE DEFINITIVE PLACENTA

As villi of the chorion laeve disappear, those attached to the decidua basalis rapidly develop to form the *mature placenta*. The cytotrophoblast shell extends laterally and penetrates deeper into maternal tissue between the anchoring villi, and increasingly complex branching villi extend in the intervillous space. Each stem villus forms the centre of the villous tree. Fetal arterioles carrying poorly oxygenated blood enter the villi and break up into an extensive arteriocapillary–venous network. The 60–70 branching villi that make up the mature placenta provide a large surface area for gaseous and metabolic exchange between fetal blood within the villi and maternal blood circulating slowly around the external surface from the intervillous space (Sheppard & Bonnar 1989) (see Fig. 29.12). (See Reflective activity Web 29.1).

## FETAL OXYGEN REQUIREMENTS

While intraplacental and fetal concentrations of oxygen increase significantly from the end of the first trimester, a $Po_2$ gradient of 13.3 mmHg persists between placenta and decidua at 16 weeks' gestation and $Po_2$, $O_2$ saturation and $O_2$ content gradients are present between fetal blood and placenta, and between placental and underlying maternal tissues (Jauniaux et al 2003). Low fetal blood $Po_2$, and $O_2$ saturation have also been found in the third trimester (Jauniaux et al 2001). The highest oxygen content is in the umbilical vein, which is 30–35 mmHg and 80–90% saturated. By the time blood reaches the left atrium, $O_2$ content has fallen to 26–28 mmHg and lower concentrations supply the lungs and lower body

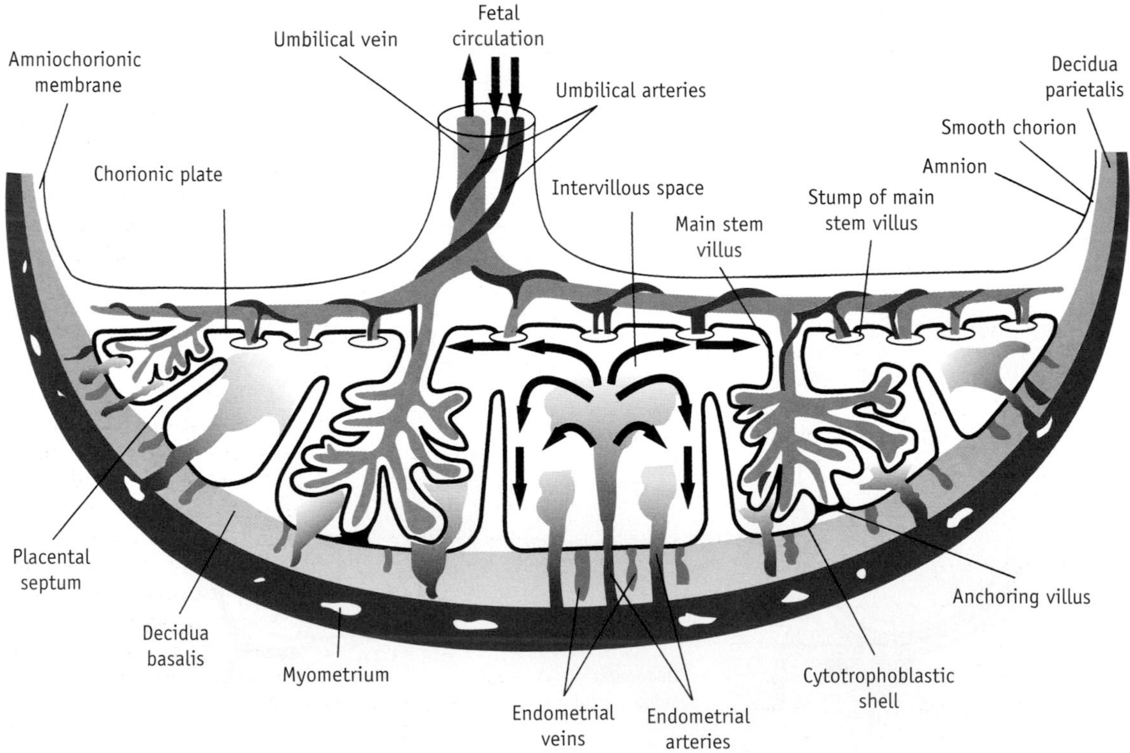


**Figure 29.12** Schematic drawing of a transverse section through a full-term placenta showing the fetoplacental and maternal–placental circulation. *(Reproduced with permission Moore & Persaud 2008:116; Fig. 7-7.)*

(Blackburn 2007). With homeostatic functions performed by maternal and placental systems, the fetus is therefore fully adapted to an aqueous environment with significantly lower oxygen concentrations than those required by maternal and placental tissues.

## FETAL REGULATION OF AMNIOTIC FLUID VOLUME

Until about 20 weeks, the dynamics of amniotic fluid volume are thought to involve a significant transmembrane pathway from maternal blood via the placenta and movement of fluid and other molecules across the fetal skin, offering no impediment to the flow of fluid into the amniotic sac. From 17 to 25 weeks' gestation, this pattern of flow diminishes, as the fetal skin begins to keratinize. During the second half of pregnancy, the fetal kidneys, lungs, gastrointestinal system and circulation make a growing contribution to the volume and circulation of amniotic fluid.

Volume increases from approximately 350–450 mL at 20 weeks, to 700–1000 mL at 36–39 weeks, and then begins to decline (Moore & Persaud 2008). Estimates of daily volumes near term suggest that fetal urine contributes 500 mL, lung fluid 300–400 mL, and 400 mL is removed by fetal swallowing (Moore & Persaud 2008). The fluid passes into the fetal circulation and waste products cross the placental membrane and enter maternal blood in the intervillous space. Through these pathways the water content of amniotic fluid is changed approximately every 3 hours (Moore & Persaud 2008).

Mechanisms regulating amniotic fluid volume are poorly understood. During the second half of pregnancy, amniotic fluid is hypo osmolar compared to maternal and fetal plasma. This osmotic gradient would be expected to drive water from the amniotic cavity into the maternal and fetal circulations via the umbilical cord, placenta and membranes. However, the precise volumes that move through these pathways remain to be confirmed (Brace 1995, Gilbert et al 1991). (See website.)

## FUNCTIONS OF AMNIOTIC FLUID

This dynamic volume of fluid provides:

- essential space for symmetric, external growth and movements of the fetus, aiding muscular development of upper and lower limbs
- fetal lung development ability
- equalization of pressure exerted by uterine contractions, preventing compression of the umbilical vessels between the fetus and the uterine wall during fetal movements and contractions
- modulation of excessive overriding of the bones of the skull, protecting underlying cerebral membranes and blood vessels, as the head is moulded during descent and rotation in the pelvic cavity.

## FETO-PLACENTAL CIRCULATION

The fetus relies on the placenta for respiration, nutrition and excretion, and fetal blood circulates throughout the placenta to realize these requirements. Fetal circulation differs from adult circulation in that blood is oxygenated in the placenta and not in the lungs. This system requires:

- larger and more numerous red cells (6–7 million/ $mm^3$)
- higher haemoglobin content (20.7 g/dL) to pick up the maximum amount of oxygen
- a modified form of haemoglobin (HbF) which is active in the slightly more acid blood
- additional fetal structures:
  - ductus arteriosus
  - ductus venosus
  - foramen ovale
  - two hypogastric arteries.

The intrauterine circulation takes shape during early embryonic formation: umbilical veins bring oxygenated blood to the primitive heart from the *chorion frondosum; vitelline veins* return blood from the yolk sac; and *cardinal veins* return blood from the rest of the body. Blood enters the heart via the sinus venous and flows through a single atrium and ventricle. When the ventricle contracts, blood is pumped through the *bulbus cordis,* passes into the dorsal aorta and eventually returns to deliver waste products to the chorion (Moore & Persaud 2008).

During fetal life, the vascular system becomes more extensive as it parallels the increasing size and complexity of individual organs and tissues. Oxygenated blood returns from a greatly enlarged placenta, via the umbilical vein. Approximately 50% of this blood enters a hepatic microcirculation and later joins the inferior vena cava via the hepatic veins. The remaining blood passes directly to the inferior vena cava, through a shunt called the *ductus venosus*. Blood flow through this vascular bypass is thought to be regulated by a physiological sphincter that responds to changing volume in the umbilical vein and helps to protect the fetus from erratic fluctuations in blood pressure (Walker 1993).

In addition to well-oxygenated blood from the placenta, the inferior vena cava receives less-oxygenated blood from the abdomen, pelvis and lower limbs, representing more than 66% of total venous return. Before entering the heart, the inferior vena cava bifurcates into two channels: the foramen ovale links it to the left atrium and a small inlet links it to the right atrium. In the left atrium, the foramen ovale ends in a one-way valve that only permits blood flow from right to left. Flow patterns in the right atrium allow 50% of oxygenated blood returning from the placenta to be shunted to the left atrium. This right-to-left flow through the foramen ovale is maintained by the larger quantity and greater speed of blood flow from the inferior vena cava on the right, compared to that entering the left atrium via the pulmonary veins from the lungs. During fetal life, lung tissue *extracts* oxygen from the low circulating blood volume entering from the right ventricle and returns poorly oxygenated blood to the left atrium. Low venous return from the lungs is actively maintained by the exposure of pulmonary vessels to blood $Po_2$, which keeps them in a state of hypoxic vasoconstriction (Moore & Persaud 2008, Walker 1993).

A small volume of well-oxygenated blood from the inferior vena cava enters the right atrium. This is mixed with poorly oxygenated blood returning from the head via the superior vena cava, which mainly enters the right ventricle through the tricuspid valve. From the right ventricle, only 10% of blood enters the lungs via pulmonary arteries. The remaining 90% is diverted into the descending aorta via a muscular artery called the *ductus arteriosus*, which connects the main pulmonary artery to the aorta. Throughout fetal life, patency and therefore relaxation of this muscular artery is actively maintained by the low fetal $Po_2$, high circulating levels of $PGE_2$ and local release of $PGI_2$ (Amash et al 2009). As a result of this shunt, most blood leaving the right ventricle perfuses the lower body and the placenta (Moore & Persaud 2008, Walker 1993).

In the left atrium, the pulmonary component combines with a much larger volume of more highly oxygenated blood from the inferior vena cava. From the left atrium, blood passes into the left ventricle. A small amount of this blood supplies the heart, two-thirds leaves via the ascending aorta to perfuse the upper part of the body with highly oxygenated blood, while the remaining one-third flows through the aortic isthmus to the descending aorta and then to the lower body, and placenta (Walker 1993). Two hypogastric arteries convey deoxygenated blood to the placenta.

Shunting of blood on the venous side by the foramen ovale and on the arterial side by the ductus arteriosus are structural devices that enable the blood to bypass the lungs and be directed to the placenta. This large volume of poorly oxygenated blood returning to the placenta flows much more rapidly than the more highly oxygenated blood supplying the upper body. The rate of flow tends to be most rapid in the descending aorta. From this vessel, blood is directly pumped into the umbilical arteries and returns for gaseous exchange in the placenta (Walker 1993) (Fig. 29.13).

During intrauterine life, the fetal–placental circulation operates as a single unit, providing a low-resistance, high-capacity reservoir in the vascular bed of the placenta, maintained by the absence of valves in the umbilical veins. From animal experiments, total fetal–placental blood volume is estimated at 100–120 mL/kg body weight, with 80–90 mL/kg representing fetal blood volume at any given time, while the remainder is contained within the umbilical–placental circulation. This additional capacity helps to protect the fetal circulation from fluctuations in blood pressure and blood flow distribution at a time when autoregulation of regional blood flow is not fully developed.

## LUNG FORMATION

Around 24 days following conception, a pouch-like laryngotracheal diverticulum arises, as a small ventral protrusion from an area of the foregut, close to that which becomes the stomach (Blackburn 2007). Once formed, the foregut elongates, separating the emerging stomach from the section that gives rise to the lungs. From an initial protrusion, the lungs take shape through a series of bifurcations beginning with the emergence of right and left lobular buds corresponding in number to those in the mature organ.

Between **5 and 26 weeks' gestation**, these branch a further 16 times, to generate the respiratory trees. All bronchial airways are formed by 16 weeks and further growth proceeds by elongation and widening of existing airways. Towards the end of this phase, each terminal bronchiole divides into two or more respiratory bronchioles, while surrounding mesodermal tissues become highly vascularized.

From **26 weeks onwards**, respiratory bronchioles continually subdivide to produce approximately 20–70 million primitive alveoli that are vascularized by a dense network of capillaries (Moore & Persaud 2008) (Figs 29.14 and 29.15).

During fetal life, these potential air spaces are filled with liquid actively secreted by the pulmonary epithelium from the surrounding circulation. Experiments have found that the volume of liquid increases from 4–6 mL/kg body weight at mid-gestation, to more than 20 mL/kg body weight near term. This liquid expansion of potential air space maintains a small distending pressure in the lumen that approximates functional residual capacity of the aerated lung in the newborn. Lung fluid also assists in the formation of surfactant-producing epithelial cells that can be identified from approximately 24 weeks' gestation.

There are a successive series of development, from changes within the lining of the bronchioles, to prepare the lungs for extrauterine breathing and gaseous exchange. From 17 weeks, the cuboidal epithelial cells provide

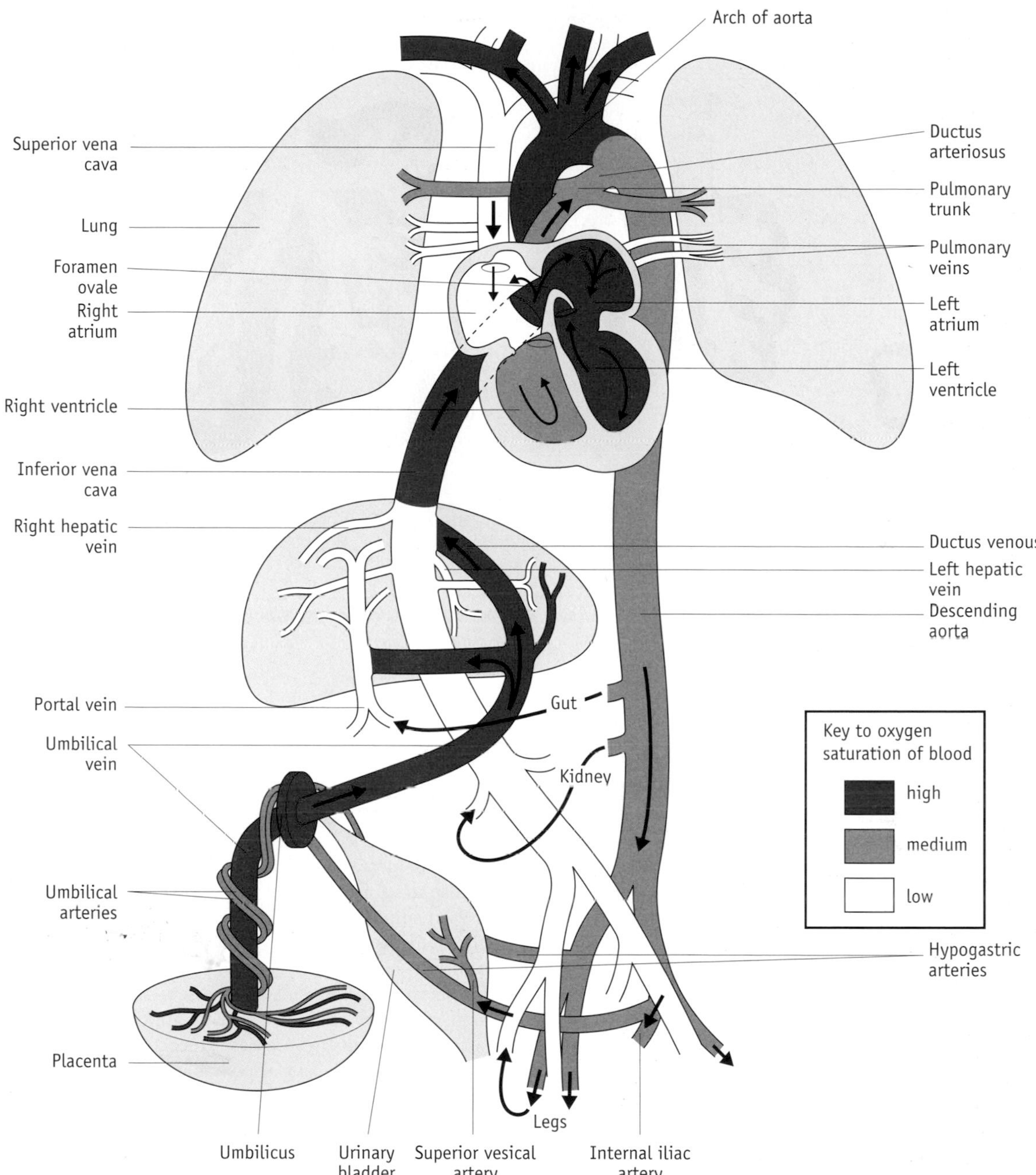


**Figure 29.13** Fetal circulation: colours indicate oxygen saturation of the blood and the arrows show the course of the blood from the placenta to the heart. *(Reproduced with permission from Moore & Persaud 2008:328; Fig. 13-46.)*

energy and act as precursors for the development of surfactant. Surfactant is crucial in reducing surface tension of the terminal sacs and stabilizing the membrane, which prevents lung collapsing following the onset of respiration (see Chapter 45 and see website for more information).

Intermittent breathing movements occur from approximately 11 weeks' gestation and from 24 weeks the pattern of this activity is integrated with circadian rhythms in heart rate, temperature, body movements and sleep that seem to be mediated by maternal melatonin which freely

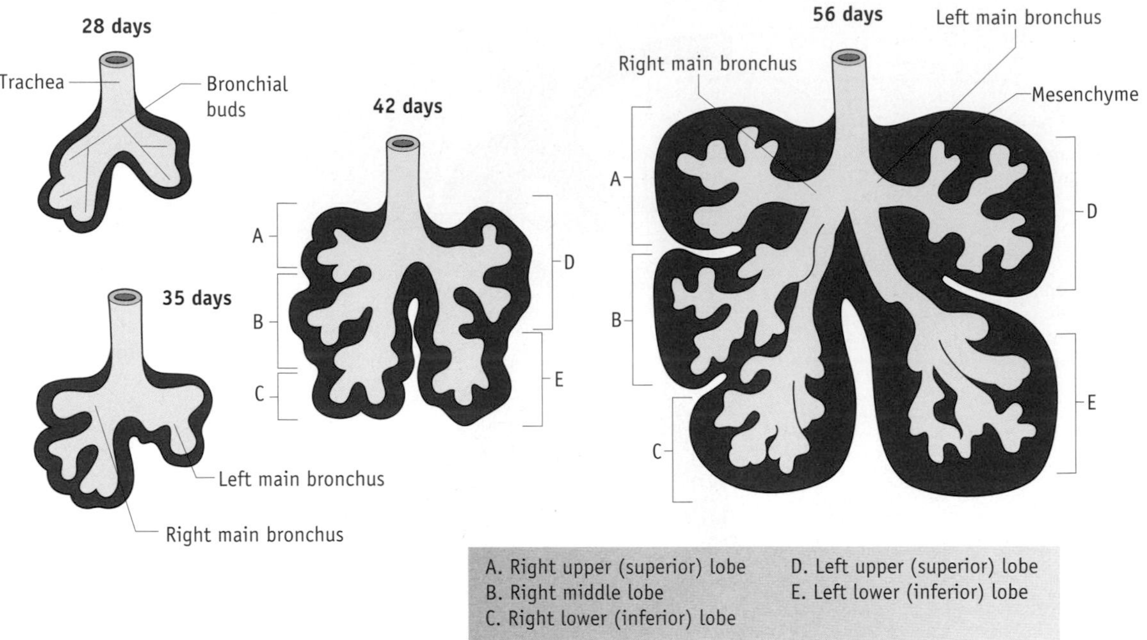


**Figure 29.14** Successive stages in development of the bronchial buds, bronchi and lungs. *(Reproduced with permission from Moore & Persaud 2008:203; Fig. 10-8.)*

crosses the placenta (Tamura et al 2008). These episodic breathing movements in utero stimulate the development of lung tissue and respiratory muscles and some experimental evidence suggests that they may increase cardiac output and blood flow to vital organs including the heart, brain and placenta. Rhythmic breathing movements are regulated by brainstem adrenergic respiratory neural networks, and adrenaline from the adrenal medualla (see website).

## Hormonal regulation of lung development and maturation

Differentiation of type II pneumocytes and production of surfactant are closely associated with increasing levels of different hormones within the fetal circulation, particularly cortisol, oestrogens, adrenaline, hPL, prolactin, triiodothyronine ($T_3$) and placental CRH (see website).

## CENTRAL ROLE OF THE ADRENAL CORTEX AND PLACENTA

Steroidogenic enzymes are present in the emerging adrenal cortex from 6–7 weeks' gestation. Synthesis of the main hormones, dehydroepiandrosterone (DHEA) and its sulphate (DHEA-S), and pregnenolone sulphate, begins from 6 weeks' gestation, while cortisol synthesis occurs between 7 and 12 weeks' gestation (Goto et al 2006, Kempna & Fluck 2008, Tsakiri et al 2002).

From 8–10 weeks' onwards, DHEA-S and pregnenolone sulphate are increasingly utilized by the placenta, as essential substrates for formation of oestrogens and progesterone (Pasqualini 2005). Transfer of maternal glucocorticoids to the fetus is regulated by a placental glucocortical 'barrier'.

Regulatory mechanisms are essential to stimulate normal placental and fetal growth and protect rapidly growing fetal organs from excess glucocorticoid exposure (Wyrwoll et al 2009). This also enables the preparation of intrauterine tissues and fetal organs for the transition from pregnancy to labour (see website).

## DEVELOPMENT OF THE ADRENAL CORTEX

The significance of the adrenal glands is indicated by their spectacular growth and secretory capacity during intrauterine life. Cells forming the cortex appear at 3–4 weeks' gestation and enlarge rapidly to equal the size of the

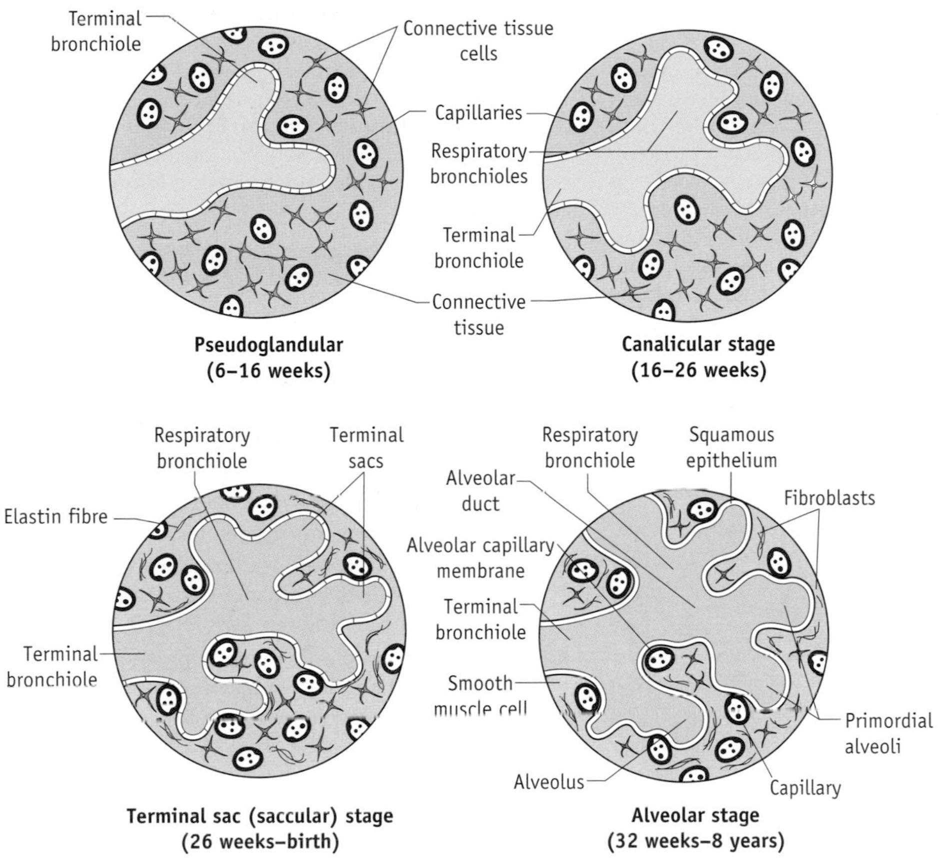


**Figure 29.15** Diagrammatic sketches of histologic sections illustrating stages of lung development from 6 weeks to 8 years. *(Reproduced with permission from Moore & Persaud 2008:204; Fig. 10-9B–D.)*

kidneys by the end of the first trimester. By 6 8 weeks' gestation, the cortex forms two distinct zones: a large inner fetal zone, an outer definitive zone that forms a thin subcapsular rim, and an indistinct transitional area between the two (Goto et al 2006, Tsakiri et al 2002). During the second trimester, the adrenals enlarge in direct proportion to the increase in total body weight. At this time, their relative weight is 35 times the adult value. In the third trimester, gland weights continue to increase but at a slower rate than the rest of the body. At term, the fetal adrenals are similar in size to those in the adult (Pearson Murphy & Branchaud 1994, Seron-Ferre & Jaffe 1981) (see website).

Adrenal growth seems to be largely regulated by hCG, ACTH, oestradiol, prolactin, melatonin and growth factors derived from within the glands, along with those from other fetal organs, including the placenta, liver and kidneys (Freemark et al 1997, Tsakiri et al 2002). Until the latter part of pregnancy, the active steroid-producing fetal zone is predominantly involved in synthesizing DHEA-S, for the placenta (Pepe & Albrecht 1990). During the last 3 months of pregnancy, maternal melatonin stimulates adrenal weight gain and synthesis of DHEA-S, while at the same time negatively regulates the process of maturation by inhibiting ACTH- and CRH-induced production of cortisol.

## ADRENAL MEDULLA

In contrast to the cortex, the chromaffin cells are formed from adjacent sympathetic ganglia that are derived from the neural crest. Unlike the cortex, this part of the gland does not become a discrete structure during fetal life. During this period, small islands of chromaffin cells are scattered throughout the cortex and larger and much more active islets form independently of the medulla, along the outside of the aorta (Mesiano & Jaffe 1997). Immature chromaffin cells have been observed from approximately 8 weeks and significant concentrations of noradrenaline have been found from 15 weeks' gestation. No degeneration has been found to occur in these cells until the postnatal period (Phillippe 1983).

Within the adrenal gland, small groups of cells containing measurable amounts of noradrenaline have been observed at 9 weeks but their content remains low until the third trimester. While noradrenaline remains predominant in the fetal response to stress, the rising capacity for cortisol production near term produces a sharp increase in the capacity of chromaffin cells to produce adrenaline. The proportion of adrenaline increases progressively from approximately 28 weeks to term, when it constitutes around 50% of total catecholamine content of the gland. As measured in amniotic fluid, catecholamine metabolites increase between the second and third trimester and plasma catecholamine concentrations rise progressively during the course of labour. These changes mediate a range of cardiovascular, metabolic and respiratory responses to labour and birth (Lagercrantz & Marcus 1992, Lagercrantz & Slotkin 1986, Phillippe 1983).

## CONCLUSION

Conditions required for implantation and formation of the distinct biological environments for embryonic and fetal formation and growth begin during the luteal phase of the cycle. The presence of the conceptus is established by hormonal communications which accelerate adaptations in central and peripheral maternal systems.

The midwife can use this knowledge to identify distinct changes that coincide with embryo formation and fetoplacental development and enhance the woman's understanding of what is unfolding to support information and advice provided.

### KEY POINTS

- Fertilization requires fusion of a healthy oocyte–cumulus complex and one out of thousands of spermatazoa, within a tight timespan.
- The process of successful fertilization,implantation and placental formation commences during the luteal phase of the cycle.
- Optimal conditions for early embryonic formation are characterized by low oxygen tension.
- The first weeks following fertilization are a time of intense local activity as organogenesis takes place, and the major organ systems are formed.
- At the end of fetoplacental development, maturational changes have taken place in organs like the lungs and liver, while the HPA axis is briefly activated to regulate the onset of labour.

## REFERENCES


Alberts B, Johnson A, Lewis J, et al: *Molecular biology of the cell*, New York, 2002, Taylor & Francis.

Amash A, Holcberg G, Sheiner E, et al: Lipopolysaccharide differently affects prostaglandin $E_2$ levels in fetal and maternal compartments of perfused human term placenta, *Prostaglandins and other Lipid Mediators* 88:18–22, 2009.

Ambrus G, Rao CV: Novel regulation of pregnant human myometrial smooth muscle cell gap junctions by human chorionic gonadotrophin, *Endocrinology* 135(6):2772–2779, 1994.

Armant DR: Blastocysts don't go it alone. Extrinsic signals fine-tune the intrinsic development program of trophoblast cells, *Developmental Biology* 280:260–280, 2005.

Bahat A, Tur-Kaspa I, Gakamsky A, et al: Thermotaxis of mammalian sperm cells: a potential navigation mechanism in the female genital tract, *Nature Medicine* 9(2):149–151, 2003.

Battista N, Pasquariello N, Di Tomaso M, et al: Interplay between endocannabinoids, steroids and cytokines in the control of human reproduction, *Journal of Neuroendocrinology* 20(Suppl 1):82–89, 2008.

Bell RJ, Eddie LW, Lester AR, et al: Relaxin in human pregnancy serum measured with a homologous radioimmunoassay, *Obstetrics and Gynecology* 69:585–589, 1987.

Blackburn ST: *Maternal fetal & neonatal physiology*, Missouri, 2007, Saunders.

Brace RA: Current topic: progress toward understanding the regulation of amniotic fluid volume: water and solute fluxes in and through the fetal membranes, *Placenta* 16:1–18, 1995.

Burton GJ, Hempstock J, Jauniaux E: Nutrition, genetics and placental development, *Placenta* 22(Suppl A):S70–S76, 2001.

Burton GJ, Watson AL, Hempstock J, et al: Uterine glands provide histotrophic nutrition for the human fetus during the first trimester of pregnancy, *Journal of Clinical Endocrinology and Metabolism* 87(6):2954–2959, 2002.

Burton GJ, Kaufmann P, Huppertz B: Anatomy and genesis of the placenta. In Neill JD, editor: *Knobil and Neill's Physiology of Reproduction*, Amsterdam, 2006, Elsevier.

Burton GJ, Jauniaux E, Charnock-Jones DS: Human early placental development: potential roles of the endometrial glands, *Placenta* 28(Suppl A):S64–S69, 2007.

Burton GJ, Woods AW, Jauniaux E, et al: Rheological and physiological consequences of conversion of the maternal spiral arteries for uteroplacental blood flow during human pregnancy, *Placenta* 30:473–482, 2009.

Calvo RM, Jauniaux E, Gulbis B, et al: Fetal tissues are exposed to biologically relevant free thyroxine concentrations during early phases of development, *Journal of Clinical Endocrinology and Metabolism* 87(4):1768–1777, 2002.

Cameo P, Srisuparp S, Strakova Z, et al: Chorionic gonadotrophin and uterine dialogue in primates, *Reproductive Biology and Endocrinology* 2:50, 2004.

Caniggia I, Winter JL: Hypoxia inducible factor-1: oxygen regulation of trophoblast differentiation in normal and pre-eclamptic pregnancies – a review, *Placenta* 23(Suppl A):S47–S57, 2002.

Caniggia I, Mostachfi H, Winter J, et al: Hypoxia-inducible factor-1 mediates the biological effects of oxygen on human trophoblast differentiation through TGF$\beta_3$, *Journal of Clinical Investigation* 105(5):577–587, 2000.

Carlson BM: *Human embryology and developmental biology*, St Louis, 1994, Mosby.

Carvajal JA, Delpiano AM, Cuello MA, et al: Brain natriuretic peptide (BNP) produced by human chorioamnion may mediate pregnancy myometrial quiescence, *Reproductive Sciences* 16(1):32–42, 2009.

Casan EM, Raga F, Polan ML: GnRH mRNA and protein expression in human preimplantation embryos, *Molecular Human Reproduction* 5(3):234–239, 1999.

Casan EM, Raga F, Bonilla-Musoles F, et al: Human oviductal gonadotrophin-releasing hormone: possible implication in fertilization, early embryonic development, and implantation, *Journal of Clinical Endocrinology and Metabolism* 85(4):1377–1381, 2000.

Chamberlain G, Broughton Pipkin F: *Clinical physiology in obstetrics*, Oxford, 1998, Blackwell Scientific.

Chapman AB, Zamudio S, Woodmansee W, et al: Systemic and renal hemodynamic changes in the luteal phase of the menstrual cycle mimic early pregnancy, *American Journal of Physiology* 273(42):F777–F782, 1997.

Chard T, Iles R, Wathen N: Why is there a peak of human chorionic gonadotrophin (HCG) in early pregnancy? *Human Reproduction* 10(7):1837–1840, 1995.

Cootauco AC, Murphy JD, Maleski J, et al: Atrial natriuretic peptide production and natriuretic peptide receptors in the human uterus and their effects on myometrial relaxation, *American Journal of Obstetrics and Gynecology* 199:429.e1–429.e6, 2008.

Davison JM, Shiells EA, Phillips PR, et al: Influence of hormonal and volume factors on altered osmoregulation of normal human pregnancy, *American Journal of Physiology* 258(27):F900–F907, 1990.

De Swiet M: The cardiovascular system. In Hytten F, Chamberlain G, editors: *Clinical physiology in obstetrics*, Oxford, 1991, Blackwell Scientific.

Douglas AJ: Baby on board: do responses to stress in the maternal brain mediate adverse pregnancy outcome? *Frontiers in Neuroendocrinology* 31(3):359–376, 2010.

Downs KM: Embryological origins of the human individual, *DNA and Cell Biology* 27(1):3–7, 2008.

Drobnis EZ, Overstreet JW: Natural history of mammalian spermatozoa in the female reproductive tract, *Oxford Reviews of Reproductive Biology* 14:1–45, 1992.

Dunstan GR, editor: *The human embryo*, Exeter, 1990, University of Exeter Press.

Ellery PM, Cindrova-Davies T, Jauniaux E, et al: Evidence for transcriptional activity in the synctiotrophoblast of the human placenta, *Placenta* 30:329–334, 2009.

Erwich JJHM, Keirse MJMC: Placental localisation of 15-hydroxyprostaglandin dehydrogenase in early and term pregnancy, *Placenta* 13:223–229, 1992.

Evans JP: The molecular basis of sperm–oocyte membrane interactions during mammalian fertilization, *Human Reproduction Update* 8(4):297–311, 2002.

Ferretti C, Bruni L, Dangles-Marie V, et al: Molecular circuits shared by placental and cancer cells, and their implications in the proliferative, invasive and migratory capacities of trophoblasts, *Human Reproduction Update* 13(2):121–141, 2007.

FitzGerald MJT, FitzGerald M: *Human embryology*, London, 1994, Baillière Tindall.

Fitzgerald JS, Poehlmann TG, Schleussner E, et al: Trophoblast invasion: the role of intracellular cytokine signalling via signal transducer and activator of transcription 3 (STAT3), *Human Reproduction Update* 14(4):335–344, 2008.

Fleming TP, Kwong WY, Poorter R, et al: The embryo and its future, *Biology of Reproduction* 71:1046–1054, 2004.

Freemark M: The fetal adrenal and the maturation of the growth hormone and prolactin axes, *Endocrinology* 140(5):1963–1965, 1999.

Freemark M, Driscoll P, Maaskant R, et al: Ontogenesis of prolactin receptors in the human fetus in early gestation, *Journal of Clinical Investigation* 99(5):1107–1117, 1997.

Fride E: Multiple roles for the endocannabinoid system during the early stages of life: pre- and postnatal development, *Journal of Neuroendocrinology* 20(s1):75–81, 2008.

Gargett CE, Lederman F, Heryonto B, et al: Focal vascular endothelial growth factor correlates with angiogenesis in human endometrium. Role of intravascular neutrophils, *Human Reproduction* 16(6):1065–1075, 2001.

Gilbert WM, Moore TR, Brace RA: Amniotic fluid volume dynamics, *Fetal Medicine Review* 3:89–104, 1991.

Glock JL, Nakajima ST, Stewart DR, et al: The relationship of corpus luteum volume to relaxin, estradiol, progesterone and human chorionic gonadotrophin levels in early normal pregnancy, *Early Pregnancy: Biology and Medicine* 1:206–211, 1995.

Goto M, Hanley KP, Marcos J, et al: In humans, early cortisol biosynthesis provides a mechanism to safeguard female sexual development, *Journal of Clinical Investigation* 116(4):953–960, 2006.

Gubbay O, Critchley HO, D Bowen JM, et al: Prolactin induces ERK phosphorylation in epithelial and CD56$^+$ natural killer cells of the human endometrium, *Journal of Clinical Endocrinology and Metabolism* 87(5):2329–2335, 2002.

Habayeb OMH, Taylor AH, Bell SC, et al: Expression of endocannabinoid system in human first trimester placenta and its role in trophoblast proliferation, *Endocrinology* 149(10):5052–5060, 2008.

Handschuh K, Guibourdenche J, Tsatsaris V, et al: Human chorionic gonadotrophin expression in human trophoblasts from early placenta: comparative study between villous and extravillous trophoblastic cells, *Placenta* 28:175–184, 2007.

Hunter RHF: *The fallopian tubes*, Berlin, 1988, Springer-Verlag.

Hustin J: The maternotrophoblast interface: uteroplacental blood flow. In Barnea ER, Hustin J, Jauniaux E, editors: *The first twelve weeks of gestation*, Berlin, 1992, Springer-Verlag.

Hustin J, Franchimont P: The endometrium and implantation. In Barnea ER, Hustin J, Jauniaux E, editors: *The first twelve weeks of gestation*, Berlin, 1992, Springer-Verlag.

Hustin J, Schaaps J-P: Echocardiographic and anatomic studies of the maternotrophoblast border during the first trimester of pregnancy, *American Journal of Obstetrics and Gynecology* 157(1):162–168, 1987.

Hustin J, Schaaps J-P, Lambotte R: Anatomical studies of the utero-placental vascularization in the first trimester of pregnancy, *Trophoblast Research* 3:49–60, 1988.

Iskaros J, Pickard M, Evans I, et al: Thyroid hormone receptor gene expression in first trimester human fetal brain, *Journal of Clinical Endocrinology and Metabolism* 85(7):2620–2623, 2000.

Islami D, Bischof P, Chardonnens D: Modulation of placental vascular endothelial growth factor by leptin and hCG, *Molecular Human Reproduction* 9(7):395–398, 2003.

Jabbour HN, Critchley HOD: Potential roles of decidual prolactin in early pregnancy, *Reproduction* 121:197–205, 2001.

Jauniaux E, Gulbis B: Embryonic physiology. In Jauniaux E, Barnea ER, Edwards RG, editors: *Embryonic medicine and therapy*, Oxford, 1997, Oxford University Press.

Jauniaux E, Gulbis B: In vivo investigation of placental transfer early in human pregnancy, *European Journal of Obstetrics and Gynecology and Reproductive Biology* 92:45–49, 2000.

Jauniaux E, Moscoso JG: Morphology and significance of the human yolk sac. In Barnea ER, Hustin J, Jauniaux E, editors: *The first twelve weeks of gestation*, Berlin, 1992, Springer-Verlag.

Jauniaux E, Gulbis B, Jurkovic D, et al: Protein and steroid levels in embryonic cavities in early human pregnancy, *Human Reproduction* 8(5):782–787, 1993.

Jauniaux E, Gulbis B, Jurkovic D, et al: Relationship between protein concentrations in embryological fluids and maternal serum and yolk sac size during human early pregnancy, *Human Reproduction* 9(1):161–166, 1994.

Jauniaux E, Watson AL, Hempstock J, et al: Onset of maternal arterial blood flow and placental oxidative stress, *American Journal of Pathology* 157(6):2111–2122, 2000.

Jauniaux E, Wilson A, Burton G: Evaluation of respiratory gases and acid-base gradients in human fetal fluids and uteroplacental tissue between 7 and 16 weeks' gestation, *American Journal of Obstetrics and Gynecology* 184(5):998–1003, 2001.

Jauniaux E, Gulbis B, Burton GJ: The human first trimester gestational sac limits rather than facilitates oxygen transfer to the foetus – a review, *Placenta* 24(Suppl A):S86–S93, 2003.

Jauniaux E, Cindrova-Davies T, Johns J, et al: Distribution and transfer pathways of antioxidant molecules inside the first trimester human gestational sac, *Journal of Clinical Endocrinology and Metabolism* 89(3):1452–1458, 2004.

Johnson MH: *Essential reproduction*, ed 6, Oxford, 2007, Blackwell Scientific.

Jones CJP: The life and death of the embryonic yolk sac. In Jauniaux E, Barnea ER, Edwards RG, editors: *Embryonic medicine and therapy*, Oxford, 1997, Oxford University Press.

Kaji K, Kudo A: The mechanism of sperm-oocyte fusion in mammals, *Reproduction* 127:423–429, 2004.

Kancheva R, Hill M, Cibula D, et al: Relationships of circulating pregnanolone isomers and their polar conjugates to the status of sex, menstrual cycle, and pregnancy, *Journal of Endocrinology* 195:67–78, 2007.

Kempna P, Fluck CE: Adrenal gland development and defects, *Best Practice & Research Clinical Endocrinology & Metabolism* 22(1):77–93, 2008.

Kikkawa F, Kajiyama H, Watanabe Y, et al: Possible involvement of placental peptidases that degrade gonadotrophin-releasing hormone(GnRH) in the dynamic pattern of placental hCG secretion via GnRH degradation, *Placenta* 23:483–489, 2002.

King AE, Critchley HO, Kelly RW: The NF-kappaβ pathway in human endometrium and first trimester decidua, *Molecular Human Reproduction* 7:175–183, 2001.

Kosaka K, Fujiwara H, Tatsumi K, et al: Human chorionic gonadotrophin (HCG) activates monocytes to produce interleukin-8 via a different pathway from luteinizing hormone/HCG receptor system, *Journal of Clinical Endocrinology and Metabolism* 87(11):5199–5208, 2002.

Kristiansson P, Wang JX: Reproductive hormones and blood pressure during pregnancy, *Human Reproduction* 16(1):13–17, 2001.

Kunz G, Noe M, Herbertz M, et al: Uterine peristalsis during the follicular phase of the menstrual cycle: effects of oestrogen, antioestrogen and oxytocin, *Human Reproduction Update* 4(5):647–654, 1998.

Lacroix M-C, Guibourdenche J, Fournier T, et al: Stimulation of human trophoblast invasion by placental growth hormone, *Endocrinology* 146(5):2434–2444, 2005.

Lagercrantz H, Marcus C: Sympathoadrenal mechanisms during development. In Polin RA, Fox WW, editors: *Fetal and neonatal physiology*, Philadelphia, 1992, Saunders.

Lagercrantz H, Slotkin TA: The 'stress' of being born, *Scientific American* 254:92–102, 1986.

Lapointe J, Kimmins S, McLaren LA, et al: Estrogen selectively up-regulates the phospholipid hydroperoxide glutathione peroxidase in the oviducts, *Endocrinology* 146(6):2583–2592, 2005.

Leese HJ: Metabolic control during preimplantation mammalian development, *Human Reproduction* 1(1):63–72, 1995.

Leese HJ, Tay JI, Reischi J, et al: Formation of fallopian tubal fluid: role of a neglected epithelium, *Reproduction* 121:339–346, 2001.

Lei ZM, Rao CV, Kornyei JL, et al: Novel expression of human chorionic gonadotrophin/luteinizing hormone receptor gene in brain, *Endocrinology* 132(5):2262–2270, 1993.

Leppens-Luisier G, Urner F, Sakkas D: Facilitated glucose transporters play a crucial role throughout mouse preimplantation embryo development, *Human Reproduction* 16(6):1229–1236, 2001.

Lessey BA: The role of the endometrium during embryo implantation, *Human Reproduction* 15(Suppl 6):39–50, 2000.

Liggins GC: The role of cortisol in preparing the fetus for birth, *Reproduction Fertility and Development* 6:141–150, 1994.

Lopata A, Oliva K, Stanton PG, et al: Analysis of chorionic gonadotrophin secreted by cultured human blastocysts, *Molecular Human Reproduction* 3(6):517–521, 1997.

Ma W, Tan J, Matsumoto H, et al: Adult tissue angiogenesis: evidence for negative regulation by estrogen in the uterus, *Molecular Endocrinology* 15(11):1983–1992, 2001.

Mark PJ, Smith JT, Waddell BJ: Placental and fetal growth retardation following partial progesterone withdrawal in rat pregnancy, *Placenta* 27:208–214, 2006.

Mesiano S, Jaffe RB: Development and functional biology of the primate fetal adrenal cortex, *Endocrine Reviews* 18(3):378–403, 1997.

Mesiano S, Jaffe RB: Human fetal adrenal cortical function in pregnancy and parturition, *Current Problems in Obstetrics, Gynaecology and Fertility* (Nov/Dec):199–220, 1999.

Moore KL, Persaud TVN: *The developing human*, Philadelphia, 2008, Saunders.

Muller-Schottle F, Classen-Linke I, Alfer J, et al: Expression of uteroglobin in the human endometrium, *Molecular Human Reproduction* 5(12):1155 1161, 1999.

Muyan M, Boime I: Secretion of chorionic gonadotrophin from human trophoblasts, *Placenta* 18:237–241, 1997.

Nagy A-M, Glinoer D, Picelli G, et al: Total amounts of circulating human gonadotrophin α and β subunits can be assessed throughout human pregnancy using immunoradiometric assays calibrated with the unaltered and thermally dissociated heterodimer, *Journal of Endocrinology* 140:513–520, 1994.

Oon VJG, Johnson MR: The regulation of the human corpus luteum steroidogenesis: a hypothesis? *Human Reproduction Update* 6(5):519–529, 2000.

Pasqualini JR: Enzymes involved in the formation and transformation of steroid hormones in the fetal and placental compartments, *Journal of Steroid Biochemistry and Molecular Biology* 97:401–415, 2005.

Pearson Murphy BE, Branchaud CL: The fetal adrenal. In Tulchinsky D, Little BA, editors: *Maternal–fetal endocrinology*, Philadelphia, 1994, Saunders.

Pepe GJ, Albrecht ED: Regulation of the primate fetal adrenal cortex, *Endocrine Reviews* 11(1):151–176, 1990.

Phillippe M: Fetal catecholamines, *American Journal of Obstetrics and Gynecology* 146(7):840–855, 1983.

Phillips RJ, Tyson-Capper AJ (nee Pollard), Bailey J, et al: Regulation of expression of the chorionic gonadotrophin/luteinizing hormone receptor gene in the human myometrium: involvement of specific protein-1 (Sp1), Sp3, Sp4, Sp-like proteins, and histone deacetylases, *Journal of Clinical Endocrinology and Metabolism* 90(6):3479–3490, 2005.

Pijnenborg R, Vercruysse L, Hanssens M: The uterine spiral arteries in human pregnancy: facts and controversies, *Placenta* 27:939–958, 2006.

Ramsey EM, Houston ML, Harris JW: Interaction of the trophoblast and maternal tissues in three closely related primate species, *American Journal of Obstetrics and Gynecology* 124(6):647–652, 1976.

Rodway MR, Rao CV: A novel perspective on the role of human chorionic gonadotrophin during pregnancy and in gestational trophoblastic disease, *Early Pregnancy: Biology and Medicine* 1:176–187, 1995.

Santoro N, Goldsmith LT, Weiss G: Hormone interactions of the corpus luteum. In Barnea ER, Cheek JH, Grudzinskas JG, et al, editors: *Implantation and early pregnancy in humans*, New York, 1994, Parthenon.

Schultz RM: Blastocyst. In Knobil E, Neill JD, editors: *Encyclopedia of Reproduction*, Vol 1, San Diego, 1998, Academic Press.

Seppala M, Taylor RN, Koistinen H, et al: Glycodelin: a major lipocalin protein of the reproductive axis with diverse actions in cell recognition and differentiation, *Endocrine Reviews* 23(4):401–430, 2002.

Seron-Ferre M, Jaffe RB: The fetal adrenal gland, *Annual Review of Physiology* 43:141–162, 1981.

Shafik A, Shafik AA, El Sibai O, et al: Specialized pacemaking cells in the human fallopian tube, *Molecular Human Reproduction* 11(7):503–505, 2005.

Sheppard BI, Bonnar J: The maternal blood supply to the placenta, *Progress in Obstetrics and Gynaecology* 7:27–30, 1989.

Simmons DM, Voss JW, Ingraham HA, et al: Pituitary cell phenotypes involve cell-specific Pit-1 mRNA translation and synergistic interactions with other classes of transcription factors, *Genes and Development* 4:695–711, 1990.

Simon C, Gimeno J, Mercader A, et al: Embryonic regulation of $\beta_3$, $\alpha_4$ and $\alpha_1$ in human endometrial cells in vitro, *Journal of Clinical Endocrinology and Metabolism* 82(8):2607–2616, 1997.

Starkey PM: The decidua and factors controlling placentation. In Redman CWG, Sargent IL, Starkey PM, editors: *The human placenta*, Oxford, 1993, Blackwell Scientific.

Strauss J, Coutifaris C: The endometrium and myometrium: regulation and dysfunction. In Yen SSC, Jaffe RB, Barbieri RL, editors: *Reproductive endocrinology*, Philadelphia, 1999, Saunders.

Symonds ME, Phillips ID, Antrhony RV, et al: Prolactin receptor gene expression and fetal adipose tissue, *Journal of Neuroendocrinology* 10:885–890, 1998.

Talbot PD, Shur BD, Myles DG: Cell adhesion and fertilization: steps in oocyte transport, sperm-zona pellucida interactions, and sperm-egg fusion, *Biology of Reproduction* 68:1–9, 2003.

Tamura H, Nakamura Y, Terron MP, et al: Melatonin and pregnancy in the human, *Reproductive Toxicology* 25:291–303, 2008.

Tarrade A, Kuen RL, Malassine A, et al: Characterization of human villous and extravillous trophoblasts isolated from first trimester placenta, *Laboratory Investigation* 81(9):1199–1211, 2001.

Telgmann R, Gellersen B: Marker genes of decidualisation: activation of the decidual prolactin gene, *Human Reproduction Update* 4:472–479, 1998.

Ticconi C, Zicari A, Belmonte A, et al: Pregnancy-promoting actions of HCG in human myometrium, and fetal membranes, *Placenta* 28(Suppl A):S137–S143, 2007.

Tosti E, Boni R: Electrical events during gamete maturation and fertilization in animals and humans, *Human Reproduction Update* 10(1):53–65, 2004.

Tsakiri SP, Chrousos GP, Margioris AN: Molecular development of the hypothalamic-pituitary-adrenal (HPA) axis. In Eugster EA, Pescovitz OH, editors: *Developmental endocrinology*, Totowa, NJ, 2002, Humana Press.

Tseng L, Zhu HH, Mazella J, et al: Relaxin stimulates glycodelin mRNA and protein concentrations in human endometrial glandular epithelial cells, *Molecular Human Reproduction* 5(4):372–375, 1999.

Vokes TJ, Weiss NM, Schreiber J, et al: Osmoregulation of thirst and vasopressin during normal menstrual cycle, *American Journal of Physiology* 254(23):R641–R647, 1988.

Walker AM: Circulatory transitions at birth and the control of neonatal circulation. In Hanson MA, Spencer JAD, Rodeck CH, editors: *Fetus and neonate: physiology and clinical applications, Vol 1, The circulation*, Cambridge, 1993, Cambridge University Press, pp 160–196.

Wang H, Guo Y, Wang D, et al: Aberrant cannabinoid signalling impairs oviduct transport of embryos, *Nature Medicine* 10(10):1074–1080, 2004.

Wang H, Xie H, Guo Y, et al: Fatty acid amide hydrolase deficiency limits early pregnancy events, *Journal of Clinical Investigation* 116(8):2122–2131, 2006.

Wildt L, Kissler S, Licht P, et al: Sperm transport in the human female genital tract and its modulation by oxytocin as assessed by hysterosalpingoscintigraphy, hysterotonography, electrohysterography and Doppler sonography, *Human Reproduction Update* 4(5):655–666, 1998.

Williams GR: Neurodevelopmental and neurophysiological actions of thyroid hormone, *Journal of Neuroendocrinology* 20:784–794, 2008.

Winter JSD: Fetal and neonatal adrenocortical physiology. In Polin RA, Fox WW, editors: *Fetal and neonatal physiology*, Philadelphia, 2004, Saunders.

Wyrwoll CS, Seckl JR, Holmes MC: Altered placental function of 11β-hydroxysteroid dehydrogenase 2 knockout mice, *Endocrinology* 150(3):1287–1293, 2009.

Zervomanolakis I, Ott HW, Seeber BE, et al: Uterine mechanisms of ipsilateral directed transport: evidence for a contribution of the utero-ovarian countercurrent system, *European Journal of Obstetrics and Gynecology and Reproductive Biology* 144S:S45–S49, 2009.

Chapter |30|

# The fetal skull

*Barbara Burden and M Susan Sapsed*

### LEARNING OUTCOMES

After reading this chapter, you will be able to:

- review the process of fetal development of the structures of the skull
- assess the structures, circumference and diameters of the fetal skull and their importance in clinical practice
- identify internal structures within the fetal skull and possible complications that can occur during the birthing process
- describe the structures of the fetal skull and evaluate how this knowledge enables midwives to assess progress during labour, and care through the neonatal period.

## INTRODUCTION

It is essential for a midwife to understand the parameters and characteristics of the fetal skull because of its significance during the mechanism of labour. Two key functions of the fetal skull are the protection of the brain, which is subjected to pressure as it descends through the birth canal during labour, and an ability to change shape, adapting to the process of labour in response to uterine contractions and the size and shape of the pelvis. By assessing the landmarks of the fetal skull, such as sutures and fontanelles, a midwife is able to diagnose the position and attitude of the fetal head in the pelvis and determine the most likely mechanism of labour and mode of delivery.

## DEVELOPMENT OF THE FETAL SKULL

As the fetus develops in utero, the mesenchyme layer surrounding the brain starts to ossify, forming the various bones of the fetal skull. This process is called intramembranous ossification and begins between 4 to 8 weeks of gestation. The initial development of the skull occurs from this intramembranous structure, derived from neural crest cells and mesoderm. The intramembranous structure is divided into two major components, the neurocranium, which forms the protective case of the skull, and the viscerocranium, forming the bones of the face.

The neurocranium can be subdivided into the chondrocranium and the dermatocranium. The chondrocranium (cartilaginous part) is formed by the fusion of cartilages, and following ossification becomes the occipital, temporal, sphenoid and ethmoid bones. The dermatocranium (membranous part) is thought to arise from the external dermal scales developed to protect the brain. This lies under the superficial layers of the skin, covering and protecting the dorsal section of the brain, giving rise to the parietal and frontal bones.

The earliest visible signs of development can be seen on ultrasonography at about 4 weeks' gestation with calcification of the membranes and the development of the occiput. This becomes easier to determine from approximately 8 weeks, when intramembranous ossification is more prominent. At 12 weeks, the outline of the individual bones become evident (Moore & Persaud 2007, Sadler 2009) (see Fig. 30.1). Ossification of the bones continues throughout pregnancy with individual bones ossifying from their centre. At term, the bones of the skull

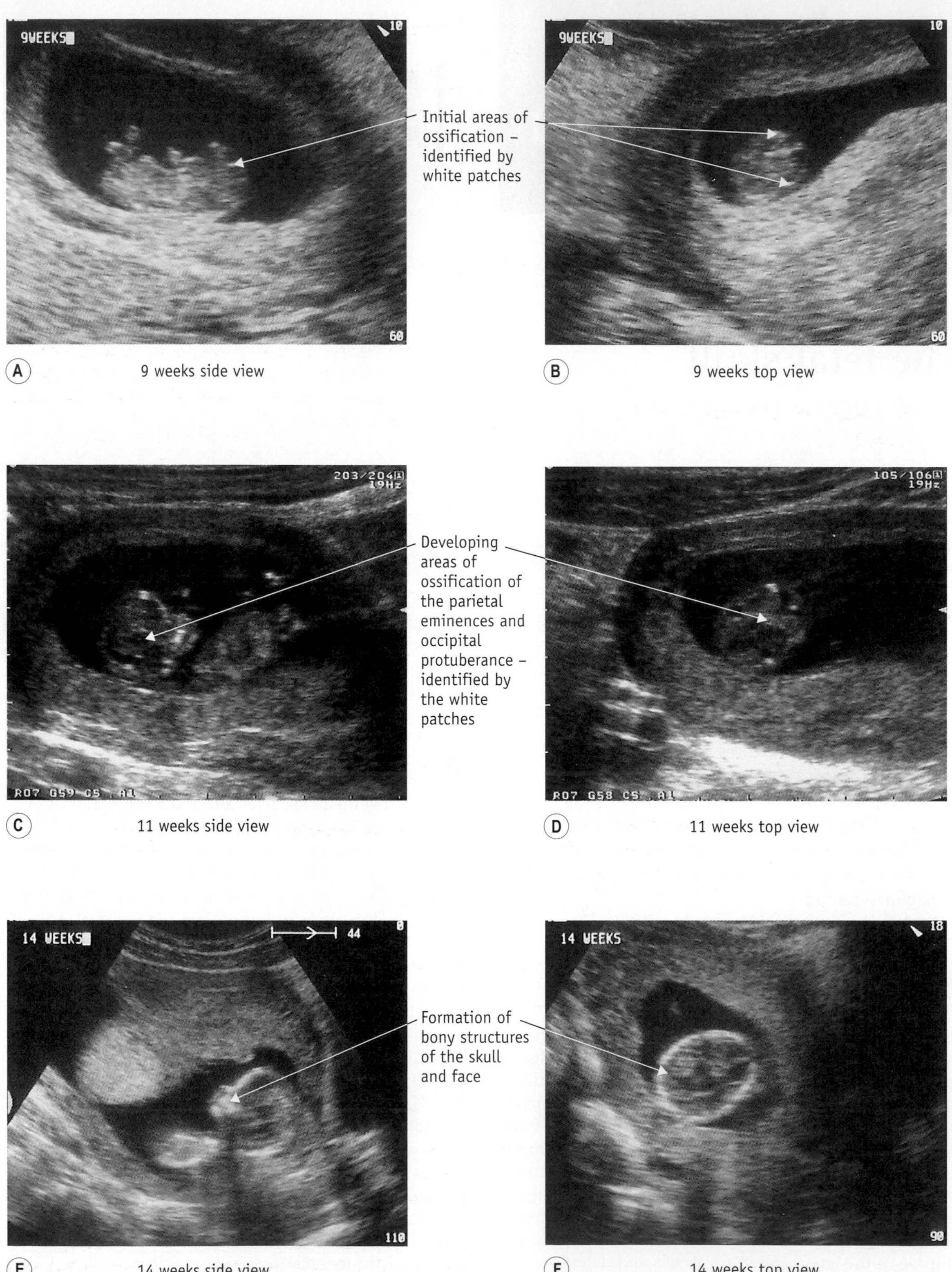


**Figure 30.1** Ultrasound images illustrating development and ossification of the fetal skull at 9, 11 and 14 weeks' gestation. *(Reproduced by kind permission of the Ultrasound Department at the Luton and Dunstable Hospital NHS Trust.)*

are thin and pliable, enabling some movement of bones to take place during labour. The two frontal bones have usually united by term.

## THE EXTERNAL STRUCTURES OF THE NEWBORN SKULL (Fig. 30.2)

Following birth, the midwife examines the external structures of the newborn head in order to identify any unusual characteristics or abnormalities in the skull structure. A baseline measurement of the newborn skull is sometimes taken during this procedure and documented within the child's neonatal records.

### Layers of the external structures of the skull

- Skin.
- Connective tissue – containing blood vessels and hair follicles. This may become oedematous during labour, resulting in a caput succedaneum.
- Aponeurosis – a fibrous sheet.
- Connective tissue – loose layer enabling movement of the scalp.
- Periosteum – a double layer of connective tissue covering and nourishing the bone. It is attached to the edges of bone.

## THE SKULL (Fig. 30.3)

The fetal skull is a complex structure consisting of 29 irregular flat bones with 22 of these paired symmetrically: 8 bones form the cranium, 14 the face, and 7 the base. Knowledge of the fetal skull in the antenatal period enables a midwife to assess the size of the fetal head in relation to the size of the pelvis, assess engagement of the fetal skull in the pelvis (Dietz & Lanzarone 2005). It also helps inform reviews of ultrasonography and pelvimetry reports.

### Sutures

The sutures of the fetal skull are soft fibrous tissues linking some bones of the skull. They enable moulding of the head to take place during labour and expansion of the brain as it develops during childhood.

The sutures of the skull are:

- frontal suture (Fig. 30.4)
- sagittal suture
- lambdoidal suture
- coronal suture.

### Fontanelles

A fontanelle is a membranous, non-ossified area of the skull where three or more sutures meet.

The significant fontanelles of the skull are:

- anterior fontanelle or bregma (Fig. 30.4)
- posterior fontanelle (Fig. 30.4)
- anterolateral or temporal fontanelles
- posterolateral or mastoid fontanelles.

### Sinuses

A sinus is a naturally occurring cavity in the body. Sinuses enable blood to circulate throughout the skull and into the brain membranes. The sinuses associated with the frontal, ethmoidal, sphenoidal and maxillary bones change shape during puberty and are thought to be associated with voice tone.

**Reflective activity 30.1**

Use the diagrams of the fetal skull in Figure 30.19 to revise the information outlined within this chapter. Photocopy the diagrams and revise the structures until you are confident that you know all of the components of the fetal skull and their application to midwifery practice.

### The bones and regions of the skull (Figs 30.3 and 30.4)

The skull is divided into three main regions:

- the vault
- the base
- the face.

The vault of the skull comprises:

- two frontal bones
- two parietal bones
- two temporal bones
- one occipital bone.

### Measurements of the fetal skull

The presentation and position of the fetal head in relation to the pelvic brim, influence the degree of flexion or extension of the head and determine the precise realignment of the skull bones during labour and delivery. To assess the skull size in relation to various diameters of the maternal pelvis, diameters of the fetal skull have been measured to correspond with common postures adopted by the fetal head as it enters the pelvic brim (Figs 30.5 and 30.6). Each

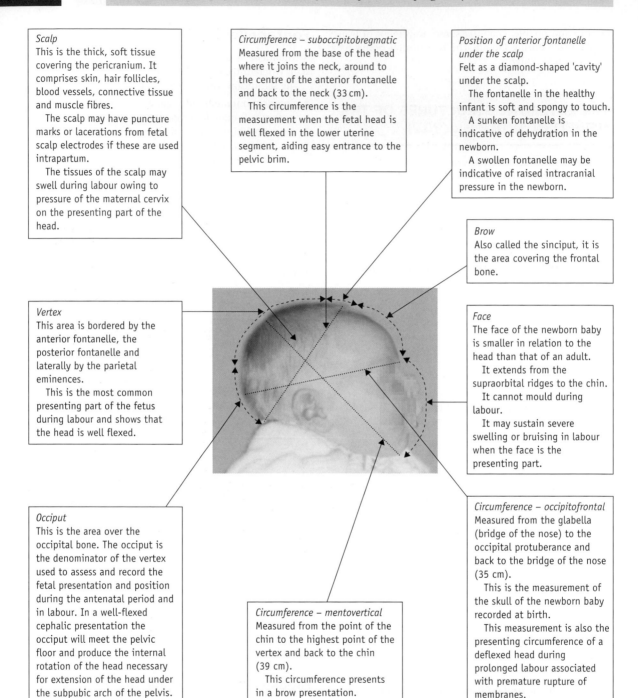

*Scalp*
This is the thick, soft tissue covering the pericranium. It comprises skin, hair follicles, blood vessels, connective tissue and muscle fibres.

The scalp may have puncture marks or lacerations from fetal scalp electrodes if these are used intrapartum.

The tissues of the scalp may swell during labour owing to pressure of the maternal cervix on the presenting part of the head.

*Circumference – suboccipitobregmatic*
Measured from the base of the head where it joins the neck, around to the centre of the anterior fontanelle and back to the neck (33 cm).

This circumference is the measurement when the fetal head is well flexed in the lower uterine segment, aiding easy entrance to the pelvic brim.

*Position of anterior fontanelle under the scalp*
Felt as a diamond-shaped 'cavity' under the scalp.

The fontanelle in the healthy infant is soft and spongy to touch.

A sunken fontanelle is indicative of dehydration in the newborn.

A swollen fontanelle may be indicative of raised intracranial pressure in the newborn.

*Brow*
Also called the sinciput, it is the area covering the frontal bone.

*Vertex*
This area is bordered by the anterior fontanelle, the posterior fontanelle and laterally by the parietal eminences.

This is the most common presenting part of the fetus during labour and shows that the head is well flexed.

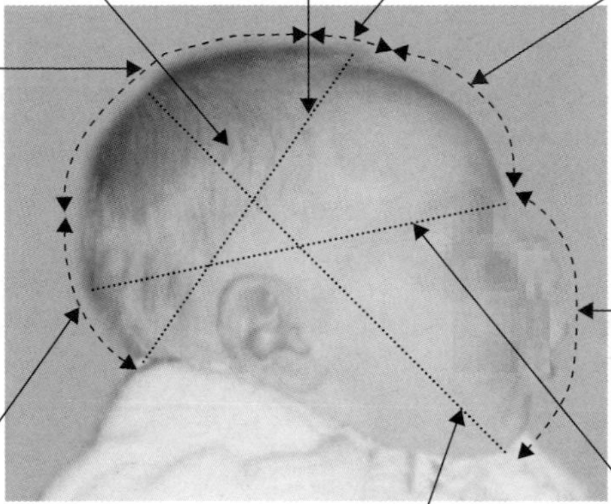

*Face*
The face of the newborn baby is smaller in relation to the head than that of an adult.

It extends from the supraorbital ridges to the chin.

It cannot mould during labour.

It may sustain severe swelling or bruising in labour when the face is the presenting part.

*Occiput*
This is the area over the occipital bone. The occiput is the denominator of the vertex used to assess and record the fetal presentation and position during the antenatal period and in labour. In a well-flexed cephalic presentation the occiput will meet the pelvic floor and produce the internal rotation of the head necessary for extension of the head under the subpubic arch of the pelvis.

*Circumference – mentovertical*
Measured from the point of the chin to the highest point of the vertex and back to the chin (39 cm).

This circumference presents in a brow presentation.

*Circumference – occipitofrontal*
Measured from the glabella (bridge of the nose) to the occipital protuberance and back to the bridge of the nose (35 cm).

This is the measurement of the skull of the newborn baby recorded at birth.

This measurement is also the presenting circumference of a deflexed head during prolonged labour associated with premature rupture of membranes.

**Figure 30.2** External structures and circumferences of the newborn skull.

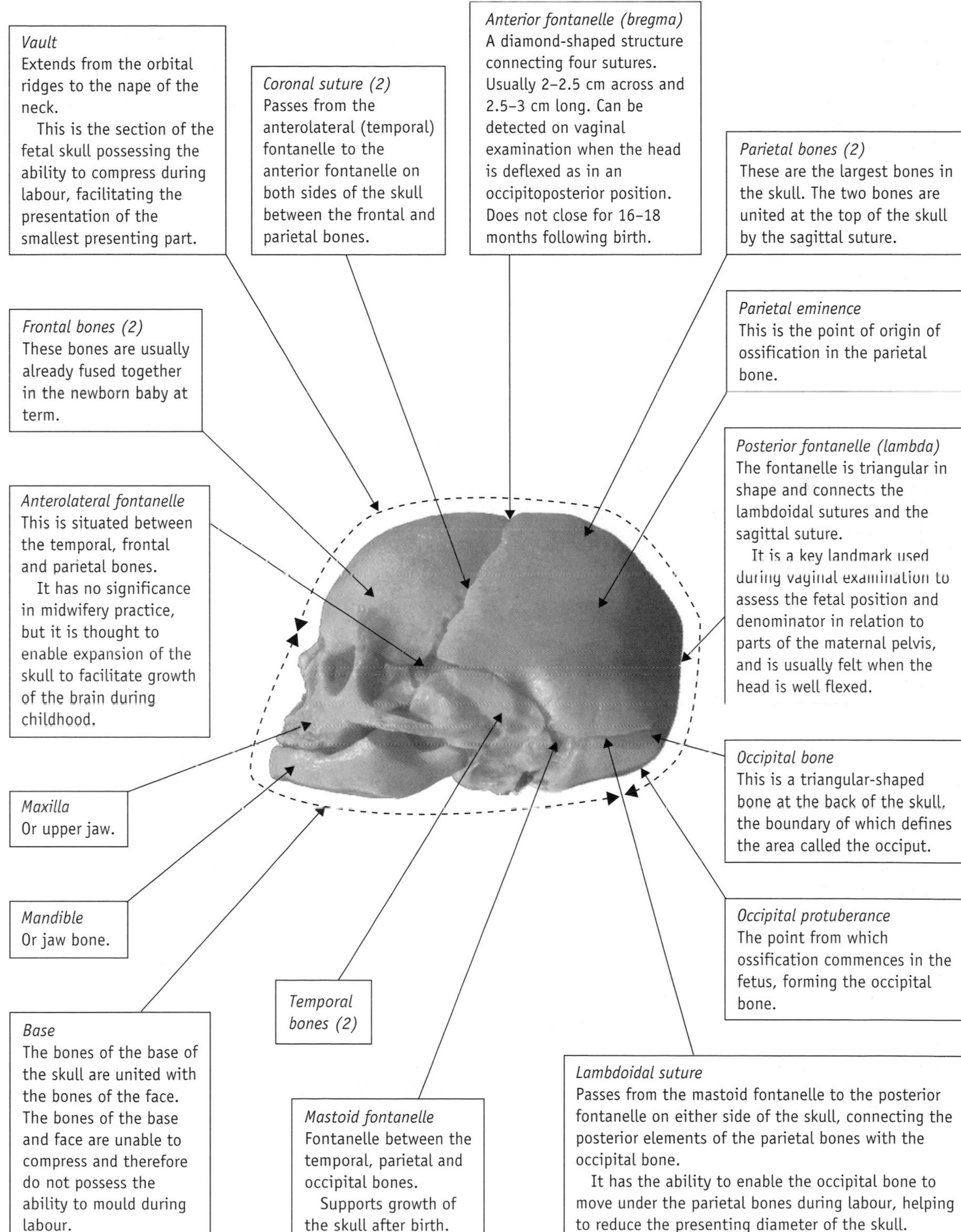

Vault
Extends from the orbital ridges to the nape of the neck.
This is the section of the fetal skull possessing the ability to compress during labour, facilitating the presentation of the smallest presenting part.
Coronal suture (2)
Passes from the anterolateral (temporal) fontanelle to the anterior fontanelle on both sides of the skull between the frontal and parietal bones.
Anterior fontanelle (bregma)
A diamond-shaped structure connecting four sutures. Usually 2–2.5 cm across and 2.5–3 cm long. Can be detected on vaginal examination when the head is deflexed as in an occipitoposterior position. Does not close for 16–18 months following birth.
Parietal bones (2)
These are the largest bones in the skull. The two bones are united at the top of the skull by the sagittal suture.
Parietal eminence
This is the point of origin of ossification in the parietal bone.
Frontal bones (2)
These bones are usually already fused together in the newborn baby at term.
Posterior fontanelle (lambda)
The fontanelle is triangular in shape and connects the lambdoidal sutures and the sagittal suture.
It is a key landmark used during vaginal examination to assess the fetal position and denominator in relation to parts of the maternal pelvis, and is usually felt when the head is well flexed.
Anterolateral fontanelle
This is situated between the temporal, frontal and parietal bones.
It has no significance in midwifery practice, but it is thought to enable expansion of the skull to facilitate growth of the brain during childhood.
Occipital bone
This is a triangular-shaped bone at the back of the skull, the boundary of which defines the area called the occiput.
Maxilla
Or upper jaw.
Mandible
Or jaw bone.
Occipital protuberance
The point from which ossification commences in the fetus, forming the occipital bone.
Temporal bones (2)
Base
The bones of the base of the skull are united with the bones of the face. The bones of the base and face are unable to compress and therefore do not possess the ability to mould during labour.
Mastoid fontanelle
Fontanelle between the temporal, parietal and occipital bones.
Supports growth of the skull after birth.
Lambdoidal suture
Passes from the mastoid fontanelle to the posterior fontanelle on either side of the skull, connecting the posterior elements of the parietal bones with the occipital bone.
It has the ability to enable the occipital bone to move under the parietal bones during labour, helping to reduce the presenting diameter of the skull.

**Figure 30.3** Characteristics of the fetal skull.

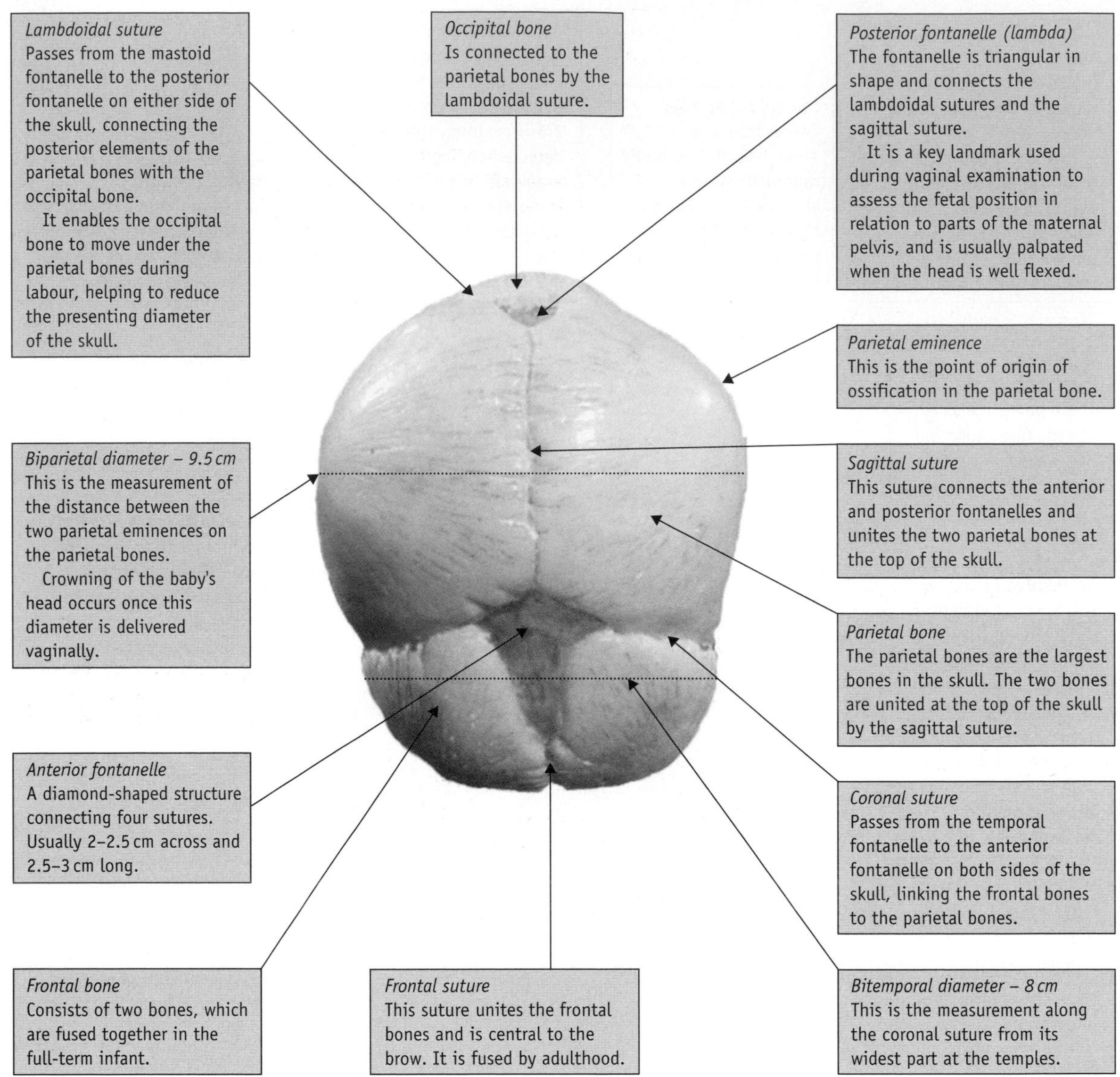

*Lambdoidal suture*
Passes from the mastoid fontanelle to the posterior fontanelle on either side of the skull, connecting the posterior elements of the parietal bones with the occipital bone.
It enables the occipital bone to move under the parietal bones during labour, helping to reduce the presenting diameter of the skull.
*Occipital bone*
Is connected to the parietal bones by the lambdoidal suture.
*Posterior fontanelle (lambda)*
The fontanelle is triangular in shape and connects the lambdoidal sutures and the sagittal suture.
It is a key landmark used during vaginal examination to assess the fetal position in relation to parts of the maternal pelvis, and is usually palpated when the head is well flexed.
*Parietal eminence*
This is the point of origin of ossification in the parietal bone.
*Biparietal diameter – 9.5 cm*
This is the measurement of the distance between the two parietal eminences on the parietal bones.
Crowning of the baby's head occurs once this diameter is delivered vaginally.
*Sagittal suture*
This suture connects the anterior and posterior fontanelles and unites the two parietal bones at the top of the skull.
*Parietal bone*
The parietal bones are the largest bones in the skull. The two bones are united at the top of the skull by the sagittal suture.
*Anterior fontanelle*
A diamond-shaped structure connecting four sutures. Usually 2–2.5 cm across and 2.5–3 cm long.
*Coronal suture*
Passes from the temporal fontanelle to the anterior fontanelle on both sides of the skull, linking the frontal bones to the parietal bones.
*Frontal bone*
Consists of two bones, which are fused together in the full-term infant.
*Frontal suture*
This suture unites the frontal bones and is central to the brow. It is fused by adulthood.
*Bitemporal diameter – 8 cm*
This is the measurement along the coronal suture from its widest part at the temples.

**Figure 30.4** The bones, sutures and fontanelles of the fetal skull.

of these diameters and degree of flexion and extension of the fetal head has a direct impact on the progress and possible outcome of labour. By understanding this, the midwife can suitably inform the mother so that decisions can be made on positions in labour, pain relief and subsequent care of the baby at delivery. It is important to remember, though, that these measurements are only an estimate and vary considerably depending on the baby's size and weight.

**Reflective activity 30.2**

When you next examine a baby, pay particular attention to the skull bones, sutures and fontanelles, which can easily be felt under the scalp. Note the degree of tension of the anterior fontanelle to assess the well being of the newborn. Familiarize yourself with the importance of these structures within midwifery practice.

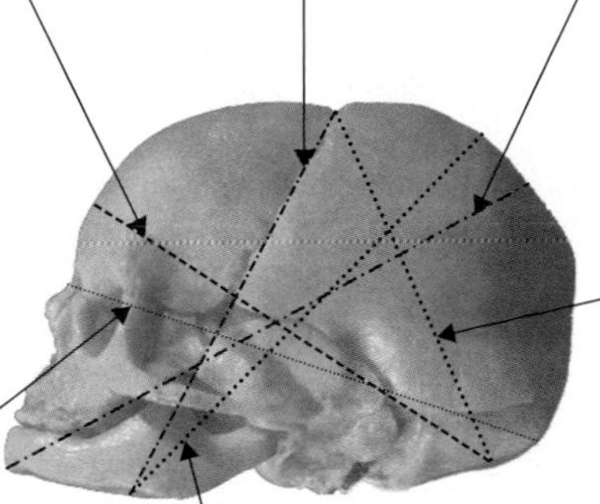

*Submentobregmatic – 9.5 cm*
Measured from the junction of the chin with the neck to the centre of the anterior fontanelle.
This diameter engages when the head is fully extended in a face presentation.
*Suboccipitofrontal – 10 cm*
Measured from the junction of the head with the neck just below the occipital protuberance to the centre of the frontal suture.
This diameter presents when the fetal head is almost completely flexed and engages in the pelvis in a vertex presentation.
May result in normal moulding of the skull and possible caput succedaneum.
*Mentovertical – 13.5 cm*
Measured from the point of the chin to the central point of the top of the head at the vertex.
This diameter presents in a brow presentation where the head is midway between flexion and extension.
*Suboccipitobregmatic – 9.5 cm*
Measured from the junction of the head with the neck just below the occipital protuberance to the centre of the anterior fontanelle.
This diameter presents when the fetal head is flexed and engages in the pelvis in a vertex presentation. This is the optimum diameter and shape for dilatation of the cervix in labour.
May result in normal moulding of the skull and possible caput succedaneum.
*Occipitofrontal – 11.5 cm*
Measured from the glabella (bridge of the nose) to the occipital protuberance.
This diameter presents in an occipitoposterior or occipitolateral position when there is insufficient flexion of the head. The outcome at birth may be a face-to-pubes delivery of the head following a persistent occipitoposterior position.
*Submentovertical – 11 cm*
Measured from the junction of the chin with the neck to the highest point on the vertex.
This diameter presents in a face presentation when the head is not fully extended.


**Figure 30.5** Diameters of the fetal skull.

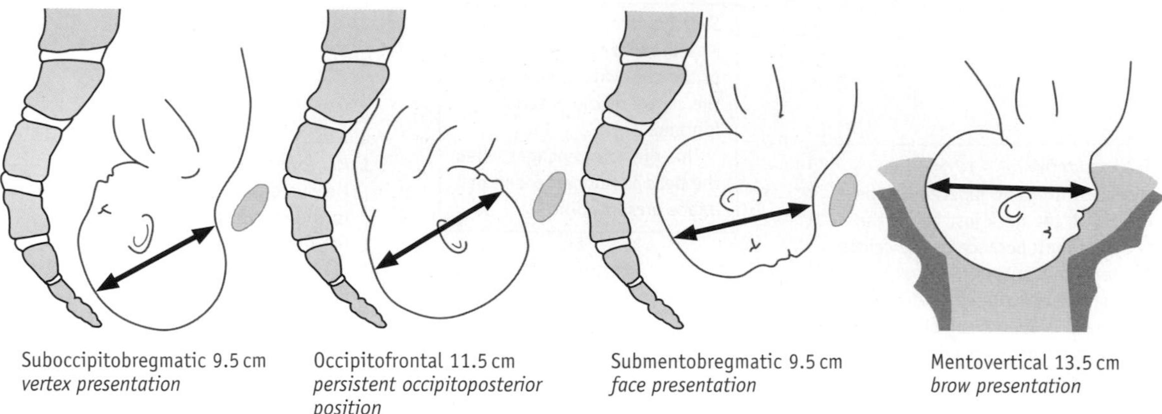


**Figure 30.6** Diameters of the fetal head in relation to the maternal pelvis.

## INTERNAL STRUCTURES OF THE FETAL SKULL

### The anatomy of the brain

The internal structures of the fetal skull, although protected by the cranium, are at risk because of the skull's ability to change shape during labour and birth. Altering the shape of the skull can result in overstretching of the internal structures and tearing of tissues or rupture of blood vessels.

#### Regions of the cerebrum (Fig. 30.7)

The regions of the cerebrum are divided according to the bones under which they lie:

- parietal lobe
- temporal lobe
- frontal lobe
- occipital lobe.

#### Meninges of the brain (Figs 30.8 and 30.9)

The three membranous coverings of the brain are called:

- dura mater
- arachnoid mater
- pia mater.

## MOULDING OF THE FETAL SKULL DURING LABOUR

The fetal skull has a unique ability to flex during birth, while adapting to prolonged compression, to enhance its passage through the birth canal. This adaptation process is termed *moulding*, a process during which bones of the skull override each other as a result of pelvic girdle pressure (Fig. 30.10).

Moulding can increase or reduce the diameters of the skull by up to 1.5 cm. In normal moulding, the frontal bones move under the anterior aspects of the parietal bones, with the occiput moving under the parietal bones at the rear. This enables the skull to change shape but not volume. Where one diameter is decreased, another will be increased to accommodate the volume (see Table 30.1 and Figs 30.11 and 30.12). Where there is extreme or rapid moulding or abnormal compression of the fetal

**Table 30.1 Variations in the diameters of the fetal skull due to compression and moulding**

| Presentation | Effect on diameter |
|---|---|
| Vertex presentation with good flexion | Suboccipitobregmatic decreased<br>Biparietal decreased<br>Mentovertical increased |
| Persistent occipitoposterior position of the vertex (POP) | Occipitofrontal decreased<br>Biparietal decreased<br>Submentobregmatic increased |
| Face presentation | Submentobregmatic decreased<br>Biparietal decreased<br>Occipitofrontal increased |
| Brow presentation | Mentovertical decreased<br>Biparietal probably decreased<br>Suboccipitobregmatic increased |

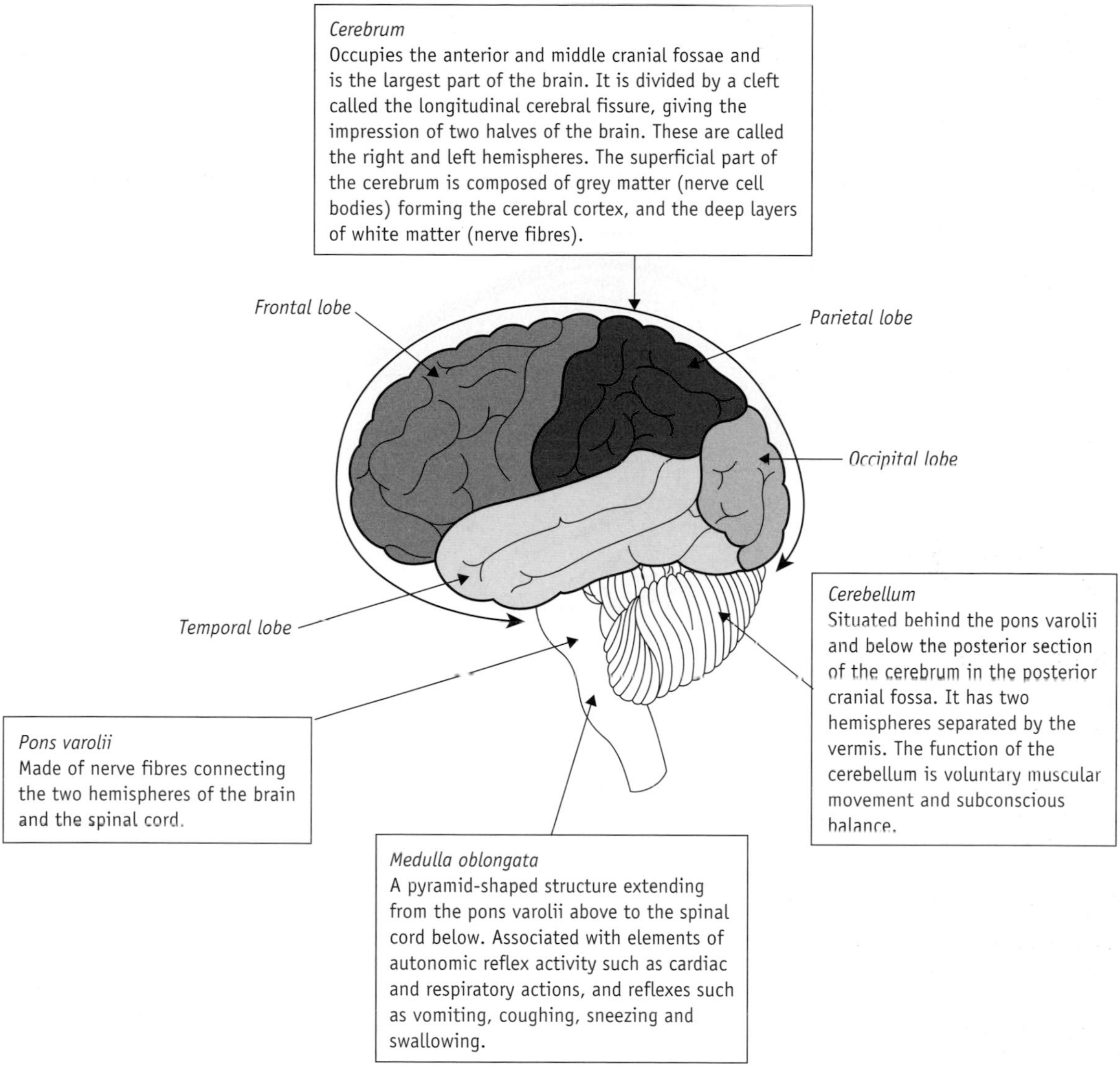

*Cerebrum*
Occupies the anterior and middle cranial fossae and is the largest part of the brain. It is divided by a cleft called the longitudinal cerebral fissure, giving the impression of two halves of the brain. These are called the right and left hemispheres. The superficial part of the cerebrum is composed of grey matter (nerve cell bodies) forming the cerebral cortex, and the deep layers of white matter (nerve fibres).

*Frontal lobe*

*Parietal lobe*

*Occipital lobe*

*Temporal lobe*

*Cerebellum*
Situated behind the pons varolii and below the posterior section of the cerebrum in the posterior cranial fossa. It has two hemispheres separated by the vermis. The function of the cerebellum is voluntary muscular movement and subconscious balance.

*Pons varolii*
Made of nerve fibres connecting the two hemispheres of the brain and the spinal cord.

*Medulla oblongata*
A pyramid-shaped structure extending from the pons varolii above to the spinal cord below. Associated with elements of autonomic reflex activity such as cardiac and respiratory actions, and reflexes such as vomiting, coughing, sneezing and swallowing.

**Figure 30.7** External structures of the brain.

skull, a tear in the *falx cerebri* or *tentorium cerebelli* can occur.

The midwife must record the degree of moulding present at birth. During the neonatal examination, the midwife reassesses moulding to ensure it is decreasing, and this may include taking measurements of the occipitofrontal circumference. Posterior moulding reduces within a few hours of birth, whereas anterior moulding is visible longer, decreasing over the first 48 hours of life.

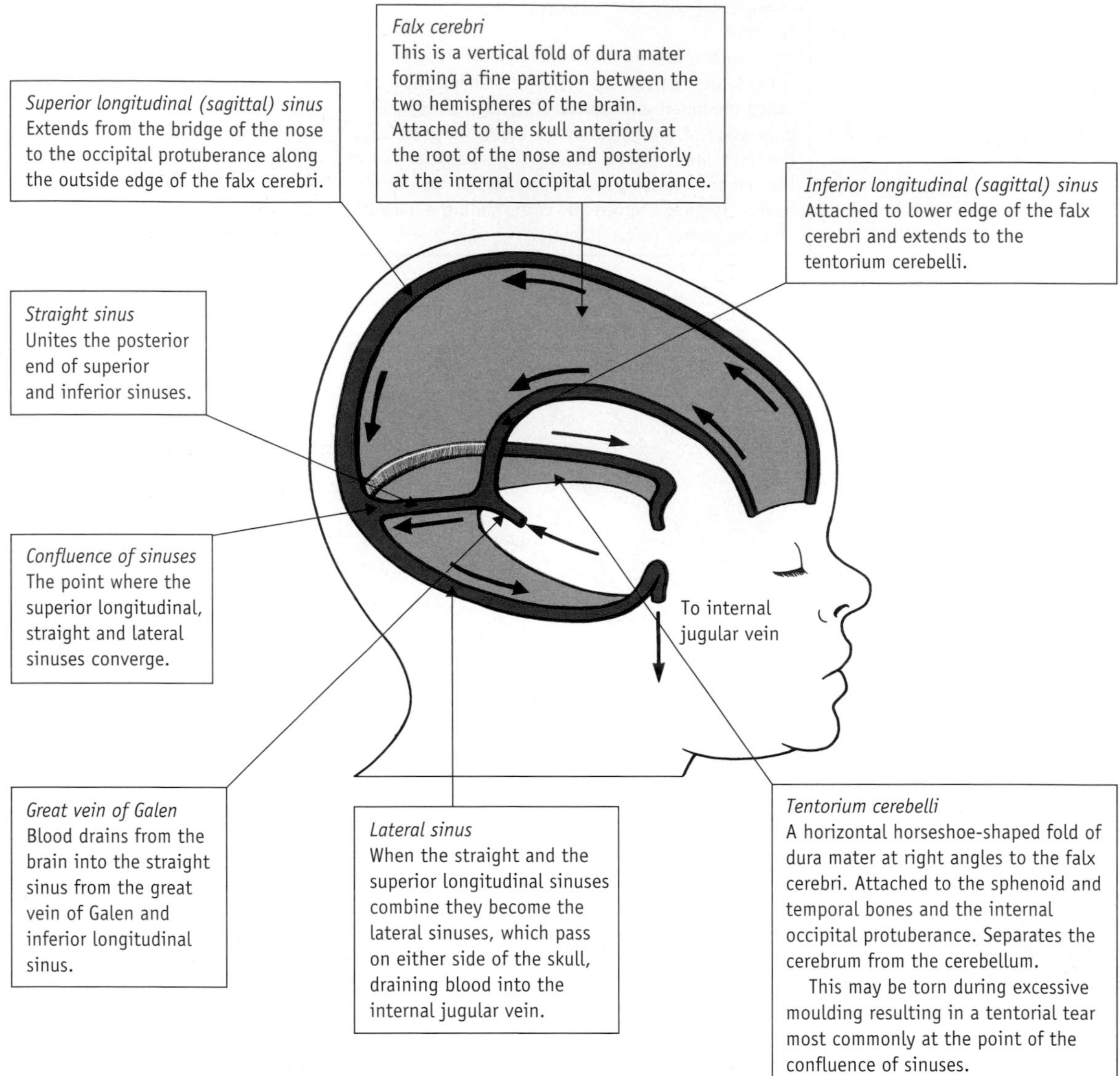

Falx cerebri
This is a vertical fold of dura mater forming a fine partition between the two hemispheres of the brain. Attached to the skull anteriorly at the root of the nose and posteriorly at the internal occipital protuberance.
Superior longitudinal (sagittal) sinus
Extends from the bridge of the nose to the occipital protuberance along the outside edge of the falx cerebri.
Inferior longitudinal (sagittal) sinus
Attached to lower edge of the falx cerebri and extends to the tentorium cerebelli.
Straight sinus
Unites the posterior end of superior and inferior sinuses.
Confluence of sinuses
The point where the superior longitudinal, straight and lateral sinuses converge.
To internal jugular vein
Great vein of Galen
Blood drains from the brain into the straight sinus from the great vein of Galen and inferior longitudinal sinus.
Lateral sinus
When the straight and the superior longitudinal sinuses combine they become the lateral sinuses, which pass on either side of the skull, draining blood into the internal jugular vein.
Tentorium cerebelli
A horizontal horseshoe-shaped fold of dura mater at right angles to the falx cerebri. Attached to the sphenoid and temporal bones and the internal occipital protuberance. Separates the cerebrum from the cerebellum.
This may be torn during excessive moulding resulting in a tentorial tear most commonly at the point of the confluence of sinuses.


**Figure 30.8** The sinuses and dura mater folds of the brain.

## INJURIES TO THE FETAL SKULL AND SURROUNDING TISSUES

### Caput succedaneum

A caput succedaneum is an oedematous swelling within the superficial connective tissue layer of the scalp (see Figs 30.13 and 30.14). The swelling results from the pressure exerted on the fetal head by the cervix during labour. Oedema collects in the unsupported section of the fetal head, which protrudes through the opening developed by the dilating cervix. The size of the swelling depends on the stage of cervical dilatation, and at full dilatation it may cover an extensive section of the presenting part. Not all babies develop caput, as factors such as duration of labour, strength of contractions and descent of the presenting part, all influence its development.

#### Characteristics of caput succedaneum

- Present at birth.
- Moulding of the skull is present.
- Usually a soft swelling that pits on pressure.

Parietal bone
Periosteum
Sagittal suture
Superior sagittal sinus

*Pia mater*
Contains minute blood vessels and connective tissue completely covering the surface of the brain.

*Dura mater*
A double tough fibrous membrane covering the outer surface of the brain and inner surface of the skull bones.

*Arachnoid mater*
Lies between the dura mater and the pia mater; all three continue down the spinal cord.

*Subdural space*
Space between the dura and arachnoid maters.

*Subarachnoid space*
Space between the arachnoid and the pia maters that contains cerebrospinal fluid.

Cerebrum
Pons varolii
Cerebellum

*Falx cerebri*
*Inferior sagittal sinus*
*Tentorium cerebelli*
*Lateral sinus*
*Medulla oblongata*

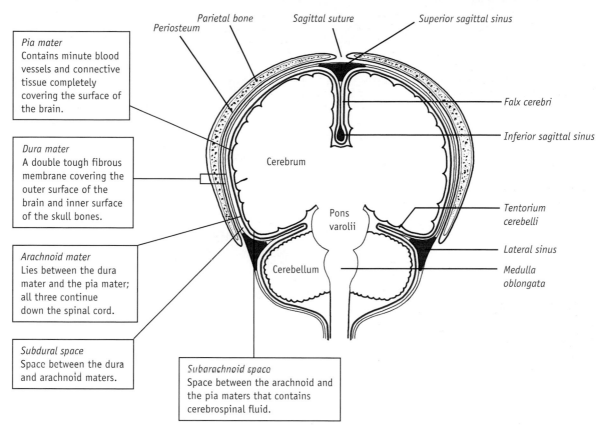

**Figure 30.9** Coronal section through the fetal head showing the internal structures of the brain.

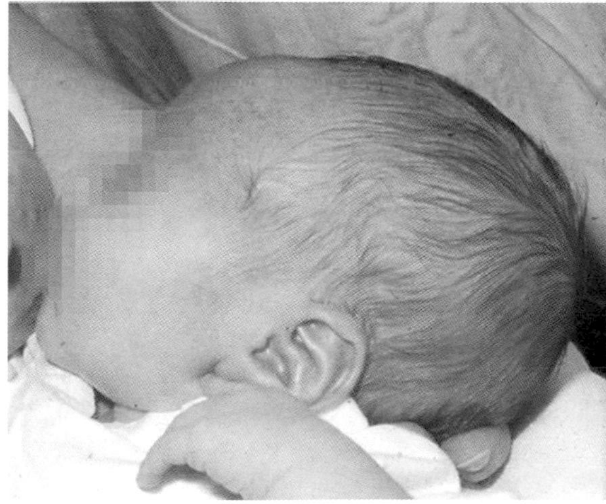

**Figure 30.10** Normal moulding.

- May cross suture lines.
- Tends to decrease in size after delivery.
- No treatment is required as it generally disappears within 24–48 hours as the fluid is reabsorbed.

## Cephalhaematoma

A cephalhaematoma is bleeding between the periosteum and the bone of the fetal skull (Figs 30.15 and 30.16). It is caused by friction of the skull against the pelvis or forceps during labour, and is associated with asynclitism of the fetal skull (the sideways rocking mechanism of the fetal head as it descends), or trauma following a vacuum extraction. Injury to the fetal skull results in the periosteum separating from the underlying bone with subsequent bleeding between layers. The resulting swelling is confined to the area of the affected skull bone by the periosteum layer. A cephalhaematoma can be present in more than one bone but occurrs most commonly in the parietal bones. The affected area is initially soft, but as osmosis occurs, fluid is removed and the area becomes firm.

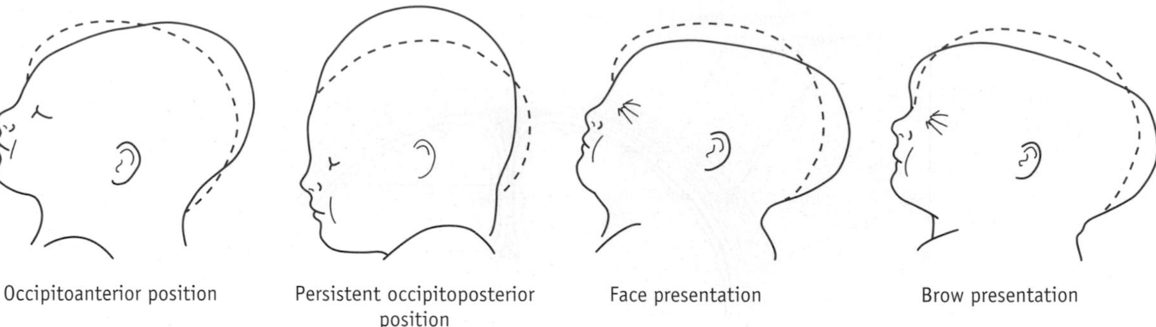


**Figure 30.11** Moulding of the head.

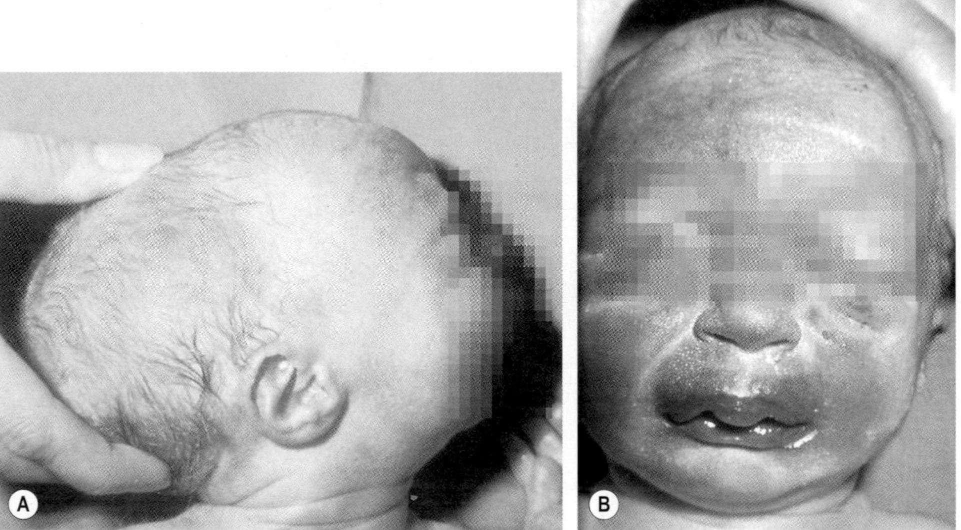


**Figure 30.12** Moulding following face presentation and delivery: **A**. side view; **B.** front view.

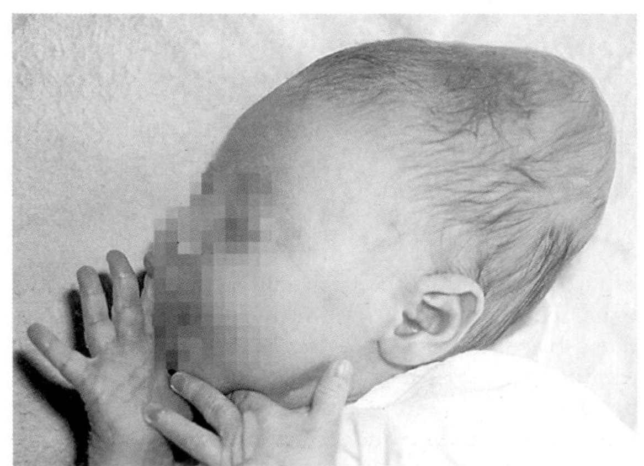

**Figure 30.13** A neonate with caput succedaneum.

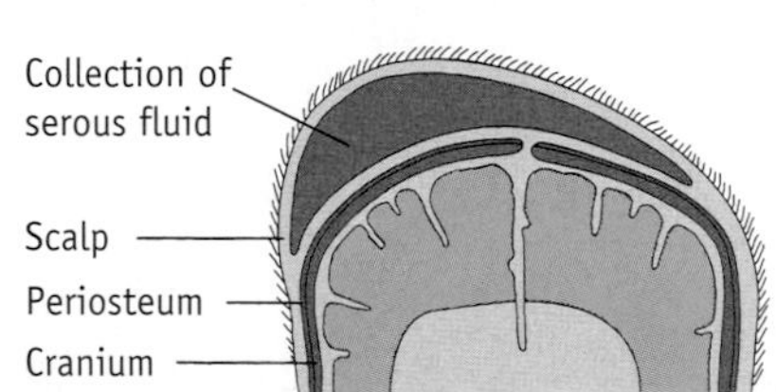


**Figure 30.14** Caput succedaneum.

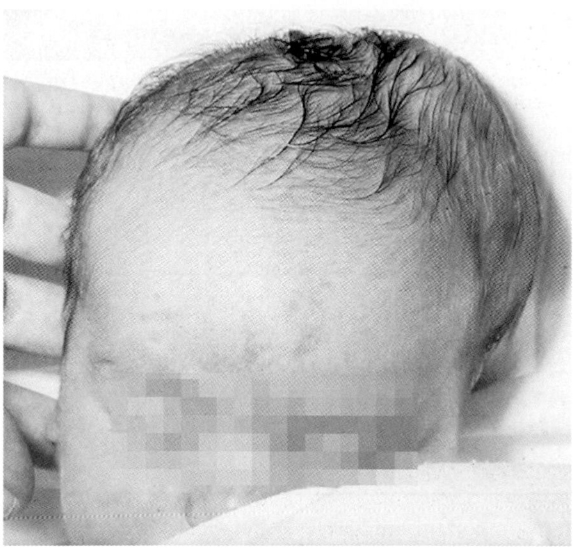

Figure 30.15 A neonate with cephalhaematoma.

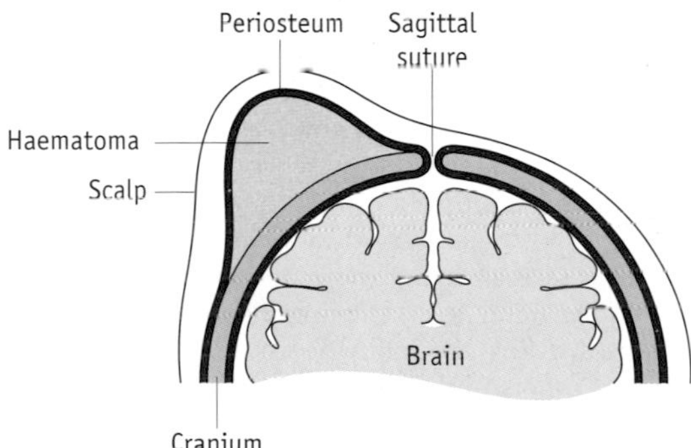


Figure 30.16 Cephalhaematoma.

### Characteristics of cephalhaematoma

- Appears 12–72 hours following delivery.
- Tends to enlarge following delivery.
- Is circumscribed and does not pit on pressure.
- May be bilateral.
- Can persist for weeks and in rare cases months.
- May contribute to jaundice.

Treatment for this condition is rare, as most cephalhaematomas disperse naturally. The neonate is usually unperturbed by the injury or slightly irritable and requiring gentle handling. As with any blood loss, the baby must be monitored for signs of anaemia and jaundice as lysis of blood occurs, and vitamin K is administered to increase prothrombin levels and assist with clotting.

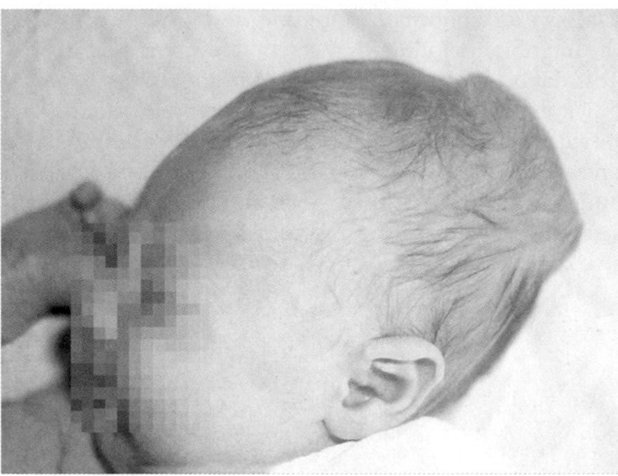

Figure 30.17 A ventouse 'chignon'.

### Lacerations

Lacerations to the scalp or face can result from fetal scalp electrodes, fetal blood monitoring or instrumental delivery. They usually require little or no treatment and heal quickly. The aim of neonatal care in this instance involves prevention and detection of infection and promotion of wound healing.

### Chignon

A chignon may result following application of a vacuum extraction cup to the fetal scalp during delivery (Fig. 30.17). The vacuum cup is applied to the scalp and suction applied, drawing the scalp into the cup. Any slight movement of the scalp layers results in the area under the cup becoming oedematous and bruised. The result is an oedematous structure the same size and shape as the vacuum cup. This condition usually disappears within a week following delivery. In rare cases, vacuum extraction has been associated with *subaponeurotic haemorrhage*, when bleeding occurs below the epicranial aponeurosis. Bleeding in this instance may be extensive and so admission to a neonatal unit for observation and treatment is necessary.

## INTERNAL INJURIES

### Tentorial tear

The tentorium cerebelli is a fold of dura mater within which are present the venous sinuses containing blood being removed from the brain. On rare occasions, the fetal head can be compromised by a difficult delivery or excessive or abnormal moulding, resulting in tearing of the membranes followed by cerebral bleeding (Fig. 30.18). This damage is often labelled as a *tentorial tear*.

The baby presents with signs of cerebral irritation and raised intracranial pressure, including a tense, expanded anterior fontanelle, asphyxia (bradycardia and apnoea), and convulsions. In these instances, the midwife must seek medical aid and arrange transfer to a neonatal intensive care unit for observation (see Ch. 48).

**Reflective activity 30.3**

Revise the internal structures of the fetal skull.

Visit your local neonatal intensive care unit to discuss the current treatment and care required by a baby with a tentorial tear.

Make notes on the advice given, including signs and symptoms to enable you to detect this condition and current patterns of care available for this baby.

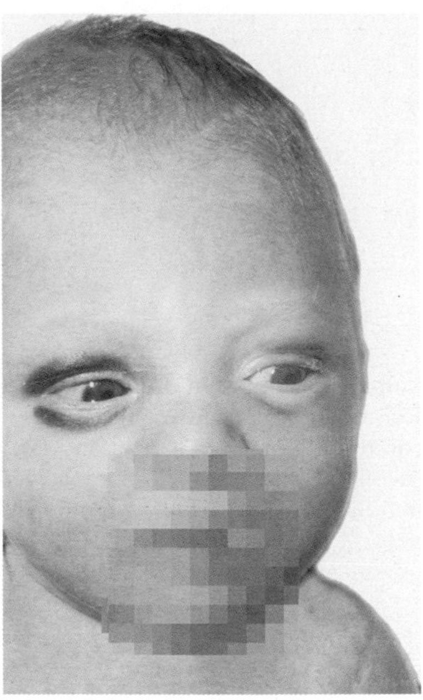

**Figure 30.18** External signs of cerebral bleeding.

## THE RELEVANCE OF THE FETAL SKULL TO PARENTS

It is important midwives share their knowledge with parents in order to expand understanding of the needs of their baby. This commences in the antenatal period when the midwife discusses the nutritional needs of the fetus during development and growth, and explains the link between the mother's pelvis and the fetal skull during labour.

Immediately following delivery, during examination of the neonate, the midwife can point out to parents the key features of the skull and their significance, to include fontanelles and sutures, and the presence of any deviations from normal, for example a caput.

During the postnatal period, it is important that the midwife discusses checking the anterior fontanelle as a measure of the neonate's wellbeing. Box 30.1 provides a useful checklist for the midwife to use in educating mothers and others in the care of the baby.

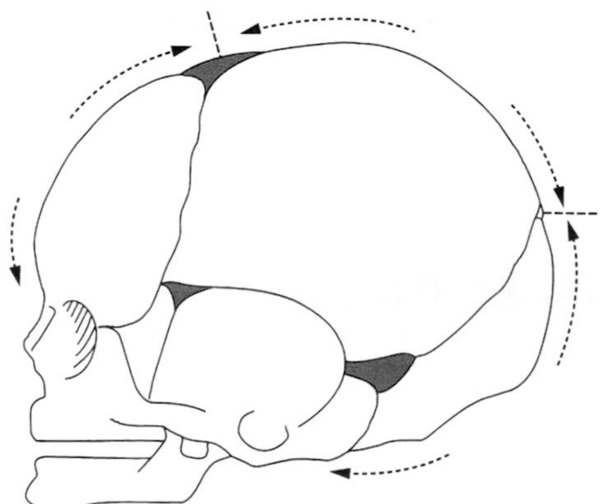

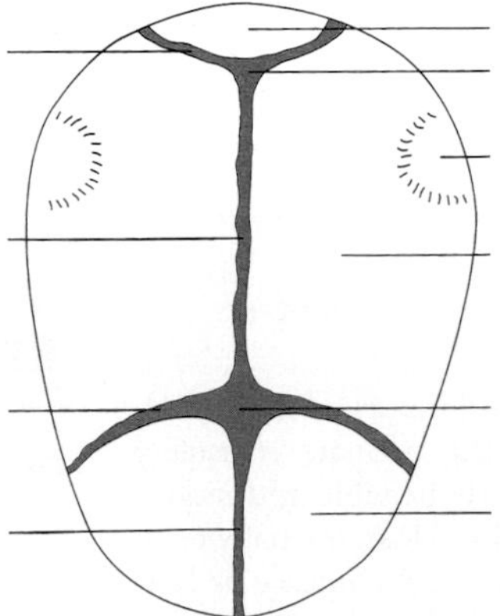

**Figure 30.19** Diagrams of the fetal skull.

**Box 30.1 Helpful information points for parents**

- Handle the head of the newborn carefully, to avoid injury.
- Do not shake the baby as damage can occur to the internal structures of the skull.
- Support the baby's head for 3 months until the baby has developed some control over movement.
- The top of the head of the baby should be washed carefully because of the soft anterior fontanelle.
- Babies lose most of their heat through the head, so in cold environments their head should be covered.
- Observe the anterior fontanelle for signs of dehydration in the newborn (indented) but remember to allow time for the baby to absorb a feed once fed. The anterior fontanelle (see Fig. 30.2) is diamond shaped and feels soft and spongy to touch in a normal healthy baby.
- Injuries to the baby's head should be reported immediately to a doctor so assessment can take place.
- A caput succedaneum usually disappears within 48 hours.
- A cephalhaematoma is absorbed within 1–4 weeks.

## CONCLUSION

Knowledge of the anatomy of the brain and fetal skull enables practitioners to understand the role they play during labour and birth, helping them to assess, prevent, predict and diagnose potential and actual morbidity, while understanding the process of natural changes within the skull that help facilitate the birth of a baby.

Following birth, the midwife uses skills of observation and diagnosis to ensure the baby's health and wellbeing. Knowledge of the structures outlined in this chapter enable the midwife to provide health promotion information and advice to parents, on both the process and outcome of birth, and the subsequent care their new baby requires.

## KEY POINTS

- It is important for midwives to be conversant with the structure and development of the fetal brain and skull.
- The fetal skull impacts upon labour, influencing its duration, pain relief required and outcome.
- Labour impacts upon the fetal skull by influencing the amount and type of moulding and internal injuries that occur during birth.
- The midwife must anticipate and assess injuries relating to the fetal skull, including the presence of caput succedaneum, cephalhaematoma, chignon, and scalp electrode injury. Assessment must include consideration of injuries relating to internal structures of the skull such as tentorial tears.
- Midwives use their knowledge to inform practice and assist families in developing knowledge and confidence in caring for their baby.

## REFERENCES


Dietz H, Lanzarone V: Measuring engagement of the fetal head: validity and reproducibility of a new ultrasound technique, *Ultrasound in Obstetrics and Gynecology* 25(2):165–168, 2005.

Moore K, Persaud T: *Before we are born: essentials of embryology and birth defects*, ed 7, London, 2007, WB Saunders.

Sadler T: Langman's medical embryology, ed 11, London, 2009, Lippincott Williams & Wilkins.

# Part | 5 |

# Pregnancy

Chapter |31|

# Maternal and fetal responses to pregnancy

*Mary McNabb*

## LEARNING OUTCOMES

After reading this chapter, you will be able to:

- understand the extensive adaptations in maternal organ and neuroendocrine homeostatic systems to different phases of the fertile cycle
- explore the complex interactions between maternal, embryonic and fetoplacental compartments that coordinate maternal adaptations in reproductive and non-reproductive organ systems at different phases of the fertile cycle.

## INTRODUCTION

In healthy, non-pregnant women, cyclical variations occur in a range of homeostatic mechanisms across the ovarian cycle, including thirst, fluid balance, appetite, temperature, cardiovascular, haemodynamic, metabolic and respiratory regulation. Following fertilization, luteal changes are accentuated and other physiological and behavioural adaptations unfold in response to distinct neurohormonal interactions that characterize successive phases of pregnancy and lactation. These altered regulatory mechanisms accommodate changing maternal needs and those of the conceptus, during implantation, and embryo formation, while changes occur in a variety of maternal systems to anticipate the distinct needs of the fetus and neonate.

Detailed information on the time course of specific changes and improved understanding of the coordinating factors have increased the potential number of tools to measure key adaptations and assess maternal health. For example, higher plasma concentrations of progesterone and relaxin in early pregnancy are associated with lower mean systolic blood pressure in the second and third trimester, and a positive correlation exists between the extent of plasma volume expansion and fetal growth, reduced risk of pregnancy complications, and pre-term labour (Khraibi et al 2003, Kristiansson & Wang 2001, Steer 2000). Some pre-existing and potential maternal health problems in early pregnancy may be identified through assessment of different hormone levels; and raised body mass index (BMI) (Duvekot et al 1995, Lain et al 2008, Maccarrone & Finazzi-Agro 2004).

This chapter will outline the time course and regulation of adaptive responses of maternal cardiovascular, renal and haemodynamic systems to pregnancy; adaptive responses of maternal hypothalamic–pituitary regulation of prolactin and growth hormone, and adaptive responses of maternal hypothalamic–pituitary–adrenal (HPA) axis to early and late pregnancy (Brunton et al 2008, Douglas 2010). It will conclude by examining the time course and regulation of the adaptive response of the uterus and mammary gland during pregnancy. See also website for more information.

## PULMONARY AND CARDIOVASCULAR ADAPTATIONS

During the infertile cycle, regulation of fluid balance, cardiovascular volume and blood pressure varies during different phases (Chapman et al 1997). This includes some degree of hyperventilation and changing alveolar and arterial tensions of carbon dioxide ($CO_2$) levels influenced by oestrogens and progesterone (see website).

When conception occurs, hyperventilation increases and the magnitude of decline in $P\text{CO}_2$ correlates with

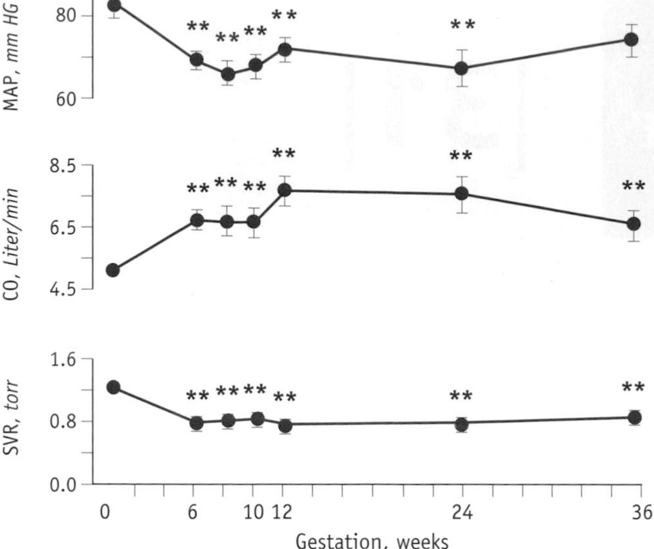


**Figure 31.1** Systemic haemodynamic changes before and during pregnancy. Mean arterial pressure (MAP) decreases and cardiac output (CO) increases significantly by 6 weeks' gestation in association with a decline in systemic vascular resistance (SVR). *(Reproduced with permission from Chapman et al 1998: Fig. 1; 2059.)*

arterial concentrations of progesterone (Chapman et al 1998, Jensen et al 2005).

During the luteal phase, mean arterial pressure (MAP) declines significantly, leading to a reflexive rise in cardiac output, while blood volume remains constant (Chapman et al 1997, Williams et al 2001). In most studies, systolic blood pressure is slightly raised compared to the follicular phase, while diastolic pressure is 5% lower. Following conception, the largest change in blood pressure occurs before 8 weeks' gestation. At this point, 80–90% of the total pregnancy-related fall of around 10 mmHg in MAP has already taken place (Duvekot & Peeters 1998). After 8 weeks, MAP continues to fall, reaching its lowest level by 24 weeks (Robson et al 1989). This pregnancy-related decline in MAP is largely due to the fall in diastolic pressure that begins during the luteal phase (Duvekot & Peeters 1998). Systolic blood pressure remains constant until 20 weeks, rising significantly during the second half of pregnancy, while diastolic pressure reaches its lowest point at 24 weeks and rises significantly for the remainder of pregnancy (Mabie et al 1994, Volman et al 2007) (see Figs 31.1 and 31.2).

## ADAPTATIONS IN FLUID REGULATION

Osmotic thresholds for thirst and vasopressin secretion decline during the luteal phase (see website) leading to a comparable reduction in plasma osmolality, through a fall in plasma sodium and its associated *anions*, primarily chloride and bicarbonate (Chapman et al 1997, Vokes et al 1988). When conception occurs, plasma osmolality continues to decline to 8–10 mOsmol/kg below mid-follicular values by 10 weeks' gestation, and this new set-point for thirst and vasopressin secretion is maintained throughout pregnancy and labour (Chapman et al 1998, Davison et al 1981). These changes are stimulated by a primary renal and systemic vasodilation, which creates a fall in total vascular resistance (Fig. 31.3).

In the absence of any increase in plasma volume, the post-ovulatory fall in renal and systemic vascular resistance initiates a decline in ventricular afterload. This stimulates a reflex rise in cardiac output followed by a significant expansion in plasma volume by 6 weeks' gestation, increasing rapidly to around 45–50% of non-pregnant values by 36 weeks (Chapman et al 1998). The fall in systemic vascular resistance from the luteal phase stimulates renal sodium and water retention, by activating fluid-retaining components of the renin–angiotensin–aldosterone system (RAAS) while blunting its vasoconstrictive effects (Chapman et al 1997, Chidambaram et al 2002, Sealey et al 1987).

When conception occurs, *plasma renin* activity, *aldosterone* and *atrial natriuretic peptide* (ANP) increase significantly by 6 weeks' gestation (Chapman et al 1997, 1998, Sealey et al 1985). Despite higher basal activity of the RAAS during pregnancy, the early fall in plasma sodium sets a lower response threshold, and renal reactions to natriuretic stimuli like ANP and vascular responses to vasoconstrictor components, notably *vasopressin* and *angiotensin II*, are significantly blunted, as occurs during the luteal phase.

These responses are largely mediated by rising levels of *hCG, oestrogens* and *progesterone* (Fig. 31.4). Oestrogens stimulate hepatic synthesis of angiotensinogen (renin substrate) and promote formation of angiotensin-(1-7)

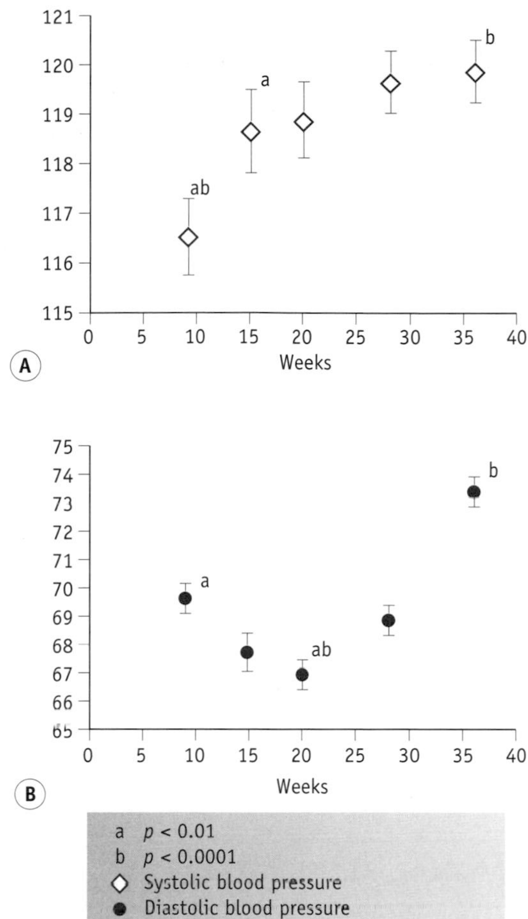


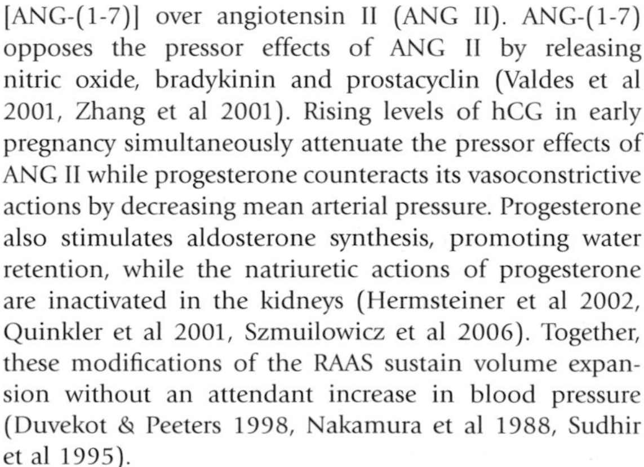


**Figure 31.2** Changes in (**A**) systolic and (**B**) diastolic blood pressure from 8 weeks' gestation *(Reproduced from Kristiansson & Wang 2001; Figs 1 and 2: 15, with kind permission of OUP. www.oup.com)*

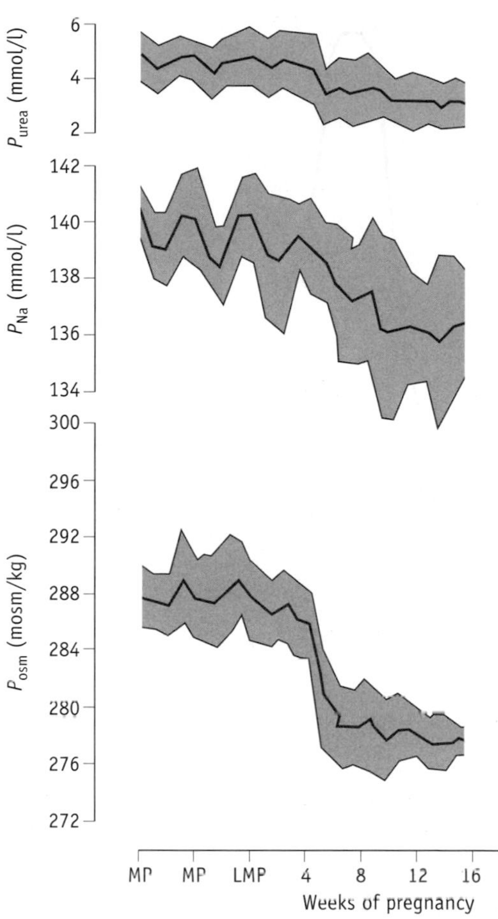


**Figure 31.3** Mean values (±SD) for plasma urea ($P_{urea}$), sodium ($P_{Na}$) and osmolality ($P_{osm}$) measured at weekly intervals during the infertile cycle and following conception to 16 weeks' gestation *(Reproduced with permission from Baylis & Davison 1998; Fig. 10.17; 284.)*

[ANG-(1-7)] over angiotensin II (ANG II). ANG-(1-7) opposes the pressor effects of ANG II by releasing nitric oxide, bradykinin and prostacyclin (Valdes et al 2001, Zhang et al 2001). Rising levels of hCG in early pregnancy simultaneously attenuate the pressor effects of ANG II while progesterone counteracts its vasoconstrictive actions by decreasing mean arterial pressure. Progesterone also stimulates aldosterone synthesis, promoting water retention, while the natriuretic actions of progesterone are inactivated in the kidneys (Hermsteiner et al 2002, Quinkler et al 2001, Szmuilowicz et al 2006). Together, these modifications of the RAAS sustain volume expansion without an attendant increase in blood pressure (Duvekot & Peeters 1998, Nakamura et al 1988, Sudhir et al 1995).

## RENAL HAEMODYNAMIC ADAPTATIONS

Although the kidneys constitute less than 0.5% of total body weight, in resting non-pregnant adults, blood flow is equal to 25% of cardiac output, reflecting their key role in regulating fluid and electrolyte balance (Stanton & Koeppen 1993). From the mid-luteal phase of the cycle, significant changes occur in renal haemodynamics, as vascular resistance declines, while plasma flow and glomerular filtration rate increase significantly, by 6 weeks' gestation, compared to values obtained during the mid-follicular phase of the cycle. Minimal renal vascular resistance occurs at 8 weeks' gestation and this coincides with

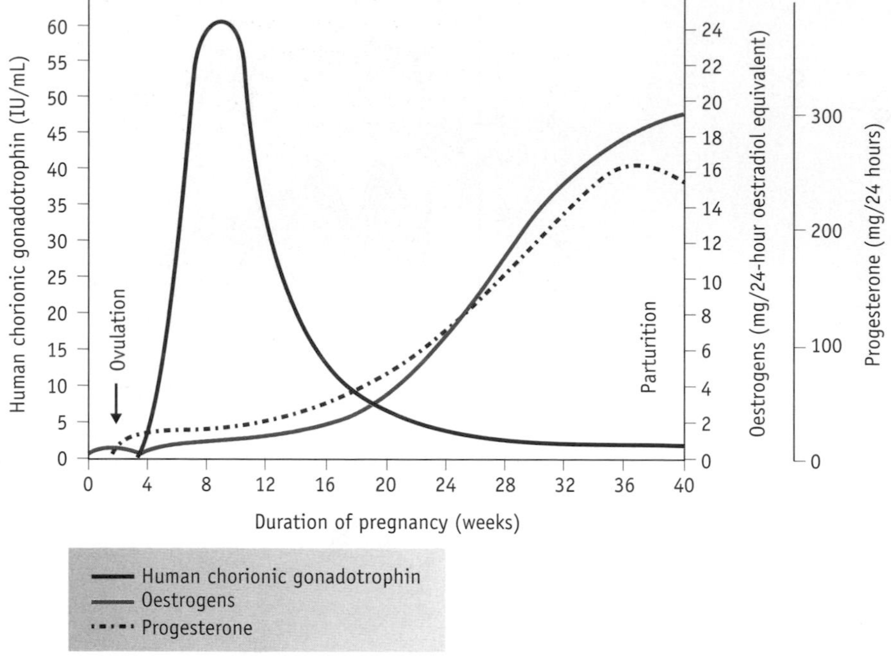


**Figure 31.4** Patterns of release of human chorionic gonadotrophin, progesterone and oestrogens from ovulation to birth *(Reproduced with permission from Blackburn 2007:100.)*

a peak rise in plasma flow of around 70%, which remains at slightly lower values for the remainder of pregnancy (Baylis & Davison 1998, Chapman et al 1998, Conrad & Novak 2004) (Fig. 31.5).

These findings suggest that hormonal changes in the corpus luteum, before and after conception, stimulate a primary fall in renal and systemic vascular resistance that initiates a chain of events leading to an early rise in cardiac output, renal sodium and water retention, despite the increase in glomerular filtration rate, leading to an expansion in plasma volume, before any increase in basal metabolic rate (Spaanderman et al 2000). A primary reduction in vascular resistance of non-reproductive organs may be initiated in preparation for the dramatic increase in utero-placental blood flow during the second and third trimesters.

Considerable evidence suggests that the luteal decline in vascular resistance and plasma osmolality and the subsequent rise in plasma volume and total body water are positive indicators of maternal adaptations to pregnancy and long-term health, because of their strong association with increased fetal growth, reduced perinatal mortality and risk of cardiovascular disease in later life (Churchill et al 1997, Conrad et al 2001, Duvekot et al 1995, Steer et al 1995) (see website).

## HORMONAL REGULATION

Current findings suggest that the renal and systemic fall in vascular resistance and the rise in cardiac output are stimulated by the post-ovulatory increase in *relaxin, oestrogens* and *progesterone* from the corpus luteum followed by a significant rise in adrenomedullin, a long-lasting vaso-relaxant, from a variety of tissues by 8 weeks' gestation (Conrad et al 2001, Di Iorio et al 1999, Hermsteiner et al 2002, Nakamura et al 1988, Novak et al 2001, Sudhir et al 1995).

In pregnancy, relaxin is detectable in the peripheral circulation 6 days after the midcycle LH/FSH surge. By 11 days, concentrations are significantly higher in fertile than in non-fertile cycles and concentrations increase rapidly up to 20 weeks' gestation (Johnson et al 1991, Stewart et al 1993). Limited human studies have demonstrated that higher plasma concentrations of relaxin and progesterone in early pregnancy are associated with lower mean systolic blood pressure in late pregnancy (Kristiansson & Wang 2001). Recent evidence suggests that while oestrogens have a stimulatory effect on cardiac output and oestrogens and progesterone stimulate systemic and uterine vasodilation, neither hormone seems to influence renal

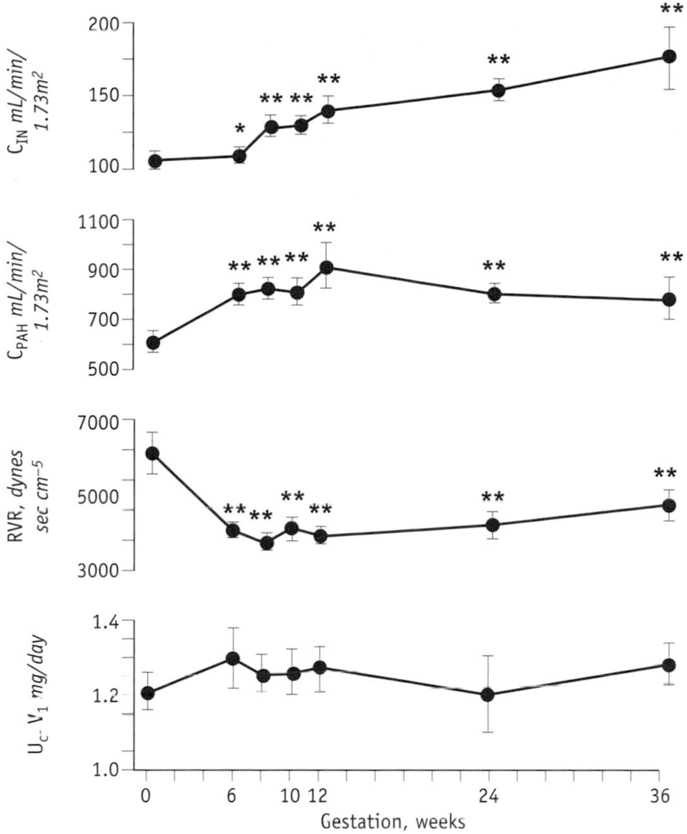


**Figure 31.5** Renal haemodynamic changes before and during pregnancy. Changes in glomerular filtration rate, effective renal plasma flow and renal vascular resistance from mid-follicular phase until 36 weeks' gestation. *(Reproduced with permission from Chapman et al 1998: Fig. 3; 2059.)*

blood vessels, which show a marked degree of dilation following ovulation (Chapman et al 1997, Nakamura et al 1988, Sudhir et al 1995) (Fig. 31.6).

## CARDIOVASCULAR ADAPTATIONS

The maternal cardiovascular system undergoes an extensive expansion in response to pregnancy. The first event is decreased vascular resistance of non-reproductive organs, leading to a profound fall in systemic vascular resistance, which reaches its lowest point at the end of the first trimester (Poppas et al 1997). By reducing cardiac afterload, this primary adaptation stimulates an overall rise of approximately 40–50% in cardiac output (Duvekot et al 1995, Volman et al 2007). Longitudinal studies suggest that cardiac output rises significantly during the first trimester, and peaks at 20 to 32 weeks, with no significant changes thereafter, or continues to show further small rises until term (Chapman et al 1997, Desai et al 2004, Duvekot & Peeters 1998, Mabie et al 1994, Volman et al 2007). Measures of the pattern and relative contribution of heart rate (HR) and stroke volume (SV) to increased cardiac output suggest that HR rises progressively until 38 weeks while SV increases significantly by 8 weeks and rises further to reach maximum values between 20 and 37 weeks and declines slightly over the remainder of pregnancy (Desai et al 2004, Robson et al 1989, Volman et al 2007).

Stroke volume increases significantly by 8 weeks, peaks at 16–22 weeks and plateaus or shows further small increases during the third trimester (Volman et al 2007). This represents a rise of 21–22% over pre-pregnancy values. In different studies, HR has been found to increase significantly above pre-pregnancy values by 5 and 16 weeks' gestation. Data on the remainder of pregnancy suggest that the increase peaks at 31–36 weeks and shows no significant change or a slight decline thereafter. Current evidence indicates that HR may increase by between 11% and 17% over pre-pregnancy values (Capeless & Clapp 1989, Duvekot et al 1993, Robson et al 1989, Volman et al 2007) (see website).

### Peripheral arterial vasodilatation

Cardiac output rises in early pregnancy, in response to a fall in systemic vascular resistance that reduces afterload

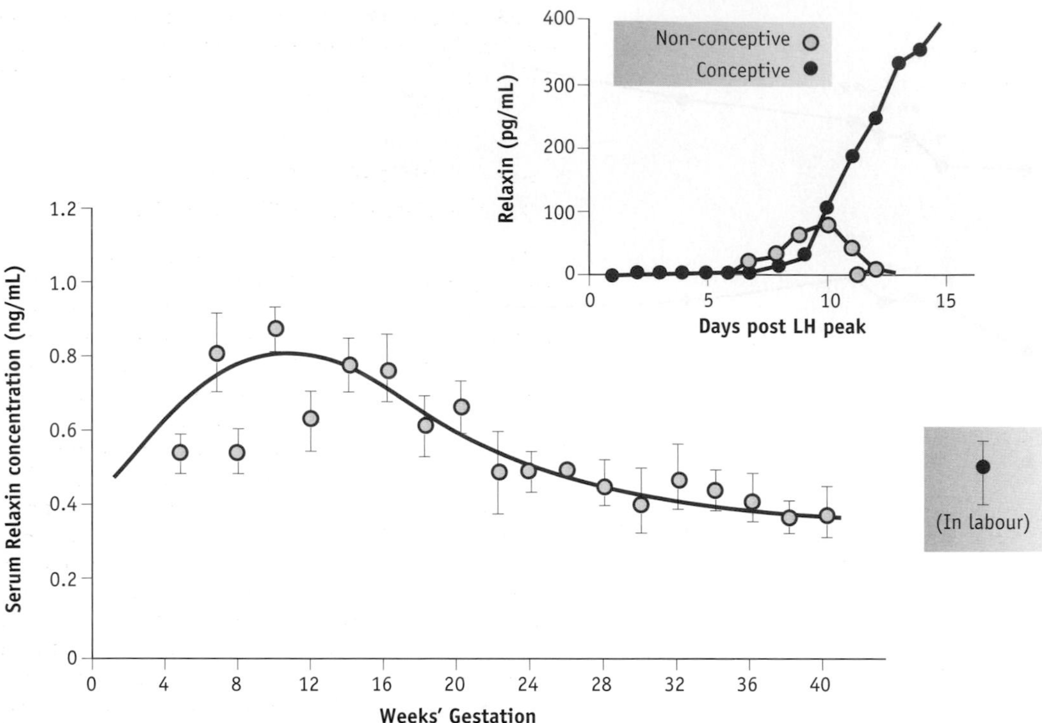


**Figure 31.6** Serum relaxin concentrations from ovulation in a non-conceptive and a conceptive cycle. *(Reproduced with permission from Jaffe 1999: Fig. 27-16; 775.)*

in the myocardial fibres during left ventricular ejection. Decreases in both MAP and total peripheral resistance are evident at 8 weeks' gestation and reach their lowest point by the middle of pregnancy, before returning to similar or slightly above pre-pregnancy values at term (Desai et al 2004). The decline in peripheral vascular resistance is brought about by early reduced vasomotor tone; remodelling of resistance-sized arteries; relaxation of systemic, renal and pulmonary vascular tone and development of new vascular beds in the placenta during the second trimester (Conrad & Novak 2004, Kelly et al 2004, Schrier & Briner 1991).

The initial fall is induced during the luteal phase by rising levels of oestrogens and progesterone. Progesterone has been shown to reduce muscle tone in the vasculature (Magness & Rosenfeld 1989, Omar et al 1995). When fertilization occurs, the further fall in peripheral vascular resistance creates a state of relative hypovolaemia, causing a reflexive increase in stroke volume and heart rate (Clapp et al 1988, Davison & Noble 1981, Duvekot et al 1993, Schrier & Briner 1991).

The compensatory rise in cardiac output produces a rise in vascular filling state characterized by a rise in left atrial diameter, a rise in glomerular filtration rate and little change in plasma renin, between 5 and 8 weeks' gestation (Duvekot et al 1995). Studies have demonstrated that the fall in vascular resistance precedes the rise in circulating blood volume during pregnancy. This suggests that systemic vasodilatation is a primary adaptation to pregnancy that initiates a rise in cardiac output and maintains overall tissue perfusion and blood pressure, prior to significant increases in circulating blood volume (Capeless & Clapp 1989, Phippard et al 1986) (Fig. 31.7).

## Blood volume

The increase in blood volume is composed of a maximum rise of 45–50% in plasma volume and a 20% rise in red cell volume above non-pregnant values. The time course of the increase in plasma volume differs from the rise in red cell mass. Plasma volume begins to increase in the first trimester, increases more rapidly in the second, only slightly during the remainder of pregnancy and is reversed following birth. In contrast, expansion in red cell mass begins in the second trimester and achieves highest increases in the third.

Because of the different pace at which these changes proceed, haemoglobin concentration and haematocrit decline progressively until about 30 weeks' gestation. From then onwards, this trend is reversed, since increases

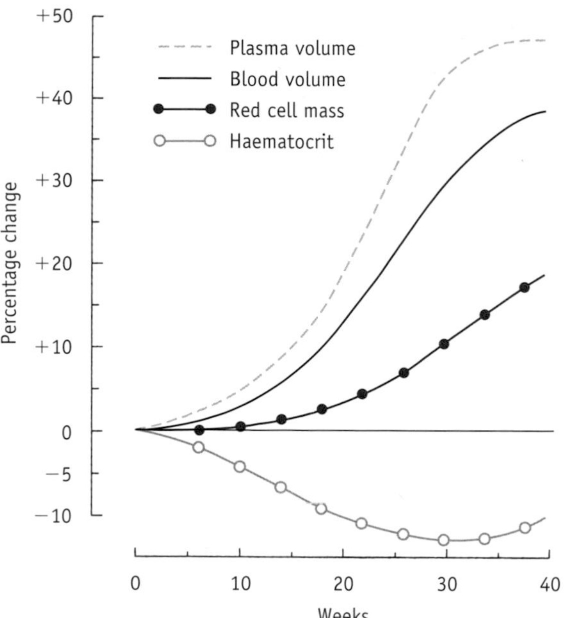


**Figure 31.7** Changes in plasma volume, blood volume, red cell mass and haematocrit during normal pregnancy, expressed as a percentage of pre-pregnancy levels. *(Reproduced with permission from Rosso 1990:25.)*

in red cell volume outstrip plasma volume expansion during the last trimester.

## ADAPTATIONS IN THE VASCULAR RENIN–ANGIOTENSIN–ALDOSTERONE SYSTEM

Current evidence suggests that plasma volume expansion is primarily stimulated by the decline in total peripheral vascular resistance, which activates multiple changes in different components of the maternal vascular renin–angiotensin–aldosterone system (August et al 1995, Irani & Xia 2008, Joyner et al 2007, Skinner 1993).

Angiotensinogen or renin substrate increases very early in pregnancy and closely mirrors levels of oestrogens in individual women (Skinner 1993). During pregnancy, placental oestrogens are largely converted in a series of enzymatic transformations from *dehydroepiandrosterone* (DHEA-S) and related androgens in the fetal zone of the adrenal glands and the fetal liver (Pasqualini 2005). When these androgens reach the placenta and membranes, they undergo enzymatic conversion to a form that serves as substrate for the synthesis of oestrogens (Ticconi et al 2006). Rising concentrations of oestrogens in the maternal circulation and the simultaneous fall in mean arterial pressure stimulates renal production of renin, and oestrogens provide the main stimulus for hepatic production of angiotensinogen, which acts as a substrate for renin (Romen et al 1991).

### Renin, angiotensins and angiotensin-converting enzymes

Renin is a proteolytic enzyme synthesized and released mainly by specialized smooth muscle cells of afferent arterioles entering the glomeruli of the kidney, in response to low blood pressure, low circulating levels of sodium chloride, a rise in effective renal plasma flow and rising levels of oestrogens (Irani & Xia 2008, Romen et al 1991, Valdes 2001). In pregnancy, plasma renin remains fairly stable between 5 and 10 weeks and measures of active renin show a modest rise after 20 weeks' gestation (Duvekot et al 1995, Skinner 1993). On reaching the bloodstream, renin cleaves off part of angiotensinogen, triggering an enzymatic cascade that initially forms a biologically inactive peptide called *angiotensin I* (ANG I). In pregnancy, the next phase involves an oestrogen-induced downregulation of *angiotensin-converting enzyme* (ACE), which circulates in plasma and is found in most tissues but particularly high activities of the enzyme have been found in the lungs (Valdes et al 2001). This glycoprotein cleaves off part of ANG I to form the biologically active peptide, *ANG II*. Within the kidneys, ANG II stimulates increased fluid reabsorption in the proximal tubular cells, by enhancing reabsorption of bicarbonate. Within the adrenals, ANG II stimulates cells in the outer zone of the cortex to secrete aldosterone. In the non-pregnant state, ANG II also acts on peripheral arterioles as a potent vasoconstrictor (Skinner 1993).

During pregnancy, the vasodilatory peptide ANG-(1-7) is formed from ANG II, by angiotensin-converting enzyme 2 (ACE2), and from the biologically inactive peptide ANG I in the vasculature (Heitsch et al 2001). Current evidence shows a progressive rise in urinary excretion of ANG-(1-7) from 6 weeks' gestation (Brosnihan et al 2003, Valdes et al 2001). Although plasma levels of ANG II are double those in the non-pregnant state by the second week of pregnancy, its pressor effects are attenuated by hCG, ANG-(1-7) and by an oestrogen-induced rise in endothelial production of nitric oxide and prostacyclin (Cook & Trundinger 1993, Heitsch et al 2001, Krane & Hamrahian 2007, Skinner 1993, Weiner et al 1994). Oestrogens also inhibit adrenal receptors for ANG II, reducing its stimulatory effect on aldosterone (Wu et al 2003).

### Aldosterone, progesterone and deoxycorticosterone

Aldosterone reduces sodium excretion primarily by acting on distal portions of the renal tubules, where it stimulates

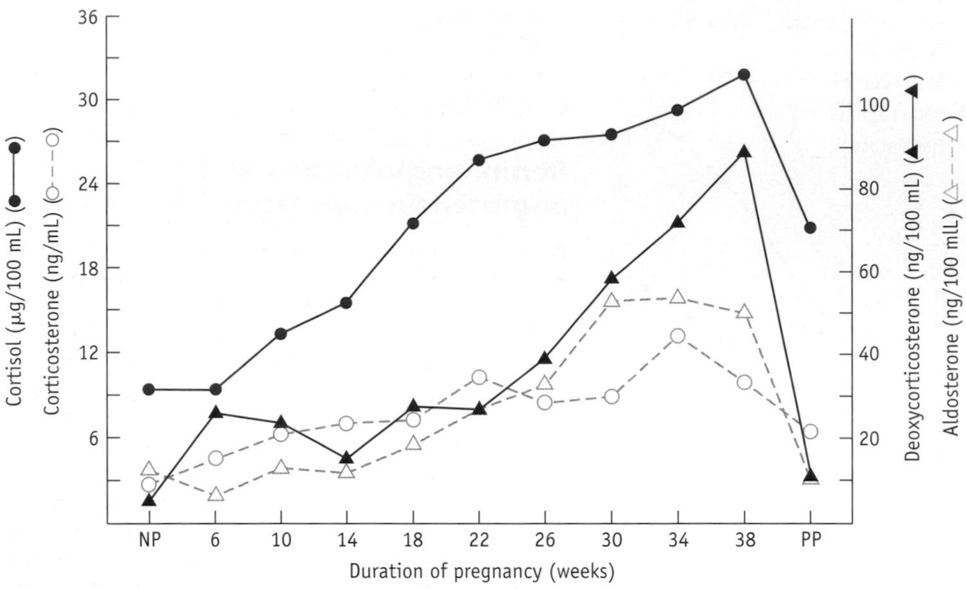


**Figure 31.8** Mean adrenocorticosteroid levels in 11 women throughout pregnancy and postpartum (PP) compared to levels in non-pregnant (NP) women. *(Reproduced from Wintour et al 1978:399, with kind permission of OUP. www.oup.com)*

reabsorption of sodium ions. Plasma levels increase significantly by 12 weeks' gestation and reach a plateau at 30 weeks that is three to five times higher than non-pregnant values. During the first half of pregnancy, effective renal plasma flow increases by 70–80%, and then declines slightly in the third trimester but remains 50–60% above non-pregnant values, which is greater than occurs in any other physiological state. The resulting increase in glomerular filtration rate increases the sodium load from 20,000 to 30,000 mmol/day (Skinner 1993). In pregnancy, aldosterone plays a key role in stimulating sodium retention (Quinkler et al 2001).

In the non-pregnant state, progesterone acts to enhance the excretion of sodium by decreasing its reabsorption in the proximal tubules and by blocking the increased reabsorption of sodium by aldosterone, in the distal tubules. Although progesterone concentrations exceed those of aldosterone at least 50-fold during pregnancy, the renal activity of aldosterone is preserved by the enzymatic conversion of progesterone to a number of different metabolites (Quinkler et al 2001). Current findings suggest that progesterone is effectively converted to various metabolites in the kidneys, which reduces its binding to mineralocorticoid receptors, thereby attenuating its capacity to competitively inhibit aldosterone (Quinkler et al 2001). Some of the increase in progesterone is also converted to *deoxycorticosterone* (DOC), which acts on the distal tubules to promote the reabsorption of sodium. Rising levels of DOC occur by approximately 8 weeks' gestation and increase 10–15-fold, to a peak of approximately 100 mg/dL at term, which is higher than aldosterone. However, the salt-retaining properties of this hormone are 30–50 times less potent than aldosterone (Nolten & Rueckert 1981, Skinner 1993) (Fig. 31.8).

## Atrial natriuretic peptide

*Atrial natriuretic peptide* (ANP) is a diuretic, natriuretic and vasodilator hormone, produced in the atrial chambers of the heart. Outside of pregnancy, secretion is primarily stimulated by stretching of the atrial wall that accompanies volume expansion or increases in blood pressure. ANP acts in a variety of ways to decrease fluid intake, promote salt and water excretion, and counter all components of the RAAS (Cootauco et al 2008, Duvekot & Peeters 1998, Kaufman 1995). Within the kidneys, ANP directly inhibits renin production and tubular reabsorption of sodium, and production of aldosterone, in the adrenals. In vitro studies have also shown that ANP produces marked relaxation of vascular smooth muscle and antagonizes the vasoconstrictive effects of ANG II (Cootauco et al 2008, Steegers 1991).

Conflicting evidence currently exists on the pattern of ANP secretion during normal pregnancy and the extent to which its actions are blunted. Plasma levels have been reported to decline from 20 weeks' gestation, reach lowest levels at 36 weeks and return to non-pregnant values by 12 weeks' postpartum (Thomsen et al 1993). Other studies have reported a modest rise with advancing gestation, declining at term or at placental separation and then falling significantly by 72 hours postpartum (Lowe et al 1992, Yoshimura et al 1994).

All experimental evidence indicates that atrial, renal and adrenal responsiveness to ANP is blunted during pregnancy. Oestrogens and progesterone reduce ANP receptors in the zona glomerulosa, thereby inhibiting its aldosterone-suppressant effects, while the kidneys display a blunted response to the diuretic effects of both ANP and nitric oxide (Knight et al 2006, Vaillancourt et al 1997). At the same time, the pregnancy-induced rise in nitric oxide blunts the activity of atrial volume receptors, which attenuates the reduction in renal tubular sodium reabsorption, thus facilitating the expansion in extracellular fluid volume (Tam & Kaufman 2002). These regulatory mechanisms persist until late pregnancy, when ANP responsiveness to intravenous volume expansion is enhanced (Lowe et al 1992). Experimental evidence suggests that activation of the cardiac oxytocin system induces a rapid rise in ANP, which may stimulate the rapid diuresis that occurs postpartum (Mukaddam-Daher et al 2002, Yosimura et al 1994).

## Erythropoiesis

The increase in red cell mass during pregnancy is stimulated by *erythropoietin*. This glycoprotein hormone is synthesized in ground tissue, in the kidneys and to a lesser extent in the liver. Levels of serum immunoreactive erythropoietin remain at non-pregnant values during the first trimester, begin to rise during the second and reach maximum levels during the third trimester. Within the bone marrow, erythropoietin acts on erythrocyte colony-forming cells. These give rise to increasing numbers of mature erythrocytes within 2 days of increased levels of erythropoietin within the circulation.

At present, the precise mechanisms involved in stimulating erythropoietin during pregnancy remain unclear. The evidence suggests that components of the maternal plasma renin–angiotensin system may be involved. Angiotensinogen and erythropoietin share a number of similarities. Both compete for specific binding to erythropoietin receptors on human bone marrow cells, and bone marrow cells show binding of angiotensinogen that is inhibited by erythropoietin. This evidence suggests that angiotensinogen is a precursor for erythropoietin. While both components are increased in the maternal circulation during pregnancy, the timing and possible interactions between these components and erythropoietin remain to be clarified. A number of pregnancy hormones have stimulatory and inhibitory influences on the actions of erythropoietin. Progesterone partly prevents the inhibitory influence of oestrogen on stem cell utilization of erythropoietin, while placental lactogen and prolactin enhance the stimulatory action of erythropoietin on red cell production. At present, however, the relative significance of these hormonal actions remains unclear (Beguin et al 1990).

## VENTILATION

Extensive anatomical and functional changes occur in the respiratory system. These accommodate both the progressive increase in gas exchange required by the rising blood volume and the growing space occupied by the uterus. From early pregnancy onwards, the overall shape of the chest alters, by a flaring of the lower ribs that seems to occur independently of any mechanical pressure from the growing uterus. This progressively increases the subcostal angle, from 68 degrees in early pregnancy to 103 degrees at term, and increases the transverse diameter of the chest by approximately 2 cm. Because of the flaring of the lower ribs, the diaphragm rises by a maximum of 4 cm while its contribution to the respiratory effort increases and shows no evidence of being impeded by the uterus. Studies on diaphragmatic movements during respiration – either sitting or lying down – have found them to be larger than in the non-pregnant state. This implies that breathing during pregnancy is more diaphragmatic than costal (de Swiet 1991a, Romen et al 1991) (Fig. 31.9).

The main functional change that occurs within the lungs is the gradual increase in the amount of air that is inspired or expired with a normal breath. This functional capacity (tidal volume) increases from 500 mL in the non-pregnant state to approximately 700 mL at term. As a result of this change, women breathe more deeply during pregnancy than in the non-pregnant state (Fig. 31.10).

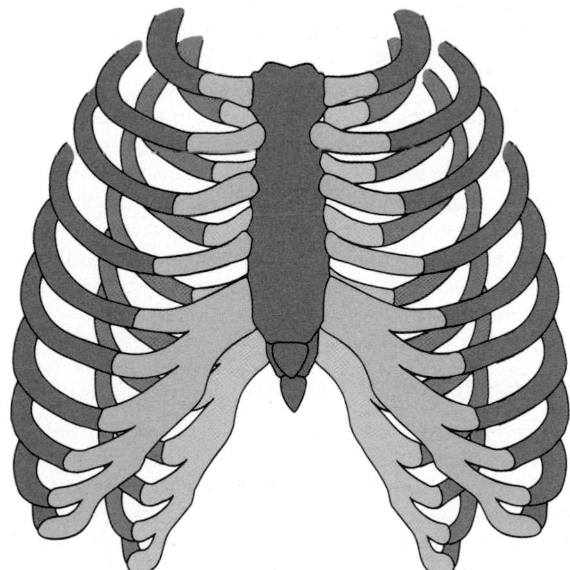

**Figure 31.9** The ribcage in pregnancy (**coloured**) and the non-pregnancy state (**grey**) showing the increased subcostal angle, the increased transverse diameter and the raised diaphragm in pregnancy. *(Reproduced with permission from de Swiet 1991a:88.)*

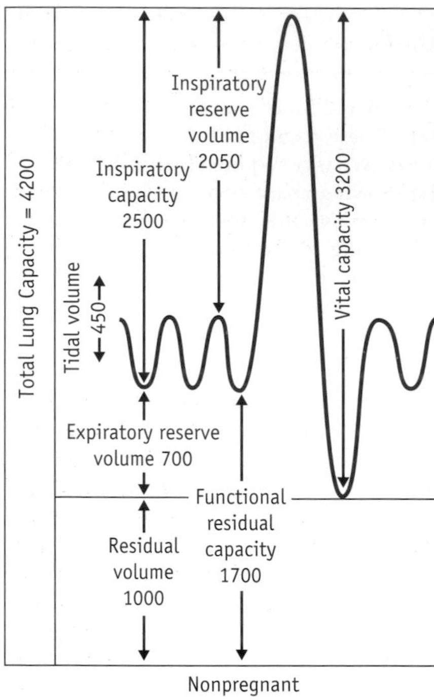


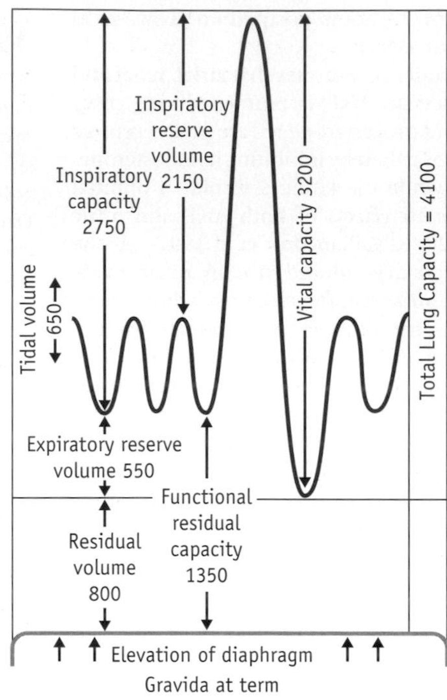


**Figure 31.10** Lung volume changes in pregnancy. *(Reproduced with permission from Blackburn 2007:316.)*

Since the maximum amount of air that can be expired forcibly after maximum inspiration only increases by 100–200 mL, the increase in tidal volume is produced at the expense of the expiratory reserve volume. This means that a smaller amount of air remains in the lungs at the end of quiet expiration. As less residual air is mixed with the next inspiration of fresh air, this results in lower levels of $P\text{CO}_2$ that bring about a reciprocal rise in $P\text{O}_2$. $P\text{CO}_2$ declines from approximately 39 mmHg in the non-pregnant state to 31 mmHg during pregnancy, while $P\text{O}_2$ increases from 93.4 to 101.8 mmHg, over the same period (de Swiet 1991a).

## Oxygen consumption

The progressive increases in cardiac output and pulmonary ventilation are proportionately greater than those occurring in maternal and fetal oxygen consumption during pregnancy. Oxygen consumption shows a linear increase with body weight as pregnancy advances, increasing to 38 mL/min (15%) above average values in the non-pregnant state (de Swiet 1991a). It is composed of the overall increase in tissue mass, higher metabolic rate of fetal and placental tissue, along with that of some maternal organs, particularly the heart, lungs and kidneys (Fig. 31.11).

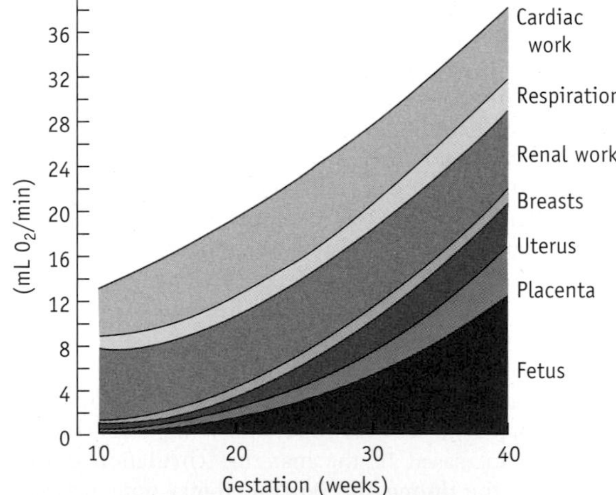


**Figure 31.11** Partition of the increased oxygen consumption in pregnancy among the organs concerned. *(Reproduced with permission from de Swiet, 1991a:91.)*

The increase in oxygen consumption is facilitated by a 40–50% increase in ventilation and by an 18% increase in the oxygen-carrying capacity of the blood. Because of this relative oversupply of oxygen, higher concentrations are returned to the heart from the venous circulation, making the arteriovenous oxygen difference significantly smaller than in the non-pregnant state. The extent of the arteriovenous oxygen difference is smallest in early pregnancy and does not reach average non-pregnant values until term (de Swiet 1991a).

The increase in ventilation during pregnancy reduces alveolar and plasma concentrations of carbon dioxide. Studies have demonstrated that arterial partial pressure of carbon dioxide ($P\text{CO}_2$) is about 30 mmHg in late pregnancy, compared to 39 mmHg during the follicular phase of the cycle. Since fetal $P\text{CO}_2$ remains at approximately 41 mmHg, the lower levels in the maternal circulation encourage the diffusion of $CO_2$ from fetal blood, across the placental membranes.

**Reflective activity 31.1**

Consider the changes that occur in maternal organ systems. How would you use this information to assess maternal health and fetal growth.

## THE MAMMARY GLANDS/BREASTS

See Chapter 43.

## UTERINE ADAPTATIONS

The uterus changes from being a small pelvic organ, with a cavity of around 10 mL and weighing approximately 50 g. By 36 weeks, its weight has increased to an estimated 1100 g, representing almost a 20-fold increase in mass, and its average volume is 5 litres. It is then in contact with the anterior abdominal wall and extends as far as the xiphisternum. During pregnancy, the uterus is a central recipient of the increases in circulating blood volume. In the follicular phase of the cycle, uterine blood flow is approximately 45 mL/min (Burton et al 2009). This changes very little during early pregnancy, but rises sharply from about 20 weeks, to reach approximately 750 mL/min at term, when it receives nearly 20% of total cardiac output (Burton et al 2009, Steer 1991).

Uterine growth is characterized by a highly regulated process of myometrial cell differentiation:

- proliferation and reduced apoptosis in early pregnancy
- hypertrophy of existing cells and increased matrix elaboration during the remainder of pregnancy (Shynlova et al 2009).

Growth is stimulated by hCG, progesterone, growth factors, oestrogens and oxytocin, and by progressive distension exerted by the fetus, placenta and amniotic fluid, particularly during the third trimester. These factors promote synthesis of structural and contractile proteins (Blackburn 2007, Shynlova et al 2009, Ticconi et al 2006 (see website). During the first few months of pregnancy, growth is accompanied by increasing thickness of the myometrium in the corpus and the fundus. As the organ increases in length from around 12 weeks, the isthmus is gradually formed as an area with reduced density of muscle fibres (Steer 1991).

### Myometrial changes

The bundles of smooth muscle fibres within the uterus are arranged in three or four layers embedded in a matrix of connective tissue and ground substance. The former acts as intramuscular tendons while the latter transmits contractile forces from individual cells along the muscle bundle during labour (Blackburn 2007). Two outer layers contain longitudinal and circular fibres that are partly continuous with the supporting ligaments. The middle layers that hold the vascular supply have a criss-cross pattern of fibres that run in all directions. Finally, the inner layer is composed of longitudinal fibres and covers the decidua (Steer 1991) (see website).

The smooth muscle forming the myometrium does not have the precise transverse alignment of thick and thin filaments that characterizes the organization of skeletal fibres. Filaments of smooth muscle are situated in random bundles throughout the cells, and myosin filaments are arranged alongside actin in uninterrupted unidirectional order. In addition to these main contractile filaments, smooth muscle also contains intermediate filaments. These are attached to all areas of cell membrane, which allows them to form networks across the cell. As a result of this organization, contractions can generate force in any direction and also produce a much greater degree of shortening than in skeletal muscle. For most of pregnancy, this action remains local, as few intracellular connections are formed and quiescence is actively maintained, by hormonal mechanisms that regulate the process of differentiation, until the last few weeks of pregnancy (Blackburn 2007, Shynlova et al 2009) (see website).

## CONCLUSION

The adaptations of pregnancy affect all systems of the body, and are regulated by a complex series of neurohormonal interactions between maternal reproductive organ systems and the fetoplacental unit. This chapter has identified the time course of key changes to enable midwives to look for the characteristic features of each trimester.

## KEY POINTS

- Pregnancy is a progressive period of structural and functional adaptations in all organ systems.
- These changes are regulated by neurohormonal interactions between maternal organs of reproduction and the conceptus.
- Neurohormonal regulation of maternal adaptations are critical to a successful pregnancy, the onset of labour at term, and the shift from placental to mammary nutrition immediately after birth.

## REFERENCES


August P, Mueller FB, Sealey JE, et al: Role of renin-angiotensin system in blood pressure regulation in pregnancy, *Lancet* 345:896–897, 1995.

Baylis C, Davison J: The urinary system. In Chamberlain G, Broughton Pipkin F, editors: *Clinical physiology in obstetrics*, Oxford, 1998, Blackwell Science, pp 263–307.

Beguin Y, Lipscei G, Oris R, et al: Serum immunoreactive erythropoietin during pregnancy and in the early postpartum, *British Journal of Haematology* 76:545–549, 1990.

Blackburn S: *Maternal, fetal & neonatal physiology*, Missouri, 2007, Saunders Elsevier.

Brosnihan KB, Neves LAA, Joyner J-N, et al: Enhanced renal immunocytochemical expression of ANG-(1-7) and ACE2 during pregnancy, *Hypertension* 42(2):749–753, 2003.

Brunton PJ, Russell JA, Douglas AJ: Adaptive responses of the maternal-hypothalamic-pituitary-adrenal axis during pregnancy and lactation, *Journal of Neuroendocrinology* 20:764–776, 2008.

Burton GJ, Woods AW, Jauniaux E, et al: Rheological and physiological consequences of conversion of the maternal spiral arteries for uteroplacental blood flow during human pregnancy, *Placenta* 30:473–482, 2009.

Capeless EL, Clapp JF: Cardiovascular changes in early pregnancy, *American Journal of Obstetrics and Gynecology* 161(6):1449–1452, 1989.

Chapman AB, Zamudio S, Woodmansee W, et al: Systemic and renal haemodynamic changes in the luteal phase of the menstrual cycle mimic early pregnancy, *American Journal of Physiology* 273(42):F777–F782, 1997.

Chapman AB, Abraham WT, Zamudio S, et al: Temporal relationships between hormonal and hemodynamic changes in early pregnancy, *Kidney International* 54:2056–2063, 1998.

Chidambaram M, Duncan JA, Lai VS: Variation in the renin angiotensin system throughout the normal menstrual cycle, *Journal of the American Society of Nephrology* 13:446-452, 2002.

Churchill D, Perry IJ, Beevers DG: Ambulatory blood pressure in pregnancy and fetal growth, *Lancet* 349:7–10, 1997.

Clapp JF, Seaward BL, Sleamaker RH, et al: Maternal physiologic adaptations to early pregnancy, *American Journal of Obstetrics and Gynecology* 159(6):1456–1460, 1988.

Conrad KP, Novak J: Emerging role of relaxin in renal and cardiovascular function, *American Journal of Physiology* 287:R250–R261, 2004.

Conrad KP, Danielson LA, Novak JN, et al: Is relaxin the 'elusive' vasodilator of pregnancy? In Tregear GW, Ivell R, Bathgate RA, et al, editors: *Relaxin 2000*, Dordrecht, 2001, Kluwer Academic Press, pp 169–176.

Cook C, Trundinger B: Angiotensin sensitivity predicts aspirin benefit in placental insufficiency, *British Journal of Obstetrics and Gynaecology* 100:46–50, 1993.

Cootauco AC, Murphy JD, Maleski J, et al: Atrial natriuretic peptide production and natriuretic peptide receptors in the human uterus and their effects on myometrial relaxation, *American Journal of Obstetrics and Gynaecology* 199:429.e1–429.e6, 2008.

Davison JM, Noble MCB: Serial changes in 24 hour creatinine clearance during normal menstrual cycles and the first trimester of pregnancy, *British Journal of Obstetrics and Gynaecology* 88:10–17, 1981.

Davison JM, Vallotton MB, Lindheimer MD: Plasma osmolality and urinary concentration and dilution during and after pregnancy: evidence that lateral recumbency inhibits maximal urinary concentrating ability, *British Journal of Obstetrics and Gynaecology* 88:427–479, 1981.

Desai DK Modley J, Naidoo DP: Echocardiographic assessment of cardiovascular hemodynamics in normal pregnancy, *Obstetrics and Gynaecology* 104:20–29, 2004.

de Swiet M: The respiratory system. In Hytten F, Chamberlain G, editors: *Clinical physiology in obstetrics*, Oxford, 1991a, Blackwell Scientific, pp 83–100.

Di Iorio R, Marinoni E, Letizia C, et al: Adrenomedullin production is increased in normal human pregnancy, *European Journal Endocrinology* 140:201–206, 1999.

Douglas AJ: Baby on board: do responses to stress in the maternal brain mediate adverse pregnancy outcome? *Frontiers in Neuroendocrinology* 31(3):359–376, 2010.

Duvekot JJ, Peeters LLH: Very early changes in cardiovascular physiology. In Chamberlain G, Broughton Pipkin F, editors: *Clinical physiology in obstetrics*, Oxford, 1998, Blackwell Science, pp 3–32.

Duvekot JJ, Cheriex EC, Pieters FAA: Early pregnancy changes in hemodynamics and volume homeostasis are consecutive adjustments triggered by a primary fall in systemic vascular tone, *American Journal of Obstetrics and Gynecology* 169(6):1382–1392, 1993.

Duvekot JJ, Cheriex EC, Pieters FAA, et al: Maternal volume homeostasis in early pregnancy in relation to fetal growth restriction, *Obstetrics and Gynecology* 85(3):361–367, 1995.

Heitsch H, Brovkovych S, Malinski T, et al: Angiotensin-(1-7) stimulated nitric oxide and superoxide release from endothelial cells, *Hypertension* 37:72–76, 2001.

Hermsteiner M, Zoltan DR, Kunzel W: Human chorionic gonadotrophin attenuates the vascular response to angiotensin II, *European Journal of Obstetrics and Gynaecology and Reproductive Biology* 102:148–154, 2002.

Irani RA, Xia Y: The functional role of the renin-angiotensin system in pregnancy and preeclampsia, *Placenta* 29:763–771, 2008.

Jaffe RB: Neuroendocrine-metabolic regulation of pregnancy. In Yen SSC, Jaffe RB, Barbieri RL, editors: *Reproductive Endocrinology*, Philadelphia, 1999, Saunders, p 775.

Jensen D, Wolfe LA, Slatkovska L, et al: Effects of human pregnancy on the ventilatory chemoreflex response to carbon dioxide, *American Journal of Physiology* 288:R1369–R1375, 2005.

Johnson MR, Okokon E ,Collins WP, et al: The effect of human chorionic gonadotrophin and pregnancy on the circulating level of relaxin, *Journal of Clinical Endocrinology and Metabolism* 72(5):1042–1047, 1991.

Joyner J, Neves LAA, Granger JP, et al: Temporal-spatial expression of ANG-(1-7) and angiotensin-converting enzyme 2 in the kidney of normal and hypertensive rats, *American Journal of Physiology* 293:R169–R177, 2007.

Kaufman S: Control of intravascular volume during pregnancy, *Clinical Experimental Pharmacological Physiology* 22:157–163, 1995.

Kelly BA, Bond BC, Poston L: Aortic adaptation to pregnancy: elevated expression of matrix metalloproteinases-2 and -3 in rat gestation, *Molecular Human Reproduction* 10(5):331–337, 2004.

Khraibi AA, Yu T, Tang D: Role of nitric oxide in the natriuretic and diuretic responses in pregnant rats, *American Journal of Physiology* 285:F938–F944, 2003.

Knight S, Snellen H, Humphreys M, et al: Increased renal phosphodiesterase-5 activity mediates the blunted natriuretic response to ANP in the pregnant rat, *American Journal of Physiology* 292:F655–F659, 2006.

Krane NK, Hamrahian M: Pregnancy: kidney diseases and hypertension, *American Journal of Kidney Disease* 49(2):336–345, 2007.

Kristiansson P, Wang JX: Reproductive hormones and blood pressure during pregnancy, *Human Reproduction* 16(1):13–17, 2001.

Lain KY, Daftary AR, Ness RB: First trimester adipocytokine concentrations and risk of developing gestational diabetes later in pregnancy, *Clinical Endocrinology* 69(3):407–411, 2008.

Lowe SA, Macdonald GJ, Brown MA: Atrial natriuretic peptide in pregnancy: response to oral sodium supplementation, *Clinical and Experimental Pharmacological & Physiology* 19:607–612, 1992.

Mabie W, DiSessa TG, Crocker LG, et al: A longitudinal study of cardiac output in normal human pregnancy, *American Journal of Obstetrics and Gynecology* 170(3):849–856, 1994.

Maccarrone M, Finazzi-Agro A: Anandamide hydrolase: a guardian angel of human reproduction, *Trends in Pharmacological Sciences* 25(7):353–357, 2004.

Magness RR, Rosenfeld CR: Local and systemic estradiol-17β: effects on uterine and systemic vasodilation, *American Journal of Physiology* 256:E536–E542, 1989.

Mukaddam-Daher S, Jankowski M, Wang D, et al: Regulation of cardiac oxytocin system and natriuretic peptide during rat gestation and postpartum, *Journal of Endocrinology* 175:211–216, 2002.

Nakamura T, Matsui K, Ito M, et al: Effect of pregnancy and hormone treatments on pressor responses to angiotensin II in conscious rats, *American Journal of Obstetrics and Gynecology* 159(5):989–995, 1988.

Nolten WE, Rueckert PA: Elevated free cortisol index in pregnancy: possible regulatory mechanisms, *American Journal of Obstetrics and Gynecology* 139(4):492–498, 1981.

Novak J, Danielson LA, Kerchner LJ, et al: Relaxin is essential for renal vasodilation during pregnancy in conscious rats, *Journal of Clinical Investigation* 107(11):1469–1475, 2001.

Omar HA, Ramirez R, Gibson M: Properties of a progesterone-induced relaxation in human placental arteries and veins, *Journal of Clinical Endocrinology and Metabolism* 80(2):370–373, 1995.

Pasqualini JR: Enzymes involved in the formation and transformation of steroid hormones in the fetal and placental compartments, *Journal of Steroid Biochemistry and Molecular Biology* 97:401–415, 2005.

Phippard AF, Horvath JS, Glynn EM: Circulatory adaptations to pregnancy – serial studies of haemodynamics, blood volume, renin and aldosterone in the baboon, *Journal of Hypertension* 4:773–779, 1986.

Poppas A, Shroff SG, Korcarz CE, et al: Serial assessment of cardiovascular system in normal pregnancy: role of arterial compliance and pulsatile arterial load, *Circulation* 95:2407–2415, 1997.

Quinkler M, Johanssen S, Bumke-Vogt C, et al: Enzyme-mediated protection of the mineralocorticoid receptor against progesterone in the human kidney, *Molecular Cellular Endocrinology* 171:21–24, 2001.

Robson SC, Hunter S, Boys RJ, et al: Serial study of factors influencing changes in cardiac output during human pregnancy, *American Journal of Physiology* 256:H1060–H1065, 1989.

Romen Y, Masaki DI, Mittelmark RA: Physiological and endocrine adjustments to pregnancy. In Mittelmark RA, Wiswell RA, editors: *Exercise in pregnancy*, Baltimore, 1991, Williams and Wilkins, pp 9–29.

Rosso P: *Nutrition and metabolism in pregnancy*, New York, 1990, Oxford University Press.

Schrier RW, Briner VA: Peripheral arterial vasodilation hypothesis of sodium and water retention in pregnancy: implications for pathogenesis of pre-eclampsia, *Obstetrics and Gynecology* 77(4):632–639, 1991.

Sealey JE, Atlas SA, Glorioso N, et al: Cyclical secretion of prorenin during the menstrual cycle: synchronization with luteinizing hormone and progesterone, *Proceedings of the National Academy of Science USA* 82:8705–8709, 1985.

Sealey JE, Cholst I, Glorioso N, et al: Sequential changes in plasma luteinizing hormone and plasma prorenin during the menstrual cycle, *Journal of Clinical Endocrinology and Metabolism* 65(1):1–5, 1987.

Shynlova O, Tsui P, Jaffer S, et al: Integration of endocrine and mechanical signals in the regulation of myometrial functions during pregnancy and labour, *European Journal of Obstetrics & Gynaecology and Reproductive Biology* 1445:S2–S10, 2009.

Skinner SL: The renin system in fertility and normal human pregnancy. In Robertson JIS, Nicholls MG, editors: *The renin–angiotensin system*, Vol 1, London, 1993, Gower Medical, pp 50.1–50.16.

Spaanderman MEA, Meertens M, Van Bussell M, et al: Cardiac output increases independently of basal metabolic rate in early pregnancy, *American Journal of Physiology* 278:H1585–H1588, 2000.

Stanton BA, Koeppen BM: The kidney. In Berne RM, Levy MN, editors: *Physiology*, St Louis, 1993, Mosby Year Book.

Steegers EAP: Atrial natriuretic peptide during human pregnancy and puerperium, *Fetal Medicine Review* 3:185–196, 1991.

Steer PJ: The genital system. In Hytten F, Chamberlain G, editors: *Clinical Physiology in Obstetrics*, Oxford, 1991, Blackwell Scientific, pp 303–344.

Steer PJ: Maternal hemoglobin concentration and birth weight, *American Journal of Clinical Nutrition* 71(5):1285S–1287S, 2000.

Steer P, Ash Alam M, Wadsworth J, et al: Relation between maternal haemoglobin concentration and birth weight in different ethnic groups, *British Medical Journal* 310:489–491, 1995.

Stewart DR ,Overstreet JW, Nakajima ST, et al: Enhanced ovarian steroid secretion before implantation in early human pregnancy, *Journal of Clinical Endocrinology and Metabolism* 76(6):1470–1476, 1993.

Sudhir K, Chou TM, Mullen WL, et al: Mechanisms of oestrogen induced vasodilation: in vivo studies in canine coronary conductance and resistance arteries, *Journal of the American College of Cardiology* 26:807–814, 1995.

Szmuilowicz ED, Adler GK, Williams JS, et al: Relationship between aldosterone and progesterone in the human menstrual cycle, *Journal of Clinical Endocrinology and Metabolism* 91(10):3981–3987, 2006.

Tam S, Kaufman S: NOS inhibition restores renal responses to atrial distension during pregnancy, *American Journal of Physiology* 282:R1364–R1367, 2002.

Thomsen JK, Fogh-Andersen N, Jaszczak P, et al: Atrial natriuretic peptide (ANP) decrease during normal pregnancy as related to hemodynamic changes and volume regulation, *Acta Obstetricia et Gynecologica Scandinavica* 72:103–110, 1993.

Ticconi C, Belmonte A, Piccione E, et al: Feto-placental communication system with the myometrium in pregnancy and parturition: the role of hormones, neurohormones, inflammatory mediators, and locally active factors, *Journal of Maternal-Fetal & Neonatal Medicine* 19(3):125–133, 2006.

Vaillancourt P, Omer S, Palfree R, et al: Downregulation of adrenal atrial natriuretic peptide receptor mRNAs and proteins by pregnancy in the rat, *Journal of Endocrinology* 155:523–530, 1997.

Valdes G, Germain AM, Corthorn J, et al: Urinary vasodilator and vasoconstrictor angiotensins during menstrual cycle, pregnancy, and lactation, *Endocrine* 16(2):117–122, 2001.

Vokes TJ, Weiss NM, Schrieiber J, et al: Osmoregulation of thirst and vasopressin during normal menstrual cycle, *American Journal of Physiology* 254(23):R641–R647, 1988.

Volman MNM, Rep A, Kadzinska I, et al: Haemodynamic changes in the second half of pregnancy: a longitudinal, noninvasive study with thoracic electrical bioimpedance, *BJOG* 114(5):576–581, 2007.

Weiner CP, Lizasoain I, Baylis SA, et al: Induction of calcium dependent nitric oxide synthases by sex hormones, *Proceedings of the National Academy of Science USA* 91:5212–5216, 1994.

Williams MR, Westerman RA, Kingwell BA: Variations in endothelial function and arterial compliance during the menstrual cycle, *Journal of Clinical Endocrinology and Metabolism* 86(11):5389–5395, 2001.

Wintour EM, Coghlan JP, Oddie CJ, et al: A sequential study of adrenocorticosteroid level in human pregnancy, *Clinical and Experimental Pharmacology & Physiology* 5(4):399–403, 1978.

Wu Z, Zheng W, Sandberg K: Estrogen regulates adrenal angiotensin type 1 receptors by modulating adrenal angiotensin levels, *Endocrinology* 144(4):1350–1356, 2003.

Yoshimura T, Yoshimura M, Yasue H, et al: Plasma concentration of atrial natriuretic peptide and brain natriuretic peptide during normal human pregnancy and the postpartum period, *Journal of Endocrinology* 140:393–397, 1994.

Zhang Y, Stewart KG, Davidge ST: Endogenous estrogen mediates vascular reactivity and distensibility in pregnant rat mesenteric arteries, *American Journal of Physiology* 280:H956–H961, 2001.

Chapter 32

# Confirming pregnancy and care of the pregnant woman

*Kuldip K. Bharj and Anne Marie Henshaw*

## LEARNING OUTCOMES

After reading this chapter, you will be able to:

- discuss the role of the midwife in the provision of woman-centred care during pregnancy giving due consideration to women's physiological, educational, psychological and socioeconomic needs as well as recognizing the importance of culture, ethnicity, age, disability and sexual orientation in the provision of responsive care
- describe the physical and biochemical assessments that may enable the diagnosis and confirmation of pregnancy
- discuss opportunities for women to make early contact with the maternity service and discuss the purpose of the initial visit, identifying the importance of taking a comprehensive antenatal history, and consider the relevance of the information obtained in determining future care and the options for place of birth
- examine the physiological changes during pregnancy that might lead to disturbance and discomfort within the various body systems and discuss their implications and the ways in which these may be alleviated or minimized
- describe the physical examination, including the abdominal examination, undertaken during initial and subsequent antenatal visits and discuss the relevance of the information obtained in planning prospective care
- discuss the psychological needs of women during pregnancy and explore the role of the midwife in supporting women during their transition into pregnancy, childbirth and early parenting
- recognize the importance of health education and promotion during the antenatal period to maintain and/or improve the woman and her baby's health
- describe the signs and symptoms of pelvic girdle pain and discuss its possible physical and psychological effects and its management during the antenatal, intranatal and postnatal period
- appreciate the importance of effective communication with women and their families during the antenatal period to provide sensitive and responsive care and to develop positive relationships with them.

## INTRODUCTION

This chapter focuses upon the care and services provided and delivered to women during the antenatal period from the point at which a woman believes she may be pregnant to the onset of labour. During this period, pregnant women experience major physiological and psychological changes facilitating adaptation and preparation for birthing and transition to parenting (Coad & Dunstall 2005, Stables & Rankin 2005). Midwives are key professionals who deliver care to the women and their families. They work in partnership with women to assess women's individual needs and to plan and implement the most appropriate care.

## CONFIRMATION OF PREGNANCY

Many women of childbearing age who are sexually active may suspect that they are pregnant, especially if their menstrual period is delayed and/or other symptoms of pregnancy, such as nausea or vomiting, are experienced. Often, many women say that they 'just feel different'. Women may choose to confirm their pregnancy either by using a home pregnancy test or by seeking diagnosis through their midwife or general practitioner (GP). Confirmation of pregnancy is established by a detailed history and a clinical examination based on the signs and symptoms of pregnancy, resulting from the physiological alteration in the body's systems and organs. These include amenorrhoea; breast changes and tenderness; nausea and vomiting; increased frequency of micturition; enlargement of the uterus; and skin changes. These signs and symptoms become obvious to the woman as her pregnancy advances, but as some of these symptoms and signs may be found in other conditions not associated with pregnancy, it is important that the midwife is aware of these conditions, as she may need to refer the woman for further investigations or specialist advice.

**Reflective activity 32.1**

When you next undertake a 'booking' interview, discuss with the woman, and, if appropriate, her partner:

- What made her suspect that she was pregnant?
- How did she confirm the pregnancy? Did she use a home test?
- How many weeks pregnant was she when the pregnancy was confirmed?
- How, and at what gestation, did she make contact with her midwife and/or GP?

Signs and symptoms of pregnancy may be considered as presumptive, probable and positive, as illustrated in Table 32.1.

### First 4 weeks

**Amenorrhoea:** Following implantation of the fertilized ovum, the endometrium undergoes decidual change and normally menstruation does not occur throughout pregnancy.

Amenorrhoea almost invariably accompanies pregnancy and, in a sexually active woman who has previously menstruated regularly, can be considered to be due to pregnancy unless this is disproved. However, the possibility of secondary amenorrhoea should be considered.

**Breast changes:** Discomfort, tenderness or tingling and a feeling of fullness of the breasts may be noticed as early as the third or fourth week of pregnancy, as the blood supply to the breasts increases.

**Nausea and vomiting:** These are common symptoms, with nausea affecting about 70% to 85% of pregnant women and vomiting approximately 50% (Gadsby et al 1993, Lacroix et al 2000, Whitehead et al 1992). Of the women who experience nausea, only a small percentage experience it in the morning but many suffer from it throughout the day. Vomiting, however, is also a feature of a variety of conditions, such as gastroenteritis, urinary tract infection and hydatidiform mole, and these should be ruled out.

### Around 8 weeks

**Nausea and vomiting:** These usually persist in those women who are affected.

**Frequency of micturition:** This is due to increased vascularity of the bladder and lasts until about the 16th week of pregnancy, when the gravid uterus rises out of the pelvic girdle.

**Breast changes:** The breasts enlarge and the superficial veins on both the chest and breasts dilate. The enlarged breasts may be painful.

### Around 12 weeks

**Nausea and vomiting:** These may decrease, and, for some women, cease altogether. The mean duration of nausea is about 34.6 days and in about 50% of women it lasts until 14 weeks' gestation (Lacroix et al 2000).

**Enlarged uterus:** The enlarged uterus is just palpable above the symphysis pubis at about 12 weeks. Other reasons for an enlarged uterus include tumours such as ovarian cysts or fibroids. Ascites may be mistaken for a pregnant uterus.

**Skin changes:** Pigmentation of the skin occurs and is especially pronounced in brunettes. Areas of increased pigmentation include the nipples and areola; the linea nigra, which is the line of pigmentation from the symphysis pubis to the umbilicus; and, rarely, chloasma, which is sometimes referred to as the 'mask of pregnancy' (see website). The nipples become more prominent and Montgomery's tubercles are visible on the areola.

### Around 16 weeks

**Colostrum:** The breasts may begin to secrete colostrum, which persists throughout pregnancy and for the first few days after delivery until milk is produced. A secondary areola may appear in brunettes.

**Quickening:** The first fetal movements may be felt by primigravidae at 19+ weeks and by multigravidae at 17+ weeks. The time scale over which fetal movements are first

**Table 32.1 Signs and symptoms of pregnancy**

| Time – weeks of gestation | Presumptive signs | Probable signs | Positive signs | Differential diagnosis |
|---|---|---|---|---|
| 4+ | Amenorrhoea | | | Emotional disturbance<br>Illness such as tuberculosis or thyrotoxicosis<br>Hormonal imbalance |
| 4 onwards | | | Presence of human chorionic gonadotrophin (hCG) in blood and urine | Hydatidiform mole |
| 4–14 | Nausea and vomiting | | | Gastroenteritis<br>Urinary tract infection<br>Hydatidiform mole |
| 3–4+ | Breast changes | | | |
| 5–6 | | | Visualization of gestational sac and pulsation of fetal heart on ultrasound | |
| 6–10 | | Hegar's sign – softening of the vagina and cervix | | |
| First 12 | Frequency of micturition | | | Urinary tract infection |
| 6–12 | Skin changes | | | |
| 8 onwards | | Goodell's sign – softening of the cervix and vagina – accompanied by increased leukorrhoeal discharge<br>Osiander's sign – pulsation of the uterine arteries through the lateral fornices<br>Chadwick's sign – lilac discoloration of the vaginal mucous membrane<br>Changes in the uterus – size increases and the shape changes | | Pelvic congestion |
| 10 | | | Fetal heart sounds audible with Sonicaid | |
| 14–16 | | | Fetal skeleton visible on radiological examination, although unlikely to be used because of the risks of irradiation | |
| 16 onwards | Quickening – first fetal movements felt by the woman | | | Intestinal movement possibly due to wind |
| 16 | | Colostrum may be expressed from the breasts<br>Uterine souffle<br>Abdominal enlargement | | Increased blood flow to uterus in, for example, ovarian tumours |
| 16–28 | Internal ballottement | | | |
| From 20 | Braxton Hicks contractions | | | |
| From 22 | | Fetal parts felt by examiner | | |
| 24 | | Fetal heart audible with Pinard's stethoscope | | |

felt by the mother ranges from 15 to 22 weeks in primigravidae and from 14 to 22 weeks in multigravidae (O'Dowd & O'Dowd 1985). Quickening, often described as 'flutters', or a feeling of 'bubbles coming to the surface' rather than recognizable movements, is an unreliable indicator of gestational age as sometimes these feelings can be attributed to flatulence.

### Around 20 weeks

For 90% of women, nausea and vomiting have usually diminished by 22 weeks' gestation (Lacroix et al 2000). The secondary areola, if not already present, may appear. The fundus of the uterus is normally palpated just below the umbilicus.

### Around 24 weeks

The fundus can be felt just above the umbilicus and the fetal parts and movements may be felt on abdominal palpation. The fetal heart sounds may be heard with a fetal stethoscope and at 24 weeks the fetus is considered to be capable of an independent existence.

### From 28 to 40 weeks

The fundus continues to rise until 36 weeks, when it reaches the xiphisternum and remains at that level until the fetal head engages. Braxton Hicks contractions, painless irregular uterine contractions, may be palpated from about 16 weeks and these persist until the end of pregnancy.

When engagement occurs from 36 weeks, the fundus descends slightly, causing, together with the increased flexion of the fetus, a relief of pressure which is experienced by the woman in the form of *'lightening'*. This may not occur in multigravidae as the head often does not engage until labour is established. This lightening allows the woman to breathe with more comfort; however, the descent of the head may cause pressure on the bladder, resulting in increased frequency of micturition.

## Signs of pregnancy found by vaginal examination

It is now uncommon to undertake a vaginal examination in early pregnancy; however, if performed, the following signs of pregnancy may be observed:

- *Goodell's sign*. This is softening, and increasing vascularity, of the cervix and vagina and is accompanied by increased leukorrhoeal discharge (Blackburn 2007).
- *Hegar's sign*. The softening and increased compressibility of the lower uterine segment makes it possible, on bimanual examination, for the fingers in the anterior fornix and those on the abdomen almost to meet (Blackburn 2007).
- *Osiander's sign*. The increased pulsation of the uterine arteries through the lateral fornices can be detected.
- *Chadwick's sign* – a purplish discoloration of the vaginal and cervical mucous membrane resulting from increased vascularity of those tissues (Blackburn 2007).
- *Enlargement of the uterus* is noted and compared with the period of gestation.
- *Internal ballottement of the fetus* may be possible from 16 weeks' gestation. With two fingers in the anterior fornix, the uterus is given a sharp tap. The fetus is pushed upwards and a slight impact on the fingers may be felt when the fetus returns to its original position.

## Positive signs of pregnancy

Although there are many physical changes experienced by the woman which might suggest pregnancy, there are a number of positive signs that will confirm pregnancy:

1. *Fetal heart sounds*: which may be detected from 10 weeks' gestation using Sonicaid ultrasonic equipment and from 24 weeks' gestation can be heard with the Pinard fetal stethoscope.
2. *Fetal movements*: felt by the examiner.
3. *Palpation of fetal parts*: felt by the examiner.
4. *Fetal skeleton*: is visible on radiological assessment at 14–16 weeks, although X-rays are now rarely used because of the risks of damage to the developing fetus through irradiation.
5. *Gestational sac*: may be visualized by ultrasonography at about 5 weeks and the fetal heart may be seen pulsating at 6 weeks using abdominal ultrasound. Vaginal ultrasound scanning may detect these a week earlier (Chudleigh & Pearce 1994). A viable intrauterine pregnancy is confirmed when fetal heart pulsations can be seen in the gestational sac in the uterus.

## Laboratory diagnosis of pregnancy

Chorionic tissue, which later forms the placenta, starts producing the hormone *human chorionic gonadotrophin* (hCG), which is excreted in the urine. This hormone is usually detected in the urine from the time of the first missed period. Immunological tests depend on the detection of hCG in the urine. Pregnancy tests fall into three categories with varying sensitivities to hCG:

- *Direct latex agglutination tests* (Fig. 32.1), where a small amount of latex particle reagent is placed on a dark glass slide; the latex particles are coated with antibodies which will bind to hCG. The reagent is milky in appearance, but when urine with hCG is added, the antibodies bind to the hCG, causing the particles to agglutinate. The liquid changes to a granular consistency, indicating a positive test result. Where no hCG is present, agglutination does not occur and the liquid remains milky (Wheeler 1999).

- *Monoclonal antibody tests/indirect agglutination tests.* Latex particles or red blood cells are coated with hCG. When the antibody solution is added, the particles or cells agglutinate. When urine containing hCG is added, the hormone binds to the antibodies, preventing them attaching to the hCG on the cells, and no agglutination occurs (Wheeler 1999).
- *The wick or cassette method* (Fig. 32.2). This may be a simple dipstick test with an absorbent wick on a cardboard or plastic backing, or a more sophisticated wick enclosed in a case to give a cassette-type test as with home pregnancy tests; it may also contain a control window. The absorbent wick is passed through the urine stream or dipped into the urine, or drops of urine are placed upon the sample window. Antibodies labelled with a coloured dye placed between the application area and the result area bind to the hCG. As the urine is absorbed, it travels along the wick to the result area – this appears as a coloured band. The excess urine moves further along the wick to the control panel, where it is bound to another antibody and a further coloured band is displayed. When hCG is present and the test is performed correctly, the result window and the control window will show coloured bands. If hCG is not present, no band will be visible in the result window, only in the control window. If the control window is blank, the test has not been performed correctly and should be repeated.

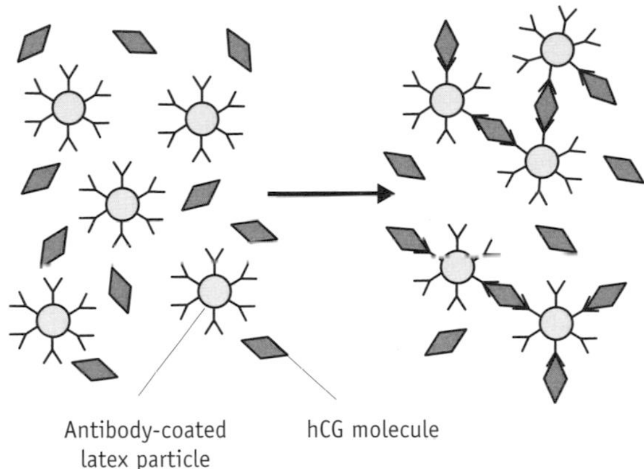


**Figure 32.1** The principle of direct latex agglutination tests. *(From Wheeler 1999.)*

Up to 40 types of laboratory test kit are available in the UK (Wheeler 1999). These have a wide range of different sensitivities, from 20 to 1000 IU/L of hCG.

Home pregnancy tests have a more consistent range of sensitivity, from 25 to 50 IU/L, take from 1 minute to obtain a result, appear easy to use and manufacturers claim a 99% accuracy rate. However, an American meta-analysis of the efficiency, sensitivity and specificity of tests highlighted that the diagnostic efficiency of home pregnancy tests is affected by the characteristics of the users (Bastian et al 1998). False negative results arose from testing before the recommended number of days from the last menstrual period, or from a failure to read or follow the instructions. Therefore, a negative result in a woman who does not menstruate within a week should be treated with caution. The test should be repeated and laboratory confirmation sought if doubt of pregnancy exists.

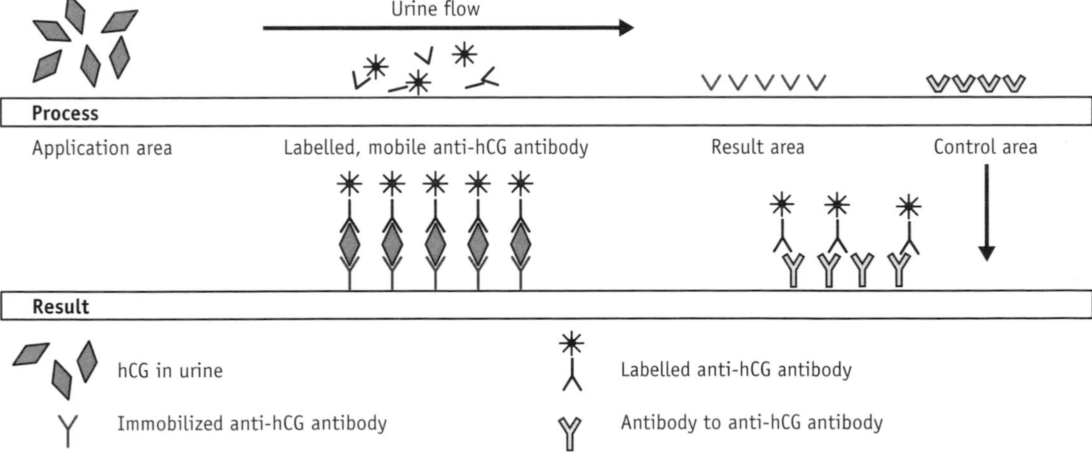


**Figure 32.2** The principle of the wick test as used in dipstick and cassette devices. *(From Wheeler 1999.)*

The advantages of using home pregnancy tests are that they can confirm pregnancy in the privacy of the home. This enables a woman to be the first to have the information and it provides a quick result at an early point in the pregnancy. However, given the varying sensitivities of home and laboratory tests, it is possible that a woman may receive a positive diagnosis of pregnancy using a home pregnancy test and a negative result from a laboratory test. This may cause anxiety and confusion. If this happens, the midwife needs to ask the laboratory which test they are using and its sensitivity. A repeat test may then be requested, to confirm pregnancy. It is also possible that spontaneous miscarriage could have occurred between the two tests.

Following confirmation of pregnancy, women are encouraged to contact their midwife or doctor to commence their antenatal care.

### Pseudocyesis

This is a phantom or false pregnancy and may occur in women with an intense desire to become pregnant. Amenorrhoea will be present. The woman will complain of all the subjective symptoms of pregnancy, usually in a bizarre order; the abdomen may be distended and the breasts may secrete a cloudy liquid. However, she is not pregnant. The signs on which a certain diagnosis of pregnancy can be made – namely, palpation of the fetus or hearing the fetal heart – are not present. Referral to a psychologist or psychiatrist may be required.

## ANTENATAL CARE

Over the past two centuries, antenatal services have seen major developments in terms of their provision and delivery. Contemporary antenatal services have quality at their heart, with patient safety, patient experience and effectiveness of care as their central tenets (DH 2008). All women seek a healthy outcome to their pregnancy; they want high-quality, personalized care coupled with greater information so that they can make informed choice about the place and nature of their care and are more in control of the care that they receive (Redshaw et al 2007).

The UK maternity services aim to provide a world-class service to women and their families, with the overall vision for the services to be flexible and individualized. Services should be designed to fit around the needs of the woman, baby and family circumstances, with due consideration being given to factors that may render some women and their families to become vulnerable and disadvantaged. Pregnancy is a normal physiological process for the majority of women. Women and their families need support to have as normal a pregnancy and birth as possible, with medical intervention being offered only if it is of benefit. However, in some circumstances, both midwifery and obstetric care are indicated and care should be based on providing good clinical and psychological outcomes for the woman and her baby (DH 2007a, DH & DfES 2004, NICE 2008).

### Aims of antenatal care

The overall purpose of antenatal care is to work with women to improve and maintain maternal and fetal health by monitoring the progress of pregnancy to confirm normality and detect any deviation early so that corrective care can be provided. The aims of antenatal care are to:

- facilitate the development of partnership between the woman and the professionals involved in her care
- exchange information about all aspects of care with the woman and her family, enabling them to make informed decisions about pregnancy, birth and parenting
- increase the woman's understanding of public health issues in order to maintain and promote her health, and make positive lifestyle choices during childbirth and onwards
- regularly monitor maternal and fetal health in pregnancy to confirm normality and to detect early any complications of pregnancy and refer women to appropriate healthcare professionals from the multidisciplinary team
- prepare the woman and her family for the physical, psychological and emotional adaptation to pregnancy as well as for safe birth, where possible drawing up a birth plan to facilitate a fulfilling experience for them
- afford opportunities for the woman and her family to increase their knowledge of aspects essential for childbirth and for early parenthood
- provide evidence-based information for the woman and her family, supporting them to make informed choice about methods of infant feeding
- prepare for the period following birth, including family planning advice.

### Care during pregnancy

It is important that women seek professional healthcare early in pregnancy – that is, within the first 12 weeks of pregnancy (HM Treasury 2007, Lewis 2007, NICE 2008) – so that they can obtain and use evidence-based information to plan their pregnancy and to benefit from antenatal screening and health promotion activities (DH 2007a, DH & DfES 2004, NICE 2008). With early information about the available models of antenatal care, women, in partnership with healthcare professionals, can make decisions about the most appropriate pathway of their care best suited to their personal, social and obstetric circumstances.

Where women seek care at a later stage in pregnancy, they will have reduced access to antenatal care. It is likely that the woman will have reduced options in terms of antenatal screening tests. Some investigations, such as serum screening for Down syndrome (see Ch. 26), are accurate only if carried out at specific times, in this case between 15 and 18 weeks. Early detection of these conditions enables further investigations, such as ultrasound scan or amniocentesis, to be carried out at the optimum time.

Early access to antenatal care enables healthcare professionals to obtain baseline measures, facilitating accurate monitoring of the effect of physiological changes on vital systems and organs of the body and early detection of any complications. For example, the recording of the blood pressure in the first trimester of pregnancy provides a baseline against which the physiological changes in the blood pressure can be assessed. In some cases, complications may have already arisen by the time the woman seeks antenatal care.

The woman should be able to choose whether her first contact in pregnancy is with a midwife or her GP (DH 2007a). That said, antenatal services vary; in many parts of the UK, the first point of contact for maternity services is the woman's GP (CHAI 2008, Redshaw et al 2007), but services are working towards the midwife being the first point of contact in the community setting.

To achieve the principles of antenatal care, pregnant women require evidence-based information. Evidence suggests that women desire accurate and timely information about pregnancy and childbirth so that they can develop their knowledge and understanding of pregnancy, childbirth and related issues, enabling them to make informed decisions about the care they want and prefer (Bharj 2007, Kirkham & Stapleton 2001, Mander 2001, Singh & Newburn 2000). Women need information which is based upon current evidence that is clearly understood and in a format they can easily access. When offering information, healthcare professionals must take into account the requirements of women who have physical and sensory learning disabilities and women whose competence in speaking and reading English is low, exploring appropriate ways of exchanging meaningful information.

Midwives are key healthcare professionals who work with women to support them to make informed choices regarding preferred arrangements for antenatal care, place of birth and postnatal care. Midwives should be friendly, kind, caring, approachable, non-judgemental, have time for women, be respectful, good communicators, providing support and companionship (Bharj & Chesney 2009, Nicholls & Webb 2006). These attributes are essential for the development of the woman–midwife relationship. Many worldwide studies highlight that all women perceive the woman–midwife relationship to be central to their pregnancy, childbirth and postnatal experiences (Anderson 2000, Bharj 2007, Davies 2000, Edwards 2005, Kirkham 2000, Lundgren & Berg 2007, Walsh 1999). Midwives therefore play an essential role in the life of women during their most significant period and have the power to either augment or mar women's experiences of pregnancy and childbirth.

**Reflective activity 32.2**

Reflect upon the discussions you have had, or have observed, with women during the initial visit. Do you think that you provided sufficient information for the woman to make informed decisions about patterns of antenatal care, home birth and who she would wish to see during the antenatal period?

## Outline of present pattern of maternity services in England

There are a wide range of models of care operating across the UK because of the geographical and demographic variations (Green et al 1998, Wraight et al 1993). The organization of maternity services varies throughout the UK. The maternity and obstetric units are formed as a part of larger district or regional general hospitals and the maternity and midwifery services are normally provided through such units and are integrated within the community and hospital. Midwifery units are designed and staffed according to the birth rates, therefore, the sizes of the units are variable dependent on the birth rates. Some NHS hospitals provide tertiary maternity and neonatal services for part of the regions. Generally, midwifery staff are employed by an acute maternity unit and may work either in the community or in the hospital, or, in some models of care, in both.

### Birth settings

There are four different birth settings: 'consultant-led obstetric units' (CLU), 'midwifery-led units' (MLU), 'home', and 'free-standing maternity units' (FMU) (Hall 2003) (for choices of place of birth, see Ch. 34). CLUs are usually attached to the district or regional units and deliver care both for women who have complex healthcare needs and for those with no complications of pregnancy, labour and birth. CLUs are staffed by midwives and obstetricians. Women are normally referred to an obstetrician who becomes the lead professional for the duration of their childbirth continuum. Women with complex healthcare needs may access all their care in the antenatal, intranatal and postnatal period within these settings.

Some women with less complex healthcare needs may access some of their care in the hospital setting and some in the community setting. Some women who have had uncomplicated pregnancies and who are at low risk of developing complications during labour and/or birth choose to labour and birth within a CLU with a midwife as lead professional rather than an obstetrician. A full range of obstetric facilities (such as anaesthesia, surgery, blood transfusion and neonatal intensive care) are readily available in CLUs.

MLUs, sometimes known as 'low-risk maternity units' (Hall 2003), are often located close to, but separate from, CLUs. These units normally aim to provide care to women with uncomplicated pregnancies; the women, however, have to meet the criteria for the unit throughout pregnancy, labour and birth. MLUs are staffed predominantly by midwives, although they may be jointly run by midwives and GPs. If a deviation from normal is detected during pregnancy, labour or birth, the woman will be referred to an obstetrician, or, if appropriate, a GP, and may have to transfer place of care to the CLU. Normally, women access the majority of their antenatal care in the community setting with minimal care in the hospital setting.

Women may choose to have their babies at home instead of a hospital setting (see Ch. 34). Each of the midwifery units in the UK has its own arrangements for providing a home birth service and its own guidelines and attitudes towards these. The provision of this service depends on local resources, local practices and policies, and the beliefs, skills and commitment of individual practitioners providing the service. Women who choose to have a home birth are normally given care in the community by the lead professional who may be either a midwife or GP. In circumstances where the maternity needs of the woman cannot be managed in the home setting, then she and/or her baby is transferred to the nearest CLU.

The purpose of the FMUs is to offer a 'home-like' environment within an institutional setting. The philosophy and the kind of care offered by an FMU are very similar to those of the MLUs and the main difference is that the FMU is geographically situated away from the CLU. Generally, women who access care at these settings have to fit in with the guidelines and protocols of these units and are normally those women who are less likely to require interventions. Should an intervention be required for a woman, a decision will need to be made about transferring to the CLU.

To meet the maternity needs of the local populations, two things have happened concomitantly in some areas of England. The move to centralize maternity services has seen a number of mergers and, at the same time, there have appeared a small number of new community units or birth centres to provide a limited service for women who would otherwise have to travel long distances to have their babies in large obstetric units (for example, see Kirkham 2003).

## Team midwifery

Maternity services for women in the NHS are normally provided by a multiprofessional team comprising community midwives, GPs, and hospital-based midwives or doctors in the antenatal period and usually by hospital-based midwives or doctors in the intrapartum period (unless they have a home birth) and by midwives and the GPs in the postnatal period. However, many maternity units are maximizing a multiprofessional approach to service provision and delivery and are collaborating with other relevant healthcare professionals to develop a multi-agency integrated care pathway, involving shared care, for example, with the drug and alcohol treatment services. This collaborative approach to care has improved the experience and outcome for women and babies.

A variety of approaches to *team midwifery* are emerging; they strive to provide choice and continuity and these include team midwifery normally based in the community, *one-to-one midwifery practice* care for women (Green et al 1998, Page et al 2000), that is, a complete episode of care from the booking interview to transfer to the health visitor following birth, including intrapartum care. Other approaches include *caseload midwifery*, or, as it is sometimes referred to, *midwifery group practice*. This comprises a small number of midwives organized into a team who are responsible for the delivery of full range of maternity care (SNMAC 1998). The midwives in the team are each responsible for approximately 30–40 women in a year.

While many parts of the UK have some sort of team arrangement for providing maternity services, these teams may vary from two or three midwives to over 30. There is no agreed definition of teams (RCM 2000, SNMAC 1998, Wraight et al 1993) though teams are responsible for providing care in the hospital setting, community settings, or both. There are four possible options of care:

- a team of community midwives with support from the GP deliver antenatal and postnatal care in the community setting and also provide care during labour and birth at home
- most of the antenatal and postnatal care is provided in the community with some hospital visits in the antenatal period, particularly for routine scans, antenatal screening, obstetric and any medical care; intrapartum care is in the hospital setting by team midwives and then early transfer home
- antenatal care is shared by the hospital and community and is determined by the health needs of the woman; intranatal care is given in the hospital by hospital midwives and then postnatal care in the community setting by community midwives
- antenatal and intrapartum care are offered in the hospital setting together with specialized services and then postnatal care is determined by the woman's health needs (Perkins & Unell 1997).

The type of care offered is dependent on the health needs of the woman and local practices and protocols.

Where women do not have any perceived complications in the antenatal and intrapartum period, they may choose to have all their care in the community setting or a mixture of both community and hospital. However, those women who have or develop complications in pregnancy or the intrapartum period access services in the hospital setting.

Increasingly there are developments where the NHS is collaborating with the local authority to offer maternity services from children's centres. In addition to this, some midwives are seconded to specialist outreach services, particularly *Sure Start* (integrated health, education and welfare support services for children under 4 and their families) and smoking cessation services.

In many areas, antenatal day assessment units have been developed to provide outpatient care. In circumstances where complications arise, such as moderate pregnancy-induced hypertension, the pregnant women can be referred to the antenatal assessment unit, where her and her baby's health may be assessed and monitored. Referral to such units can be made by the women themselves, by midwives or by other healthcare professionals.

### Domiciliary in and out scheme (DOMINO scheme)

A domiciliary in and out scheme (DOMINO scheme) is offered in some areas for women who wish for community-based care (Wardle et al 1997). Within this model, antenatal care is delivered by a community midwife as it would be for a home birth. The community midwife provides care at home during labour, and continues care when the woman is transferred into hospital for birth. Following birth, the woman and her baby, when healthy, are transferred home with postnatal care provided by the community midwife.

### Independent midwifery services

Independent midwives are currently in the minority, delivering around 500 births per year in the UK. The midwives are self-employed and offer themselves for service to individual women. Their education and governance is the same as that of any other practising midwife within the UK and within the same regulatory body and with Supervision of Midwives. The main differences are that they set up their protocols for practice, using evidence-based practice, and usually offer a home birth service, meeting women's individual requirements; and usually practise in small groups of two or three or in some cases single-handedly. Some midwives have honorary contracts with their local hospitals and offer a DOMINO service, though where midwives are unable to secure contracts, when a woman booked with them requires medical services, the independent midwife can only accompany her to hospital as a friend or doula.

### Place of birth

During pregnancy, women need unbiased information to consider where they wish to give birth. This is discussed in more detail in Chapter 34. The most common place of birth continues to remain the hospital setting and the rate of home births has not changed significantly over the past few decades, despite calls for increasing women's choice in the place of birth (DH 2007a). Although the rate of home birth remains low, there are marked geographical variations. This appears to depend on midwives and doctors supporting the idea of healthy women having their babies at home. Where this was the case, the numbers of women having home births increased (Sandall et al 2001).

## Pattern of care

Historically, irrespective of their personal needs, individual risk status or parity, all pregnant women were encouraged to routinely attend an antenatal clinic every 4 weeks up to 28 weeks' gestation, then 2-weekly up to 36 weeks, and then weekly thereafter. Evidence in the 1980s suggested that healthy women were at no greater risk of maternal or perinatal mortality if they attended fewer antenatal visits than the historical pattern of care (Hall et al 1985) and in 1982 the Royal College of Obstetricians and Gynaecologists (RCOG) recommended that maternity care providers should reduce the number of antenatal visits for women who do not have any complications of pregnancy from the historical pattern of 14–16 visits for all women to five to seven visits for multiparous women and eight or nine visits for primiparous women (RCOG 1982). This recommendation was not widely implemented until it was reiterated in the 'Changing childbirth' report (DH 1993), where it was suggested that many existing maternity care practices, such as the frequency and timing of antenatal care, had continued as a result of tradition and ritual rather than as a result of evidence of effectiveness. More recently, the NICE guidance (2008) recommended that for nulliparous women with uncomplicated pregnancies, ten antenatal appointments 'should be adequate', and that for parous women with uncomplicated pregnancies, seven antenatal appointments 'should be adequate'. However, 25% of women have reported receiving fewer than the recommended number of antenatal visits (CHAI 2008). Whilst it is acknowledged that a reduction in the frequency of antenatal appointments does not result in an increase in adverse biological maternal and perinatal outcomes (Villar et al 2001), it is not clear whether a reduction in the frequency of antenatal visits affects women's satisfaction with antenatal care and the social support that they may require. Nevertheless, it is essential that the number of antenatal visits should be tailored to meet women's individualized health needs instead of attending antenatal appointments in a ritualistic pattern.

Throughout the childbearing period, all women should be provided with the opportunity to discuss issues and to ask questions (NICE 2008). To enable women to make informed choices about their care, midwives need to work in partnership with women and their families to develop and maintain relationships based upon effective communication skills, empathy and trust (Berry 2007). To communicate effectively and discuss matters fully with women, antenatal appointments need to be structured in such a way as to ensure the woman has sufficient time to make informed decisions (NICE 2008) and midwives need to develop the knowledge required to ensure they are able to offer up-to-date, consistent, evidence-based information and clear explanations, using terminology that women and their families are able to understand. Adjustments may need to be made to ensure that women with additional communication needs are able to access information in a format they are able to understand. This may include using interpreters, online resources or DVDs as well as leaflets and books to support discussions.

## THE FIRST ANTENATAL VISIT

The first antenatal visit and taking of the woman's history may occur in the woman's home, a health centre or GP surgery, or at the first visit to the hospital antenatal clinic. If a combined approach is taken, this will reduce the visits that the woman may have to make.

Women may feel apprehensive at their first visit, especially if they have not previously met the midwives or medical staff. Good communication skills and a non-judgemental attitude are important to enable women to feel at ease in discussing very intimate personal details. A warm, friendly greeting and a pleasant, comfortable environment can also help to put women at their ease. Whilst many women may be rather apprehensive at the first visit, young teenagers, women who are less proficient in speaking English and those who are unhappy about their pregnancy may feel especially vulnerable. Interpreters are required for women who have limited fluency in speaking English and, where possible, such women should be given information in formats that enable them to access and understand the information easily – for example, written information in their own language, audiovisual tapes or in braille. In many large cities where the number of teenage pregnancies is high, special 'teenagers' clinics' or clubs may be provided to meet their particular needs.

Whatever the background of the woman, or her reactions to her pregnancy, building a positive relationship with her is one of the midwife's most important aims during this first antenatal visit. This provides a foundation upon which the trust between a midwife and a woman will be built during the rest of the pregnancy. The woman needs open communication with a midwife who is well informed and committed to supporting her as an individual, encouraging the development of mutual respect, trust and partnership (Nicholls & Webb 2006, Redshaw et al 2007). There is growing evidence of women's views of the maternity services that consistently highlights the importance of the quality of the women's relationship with their midwife and the importance of this relationship in their satisfaction levels (CHAI 2008, Redshaw et al 2007).

The importance at the beginning of the interview is for the woman to establish confidence in the midwife, and so the purpose and process of the interview and issues such as confidentiality must be addressed initially. The woman needs to understand the midwife's professional responsibilities, in terms of information which may be shared, and which may need to be discussed with other members of the team. Similarly, the midwife needs to ensure that a woman's request that information is kept confidential is respected.

### History taking

When the history is taken at home or in a community clinic, the woman is likely to be more at ease. If the interview takes place in the hospital, the midwife should prepare the interview room to be as pleasant and non-clinical as possible in order to facilitate communication and the development of a relationship of mutual trust. The midwife must also provide privacy and sufficient time for the interview, and make this clear to the woman.

During early pregnancy the woman may be experiencing nausea and fatigue and will appreciate not having to travel to attend a busy clinic amongst strangers. Any problems can usually be discussed in private and the midwife can give information and offer advice as appropriate. When other members of the family are present during this initial assessment, this gives the midwife the opportunity to meet them, but she should also be sensitive that there may be information that the woman considers private or confidential and would prefer not to discuss in their presence. Some time alone spent between the midwife and woman is essential and this should be facilitated.

The interview should be a two-way process of interaction between the woman and midwife. It involves assessment of the woman's social, psychological, emotional and physical condition as well as obtaining information about the present and previous pregnancies, and the medical and family history. Care can then be planned in conjunction with the woman to meet her specific needs and wishes.

An antenatal booking interview should comprise more than merely recording an obstetric history; it should be about communicating information and promoting a relationship between the woman and the midwife (Methven 1982a,1982b). Factors conducive to a more relaxed atmosphere and which promote communication should be considered, for example, the environment of the setting where the history is going to be taken, arrangements of the furniture in the room, body language and interpersonal skills. A few minutes spent by the midwife in introducing herself and talking informally enable the woman to settle down and relax before personal issues are discussed. A skilled midwife can elicit most of the information required from the woman in a pleasant conversational manner without the woman realizing that she is being closely questioned. Open rather than closed questions should be employed because these encourage free responses and promote two-way interaction between the woman and midwife. During the interview the midwife should be sensitive to the woman's attitude to her pregnancy and, if possible, to that of her partner. Unusually adverse attitudes and body language should be noted and counselling and support given as required.

## Personal details

The woman's full name, marital status, address, telephone number, age, date of birth, race, religion and occupation (and that of her partner) are accurately recorded. Information regarding the woman's marital status is elicited to determine if the woman is in a stable relationship or if the woman is alone and may need additional support from the midwife and other agencies.

The woman's ethnicity is ascertained because some medical and obstetric conditions are more likely to occur in certain ethnic groups and appropriate diagnostic tests are required. However, asking about ethnicity is complex (Dyson 2005) and midwives need to develop competence in accomplishing this sensitively. The religion of the woman is recorded because of the special requirements and rituals which may be practised and affect the mother and her baby. Occupation gives an indication of socioeconomic status. Women in socioeconomic groups IV and V (see website) may experience social and economic inequalities. These wider determinants of health coupled with poverty are most likely to adversely affect their or their fetus's/baby's health and clinical outcomes (Lewis 2007, Palmer et al 2008). The midwife needs to work with other agencies to provide the woman and her family with appropriate support to promote and improve her health.

## Present pregnancy

The date of the first day of the last menstrual period (LMP) is ascertained, care being taken to check that this was the last *normal* menstrual period. Some women have a slight blood loss when the fertilized ovum embeds into the decidual lining of the uterus and many mistake this for the last period. Pregnancy has been assumed to last 280 days, and to overcome the irregularity of the calendar a working rule of thumb was devised by Naegele. By counting forwards 9 months and adding 7 days from the first day of the last normal menstrual period, it is possible to arrive at an estimated date of delivery (EDD); alternatively, count back 3 months and add 7 days. This method of calculating the EDD is known as *Naegele's rule*. However, as February is a short month and the remaining months have 30 or 31 days, from 280 to 283 days may be added to the date of the LMP. Rosser (2000) states that it is unclear whether the length of pregnancy is affected by social, ethnic or obstetric factors. It is important to explain that it is quite normal for the actual day of delivery to be up to 2 weeks before or after the EDD.

**Table 32.2 Calculation of the EDD**

| Cycle 28 days | Cycle 33 days | Cycle 23 days |
|---|---|---|
| LMP: 12 Aug 2010 | LMP: 12 Aug 2010 | LMP: 12 Aug 2010 |
| +7 days +9 months | +7 days +5 days +9 months | +7 days −5 days +9 months |
| EDD: 19 May 2011 | EDD: 24 May 2011 | EDD: 14 May 2011 |

Details of the woman's menstrual history should be sought: the age at which menstruation began; the duration of the periods; and the number of days in the cycle. Conception occurs shortly after ovulation. With a regular cycle of about 28 days, the standard calculation is reasonably accurate to within a few days, provided that the woman knows the date of her last normal menstrual period.

In a 35-day cycle, however, ovulation would occur 21 days after the period; in a 21-day cycle, only 7 days after. Adjustments may be made, therefore, when the woman has a regular long or short cycle. If the cycle is long (for example, 33 days), the days in excess of 28 are added when calculating the EDD (Table 32.2). With a regular short cycle, such as 23 days, the number of days less than 28 is subtracted from the EDD.

The calculation is difficult if the woman does not know the date of her last menstrual period, cycles are irregular, or a normal cycle has not resumed since taking the oral contraceptive pill or following a previous birth. If the woman has a good idea of when conception occurred, the EDD can be calculated by adding 38 weeks to this date, or subtracting 7 days from 9 months.

Women should be asked to note the date when fetal movements are first felt. Primigravidae normally become aware of fetal movements between 18 and 20 weeks, whereas multigravidae recognize the sensation a little earlier, between 16 and 18 weeks. This may be used to confirm the expected date of delivery, although with the widespread use of ultrasound in the UK, the gestational age is usually established during ultrasound examination (see Ch. 33). A dating ultrasound offered to a woman between 10 and 13 weeks of pregnancy normally measures the crown–rump length (CRL) and for pregnancies beyond

14 weeks the fetal gestational age is determined by the measurement of the head circumference or biparietal diameter (BPD) (NICE 2008).

Although the use of ultrasound to estimate gestational age is very useful, some women may find it distressing if there are discrepancies between the date estimated by Naegele's rule and that given following ultrasound examination, especially those who are certain of the date of conception or who have a regular cycle and are certain of the date of the first day of their last menstrual period. In most cases it would be inappropriate to alter the expected date of delivery without the mother's agreement, especially when there is less than 10–14 days' discrepancy with the previously given date (Proud 1997).

Other pregnancy symptoms such as breast changes, nausea and vomiting, and increased frequency of micturition are noted. Nausea and vomiting may range from occasional slight nausea to frequent severe vomiting with ketosis, when immediate medical treatment is necessary (see Ch. 53). Any history of bleeding per vaginam since the last normal menstrual period is recorded and the woman is requested to seek medical attention immediately should further bleeding occur (see Ch. 54).

In the first trimester of pregnancy a woman is quite likely to feel tired, perhaps nauseated and generally rather off-colour. A caring, approachable midwife who provides support, encourages the woman to express any worries and ask questions, and gives clear information, can be a great help to the woman at this time.

## Previous pregnancies

It is necessary to ask about all previous pregnancies, including miscarriages or terminations of pregnancy. If the woman has had a miscarriage, she is asked at what stage in pregnancy it occurred, whether she knows of any possible cause, if she was transferred to hospital, and, if so, whether she needed either an operation to remove retained products of conception, or a blood transfusion, or both.

Similar questions are asked about terminations of pregnancy, including the reason for termination and how it was performed. Some women may not wish this information to be recorded in handheld notes and their autonomy should be respected; however, the information should be recorded within hospital notes, and the reasons for this discussed with the woman.

Details of all pregnancies, labours and puerperia are essential:

- Was the pregnancy uncomplicated or complicated – for example, did the woman experience vomiting, hypertension or haemorrhage?
- Was the birth of baby at term and were there any complications?
- What was the length of the labour?
- Was the baby born in hospital or at home?
- Was the birth of the baby with or without assistance – for example, was the birth assisted with a forceps, ventouse extraction or a caesarean section? If so, why was the intervention required?
- Did she have a normal healthy baby and was the baby well at birth? And now?
- If the baby died, she is asked if she knows why, and what happened. This information is important to record, as the reasons for the baby's demise may indicate risks to the current pregnancy.
- The birthweight of any previous baby is important, since this gives some indication of the capacity of the woman's pelvis.
- Was the woman unwell after her baby's birth, or were there any problems such as haemorrhage or any other complications?
- She is asked if she breastfed her baby, if this was an enjoyable experience, and for how long she was able to breastfeed. Her previous experience may influence how she intends to feed her expected baby (Foster et al 1997). If she fed artificially, the reasons for this are explored. The midwife will ensure that the woman is fully informed of the health benefits of breastfeeding, to both herself and her baby, to enable her to make an informed choice of feeding method, and she is asked how lactation was suppressed.

All pregnancies are dealt with in chronological order. If the history reveals any obstetric or paediatric complications and previous notes are not accessible, the information should be sought from the hospital where care was delivered.

This is a useful part of the interview, as this may be the first opportunity that the woman has had for reviewing and reflecting on her previous childbirth experiences, and this provides a forum for clarifying management of problems both previously and in the future.

## Medical and surgical history

This includes enquiry about any illness, operation or accident which could complicate pregnancy. It is necessary to ask by name about rheumatic fever; chorea; cardiac, respiratory and renal diseases; thyrotoxicosis; diabetes; hypertension; thromboembolic disorders; tuberculosis; epilepsy; and mental illness.

A history of mental illness, especially postnatal depression or puerperal psychosis, is of significance because such conditions may recur in a subsequent pregnancy. The woman is asked about infectious diseases of childhood and whether she has had rubella or been vaccinated against the disease. A blood test will confirm whether or not she is immune, and if non-immune, she is advised to avoid contact with the disease, as rubella virus, if contracted in pregnancy, can cross the placenta and cause fetal abnormality.

Operations on the uterus or the pelvic floor are significant. Following caesarean section or myomectomy, there may be a weakened uterine scar, especially if the wound was infected, and there is a slight risk that it could rupture during a subsequent pregnancy or labour. Women of childbearing age sometimes have to undergo extensive pelvic floor repair operations. If a woman has had a successful operation for the relief of stress incontinence, both the woman and the obstetrician will be concerned about the mode of delivery; sometimes, another vaginal delivery is considered inadvisable and caesarean section is planned.

Relevant accidents include those involving the spine and pelvis, particularly if a fracture has occurred and deformity resulted. Deformity of the spine or pelvis following poliomyelitis or congenital dislocation of the hip would cause similar concern, since in all these instances the bony pelvis may be asymmetrical and accordingly have a smaller capacity. Enquiry may be made about back pain or symphysis pubis dysfunction and appropriate support and advice given, and referral made if appropriate.

Details of any blood transfusions are important, including the reason and any adverse reactions.

## Drugs and medications

It is important to ask the woman whether she is taking any drugs, because many drugs which are quite safe for the woman may have a teratogenic effect on the fetus. The woman should be informed about the risk of taking over-the-counter drugs without medical advice (NICE 2008).

Drug dependency in women of childbearing age is an increasing problem (Siney 1999) and it is important that the midwife ascertains whether the woman has previously taken or is currently taking prescribed drugs and/or drugs for 'social or recreational' use. The misused substances are likely to have a detrimental effect on the health of the woman and her fetus/baby; however, this is dependent on the type, dose and the route of the drug used. Women with drug dependency are at an increased risk of developing medical and obstetrical problems than are women who do not misuse drugs, and their babies are at an increased risk of neonatal complications (DH 1998, Hepburn 1993).

Women who misuse drugs may have a multitude of social, emotional, financial and sexual health problems that necessitate multi-agency involvement to try to minimize harm to themselves, their children and families. It is essential that the approach and attitude of the midwife is caring, non-judgemental and constructively helpful when discussing health needs and the support that can be offered to the woman; otherwise the woman may reject the help that the health and other specialist services can offer.

## Smoking in pregnancy

Smoking during pregnancy is a most significant contributing factor for poor health, poor clinical outcomes and health inequalities, increasing, for example, the risk of miscarriage, placental abruption, placenta praevia, preterm birth, perinatal death, sudden unexpected death in infancy, and congenital abnormalities such as development of cleft lip and cleft palate in babies (Ananth et al 1999, Castles et al 1999, DiFranza & Lew 1995, Shah & Bracken 2000, Wyszynski et al 1997). Therefore, reducing smoking in pregnant women is an area of priority for all (DH & DfES 2004). Midwives are ideally placed to give health promotion advice to the woman and her partner on the detrimental effects of smoking on the woman, fetus and newborn baby. The initial interview and antenatal visits are ideal times to discuss whether the woman smokes, the implications of this, and whether she would like to give up smoking (NICE 2008).

Women should be encouraged to either stop or reduce smoking during pregnancy. They should be provided with unbiased and evidence-based information, aiming to encourage them to stop smoking, rather than cause fear or stress. Discussion with women's partners and enlisting their support in reducing smoking may also be beneficial. Women should be offered details of how to access local NHS Stop Smoking Services and the NHS pregnancy smoking helpline. Smoking cessation programmes in pregnancy – such as providing information on the effects of smoking, advantages of stopping, and strategies to stop, particularly with individual counselling – have shown a varied benefit in stopping smoking, increasing mean birthweight and reducing prematurity (Lumley et al 2000).

The National Institute for Health and Clinical Excellence is in the process of developing guidance on public health intervention aimed at stopping smoking in pregnancy and following childbirth (NICE 2009) that would further assist midwives and other healthcare professionals to access and utilize recommendations for good practice.

## Alcohol consumption during pregnancy

Alcohol has detrimental effects on the fetus (Gray & Henderson 2006). Women who consume high levels of alcohol before and during pregnancy and those who are alcohol dependent are more likely to have babies with varying forms of congenital abnormalities, often described as *fetal alcohol syndrome* (RCOG 2006).

The midwife should use the opportunity to take a history of alcohol use, assess the risk of alcohol dependence, or risk to the fetus from alcohol consumption, and advise and refer appropriately. There is no conclusive evidence regarding what is a safe amount of alcohol to drink during pregnancy and the advice given to the expectant mother should be based upon the current recommendation of NICE

(2008). The NICE guidance recommends that women should be advised to avoid alcohol during pregnancy where possible. If they do choose to drink, they should not drink more than 1–2 UK units once or twice a week (1 unit equals half a pint of ordinary-strength lager or beer, or one shot [25 mL] of spirit; one small [125 mL] glass of wine is equal to 1.5 UK units). However, evidence suggests that getting drunk or binge drinking (that is, more than five standard drinks or 7.5 UK units on a single occasion) may be harmful to the baby (NICE 2008).

## Diet in pregnancy

It is important to ask about the woman's diet and nutritional intake. Advice should be tailored to her individual circumstances, taking into account her cultural, faith and socioeconomic background (see Ch. 17). General advice to all women should include the need for a well-balanced diet containing proteins (beans, pulses, lentils, meat and fish), dairy products (milk, cheese, yoghurt), fruit and vegetables, carbohydrates (bread, pasta, rice and potatoes) and fibre (wholegrain flour, wholegrain bread, and fruit and vegetables) (NICE 2008).

Pregnant women should be advised to avoid foods that may place their fetus at risk of *Listeria monocytogenes* infection, for example, unpasteurized soft cheeses and mould-ripened cheeses. Raw eggs and products containing raw eggs, such as mayonnaise, should be avoided because of the risk of salmonella infection, and undercooked meats and pâtés (which may be a source of *Listeria, Escherichia coli* and *Toxoplasma*) should also be avoided. Vegetable and salad foods should be washed prior to eating, and food should be stored at the correct temperature in the refrigerator and on the appropriate shelves to reduce the risk of infections such as listeriosis, *E. coli* and toxoplasmosis.

As high intakes (more than 10 times the recommended daily allowance) of retinol – the animal form of vitamin A – may be associated with congenital abnormality, the NICE (2008) recommendation is that foods containing vitamin A, such as liver and liver products, should be avoided. Women should be informed about the importance of vitamin D for their and their fetus's health and encouraged to eat foods such as oily fish, eggs, nuts, meat and foods fortified with vitamin D.

## Family history

The woman's family medical history is important. Familial diseases such as hypertension and diabetes are sometimes discovered during routine antenatal examinations and it is useful to know the woman's medical background. It is essential to know if any near relative has pulmonary tuberculosis, since the newborn child is very vulnerable to the infection and must be protected. Arrangements are made for the child to receive BCG vaccination before leaving hospital, as well as being segregated from the infected person.

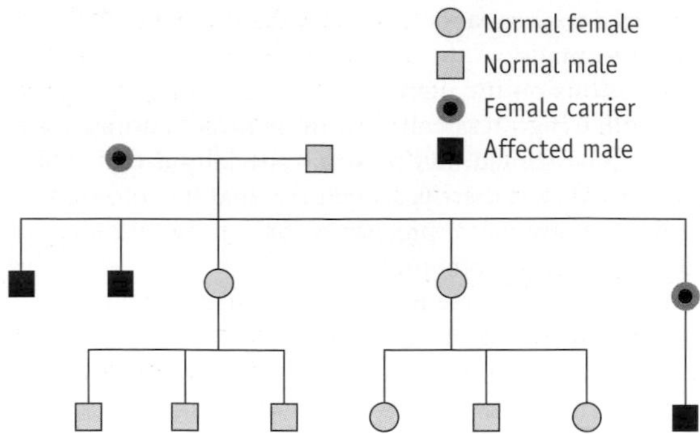


**Figure 32.3** A medical pedigree showing three generations with X-linked haemophilia.

As there is a familial tendency to produce twins, especially dizygotic twins, it is important to ask if there are twins in the family and, if so, whether they are monozygotic (identical) or dizygotic (non-identical) (Ch. 59).

The woman should be asked if there is any history of congenital abnormality in the family (Fig. 32.3) as she and her partner may need referral for genetic counselling (see Ch. 26). A number of diagnostic techniques are available for the diagnosis of congenital conditions in pregnancy and these may be discussed with the couple.

The midwife also carefully observes and enquires about the woman's reaction to her pregnancy, whether she is happy about it and coping with the initial minor disorders, or appears anxious, tense and unhappy. Guiding the conversation in a skilful, relaxed, unhurried manner and active listening and interpretation of both verbal and non-verbal communications help to elicit the woman's feelings and concerns. Appropriate support and help can then be offered.

It might appear that history taking is a lengthy procedure; however, in most cases it can be completed within 30–60 minutes, as the majority of clients are healthy young women who have never been seriously ill. This personal history provides a basis on which it is possible to assess the woman's physical, psychological and emotional health and wellbeing and, to some extent, anticipate the outcome of her pregnancy. An important aspect of this time spent taking the history is that the midwife and woman can meet and develop the relationship which has such a fundamental influence on the woman's subsequent experience of pregnancy and childbirth.

On completion, the midwife can make an holistic assessment of the woman that influences the discussion around her particular needs and wishes. The midwife gives clear, accurate information about the variety of services available to enable the woman to make informed choices. Only then can a care plan for pregnancy and childbirth be discussed, tailored and agreed to the woman's individual needs. The woman should be given appropriate literature for her reference after her visit, such as *The Pregnancy Book* (DH 2007b). A future appointment may be made with the midwife and arrangements are made for any antenatal diagnostic tests to be undertaken.

## Domestic abuse

Domestic abuse during pregnancy is of major concern; it affects the physical and mental health and safety of the woman and her fetus. (This is discussed in Chapter 23 but a brief overview is given here as part of the antenatal care routine.) Pregnancy may trigger or exacerbate abuse (Mooney 1993), and this may result in injury, obstetric complications such as miscarriage, placental abruption, antepartum haemorrhage, preterm labour, intrauterine growth restriction and stillbirth (Cokkinides et al 1999, Janssen et al 2003), as well as maternal death (Lewis 2007).

All women should be routinely asked about domestic abuse (BMA 1998, RCM 1999, RCOG 1997).The midwife may be the first point of contact for possible help for a woman who is abused, and the opportunity to initiate questions that may lead to disclosure of abuse can arise at the booking interview or during subsequent antenatal care. Suspicion may arise where the woman is always accompanied by her partner, especially where he constantly answers questions and undermines her. In addition to having an understanding of domestic abuse, including the symptoms and signs of abuse, the midwife needs to be skilled in asking difficult questions (see Ch. 23). All women should be afforded an opportunity to disclose domestic abuse in a safe environment (NICE 2008). Women who experience domestic abuse should be offered information about the choices available to them and the resources to support them. Documentation of abuse should be made with the woman's consent, but **not** in handheld records. Medical evidence of abuse may be needed should the case proceed to court. If the woman does not wish her disclosure to be recorded, her autonomy should be respected.

## Antenatal screening

At the first visit, women should be offered evidence-based information in relation to screening for fetal anomalies and assistance to make an informed choice about having or not having a scan (NICE 2008) (see Chs 26 and 33).

# SUBSEQUENT ANTENATAL APPOINTMENTS

When the woman and midwife meet for an antenatal appointment, the midwife should greet the woman in a friendly manner, introduce herself, review with the woman the purpose of the appointment, and elicit from the woman any concerns or questions she may have regarding the wellbeing of herself or her fetus, or any other issues.

Antenatal appointments offer women opportunities to discuss and ask questions about their maternity care. They also provide the midwife with an opportunity to offer women information about pregnancy, health promotion and preparation for parenthood. Issues that should be discussed during the antenatal period include infant feeding, management of breastfeeding, care of the baby, vitamin K prophylaxis and newborn screening tests, as well as information about changes that the woman may experience during the postnatal period, including 'baby blues' and postnatal depression (NICE 2008).

Details of all discussions between the woman and the maternity care provider, including information discussed, advice offered and plans of care developed, should be agreed and then recorded in the woman's handheld records, using terminology that the woman is able to understand.

Antenatal appointments may take place in a range of settings, such as the woman's home, a GP surgery, hospital or children's centre. Whilst easy access to the setting for women is essential, the midwife must carefully consider the environment in which the antenatal appointment will take place and ensure that women have the opportunity to discuss issues they regard as sensitive in a confidential manner.

## Infant feeding

An important area of discussion relates to the woman's intended method of feeding (see Ch. 43). The woman should be asked about whether in previous pregnancies she commenced breastfeeding and for how long she fed her baby. It is useful to explore whether she had any difficulty last time and/or whether she is aware of the health benefits of breastfeeding for herself and her baby.

The difficulties that women have in breastfeeding can be overcome, and the rate and duration of breastfeeding increased, if the woman has access to evidence-based information and care (see Ch. 43). During the antenatal period, women should have the opportunity to discuss in detail with a midwife how successful breastfeeding can be initiated and maintained. This can include information on analgesia in labour, offering the baby skin-to-skin contact and an early opportunity to suckle following delivery, correct 'latching' and positioning, the value of breast milk, baby-led feeding (both day and night), rooming in, and the management of common breastfeeding problems. Midwives need to be aware, when discussing infant feeding, that 'How do you intend to feed your baby – breast or bottle?' is a loaded question and the two choices should never be offered as if they are equal. Many women are unaware of the risks associated with artificial feeding and need appropriate and accurate information on which to make an informed choice. For women who have decided to breastfeed, the values of breastfeeding should be reinforced, with positive encouragement of how they can succeed. For women who express a preference for artificial feeding, the reasons for their choice should be explored and information offered to support them to make an informed choice.

## Assessments in pregnancy

### Maternal weight

Many women are concerned about their weight during pregnancy. Maternal obesity is internationally recognized as being a major cause of maternal mortality and morbidity. In the UK, the Confidential Enquiry into Maternal and Child Health (CEMACH) report 'Why mothers die 2000–2002' (Lewis 2004) identified that 35% of women who had a pregnancy-related death were obese and that obesity is related to an increase in complications during pregnancy. To identify which women may be at increased risk of complications as a result of obesity, women's body mass index (BMI) is calculated during the first antenatal appointment (see Box 32.1).

Research has identified that risk factors for maternal obesity include health inequalities and socioeconomic deprivation (Heslehurst et al 2007). During the antenatal period it is essential that healthy nutrition and weight management are discussed with pregnant women. Referral to a dietician may be appropriate. Traditionally, women were weighed during each antenatal appointment; however, it is now recommended that repeated maternal weighing, as part of routine antenatal care, should not be undertaken (NICE 2008), although some women may express a preference to be weighed in order to monitor their weight.

**Box 32.1 Calculation of body mass index (BMI)**

$$\text{BMI} = \frac{\text{Weight in kilograms}}{(\text{Height in metres})^2}$$

*Example 1* Weight 57 kg (9 stone); height 1.68 m (5′ 6″):

$$\text{BMI} = \frac{57}{1.68^2} = 20.3$$

*Example 2* Weight 64 kg (10 stone); height 1.57 m (5′ 2″):

$$\text{BMI} = \frac{64}{1.57^2} = 25.6$$

*Example 3* Weight 76 kg (12 stone); height 1.57 m (5′ 2″)

$$\text{BMI} = \frac{76}{1.57^2} = 30.7$$

| BMI score | Category |
|---|---|
| <18.5 | Underweight |
| 18.5–24.9 | Normal |
| 25.0–29.9 | Overweight |
| 30.0–34.9 | Moderately obese |
| 35.0–39.9 | Obese |
| ≥40 | Severely obese |

### Blood pressure and urinalysis

At each antenatal visit, the woman's blood pressure must be measured and a sample of her urine tested for protein (NICE 2008). These tests are performed to screen for hypertensive disorders and pre-eclampsia (see Ch. 56). The midwife needs to ensure that the results of these screening tests are accurate, as clinical decision making and subsequent care will be informed by the results. Accuracy of the results may be affected by poor technique, or the use of inaccurate or inappropriate equipment.

During antenatal appointments it is usual to measure blood pressure when the woman is sitting upright with her back supported for comfort (see Ch. 56). The woman should rest for 5 minutes prior to the measurement being taken and the midwife should instruct the woman not to talk or eat during the measurement as this may result in an inaccurate higher measurement being recorded (McAlister & Straus 2001). Tight clothing on the arm should be removed; the upper arm supported at heart level and the sphygmomanometer cuff placed at heart level. This is because measurements made with the arm lower than heart level can be 11–12 mmHg higher than those made with the arm supported and the cuff at heart level (Dougherty & Lister 2008). Conversely, if the arm is raised above heart level, the measurement may be falsely low (Beevers et al 2001). Selection of the appropriate sized cuff for the individual woman is important to obtain an accurate reading; the cuff should cover 80% of the circumference of the woman's upper arm (British Hypertensive Society 2008).

Urine testing for protein can be performed by quickly dipping a reagent strip into a sample of fresh urine. The reagent strips are impregnated with chemicals that react with abnormal substances in the urine and change colour. It is important to inform women that the urine sample should be fresh, as urine that has been stored deteriorates quickly and this can affect the final result (Higgins 2008).

To ensure reliable results, it is essential that the reagent strips are stored and used according to the manufacturer's instructions. The reagent strips usually need to be stored in a dry, dark place, so it is important to make certain that the lid is always replaced between antenatal consultations during a clinic.

During pregnancy it is common for women to report an increase in the amount of vaginal discharge they experience. This discharge may contaminate the urine sample and protein be detected in the urine. If abnormal substances are detected in the urine, culture and sensitivity testing under laboratory conditions may be indicated. For example, if a reagent stick test indicated the presence of nitrites or leucocyte esterase in the urine, culture and sensitivity testing would identify the organism and specify the most appropriate treatment (Dougherty & Lister 2008).

### Blood testing

#### *Anaemia*

During pregnancy, maternal iron requirements increase due to the requirements of the fetus and placenta and an increase in maternal red cell mass (NICE 2008). Maternal plasma volume increases by up to 50% and the red cell mass increases by up to 20%, resulting in a drop in the haemoglobin concentration in the blood which resembles iron deficiency anaemia. In addition to testing for anaemia in early pregnancy, all women should be offered testing for anaemia at 28 weeks' gestation (NICE 2008). If anaemia is detected, treatment should be considered, as treatment at this point should allow sufficient time for correction of anaemia before term. Haemoglobin levels outside the normal UK range (10.5 g per 100 mL at 28 weeks) should be investigated (NICE 2008). Irrespective of their rhesus D status, it is recommended that all women are screened for atypical red cell antibodies at 28 weeks' gestation (NICE 2008) (for further details, see Ch. 33).

## Abdominal examination

During the antenatal period, abdominal examination is carried out to determine the symphysis fundal height and, from 36 weeks' gestation, to determine the presentation of the fetus. To perform an abdominal examination, the midwife needs to be able to observe, palpate and auscultate the woman's abdomen. Some women may find the nature of this examination intimate and embarrassing. Attention to privacy and the woman's comfort should reassure the woman. Sensitive communication skills are required to enable the midwife to explain the purpose and procedure of the examination, and as the midwife performs the examination, she should ensure that the woman understands the findings by explaining them using appropriate language and terminology.

Prior to commencing the abdominal examination, the woman should be asked to empty her bladder if she has not done so recently. This is to ensure that the examination does not cause the woman undue discomfort and that a full bladder does not distort either the measurement of symphysis–fundal height or the palpation.

The woman should then lie as flat as she finds comfortable in the supine position. One or two pillows may be required for comfort and she may wish to slightly flex her legs. Some women experience a condition called supine hypotensive syndrome when lying flat on their back, which results from compression of the inferior vena cava and the abdominal aorta by the gravid uterus. Signs that a woman may be suffering from supine hypotensive syndrome include dizziness, pallor, tachycardia, sweating, nausea and hypotension. These unpleasant signs should resolve when the woman is assisted to turn onto her side and blood flow is no longer obstructed. To reduce the risk of this syndrome, the midwife should consider using a wedge, or pillows, under the woman's right side to alter the centre of gravity and reduce compression of the inferior vena cava and abdominal aorta. Only the woman's abdomen needs to be exposed, and sheets, or a blanket, can be used to cover legs if required. The midwife should wash and dry her hands prior to commencing the abdominal examination.

During the antenatal period an abdominal examination consists of the following parts:

- observation
- palpation and measurement of the **symphysis–fundal** height
- auscultation of the fetal heart.

#### *Observation*

The approximate size and shape of the uterus should be observed. The size of the uterus should correspond to the estimated period of gestation calculated by the dating scan or, if this is not available, the date of the last known menstrual period. When making this assessment, take into account the height of the woman.

If the uterus appears to be larger than that indicated by the period of gestation, the main possibilities include:

- large-for-gestational-age fetus
- multiple pregnancy
- polyhydramnios
- uterine fibroids
- hydatidiform mole (Sasaki 2003).

If the uterus appears to be smaller than that indicated by the period of gestation, the most likely causes are:

- small-for-gestational-age fetus
- oligohydramnios
- fetal death.

The gravid uterus is usually a longitudinal ovoid in shape. Sometimes, during late pregnancy, the shape of the uterus may be described as 'unusual'. This may be due to the fetus lying in either an oblique or transverse position.

Whilst observing the size and shape of the uterus, the midwife may note abdominal scars, *striae gravidarum* (also called stretch marks), or a line of dark pigmentation called the *linea nigra* which extends from the umbilicus to the pubis. If not already noted in the maternity records, the reason for abdominal scars should be ascertained and this recorded in the maternity records. Striae gravidarum may be seen as red marks if they are new or silver-coloured marks if they date from a previous pregnancy or weight gain. Fetal movements may also be observed.

### Palpation

Palpation of the abdomen should be carried out gently and smoothly using both hands, warmed. Whilst it is the pads of the fingers that are used to palpate the fetal parts, it is essential that nails are short to avoid causing the woman discomfort. Undue pressure may cause the woman pain and tightening of the abdominal muscles, as well as stimulation of uterine contractions; both of which will make the palpation more difficult. During the palpation, the midwife should position herself so that she is able to observe the woman's face for signs of discomfort, such as grimacing. If signs of discomfort are observed, the midwife should ascertain the reason for the discomfort, reassure the woman and amend her technique.

Symphysis pubis–fundal height may be estimated by palpation, or, as recommended by NICE (2008), measured using a tape measure. If the midwife is estimating the fundal height by palpation, the ulnar border of the hand is placed at the uppermost point of the fundus of the uterus and the height compared with the size expected for the period of gestation (see Fig. 32.4).

Whilst NICE currently recommends that the symphysis–fundal height is measured using a tape measure, there are some limitations to this procedure. A review of the current evidence base revealed a wide variation in accuracy and limited predictive value in the use of symphysis–fundal height measurement in detecting both small and large-for-gestational-age babies (NICE 2008). Research has also shown that clinicians are biased in their measurement of fundal height if they have knowledge of the gestational age of the pregnancy or if they use a marked tape measure (Ross 2007).

The Perinatal Institute for Maternal and Child Health (2007) recommends using a non-elastic tape measure with the centimetre markings placed on the underside next to the woman's abdomen to reduce observer error and bias. The tape measure should be secured at the top of the fundus with one hand and, with the tape measure staying in contact with the skin, the tape measure should be run along the longitudinal axis of the uterus to the top of the symphysis pubis, without correcting to the midline

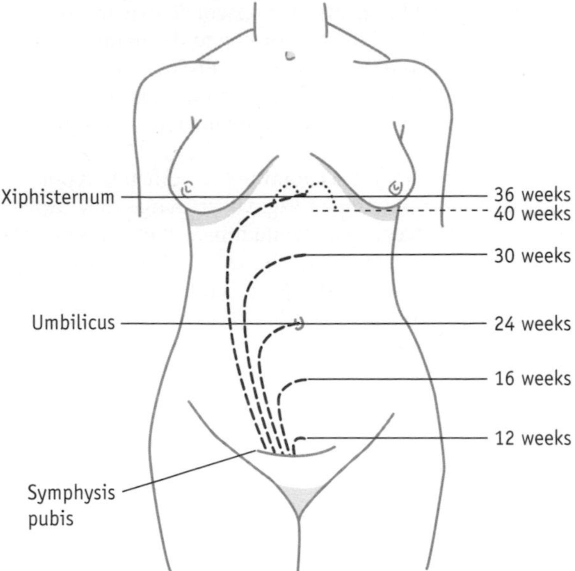


**Figure 32.4** The height of the fundus at different stages of pregnancy.

of the woman's abdomen. The measurement should be recorded in the woman's antenatal maternity record and plotted on a growth chart. Customized symphysis–fundal height charts, adjusted for maternal weight, height, parity and ethnic group, are available. If the midwife suspects that the fetus is small for gestational age, then referral should be made for ultrasound biometric testing (RCOG 2002).

From 36 weeks' gestation the abdominal examination should include palpation to determine the position of the fetus. Assessment of fetal presentation by abdominal palpation prior to 36 weeks' gestation should not be routinely offered to women because it is not always accurate, is of little predictive value and may cause unnecessary discomfort (NICE 2008).

The following terms are used in relation to the position of the fetus in utero:

- presentation
- denominator
- position
- attitude
- engagement
- lie.

The presentation of the fetus in utero is determined by the part of the fetus lying in the lower pole of the uterus (Fig. 32.5). After 36 weeks' gestation, the most common presentation is cephalic. Other possible presentations are breech, face, brow and shoulder.

The denominator is a fixed point on the presenting part which is used to indicate the position:

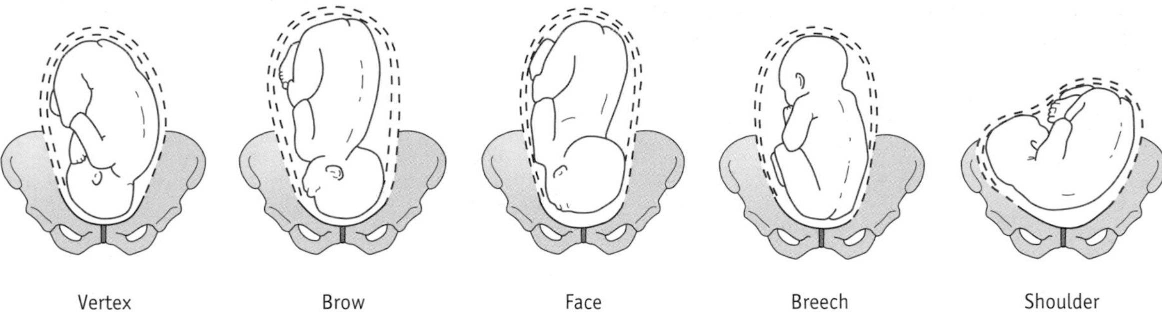


**Figure 32.5** The presentation of the fetus.

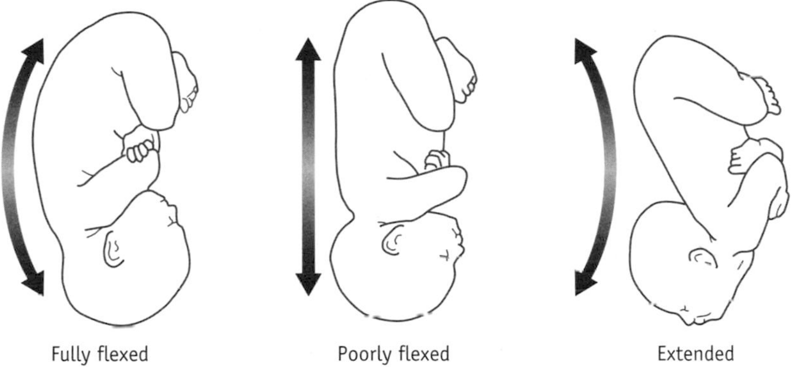


**Figure 32.6** The attitude of the fetus.

- In a cephalic presentation, the denominator is the occiput.
- In a breech presentation, the denominator is the sacrum.
- In a face presentation, the denominator is the mentum (chin).

The position of the fetus in utero is the relationship of the denominator to the six areas of the woman's pelvis (see website). The areas of the woman's pelvis are:

- left and right anterior
- left and right lateral
- left and right posterior.

In a cephalic presentation, the denominator is the occiput, so the position of the fetus is described as:

- left or right occipitoanterior (LOA, ROA)
- left or right occipitolateral (LOL, ROL)
- left or right occipitoposterior (LOP, ROP).

Anterior positions are more common than posterior positions and help to promote flexion of the fetus. In the anterior position, the fetal back is uppermost and can flex more easily against the woman's soft abdominal wall than when it lies against the woman's spinal column as occurs in a posterior position.

The attitude is the relationship of the fetal head and limbs to its body. The attitude of the fetus may be described as being fully flexed, deflexed, partially extended or completely extended (Fig. 32.6). When fully flexed, the fetal head and spine are flexed, the arms are crossed over the chest, and the legs and thighs are flexed, forming a compact ovoid which fits the uterus comfortably.

Engagement of the fetal head occurs when the transverse diameter of the fetal skull has passed through the brim of the pelvis (that is, the biparietal diameter measuring 9.5 cm) (Fig. 32.7). Engagement of the fetal head may be measured in fifths. The amount of head palpable above the brim of the pelvis is assessed and described as follows (Fig. 32.8):

5/5: Five-fifths of the fetal head are palpable above the brim of the pelvis on abdominal palpation. That is, the whole head can be palpated.

4/5: Four-fifths of the fetal head are palpable above the brim of the pelvis on abdominal palpation. One-fifth is below the pelvic brim and cannot be palpated per abdomen.

3/5: Three-fifths of the fetal head are palpable above the brim of the pelvis on abdominal palpation. Two-fifths

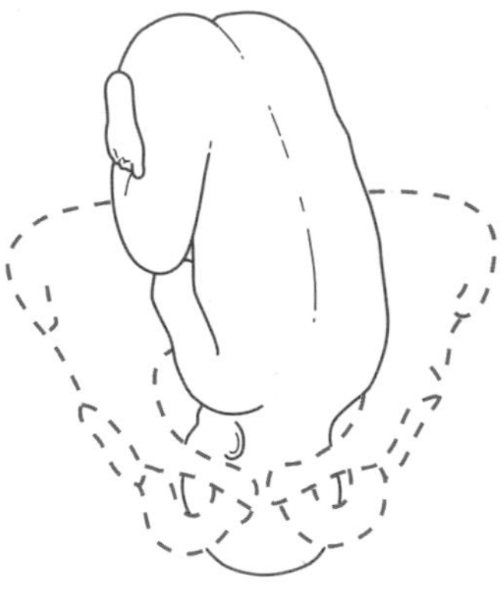

**Figure 32.7** Engagement of the fetal head.

are below the pelvic brim and cannot be palpated per abdomen.

2/5: Two-fifths of the fetal head are palpable above the brim of the pelvis on abdominal palpation. Three-fifths are below the pelvic brim and cannot be palpated per abdomen. The widest transverse diameter of the fetal head has now passed through the brim of the pelvis and the fetal head is described as being engaged.

1/5: One-fifth of the fetal head is palpable above the brim of the pelvis on abdominal palpation. Four-fifths are below the pelvic brim and cannot be palpated per abdomen. The fetal head is sometimes described as being 'deeply engaged' in the pelvis.

The lie is the relationship of the long axis of the fetus to the long axis of the uterus (Fig. 32.9). The lie of the fetus may be longitudinal, oblique or transverse. In the later weeks of pregnancy, the lie should be longitudinal.

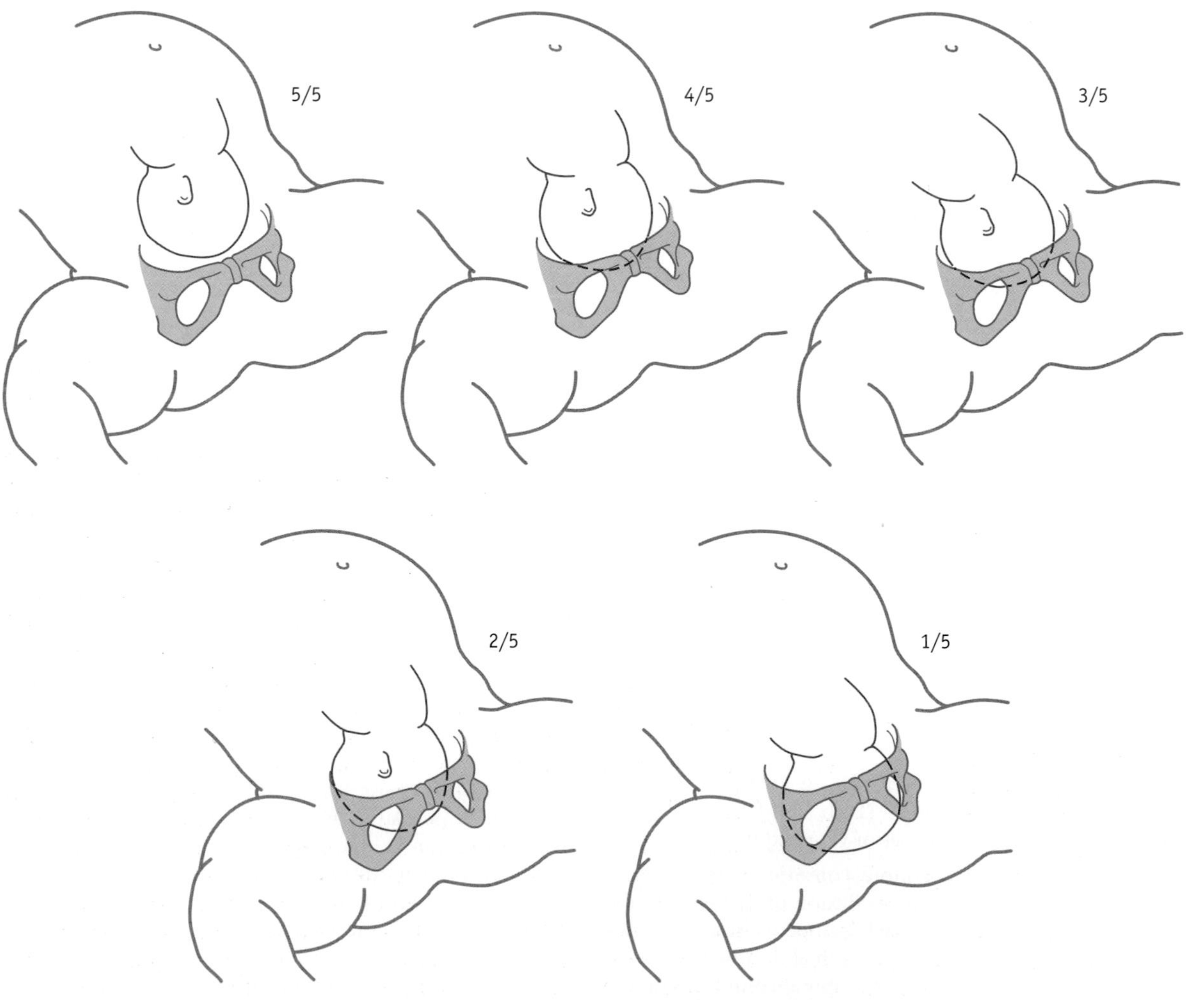

5/5
4/5
3/5
2/5
1/5

**Figure 32.8** Abdominal examination to determine the descent of the fetal head in fifths.

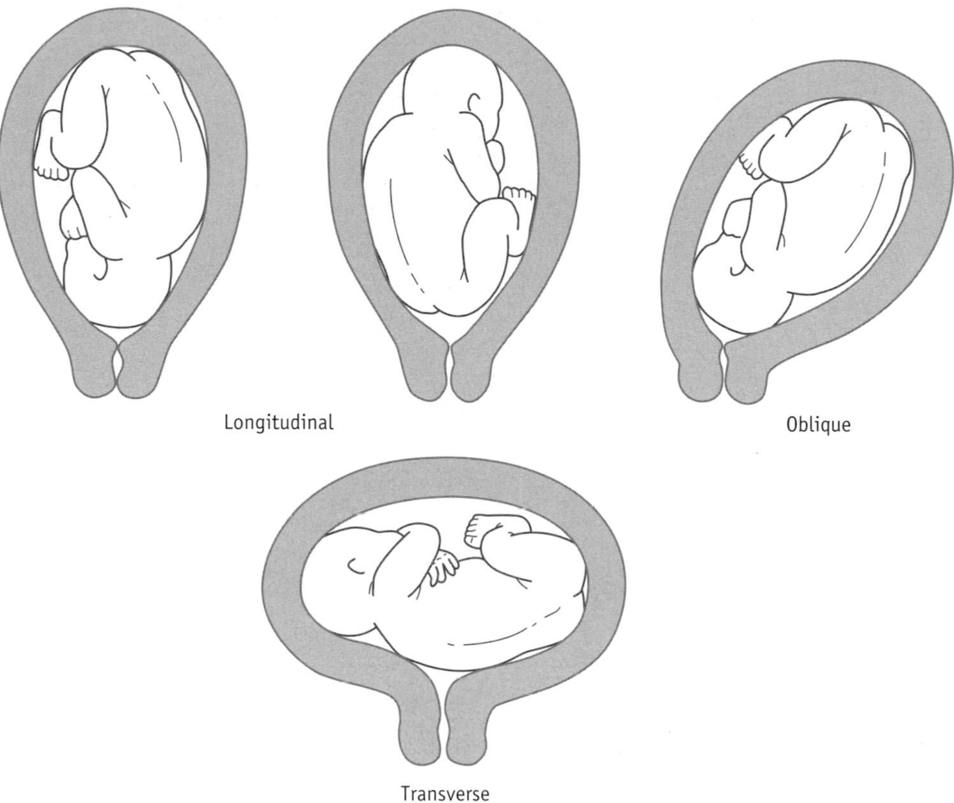


**Figure 32.9** The lie of the fetus.

To determine the presentation, position, attitude, engagement and lie of the fetus in utero by abdominal examination, the midwife will use three distinct manoeuvres:

- pelvic palpation
- fundal palpation
- lateral palpation.

For palpation of the abdomen, see Figure 32.10.

### *Pelvic palpation*

This is the most important manoeuvre in abdominal palpation as it is during the pelvic palpation that the presentation of the fetus is determined. Traditionally, midwives may have performed a fundal palpation, followed by a lateral palpation and then a deep pelvic palpation. However, for some women, palpation of the uterus may cause tightening of the uterine and abdominal muscles, which may make it very difficult to determine fetal presentation, so consideration should be given to performing the pelvic palpation first, when the muscles of the uterus and abdomen are relaxed. In addition to determining the presentation of the fetus, the attitude and degree of engagement of the fetal head may also be identified. To perform a deep pelvic palpation, the midwife stands alongside the woman, facing the woman's feet. The midwife then places one hand on each side of the uterus near the pelvic brim. The fingertips should then sink gently and smoothly into the pelvis to feel the presentation. The fetal head feels hard and round. If the fetal head is not engaged, it may be possible to ballotte it. This means that if the fetal head is given a gentle tap by an examining finger, the head floats away from the finger and then is felt to return to the examining finger. If the fingertips can sink further into the pelvis, more on one side than the other, this may mean that the head is flexed and the occiput is lying on the side into which the fingers sink more deeply. Occasionally, some midwives or obstetricians may also perform pelvic palpation using a manouevre called 'Pawlick's grip'. The thumb and first finger of the hand are spread open and placed just above the symphysis pubis with the thumb and finger tips pointing towards the woman's face. The thumb and finger then grasp the lower part of the abdomen to determine the presentation and engagement of the presenting part. Some practitioners find this manoeuvre useful if the presenting part is above the pelvic brim; however, it is unlikely that all the information required during a pelvic palpation can be ascertained

Pelvic palpation

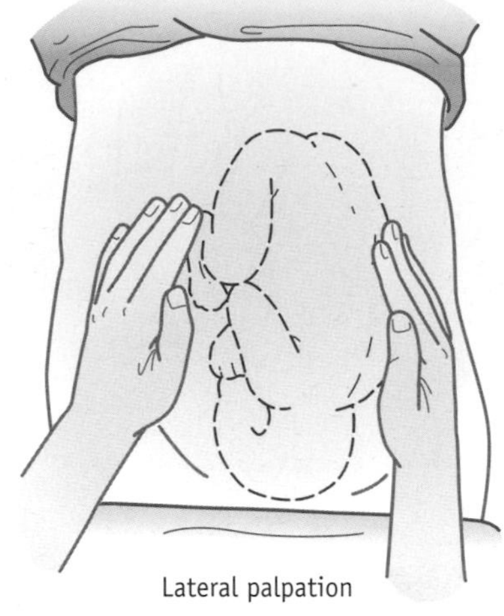


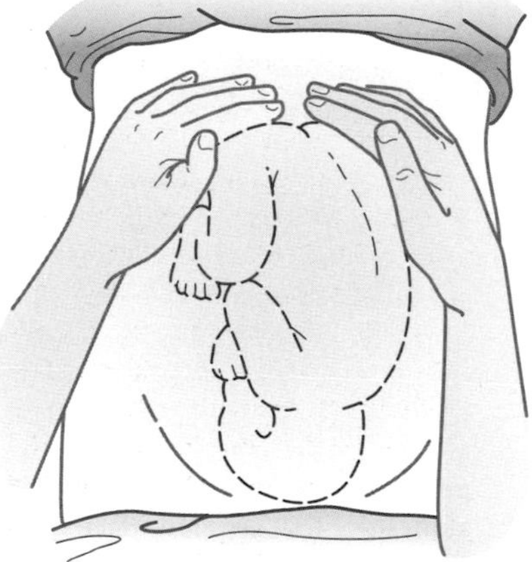

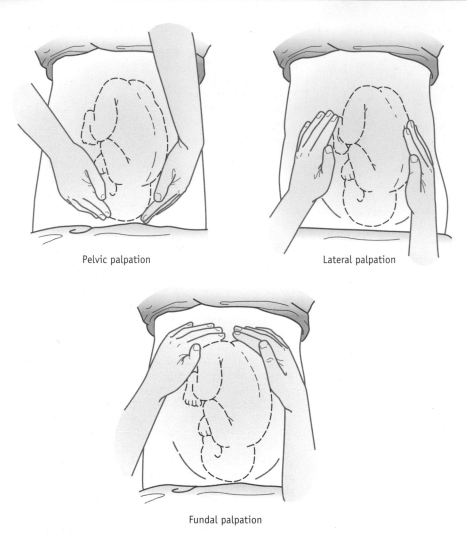


**Figure 32.10** Palpation of the abdomen.

by use of Pawlick's grip alone and deep pelvic palpation may need to be carried out in addition to Pawlick's grip. In order to minimize discomfort for the woman, it may be more prudent to perform deep pelvic palpation first.

## *Fundal palpation*

Fundal palpation is carried out to determine which part of the fetus is lying in the fundus of the uterus. Still turned to face the woman, the midwife uses both hands to gently palpate the fundus. If the fetal presentation is cephalic, then the breech will be felt in the fundus. The breech feels irregular in outline, less hard than the fetal head, and fetal lower limbs may be felt near it. If the presentation of the fetus is breech, then the fetal head will be felt in the fundus. The fetal head feels smooth, round and hard. It is usually ballottable and separated from the trunk by a groove, the fetal neck. It is possible to move the fetal head more freely than the breech, which can only be moved from side to side.

## *Lateral palpation*

Lateral palpation is carried out to determine the position of the fetal back. The midwife turns to face the woman's face. One hand is placed flat on one side of the woman's abdomen to steady it whilst the other hand gently palpates down the length of the other side of the maternal abdomen. The process is then reversed, with the hand that was being used to steady the abdomen being used to palpate the length of the abdomen and the hand that was firstly used to palpate the abdomen being used to steady the uterus. The fetal back is felt as a continuous smooth resistant object whereas the fetal limbs are felt as being small irregular objects which may move whilst they are being palpated. If the fetal back cannot be palpated but fetal limbs are felt on both sides of the midline of the uterus, the fetal position is most likely to be occipitoposterior.

### *Auscultation*

This is carried out when women visit the antenatal clinic. The early sounds are heard through ultrasound and from about 16 weeks may be heard via the electronic monitor (see Ch. 36).

Auscultation can be done with the Pinard monaural fetal stethoscope or the binaural stethoscope, and/or with an electronic fetal heart monitor. Ideally, the midwife should use the Pinard, and then the electronic monitor, as the means of monitoring the heartbeat are different, and the former is more likely to identify a true fetal heartbeat (Gibb & Arulkumaran 1997). Having palpated the abdomen, the midwife should know where to listen for the fetal heart sounds, which are heard at their maximum at a point over the fetal shoulder. When the fetus is lying in an occipitoanterior or occipitolateral position, the heart sounds are heard from the front and to the right or left according to the side on which the fetal back lies (Fig. 32.11). The fetal heart sounds like the ticking of a watch under a pillow, the rate being about double that of the woman's heartbeat observed at the wrist. The woman and her partner usually enjoy listening to their baby's heartbeat too.

A uterine souffle, caused by the flowing of blood through the uterine arteries, may be heard; this is a soft, blowing sound, the rate of which corresponds to the woman's pulse.

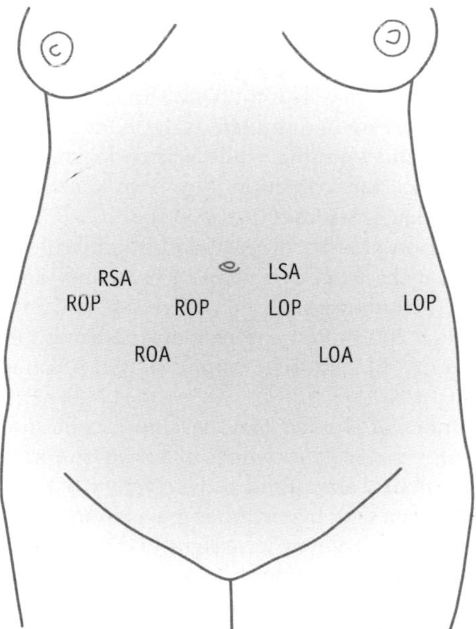


**Figure 32.11** The approximate points of the fetal heart sounds in vertex and breech presentations.

## Abdominal findings throughout pregnancy

At first, only the height of the fundus is ascertained (see Fig. 32.4).

- *Week 12* (sometimes earlier): The fundus is just palpable above the symphysis.
- *Week 16*: The fundus is halfway to the umbilicus. At this stage, a multigravida may have felt fetal movements.
- *Week 20*: The fundus reaches the lower border of the umbilicus and all women should be asked about movements. Fetal heart sounds may be audible.
- *Week 24*: The fundus reaches the upper border of the umbilicus, the fetus may just be palpable and fetal heart sounds are heard.
- *Week 28*: The fundus of the uterus is one-third of the distance from the umbilicus to the xiphisternum. The fetus is now easily palpable, very mobile and may be found in any lie, presentation or position.
- *Week 32*: The uterus is two-thirds of the distance from the umbilicus to the xiphisternum. The fetus lies longitudinally and, usually, the head presents. If the midwife finds a breech presentation, she should refer the woman to a doctor. It may be decided to turn the fetus, though the doctor will probably want to wait to see whether it turns spontaneously.
- *Week 34*: The uterus extends nearly as far as the xiphisternum. Almost always the lie is longitudinal; usually the presentation is cephalic. If the breech presents, then external cephalic version may be attempted or left to term.
- *Week 36*: The fundus reaches the xiphisternum. The presentation should be cephalic. In a primigravida the head may be engaged or engagement may occur a little later. If the head is engaged, the fundus will be lower, at about the level of a 34-week pregnancy, and the woman will have experienced 'lightening'.
- *Weeks 37–40*: The findings will all be similar except that the fetus becomes more stable and the amount of liquor diminishes slightly. The midwife must observe the woman carefully for signs of supine hypotensive syndrome during abdominal examinations, especially as pregnancy advances and the weight of the uterus increases.

## Engagement of the fetal head

There is a popular myth that engagement of the head occurs at 36 weeks in a primigravida. In about 50% of primigravidae, engagement of the head occurs between 38 and 42 weeks (Weekes & Flynn 1975), and in 80% of cases labour ensues within 14 days of the head engaging. In multigravidae, because of lax uterine and abdominal muscles, engagement may not take place until labour is established. If the head is engaged, the pelvic brim is certainly of adequate size and the probability is that the cavity and outlet are also adequate.

Engagement is often referred to as *lightening*, because of the sense of lightness women feel as the pressure is lessened on the diaphragm. In some women the head may not be engaged at term. This may be due to a full bladder or rectum or an occipitoposterior position where the presenting part tends to be deflexed. A steep angle of inclination of the pelvic brim tends to delay engagement until labour is well established. This is seen more commonly as a racial characteristic in West African and West Indian women.

If the head is high, an ultrasound scan may be performed to exclude placenta praevia. It is difficult to determine cephalopelvic disproportion prior to labour because of the factors involved in labour itself.

Following this examination, the findings are recorded and the woman is informed of these.

## Helping women to manage and cope with pregnancy changes

Most women experience physical changes during pregnancy which, although they are not life threatening, may be a source of anxiety and discomfort. These changes are sometimes referred to as 'minor disorders of pregnancy'. However, for many women, the impact of these changes is certainly not minor; they have to manage and cope with the 'minor disorders' in addition to their ongoing responsibilities for family, home and employment at a time when they may also be experiencing pregnancy-related fatigue and discomfort. It is important that the midwife treats the woman with sensitivity and respect when these changes are being discussed, offering evidence-based information and advice to support the woman at this time (NMC 2008).

**Reflective activity 32.3**

Ask a pregnant woman what it felt like when her abdomen was palpated.

When you are present at an antenatal examination, observe the verbal and non-verbal communication that occurs between the mother and the midwife, and consider the points that were particularly good as well as those that may be improved.

## CHANGES WITHIN THE SYSTEMS IN PREGNANCY

## The gastrointestinal tract

### Periodontal disease

Many women experience periodontal disease during pregnancy, resulting in local (gingival) and systemic inflammatory and immune responses (Boggess et al 2003, Mukherjee & Almas 2010). Periodontal disease has been associated with preterm birth, pre-eclampsia, second trimester miscarriage and small-for-gestational-age infants (Boggess et al 2003, Moore et al 2004), although the precise links between periodontal disease and adverse pregnancy outcome are yet unknown.

Gingivitis occurs as food debris and calcified dental plaque collect in the minute spaces between the teeth and the gum, causing irritation and inflammation. Bleeding of the gums may occur during eating, brushing or if the gums are probed. Some women may also report an increase in tooth mobility. All women should be encouraged to attend the dentist (care is free for pregnant women and for a year following the birth of the baby in the UK). Women who experience bleeding gums should be advised to use a soft toothbrush to brush their teeth.

### Nausea and vomiting

Nausea and vomiting are the most common gastrointestinal symptoms experienced in early pregnancy, with up to 85% of women experiencing nausea and 50% of women actually vomiting (Jewell & Young 2003) (see Ch. 53). Whilst the aetiology is unclear, rising levels of human chorionic gonadotrophin during pregnancy have been implicated. A review by Jewell & Young (2003) suggested that nausea is less common in women who experience miscarriage, and more common in multiple pregnancies and molar pregnancies.

Nausea and vomiting during pregnancy are often referred to as 'morning sickness', yet many women report experiencing symptoms throughout the day or in the evening rather than only in the morning. Women may become concerned about the effect of nausea and vomiting upon their pregnancy. The midwife should reassure women that there are no harmful effects upon the fetus as a result of nausea and vomiting, whilst acknowledging the detrimental impact the condition can have upon the woman's day-to-day activities (NICE 2008).

A number of non-pharmacological and pharmacological treatments for the relief of nausea in pregnancy have been suggested, including ginger, P6 acupressure and antihistamines (NICE 2008). Rest and regular small amounts of carbohydrate are thought to be helpful (Jewell & Young 2003).

A small number of women may develop a condition called *hyperemesis gravidarum*, where excessive vomiting during early pregnancy alters fluid and electrolyte balance (see Ch. 53). Women with hyperemesis gravidarum generally feel very unwell. They may have signs of dehydration, including a dry mouth and mucous membranes, and dipstick urine testing may show the presence of ketones in the urine. Admission to hospital is usually required to correct the fluid and electrolyte imbalance via intravenous fluid therapy.

### Heartburn

Heartburn is a frequent complaint during pregnancy, reported by up to 72% of women during the third trimester of pregnancy (Marrero et al 1992). Heartburn is described as a burning sensation, or discomfort, felt behind the sternum or throat. It may be accompanied by regurgitation of the acidic stomach contents into the throat or mouth, causing a bitter taste. Regurgitation may be due to the effects of progesterone relaxing the lower oesophageal sphincter, resulting in gastro-oesophageal reflux. Whilst heartburn is not associated with adverse outcomes of pregnancy, it is important to distinguish between the pain caused by heartburn and epigastric pain associated with pre-eclampsia (NICE 2008). Measuring the woman's blood pressure and testing her urine for protein enables the midwife to exclude pre-eclampsia.

Treatment of heartburn is aimed at providing relief of symptoms. An upright position, especially after meals, and sleeping in a propped-up position may resolve the symptoms of heartburn. Additionally, eating small frequent meals and reducing the quantity of high-fat foods and gastric irritants, such as caffeine and caffeine derivatives, may prove effective. Antacids may also be considered for the relief of heartburn where lifestyle and dietary modification has not been effective at relieving symptoms.

### Constipation

Constipation may occur as a result of rising progesterone levels in pregnancy, causing a reduction in gastric motility and hence increased gastric transit time. Constipation is associated with poor dietary fibre intake and may cause abdominal discomfort and pain during defecation. Constipation has also been found to be a predisposing factor for haemorrhoids (Quijano & Abalos 2005).

As a preventative measure, and for women who experience constipation, information regarding the benefits of increasing the amount of fibre and fluid within the diet should be offered. Some women may not understand which foods are high in fibre and the midwife may need to discuss how the woman's diet can be modified to include more fibre-rich foods and fluids. Many women drink carbonated drinks or drinks containing caffeine, and rather than increasing their intake of these fluids, midwives should encourage them to drink additional water or caffeine-free drinks.

If constipation is not resolved by theses simple measures, women may choose to take a fibre supplement (NICE 2008).

### Haemorrhoids

Haemorrhoids are swollen veins at, or near, the anus. The aetiology of haemorrhoids is unclear, but predisposing factors include a history of constipation, a low-fibre low-fluid diet, and bowel disease associated with an increase in intra-abdominal pressure or diarrhoea (Quijano & Abalos 2005). Haemorrhoids are normally asymptomatic, but during pregnancy they may become symptomatic as a result of altered tone and position of the pelvic floor and sphincter muscles. Some women report that haemorrhoids cause them to experience a burning sensation or itching around the anus. Intermittent bleeding of the anus and leakage of mucus, faeces or flatus have also been reported (Quijano & Abalos 2005). The symptoms of haemorrhoids are usually transient and in most cases mild, but they can cause some woman discomfort or pain. Treatment of haemorrhoids during pregnancy is aimed at relieving symptoms, especially pain control, and any corrective treatment is usually deferred until after the birth of the baby (Quijano & Abalos 2005). Women should be offered information about increasing the amount of fibre and fluid, particularly water, within their diet, as this has been shown to be an effective treatment for symptomatic haemorrhoids and bleeding (Alonso-Coello et al 2005). A fibre supplement may be considered and local ointments containing an anaesthetic are widely used although there is currently no evidence regarding their effectiveness or safety in pregnancy (NICE 2008).

## The circulatory system

### Varicose veins

Varicose veins occur when a valve within the vein weakens and allows a backflow of blood, putting more pressure on the other valves and causing blood to pool and stagnate. The vein then becomes distended and swollen near to the surface of the skin. The veins of the leg are the most commonly affected but veins in the vulva (vulval varicosities) and anus (haemorrhoids) can also be affected. During pregnancy, the veins are placed under increased pressure as a result of an increase in circulating blood volume and the effect of progesterone relaxing the muscular wall of the blood vessels (Bamigboye & Smyth 2007). Varicose veins are thought to affect up to 40% of pregnant women (Rabhi et al 2000) with multiparous women having a greater risk of developing varicose veins than primiparous women (Beebe-Dimmer et al 2005). Symptoms of varicose veins and oedema include heavy achy legs, which the woman may feel are unsightly, pain, night cramps, tingling or numbness (Bamigboye & Smyth 2007). The skin around the varicose vein may feel itchy. Some women report a burning sensation or throbbing. Carr (2006) suggests that for up to 80% of the women who develop problems with varicose veins during pregnancy, these symptoms appear during the first trimester of pregnancy. Treatment for varicose veins may be surgical removal, pharmacological treatments where liquid sclerosing drugs are injected into the affected veins to make them shrink, or non-pharmacological treatments, such as compression bandages, rest, leg elevation, exercise, immersion in water and reflexology. During pregnancy, treatment focuses upon relief of symptoms, with surgical and pharmacological treatments being deferred until after the birth. For the majority of women, the varicose veins resolve on their own within the first 3 or 4 months after the baby's birth (Bamigboye & Smyth 2007). A review by Bamigboye & Smyth (2007) exploring interventions for varicose veins and oedema during pregnancy concluded that the available evidence was insufficient to make reliable recommendations for clinical practice. The most common treatments for the relief of symptoms of varicose veins and oedema during pregnancy were found to be compression stockings and elevation of the feet, but neither of these treatments had been adequately researched (Bamigboye & Smyth 2007). The review suggested that reflexology appeared to improve the symptoms for women with leg oedema but a larger-scale study is required (Bamigboye & Smyth 2007).

## The vaginal tract

### Vaginal discharge

*Leucorrhoea* describes the change in the amount and type of vaginal discharge that many women experience during pregnancy; this often increases, and is usually white, non-offensive and non-irritant. However, if the change is associated with an itch, soreness, offensive smell, or pain when passing urine, the underlying cause should be determined (NICE 2008). It is essential that when discussing these issues with women, the midwife asks appropriate questions, in a sensitive manner, to determine which investigations and treatment may be required.

The most common causes of vaginal discharge during pregnancy are *bacterial vaginosis, vaginal trichomoniasis* and *vaginal candidiasis* (commonly called *thrush*). Bacterial vaginosis is a common condition caused by an overgrowth of bacteria within the vagina and characterized by a white–grey vaginal discharge which may smell fish-like. The discharge does not usually cause soreness or itching of the vagina or vulva.

Trichomoniasis is one of the most commonly sexually transmitted infections and is characterized by a green–yellow frothy vaginal discharge and pain on urination. The discharge may have an unpleasant or fish-like smell (see Ch. 57).

Vaginal candidiasis is caused by the yeast *Candida albicans* and is characterized by a white vaginal discharge which may smell of yeast. The discharge may be thicker than the woman's usual discharge, but in some women it is more watery.

Investigation of the cause of vaginal discharge includes taking vaginal and cervical swabs. If the test result is positive, referral to a medical practitioner will be required. This may be the woman's own GP or a sexual health clinic.

The recommended treatment of vaginal candidiasis during pregnancy is a 1-week course of a topical imidazole cream and/or vaginal pessaries (NICE 2008). As yet, the safety of oral treatments for vaginal candidiasis in pregnancy has not been ascertained and so they should not be offered to pregnant women (NICE 2008). The midwife should offer the woman information about self-help measures that may reduce the discomfort associated with vaginal candidiasis, including avoiding perfumed soaps, bubble baths and vaginal deodorants which may further irritate the sore skin of the vulva and vagina and keeping the perianal area as cool as possible by wearing loose clothing and cotton underwear. Cold compresses or ice cubes wrapped in a cloth and placed against the vulva may reduce soreness and itching. (For further information on sexually transmitted diseases, see Chapter 57.)

## The skin in pregnancy

Hyperpigmentation of the skin during pregnancy is very common, occurring in up to 90% of pregnant women. Hyperpigmentation results in a darkening of areas that are already pigmented, like the areola, nipples, vulva and perianal region. Some women also note hyperpigmentation of the skin in the inner thigh region and axilla. It is usually more noticeable in women with dark complexions. The cause of hyperpigmentation is unclear, but it is thought to be related to an increase in serum oestrogen, serum progesterone and melanocyte-stimulating hormone.

### Connective tissue changes

Approximately 90% of pregnant women experience striae gravidarum, commonly called 'stretch marks', by the end of the second trimester of pregnancy, as a result of abdominal distension, maternal weight gain, genetic predisposition and the hormonal changes that occur in pregnancy (Muallem & Rubeiz 2006). Striae gravidarum appear as red–purple linear streaks over the abdomen, thighs, arms, breasts and buttocks, and gradually fade into pale, skin- or silver-coloured streaks. Itching may accompany the striae gravidarum. A number of preventative measures, including the application of creams and oils, have been suggested as beneficial in preventing the development of striae gravidarum, but studies have shown limited effects (Muallem & Rubeiz 2006).

## The musculoskeletal system in pregnancy

### Backache

Back and pelvic pain are common in pregnancy, with up to 76% of women reporting back pain at some point during their pregnancy (Kristiansson et al 1996). It is thought that loosening of the ligaments in the pelvic area under the influence of relaxin and progesterone and altered maternal posture are the main causes of back and pelvic pain during pregnancy.

Posture is altered as pregnancy advances because the curvature of the lower spine becomes exaggerated to balance the increasing anterior weight of the gravid uterus. Many women report that back and pelvic pain are worse during the evening and in the last trimester of pregnancy, disturbing sleep and interfering with ordinary daily activities, such as walking, sitting and working (Pennick & Young 2007). A review found that pregnant-specific exercise programmes, physiotherapy and acupuncture appeared to reduce back or pelvic pain, whilst some women reported pain relief by using pillows to support their stomachs when lying down. Back strain may be reduced by women turning onto their sides when sitting up and as they swing their legs down when they get up off a couch or bed, rather than attempting to raise themselves from their back without using their arms for support (Pennick & Young 2007).

## Leg cramp

The cause of leg cramps during pregnancy is unclear. It has been suggested that leg cramps may occur as a result of either circulatory changes during pregnancy or changes in calcium and magnesium levels during pregnancy (Jewell & Young 2002). Though leg cramps do not cause any lasting damage, they can be very painful. The pain is caused by a build-up in lactic and pyruvic acid that leads to an involuntary contraction of the calf muscle. Leg cramps are often experienced during the night, so women may suddenly wake in pain; this can be extremely distressing.

During an episode of leg cramps, women may find that getting out of bed, walking around, stretching and massaging the affected muscle helps. A review by Jewell & Young (2002) found that calcium supplementation did not prevent leg cramps in pregnancy, but for some women magnesium supplementation stopped them having leg cramps altogether and for other women the frequency of attacks was reduced.

## Carpal tunnel syndrome

Carpal tunnel syndrome occurs as a result of oedema in the carpal tunnel; this compresses the median nerve, causing paraesthesia, swelling and pain in the hand or hands and impairs sensory and motor function of the hand (NICE 2008). Interventions to reduce the symptoms of carpal tunnel syndrome include wrist splints and analgesia. Referral to the physiotherapist should be considered.

## Pregnancy-related pelvic girdle pain

Pregnancy-related pelvic girdle pain affects approximately one in five pregnant women (Association of Chartered Physiotherapists in Women's Health 2007), who experience pain in the joints of the pelvis; the symphysis pubis joint at the front of the pelvis and the sacroiliac joints at the back of the pelvis. It is thought that the pain is caused by abnormal stretching of the pelvic joints during pregnancy (Wellock 2002). For non-pregnant women the average gap between the pelvic bones at the pubic joint is 4–5 mm. During pregnancy, this gap may widen by 2–3 mm (Leadbetter et al 2004). Studies have shown that many women experience significant pain without great separation of the bones and the degree of pain is unrelated to the degree of separation (Leadbetter et al 2004). Stability of the pubic joint is essential for efficient weight bearing and mobility, and instability may cause pain in the symphysis pubis; mild to severe pain in the groin, inner thigh, lower back, abdomen, perineum or leg (Leadbetter et al 2004); pain during walking or whilst performing activities that require the woman to part, or lift, her legs, such as climbing stairs, getting dressed or turning over in bed (Leadbetter et al 2004, Wellock & Crichton 2007). Women with pelvic girdle pain may be observed walking with a 'waddling' gait, whilst some women report hearing or feeling a clicking, snapping or grinding within the symphysis pubis (Leadbetter et al 2004).

In some rare cases, the gap between the pelvic bones widens by more than 10 mm, causing a partial or complete rupture of the symphysis pubis. This condition is called diastasis symphysis pubis (DSP) and may occur as a result of traumatic separation of the symphysis during a spontaneous or operative delivery or as a result of accidental injury to the pelvis during pregnancy (Leadbetter et al 2004). Whilst pelvic girdle pain may be diagnosed by taking a history of the symptoms experienced by the woman, DSP is diagnosed by X-ray.

The onset of symptoms of pelvic girdle pain may occur gradually or acutely during the second or third trimester of pregnancy, or during labour or birth. The actual incidence of SPD is unclear as many women, and their maternity care providers, may dismiss the symptoms of SPD as being the 'aches and pains' of pregnancy, thus underdiagnosing the condition. Nevertheless, SPD does have a significant impact upon women's wellbeing and quality of life. Wellock & Crichton (2007) explored the impact of pelvic girdle pain upon women's quality of life and found that the chronic pain associated with pelvic girdle pain profoundly affected all aspects of the women's daily lives and made caring for their homes, families and themselves very difficult. In particular, the women felt unable to care for their children and reported social isolation as their ability to leave the home and, in particular, get in and out of the car, was challenged as a result of pain.

During the antenatal period, the aim of management of the condition is to reduce activities which exacerbate pain. Most cases are managed conservatively and so it is important that women understand the aetiology of the condition and what lifestyle changes they may need to make. These changes may include reducing non-essential activities, and accepting help regarding childcare and household chores. Self-help measures, such as placing pillows between the knees, may make it more comfortable for women when they are side-lying in bed (Wellock & Crichton 2007).

The Pelvic Partnership (2008), a charitable organization aimed at raising awareness of the condition, suggest that women plan ahead prior to performing activities and consider:

- How they could make the activity easier?
- Do they have everything they need before they start the activity?
- Do they really need to undertake the activity at all, or could someone else help them?

Referral to an obstetric physiotherapist for a pelvic and back assessment and advice about posture and mobility should be considered. Elbow crutches or a wheelchair may be required if mobility is significantly impaired. Some women find that a trochanteric, or pelvic, support belt gives some relief of pain, but the belts do not correct pelvic asymmetry and the woman may still require analgesia.

During labour, women with pelvic girdle pain may find it difficult to move into different positions and the midwife may need to be an advocate for the woman, facilitating her to move in ways that do not exacerbate her symptoms. This may include either a lateral or a supported 'all fours' position for vaginal examinations and birth. The lateral position may be preferable for fetal blood sampling, assisted deliveries or suturing of the perineum if required. Immersion in water may be beneficial for some women, as water relieves weight bearing and allows for ease of position change, but entering and exiting a birth pool may cause pain and, in some cases, delay treatment. An individual assessment of the woman's mobility will be required prior to her entering the water.

If the woman chooses either epidural or spinal anaesthesia for labour and birth, the woman and midwife need to be aware of the possibility of the symptoms of pelvic girdle pain being masked and excessive mobilization of the joint, causing increased pain during the postpartum period. Prior to receiving either epidural or spinal anaesthesia, the range of hip abduction should be measured and recorded in the woman's notes. The midwife needs to ensure that this range is not exceeded whilst the anaesthesia is effective.

During the postnatal period, women with pelvic girdle pain may require assistance with personal hygiene and care of their baby. This may include assisting the woman to the toilet and providing aids within the shower, such as handrails and chairs. Assistance with bathing and changing the baby may be needed as well as help in handing the baby to the mother rather than the mother having to get up to attend to the baby's needs. Consideration needs to be given to the position the woman adopts to feed her baby; a lateral position may be more comfortable for women who wish to breastfeed their babies. During this period, the midwife should make an assessment of the woman's risk of being predisposed to a deep vein thrombosis. Antiembolic stockings may be worn and thromboprophylaxis prescribed if appropriate. Women with moderate to severe symptoms may need referral to an obstetric physiotherapist during the postnatal period, and if the symptoms fail to resolve, referral to an orthopaedic surgeon may need to be considered. Very rarely, pelvic suturing may be required.

## CONCLUSION

As this chapter has demonstrated, the antenatal period is a time of tremendous psychological and physical adjustment for the pregnant woman and her family. The midwife can work in partnership with the woman to increase the woman's understanding of these changes, and to help her prepare for the birth and parenthood, by offering evidence-based information and individualized plans of care and support, taking into account women's diverse, and sometimes complex, backgrounds. Many women experience physiological changes in pregnancy that may lead to disturbance and discomfort within various body systems. The midwife is ideally placed to offer women information and support to enable them to cope with these changes and the challenges they might present to them in their day-to-day life. Initial and subsequent antenatal care should be provided within an environment of respect and partnership, and the midwife should aim to make every woman feel valued and every antenatal visit positive and informative.

### KEY POINTS

- The midwife should be aware of the main pregnancy tests available to women, and the accuracy of these.
- The initial antenatal 'booking' visit is an important opportunity to assess the physical, psychological, educational and social needs of the woman, and plan care accordingly.
- The antenatal period is a time of physical, psychological and social adjustment for the woman and her family, through which the midwife can guide and assist both.
- The significance of the woman's social, family, medical and obstetric histories should be carefully

assessed in order to identify any potential problems, and highlight her individual needs throughout the antenatal period in preparation for childbirth.

- The physiological changes which are wrought by pregnancy may have effects that are uncomfortable or of concern to the woman and an important part of the midwife's role lies in assessing the changes, ensuring the woman understands why they are occurring and suggesting strategies for increasing the comfort and wellbeing of the woman and her growing fetus.
- The midwife should be conversant with the physiology of pregnancy, be able to identify when pregnancy deviates from the norm and be able to refer to the appropriate practitioner.
- The antenatal period offers an ideal opportunity for the midwife in terms of health promotion and wider public health, from advising on smoking cessation, to diet and exercise.

## REFERENCES


Alonso-Coello P, Guyatt G, Heels-Ansdell D, et al: Laxatives for the treatment of haemorrhoids. *Cochrane Database of Systematic Reviews* (4):CD004649, 2005.

Ananth CV, Smulian JC, Vintzileos AM: Incidence of placenta abruption in relation to cigarette smoking and hypertensive disorders during pregnancy: a meta-analysis of observational studies, *Obstetrics and Gynecology* 93(4):622–628, 1999.

Anderson T: Feeling safe enough to let go: the relationship between a woman and her midwife during the second stage of labour. In Kirkham M, editor: *The midwife-mother relationship*, London, 2000, Macmillan.

Association of Chartered Physiotherapists in Women's Health: *Pregnancy related pelvic girdle pain. Guidance for mothers to be and new mothers* (website). www.acpwh.org.uk/docs/ACPWH-PGP_Pat.pdf. 2007. Accessed January 2009.

Bamigboye AA, Smyth R: Interventions for varicose veins and leg oedema in pregnancy, *Cochrane Database of Systematic Reviews* (1):CD001066, 2007.

Bastian L, Nanda K, Hasselblad V, et al: Diagnostic efficiency of home pregnancy test kits, *Archives of Family Medicine* 7(5):465–469, 1998.

Beebe-Dimmer JL, Pfeifer JR, Engle JS, et al: The epidemiology of chronic venous insufficiency and varicose veins, *Annals of Epidemiology* 15(3):175–184, 2005.

Beevers G, Lip GYH, O'Brien E: Blood pressure measurement. Part 1. Sphygomomanometry: factors common to all techniques, *British Medical Journal* 322(7292):981–985, 2001.

Berry D: *Health communication: theory and practice*, Maidenhead, 2007, Open University Press.

Bharj KK: *Pakistani Muslim women birthing in northern England: exploration of experiences and context*, Unpublished thesis, Sheffield, 2007, Sheffield Hallam University.

Bharj KK, Chesney M: *Pakistani Muslim women and midwives relationship: what are the essential attributes?* In press. 2010.

Blackburn ST: *Maternal, fetal and neonatal physiology*, Philadelphia, 2007, WB Saunders.

Boggess KA, Lieff S, Murtha AP, et al: Maternal periodontal disease is associated with an increased risk for pre-eclampsia, *Obstetrics and Gynaecology* 10(2):227–231, 2003.

British Hypertensive Society: *Blood pressure measurement* (website). www.bhsoc.org/bp_monitors/BLOOD_PRESSURE_1784b.pdf. 2008. Accessed August 2008.

British Medical Association (BMA): *Domestic violence: a health care issue?* London, 1998, BMA.

Carr S: Current management of varicose veins, *Clinical Obstetrics and Gynaecology* 49(2):414–426, 2006.

Castles A, Adams EK, Melvin CL, et al: Effects of smoking during pregnancy: five meta-analyses, *American Journal of Preventive Medicine* 16(3):208–215, 1999.

Chudleigh P, Pearce M: *Obstetric ultrasound*, ed 2, Edinburgh, 1994, Churchill Livingstone.

Coad J, Dunstall M: *Anatomy and physiology for midwives*, Edinburgh, 2005, Churchillll Livingstone.

Cokkinides VE, Coker AL, Sanderson M, et al: Physical violence during pregnancy: maternal complications and birth outcomes, *Obstetrics and Gynecology* 93(5):661–666, 1999.

Commission for Healthcare Audit and Inspection (CHAI): *Towards better births: a review of maternity services in England*, London, 2008, CHAI.

Davies J: Being with women who are economically without. In Kirkham M, editor: *The midwife-mother relationship*, London, 2000, Macmillan.

Department of Health (DH): *Changing childbirth, Part 1. Report of the Expert Maternity Group*, London, 1993, HMSO.

Department of Health (DH): *Why mothers die. Report on Confidential Enquiries into Maternal Deaths in the United Kingdom 1994–1996*, London, 1998, The Stationery Office.

Department of Health (DH): *Maternity matters: choice, access and continuity of care in a safe service*, London, 2007a, The Stationery Office.

Department of Health (DH): *The pregnancy book* (website). www.dh.gov.uk/en/Publicationsandstatistics/Publications/PublicationsPolicyAndGuidance/DH_074920. 2007b. Accessed August 2008.

Department of Health (DH): *High quality care for all: NHS Next Stage Review final report*, London, 2008, The Stationery Office.

Department of Health (DH), Department for Education and Skills (DfES): *National service framework for children, young people and maternity services*, London, 2004, HMSO.

DiFranza JR, Lew RA: Effects of maternal cigarette smoking on pregnancy complications and sudden death syndrome, *Journal of Family Practice* 40(4):385–394, 1995.

Dougherty L, Lister S: *The Royal Marsden Hospital manual of clinical nursing procedures*, Chichester, 2008, Wiley-Blackwell.

Dyson S: *Ethnicity and screening for sickle cell/thalassaemia*, Oxford, 2005, Elsevier.

Edwards N: *Birthing autonomy: women's experiences of planning home births*, London, 2005, Routledge.

Foster K, Lader D, Cheesebrough S: *Infant feeding 1995*, London, 1997, Office for National Statistics.

Gadsby R, Barnie-Adshead AM, Jagger C: A prospective study of nausea and vomiting during pregnancy, *British Journal of General Practice* 43(371):245–248, 1993.

Gibb DME, Arulkumaran S: *Fetal monitoring in practice*, ed 2, London, 1997, Butterworth Heinemann.

Gray R, Henderson J: *Review of the fetal effects of prenatal alcohol exposure*, Oxford, 2006, National Perinatal Epidemiology Unit.

Green JM, Curtis P, Price H, et al: *Continuing to care, the organisation of maternity services in the UK: a structured review of evidence*, Hale, 1998, Books for Midwives.

Hall J: Free-standing maternity units in England. In Kirkham M, editor: *Birth centres, a social model for maternity services*, London, 2003, Books for Midwives.

Hall M, MacIntyre S, Porter M: *Antenatal care assessed: a case study of an innovation in Aberdeen*, Aberdeen, 1985, Aberdeen University Press.

Hepburn M: Drug use in pregnancy, *British Journal of Hospital Medicine* 49(1):51–55, 1993.

Heslehurst N, Ells LJ, Simpson H, et al: Trends in maternal obesity incidence rates, demographic predictors, and health inequalities in 36 821 women over a 15-year period, *BJOG: An International Journal of Obstetrics & Gynaecology* 114(2):187–194, 2007.

Higgins D: Patient assessment. Part 6 – urinalysis, *Nursing Times* 104(12):24–25, 2008.

H M Treasury: *Public Service Agreement 19. Ensure better health for all*, London, 2007, H M Treasury.

Janssen PA, Holt VL, Sugg NK, et al: Intimate partner violence and adverse pregnancy outcomes: a population based study, *American Journal of Obstetrics and Gynecology* 188(5):1341–1347, 2003.

Jewell D, Young G: Interventions for leg cramps in pregnancy, *Cochrane Database of Systematic Reviews* (1):CD000121, 2002.

Jewell D, Young G: Interventions for nausea and vomiting in early pregnancy, *Cochrane Database of Systematic Reviews* (4):CD000145, 2003.

Kirkham M, editor: *The midwife-mother relationship*, Basingstoke, 2000, Macmillan.

Kirkham M, editor: *Birth centres, a social model for maternity services*, London, 2003, Books for Midwives.

Kirkham M, Stapleton H, editors: *Informed choice in maternity care: an evaluation of evidence-based leaflets*. NHS Centre for Reviews and Dissemination, Report 20. York, 2001, University of York.

Kristiansson P, Svardsudd K, Von Schoultz B: Serum relaxin, symphyseal pain and back pain during pregnancy, *American Journal of Obstetricians and Gynaecology* 175(5):1342–1347, 1996.

Lacroix R, Eason E, Melzack R: Nausea and vomiting during pregnancy: a prospective study of its frequency, intensity, and patterns of change, *American Journal of Obstetrics and Gynecology* 182(4):931–937, 2000.

Leadbetter RE, Mawer D, Lindow SW: Symphysis pubis dysfunction: a review of the literature, *Journal of Maternal-Fetal and Neonatal Medicine* 16(6):349–354, 2004.

Lewis G, editor: *Confidential Enquiry into Maternal and Child Health: Improving the health of mothers, babies and children, "Why mothers die" (2000–2002). The Sixth Report of Confidential Enquiry into Maternal Deaths in United Kingdom*, London, 2004, RCOG.

Lewis G, editor: *The Confidential Enquiry into Maternal and Child Health (CEMACH). Saving mothers' lives: reviewing maternal deaths to make motherhood safer – 2003-2005 The Seventh Report on Confidential Enquiries into Maternal Deaths in the United Kingdom*, London, 2007, CEMACH.

Lumley J, Oliver S, Waters E: Interventions for promoting smoking cessation during pregnancy, *Cochrane Database of Systematic Reviews* (2):CD001055, 2000.

Lundgren I, Berg M: Central concepts in the midwife-woman relationship, *Scandinavian Journal of Caring Services* 18(2):368–375, 2007.

Mander R: *Supportive care and midwifery*, Oxford, 2001, Blackwell Science.

Marrero JM, Goggin PM, Caestecker JS: Determinants of pregnancy heartburn, *British Journal of Obstetrics and Gynaecology* 99(9):731–734, 1992.

McAlister FA, Straus SE: Evidence based treatment for hypertension, *British Medical Journal* 322(7291):908–911, 2001.

Methven RC: The antenatal booking interview: recording an obstetric history or relating with a mother-to-be? Research and the Midwife Conference Proceedings, Glasgow 1982a:63–76.

Methven RC: The antenatal booking interview: recording an obstetric history or relating with a mother-to-be? Research and the Midwife Conference Proceedings, Glasgow 1982b:77–86.

Mooney J: *The hidden figure of domestic violence in North London*, London, 1993, Islington Council.

Moore S, Ide M, Coward PY, et al: Periodontal disease and adverse pregnancy outcome, *British Dental Journal* 197(5):251–258, 2004.

Muallem MM, Rubeiz NG: Physiological and biological skin changes in pregnancy, *Clinics in Dermatology* 24(2):80–83, 2006.

Mukherjee PM, Almas K: Orthodontic considerations for gingival health during pregnancy, a review, *International Journal of Dental Hygiene* 8(1):3–9, 2010.

National Institute for Health and Clinical Excellence (NICE): *NICE clinical guideline 62. Antenatal care: routine care for the healthy pregnant woman*, London, 2008, NICE.

National Institute for Health and Clinical Excellence (NICE): *Public health guidance, draft scope on 'how to stop smoking in pregnancy and following childbirth'* (website). www.nice.org.uk/guidance/index.jsp?action=download&o=40145. 2009. Accessed February 2009.

Nicholls L, Webb C: What makes a good midwife? An integrative review of methodologically-diverse research, *Journal of Advanced Nursing* 56(4):414–429, 2006.

Nursing and Midwifery Council (NMC): *The code: standards of conduct, performance and ethics for nurses and midwives*, London, 2008, NMC.

O'Dowd M, O'Dowd T: Quickening – a re-evaluation, *British Journal of Obstetrics and Gynaecology* 92(10):1037–1039, 1985.

Page AL, Cooke P, Percival P: Providing one-to-one practice and enjoying it. In Page L, editor: *The new midwifery: science and sensitivity in practice*, London, 2000, Churchill Livingstone.

Palmer G, MacInnes T, Kenway P: *Monitoring poverty and social exclusion 2008*, York, 2008, Joseph Rowntree Foundation.

Pelvic Partnership (website). www.pelvicpartnership.org.uk/index2.html. 2008. Accessed August 2008.

Pennick VE, Young G: Interventions for preventing and treating pelvic and back pain in pregnancy, *Cochrane Database of Systematic Reviews* (2):CD001139, 2007.

Perinatal Institute for Maternal and Child Health: *Fetal growth fundal height measurements* (website). www.pi.nhs.uk/growth/fhm.htm. 2007. Accessed November 2008.

Perkins ER, Unell J: Continuity and choice in practice: a study of a community-based team midwifery scheme. In Kirkham MJ, Perkins ER, editors: *1997 Reflections on midwifery*, London, 1997, Baillière Tindall.

Proud J: *Understanding obstetric ultrasound*, ed 2, Hale, 1997, Books for Midwives.

Quijano CE, Abalos E: Conservative management of symptomatic and/or complicated haemorrhoids in pregnancy and the puerperium, *Cochrane Database of Systematic Reviews* (3):CD004077, 2005.

Rabhi Y, Charras-Arthapignet C, Gris JC, et al: Lower limb vein enlargement and spontaneous blood flow echogenicity are normal sonographic findings during pregnancy, *Journal of Clinical Ultrasound* 28(8):407–413, 2000.

Redshaw M, Rowe R, Hockley C, et al: *Recorded delivery: a national survey of women's experience of maternity care*, Oxford, 2007, National Perinatal Epidemiology Unit.

Ross MG: Clinical bias in fundal height measurement, *Obstetrics and Gynaecology* 110(4):892–899, 2007.

Rosser J: Calculating the EDD – which is more accurate, scan or LMP? *The Practising Midwife* 3(3):28–29, 2000.

Royal College of Midwives (RCM): *Domestic abuse in pregnancy*, London, 1999, RCM.

Royal College of Midwives (RCM): *Vision 2000*, London, 2000, RCM.

Royal College of Obstetricians and Gynaecologists (RCOG): *Report from the RCOG Working Party on Antenatal and Intrapartum Care*, London, 1982, RCOG.

Royal College of Obstetricians and Gynaecologists (RCOG): *Violence against women*, London, 1997, RCOG.

Royal College of Obstetricians and Gynaecologists (RCOG): *Investigation and management of the small for gestational* (website). wwwrcog.org.uk/files/rcog-comp/uploaded-files/GT31SmallgestationalAgeFetus.pdf. 2002. Accessed September 2009.

Royal College of Obstetricians and Gynaecologists (RCOG): *Alcohol consumption and the outcomes of pregnancy. RCOG Statement No 5*, London, 2006, RCOG.

Sandall J, Davies J, Warwick C: *Evaluation of the Albany Midwifery Practice*, London, 2001, Kings College Hospital.

Sasaki S: Clinical presentation and management of molar pregnancy, *Best Practice & Research. Clinical Obstetrics & Gynaecology* 17(6):885–892, 2003.

Shah NR, Bracken MB: A systematic review and meta-analysis of prospective studies on the association between maternal cigarette smoking and preterm delivery, *American Journal of Obstetrics and Gynecology* 182(2):465–472, 2000.

Siney C: *Pregnancy and drug misuse*, ed 2, Hale, 1999, Books for Midwives.

Singh D, Newburn M: *Access to maternity information and support*, London, 2000, National Childbirth Trust.

Stables D, Rankin J: *Physiology in childbearing: with anatomy and related biosciences*, ed 2, Edinburgh, 2005, WB Saunders.

Standing Nursing and Midwifery Advisory Committee (SNMAC): *Midwifery: delivering our future*, London, 1998, Department of Health.

Villar J, Carroli G, Khan-Neelofur D, et al: Patterns of routine antenatal care for low-risk pregnancy, *Cochrane Database of Systematic Reviews* (4):CD000934, 2001.

Walsh D: An ethnographic study of women's experience of partnership caseload midwifery practice: the professional as friend, *Midwifery* 15(3):165–176, 1999.

Wardle SA, Wright PJ, Court BV: Knowledge of and preference for the DOMINO delivery option, *Midwifery* 13(3):149–153, 1997.

Weekes ARL, Flynn MJ: Engagement of the fetal head in primigravidae and its relationship to the duration of gestation and time of onset of labour, *British Journal of Obstetrics and Gynaecology* 82(1):7–11, 1975.

Wellock VK: The ever-widening gap: symphysis pubis dysfunction, *British Journal of Midwifery* 10(6):348–353, 2002.

Wellock VK, Crichton MA: Understanding pregnant women's experiences of symphysis pubis dysfunction: the effect of the pain, *Evidence Based Midwifery* 5(2):40–46, 2007.

Wheeler M: Home and laboratory testing pregnancy testing kits, *Professional Nurse* 14(8):571–576, 1999.

Whitehead SA, Andrews PLR, Chamberlain GVP: Characterisation of nausea and vomiting in early pregnancy: a survey of 1000 women, *Journal of Obstetrics and Gynaecology* 12(6):364–369, 1992.

Wraight A, Ball J, Seccombe I, et al: *Mapping team midwifery*. IMS Report Series 242. Brighton, 1993, Institute of Manpower Studies, University of Sussex.

Wyszynski DF, Duffy DL, Beaty TH: Maternal cigarette smoking and oral clefts: a meta-analysis, *Cleft Palate-Craniofacial Journal* 34(3):206–210, 1997.

Chapter 33

# Antenatal investigations

Maureen Boyle

## LEARNING OUTCOMES

After reading this chapter, you will be able to:

- understand the fundamental differences between screening and diagnostic tests used during the antenatal period
- be familiar with, and be able to discuss, the range of routine and specialized tests available to the woman and her family during the antenatal period
- be aware of the research and evidence around screening and diagnostic tests, and the means by which the midwife and mother can access this information
- be conversant with the necessity and strategies for information sharing between the woman and midwife to ensure informed choice by the woman.

## INTRODUCTION

The field of antenatal investigations has grown greatly in the past few years. Tests are being offered today – and decisions from women are becoming necessary – that would have been unthinkable previously. Although NICE (2008) guidelines for antenatal care recommend a schedule of antenatal tests, there is still a wide variation in what tests are considered 'routine' in various parts of the UK. The increase in use of information technology has meant that women and their partners often have accessed much specialized information themselves, and this may shape their questions.

Therefore, midwives need to have a better-than-ever knowledge of what tests are being offered, in order that they can ensure women are making their choices based on up-to-date and comprehensive information. They also need to be effective counsellors as it is acknowledged that the skills and attitudes of midwives influence the uptake of screening tests (Heyman & Henriksen 2001, van den Berg et al 2007). The midwife should also appreciate that the complete clinical antenatal examination is one of the most effective and efficient screening and diagnostic tools, if undertaken systematically and skilfully.

## SCREENING AND DIAGNOSIS

Although the meanings of screening and diagnosis are very different, they are often confused, and the midwife must ensure that the woman fully understands the difference.

*Screening* can be defined as determining the risk or likelihood of a condition, whereas a *diagnostic test* will give a definite answer. Sometimes, action will be taken following the results of a screening test. For example, a low haemoglobin (Hb) result in pregnancy may be assumed to be caused by pregnancy-induced anaemia and iron tablets will probably be given without further investigation, although in a few rare cases the anaemia may be caused by uncommon conditions, such as chronic renal infection, which would need further investigations to obtain a diagnosis. However, it would not be cost-effective to do an infinite range of investigations for every woman who presented with a positive screening test where the usual cause can be easily treated.

Some screening tests will produce results which mean an invasive test will be necessary to obtain a diagnosis. This needs to be made clear to the woman by the midwife providing counselling – should a woman be undertaking

**Table 33.1 Common procedures used for fetal assessment**

| Test | | Time |
|---|---|---|
| Nuchal translucency (screening) | Chromosomal abnormality | 10–14 weeks |
| Chorionic villus sampling (diagnostic) | Chromosomal abnormality<br>Genetic disease<br>Metabolic disorders<br>Haemoglobinopathies<br>Infection | >10 weeks |
| Amniocentesis (diagnostic) | Chromosomal abnormality<br>Genetic disease<br>Metabolic disorders<br>Haemoglobinopathies<br>Infection | 10–14 weeks (early)<br>15–18 weeks |
| Ultrasound (screening and diagnostic) | Assess fetus (dates/growth/viability/number)<br>Diagnosis of some abnormalities (e.g. structural)<br>Screening for abnormalities (e.g. soft markers)<br>Assessment of placental site<br>Liquor volume | All gestations |
| Cordocentesis (diagnostic) | Obtain fetal blood sample | 2nd/3rd trimester |
| Doppler (screening) | Assess fetal/placental/uterine blood flow | 2nd/3rd trimester |

a serum screening for Down syndrome test if she would not undergo amniocentesis in the case of a 'high risk' result? Some tests, such as ultrasound, can be both screening and diagnostic (see Table 33.1) – for instance, a scan can diagnose a missing limb or neural tube defect, but can also discover anomalies (for example, 'soft markers') which would need further investigations to determine a diagnosis. (See the NHS screening website for the timeline for antenatal tests.)

It is obviously not enough just to have the tests explained by the midwife – the implications of both positive and negative results also need to be explored before a woman can be said to be making an informed choice. As tests become more varied and complex and midwives' time more limited, ensuring properly informed choice is becoming a greater challenge for midwives.

## BLOOD TESTS

Blood is taken from a woman during pregnancy to detect conditions which may influence her wellbeing and that of the developing fetus.

### Blood tests for assessment of maternal wellbeing

See Table 33.2 for normal blood laboratory values.

### ABO and rhesus blood grouping

Blood is typed as A, B, AB or O depending on specific agglutinogens on the erythrocytes. The rhesus factor identifies the blood group as negative or positive depending on whether the rhesus factor antigen is present. Because of the risk of anaemia, haemorrhage and shock in pregnancy and during birth, and the possible need to provide transfusion, it is important that the blood group is identified early in the pregnancy.

### Antibodies

Maternal blood is examined for the presence of antibodies, particularly rhesus antibodies if the woman is rhesus negative. If the fetus is rhesus positive, antibodies can be stimulated by the occurrence of a fetomaternal haemorrhage, when 'leaks' occur and some fetal rhesus-positive cells pass into the maternal circulation. This can happen as pregnancy progresses, during procedures such as amniocentesis, chorionic villus sampling (CVS) or external cephalic version, in situations such as an antepartum haemorrhage, or at delivery. The rhesus-negative woman may respond by producing antibodies, in this or subsequent pregnancies, which may then cross the placenta to the fetal circulation and cause haemolysis in a rhesus-positive fetus. The administration of anti-D immunoglobulin is effective in preventing the production of these antibodies (MacKenzie et al 1991). Recent guidance from NICE (2008) suggests that routine antenatal anti-D

**Table 33.2 Normal blood levels and specific diagnostic tests**

| | Non-pregnant | Pregnant |
|---|---|---|
| **General screening assays** | | |
| Haemoglobin | 12–16 g/dL | 11–13 g/dL |
| Packed cell volume (PCV) | 37–45% | 33–39% |
| Red blood cell count (RBC) | 4.2–5.4 million/mm$^3$ | 3.8–4.4 million/mm$^3$ |
| Mean corpuscular volume (MCV) | 80–100 fL | 70–90 fL |
| Mean corpuscular haemoglobin (MCH) | 27–34 fL | 23–31 fL |
| Mean corpuscular haemoglobin concentration (MCHC) | 32–35 fL | 32–35 fL |
| Reticulocyte count | 0.5–1% | 1–2% |
| White blood cells (WBC) | 4–11 × 10$^9$/L | 6–16 × 10$^9$/L |
| Platelets | 150–400 × 10$^9$/L | 150–400 × 10$^9$/L |
| C-reactive protein (CRP) | 0–7 g/L | 0–7 g/L |
| **Specific diagnostic tests** | | |
| Serum iron | 50–100 mg/dL | 30–100 mg/dL |
| Unsaturated iron binding capacity | 250–300 mg/dL | 280–400 mg/dL |
| Transferrin saturation | 25–35% | 15–30% |
| Iron stores (bone marrow) | Adequate ferritin | Unchanged |
| Serum folate | 6–16 mg/mL | 4–10 mg/mL |
| Serum vitamin $B_{12}$ | 70–85 ng/dL | 70–500 ng/dL |
| Serum ferritin | 15–300 pg/L | Unchanged |

prophylaxis should be offered to all non-sensitized, rhesus-negative women. It is crucial that careful discussion takes place regarding this prophylaxis as the woman must appreciate that she is being given a blood product. If the woman knows that the father of the child is rhesus negative also, prophylaxis will be unnecessary.

ABO incompatibility and less common antibodies such as Kell, Duffy and Kidd (Hoffbrand et al 2006) can also affect the fetus or newborn.

## Full blood count

Full blood counts are taken routinely at booking and intervals during pregnancy, to detect a pathological fall in haemoglobin (Hb) which may indicate an iron deficiency anaemia. No woman should reach term with a potentially dangerous anaemia because this exposes her to the risk of excessive blood loss at delivery. It must be remembered, however, that other rare conditions may be discovered 'accidentally'; for example, a low white cell count may lead to a diagnosis of leukaemia. It is important therefore that no abnormal result ever be disregarded.

### *Haemoglobin (Hb)*

Because of physiological changes in pregnancy, haemoglobin levels will normally reduce, with the lowest reading expected at about 34 weeks. The World Health Organization (see website) cites 11 g/dL as the lowest acceptable reading, although other authorities quote figures down to 10 g/dL. A low Hb reading needs further investigation to establish the cause, so that appropriate treatment can be commenced.

Serum ferritin levels and total iron-binding capacity (TIBC) may be assessed (McGhee 2000) and causes of insidious blood loss, such as from chronic renal infection or parasitic infestation, may be investigated.

In the past, iron supplements were routinely given to pregnant women, but this is no longer considered appropriate (NICE 2008). Measurement of serum ferritin at booking may predict those who will develop anaemia during pregnancy and therefore treatment could be commenced before the Hb becomes low (Letsky 2002).

#### Mean corpuscular volume (MCV)

The earliest effect of iron deficiency is a reduced MCV. MCV is also reduced with alpha and beta thalassaemia minor. A raised MCV is associated with folate deficiency (high alcohol intake can reduce absorption of folic acid) or $B_{12}$ deficiency.

#### Platelets

Platelets usually stay within the normal range for non-pregnant women, although levels may fall during pregnancy within this range. An abnormal fall could indicate various medical conditions and would need further investigation.

#### White cell count

The total number of white cells rises in pregnancy, mainly due to the increase of neutrophils. However, an abnormal rise could indicate an infection, and this cause needs additional exploration.

## Haemoglobinopathies

Haemoglobinopathies are a diverse group of inherited single-gene disorders involving abnormal haemoglobin patterns which constitute two major conditions: *thalassaemia (minor* or *major*) and *sickle cell* disorders: *sickle cell trait (SCT* or *HbAS); sickle cell haemoglobin C disease (HbSC)*; and *sickle cell disease/anaemia (HbSS)*.

Both sickle cell disease and thalassaemia are recessive conditions (see Ch. 26), therefore only those inheriting an affected gene from each parent will have the disease. If a woman is found to be carrying either the HbS gene or the thalassaemia trait (thalassaemia minor), it is necessary to test her partner before a prediction about the baby's condition can be made. If both parents carry the gene, prenatal diagnosis can be made by chorionic villus sampling (CVS), amniocentesis or, more rarely, cordocentesis.

Currently, in high-prevalence areas, booking bloods for all women are automatically screened by hospital laboratories. In areas considered low prevalence, the Family Origin Questionnaire (DH 2007) should be used by midwives to identify who to test (see website).

## Maternal infection screening

### Rubella

This common viral infection is a significant condition in pregnancy because of the teratogenic effect on the developing fetus caused by transplacental transmission of the virus. Detection of rubella antibodies is carried out by serological testing to identify immunity (IgM and IgG antibodies).

The majority of women in the UK are immune as a result of routine vaccination against rubella at 11–14 years of age. However, since 1988, vaccination is now by measles, mumps and rubella (MMR) vaccine, usually administered before 15 months to male and female infants. It was hoped that with a universal take-up, rubella would be eradicated altogether. However, controversies over routine vaccination for infants reported in the media may compromise this.

All pregnant women are tested for rubella immunity at antenatal booking. Some women who have previously tested as immune have been known to become infected or test as susceptible, therefore testing in the preconception period is to be advised.

If a woman is not immune and comes into contact with rubella, she may develop the disease. Rubella can cause the loss of the pregnancy or the birth of a rubella-infected baby with various physical and mental anomalies. The fetus is most vulnerable up until 16 weeks, but the infection can cross the placenta at any gestation. To avoid the danger of rubella in future pregnancies, the non-immune woman is offered vaccination in the puerperium, together with contraceptive advice for a period of 3 months.

### Hepatitis

Hepatitis means inflammation of the liver. There are several different viruses which affect the liver (A, B, C, D, E and F) but B and C are the types with the most direct relevance to midwives at present.

#### Hepatitis B (HBV)

Hepatitis B is an infectious blood-borne viral disease. It can cause a range of symptoms from very mild to life threatening. About 10% of adults infected become chronic carriers and this may then progress to serious liver disease. Transmission is by contact with body fluids or vertically to the fetus. However, although there is a high chance of perinatal transmission, interventions after birth can greatly reduce the risk of the baby becoming a chronic carrier, and therefore identification of the mother's HBV status during pregnancy is important. All pregnant women should be screened for HBV infection (NICE 2008).

Because of its high level of infectivity, all healthcare workers (especially midwives) who have contact with body fluids should be vaccinated against HBV.

#### Hepatitis C (HCV)

Although HCV is very similar to hepatitis B, many more people infected with it will become chronic carriers and develop liver damage. There is no vaccine against HCV. At present, universal antenatal screening for HCV is not undertaken, but recent research has demonstrated a 0.8% prevalence rate in inner London, and in this study the majority of the infected women had no identified risk factors (Ward et al 2000).

### Human immunodeficiency virus (HIV) infection

Department of Health (1999) guidelines state that HIV testing should be recommended to all women as part of routine antenatal testing, as there are now clearly identified strategies which can reduce transmission to the fetus. As with all tests, informed consent is necessary and the midwife must ensure her knowledge base, in this very fast-changing area, is up to date in order that she can offer explanations and answer questions. This is a condition where new research is almost continuously being published and therefore all maternity units should have an identified resource person to whom the more complex enquiries can be referred.

### Toxoplasmosis

Toxoplasmosis is a parasitic infection caused by the protozoon *Toxoplasma gondii* which may cause congenital infection in the fetus. It can be transmitted from domestic cat faeces, soil, raw meat and unpasteurized milk. Pregnant women are also advised to avoid contact with sheep during lambing (DH 2000).

The test, which examines the immunity status of the woman by looking at IgG and IgM antibodies, should be performed in a toxoplasmosis reference laboratory, as diagnosis is not straightforward. NICE (2008) does not recommend routine testing.

### Listeriosis

Listeriosis can cause upper respiratory disease, septicaemia and encephalic disease. In pregnancy it can result in preterm labour, stillbirth or meningitis (of mother or baby). It is caused by a common bacterium usually transmitted via contaminated food, and advice is given to pregnant women to specifically avoid soft cheeses and pâtés, and to ensure 'cook-chill' meals are well heated through. Pregnant women are advised to avoid contact with sheep during lambing (DH 2000). Diagnosis is made by culture of blood or cerebrospinal fluid.

### Cytomegalovirus (CMV)

Cytomegalovirus is a herpesvirus that can be passed on by many routes, including sexual activities. CMV can lie latent in maternal tissues and become reactivated during pregnancy. The presence of CMV antibodies in the blood is indicative of infection and virus-specific IgM antibody is present in acute infections. It is the most common cause of intrauterine infection, and the fetus can be assessed by amniotic fluid studies (Antsaklis et al 2000).

### Serology

Serological tests, both non-treponemal and treponemal, can be done in the antenatal period, and most women in the UK are routinely screened for syphilis at booking, as there is evidence that this is still an appropriate test (Cross et al 2005). It is possible to get false positive results with conditions such as malaria, tuberculosis and glandular fever, and those infected with pinta and yaws may test positive. Those who abuse narcotics can also test as a false positive.

## Antenatal maternal blood tests to assess the fetus

### Maternal serum screening for Down syndrome (MSSDS)

In the late 1980s, workers at St Bartholomew's Hospital, London, developed a method of screening all women for the risk factor of Down syndrome (chormosone anomaly trisomy 21) in a current pregnancy by means of a maternal blood test (Loncar et al 1995). Since then, the test has been refined, expanded and nuchal translucency (NT) ultrasound added (see Ch. 26). Combined with the mother's age (it has long been recognized that the incidence of Down syndrome increases with the age of the woman), these calculations result in an individual risk estimation.

Currently there are several variations of the test and local NHS Trust policies will determine the specific tests offered. NICE (2008) recommends the combined test between 11 weeks and 13 weeks 6 days, with the triple or quadruple test if booking later, at 15–20 weeks.

- *Triple or quadruple test*: alpha-fetoprotein, unconjugated oestriol, free beta-hCG (or total hCG) and – if quadruple – inhibin-A, done in the second trimester.
- *Integrated test*: pregnancy-associated plasma protein A (PAPP-A ) and NT in the first trimester, plus the quadruple test in the second trimester, and the results integrated to provide one result.
- *Combined test*: NT plus free beta-hCG and PAPP-A, done in the first trimester.
- *Serum integrated test*: serum only (PAPP-A in the first trimester and the quadruple test in the second trimester).

Because accurate dates are important in the assessment of serum levels, a 'dating scan' is often offered at booking, with or without the NT, if the woman plans to have serum screening. It is important the woman realizes that the outcome is only a risk assessment and if her result is considered a 'screen positive' she will probably need an amniocentesis for a diagnosis. It is obviously also possible that a 'screen negative' may well occur despite an affected fetus, and this also needs to be made clear.

An increased level of alpha-fetoprotein (AFP) has been previously used on its own as a screening test for neural tube defects (spina bifida and anencephaly), to be followed by amniocentesis to detect diagnostic levels in the amniotic fluid. Most neural tube defects are now diagnosed by ultrasound examination.

Not all pregnancies are suitable for routine MSSDS screening. Levels can be influenced by a multiple pregnancy, intrauterine bleeding, obesity or the woman being an insulin-dependent diabetic. Different values may also be necessary for IVF pregnancies (Wald et al 1999).

## ASSESSMENT OF FETAL WELLBEING

### Fetal heart rate

In looking at the fetal heart rate as an indication of fetal wellbeing, it is usual practice to assess baseline rate, variability and alteration in heart rate in reaction to stress or movement.

The fetal heart rate varies through the antenatal period, ranging between 110 and 160 beats per minute (bpm), with an average baseline of:

- 155 bpm at 20 weeks
- 144 bpm at 30 weeks
- 140 bpm at term.

During this time, variations around 20 bpm above and below these baselines are considered within normal limits and signify changes in fetal oxygenation. Tachycardia is more common in the preterm fetus, but may also indicate fetal infection, reaction to maternal medication, maternal pyrexia or tachycardia, acute blood loss, fetal anaemia, or conditions, such as Wolff–Parkinson–White disease. Tachycardia may be seen in fetal hypoxia but not usually without other indications.

Bradycardia (heart rate under 110 bpm) is most likely to be caused by hypoxia, fetal heart block, hypothermia or vagal nerve stimulation.

### Fetal movements

Monitoring fetal movements as a test of fetal wellbeing was introduced by Sadovsky in the 1970s (Sadovsky & Polishuk 1977, Sadovsky et al 1983), and this led to extensive use of the Cardiff 'Count to ten kick chart'. This required the woman to count 10 movements over a 12-hour period, with instructions to contact her GP or midwife should the 10 movements not be achieved. Despite many perceived problems (for example, non-compliance, increased anxiety), fetal movements are deemed to be an effective means of assessing wellbeing and reduced fetal activity is one of the most accurate means of identifying the fetus at risk of intrauterine death (Heazell & Froen 2008, James 2002); however, NICE (2008) suggests routine fetal movement counting should not be offered.

Maternity services have a variety of approaches and some still use 'kick charts'. Whatever system is in place, it is important to encourage the woman to become familiar with her own baby's pattern of movement, and for her to be aware of what actions she should take should there be a significant change in the movements.

## ULTRASOUND

Today, ultrasound scanning (USS) (Fig. 33.1) is routine in antenatal care for women, as well as being an integral part of many of the specialized investigations. Ultrasound imaging is a non-invasive (when done with an abdominal transducer) screening and diagnostic technique using sound waves with a frequency well above the range of human hearing. (See website for background and method.) Although at present the usual method of ultrasound scanning is abdominal, vaginal ultrasound, using a special probe, is becoming more common in early pregnancy.

Ultrasound scans can be performed for a variety of reasons, from the earliest gestation up to and including when in labour, as well as postnatally to detect complications in the mother (for example, retained products) or to assess the baby. However, antenatal USS is most common, and it is important to remember that a scan for any reason during this period may result in findings apart from the purpose for which it was being done – for instance, a scan to assess the placental site may result in the discovery of

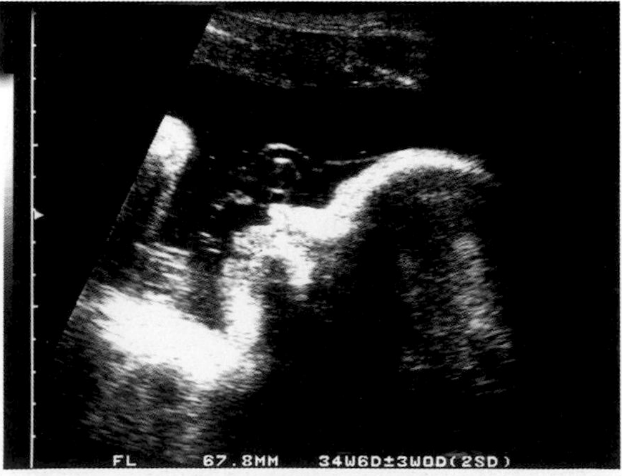


**Figure 33.1** Ultrasound scan.

a fetal abnormality. A woman undergoing ultrasound scanning should be aware of a scan's capabilities, that a raised BMI can make ultrasound difficult and therefore less accurate, and that the finding of no abnormalities on USS is not a guarantee of no problems.

**Reflective activity 33.1**

With the woman's and ultrasonographer's permission, sit in on some ultrasound scans at various gestations in pregnancy, so you can become familiar with the findings of the ultrasonographer and with the questions women may ask.

## Indications for first trimester ultrasound

### Booking/early/dating scans

Historically, first trimester scans were only routinely offered to women unsure of their last menstrual period, and therefore an estimated delivery date (EDD) was able to be calculated from fetal measurements taken during scanning. However, with the increase in MSSDS and NT, a 'dating' scan is often routinely offered to ensure accurate timing of the tests.

Parameters that may be used to determine gestational age are crown–rump length, biparietal diameter, femur length, and head circumference. The gestational sac is sometimes assessed early in the first trimester to confirm an intrauterine pregnancy, to calculate the gestational age before the fetus is visible, or to diagnose an anembryonic pregnancy (no embryonic tissue).

For accuracy, the measurements to assess gestational age should be done in the first or early second trimester, as prediction of gestational age by ultrasound scan cannot be accurately made after 24 weeks, because of the wide spread of normal measurements. Measurements will be recorded, to act as a baseline in case fetal growth needs to be monitored later in pregnancy.

### Diagnosis of pregnancy

The embryonic sac may be identified as early as 5 weeks' gestation using a transabdominal probe, and at 4 weeks with a transvaginal probe. Fetal heart movements can be visualized at 6–7 weeks' gestation and lack of fetal heart movement is a reliable method of diagnosing fetal death after this time. Actual movements of the fetus can be observed from 8–9 weeks. Doppler ultrasound equipment which produces amplified sound waves (that is, Sonicaid/Doptone) may be used to hear the fetal heart after about 12 weeks' gestation, but failure to hear the fetal heart should not be assumed to indicate fetal death. Fetal viability should be checked by an ultrasound scan.

### Ectopic pregnancy

This may be detected by ultrasound scan, the transvaginal route being more accurate than the abdominal route (Chudleigh & Thilaganathan 2004). Diagnosis is not always easy, but identification of high-risk groups, clinical examination and biochemical tests usually assist the diagnosis.

### Miscarriage/missed abortion/ vaginal bleeding

If a woman reports no longer 'feeling pregnant', or there are no signs of expected growth, an ultrasound scan may show the fetal sac failing to grow and a visible fetal pole but no fetal heartbeat. During research, some hospitals have shown that if a scan is done routinely at 11–14 weeks, a rate of 2–3% missed miscarriages may be identified. An advantage of a routine early scan may be the avoidance of traumatic bleeding and possible emergency admission for these women (Economides et al 1999).

Vaginal bleeding is not uncommon in early pregnancy and often the cause is never determined. Ultrasound is extremely valuable in assessing fetal viability when bleeding occurs, to determine what action, if any, should be taken.

### Hydatidiform mole

Ultrasound scan confirms the diagnosis following clinical signs such as painless vaginal bleeding, a large-for-dates uterus, hyperemesis gravidarum, and absence of fetal heart sounds by 14 weeks' gestation using Doppler ultrasound.

### Cervical incompetence

In some cases, serial ultrasound from about 14 weeks can assess the condition of the cervical canal and detect shortening (Zlatnik et al 2000).

### Multiple pregnancy

Multiple pregnancy can be identified by ultrasound from 4 weeks transvaginally, and 5 weeks abdominally. Initially it is suspected when more than one fetal sac is seen; the presence of two (or more) viable fetuses confirms the diagnosis.

Many twin pregnancies result in a singleton birth. Since the increased number of first trimester ultrasound scans, the 'vanishing twin' syndrome has been described, where twins are seen on an early scan but one is then lost – this is sometimes associated with vaginal bleeding, but often not (see Ch. 59). The figures for this are uncertain and range between 20% and 50% of twin pregnancies.

### Nuchal translucency (see Ch. 26)

It is suggested that by examining fetal anatomy as well as measuring nuchal translucency at 12–13 weeks, the majority of structural and chromosomal abnormalities can be detected. However, significant defects can be missed (such as some heart and spine abnormalities); therefore, a later scan would also be recommended (Economides et al 1999).

## Indications for second trimester ultrasound

Since the 1980s, women have been offered routine ultrasound assessment between 18 and 20 weeks' gestation, often called the 'anomaly', 'mid-pregnancy' or 'mid-trimester' scan. By this time, most fetal organs are formed and many abnormalities can be seen. However, it must be stressed that not all structures and their functions can be assessed – some may need later scans and many abnormalities may not be able to be assessed by ultrasound at all. In spite of this, women frequently see this routine scan as a signal that 'everything is alright' and a guarantee of a problem-free pregnancy and baby, which can be a very misleading assumption.

### Estimation of fetal age

If an earlier scan has not been done, the accuracy of the gestational age by dates can be confirmed by fetal measurements. These measurements are recorded at this time as a baseline to use if there is a suspected IUGR (intrauterine growth restriction) later in pregnancy.

### Placental location

During all ultrasound examinations, identification of the placenta is made, but it is routinely done during this scan. If the placental site is low in the mid-trimester scan, depending on its position (NICE 2008), a repeat scan is usually offered in the third trimester, and the woman is advised as to what to do in the case of bleeding prior to this. Only a minority of placentae will fail to become fundal by 32 weeks (Chudleigh & Thilaganathan 2004), but if the placenta remains partially or wholly in the lower uterine segment it is a placenta praevia and appropriate care must be instigated.

### Identification of fetal anomalies

Although fetal anomalies can be detected during any ultrasound scan, the mid-trimester scan is used routinely for this examination.

Fetal anatomy is assessed and many conditions, mainly structural, can be diagnosed (although some may need referral to a specialist centre for a definitive diagnosis). In addition, the ultrasonographer can also note any 'soft markers' – for example, extra digits, choroid plexus cysts or talipes. These can be benign anomalies which either disappear (for example, most choroid plexus cysts) or can be easily treated after birth. However, they can also be a manifestation of more serious underlying conditions, such as a chromosomal abnormality. An amniocentesis may be offered to exclude this. The use of soft markers is a controversial subject and can be a cause of great anxiety for many (Loughna 2006, Weisz et al 2007).

## Indications for third trimester ultrasound

### Assessment of fetal growth

Fetal growth is assessed clinically at every antenatal visit. If the midwife or doctor feels growth is suboptimal, a referral for ultrasound assessment is usually made, to confirm the clinical findings.

To assess fetal growth by ultrasound, the age of the fetus must be accurately established before 24 weeks' gestation. Fetal growth may be monitored by serial ultrasound measurements of various parameters, every 2–4 weeks. Measurements of head and abdominal circumference are commonly used to estimate the growth in small-for-gestational-age fetuses, both asymmetrical and symmetrical, and large-for-gestational-age fetuses. In a fetus with symmetrical IUGR, the normal growth shows deviation below the 5th (or 10th) centile. In the asymmetrical condition, the abdominal circumference growth is slow and may stop, and eventually the head circumference growth also slows. IUGR can be diagnosed by plotting serial scans along centile lines previously defined as the normal growth pattern for that population. If IUGR occurs, a fall-off of growth can be seen (Fig. 33.2). Growth acceleration (large abdominal circumference) above the 90th centile may be due to maternal diabetes mellitus, especially if associated with polyhydramnios and a large placenta.

### Estimation of fetal weight

Estimation of fetal weight can be made by using measurements obtained during ultrasound assessment. For the preterm fetus, and especially very preterm and multiples, ultrasound estimation of weight is the method of choice. This may provide vital information when consideration is being given to expediting a premature delivery.

However, at term it has been shown that parous women can often estimate the weight of the fetus as accurately as professionals using palpation (Diase & Monga 2002, Herrero & Fitzsimmons 1999). Clinical assessment can also be as accurate as ultrasound (Baum et al 2002) in estimating fetal weight around term – however, research studying this has specified using experienced professionals to do the assessments. It may be that a generation of practitioners, who are becoming increasingly dependent upon ultrasound in their practice, may not be able to

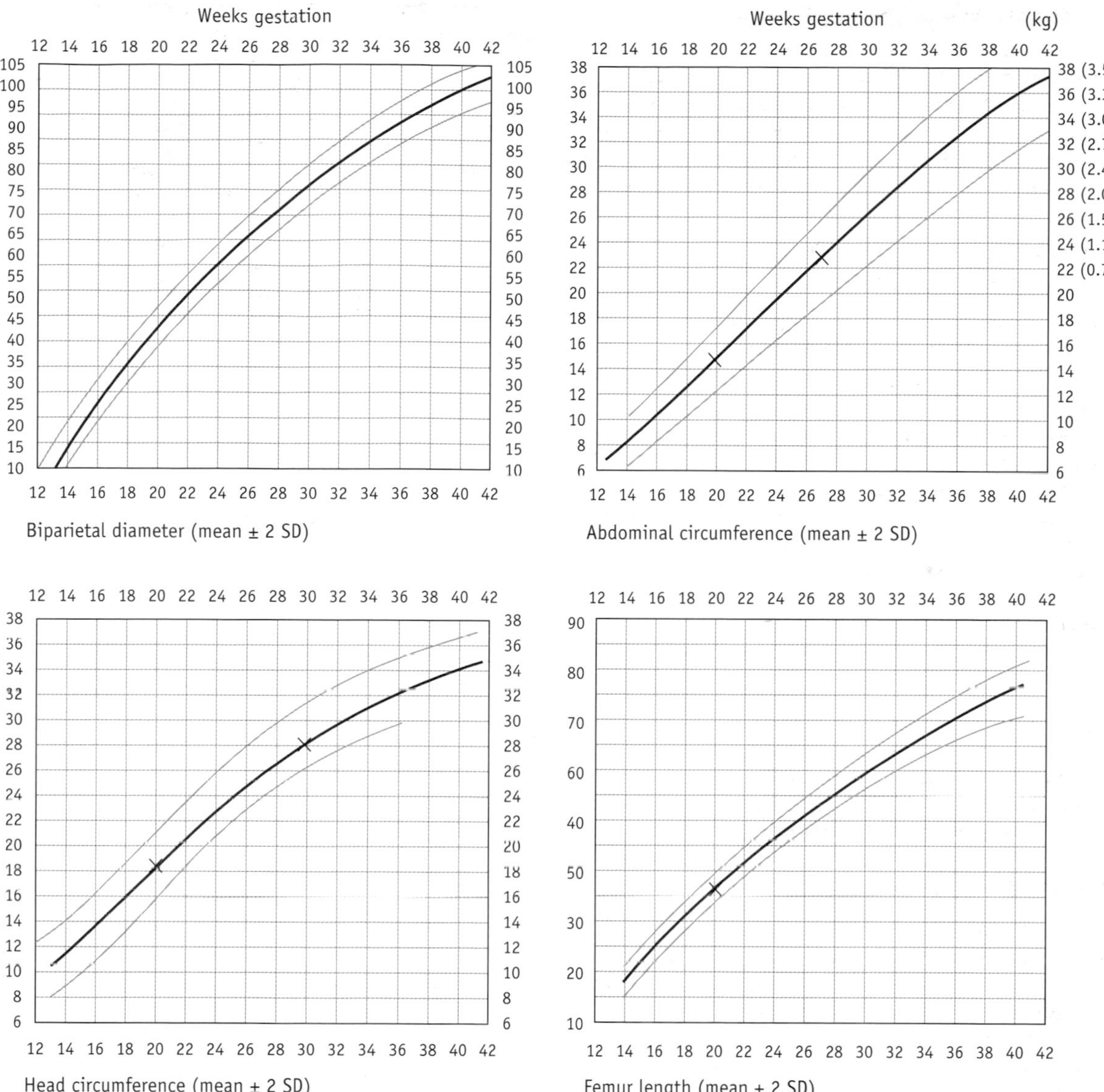


**Figure 33.2** Ultrasound scan centile graphs to indicate 'fall-off' of growth of a 30-week fetus.

replicate this research in the future. Since there will always be situations where ultrasound cannot be accessed, it is a reminder for all midwives to maintain their clinical skills of palpation and weight estimation.

> **Reflective activity 33.2**
>
> When carrying out an antenatal check in late pregnancy or when caring for a woman in labour, try to estimate the fetal weight during your routine palpations. Check after the birth to assess your skill.

## Malpresentations/malpositions

Late in the third trimester an ultrasound scan can be used to confirm clinical findings regarding the presentation and position of the fetus (or each fetus in the case of a multiple pregnancy). This information can be used to help decision making if there is a question over the mode of delivery.

Ultrasound will also be used to guide the clinician if external cephalic version (ECV) is undertaken to turn a breech presentation.

## Additional fetal assessment

### Doppler ultrasound

As well as being used to monitor the fetal heart (for example, Sonicaid), this technique is also used to measure blood flow in the fetal and uterine/placental vessels from a waveform recording on a monitor screen. The blood flow pattern will change as an adaptation to poor placental function, so it is thought that alterations in the fetal umbilical blood flow may occur in early fetal compromise. Women will be referred for Doppler assessment in the second and third trimester because of oligohydramnios, differing growth in multiple pregnancies, IUGR (or a history of IUGR in a previous pregnancy) or maternal conditions (such as hypertensive disorders of pregnancy). It may also form part of post-dates assessment (NICE 2008).

### Amniotic fluid measurement

As a routine clinical assessment during palpation in the second and third trimester, amniotic fluid quantity may be estimated to be reduced (oligohydramnios) or increased (polyhydramnios). Both these conditions, if suspected, need to be referred for ultrasound evaluation. Oligohydramnios may be associated with various fetal abnormalities, or with fetal compromise. Polyhydramnios may also be associated with fetal abnormality (for example, oesophageal atresia), or associated with maternal disease (such as diabetes mellitus) and a large fetus. All these conditions will need expert assessment, especially in determining timing and mode of delivery and planning aftercare. Amniotic fluid volume will also be observed as part of the assessment of fetal wellbeing for a woman with a medical condition (for example, pre-eclampsia) or as part of a post-term assessment.

See website for additional uses for ultrasound and for information on radiological and magnetic visualization techniques.

## INVASIVE TESTS

## Chorionic villus sampling (CVS)

Chorionic villus sampling can be undertaken at any gestation, but is used primarily as a first trimester test. Under continuous ultrasound visualization of the placenta, chorionic villi are obtained, usually by syringe, and these can be analysed for fetal chromosomal abnormalities. A provisional result is usually available within a few days. Depending on the position of the placenta, the procedure can be done either transabdominally or via the cervix.

The advantage of an early diagnostic test for chromosomal abnormality is that the woman would probably have the option of a first trimester termination, if that was her decision. Disadvantages include a rate of pregnancy loss usually quoted at about 2% although it has been suggested that rates of loss are reducing substantially (Evans & Andriole 2008). Difficulty in analysing the miscarriage rate is, however, complicated by the higher rate of spontaneous miscarriage in the first trimester. There is also a risk of results failure and studies have indicated a link between CVS and limb abnormality, probably restricted to procedures undertaken before 10 weeks' gestation (RCOG 2005).

Following the procedure, rhesus-negative women will be given anti-D immunoglobulin to prevent possible isoimmunization.

## Amniocentesis

Amniotic fluid can be used to test for fetal conditions such as chromosomal abnormalities, genetic diseases, or some fetal infections.

In the UK, amniocentesis is usually performed at about 15–18 weeks' gestation (see website for information on 'early' amniocentesis) using ultrasound to visualize the uterus and its contents. A fine needle is passed through the abdominal wall into the uterus and about 20 mL of amniotic fluid is extracted. The fetal cells in the amniotic fluid must be cultured and the time taken for their growth (about 2–3 weeks) accounts for the wait for a diagnosis, which women find so difficult. There may be a possibility in the future of routinely using DNA analysis for all tests done on amniotic fluid, which would give a much quicker result .

Some amniocentesis will fail to give a result when the fetal cells do not grow, and the woman must be aware of this small risk (about 1:500), as well as the other disadvantages, before she can make an informed choice to have an amniocentesis. After the procedure, the fetal heart is auscultated or visualized on ultrasound and the woman should be allowed to hear/see this. She will usually be advised to rest for that day and avoid strenuous activity for a few days. Rhesus-negative women will receive anti-D immunoglobulin to prevent possible rhesus isoimmunization.

The risk of pregnancy loss following amniocentesis is about 0.5–1% but this can vary according to operator and centre. There is also a risk of infection following any invasive procedure.

Some tests on amniotic fluid, such as diagnosis of neural tube defects (which is now done by ultrasound) or assessing the lecithin:sphingomyelin ratio for fetal pulmonary maturity, are now no longer considered a reason for an invasive test.

## Cordocentesis

This is an invasive investigation performed under ultrasound imaging, whereby a sample of fetal blood is obtained from the umbilical cord or intrahepatic vein, usually in the second or third trimester of pregnancy. The site of sampling is selected on considerations of accessibility, quality of visualization, gestational age and safety. The investigation was developed from a number of earlier interventions, including fetoscopy, for the purpose of antenatal diagnosis.

Cordocentesis carries a risk of miscarriage and also a risk of maternal infection and haemorrhage.

## CONCLUSION

The suggestion of even a minor defect in the fetus can cause extreme anxiety for parents, especially as, even if all further tests show no abnormality, no professional can guarantee a 'perfect' baby.

There is some evidence that the anxiety engendered on identification of a potential problem does not go away even after a reassuring diagnosis (Lawrence 1999), and also that maternal anxiety during pregnancy may affect the physiological development of the fetus (Teixeira et al 1999).

However, the concept of prenatal screening is popular with most women and the ability to identify many abnormal fetuses leads to women having a choice of terminating the pregnancy. There are also many healthy children – and their mothers – alive today because of the provision of the tests described in this chapter.

The midwife's role is to ensure that the woman receives accurate, evidence-based and up-to-date information in language she can understand, in order to make an informed decision. Where possible, the midwife should provide written information to support any discussions, and should also be aware of other sources of information which may be helpful, such as through the Internet and through voluntary groups. Whatever range of tests the woman and her family choose to access, for whatever reasons, the midwife should continue to provide support and respect throughout her care.

## KEY POINTS

- Investigations offered to women in the antenatal period have increased in number and complexity.
- Midwives need to keep up to date in the changing field of antenatal investigations, and have access to contemporary sources of information.
- Antenatal tests, and their potential consequences, need to be fully understood by the woman before they are undertaken. Written information should support any verbal discussion where possible.
- The wellbeing of mother and baby, and the successful outcome of a pregnancy, can be dependent on antenatal investigations.

## REFERENCES


Antsaklis A, Dkalaki G, Mesogitis S, et al: Prenatal diagnosis of fetal primary CMV infection, *BJOG: An International Journal of Obstetrics and Gynaecology* 107(1):84–88, 2000.

Baum J, Gussman D, Wirth J: Clinical and patient estimation of fetal weight vs. ultrasound estimation, *Journal of the American Medical Association* 287:1556–1560, 2002.

Chudleigh T, Thilaganathan B: *Obstetric ultrasound: how, why and when*, ed 3, Edinburgh, 2004, Elsevier.

Cross A, Luck S, Patey R, et al: Syphilis in London circa 2004: new challenges from an old disease, *Archives of Disease in Childhood* 90(10):1045–1046, 2005.

Department of Health (DH): *Targets aimed at reducing the number of children born with HIV: report from an Expert Group*, London, 1999, DH.

Department of Health (DH): *Advice to pregnant women during the lambing season*, London, 2000, DH.

Department of Health (DH): *Family origin questionnaire, NHS antenatal and newborn screening programmes*, London, 2007, DH.

Diase K, Monga M: Maternal estimates of neonatal birth weight in diabetic patients, *Southern Medical Journal* 95(1):92–94, 2002.

Economides D, Whitlow B, Braithwaite J: Ultrasonography in the detection of fetal anomalies in early pregnancy, *British Journal of Obstetrics and Gynaecology* 106(6):516–523, 1999.

Evans M, Andriole S: Chorionic villus sampling and amniocenesis in 2008, *Current Opinion in Obstetrics & Gynecology* 20(2):164–168, 2008.

Heazell A, Froen J: Methods of fetal movement counting and the detection of fetal compromise, *Journal of Obstetrics and Gynaecology* 28(2):147–154, 2008.

Herrero R, Fitzsimmons J: Estimated fetal weight: maternal vs physician estimate, *Journal of Reproductive Medicine* 44(8):674–678, 1999.

Heyman B, Henriksen M: *Risk, age & pregnancy: a case study of prenatal genetic screening and testing*, New York, 2001, Palgrave.

Hoffbrand A, Moss P, Pettit J: *Essential haematology*, ed 5, London, 2006, Blackwell Scientific.

James D: Assessing fetal health, *Current Obstetrics & Gynaecology* 12(5):243–249, 2002.

Lawrence S: Counselling for Down syndrome screening, *British Journal of Midwifery* 7(6):368–370, 1999.

Letsky E: Blood volume, haematinics, anaemia. Chapter 2. In de Swiet M, editor: *Medical disorders in obstetric practice*, ed 4, Oxford, 2002, Blackwell.

Loncar J, Barnabei J, Larsen J: Advent of maternal serum markers for Down syndrome screening, *Obstetrical & Gynecological Survey* 50(4):316–320, 1995.

Loughna P: Soft markers for congenital anomaly, *Current Obstetrics & Gynaecology* 16(2):107–110, 2006.

MacKenzie I, Selinger M, Bowell P: Management of red cell isoimmunisation in the 1990s. In Studd J, editor: *Progress in obstetrics and gynaecology*, Vol. 9, Edinburgh, 1991, Churchill Livingstone.

McGhee M: *A guide to laboratory investigations*, ed 3, Oxford, 2000, Radcliffe.

National Institute for Clinical Excellence (NICE): *Antenatal care: routine care for the healthy pregnant woman*, NICE clinical guideline 62, London, 2008, NICE.

Royal College of Obstetricians & Gynaecologists (RCOG): *Anmiocentesis and chorionic villus sampling*, Guideline No. 8, London, 2005, RCOG.

Sadovsky E, Polishuk WZ: Fetal movements in utero: nature, assessment, prognostic value, timing of delivery, *Obstetrics and Gynecology* 50(1):49–55, 1977.

Sadovsky E, Ohel G, Havazeleth H, et al: The definition and the significance of decreased fetal movements, *Acta Obstetricia et Gynecologica Scandinavica* 62(5):409–413, 1983.

Teixeira J, Fisk N, Glover V: Association between maternal anxiety in pregnancy and increased uterine artery resistance index: cohort based study, *British Medical Journal* 318(7177):153–157, 1999.

Van den Berg M, Timmermans D, Kleinveld J, et al: Are counsellors' attitudes influencing pregnant women's attitudes and decisions on prenatal screening? *Prenatal Diagnosis* 27(6):518–524, 2007.

Wald N, White N, Morris J, et al: Serum markers for Down's syndrome in women who have had IVF: implications for antenatal screening, *British Journal of Obstetrics and Gynaecology* 106(12):1304–1306, 1999.

Ward C, Tudor-Williams F, Cotzias T, et al: Prevalence of hepatitis C among pregnant women attending an inner London obstetrics department: uptake and acceptability of named antenatal testing, *Gut* 47(2):277–280, 2000.

Weisz B, Pandya P, David A, et al: Ultrasound findings after screening for Down syndrome using the integrated test, *Obstetrics & Gynecology* 109(5):1046–1052, 2007

Zlatnik F, Yankowitz J, Whitham J, et al: Vaginal ultrasound as an adjunct to cervical digital examination in women at risk of early delivery, *Gynecologic & Obstetric Investigation* 51(1):12–16, 2000.

Chapter |34|

# The choice agenda and place of birth and care

*Tina Heptinstall and Liz Gale*

**LEARNING OUTCOMES**

By the end of this chapter, the reader will be able to:

- appreciate the complexities surrounding the concept of 'choice' and how this may be perceived by women and midwives
- evaluate the meanings of choice in the context of birth at home, within birth centres, midwifery-led units and obstetric consultant-led units.

An explicit choice agenda has been evident in Government maternity services policy since the landmark document *Changing childbirth* (DH 1993). This is also an integral theme in the subsequent documents *The national service framework for children, young people and the maternity services* (DH 2004) and *Making it better: for mother and baby* (DH 2007a). In the policy document *Maternity matters* it is stated that:

> '... *four national choice guarantees [choice of how to access maternity care, type of antenatal care, place of birth and postnatal care] will be available for all women by the end of 2009 and women and their partners will have opportunities to make well-informed decisions about their care throughout pregnancy, birth and postnatally*'
>
> (DH 2007b:5)

While midwives aim to give women choices and women are encouraged to make them, the concept of choice is not straightforward, particularly around the choice of place of birth. Choices are relative and are not solely made by what is on offer in any specific place or at any particular time; choices are influenced by the values and beliefs of women, midwives and doctors (Edwards 2005). The concept of choice also needs to be viewed against a backdrop of consumerism, information giving, risk, litigation and maternity services resources. An offer of choice must be matched with having the capacity to provide that choice. This applies to the choice of a hospital birth with availability of epidural anaesthesia or water birth, a freestanding birth centre or birth at home.

Some aspects of maternity care are often not actively chosen by women; antenatal ultrasound scanning and screening for fetal abnormalities have become so commonplace and 'normalized' that they are often perceived as part of a package of care and are rarely contested. Paradoxically, women may be perceived as more 'difficult' or 'demanding' if they choose *not* to have something rather than making a choice from a list of options given to them. It is self-evident that women need to be informed in order to make choices, but decisions around pregnancy, place of birth, labour, infant feeding and motherhood are shaped by a range of factors, many of which are influential before women even become pregnant. In the UK, hospital birth is the norm, reinforced by the processes of socialization, cultural imagery around labour and birth, and the language of safety and risk; therefore choices are set within this context.

In the context of choice and place of birth, Knightly (2007) comments that people are overloaded with information, especially from the media. In a sophisticated media age characterized by the swiftness of sound bites, it is difficult to get messages across based on 'evidence'. The increasing evidence and government support of the suitability of birth at home or in midwife-led units needs to be matched with the messages conveyed in the media. The overriding notion that hospital birth is safe is supported by portrayals in popular culture of home birth as risky and fraught with danger.

Information giving by midwives and doctors is not a neutral activity; information is often framed in such a way as to maintain organizational and cultural norms and to encourage women to make certain approved or 'right' choices. This control by midwives has been referred to as 'professional dominance' (Stapleton et al 2002a), 'strategic communication' (Hindley & Thomson 2005) and 'protective steering' (Levy 2004).

In their study on the use of evidence-based leaflets on informed choice (MIDIRS Informed Choice leaflets), Stapleton et al (2002b) found that a minority of women were satisfied with the way information was presented. However, this mode of information giving, combined with few opportunities to discuss the leaflets, did not promote informed choice and active decision-making. Women generally complied with the 'professionally defined right choices' (Stapleton et al 2002b). Although the midwives in this study were positive about the leaflets, they exercised power in deciding to whom they would offer the leaflets, based on their perceptions of how realistic the choices were or whether women would understand or use them. Stapleton et al (2002b) argued that midwives are influenced by the cultural norms of their working environment, particularly power hierarchies, the use of technological interventions and the fear of litigation. They concluded that, 'the culture into which the leaflets were introduced supported existing normative patterns of care and this ensured informed compliance rather than informed choice' (Stapleton et al 2002b:639).

Information giving is not just about the transmission of objective 'facts' or even 'evidence'; it is also about a dialogue concerning what is actually going on, particularly when things change during pregnancy, labour and birth. It is about relationships, communication and trust that involves active engagement with women in decision making (Leap & Edwards 2006, Pairman 2006, Rosser 2003). Enhancing these factors presents a challenge to the dominant culture of fear, litigation and defensive practice, and where they are lacking, dissatisfaction is greater (Symon 2002).

Clearly, 'choice' is the touchstone of the maternity services and NHS Trusts and midwives are exhorted to provide more choices, including where women can give birth to their babies (DH 2004, NICE 2007). For some women the most appropriate place for their needs will be consultant-led care within a hospital, but not all women. Yet, in the UK, 96% of women have their babies in hospital, with the remainder born either in midwifery-led units (either attached to a consultant unit or 'freestanding'), birth centres or at home, with some regional differences (Birthchoice UK 2008). The Healthcare Commission report *Towards better birth, a review of maternity services in England* reported that around half of the women surveyed were offered a choice of where to have their baby and that up to a third of women would have liked more information around place of birth (Healthcare Commission 2008).

Arguments about risk and place of birth are usually constructed around medical/obstetric risk and issues of safety; social and physiological factors are rarely considered, particularly where an out-of-hospital birth may be appropriate for many women. Discussions around suitability for home birth or midwifery-led care away from consultant units are often framed around exclusion rather than inclusion criteria; why, for example, a woman should *not* have a home birth, rather than why she should have one. This approach reinforces hospital birth as the benchmark for the usual place of birth and this tradition of hospital birth has led to the institutionalization of birth in the UK (Leap & Edwards 2006). While there has been a rise in the number of midwifery-led units or birth centres, these remain small in number and are periodically closed or under threat of closure, primarily due to financial constraints, particularly shortages of midwives. The challenge for midwives is to balance the positive and persuasive arguments of 'normality' and 'small is beautiful' (Downe 2008, Kirkham 2003, Walsh 2007) with the current political climate of 'risk', reorganization, 'rationalization' and centralization of maternity services within the NHS.

Some authors urge caution against the polarization of home versus hospital in debates about the place of birth (Knightly 2007, Leap & Edwards 2006). What really matters is how maternity services can be organized to meet the needs of women; how a variety of services can be sustained within financial constraints; and how midwives can provide appropriate care as well as gaining personal and professional satisfaction and a work–life balance. For women, Leap and Edwards (2006) conclude:

> *'The overall goal has to be that women are enabled to make decisions that make them feel more powerful, wherever they are and with whoever attends them when they give birth. They can only feel safe, secure and protected if they know that their concerns will be respected and their integrity and autonomy will be preserved.'*
>
> (Leap & Edwards 2006:103)

**Reflective activity 34.1**

Attend and observe the initial antenatal (booking) visit for a woman and consider the options that are given to the woman about her choices for place of birth.

Is this the best time to offer this discussion or are there other ways and times of presenting options to women for their birth care?

For some women who have pre-existing medical or psychiatric conditions or develop complications during pregnancy and labour, consultant-led care and hospital birth are appropriate; this point has been clearly stated in the document *Saving mothers' lives: reviewing maternal deaths to make motherhood safer 2003–2005* (Lewis 2007). The majority of women do not usually require that type of care. Women who do not require expert obstetric interventions may have less favourable outcomes by being in a consultant-led unit that is often characterized by interventions to control labour and bring it to a 'timely' end. This can result in a 'cascade of intervention', a term first coined by Sally Inch (1990).

Although the NICE (2007) guidelines recommend offering low-risk mothers the choice of where they plan to have their babies, the guideline development group claim that they were 'unable to determine whether planning birth in a non-obstetric setting is as safe as birth in an obstetric unit' (NCC-WCH 2007). The National Childbirth Trust dispute this statement in their own review of the same papers on home birth (Gyte & Dodwell 2007). However, Gyte and Dodwell (2007) did not find evidence to suggest that hospital birth is any safer than home birth for low-risk women, echoing the conclusions of previous studies (Chamberlain et al 1997, Olsen & Jewell 1998). Further research into outcomes of planned births at home, in midwifery-led units or in hospital is being conducted by the National Perinatal Epidemiology Unit, Oxford, in their Birthplace in England research programme. This will report at a later date on 'wellbeing, safety and quality, women's experience of care, the process of transfer from planned place of birth, and the cost-effectiveness of different systems for care' (NPEU 2008).

A significant challenge to the prevailing dominant cultural and social practice of hospital being the most appropriate place for birth is the birth centre. Birth centres may be either low-risk maternity units attached to hospitals with access to obstetric consultants or geographically separate from the hospital, often referred to as freestanding birth centres. However, the term 'birth centre' is generally considered to refer to more than just a building or a physically attractive space. It is about a social model of midwifery care that supports a philosophy that considers that a woman has the ability to give birth to and nurture her baby, at her own pace and without intervention, supported by skilled and sensitive midwives (Kirkham 2003, Walsh 2007). The philosophy clearly places the individual characteristics of the midwife as central to the successful working of a birth centre. This, together with clear policies on when medical opinion needs to be sought, should ensure that the birth centre maintains its focus on normality rather than becoming a satellite of the consultant-led unit.

For stand-alone units, the confidence and expertise of the midwives in dealing with both normal births and the rare but potential emergencies are paramount. Admission criteria for stand-alone birth centres are similar to those used for home birth. Birth centres pride themselves on providing a 'home from home' environment and rarely have any more equipment than community midwives carry in their cars. It is interesting that women appear to be more prepared to deliver in a birth centre than in their own homes; nationally, 16% have their babies in birth centres compared with a 2% homebirth rate (Bainbridge 2006). Birth centre studies demonstrate potential savings to the NHS in lower uses of resources associated with intrapartum care (Ratcliffe 2003) and positive health and social outcomes (Kirkham 2003). It may be that women perceive birth centres to be more appropriate or safer than home. It is possible that culturally, women expect to give birth in an institution and birth centres are perceived as a 'halfway house' between hospital birth and home birth. Yet Barber et al (2007) found that most women gave birth in hospital. In their BirthPlace Choices project on the south coast of England, Barber et al (2007) investigated the influence of providing women with information and introducing educational strategies around the place of birth. They found that the women in the survey said that, given the choice, they would opt for out-of-hospital births, yet the majority still gave birth in the hospital labour ward.

While the choice of birth 'at home supported by a midwife' (DH 2007a) is an option for women, the numbers of women giving birth at home have been persistently low throughout the UK over the past few decades, although these range from 0.0% to 10% dependent on location (Birthchoice UK 2008). Edwards (2005) considers that home birth, while supported by government and local policies, remains a contested area. One of the critical reasons for women choosing and midwives supporting home birth is that women can exercise more control over the birth process. It may be the alterations that occur in the balance of power, when a midwife becomes a visitor within the woman's own home, which helps to promote this empowerment. In common with birth centre practice, successful outcomes are influenced by both the attitudes and skills of the attending midwife, who needs to be equally confident in the woman's ability to give birth to her own baby as in her own skills to be more directive and make referrals should this becomes necessary.

Further evidence of the importance of this partnership comes from some Dutch research. The Netherlands have a much higher homebirth rate than the UK; women book with a midwife who then supports them through the labour either at home or in the hospital. Van der Hulst (1999) found an increase in relational care between the midwife and the mother during home births in comparison to hospital births. Midwives spent more time with and were more attentive to labouring women within the home environment. Home birth undertaken by midwives who do not feel comfortable doing so may equate to a 'hospital birth' undertaken at home. For some women, the choice of home birth is as much about the people she wants with her during her labour as the place of birth.

In most areas, the decision on where to give birth is often expected to be made at the initial antenatal (booking) visit. This may discourage a woman from fully considering her range of options as her pregnancy progresses or in light of further information from other women or midwives. However, midwives in the Albany Midwifery Practice, an NHS midwifery group practice in South East London, undertook home labour assessments and the decision on where the woman wants to give birth is made at that point (Reed 2002). A midwife known to the woman would remain with her and support her to give birth at home, unless the woman chose to go to hospital or the midwife and the woman consider it appropriate so to do.

Transfer to hospital for women who have originally planned a home birth is often constructed as a 'failed home birth'. The use of such terminology not only is demeaning to the woman but also ignores the role of the midwife in providing continuity of care regardless of the actual place of birth. The example set by the Albany midwives, and other caseload or group practices, demonstrates the benefits and flexibility of following the mother to wherever is the appropriate place for her to have her baby – the birth is a success in itself; an 'everyday miracle' (Reed 2002:263).

Choices for women are enhanced through continuity of care schemes where women can develop meaningful relationships with midwives over a period of time (Gamble et al 2007, Page 1995, Sandall et al 2001). Caroline Flint's pioneering 'Know your midwife' scheme in the mid 1980s (Flint et al 1989) was a catalyst for further change in the organization of midwifery care throughout the 1990s when schemes were developed around the concept of continuity of carer and 'knowing your midwife'. Those midwives who work in a caseload team approach rather than a reciprocal arrangement with another midwife argue that it is the shared philosophy and attitude of the team rather than 'knowing' the individual midwife that influences the relationship (Edwards 2005).

Reflecting on the significance of the concept of continuity, Lee (1997) suggested that the concept is not clear and has a range of meanings, not least to women who receive care from midwives. Furthermore, there is little consensus regarding the term 'named midwife' and the meanings of 'care', 'carer', 'team', 'caseload' and women 'knowing' a midwife. In conclusion, Lee (1997) suggests that what women want is *good* care and that midwives should organize care in ways that increase the power of women, particularly the most vulnerable.

The caseload model is frequently used by independent self-employed midwives, working outside of the NHS in a private financial agreement with the expectant mother. Women receive one-to-one care from a known midwife. The situation for independent midwives changed after 2002, when the last commercial insurance product was withdrawn from the market. Thus, most independent midwives practise without professional indemnity insurance, thus posing a potential discouragement to prospective clients (Independent Midwives Association 2008). The threat to independent midwifery raises significant issues around the professional autonomy of midwives and the choices available to women (Anderson 2007).

**Reflective activity 34.2**

Consider the options for a woman who wishes to give birth at home but who has a medical condition where this choice could pose a risk. What options may be offered to ensure safety of care?

In summary, women's decisions about where to give birth are probably not based on objective statistical risk but rather on women's own understandings of that risk. They are influenced by a range of social and cultural factors, alongside the ways in which midwives present information about the place of birth. Ideally, midwifery care will follow the woman regardless of whether she needs or wants to give birth in hospital, at home or in a birth centre. Increasingly, midwives should encourage women to see birth out of hospital as a safe choice for uncomplicated childbirth. Final decisions about the place of birth can be left for the woman to make during labour, thereby ensuring that she keeps all her options open. This means that midwives may move more freely between hospitals and the community.

## KEY POINTS

- The concept of 'choice' around place of birth is complex; women are influenced by a wide range of social and cultural factors.
- Information giving by midwives is one factor which in turn, is influenced by organizational cultures and dominant obstetric ideologies around birth.
- Hospital birth has not been proven to be safer than birth at home, so doctors, midwives and women need to continue to rethink the concept of 'risk' as applied to home birth.
- Whether birth takes place at home or in hospital, the experience can be an empowering and positive one for both mother and midwife.

## REFERENCES


Anderson T: Is this the end of independent midwifery? *The Practising Midwife* 10(2):4, 2007.

Bainbridge J: Birth centres: what price maternal choice and professional autonomy? *British Journal of Midwifery* 14(1):40, 2006.

Barber T, Rogers J, Marsh S: Increasing out-of-hospital birth: what needs to change? *British Journal of Midwifery* 15(1):16–20, 2007.

Birthchoice UK: *How to find out about your nearest maternity units* (website) <www.birthchoiceuk.com>. 2008. Accessed January 6, 2009.

Chamberlain G, Wraight A, Cowley P: *Home births: the report of the confidential enquiry by the National Birthday Trust Fund*, Carnforth, 1997, Parthenon Publishing Group.

Department of Health (DH): *Changing childbirth: the report of the Expert Maternity Group*, London, 1993, HMSO.

Department of Health (DH): *The national service framework for children, young people and the maternity services. Standard 11 Maternity services*, London, 2004, DH.

Department of Health (DH): *Making it better: for mother and baby. Clinical case for change*, London, 2007a, DH.

Department of Health (DH): *Maternity matters: choice, access and continuity of care in a safe service*, London, 2007b, DH.

Downe S: *Normal childbirth: evidence and debate*, ed 2, Edinburgh, 2008, Churchill Livingstone.

Edwards NP: *Birthing autonomy: women's experiences of planning home birth*, Abingdon, 2005, Routledge.

Flint C, Poulengeris P, Grant A: The 'know your midwife' scheme – a randomised controlled trial of continuity of care by a team of midwives, *Midwifery* 5:11–16, 1989.

Gamble J, Creedy DK, Teakle B: Women's expectations of maternity services: a community-based survey, *Women and Birth* 20(3):115–120, 2007.

Gyte G, Dodwell M: Safety of planned home birth: an NCT review of evidence, *New Digest* 40:20–29, 2007.

Healthcare Commission: *Towards better births: a review of maternity services in England* (website). <www.healthcarecommission.org.uk/_db/_documents/Towards_better_births_200807221338.pdf>. 2008. Accessed August 26, 2008.

Hindley C, Thomson AM: The rhetoric of informed choice: perspectives from midwives on intrapartum fetal heart rate monitoring, *Health Expectations* 8:306–314, 2005.

Inch S: *Birthrights: a parents' guide to modern childbirth*, ed 2, Oxford, 1990, Green Print.

Independent Midwives Association (IMA): *Facts and background* (website). <www.saveindependentmidwifery.org/content/view/20/38/>. 2008. Accessed August 27, 2008.

Kirkham M: *Birth centres: a social model for maternity care*, Oxford, 2003, Books for Midwives.

Knightly R: Delivering choice: where to birth, *British Journal of Midwifery* 15(8):475–478, 2007.

Leap N, Edwards N: The politics of involving women in decision making. In Page LA, McCandlish R, editors: *The new midwifery: science and sensitivity in practice*, ed 2, Edinburgh, 2006, Churchill Livingstone.

Lee G: The concept of continuity – what does it mean? In Kirkham MJ, Perkins ER, editors: *Reflections on midwifery*, London, 1997, Baillière Tindall.

Levy V: How midwives use protective steering to facilitate informed choice in pregnancy. In Kirkham M, editor: *Informed choice in maternity care*, Basingstoke, 2004, Palgrave.

Lewis G, editor: *The Confidential Enquiry into Maternal and Child Health (CEMACH). Saving mothers' lives: reviewing maternal deaths to make motherhood safer 2003–2005. The Seventh Report on Confidential Enquiries into Maternal Deaths in the UK*, London, 2007, CEMACH.

National Collaborating Centre for Women's and Children's Health (NCC-WCH): *NICE clinical guideline 55. Intrapartum care: care of healthy women and their babies during childbirth*, London, 2007, RCOG.

National Institute for Health and Clinical Excellence (NICE): *Intrapartum care: care of healthy women and their babies during childbirth*, London, 2007, NICE.

National Perinatal Epidemiology Unit (NPEU): *Birthplace in England Research Programme* (website). <www.npeu.ox.ac.uk/birthplace/>. 2008. Accessed July 21, 2008.

Olsen O, Jewell MD: Home versus hospital birth. *Cochrane Database of Systematic Reviews* Issue 3. Art. No.: CD000352. DOI: 10.1002/14651858.CD000352, 1998.

Page L: *Effective group practice in midwifery: working with women*, Oxford, 1995, Blackwell Science.

Pairman S: Midwifery partnerships: working 'with' women. In Page LA, McCandlish R, editors: *The new midwifery: science and sensitivity in practice*, Edinburgh, 2006, Churchill Livingstone.

Ratcliffe J: The economic implications of the Edgware birth centre. In Kirkham M, editor: *Birth centres: a social model for maternity care*, Oxford, 2003, Books for Midwives.

Reed B: The Albany Midwifery Practice (2), *MIDIRS Midwifery Digest* 12(2):261–264, 2002.

Rosser J: How do the Albany midwives do it? Evaluation of the Albany Midwifery Practice, *MIDIRS Midwifery Digest* 13(2):251–257, 2003.

Sandall J, Davies J, Warwick C: *Evaluation of the Albany Midwifery Practice. Final report*, London, 2001, Nightingale School of Nursing and Midwifery, King's College.

Stapleton H, Kirkham M, Curtis P, et al: Framing information in antenatal care, *British Journal of Midwifery* 10(4):197–201, 2002a.

Stapleton H, Kirkham M, Thomas G: Qualitative study of evidence based leaflets in maternity care, *British Medical Journal* 324:639–642, 2002b.

Symon A: The midwife and the legal environment. In Wilson JH, Symon A, editors: *Clinical risk management in midwifery: the right to a perfect baby*, Oxford, 2002, Books for Midwives.

Van der Hulst LAM: Relational care of Dutch midwives, *Health and Social Care in the Community* 7(4):242–247, 1999.

Walsh D: Improving maternity services: small is beautiful – lessons from a birth centre, Oxford, 2007, Radcliffe Publishing.

# Part | 6 |

# Labour and birth

Chapter |35|

# Physiological changes from late pregnancy until the onset of lactation

Mary McNabb

## LEARNING OUTCOMES

After reading this chapter, you will be able to

- understand the significance of the extensive transformations in maternal brain capacities from late pregnancy to weaning
- analyse maternal–fetoplacental neurohormonal interactions that coordinate fetal maturational changes for extrauterine life, with the maternal transition from pregnancy to labour
- understand key regulatory systems that initiate coordinated changes in maternal reproductive organs from late pregnancy to birth
- appreciate the significance of a place of safety and security, to promote spontaneous vaginal birth, affiliative behaviours, suckling and lactation.

## INTRODUCTION

Over the last 4 weeks of pregnancy, all women experience significant emotional and cognitive changes associated with 'nesting' and other signs of the emergence of maternal responsiveness and affiliation (Brunton & Russell 2008, Grattan 2002, Neumann 2009). At the same time, maternal pain threshold rises, the hypothalamic–pituitary axis (HPA) becomes hyporesponsive to various stressors, and women often experience periods of heightened apprehension relating to fetal and neonatal wellbeing (Douglas 2010, Douglas et al 2005, Gintzler & Liu 2001, Kask et al 2008, Neumann 2009, Russell & Brunton 2006).

During late pregnancy and lactation, anxiety behaviours in response to stressful stimuli are attenuated by central oxytocin and prolactin, while aggressive defensive behaviours and reduced fearfulness in response to perceived threats to the fetus and neonate increase from late pregnancy to advanced labour and peak during lactation (Kinsley 2008, Neumann 2009) (see website). Several neurotransmitters and neuropeptides are implicated in regulating maternal aggression, including local release of oxytocin within selected areas of the hypothalamus during and after birth (Brunton & Russell 2008, Neumann 2009, Russell & Brunton 2009).

Maternal brain adaptations are driven by a cascade of transformations beginning during late pregnancy, and continuing during labour and following birth. These are regulated by vaginocervical stimulation during contractions, and maternal–infant sensory interactions and suckling from birth until weaning (see website).

Current findings on the affective and behavioural manifestations of these altered patterns of neuronal interactions provide insights into the sensibilities and vulnerabilities of mothers, before, during and after birth (Neumann 2009). A variety of studies indicate that maternal and neonatal outcomes are positively influenced by women's chosen place of birth; emotional security and seclusion during labour; vaginal birth; and undisturbed maternal–infant sensory contact, particularly during the first hours of extrauterine life (DeVries 2002, Erlandsson & Fagerberg 2005, Hodnett et al 2008, Johnson & Davis 2005, Klein et al 1995, Swain et al 2008).

## ACQUIRING BRAIN CAPACITIES FOR MOTHERING

Between mid-pregnancy and the first few days after birth, the maternal hypothalamus and limbic system are exposed to a progressive increase in placental steroid and peptide hormones, and a selective increase in their multiple receptor concentrations.

This includes central and peripheral levels of *oestrogens, progesterone, placental lactogen (hPL),* and *prolactin* (see website).

## Maternal HPA axis, social aggression and anxiety-related behaviours

Evidence from human and animal studies indicate that pregnancy and lactation are characterized by an enhanced parasympathetic tone, suppression of sympathetic responses to stressful stimuli, and attenuated response of the hypothalamic–pituitary–adrenal (HPA) axis to various stressors (Brunton et al 2008, Douglas 2010). This is manifested by the woman's different responses to stressors and perceived dangers to herself and her baby. A key regulator of maternal anxiety postpartum appears to be physical separation of mother and infant (see website).

## Brain mechanisms underlying neuroendocrine and behavioural adaptations

See website.

## Prolactin – maternal stress and anxiety

In humans, levels of prolactin and hPL rise throughout pregnancy. During advanced labour, prolactin levels decline rapidly but rise again soon after birth (see website). Following placental separation, hPL disappears from the maternal circulation, but suckling provides the stimulus for ongoing prolactin secretion that peaks within the first 3 months of human lactation (Diaz et al 1989, Grattan 2002).

Prolactin has been found to initiate key elements in the repertoire of behaviours involved in nest-building during late pregnancy and nurturing, protecting and nourishing the infant during lactation (Lucas et al 1998): reduction of maternal fearfulness and anxiety, and reduced anxiety and stress during lactation (see website).

## The maternal emotional brain – oxytocin and prolactin

In pregnancy, magnocellular oxytocin neurons in the supraoptic nucleus (SON) and paraventricular nucleus (PVN) are restrained from premature activation, to prevent pre-term labour and preserve accumulating oxytocin stores in the neurohypophysis, in preparation for labour, birth and the onset of lactation (Higuchi & Okere 2002, Russell & Brunton 2006, 2009, Russell et al 2003) (see website).

## Gestational analgesia

A significant rise in maternal pain threshold occurs between late pregnancy and 24 hours following birth (Gintzler & Liu 2001, Whipple et al 1990). Maternal pain threshold rises gradually from 30 weeks' gestation, accelerates during the last 3–4 weeks of pregnancy, rises further during labour, and then falls precipitously within 24 hours of birth (Gintzler & Liu 2001, Ohel et al 2007). Evidence indicates that placental steroids augment pelvic afferent tone. These nerves entering the spinal cord from the cervix and uterus activate multiple analgesic synergies between spinal $\kappa/\delta$ opioid systems, non-opioid peptides and spinal noradrenergic pathways descending from the brainstem (Liu & Gintzler 2003) (see website).

Painless nocturnal contractions occur in women from around 30 weeks' gestation, coinciding with higher circulating levels of oxytocin and melatonin, and a lower oestrogen/progesterone ratio, which increases myometrial sensitivity to oxytocin during the early hours of darkness (Fuchs et al 1992, Murphy Goodwin 1999, Sharkey et al 2009).

## Neuroendocrine and central oxytocin systems – late pregnancy to weaning

There are complex anatomical and physiological adaptations during the last few weeks of pregnancy and through labour through to the process of weaning.

During pregnancy, secretion of oxytocin and secretory response of magnocellular neurons to various physiological stimuli are progressively restrained at several levels by opioid systems which are largely stimulated by allopregnanolone – a neurosteroid metabolite of progesterone (Brunton & Russell 2008, Douglas 2010, Higuchi & Okere 2002, Russell & Brunton 2009). In late pregnancy, brainstem and forebrain neuronal projections to the SON and PVN are activated in preparation for labour, birth, the induction of maternal behaviours and lactation (de Kock et al 2003, Douglas et al 2002, Ortiz-Miranda et al 2005; Russell et al 2003) (see website).

### Central oxytocin

A distinct and independently regulated oxytocin system exists within the brain which is highly activated during the peripartum period. Central oxytocin acts as a neurotransmitter within PVN neurons that project to the forebrain, limbic system and autonomic centres in the brainstem and spinal cord (Neumann 2009, Russell & Brunton 2009). Oxytocin is also released in much larger quantities from soma and dendrites of magnocellular neurons within the SON, PVN and other associated nuclei throughout labour and lactation (Russell et al 2003) (see website).

## MYOMETRIAL QUIESCENCE

Throughout pregnancy, the smooth muscle of the myometrium undergoes a series of adaptations that facilitate proliferation and hypertrophy while the capacity for contractility is deactivated (Shynlova et al 2009). This state of quiescence facilitates implantation, placental formation, subsequent growth of the fetus and placenta, and the progressive accumulation of amniotic fluid (Price & Lopez Bernal 2001).

An array of factors maintain uterine quiescence until the end of pregnancy, including human chorionic gonadotrophin (hCG), progesterone, corticotrophin-releasing hormone (CRH), relaxin, nitric oxide and melatonin. hCG inhibits formation of gap junctions; oxytocin stimulates contractions and stimulates enzymes that synthesize relaxatory prostaglandins, until receptor concentrations for hCG decline with the onset of labour (Sparey et al 1999, Ticconi et al 2006, Zuo et al 1994).

Localized myometrial contractions occur spontaneously in response to uterine distension, towards the end of pregnancy, when uterine growth declines relative to the fetus (Shynlova et al 2009). This increases uterine wall stretch, facilitating a pre-labour rise in myometrial oxytocin receptors. Prostacyclin increases the expression of gap-junction and contractile proteins, and melatonin receptor expression declines relative to non-pregnant values, attenuating its suppressive effects on myometrial oxytocin receptors (Fetalvero et al 2008, Lindstrom & Bennett 2005, Terzidou et al 2005).

### Placental steroids

Plasma concentrations of oestrogens and progesterone increase progressively throughout pregnancy and labour, but target tissue responsiveness is controlled by changes in expression and activation of their nuclear and non-nuclear receptor subtypes, and by pregnancy-induced expression of progesterone metabolites, which maintain uterine quiescence by binding directly to membrane-bound receptors and inhibiting signalling pathways (Condon et al 2003, Mesiano 2001, Mesiano et al 2002, Mesiano & Welsh 2007, Sheehan et al 2005). The capacity of progesterone to maintain uterine quiescence is also enhanced by functional inactivation of sympathetic nerves in the myometrium and increased receptors for peptides and neurotransmitters that promote relaxation and inhibit the contractile effects of oxytocin (Casey et al 1997, Dong et al 1999, 2003, Ferguson et al 1998, Grammatopoulos et al 1996, Owman 1981, Price & Lopes Bernal 2001) (see website).

This complex balance between the oestrogen and progesterone ratios ensures that there is less myometrial responsiveness, desensitizing it to oestrogen-induced formation of gap junctions, contraction-associated proteins and responsiveness to oxytocin. At the same time, oestrogens *increase* myometrial responsiveness to the progesterone receptor, subtype B (PR-B) (Mesiano 2001, Mesiano et al 2002, Mesiano & Welsh 2007) (see website). Progesterone contributes to myometrial quiescence by modulating the expression of genes that encode a number of contraction-associated proteins, including oxytocin receptors and formation of myometrial gap-junctions, until the end of pregnancy (Mesiano et al 2002, Mesiano & Welsh 2007).

For most of pregnancy, myometrial contractions remain localized, since few intracellular connections are formed until the last trimester (see website).

### Placenta and fetal membranes

During pregnancy, spontaneous, oxytocin- and prostaglandin-induced myometrial contractions are inhibited by the placenta and chorioamniotic membranes surrounding the uterus. The placenta produces atrial natriuretic peptide (ANP), while the chorion and amnion produce brain natriuretic peptide (BNP). Both peptides inhibit oxytocin-induced contractions (Carvajal et al 2006, 2009; Cootauco et al 2008). These are ideally positioned to protect the fetus from oxytocin and other inflammatory mediators, with the capacity to stimulate myometrial contractility (Keelan et al 2003) (see website).

Amnion, chorion and decidua also express enzymes to synthesize and metabolize oestrogens and progesterone. Current evidence suggests that the dominance of PR-B is maintained in these tissues until the end of pregnancy, when enzymatic changes stimulate concurrent increases in the most biologically active oestrogen and the most inactive progestogen (Blanks et al 2003). The fetoplacental membranes and maternal decidual tissues therefore establish endocrine–paracrine networks regulating the length of gestation and the onset of labour (Chibbar et al 1995, Cootauco et al 2008, Henderson & Wilson 2001, Jaffe 2001, Rehman et al 2007, Smith 2007, Ticconi et al 2006).

## FROM PREGNANCY TO LABOUR

### Fetal preparations for labour and lactation

The progressive nocturnal rhythm in uterine activity during the last trimester gradually shifts the fetus towards the lower pole of the uterus and the presenting part descends into the pelvis. This helps the fetus to increase flexion and descent, and follow the curve of Carus. Activation of the fetal HPA axis during the third trimester produces physiological increases in cortisol, which interacts with other hormones to induce maturational changes in organs like the lungs, liver, pancreas and gut, thyroid axis, and thermogenic proteins in brown adipose tissue (Fowden et al 1995, Freemark 1999, Garbrecht et al 2006, Liggins 1994). In the brain, catecholaminergic neurons have a key role in cortical differentiation and maturation of respiratory neural networks in the brainstem (Fujii et al 2006). Cortisol and adrenaline also stimulate a gradual increase in blood pressure, in preparation for pulmonary expansion and cessation of the fetoplacental circulation soon after birth (see website).

During the last couple of days before the onset of labour, fetal breathing activity is reduced and lung fluid is produced at a gradually decreasing rate (Bland 2001). Fetal breathing may be depressed by endogenous opioids and rising concentrations of prostaglandin $E_2$ ($PGE_2$), while the decline in lung liquid volume is associated with increased production of cortisol and catecholamines, from late pregnancy to birth (Jain & Duddell 2006, Lagercrantz & Herlenius 2002). It is suggested that the fetal brain is protected from reduced oxygen and glucose supplies around the time of birth, by an increase in central oxytocin, beginning just before the onset of labour and peaking around 2 hours before birth (Brown & Grattan 2007). The fetal brain is exposed to elevated levels of oxytocin, which triggers a transient but significant switch of the GABA neurotransmitter, from excitatory to inhibitory. This reduces nutrient and oxygen requirements of the brain during transition to air-breathing and suckling (Khazipov et al 2008, Tyzio et al 2006). Current evidence suggests that the oxytocin is derived from both mother and fetus (Khazipov et al 2008).

## The fetal adreno-placental 'clock'

Duration of pregnancy is strongly associated with the rising profile of placental CRH in the maternal circulation (Smith 2007, Tyson et al 2009). CRH levels rise exponentially in maternal and fetal circulatory systems during the last 12 weeks of pregnancy, peak during labour, and fall precipitously following birth (Chan et al 1993, Goland et al 1986). In individual women, the exponential increase tends to mirror the duration of pregnancy: women who give birth prematurely have higher mid-pregnancy levels of CRH than those who give birth at term (McLean et al 1995, Smith 2007). The bioavailability of CRH is regulated by a circulating binding protein, which declines at the end of pregnancy, further increasing maternal and fetal tissue exposure to CRH (Grammatopoulos 2008) (Fig. 35.1).

During pregnancy and labour, placental CRH targets a number of maternal, placental and fetal organ systems. In

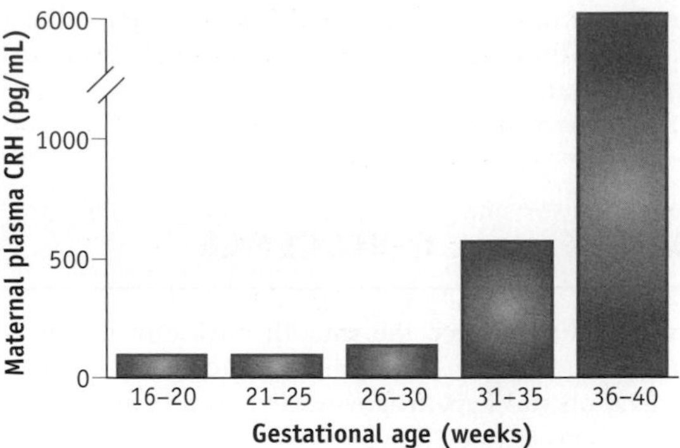


**Figure 35.1** Mean plasma CRH concentrations in eight women followed sequentially during the second half of pregnancy. *(Reproduced with permission from Goland et al 1994:1289.)*

the fetal compartment, CRH receptors have been identified in the pituitary gland, adrenal cortex, lungs, placenta and membranes (Grammatopoulos 2007, 2008). In the adrenals, placental CRH directly stimulates the fetal zone to produce DHEA-S and the definitive zone to produce cortisol, in a dose-dependent manner (Rehman et al 2007). The maternal pituitary–adrenal axis is also a target organ for CRH, while the myometrium is both a source and target for CRH and a related family of urocortin peptides (Goland et al 1994, Grammatopoulos 2007, Markovic et al 2007, Smith 2007) (see website).

### Myometrial actions of placental CRH

During pregnancy, human myometrial cells express a large number of CRH and CRH-related urocortin peptides, and their major receptor subtypes CRH-R1 and CRH-R2 (see website).

As term approaches, oxytocin and inflammatory cytokines also stimulate expression of many variants of the CRH-R1 receptor with reduced signalling capacities (Grammatopoulos & Hillhouse 1999, Hillhouse & Grammatopoulos 2001). Recent work suggests that expression of CRH-R1 variants with reduced signalling capacity are only increased in the lower uterine segment with the onset of labour (Markovic et al 2007).

In contrast to CRH-R1, activation of CRH-R2 stimulates signalling pathways that enhance myometrial contractility. Recent experiments on gene profiles in different regions of the uterus have identified expression of fundal genes for CRH-R2 that increase significantly during labour (Grammatopoulos 2008, Stevens & Challis 1998). These findings indicate that dynamic changes in the balance of myometrial CRH-R1 receptor subtypes at term stimulate concomitant physiological changes in the fundus and lower uterine segment from late pregnancy to birth. While muscles in the upper segment generate coordinated forceful contractions, those in the lower segment have reduced stimulatory influences, which facilitates increased contractility of the fundus, elongation of the lower segment over the presenting part and progressive cervical dilation, as labour advances (Bukowski et al 2006).

### CRH activity in placenta and membranes

The placenta and membranes also express two major CRH receptor subtypes: CRH-R1 and CRH-R2. In the placenta, the CRH-R1 subtype seems to increase expression of type 2 cyclo-oxygenase (COX-2), which stimulates biosynthesis of prostaglandin precursors and decreases expression of prostaglandin dehydrogenase (PGDH) – the key enzyme produced by the placenta and membranes that metabolizes active primary prostaglandins to an inactive form and inhibits production of progesterone (Amash et al 2009, Gao et al 2008, Grammatopoulos 2008) (see website).

## Uterine oxytocin receptors

During pregnancy, myometrial receptors for oxytocin (OTR) increase from 27.6 fmol/mg DNA in the non-pregnant state to 171.6 fmol/mg DNA at mid-gestation, and 1391 fmol/mg DNA at term (Fuchs et al 1984). This represents a 50-fold increase within the uterus *before* the onset of labour (see website).

Maximum receptor concentrations have been found in early labour at term, 3583 fmol/mg DNA – significantly higher than before labour begins (Fuchs et al 1982). Concentrations of decidual receptors are relatively low in mid-pregnancy and reach maximal values following the onset of labour. Within the fetal membranes, increased OTR binding has been found between late pregnancy and labour, with highest increases in the amnion (Takemura et al 1994). Myometrial receptor concentrations are highest in the fundus and corpus, significantly lower in the lower segment, and lowest in the cervix, while decidual receptors are highest in sections surrounding the corpus and lowest around the lower segment (Blanks et al 2003).

During early labour, myometrial receptor concentrations are uniformly high in the upper segment and progressively lower in the isthmus and cervix, while those in the decidua are highest in the corpus, followed by the fundus and the isthmus (Fuchs et al 1984, Fuchs & Fuchs 1991, Hirst et al 1993) (see website).

There is an important role for *gap junctions* in coordinating cellular responsiveness to oxytocin. At term, higher concentrations of myometrial gap-junctions occur in the fundus compared to the lower segment, and the difference becomes increasingly pronounced during labour. This creates increasing *fundal dominance* during the course of labour and regulates progressive conductance of electrical activity, from fundus to cervix, to propagate multicellular synchronization of myometrial responsiveness to neuroendocrine, pulsatile and intrauterine oxytocin systems (Blanks et al 2003, Fuchs et al 1991, Kimura et al 1996, Russell et al 2003, Shmygol et al 2006).

During spontaneous labour, myometrial and decidual OTR concentrations decline significantly in advanced labour, particularly in the lower segment (Fuchs et al 1984). While findings in the lower segment are unreliable because of progressive incorporation of the cervix into the lower segment, available evidence suggests that oxytocin receptor mRNA significantly declines in the lower segment with increasing duration of labour. In spontaneous labour, the decline occurs gradually over 12–16 hours, but in oxytocin-induced and oxytocin-augmented labour, it is much steeper, especially when the infusion is constant rather than pulsatile (Phaneuf et al 2000, Robinson et al 2003, Willcourt et al 1994) (see website).

## Nocturnal myometrial activation and cervical ripening

The uterus has a well-defined 24-hour rhythm of contractility and electrical and endocrine activation (Schlabritz-Loutsevitch et al 2003). In human pregnancy, increased contractile activity has been observed between 20:30 and 02:00 from 24 weeks' gestation (Fuchs et al 1992, Germain et al 1993, Moore et al 1994, Sharkey et al 2009). Current research suggests the emergence of a nocturnal surge in rhythmic myometrial contractions is a key indication of uterine activation in preparation for the shift from pregnancy to labour. Nocturnal surges in oestradiol, melatonin and oxytocin occur from around 35–36 weeks' gestation and these coincide with the 24-hour rhythm of spontaneous birth (Fuchs et al 1992, Schlabritz-Loutsevitch et al 2003, Tamura et al 2008). The nocturnal surge in oestriol, which originates almost exclusively from fetal adrenal DHEA-S, occurs from 35 weeks' gestation; nocturnal plasma melatonin rises from 36 weeks' gestation and nocturnal peaks in plasma concentrations of oxytocin occur from 37–39 weeks' gestation (Fuchs et al 1991, 1992, Germain et al 1993, Moore et al 1994, Murphy Goodwin 1999, Schlabritz-Loutsevitch et al 2003, Tamura et al 2008). Oestradiol and melatonin increase gap junctions and oxytocin receptors, and melatonin also synergizes with oxytocin, increasing oxytocin-induced contractility in a dose-dependent manner (Sharkey et al 2009).

From approximately 36 weeks onwards, structural alterations become more apparent in cervical stroma and mucosal tissues, which alters its dimensions in relation to the lower uterine segment (House et al 2009). Within cervical connective tissue, alterations occur in the composition and concentration of the gel-like material called ground substance (proteoglycans) in which connective tissue cells and fibres are embedded. At the same time, an increase occurs in enzymes that degrade collagen. The concentration of ground substance relative to collagen is thought to reach a maximum during cervical softening prior to the onset of labour. This overall increase is characterized by the emergence of a higher proportion of molecules with a weaker affinity for collagen fibrils (see website).

## Cervical and uterine muscles

During late pregnancy and the latent phase of labour, myometrial components of the cervix contract in characteristic short, high-frequency pressure increases, that are independent of the rest of the uterus, until the onset of established labour (Rudel & Pajntar 1999). These contractions may stimulate local connective tissue changes associated with cervical ripening (Olah et al 1993, Pajntar 1994). In primiparous women, softening of cervical tissue proceeds alongside effacement and is thought to occur in response to increased formation of gap junctions between adjacent cells, in the myometrium of the uterine cavity. *Gap junctions* are composed of symmetrical portions of plasma membrane from adjacent cells. These form intercellular channels for passage of ions and small molecules, facilitating rapid intracellular transmission of electrical impulses and chemical signals between cells. Gap junctions emerge in late pregnancy and undergo further increases in size and number during early labour. Formation and permeability of gap junctions are stimulated by oestrogens, prostaglandins and melatonin, and inhibited by progesterone, hCG and relaxin (Ambrus & Rao 1994, Burghardt et al 1993, Chow & Lye 1994, Sharkey et al 2009). Before labour begins, myometrial expression of gap junctions is much higher in the fundus than in the lower segment and this difference accelerates during the course of labour (Sparey et al 1999).

By facilitating the propagation of action potentials from cell to cell, gap junctions synchronize myometrial activity. Tension is transmitted from the myometrium by the outer layer of muscle that extends along the periphery of the supravaginal portion of the cervix (Pajntar 1994). This facilitates stretching of the lower uterine segment, which elongates as pressure is exerted by the fetus during descent into the pelvis. These combined forces seem to produce a differential rate of tissue uptake in the cervix and the adjacent lower segment of the uterus. Maximum uptake occurs at the lower peripheral end of the cervix, producing a gradual upward movement of soft cervical tissue that eventually merges with the lower segment (Gee & Olah 1993, Havelock et al 2005) (Fig. 35.2).

In a recent study on women following induction and augmentation of labour, a number of significant features were associated with the presence or absence of cervical contractions in response to myometrial activity. Cervical contractions predominantly occurred in women with lower measures of cervical effacement and dilatation and a longer latent phase, compared to those in whom cervical contractions were absent (Rudel & Pajmtar 1999). These indicate the importance of coordinated changes, from the fundus to the cervix, during the transition from pregnancy to labour (Havelock et al 2005, Olah et al 1993, Pajntar 1994, Rudel & Pajntar 1999).

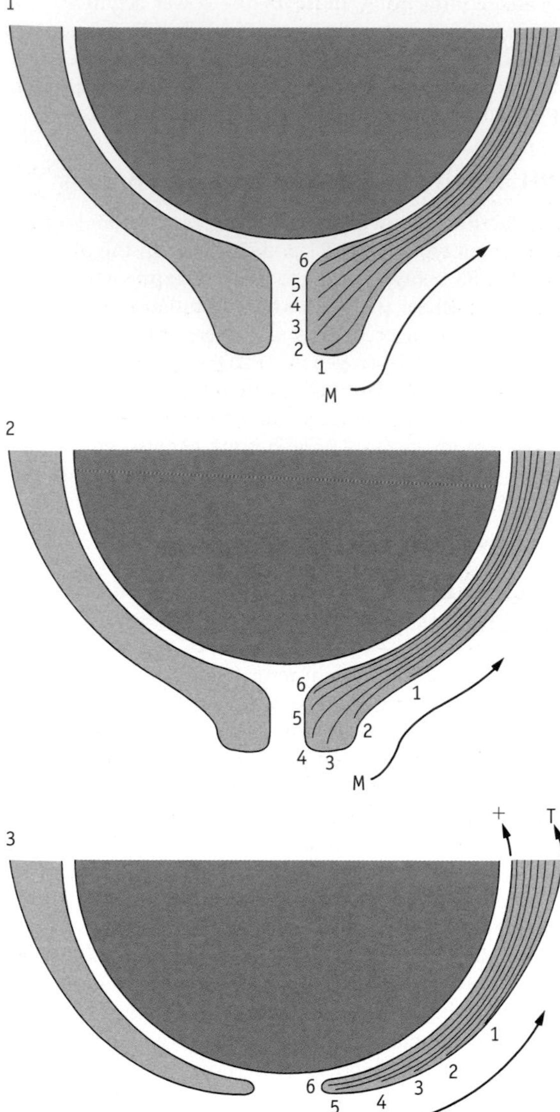


**Figure 35.2** Diagram representing a hypothesis concerning differential movement of tissue planes at the time of cervical effacement and dilatation. M, direction of movement of collagen bundles; T, +, differential tension across the myometrium. *(Reproduced with permission from Gee 1981, Fig. 14.5.)*

## Uterocervical changes and inflammation

Local pro-inflammatory changes accompany the remodelling and stretching of uterine muscle and cervical connective tissue during the latter part of pregnancy. The progressive release of inflammatory mediators like *nuclear factor kappa B (NF-κB)*, *cytokines* and *interleukins* seems to gradually overwhelm the selective suppression of inflammatory and immune responses established from the beginning of pregnancy by progesterone, prolactin and cortisol (Gubbay et al 2002, Johnson et al 2008, Lindstrom & Bennett 2005, Pepe & Albrecht 1995, Rosen et al 1998, Shynlova et al 2009, Vaisanen-Tommiska et al 2003). Remodelling of the cervical connective tissue; stretching of the lower uterine segment and of the fetal membranes overlying the cervix, produce local alterations in the relative activity of mediators of inflammatory and anti-inflammatory reactions (Allport et al 2001, Bennett et al 2001, Moore et al 2006, Vaisanen-Tommiska et al 2003).

These include increased concentrations of a key cytokine, *interleukin (IL)-8*, in the cervix and lower uterine segment with cervical ripening; higher concentrations of enzymes that synthesize prostacyclin, $PGE_2$ and $PGF_{2\alpha}$ in the lower segment compared to the fundus, before and during labour; raised cervical production of cytokines and nitric oxide (NO) at term and during labour; increased expression of NF-κB and *decreased* expression of glucocorticoid receptors in cervical tissue from late pregnancy to birth; and downregulation of *placental cortisol receptors* (Allport et al 2001, Bennett et al 2001, Johnson et al 2008, Keelan et al 2003, Lindstrom & Bennett 2005, Norman et al 1998, Sparey et al 1999). The COX-2 enzymes that stimulate prostaglandin synthesis are activated in cervical tissue by *NO* and *NF-κB*. The higher concentrations of these enzymes in the lower compared with the upper segment before labour may also increase collagenolytic activity of cervical tissue, thus contributing to cervical ripening. With the onset of labour, these enzymes increase further in the lower but not the upper segment, which suggests that prostaglandins may actively promote relaxation of the lower uterine segment throughout the course of labour (Myatt &Lye 2004, Sparey et al 1999, Zuo et al 1994).

## Remodelling gestational tissues

Fetal membranes consist of amnion and chorion layers connnected by an *extracellular matrix (ECM)* of collagen fibres that provides the main tensile strength of the membranes. Current findings suggest that membranes undergo a regulated process of tissue remodelling similar to the cervix, from late pregnancy to birth (Moore et al 2006). In the cervix and membranes, remodelling and maturation processes involve changes in collagen fibres.

The amnion lies in direct contact with amniotic fluid, which contains elevated concentrations of pro- and anti-inflammatory cytokines from early pregnancy (Keelan et al 2003). During the third trimester, surfactant proteins and phospholipids also enter amniotic fluid in increasing quantities and these have macrophage-activating properties that stimulate NF-κB activity, which regulates expression of *MMP enzymes*. Cytokines stimulate the prostaglandin H synthase 2 enzyme, which stimulates synthesis of prostaglandins, and concentrations of $PGF_{2\alpha}$ increase significantly in the amnion from around 38 weeks' gestation (Keelan et al 2003, Lee et al 2008, Smith 2007). NO has been found to stimulate release of $PGE_2$ in amnion-like cells and fetal membranes, and recent evidence suggests that oxytocin is involved in stimulating the release of NO and pro-inflammatory cytokines from fetal membranes during labour (Ticconi et al 2004).

The amnion is separated from the myometrium by the chorion and decidua. Research findings suggest that the chorion, decidua and placenta produce anti-inflammatory cytokines and the placenta and chorion also produce the enzyme *prostaglandin dehydrogenase* (PGDH) which is a potent inactivator of prostaglandins (Amash et al 2009, Keelan et al 2003). Late in pregnancy, chorionic PGDH activity declines while the expression of the inducible isoform of the *prostaglandin-generating enzyme COX-2* increases significantly in the adjacent amnion (Ticconi et al 2006). Many anti-inflammatory cytokines are produced in the decidua, which decrease local prostaglandin production, and their levels remain elevated following the onset of labour, while those in the placenta seem to decline during the course of labour (Keelan et al 2003) (see website).

## FROM LATE PREGNANCY TO BIRTH

The transition from nocturnal myometrial contractions to the onset of labour extends from around 30 weeks' gestation, particularly in primigravid women. During this period, cervical tissues become less resistant, interrelated anatomical changes occur in the cervix and lower uterine segment, and the myometrium is activated nocturnally by episodes of rhythmic contractions (House et al 2009). Progesterone dominance declines within uterine tissues and related forces that promote myometrial quiescence and inhibit multicellular interactions are progressively modulated, in a region-specific manner, within the myometrium and surrounding intrauterine tissues, from late pregnancy to birth (Bukowski et al 2006, Henderson & Wilson 2001, Mesiano & Welsh 2007, Sparey et al 1999).

From around 32 weeks, the onset of increased nocturnal release of oxytocin coincides with the decrease in the plasma oestrogen/progesterone ratio and the rise in oxytocin receptor density in the uterus. Under these conditions, a small rise in the pulsatile release of oxytocin seems to stimulate episodes of uterine contractions during the hours of darkness (Fuchs et al 1991, Germain et al 1993, Moore et al 1994). Expression of oestrogen-, melatonin- and prostacyclin-induced gap-junction proteins in the myometrium also increases from around 37 weeks, particularly in the fundus, and these provide low-resistance pathways between smooth muscle cells that increase the coordination of contractile activity throughout the uterus (Chow & Lye 1994, Fetalvero et al 2008, Sharkey et al 2009) (see website).

These dynamic changes progressively generate functionally distinct sections of the uterus from late pregnancy to birth. Towards the end of pregnancy, the recurring episodes of nocturnal contractions become stronger and more frequent, until the functionally differentiated myometrium expresses its intrinsic capacity to propagate progressively stronger contractions from the fundus to the cervix during labour and birth (Bukowski et al 2006, Sparey et al 1999, Ticconi et al 2006).

## Maternal–fetal readiness for labour

In women, the transition from nocturnal rhythms in uterine contractions to latent labour is highly variable and is influenced by a host of additional factors, including maternal cognitive activity, fetal position and emotional readiness for labour (Wuitchik et al 1989). Throughout the last 4 weeks of pregnancy, physiological adaptations seem to be enhanced when women take time out in the evenings for relaxation, to enhance the duration of sleep (Lee & Gay 2004). Using favoured ways of relaxing in late pregnancy, particularly during the early hours of darkness, facilitates the nocturnal rise in oxytocin and melatonin, which regulate the physiological increase in myometrial activity (Fuchs et al 1992, Sharkey et al 2009). This phase of preparatory changes in uterine smooth muscle and cervical tissue accelerates at term, and the onset of spontaneous labour indicates the combined readiness of maternal and fetal organ systems for labour and birth (Majzoub & Karalis 1999).

Reduced cognitive stimulation, relaxation and sleep are key elements of preparation because of the positive association between low cognitive activation and expressions of maternal love; sleep duration in late pregnancy and shorter duration of labour; and the positive association between chronic anxiety, heightened levels of fear, pain perception and labour complications (Bartels & Zeki 2004, Haddad et al 1985, Lee & Gay 2004, Saisto et al 2001). Research evidence also indicates that low cognitive anxiety enables women to experience less discomfort during latent labour, suggesting that the absence of fear modulates maternal pain perception (Wuitchik et al 1989). Once established labour begins, mothers need to be with their trusted companion, who maintains a quiet, warm, low-lit environment and communicates with minimal cognitive stimulation (Hodnett et al 2008). These conditions are conducive to the release of central oxytocin, which induces a timeless hypnotic state that deepens as labour progresses. Maintaining a calm, secure, low-lit environment also prevents a stress-induced rise in *catecholamines*, which have been shown to inhibit oxytocin and attenuate uterine contractions (Levinson & Shnider 1979, Peled 1993).

## Neuroendocrine oxytocin

The release of oxytocin from the neurohypophysis during labour occurs in response to neuronal feedback to the brainstem from the uterus, cervix and vagina. During late pregnancy and labour, innervation is low in the body of the uterus and significantly higher in the cervix, vagina and adjacent parts of the pelvic cavity. Stretching and distension of these areas activates sensory afferent nerve pathways that transmit signals via the spinal cord and brainstem to oxytocin neurons in the hypothalamus. These respond with discrete bursts of accelerated discharge that transport the stored hormone along axons of hypothalamic neurons that each give rise to numerous varicosities or large vesicles in the neurohypophysis. From here, oxytocin is released intermittently into the general circulation (Rossoni et al 2008) (Fig. 35.3).

Throughout labour and birth, increasing vaginocervical stimulation produced by downward pressure of the fetus transmits nerve impulses via the vagal and pelvic nerves, through spinal and brainstem pathways, to the hypothalamus (Russell et al 2003). These recurring episodes of sensory stimulation trigger characteristic bursts of magnocellular oxytocin neurons, resulting in minute-to-minute variation in plasma oxytocin levels during spontaneous labour (Fuchs et al 1991). As illustrated in Figure 35.4, pulse frequency increases significantly during labour but pulse amplitude remains low until the active phase, when it rises sharply, particularly during the final moments around birth. After birth, this pattern of oxytocin release accelerates in response to sensory contact and suckling, and peaks during the middle of lactation (Fuchs et al 1991, Johnston & Amico 1986, Rossoni et al 2008) (see website).

Oxytocin receptors are regulated by *oxytocinase*, an enzyme that rapidly degrades oxytocin. Placental oxytocinase is released into the maternal circulation during pregnancy and reaches highest levels just before the onset of labour (Ito et al 2001, Nomura et al 2005). This enzyme prevents receptor desensitization during prolonged oxytocin release, as happens during labour and lactation. Oxytocinase may also suppress the pain of uterine contractions before and after birth, by rapidly inactivating oxytocin following its release (see website). Because of the increase in oxytocinase before the onset of labour, receptor concentrations remain elevated for approximately 20 hours of labour, before they begin to decline (Ito et al 2001).

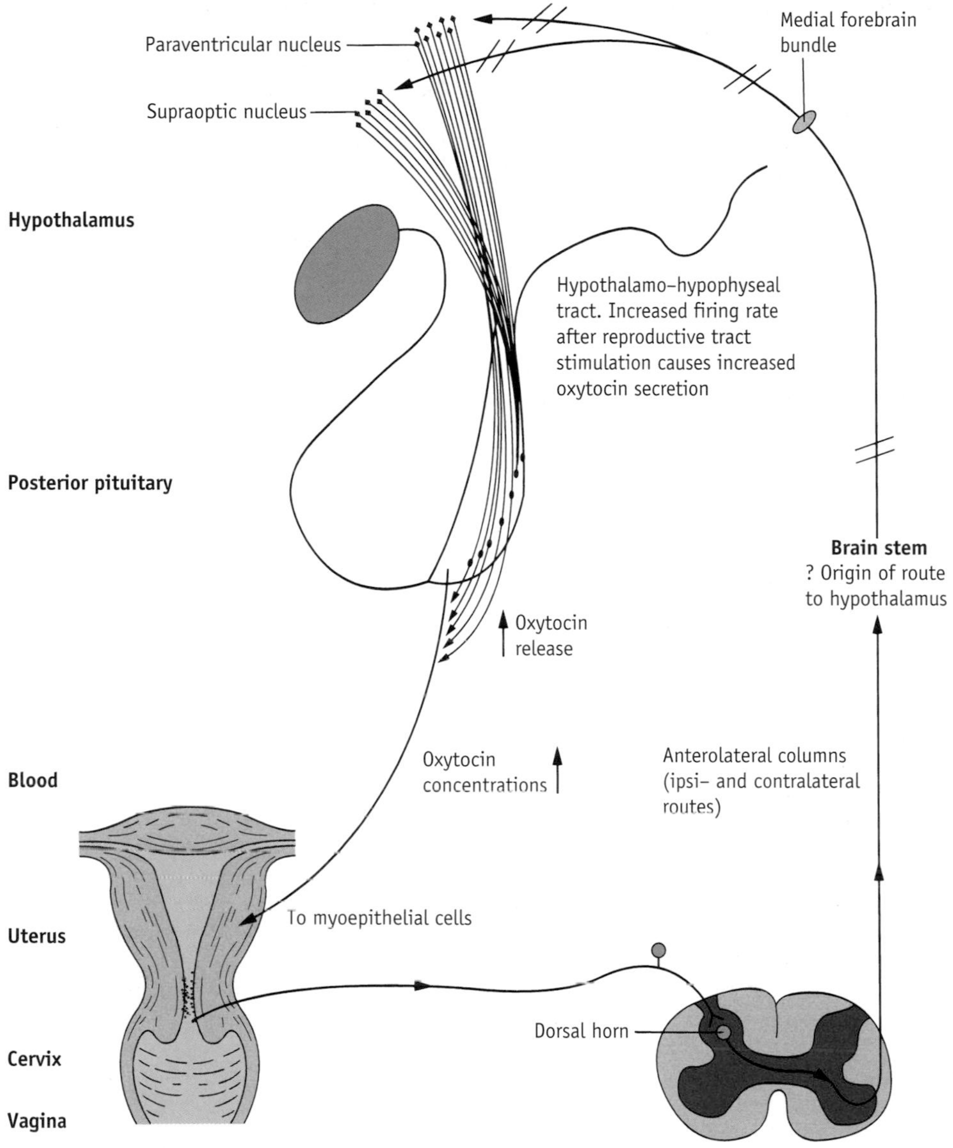


**Figure 35.3** The neuroendocrine reflex underlying oxytocin synthesis and secretion. Stretching of the cervix and lower segment (black line) activates the reflex leading to oxytocin release (red line) *(Reproduced with permission from Johnson 2007: 248.)*

## Towards the expulsive phase

Just before the cervix has been fully incorporated into the lower segment, the frequency of contractions may slow down, particularly in primigravid women. When maternal and fetal events are not completely synchronized, this presents as a slowing down of the labour process and may require experimenting with different maternal positions to allow the fetus to fully descend into the pelvic outlet. A slow pace of descent allows the simultaneous surge in fetal adrenaline to complete the removal of lung liquid which enhances respiratory adaptations immediately following birth (Bland 2001).

In biological terms, the expulsive phase is reached when the cervix has become incorporated into the lower uterine segment, which becomes progressively thinner, as expulsive contractions set up positive afferent nerve pathways to the hypothalamus. This reflexive mechanism stimulates

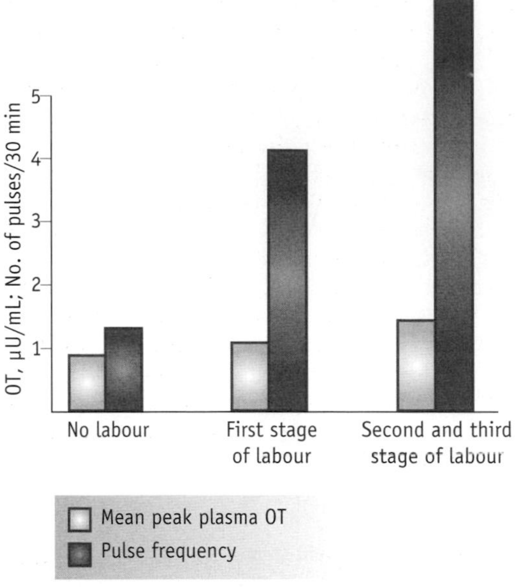


**Figure 35.4** Mean oxytocin pulse frequency and amplitude determined in women at term, not in labour (n = 11), during the first stage of labour (n = 13) and combined second and third stages (n = 8). n = number in each group. *(Reproduced with permission from Fuchs et al 1991:1520.)*

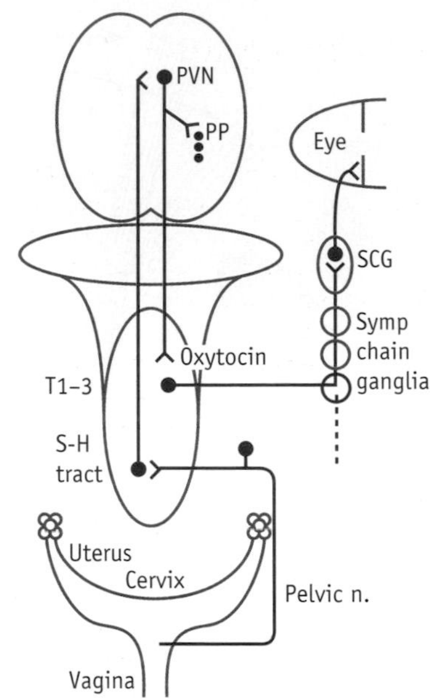


**Figure 35.5** Schematic view of the pathway mediating the reflexive release of oxytocin in response to vaginocervical stimulation and the pathway mediating the pupil dilation response to vaginocervical stimulation. *(Reproduced with permission from Komisaruk & Sansone 2003:247.)*

increased central release of oxytocin, and, with increasing flexion and anterior rotation of the fetal head, pressure from the vertex against the gutter-shaped pelvic floor muscles stimulates their stretch receptors that activate both neuroendocrine and neurotransmitter oxytocin systems (Sansone et al 2002). During the expulsive phase, vaginocervical stretch activates magnocellular and parvocellular neurons. The former release oxytocin in characteristic pulses into the systemic circulation, while the latter release oxytocin into the spinal cord, which stimulates sympathetic neurons that project to radial muscles of the iris, producing dilation of the pupils (Komisaruk & Sansone 2003) (Fig. 35.5).

Unresolved anxieties or perceived threats or dangers may stimulate catecholamines, particularly adrenaline, which inhibits the pulsatile release of oxytocin, leading to a decline or cessation of uterine contractions, excessive blood loss following birth, and delay in the onset of suckling and lactation (Chen et al 1998, Levison & Shnider 1979, Odent 1992, Peled 1993). Current evidence suggests that a private, warm, low-lit environment will enhance oxytocin secretion and minimize the rise in maternal cortisol and catecholamines activated by heightened fear and anxiety that may occur just before expulsive contractions begin (Chen et al 1998, Levinson & Shnider 1979, Wuitchik et al 1989).

The expulsive phase is accompanied by a physiological increase in maternal catecholamine levels, particularly noradrenaline. This rise increases cardiac output and pulmonary circulation, providing the physical energy that usually coincides with the final moments of labour (Odent 1987). Many women find that they focus on rhythmic breathing during the expulsive phase and this 'hypnotic-like' state enables them to follow their bodies' expulsive efforts. This encourages the woman to move the rest of the fetal body down the birth canal, without undue stress on herself or her baby.

## Spontaneous maternal breathing

To maintain uterine blood flow and adequate oxygenation to the fetus during the expulsive phase, maternal hyperventilation and breath-holding need to be avoided. Over prolonged periods, breath-holding (*Valsalva manoeuvre*) increases intrathoracic pressure, which reduces venous return to the heart. Consequently, cardiac output falls and blood pressure drops, leading to a reduction in uteroplacental perfusion (Blackburn 2007). In a recent randomized study comparing Valsalva and spontaneous pushing, the expulsive phase of labour was shorter and umbilical arterial pH, $Po_2$ and Apgar scores were higher in the spontaneous pushing group (Yildirim & Beji 2008).

## FETAL RESPONSES TO LABOUR AND BIRTH

Labour and birth induce increased secretion of *adrenomedullin, catecholamines, cortisol* and *thyroid-stimulating hormone (TSH)*. Adrenomedullin is a potent vasodilator of the pulmonary circulation which facilitates a rapid increase in pulmonary blood flow at birth (Boldt et al 1998). Free cortisol levels double in association with labour, rising further in the 1–2 hours following birth. As well as stimulating maturational changes in key organ systems, cortisol induces increased deiodination of *thyroxine* ($T_4$) to produce *triiodothyronine* ($T_3$). This works in conjunction with the dramatic surge in *thyroid-stimulating hormone (TSH)* at birth, stimulating striking increases in $T_3$ during the first 24 hours of neonatal life, which is particularly important for regulating thermogenesis (Nathanielsz et al 2003, Pearson Murphy & Branchaud 1994).

In the fetus, catecholamine levels rise throughout labour, reaching 20-times adult resting values immediately following birth. The intermittent squeezing of the fetal head during human labour triggers a rapid surge in catecholamine release (see website).

### Cardiovascular responses

Contractions induce transient reductions in uteroplacental perfusion that alter the pattern of fetoplacental circulation. Ultrasonic studies suggest that at the beginning of a uterine contraction, maternal venous outflow is halted and the content of the uterine veins is expressed into the maternal circulation. Simultaneously, arterial inflow that coincides with the onset of contractions is retained within the intervillous space. During contractions, this blood forms an increased pool that creates marked distension and vascular engorgement in the intervillous space. Transient reduction in uteroplacental perfusion during contractions may be partly compensated by the increased volume of maternal blood made available for gaseous exchange. To ensure the perfusion of the placenta, maternal blood pressure and cardiac output also rise in response to contractions. During the phase of uterine relaxation following each contraction, an increased blood flow has been observed, which may also compensate for decreased oxygen delivery during the preceding contraction (Bleker et al 1975, Robson et al 1987).

The circulation of a healthy fetus in spontaneous labour is not thought to be compromised by contractions. The umbilical circulation does not seem to be altered by changes in intrauterine pressure or by short-term changes in fetal–placental or maternal–placental blood flow that accompany contractions. Fetal cardiac output rises in response to increased intrauterine pressure during contractions, allowing fetal blood pressure to maintain a relatively constant pressure difference between the inside and outside of its vascular system. Concurrently, raised levels of fetal adrenaline specifically act to facilitate increases in heart rate and blood pressure, both of which serve to increase the rate of fetoplacental blood flow between contractions (see website).

The effect of fetal head pressure and the resulting catecholamines activates the parasympathetic system and inhibits cardiac pacemakers, resulting in decreased cardiac output, slowing of the heart rate and reduced blood pressure. Slowing of the heart rate during contractions reduces the oxygen requirements of cardiac muscle. Parasympathetic influences on heart rate can be counteracted by adrenaline but not by noradrenaline. In the fetus at term, sufficient levels of adrenaline may be released to produce variable increases or decreases in heart rate, in response to uterine contractions (see website).

## BIRTH AND PLACENTAL SEPARATION

As the fetus leaves the uterine cavity, the surface area of the contracting uterus declines rapidly to produce a uterine diameter of around 10 cm. This reduction encompasses the site of placental attachment to the decidual lining, leading to compression of placental tissue and uteroplacental blood vessels, including approximately 100 spiral arteries that have supplied the placenta at a rate of 500–800 mL/min throughout the course of labour (Letsky 1998). Tonic myometrial compression of these blood vessels following birth is greatly facilitated by placental-induced adaptations in the constituents of decidual and myometrial segments of the spiral arteries (Kawamata et al 2007). During the first and second trimesters, structural transformations of the vessel walls replace elastic lamina and smooth muscle layers with a matrix containing fibrin (Matijevic et al 1996).

When the mother is free to reach down and take the baby into her arms at birth, she brings herself into an upright position. This prevents compression of uterine blood flow returning to the heart via the inferior vena cava and allows gravity to assist the process of placental ejection, while the sight, sounds and sensory contact between mother and infant stimulate a significant increase in central and peripheral release of oxytocin, as opioid restraint on maternal oxytocin neurons is removed immediately after birth. Basal levels of oxytocin rise significantly and sensory stimulation and suckling increase pulse frequency and amplitude of oxytocin release, compared to labour and birth (Matthiesen et al 2001).

The enhanced release of oxytocin into the peripheral circulation following birth stimulates tonic contraction and retraction of the myometrium, which squeezes the spongy placental tissue and forces blood in the collapsing intervillous spaces back into the veins of the decidua

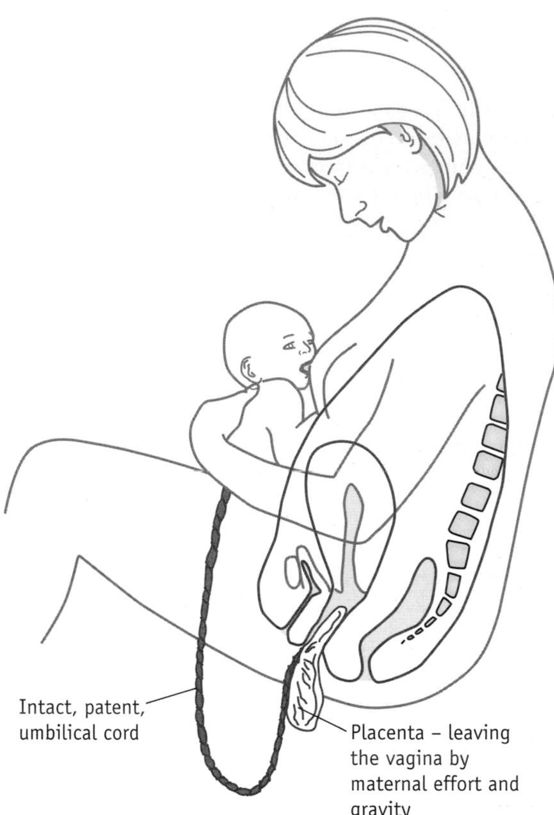


**Figure 35.6** Maternal–infant sensory contact, placental separation and the transition from placental to mammary nutrition. *(Reproduced with permission from Inch 1989.)*

(Kawamata et al 2007, Shynlova et al 2009). The uninterrupted flow of blood through the intact umbilical cord further reduces placental size, by transferring approximately 120 mL of blood into the neonatal circulation (Dunn 1985). As illustrated in Figure 35.6, the intact cord continues to provide oxygenated blood to the infant as placental separation is progressing. This allows volume adjustments to supply new capillary beds, which are opened by the dramatic fall in pulmonary vascular resistance following the rise in $P\text{O}_2$ as lung capillaries dilate with the onset of ventilation immediately following birth (Boldt et al 1998, Dunn 1985).

With sustained myometrial contraction, the congested decidual veins are severed and sealed by the shearing forces of the criss-cross network of muscle fibres surrounding them. As illustrated in Figure 35.7, the placenta is simultaneously torn from the uterine wall, at the line of the decidua basalis, and falls into the uterine cavity, peeling off the membranes as it descends towards the cervix, and falls into the vagina (Benirschke 1992). Placental separation leaves behind a surface wound of 300 cm$^2$ containing approximately 100 severed arteries in which maternal blood coagulates rapidly because of a major increase in the concentration of several coagulation factors and decreased fibrinolytic activity which characterizes pregnancy, labour and the first couple of hours following birth (Letsky 1998). Pregnancy is also accompanied by marked increases in *clotting factors VII, VIII, X* and *XII* and by a significant rise in vascular and placental *plasminogen activator inhibitors (PAIs)* leading to a marked increase in plasma fibrinogen by the third trimester (Dalaker 1986, Letsky 1998).

Before and after birth, these systemic haemostatic changes are accompanied by a local activation of *clotting factors V* and *VIII* and increased levels of *fibrinogen,* which results in a pronounced shortening of whole blood clotting time that is more pronounced in uterine than in peripheral blood. Because of their combined effects, torn blood vessels are sealed and the site of placental separation is rapidly covered by a fibrin mesh that represents 5–15% of total circulating fibrinogen (Letsky 1998). Prostaglandin metabolites are simultaneously released into the general circulation from the torn surface tissues of the decidua basalis at the site of separation where they stimulate *sustained* uterine contractions (Noort et al 1989).

When women do not experience prolonged stress-induced catecholamine release or severe vaginal or perineal laceration during labour and birth, immediate blood loss from the vagina constitutes a small proportion of the increase in plasma and red cell volume that occurs during pregnancy. Under these conditions, most of the pregnancy-induced increase in blood volume is lost over a longer time period, through diuresis during the first 48 hours and lochia discharge from the placental site over the first 2 months postpartum (Hytten 1995). While visual estimates of blood loss within the first hour following birth are highly inaccurate, the significance of estimated blood loss at birth needs to be judged in relation to the expansion in blood volume during pregnancy (Bloomfield & Gordon 1990, Gyte 1992).

## FROM FETUS TO NEONATE

Until birth, the fetus is essentially a parenterally nourished organism receiving a fairly constant supply of simple nutrients from the maternal circulation across the fetoplacental barrier. During this period of enhanced anabolic metabolism, the maternal circulation supplies the placenta with glucose, amino acids and relatively smaller amounts of essential and non-essential fatty acids for selective uptake and transfer to the fetus (Hay 1995, Herrera 2000). Soon after birth, placental transfer of nutrients and gaseous exchange between maternal and fetal circulatory systems ends along with placental hormonal interactions with the fetal adrenal gland (Ben-Davis et al 2007) (see website).

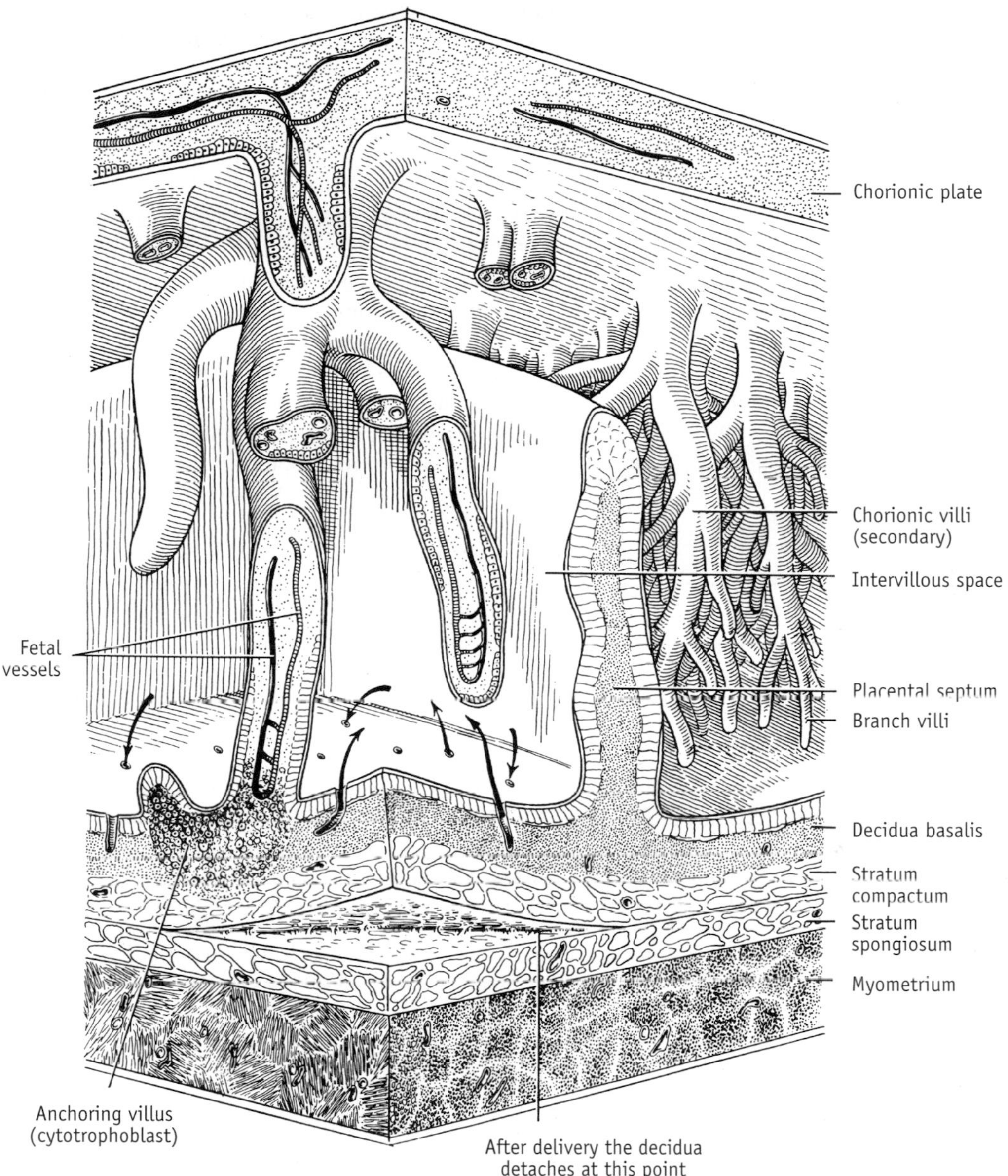


**Figure 35.7** Diagrammatic representation of placental, decidual and myometrial tissue near term, illustrating the line of placental separation. Arrows indicate blood flow from uteroplacental arteries to the intervillous space and back to the uteroplacental veins *(Reproduced with permission from Blackburn 2007; Fig. 3-11; 93.)*

The expression of innate mother–infant interactions, particularly during the early weeks after birth, is critical for the infant's long-term general health and emotional well-being (Moriceau & Sullivan 2006, Neumann 2009, Stern 1997). Close body contact reduces energy loss, regulates homeostatic mechanisms, promotes a physiological increase in glucocorticoid and mineralocorticoid brain receptors, and prevents a rise in the infant's stress axis, which is highly sensitive to periods of separation, particularly during the first 3 days after birth (Bystrova et al 2003, Christensson et al 1995, Hofer 1994, Sarrieau et al 1988).

## Initiation of maternal behaviour and attachment

Following spontaneous vaginal birth, mother and baby are in an ideal state to develop the relationship needed to initiate bonding and lactation. This includes an oxytocin-induced synaptic reorganization of the hippocampus, which improves maternal spatial memory, enabling the mother to develop a 'laser-like' focus for everything relating to the needs of her infant (Kinsley 2008, Monks et al 2003, Pedersen & Boccia 2002, Tomizawa et al 2003) (see website).

Women's stated preference for intimate 'social affection' over participating in large social groups is mediated by suckling-induced activation of the *mesocorticolimbic dopamine system*, which seems to be regulated by oxytocin (see website). The pleasurable effects of intimate contact between mother and infant set up the desire for further maternal stimulation and infant suckling, which reinforces and strengthens the maternal–infant bond, partly by increasing central oxytocin receptors and release of oxytocin into the central nervous system (see website).

## CONCLUSION

The physiology of late pregnancy and labour is characterized by a complex interplay between maternal–fetoplacental systems that is finely regulated by neurohormonal systems. It is essential that midwives are knowledgeable about recent findings regarding the onset and processes of labour, and the onset of lactation, to provide care that complements the unfolding processes involved.

### KEY POINTS

- The neurohormonal basis of labour commences during the last trimester of pregnancy.
- Processes of preparation for, initiation and continuation of labour are controlled by maternal and fetoplacental systems.
- A good understanding of current findings aids in the provision of care to complement the dynamic changes that occur from late pregnancy until the onset of lactation.
- Current evidence suggests that a peaceful, quiet and private birthing environment is important to facilitate spontaneous, labour, birth and early contact.

## REFERENCES


Allport VC, Pieber D, Slater DM, et al: Human labour is associated with nuclear factor-κB activity which mediates cyclo-oxygenase-2 expression and is involved with the 'functional progesterone withdrawal', *Molecular Human Reproduction* 7(6):581–586, 2001.

Amash A, Holcberg G, Sheiner E, et al: Lipopolysaccharide differently affects prostaglandin $E_2$ levels in fetal and maternal compartments of perfused human term placenta, *Prostaglandins and Other Lipid Mediators* 88:18–22, 2009.

Ambrus G, Rao CV: Novel regulation of pregnant human myometrial smooth muscle cell gap junctions by human chorionic gonadotrophin, *Endocrinology* 135(6):2772–2779, 1994.

Bartels A, Zeki S: The neural correlates of maternal and romantic love, *NeuroImage* 21:1155–1166, 2004.

Ben-Davis S, Zuckerman-Levin N, Epelman M, et al: Parturition itself is the basis for fetal adrenal involution, *Journal of Clinical Endocrinology and Metabolism* 92(1):93–97, 2007.

Benirschke K: Placental separation at birth. In Polin RA, Fox WW, editors: *Fetal and neonatal physiology*, Philadelphia, 1992, Saunders, pp 95–96.

Bennett P, Allport V, Loudon J, et al: Prostaglandins, the fetal membranes and the cervix, *Frontiers of Hormone Research* 27:147–164, 2001.

Blackburn ST: *Maternal, fetal & neonatal physiology*, Missouri, 2007, Saunders.

Bland RD: Loss of liquid from the lung lumen in labour: more than a simple 'squeeze', *American Journal of Physiology* 280(4):L602–L605, 2001.

Blanks AM, Vatish M, Allen MJ, et al: Paracrine oxytocin and estradiol demonstrate a spatial increase in human intrauterine tissues with labour, *Journal of Clinical Endocrinology and Metabolism* 88(7):3392–3400, 2003.

Bleker OP, Kloosterman GJ, Mieras DJ, et al: Intervillous space during uterine contractions in human subjects: an ultrasonic study, *American Journal of Obstetrics and Gynecology* 123(7):697–699, 1975.

Bloomfield TH, Gordon H: Reaction to blood loss at delivery, *Journal of Obstetrics and Gynecology* 10(Suppl 2):S13–S16, 1990.

Boldt T, Luuhleainen P, Tyhrquist F, et al: Birth stress increases adrenomedullin in the newborn, *Acta Paediatrica* 87(1):93–94, 1998.

Brown CH, Grattan DR: Does maternal oxytocin protect the fetal brain? *Trends in Endocrinology and Metabolism* 18(6):225–226, 2007.

Brunton PA, Russell JA: The expectant brain: adapting for motherhood, *Nature Reviews. Neuroscience* 9:11–25, 2008.

Brunton PA, Russell JA, Douglas AJ, et al: Adaptive responses of the maternal hypothalamic-pituitary-adrenal axis during pregnancy and lactation, *Journal of Neuroendocrinology* 20:764–776, 2008.

Bukowski R, Hankins GDV, Saade GR, et al: Labour-associated gene expression in the human uterine fundus, lower segment and cervix, *PLoS Medicine* 3(6):918–928, 2006.

Burghardt RC, Barhoumi R, Dookwah H: Endocrine regulation of myometrial gap junctions and their role in parturition, *Seminars in Reproductive Endocrinology* 11(3):250–260, 1993.

Bystrova K, Widstrom A-M, Mattheisen A-S, et al: Skin-to-skin contact may reduce negative consequences of 'the stress of being born': a study on temperature in newborn infants, subjected to different ward routines in St Petersburg, *Acta Paediatrica* 92(3):320–326, 2003.

Carvajal JA, Vidal RJ, Cuello MA, et al: Mechanisms of paracrine regulation by fetal membranes of human uterine quiescence, *Journal of the Society for Gynaecological Investigation* 13(5):343–349, 2006.

Carvajal JA, Delpiano AM, Cuello MA, et al: Brain natriuretic peptide (BNP) produced by human chorioamnion may mediate pregnancy myometrial quiescence, *Reproductive Sciences* 16(1):32–42, 2009.

Casey ML, Smith J, Alsabrook G, et al: Activation of adenylyl cyclase in human myometrial smooth muscle cells by neuropeptides, *Journal of Clinical Endocrinology and Metabolism* 82(9):3087–3092, 1997.

Chan E-C, Smith R, Lewin T, et al: Plasma corticotrophin-releasing hormone, β-endorphin and cortisol inter-relationships during human pregnancy, *Acta Endocrinologica* 128:339–344, 1993.

Chen DC, Nommsen-Rivers L, Dewey KG, et al: Stress during labour and delivery and early lactation performance, *American Journal of Clinical Nutrition* 68(2):335–344, 1998.

Chibbar R, Wong S, Miller FD, et al: Estrogen stimulates oxytocin gene expression in human chorio-decidua, *Journal of Clinical Endocrinology and Metabolism* 80(2):567–572, 1995.

Chow L, Lye SJ: Expression of the gap junction protein connexin-43 is increased in the human myometrium toward term and with the onset of labour, *American Journal of Obstetrics and Gynecology* 170(3):788–795, 1994.

Christensson K, Cabrera T, Christensson E, et al: Separation distress call in the human neonate in the absence of maternal body contact, *Acta Paediatrica* 84(5):468–473, 1995.

Condon JC, Jeyasuria P, Faust JM, et al: A decline in the levels of progesterone receptor coactivators in the pregnant uterus at term may antagonize progesterone receptor function and contribute to the initiation of parturition, *Proceedings of the National Academy of Sciences of the United States of America* 100(16):9518–9523, 2003.

Cootauco AC, Murphy JD, Maleski J, et al: Atrial natriuretic peptide production and natriuretic peptide receptors in the human uterus and their effects on myometrial relaxation, *American Journal of Obstetrics and Gynecology* 199:429.e1–429.e6, 2008.

Dalaker K: Clotting factor VII during pregnancy, delivery and puerperium, *British Journal of Obstetrics and Gynaecology* 93:17–21, 1986.

de Kock CPJ, Wierda KDB, Bosman LWJM, et al: Somatodendritic secretion in oxytocin neurons is upregulated during the female reproductive cycle, *Journal of Neuroscience* 23(7):2726–2734, 2003.

de Vries AC: Interaction among social environment, the hypothalamic-pituitary-adrenal axis, and behavior, *Hormones and Behavior* 41:405–413, 2002.

Diaz S, Seron-Ferre M, Cardenas H, et al: Circadian variation of basal plasma prolactin, prolactin response to suckling, and length of amenorrhoea in nursing women, *Journal of Clinical Endocrinology and Metabolism* 68(5):946–955, 1989.

Dong Y-L, Fang L, Kondapaka S, et al: Involvement of calcitonin gene-related peptide in the modulation of human myometrial contractility during pregnancy, *Journal of Clinical Investigation* 104(5):559–565, 1999.

Dong Y-L, Wimalawansa SJ, Yallampalli C: Effects of steroid hormones on calcitonin gene-related peptide receptors in cultural human myometrium, *American Journal of Obstetrics and Gynecology* 188(2):466–472, 2003.

Douglas AJ: Baby on board: do responses to stress in the maternal brain mediate adverse pregnancy outcome? *Frontiers in Neuroendocrinology* 31(3):359–376, 2010.

Douglas AJ, Bicknell RJ, Leng G, et al: β-Endorphin cells in the arcuate nucleus: projections to the supraoptic nucleus and changes in expression during pregnancy and parturition, *Journal of Neuroendocrinology* 14:768–777, 2002.

Douglas AJ, Meddle SL, Toschi N, et al: Reduced activity of the noradrenergic system in the paraventricular nucleus at the end of pregnancy: implications for stress hyporesponsiveness, *Journal of Neuroendocrinology* 17:40–48, 2005.

Dunn P: The third stage and fetal adaptation. In Clinch J, Matthews T, editors: *Perinatal Medicine*, Lancaster, 1985, MIT Press, pp 47–54.

Erlandsson K, Fagerberg I: Mothers' lived experiences of co-care and part-care after birth, and their strong desire to be close to their baby, *Midwifery* 21:131–138, 2005.

Ferguson JE, Seaner RM, Bruns DE, et al: Expression and specific immunolocalization of the human parathyroid hormone/parathyroid hormone-related protein receptor in the uteroplacental unit, *American Journal of Obstetrics and Gynecology* 179(2):321–329, 1998.

Fetalvero KM, Zhang P, Shyu M, et al: Prostacyclin primes pregnant human myometrium for an enhanced contractile response in parturition, *Journal of Clinical Investigation* 118(12):3966–3979, 2008.

Fowden AL, Apatu RSK, Silver M: The glucogenic capacity of the fetal pig: developmental regulation by cortisol, *Experimental Physiology* 80:457–467, 1995.

Freemark M: The fetal adrenal and the maturation of the growth hormone and prolactin axes, *Endocrinology* 140(5):1963–1965, 1999.

Fuchs A-R, Fuchs F: Physiology of parturition. In Gabbe SG, editor: *Obstetrics, normal and problem pregnancies*, New York, 1991, Churchill Livingstone, pp 147–174.

Fuchs A-R, Fuchs F, Husslein P, et al: Oxytocin receptors and human parturition: a dual role for oxytocin in the initiation of labour, *Science* 215:1396–1398, 1982.

Fuchs A-R, Fuchs F, Husslein P, et al: Oxytocin receptors in the human uterus during pregnancy and parturition, *American Journal of Obstetrics and Gynecology* 150(6):734–741, 1984.

Fuchs A-R, Romero R, Keefe D, et al: Oxytocin secretion and human parturition: pulse frequency and duration increase during spontaneous labour, *American Journal of Obstetrics and Gynecology* 165(5):1515–1523, 1991.

Fuchs A-R, Behrens O, Liu H-C: Correlation of nocturnal increase in plasma oxytocin with a decrease in plasma estradiol/progesterone ratio in late pregnancy, *American Journal of Obstetrics and Gynecology* 167(6):1559–1563, 1992.

Fujii M, Umezawa K, Arta A: Adrenaline contributes to prenatal respiratory maturation in rat medulla-spinal cord preparation. *Brain Research* 1090:45–50, 2006.

Gao L, Liu C, Xu C, et al: Differential regulation of prostaglandin production mediated by corticotrophin-releasing hormone receptor type 1 and 2 in cultured placental trophoblasts, *Endocrinology* 149(6):2866–2876, 2008.

Garbrecht MR, Klein JM, Schmidt TJ, et al: Glucocorticoid metabolism in the human fetal lung: implications for lung development and the pulmonary surfactant system, *Biology of the Neonate* 89:109–119, 2006.

Gee H: *Uterine activity and cervical resistance determining cervical change in labour*, MD Thesis, Liverpool, 1981, University of Liverpool.

Gee H, Olah KS: Failure to progress in labour. In Studd J, editor: *Progress in obstetrics and gynaecology*, Vol 10, Edinburgh, 1993, Churchill Livingstone, pp 159–181.

Germain AM, Valenzuela GJ, Ivankovic M, et al: Relationship of circadian rhythms of uterine activity with term and preterm delivery, *American Journal of Obstetrics and Gynecology* 168(4):1271–1277, 1993.

Gintzler AR, Liu N-J: The maternal spinal cord: biochemical and physiological correlates of steroid-activated antinociceptive processes, *Progress in Brain Research* 133:83–97, 2001.

Goland RS, Wardlaw SL, Stark RI, et al: High levels of corticotrophin-releasing hormone immunoreactivity in maternal and fetal plasma during pregnancy, *Journal of Clinical Endocrinology and Metabolism* 63(5):1199–1203, 1986.

Goland RS, Jozak RN, Conwell I: Placental corticotrophin-releasing hormone and the hypercortisolism of pregnancy, *American Journal of Obstetrics and Gynecology* 171(4):1287–1291, 1994.

Grammatopoulos DK: The role of CRH receptors and their agonists in myometrial contractility and quiescence during pregnancy and labour, *Frontiers in Bioscience* 12:561–571, 2007.

Grammatopoulos D: Placental corticotrophin-releasing hormone and its receptors in human pregnancy and labour: still a scientific enigma, *Journal of Neuroendocrinology* 20:432–438, 2008.

Grammatopoulos DK, Hillhouse EW: Activation of protein kinase C by oxytocin inhibits the biological activity of the human myometrial corticotrophin-releasing hormone receptor at term, *Endocrinology* 140(2):585–594, 1999.

Grammatopoulos D, Stirrat GM, Williams SA, et al: The biological activity of the corticotrophin-releasing hormone receptor–adenylate cyclase complex in human myometrium is reduced at the end of pregnancy, *Journal of Clinical Endocrinology and Metabolism* 81(2):745–751, 1996.

Grattan DR: Behavioural significance of prolactin signalling in the central nervous system during pregnancy and lactation, *Reproduction* 123:497–506, 2002.

Gubbay O, Critchley HO, Bowen JM, et al: Prolactin induces ERK phosphorylation in epithelial and $CD56^+$ natural killer cells of the human endometrium, *Journal of Clinical Endocrinology and Metabolism* 87(5):2329–2335, 2002.

Gyte G: The significance of blood loss at delivery, *MIDIRS Midwifery Digest* 2(1):88–92, 1992.

Haddad PF, Morris NF, Spielberge CD: Anxiety in pregnancy and its relation to use of oxytocin and analgesia in labour, *Journal of Obstetrics and Gynaecology* 6:77–81, 1985.

Havelock JC, Keller P, Muleba N, et al: Human myometrial gene expression before and during parturition, *Biology of Reproduction* 72:707–719, 2005.

Hay WW: Metabolic interrelationships of placenta and fetus, *Placenta* 16(1):19–30, 1995.

Henderson D, Wilson T: Reduced binding of progesterone receptor to its nuclear response element after human labour onset, *American Journal of Obstetrics and Gynecology* 185(3):579–585, 2001.

Herrera E: Metabolic adaptations in pregnancy and their implications for the availability of substrates to the fetus, *European Journal of Clinical Nutrition* 54(Suppl 1):S47–S51, 2000.

Higuchi T, Okere CO: Role of supraoptic nucleus in regulation of parturition and milk ejection revisited, *Microscopy Research and Technique* 56:113–121, 2002.

Hillhouse EW, Grammatopoulos DK: Control of intracellular signalling by corticotrophin-releasing hormone in human myometrium, *Frontiers of Hormone Research* 27:66–74, 2001.

Hirst JJ, Chibbar R, Mitchell BF: Role of oxytocin in the regulation of uterine activity during pregnancy and in the initiation of labour, *Seminars in Reproductive Endocrinology* 11(3):219 233, 1993.

Hodnett ED, Gates S, Hofmeyr GJ, et al: Continuous support for women during childbirth (Cochrane Review). In: *The Cochrane Library*, Issue 1, Chichester, 2008, John Wiley.

Hofer MA: Early relationships as regulators of infant physiology and behaviour, *Acta Paediatrica* 397:9–18, 1994.

House M, Bhadelia RA, Myers K, et al: Magnetic resonance imaging of three-dimensional cervical anatomy in the second and third trimester, *European Journal of Obstetrics and Gynaecology and Reproductive Biology* 144S:S65–S69, 2009.

Hytten F: *The clinical physiology of the puerperium*, London, 1995, Farrand Press.

Inch S: *Birthrights*, London, 1989, Merlin Press.

Ito T, Nomura S, Okada M, et al: Transcriptional regulation of human placental leucine aminopeptidase/oxytocinase gene, *Molecular Human Reproduction* 7(9):887–894, 2001.

Jaffe RB: Role of the human fetal adrenal gland in the initiation of parturition, *Frontiers of Hormone Research* 27:75–85, 2001.

Jain L, Dudell GG: Respiratory transition in infants delivered by cesarean section, *Seminars in Perinatology* 30:296–304, 2006.

Johnson KC, Davis B-A: Outcomes of planned home births with certified professional midwives: large prospective study in North America, *British Medical Journal* 330:1416–1422, 2005.

Johnson MH: *Essential Reproduction*, ed 6, Oxford, 2007, Blackwell Scientific.

Johnson RF, Rennie N, Murphy V, et al: Expression of glucocorticoid receptor messenger ribonucleic acid transcripts in the human placenta at term, *Journal of Clinical Endocrinology and Metabolism* 93(12):4887–4893, 2008.

Johnston JM, Amico JA: A prospective longitudinal study of the release of oxytocin and prolactin in response to infant suckling in long term lactation, *Journal of Clinical Endocrinology and Metabolism* 62(4):653–657, 1986.

Kask K , Backstrom T, Gulinello M, et al: Lower level of prepulse inhibition of startle response in pregnant women compared to postpartum women, *Psychoneuroendocrinology* 33:100–107, 2008.

Kawamata M, Tonomura Y, Kimura T, et al: Oxytocin-induced phasic and tonic contractions are modulated by contractile machinery rather than the quantity of oxytocin receptor, *American Journal of Physiology* 292:E992–E999, 2007.

Keelan JA, Blumenstein M, Helliwell RJA, et al: Cytokines, prostaglandins and parturition – a review, *Placenta* 17(Suppl A):S33–S46, 2003.

Khazipov R, Tyzio R, Ben-Air Y: Effects of oxytocin on GABA signalling in the foetal brain during delivery, *Progress in Brain Research* 170:243–257, 2008.

Kimura T, Takemura M, Nomura S, et al: Expression of oxytocin receptor in human pregnant myometrium, *Endocrinology* 137(2):780–785, 1996.

Kinsley CH: The neuroplastic maternal brain, *Hormones and Behavior* 54:1–4, 2008.

Klein DF, Skrobala AM, Garfield RS: Preliminary look at the effects of pregnancy on the course of panic disorders, *Anxiety* 1:227–232, 1995.

Komisaruk BR, Sansone G: Neural pathways mediate vaginal function: the vagus nerves and spinal cord oxytocin, *Scandanavian Journal of Psychology* 44:241–250, 2003.

Lagercrantz H, Herlenius E: Neurotransmitters and neuromodulators. In Lagercrantz H, Hanson M, Evrard P, et al, editors: *The Newborn Brain*, Cambridge, 2002, Cambridge University Press, pp 139–165.

Lee KA, Gay CL: Sleep in late pregnancy predicts length and type of delivery, *American Journal of Obstetrics and Gynaecology* 191:2041–2046, 2004.

Lee SE, Romero R, Park I-S, et al: Amniotic fluid prostaglandin concentrations increase before the onset of spontaneous labour, *Journal of Maternal-Fetal & Neonatal Medicine* 21(2):89–94, 2008.

Letsky EA: The haematological system. In Chamberlain G, Broughton Pipkin F, editors: *Clinical physiology in obstetrics*, Oxford, 1998, Blackwell Science, pp 71–110.

Levinson G, Shnider SM: Catecholamines: the effects of maternal fear and its treatment on uterine function and circulation, *Birth and the Family Journal* 6(3):167–174, 1979.

Liggins GC: The role of cortisol in preparing the fetus for birth, *Reproduction Fertility and Development* 6:141–150, 1994.

Lindstrom TM, Bennett PR: The role of nuclear factor kappa B in human labour, *Reproduction* 130:569–581, 2005.

Liu N-J, Gintzler AR: Facilitative interactions between vasoactive intestinal polypeptide and receptor type-selective opioids; implications for sensory afferent regulation of spinal opioid action, *Brain Research* 959:103–110, 2003.

Lucas BK, Ormandy CJ, Binart N, et al: Null mutation of the prolactin receptor gene produces a defect in maternal behaviour, *Endocrinology* 139(10):4102–4107, 1998.

McLean M, Bistits A, Davies J, et al: A placental clock controlling the length of human pregnancy, *Nature Medicine* 1(5):460–463, 1995.

Majzoub JA, Karalis KP: Placental corticotrophin-releasing hormone: function and regulation, *American Journal of Obstetrics and Gynecology* 180(1):S242–S246, 1999.

Markovic D, Vatish M, Giu M, et al: The onset of labour alters corticotrophin-releasing hormone type 1 receptor variant expression in human myometrium: putative role of interleukin-1β, *Endocrinology* 148(7):3205–3213, 2007.

Matijevic R, Meekins JW, McFaden IR, et al: Physiological changes of spiral arteries and blood flow in the placental bed during early pregnancy, *Contemporary Reviews in Obstetrics and Gynaecology* 8:127–131, 1996.

Matthiesen A-S, Ransjo-Arvidson A-BR, Nissen E, et al: Postpartum maternal oxytocin release by newborns: effects of infant hand massage and suckling, *Birth* 28(1):13–19, 2001.

Mesiano S: Roles of estrogen and progesterone in human parturition, *Frontiers of Hormone Research* 27:75–85, 2001.

Mesiano S, Welsh TN: Steroid hormone control of myometrial contractility and parturition, *Seminars in Cell and Developmental Biology* 18:321–331, 2007.

Mesiano S, Chan E-C, Fitter JT, et al: Progesterone withdrawal and estrogen activation in human parturition are coordinated by progesterone receptor A expression in the myometrium, *Journal of Clinical Endocrinology and Metabolism* 87(6):2924–2930, 2002.

Monks DA, Lonstein JS, Breedlove SM: Got milk? Oxytocin triggers hippocampal plasticity, *Nature Neuroscience* 6(4):327–328, 2003.

Moore TR, Iams JD, Creasy RK, et al: Diurnal and gestational patterns of uterine activity in normal human pregnancy, *Obstetrics and Gynecology* 83(4):517–523, 1994.

Moore RM, Mansour JM, Redline RW, et al: The physiology of fetal membrane rupture: insights gained from the determination of physical properties, *Placenta* 27:1037–1051, 2006.

Moriceau S, Sullivan RM: Maternal presence serves as a switch between learning fear and attraction in infancy, *Nature Neuroscience* 9(8):1004–1006, 2006.

Murphy Goodwin T: A role for estradiol in human labour, term and preterm, *American Journal of Obstetrics and Gynaecology* 180(1):S208–S213, 1999.

Myatt L, Lye SJ: Expression, localization and function of prostaglandin receptors in myometrium, *Prostaglandins, Leukotrienes and Essential Fatty Acids* 70:1337–1348, 2004.

Nathanielsz PW, Berghorn KA, Derks JB, et al: Life before birth: effects of cortisol on future cardiovascular and metabolic function, *Acta Paediatrica* 92:766–772, 2003.

Neumann ID: The advantage of living social: brain neuropeptides mediate the beneficial consequences of sex and motherhood, *Frontiers in Neuroendocrinology* 30:483–496, 2009.

Nomura S, Ito T, Yamamoto E, et al: Gene regulation and physiological function of placenta leucine aminopeptidase/oxytocinase during pregnancy, *Biochimica et Biophysica Acta* 1751:19–25, 2005.

Norman JE, Thompson AJ, Greer IA: Cervical ripening after nitric oxide, *Human Reproduction* 13:251–252, 1998.

Noort WA, van Bulck B, Vereecken A, et al: Changes in plasma levels of $PGF_{2\alpha}$ and $PGI_2$ metabolites at and after delivery at term, *Prostaglandins* 37(1):3–12, 1989.

Odent M: The fetus ejection reflex, *Birth* 14(2):104–108, 1987.

Odent M: *The nature of birth and breastfeeding*, Westport, 1992, Bergin & Garvey.

Ohel I, Walfisch A, Shitenberg D, et al: A rise in pain threshold during labour: a prospective clinical trial, *Pain* 132:S104–S108, 2007.

Olah KS, Gee H, Brown JS: Cervical contractions: the response of the cervix to oxytocic stimulation in the latent phase of labour, *British Journal of Obstetrics and Gynaecology* 100:635–640, 1993.

Ortiz-Miranda S, Dayanithi G, Custer E, et al: Micro-opioid receptor preferentially inhibits oxytocin release from neurohypophysial terminals by blocking R-type Ca2+ channels, *Journal of Neuroendocrinology* 17:583–590, 2005.

Owman C: Pregnancy induces degenerative and regenerative changes in the autonomic innervation of the female reproductive tract. In Elliot K, Lawrence G, editors: *Development of the autonomic nervous system*, London, 1981, Pitman Medical, pp 252–279.

Pajntar M: The smooth muscles of the cervix in labour, *European Journal of Obstetrics and Gynaecology and Reproductive Biology* 55(1):9–12, 1994.

Pearson Murphy BE, Branchaud CL: The fetal adrenal. In Tulchinsky D, Little AB, editors: *Maternal–fetal endocrinology*, Philadelphia, 1994, Saunders, pp 275–295.

Pedersen CT, Boccia ML: Oxytocin links mothering received, mothering bestowed and adult stress responses, *Stress* 5(4):259–367, 2002.

Peled G: Birth and the Gulf War, *MIDIRS Midwifery Digest* 3(1):54, 1993.

Pepe GJ, Albrecht ED: Actions of placental and fetal adrenal steroid hormones in primate pregnancy, *Endocrine Reviews* 16(5):608–648, 1995.

Phaneuf S, Rodriguez Linares B, TanbyRaja RL, et al: Loss of myometrial oxytocin receptors during oxytocin-induced and oxytocin-augmented labour, *Journal of Reproduction and Fertility* 120:91–97, 2000.

Price SA, Lopez Bernal A: Uterine quiescence: the role of cyclic AMP, *Experimental Physiology* 86(2):265–272, 2001.

Rehman K, Sirianni R, Parker R, et al: The regulation of adrenocorticotrophic hormone receptor by corticotrophin-releasing hormone in human fetal adrenal definitive/transitional zone cells, *Reproductive Sciences* 14(6):578–587, 2007.

Robinson C, Schumann R, Zhang P, et al: Oxytocin-induced desensitization of the oxytocin receptor, *American Journal of Obstetrics and Gynaecology* 188(2):497–502, 2003.

Robson SC, Dunlop W, Boys RJ, et al: Cardiac output during labour, *British Medical Journal* 295(6607):1169–1172, 1987.

Rosen T, Krikun G, Ma Y, et al: Chronic antagonism of nuclear factor-κB activity in cytotrophoblasts by dexamethasone: a potential mechanism for anti-inflammatory action of glucocorticoids in human placenta, *Journal of Clinical Endocrinology and Metabolism* 83(10):3647–3652, 1998.

Rossoni E, Feng J, Tirozzi B, et al: Emergent synchronous bursting of oxytocin neuronal network, *PLoS Computational Biology* 4(7):e1000123, 2008.

Rudel D, Pajntar M: Contractions of the cervix in the latent phase of labour, *Contemporary Reviews in Obstetrics and Gynaecology* 11(4):271–279, 1999.

Russell JA, Brunton PJ: Neuroactive steroids attenuate oxytocin stress responses in late pregnancy, *Neuroscience* 138:879–889, 2006.

Russell JA, Brunton PJ: Oxytocin (peripheral/central actions and their regulation). In Bloom F, Squire LF, Spitzer N, editors: *Encyclopedia of neuroscience*, Amsterdam, 2009, Elsevier, pp 337–347.

Russell JA, Leng G, Douglas AJ: The magnocellular oxytocin system, the fount of maternity: adaptations in pregnancy, *Frontiers in Neuroendocrinology* 249(1):27–61, 2003.

Saisto T, Kaaja R, Ylikorkala O, et al: Reduced pain tolerance during and after pregnancy in women suffering from fear of labour, *Pain* 93:123–127, 2001.

Sansone GR, Gerdes CA, Steinman JL, et al: Vaginocervical stimulation releases oxytocin within the spinal cord in rats, *Neuroendocrinology* 75:306–315, 2002.

Sarrieau A, Sharma S, Meaney MJ: Postnatal development and environmental regulation of hippocampal glucocorticoid and mineralocorticoid receptors, *Brain Research* 471:158–162, 1988.

Schlabritz-Loutsevitch N, Middendorf HR, Muller D, et al: The human myometrium as a target for melatonin, *Journal of Clinical Endocrinology and Metabolism* 88(2):908–913, 2003.

Sharkey JT, Puttaramu R, Word A, et al: Melatonin synergizes with oxytocin to enhance contractility of human myometrial smooth muscle cells, *Journal of Clinical Endocrinology and Metabolism* 94(2):421–427, 2009.

Sheehan PM, Rice GE, Moses EK, et al: 5β-reductase decrease in association with human parturition at term, *Molecular Human Reproduction* 11(7):495–501, 2005.

Shmygol A, Gullam J, Blanks A, et al: Multiple mechanisms involved in oxytocin-induced modulation of myometrial contractility, *Acta Pharmacologica Sinica* 27(7):827–832, 2006.

Shynlova O, Tsui P, Jaffer S, et al: Integration of endocrine and mechanical signals in the regulation of myometrial functions during pregnancy and labour, *European Journal of Obstetrics & Gynaecology and Reproductive Biology* 144(Suppl 1):S2–S10, 2009.

Shynlova O, Tsui P, Jaffer S: Integration of endocrine and mechanical signals in the regulation of myometrial functions during pregnancy and labour, *European Journal of Obstetrics & Gynaecology and Reproductive Biology* 1445:S2–S10, 2009.

Smith R: Parturition, *New England Journal of Medicine* 356:271–283, 2007.

Sparey C, Robson SC, Bailey J, et al: The differential expression of myometrial connexin-43, cycloxygenase-1 and -2, and Gs alpha proteins in the upper and lower segments of the human uterus during pregnancy and labour, *Journal of Clinical Endocrinology and Metabolism* 84(5):1705–1710, 1999.

Stern JM: Offspring-induced nurturance: animal–human parallels, *Developmental Psychobiology* 31:19–37, 1997.

Stevens MY, Challis JRG: Corticotrophin-releasing hormone receptor subtype 1 is significantly up-regulated at the time of labour in the human myometrium, *Journal of Clinical Endocrinology and Metabolism* 83(11):4107–4115, 1998.

Swain JE, Tasgin E, Mayes LC, et al: Maternal brain response to own baby-cry is affected by cesarean section delivery, *Journal Child Psychology and Psychiatry* 49(10):1042–1052, 2008.

Takemura M, Kimura T, Nomura S, et al: Expression and localization of human oxytocin receptor mRNA and its protein in chorion and decidua during parturition, *Journal of Clinical Investigation* 93:2319–2323, 1994.

Tamura H, Nakamura Y, Terron MP, et al: Melatonin and pregnancy in the human, *Reproductive Toxicology* 25:291–303, 2008.

Terzidou V, Soporanna SR, Kim LU, et al: Mechanical stretch up-regulates the human oxytocin receptor in primary human uterine myocytes, *Journal of Clinical Endocrinology and Metabolism* 90(1):237–246, 2005.

Ticconi C, Zicari A, Realacci M, et al: Oxytocin modulates nitric oxide generation by human fetal membranes at term pregnancy, *American Journal of Reproductive Immunology* 52:185–191, 2004.

Ticconi C, Belmonte A, Piccione E, et al: Feto-placental communication system with the myometrium in pregnancy and parturition: the role of hormones, neurohormones, inflammatory mediators, and locally active factors, *Journal of Maternal-Fetal & Neonatal Medicine* 19(3):125–133, 2006.

Tomizawa K, Iga N, Lu Y-F, et al: Oxytocin improves long-lasting spatial memory during motherhood through MAP kinase cascade, *Nature Neuroscience* 6(4):384–390, 2003.

Tyson EK, Smith R, Read M: Evidence that corticotrophin-releasing hormone modulates myometrial contractility during human pregnancy, *Endocrinology* 150(12):5617–5625, 2009.

Tyzio R, Cossart R, Khalilov I, et al: Maternal oxytocin triggers a transient inhibitory switch in GABA signalling in the fetal brain during delivery, *Science* 314:1788–1792, 2006.

Vaisanen-Tommiska M, Nuutila M, Aittomaki K, et al: Nitric oxide metabolites in cervical fluid during pregnancy: further evidence for the role of cervical nitric oxide in cervical ripening, *American Journal of Obstetrics and Gynecology* 188(5):779–785, 2003.

Whipple B, Josimovich JB, Komisaruk BR: Sensory thresholds during the antepartum, intrapartum, and postpartum periods, *International Journal of Nursing Studies* 27(3):213–221, 1990.

Willcourt RJ, Pager D, Wendel J, et al: Induction of labour with pulsatile oxytocin by computer-controlled pump, *American Journal of Obstetrics and Gynecology* 170(2):603–608, 1994.

Wuitchik M, Bakal D, Lipshitz J: The clinical significance of pain and cognitive activity in latent labour, *Obstetrics and Gynecology* 73(1):35–42, 1989.

Yildirim G, Beji NK: Effects of pushing techniques in birth on mother and fetus: a randomized study, *Birth* 35:25–30, 2008.

Zuo J, Lei ZM, Rao CV, et al: Differential cycloxygenase-1 and -2 gene expression in human myometria from preterm and term deliveries, *Journal of Clinical Endocrinology and Metabolism* 79(3):894–899, 1994.

Chapter |36|

# Care in the first stage of labour

Denis Walsh

## LEARNING OUTCOMES

After reading this chapter, you will be able to:

- understand the importance of the context of childbirth
- recognize the onset of labour and appreciate the normal physiology of labour
- provide evidence-based care appropriate to the needs of the woman and her baby
- understand principles such as woman-centred care
- have insight into the key roles of environment and relationships with carers
- have an awareness of the holistic elements of labour care.

## INTRODUCTION

Labour and birth are an amazing integration of powerful physiological and psychological forces that bring a new human life into the world. It is difficult not to devalue labour and birth when it is analysed, dissected and examined in order to make it understood, as it works best as a coherent whole. There are key physical, emotional and social dimensions to the process of labour, in that the arrival of a baby heralds the birth or extension of a family. Throughout history, labour and birth had special meaning for every culture and their occurrence is often marked by spiritual and cultural symbols (Kitzinger 2000). In the UK today, such rituals have been marginalized by the medical environment in which most parturition takes place, with about 95% of births occurring in consultant units, 2.5% at home (Richardson & Mmata 2007) and 2.5% in free-standing midwifery-led units (Walsh 2007a). For the midwife, a holistic understanding of labour and birth requires an awareness of the physiological/psychological changes and ability to see these remarkable events as deeply social and even political. This perspective has, as a starting point, *a profound respect for and trust in women's innate ability to birth without technology or medical intervention*. The chapter will attempt to describe the changes, the events and the care from these philosophical positions.

Two birth stories (Case scenarios 36.1 and 36.2) reveal the complexity of labour and birth.

The midwife's description of these births shows how the experience of labour can vary for different women. The time spans were different – the first in excess of 24 hours and the second had a 'rest phase' of 4 hours prior to the birth. The women adapted to their experience in contrasting ways – one confident and controlled, the other feeling swamped by the power of her labour. In neither case is the midwife's role described, but different strategies of support would have been required to care appropriately for each woman.

Other aspects are key to assisting our understanding of these births. Both babies were born at home. Both women had people in attendance whom they knew and had chosen to be there. Neither woman had any drugs, nor common birth interventions. They did it 'naturally'. Their births were not typical of 21st-century childbirth experience in the UK. More typically, childbirth occurs in hospital with carers who have not been previously met, using routine interventions including continuous electronic fetal monitoring. One in three results in an instrumental vaginal delivery or a caesarean section (Richardson & Mmata 2007). It could be argued that normal labour and birth is under threat, with only about 47% of women in

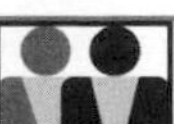

**Case scenario 36.1**

**Emily's birth story**

Emily was a 'no-nonsense' sort of person. She approached the birth of her first baby in a straightforward way. 'I'll know what to do at the time', she kept telling me. 'You just tag along and I'll ask if I need anything.' She called me out one Sunday morning and when I arrived told me her labour had started, and although she didn't want me to do anything, she asked me to stay for a few hours. Later, she said I could go as she had hours to go yet. She called me again early the next morning and said it was time for the baby to come. I drove over to her house, and 2 hours later her son was born into the birthing pool and there were tears all round. Emily was in tune with her body. She understood it and how the birth process would go for her far better than I did.

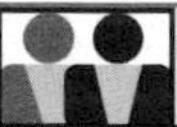

**Case scenario 36.2**

**Judy's birth story**

Judy just avoided induction of labour because she was 13 days past her due date when her waters broke. The contractions arrived 8 hours later and were huge from the start. Despite fantastic support from Ben, her partner, she felt out of control with the labour's intensity. Her cervix was 7 cm dilated when she requested a vaginal examination 2 hours later. After an hour, her contractions became even more intense and I suspected she was approaching the pushing phase. Then suddenly, everything stopped. She dozed on and off for 4 hours, when suddenly she was bearing down and the baby was born within two contractions. Judy felt traumatized by her rollercoaster ride, which she felt swept along by.

England having a drug-free normal birth (Richardson & Mmata 2007).

Being in hospital requires conforming to an environment where the woman inevitably becomes a 'patient' and carers assume the status of experts. Labour is expected to conform to protocols and policies designed for the 'average', triggering a range of interventions if deviation occurs from this 'average'. This chapter explores normal labour and birth from the perspective of non-intervention, viewing the birth environment as crucial to physiological processes. Having a baby in hospital may be viewed as a 'care intervention', likely to upset a delicate balance of physical, psychological and social processes that need to work in harmony for birth to be humane and life-enhancing.

## THE CONTINUUM OF LABOUR

Labour has been traditionally divided into stages but this demarcation has its origins in a preoccupation with the time duration of each stage and its historical link to complications for the mother and baby. When learning about labour, practitioners are introduced to notions of time at the outset, which is consistent with a biomedical understanding of parturition that anticipates pathology in an effort to treat it as early as possible.

An alternative approach is beginning to gain exposure through the writings of midwives like Downe & McCourt (2008), where labour is a continuum from onset to completion, characterized by particular physiological and psychological behaviours at various points on that continuum. Some of these behaviours are anatomical changes, for example, changes in the cervix; some are physiological, such as release of body hormones; and some psychological, such as an alertness and focusing just prior to birth.

Individual behaviours and responses vary, and the importance of knowing and intuitively connecting with women is a key challenge for the midwife and allows care to be appropriate and tailored to individual need.

Although the demarcations of the stages of labour in the traditional biomedical model are intended to aid clarity in understanding physiology and care for the professional caregiver, they may also effectively silence the woman and discredit her version of events. For the woman, labour is a continuing physiological, psychological and emotional experience, the culmination and main focal point of the reproductive process, where artificial compartmentalization may be neither relevant nor important. The significance of labour, a biologically and socially creative life event, is reflected in the minutiae of detail women can recall about their particular labour(s). Events that are relatively common and usual from a midwife's perspective, acquire much meaning and importance in the eyes of the woman and her family. To maximize the potential for a satisfactory outcome of labour, it is therefore essential that women's stories and details of events are listened to and valued.

**Reflective activity 36.1**

Ask your mother about your birth and note the phrases she uses to describe it, the memories that have stayed with her and the overall impression of the experiences that she communicates to you. If you are not able to do this, ask another woman that you know well to talk about her birth experience.

If the midwife anticipates a normal outcome to labour and birth, and trusts the woman's physiology will function optimally, this can impact positively on the woman's own attitude. Women with an optimistic demeanour towards childbirth have better experiences and outcomes than

**Table 36.1 Approximate time taken for each stage of labour**

| | Primigravidae | Multigravidae |
|---|---|---|
| First stage | 12–14 hours | 6–10 hours |
| Second stage | 60 minutes | Up to 30 minutes |
| Third stage | 20–30 minutes, or 5–15 minutes with active management | 20–30 minutes, or 5–15 minutes with active management |

those beset by anxiety and fear of what could go wrong (Green et al 1998). Midwives play a key role in empowering women as they approach childbirth.

## CHARACTERISTICS OF LABOUR

Normal labour naturally follows a sequential pattern that involves painful regular uterine contractions stimulating progressive effacement and dilatation of the cervix with descent of the fetus through the pelvis, culminating in the spontaneous vaginal birth of the baby, followed by the expulsion of the placenta and membranes. This traditional and orthodox biomedical definition of normal labour divides labour into three stages, and designates maximum time frames, depending on a woman's parity, as shown in Table 36.1:

- *First stage:* from the onset of regular uterine contractions, accompanied by effacement of the cervix and dilatation of the os, to full dilatation of the os uteri.
- *Second stage:* from full dilatation of the os uteri to the birth of the baby.
- *Third stage*: from the birth of the baby to the expulsion of the placenta and membranes.

The social model is more holistic and has contrasting values to the biomedical model (Table 36.2).

The alternative values of the social model mean that the *strenuous work* of labour is acknowledged as fundamental. Gould (2000) acknowledged this along with the crucial role of *movement*. This highlights the courage and perseverance demonstrated by women as they 'work' during labour and the importance of an environment where movement will be facilitated.

## PHYSIOLOGY OF LABOUR

Several physiological factors integrate as labour develops (Box 36.1), and these will be examined in turn.

**Table 36.2 Medical and social model**

| Medical model | V | Social model |
|---|---|---|
| Body as machine | | Whole person |
| Reductionism – powers, passages, passenger | | Integrate – physiology, psychosocial, spiritual |
| Control and subjugate | | Respect and empower |
| Expertise/objective | | Relational/subjective |
| Environment peripheral | | Environment central |
| Anticipate pathology | | Anticipate normality |
| Technology as master | | Technology as servant |
| Homogenization | | Celebrate difference |
| Evidence | | Intuition |
| Safety | | Self-actualization |

(Walsh & Newburn 2002)

**Box 36.1 Summary of the physiological changes in the first stage of labour**

- *Completion of effacement of the cervix and dilatation of the os uteri caused by uterine activity:*
  - Contraction and retraction of uterine muscles
  - Fundal dominance
  - Active upper uterine segment, passive lower segment
  - Formation of the retraction ring
  - Polarity of the uterus
  - Intensity or amplitude of contractions
  - Resting tone
- Formation of the bag of *forewaters* and the *hindwaters*
- *Rupture* of the membranes
- *Show*

### Cervical effacement and dilatation

These occur as a result of contraction and retraction of the uterine muscle.

*Effacement* (taking up) of the cervix may start in the latter 2 or 3 weeks of pregnancy and occurs as a result of changes in the solubility of collagen present in cervical tissue. This is influenced by alterations in hormone activity, particularly oestradiol, progesterone, relaxin, prostacyclin and prostaglandins (Blackburn 2007). Braxton Hicks contractions, which become stronger in the final weeks of pregnancy, may also enhance the process. Effacement is completed in labour, the cervix becomes shorter and dilates slightly, becoming funnel shaped as the internal os opens to form part of the lower uterine segment (see Fig. 36.1).

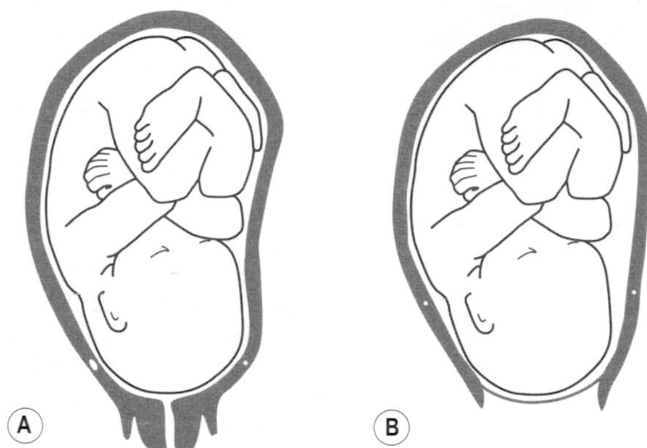


**Figure 36.1** The uterus, showing: **A.** cervix before effacement; and **B.** effacement and dilatation of the cervix and the stretched lower uterine segment.

Progressive dilatation of the cervix (see Fig. 36.2) is a definitive sign of labour.

When the cervix is dilated sufficiently to allow the fetal head to pass through, full dilatation has been achieved. Although this is usually 10 cm, it may be more or less depending on the size of the fetal head.

In primigravidae, effacement of the cervix usually precedes dilatation; however, in multigravidae, effacement and dilatation of the cervix normally occur simultaneously (see Fig. 36.2).

## Uterine contractions

Uterine contractions are responsible for achieving progressive effacement and dilatation of the cervix and for the descent and expulsion of the fetus in labour. Contractions of the uterus in labour are:

- involuntary
- intermittent and regular
- in almost all labours, painful.

The pain may be due in part to ischaemia developing in the muscle fibres during contractions. The backache which may accompany cervical dilatation is caused by

A 1

Cervical canal before effacement (Before labour)

2

Partial effacement

B 1

3

Cervix effaced and dilating

4

Cervix nearly fully dilated

2

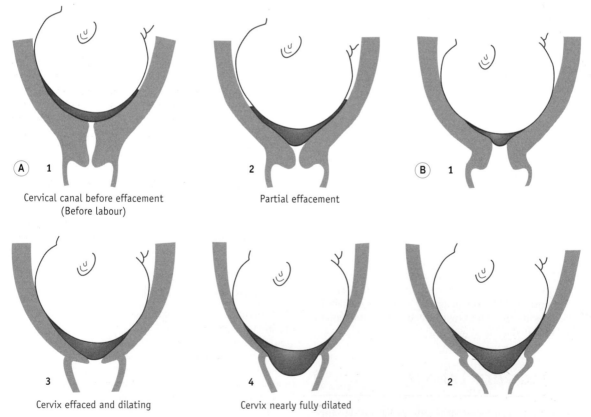

**Figure 36.2** Effacement and dilatation of the cervix: **A.** in a primigravida; **B.** occurring simultaneously in a multigravida.

stimulation of sensory fibres which pass via the sympathetic nerves to the sacral plexus.

## Coordination of contractions

Contractions start from the cornua of the uterus, passing in waves, inwards and downwards. In normal uterine action, the intensity is greatest in the upper uterine segment and lessens as the contraction passes down the uterus. This is called *fundal dominance*. The upper segment of the uterus contracts and retracts powerfully, whereas the lower segment contracts only slightly and dilates. Between contractions the uterus relaxes.

The coordinated uterine activity characteristic of normal labour occurs as a result of near-simultaneous contraction of all myometrial cells. During pregnancy, increasing numbers of gap junctions form between the cells of the myometrium. These low-resistance communication channels enhance electrical conduction velocity and facilitate the coordination of myometrial contraction (Blackburn 2007).

## Retraction

Retraction is a state of permanent shortening of the muscle fibres and occurs with each contraction (see Fig. 36.3).

The muscle fibres gradually become shorter and thicker, especially in the upper uterine segment. This exerts a pull on the less-active lower uterine segment, the maximum pull being directed towards the weakest point, the cervix, and the os uteri. Hence the cervix is gradually 'taken up', or effaced, and the upward pull then dilates the os uteri.

As the space within the upper uterine segment diminishes with the contraction and retraction of the muscle fibres, the fetus is forced down into the lower segment and the presenting part exerts pressure on the os uteri. This aids dilatation, and also causes a reflex release of oxytocin from the posterior pituitary gland, promoting further uterine action. A ridge gradually forms between the thick, retracted muscle fibres of the upper uterine segment and the thin, distended lower segment. This is called a *retraction ring* – a normal physiological occurrence in every labour.

## Polarity

The rhythmical coordination (*polarity*) between the upper and lower segments is balanced and harmonious in normal labour. While the upper segment contracts powerfully and retracts, the lower segment contracts only slightly and dilates.

## Intensity or amplitude

Contractions cause a rise in intrauterine pressure – the *intensity* or *amplitude* of contractions – which can be measured by placing a fine catheter into the uterus and attaching it to a pressure-recording apparatus. Each contraction rises rapidly to a peak and then slowly declines to the resting tone. In early labour the contractions are weak, with an amplitude of about 20 mmHg, last 20–30 seconds and occur without any particular pattern. As labour progresses, the contractions become stronger, longer and more frequent. At the end of the first stage they are strong, with an amplitude of 60 mmHg, last 45–60 seconds and occur every 2–3 minutes.

## Resting tone

The uterus is never completely relaxed, and between contractions a measured resting tone is usually 4–10 mmHg. During contractions the blood flow to the placenta is curtailed; thus, oxygen and carbon dioxide exchange in the intervillous spaces is impeded. The period of relaxation between contractions when the uterus has a low resting tone is therefore vital for adequate fetal oxygenation.

## Formation of the forewaters and hindwaters (Fig. 36.4)

As the lower uterine segment stretches and cervical effacement commences, some chorion becomes detached from

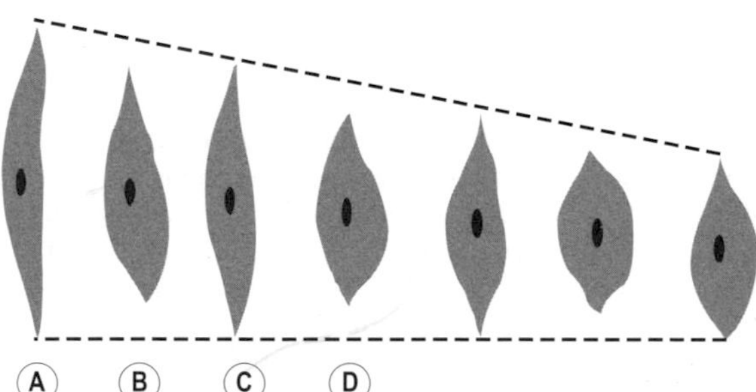


**Figure 36.3** Retraction of the uterine muscle fibres: **A.** relaxed; **B.** contracted; **C.** relaxed but retracted; **D.** contracted but shorter and thicker than those in B.

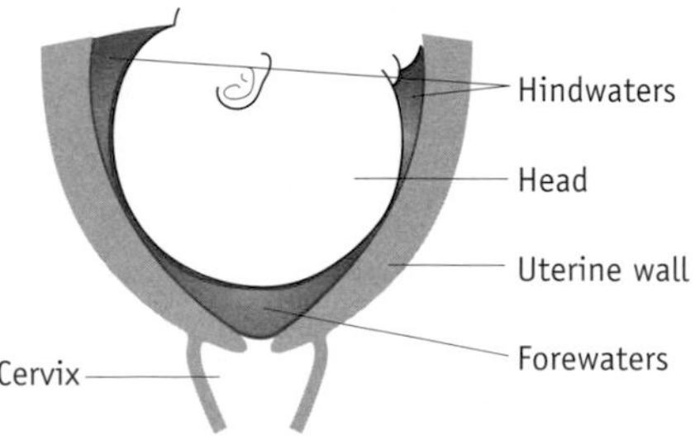


**Figure 36.4** Formation of hindwaters and forewaters.

the decidua and both membranes form a small bag containing amniotic fluid, which protrudes into the cervix. When the fetal head descends onto the cervix, it separates the small bag of amniotic fluid in front, the *forewaters*, from the remainder, the *hindwaters*. The forewaters aid effacement of the cervix and early dilatation of the os uteri, and the hindwaters help to equalize the pressure in the uterus during uterine contractions, providing some protection to the fetus and placenta.

## Rupture of the membranes

The membranes are thought to rupture as a result of increased production of prostaglandin $E_2$ in the amnion in labour (McCoshen et al 1990) and the force of the uterine contractions, causing an increase in the fluid pressure inside the forewaters and a lessening of the support as the cervix dilates. In normal labour the membranes usually rupture during the second stage of labour.

## Show

The 'show' is the *operculum* from the cervical canal passed per vaginam in labour, displaced when effacement of the cervix and dilatation of the os uteri occur. It is usually mucoid and slightly streaked with blood due to some separation of the chorion from the decidua around the cervix.

There is increasingly awareness of the relationship between oxytocin release and the level of catecholamines (see Ch. 35). Anxiety and fear stimulate the release of adrenaline (epinephrine) and noradrenaline (norepinephrine), and inhibit oxytocin; hence the importance of birth environment and birth relationships in promoting calm and confidence in birthing women.

# CARE DURING THE FIRST STAGE OF LABOUR

The aims of midwifery care in labour are to achieve a safe labour and birth for mother and baby, and a pleasurable, fulfilling experience of childbirth for the mother and her partner.

Now that deaths in childbirth for women and babies in the western world are rare, women's experience of childbirth has taken on greater significance and has become a major focus for the professionals assisting childbirth. Most early research on labour and birth did not explore women's experiences and was based around professionals' priorities and their interests. Recent studies have determined women's views on various aspects of care (Lally et al 2008, Redshaw et al 2007, Rudman et al 2007) and these can be summarized under the following themes:

- information that is full, accurate, evidence-based, individualized
- choice
- control
- continuity.

These themes should underpin the philosophy of care and its application, helping to define woman-centred care, as described and endorsed in maternity care policy at government level (DH 2007a, 2007b).

In order to provide woman-centred care, the midwife should:

1. assess the needs and expectations of each individual woman regarding labour and birth
2. plan care with each woman in labour, tailored to meet her specific needs and expectations
3. put the care plan into practice
4. evaluate the care given to measure its effectiveness.

## Partnership in care

The relationship between the woman and her midwife is ideally a partnership (Pairman 2000) which should begin in pregnancy, and has been described as 'skilled companionship' or the 'professional friend' in its intimacy and reciprocity (Page 1995). The partnership ethos requires a social rather than medical model of maternity care, endorsing the involvement of the woman and her partner in decision-making, and requiring the woman to be able to voice her needs and wishes freely. The midwife should strive to build a relationship of mutual trust and create an environment in which expectations, wishes, fears and anxieties can be readily discussed. This requires good communication, which results from a two-way interaction between equals.

## Emotional and psychological care

The midwife needs to have a good understanding of a woman's feelings in labour. Attitudes and reactions to childbirth vary considerably and are influenced by differing social, cultural and religious factors. For a multigravida, previous experience of birth will also be important.

Many women anticipate labour with mixed feelings of fear and excitement. Some may eagerly anticipate the birth, confident in their ability to cope, seeing birth as an emotionally fulfilling and enriching experience involving all immediate family members. They may have attended teaching sessions for natural or active childbirth and have a particular plan of action for their labour. Others may be excited at the prospect of actually seeing their baby, yet fearful of labour and anxious about their ability to cope with pain and 'perform' well. Some expect labour to be painful and unpleasant, controlled by obstetricians and midwives to be achieved with as little pain and active participation as possible.

The woman may be apprehensive about entering an unknown, and perhaps threatening, hospital environment and concerned about relinquishing her personal autonomy and identity. Alternatively, expectations of labour may be unrealistic, and may be unfulfilled, leading to feelings of disappointment, failure or loss. Multigravidae are often anxious about children they have left at home. The midwife can do much to alleviate these worries.

Birth partners may also have particular concerns which they feel unable to share. Reservations may be influenced by the role society attributes to gender – a man being expected to be strong and able to cope; or may be due to fear of the unknown and concern for someone who is loved. With a partnership and individual approach to care, particularly if established during the antenatal period, the midwife has a valuable opportunity to encourage the couple to voice their particular needs and anxieties, and explore and agree ways of dealing with them. Whatever the needs of the individual couple, they are usually influenced by the desire to do what is best for their baby and, if they are confident that the midwife will respect and comply with their wishes in normal circumstances, they will usually readily agree to modify expectations should problems arise.

Throughout labour there should be a free flow of information between the woman, her partner and the midwife, particularly in relation to examinations and their findings. Being fully informed and involved in decision-making helps the woman to retain a sense of autonomy and control (Healthcare Commission 2008). The midwife should be aware that not all individuals may feel sufficiently secure or freely able to express fears or anxieties during labour. Circumstances such as an unwanted pregnancy, fear or previously poor relationships with professional caregivers may engender feelings of unhappiness, hostility and resentment. The midwife needs to be particularly sensitive to non-verbal indicators of such feelings and give the necessary help and support needed by the woman.

## The role of the birth supporter

Evidence from a number of studies indicates the positive effect of continuous support in labour (Hodnett et al 2008a). Although it is usual in the UK for a couple to support each other in labour, some women may choose to have a relative, friend, or labour supporter from a voluntary organization, such as the National Childbirth Trust (NCT), as labour companions. Whoever has been chosen, the midwife should explore with supporters their experiences of childbirth, their role expectations during labour and their ability to undertake the supporter role. It has been suggested that if chosen supporters have had negative childbirth experiences, these need to be addressed by the midwife if they are not to hinder the supporting relationship with the woman.

The midwife involves the birth supporter as part of the team, with a defined role, which can include massaging back, abdomen or legs, helping with breathing awareness and relaxation, and offering drinks and other means of sustenance. Such activities, during a highly anxious time, can be very valuable in helping the partner to feel usefully occupied and involved in the birthing event.

The midwife must be sensitive to the possible need for personal space and privacy and should judge when, and if, it is appropriate to leave the woman and partner alone. This is usually more acceptable in early labour but less so when labour is strong and well advanced, when to be left alone might be frightening. If the midwife must leave for a short period, she must ensure that the couple can summon help if necessary. The midwife must also be sensitive to the emotional needs of the partner and other members of staff and recognize that, particularly during a long labour, a short break may be beneficial in helping to replenish energy levels.

## Advocacy

For some women, fear of the unknown, being cared for in hospital by unfamiliar people, greater pain than expected or the effect of analgesic drugs can cause feelings of vulnerability, loss of personal identity, and powerlessness. This may be magnified for women for whom English is not their first language. Vulnerable individuals can lose the ability to adequately express their needs, wishes, values and choices and adopt a passive recipient role. The midwife may need to act as advocate, in order to ensure that personal needs are met (Walsh 2007b). This includes informing, supporting and protecting women, acting as intermediary between them and obstetric and other professional colleagues, and facilitating informed choice. In order to achieve this, the midwife must be professionally confident, have a clear awareness of the woman's needs, and be able to communicate these to other colleagues to ensure effective collaboration. Developing and trusting *intuition* is central to this activity. The midwife's rapport and connectedness with the woman for whom she is caring mean that appropriate decision-making and a facilitatory birth environment is more likely (Walsh 2007a). Using these skills, the midwife is more able to empower the woman and her partner so that they feel sufficiently informed and confident to participate in decision-making during this important life experience.

## BIRTH ENVIRONMENT

Practitioners of normal birth and women themselves know how significant the birth environment is for the experience and outcomes of birth, including the birth setting, the relational components of care, and congruence of values about birth.

## Home

Home birth has long generated an intense debate, and birth at home has become a rallying point for midwives and women who endorse childbirth's essential normality against those who can only view its normality retrospectively. Tew (1998) first challenged the dominant 1970's/1980's view that the safest environment for birth was hospital. She exposed the fundamental flaw of assigning a single cause (hospitalization of birth) to a discrete effect (lowering perinatal mortality rates) without consideration of alternative explanations. This spurious logic had led to a nationwide movement of birth to hospitals over 20 years before an alternative explanation gained credibility – that the fall was due to the dramatic improvement in the general health of women in the post-war period coupled with an even more dramatic rise in living standards (Campbell & McFarlane 1994, Tew 1998).

It is now acknowledged that current evidence does not provide justification for requiring that all women give birth in hospital (Olsen & Jewell 2006) and that women should be offered an explicit choice when they become pregnant of where they want to have their baby (DH 2007a). A comprehensive literature review of home birth research, which included 26 studies from many parts of the developed world, concluded that 'studies demonstrate remarkably consistency in the generally favourable results of maternal and neonatal outcomes, both over time and among diverse population groups' (Fullerton & Young 2007:323). The outcomes were also favourable when viewed in comparison to various reference groups (birth-centre births, planned hospital births).

Randomized controlled trials (RCTs) have demonstrated clear benefit in a number of associated elements of the home birth 'package of care', including continuity of care during labour and birth (Hodnett et al 2008) and midwife-led care (Hatem et al 2008), both of which are probably universal aspects of home birth provision.

Though official UK government policy up to the present is to offer women a choice about place of birth, the UK home birth rate remains just above 2%, compared with 25% in the early 1960s (Chamberlain et al 1997). There are anecdotal stories of women either being discouraged from choosing the home birth option or being told that staff shortages may impact on the availability of midwives.

One practical measure to reduce the bias to hospital birth may be to keep the option for home birth open until labour begins. Requiring a firm decision in early pregnancy regarding home birth may be problematic. Some women:

- may develop complications during pregnancy which require hospital care
- have access to midwifery support at home in early labour and may prefer to stay there rather than face an uncomfortable journey to hospital.

## Birth centres or midwifery-led units

Free-standing birth centres as an option for women are especially relevant now (see Chs 32 & 34). Maternity services across the UK are merging, driven by the growth of neonatal tertiary referral centres and by rationalizing of management and clinical structures of individual hospitals that are no longer seen as cost-effective if they remain separate. These pressures are leading to stakeholders choosing to combine birth facilities on one site with neonatal services or retain present infrastructures and open midwifery-led units or birthing units (DH 2007b). The current trend appears to favour the first option, potentially resulting in further centralization of birth, in some areas up to 10,000 births per year in a single hospital, mirroring the controversial process in the 1980s, during which many small hospitals and isolated GP units closed, since lamented by midwives and user lobby groups.

Research and evaluation is needed to establish whether expansion is appropriate, as currently, service providers and clinicians are drawing from a pool of methodologically flawed papers. There are currently no RCTs and a paucity of good-quality research on free-standing birth centres or midwifery-led units. A structured review found these environments lowered childbirth interventions but methodological weaknesses in all studies made conclusions tentative (Walsh & Downe 2004), findings echoed by Stewart et al's (2005) commissioned review. This model, endorsed by the Department of Health in England, reflects policy thinking that free-standing birth centres would be unlikely to have worse outcomes than home birth (DH 2007a).

Evaluations of integrated birth centres or alongside midwifery-led units have shown no statistical difference in perinatal mortality, suggesting encouraging results for the reduction in some labour interventions (Hodnett et al 2010). Debate continues regarding the noted non-significant trend in some of the studies of higher perinatal mortality for first-time mothers (Fahy 2005, Tracey et al 2007). This is unlikely to be resolved until contextual studies exploring the interface at transfer or impact of contrasting philosophies is examined in depth.

**Reflective activity 36.2**

During your course/practice, search out opportunities to see birth in environments alternative to hospital, such as in women's homes, birth centres or in midwifery-led units.

Qualitative literature on home birth and free-standing birth centres highlights two other aspects of care: how temporality is enacted and how smallness of scale impacts on the ethos and ambience of care. The regulatory effect of clock time is less evident both at home and in birth centres. Labour rhythms rather than labour progress tend to be emphasized by staff and there is usually greater flexibility with the application of the labour record, the partogram (Fig. 36.5). Part of the reason for this lies in the absence of an organizational imperative to 'get women through the system' (Walsh 2006a). Small numbers of women birthing mean less stress on organizational processes and a more relaxed ambience in the setting. This appears to suit women and staff well, suggesting attunement to labour physiology, inherently manifesting as biological rhythms based on hormonal pulses of activity, rather than regular clock time rhythms (Adam 1995). This increases the perception of clinical

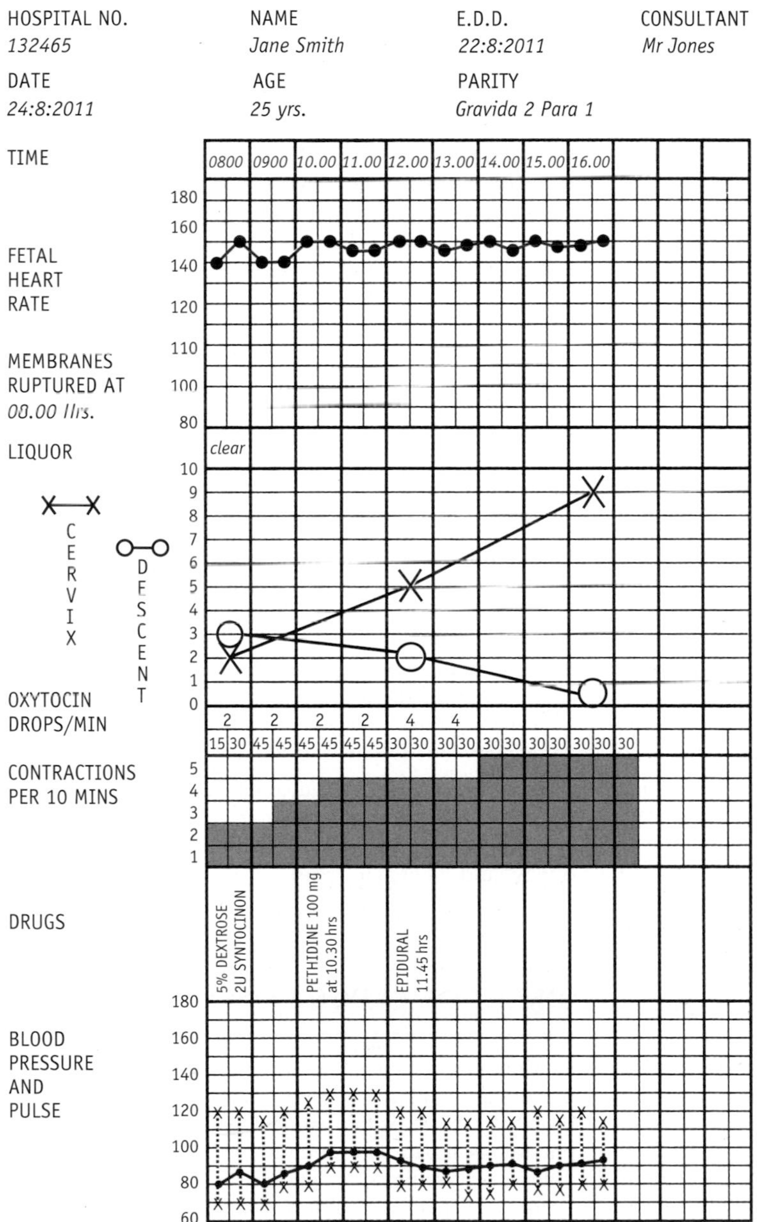


**Figure 36.5** A partogram.

freedom, satisfaction and feeling of belonging for midwives (Walsh 2006b).

Significant research undertaken into different organizational models of midwifery care including teams, caseloads and midwifery group practices has been premised on the principle that women benefit from establishing an ongoing relationship with their carers rather than being cared for by strangers within a fragmented model. Common sense may suggest that journeying through such significant rites of passage in the experience of childbirth is best done in the company of known carers. Even without the studies, it could be argued that indigenous birth practices have much to inform maternity care in the west. For thousands of years, traditional birth attendants working with local women have harnessed the power of known birth companions in facilitating birth for the uninitiated woman. Western-style birth lost this crucial dimension when birth was hospitalized and supported by professionals who were usually unknown to labouring women. After the advent of doulas in US hospitals in the late 1970s, recognition was given to this fundamental aspect of labour care.

Doula studies examined the value of being supported throughout the entire labour and this aspect of care has now been extensively researched. A systematic review of nine RCTs (Hodnett et al 2007) concluded that continuous support during labour:

- reduced caesarean sections, pharmacological analgesia, assisted vaginal birth, low Apgar scores and labour length
- resulted in women experiencing more positive births
- could provide the most effective support from those not employed by the institution
- will be less effective in a highly medicalized environment.

A review of eight studies of labour support provided by five different categories of persons concluded that care by *known*, untrained laywomen, starting in early labour, was most effective (Rosen 2004). A study echoing childbirth physiology found that oxytocin was released in women exposed to stress and this triggered 'tending' and 'befriending' behaviours rather than the classical (male) response of 'fight and flight'. In a further mirroring of the hormonal cascade of labour, endogenous opiates, also released during the experience of stress, augment these effects (Taylor et al 2000).

The *number* of carers a woman has during her period of continuous support may also be relevant to outcome, as caesarean section rates appear to increase in direct line with increasing number of carers. Keeping the number of changes of labour support persons to a minimum has been recommended (Gagnon et al 2007).

Midwives have argued for decades to provide continuous support in labour so that they can genuinely be 'with woman'. It is likely that this organizational aspect alone would increase normal birth rates substantially. Yet achieving this goal remains an objective rather than an imperative for most maternity services.

Continuity has been the subject of research and debate in midwifery for two decades. Examination of wider health literature reveals that continuity has been of interest for many other areas, summarized by Haggerty et al (2003) as being centred on:

- informational continuity (patient story available to all relevant agencies)
- management continuity (consistent, coherent care)
- relational continuity (known carers).

All three contribute to a better patient experience and, arguably, better care. Midwifery care has focused more on *relational continuity*, possibly believing that the other two will follow, though this may not be the case. A case can be made for this focus because of the unique features of the midwife/woman relationship: its biologically determined longevity, its journey through a major rites of passage experience, and the intimate nature of its focus.

There are many organizational variants of continuity of care in midwifery services, including: named midwife, teams, caseloads, group practices. Research has suggested:

- Teams should number no more than six because, as numbers increase, 'a known midwife' becomes 'someone met once or twice' to eventually 'someone spoken of by a colleague' and continuity becomes meaningless (Flint 1993).
- Continuity needs differ depending on phases of care. Keeping the number of carers to a minimum may be more important for labour and the postnatal period than antenatally (Green et al 1998).
- Continuity between phases, especially having a known midwife for labour, is highly valued by women (Walsh 1999) and reduces labour interventions (NSCCRT 2000, Page et al 1999).

In relation to clinical outcomes and satisfaction with care, team and continuity variants generally reduce interventions, including epidural, induction of labour, episiotomy and neonatal resuscitation rates, and improve satisfaction.

## ONSET OF LABOUR

Physiological changes occuring in late pregnancy are described in Chapter 35 and lead to signs heralding the onset of labour. Some women will follow a particular physiological pattern, but allowance should be made for individual variations, which may be associated with differences in pain perception and response, parity, and expectations of labour. These factors must be considered by the midwife in assisting the woman to recognize when she is in labour.

## Uterine contractions

Women become aware of the painless, irregular, *Braxton Hicks* contractions of pregnancy which increase as pregnancy advances. In labour these become regular and painful. Initially the woman may experience minimal discomfort and complain of sacral and/or lower abdominal pain, not necessarily immediately associated with labour. Such discomfort may later be noted to coincide with tightening or tension of the abdomen, occurring at regular intervals of 20–30 minutes and lasting 20–30 seconds. These uterine contractions can be paplpated by the midwife on abdominal palpation. As labour progresses, contractions become longer, stronger and more frequent, resulting in progressive effacement and dilatation of the cervix.

## Show

This mucoid, often blood-stained, discharge is passed per vaginam, representing the passage of the operculum which previously occupied the cervical canal. This is indicative of a degree of cervical activity – that is, softening and stretching of tissues, causing separation of the membranes from the decidua around the opening of the internal os. The show is often the first sign that labour is imminent or has started.

## Rupture of the membranes

Rupture of the membranes can occur before labour or at any time during labour (see Ch. 35). Although significant, it is not a true sign of labour unless accompanied by dilatation of the cervix. An estimated 6–19% of women at term will experience spontaneous rupture of the membranes before labour starts (Tan & Hannah 2002) and in 85% of women the membranes rupture spontaneously at a cervical dilatation of 9 cm or more (Schwarcz et al 1977). The amount of amniotic fluid lost when the membranes rupture depends largely on how effectively the fetal presentation assists in the formation of the forewaters. In the presence of a normal amount of amniotic fluid, if the head is not engaged in the pelvis and the presenting part is not well applied to the os uteri, rupture of the membranes is easily recognized by a significant loss of fluid. If the presenting part is engaged and well applied, rupture of the forewaters may result in minimal fluid loss. This is usually followed by further seepage of amniotic fluid, which may be mistaken for urinary incontinence (not uncommon in late pregnancy). Usually the woman's history or evidence of amniotic fluid confirms the rupture of the membranes.

## Contact with the midwife

Changing patterns of care reflect recent research highlighting the importance of consistent advice and continuity of care for this early phase of labour (Walsh 2007b). The woman should therefore be advised to contact the midwife when regular contractions are recognized, the membranes rupture, or if she is concerned for any reason.

Clear and written instructions, given well in advance of the expected date of birth, including relevant telephone numbers of the community or team midwives and their location, are necessary and useful for anxious partners/birth supporters.

If the woman does not know the midwife, the midwife must be aware of the sensitivity of the first meeting and the importance of the initial interaction with the woman, which forms the basis for their future relationship. Women experience a variety of conflicting emotions and it is important that at the initial meeting, the midwife makes a rapid assessment of the woman and context in order to prioritize her care.

Information should be calmly and sensitively sought, allowing sufficient time for the woman to express her feelings and identify needs. In particular, a woman's story of how labour started should be validated, not dismissed as not fitting with what the textbooks say (Gross et al 2003). The midwife can achieve a relaxed, confident and reassuring approach, while acquiring the necessary information and enabling the woman's verbal contribution to be valued, fostering the desired supportive partnership in care.

Prior to examining the woman, the midwife should review the woman's notes and ensure that all required information is present. The birth plan should indicate the special needs and wishes of the woman and her partner and can assist in providing continuity of care and may provide reassurance to the woman that her particular needs and wishes are recorded for staff caring for her to see. Such plans may also be instrumental in enabling the woman to retain control of labour events and can provide the midwife with a valuable opportunity for health education in relation to birth.

# OBSERVATIONS

## General examination

The midwife assesses the woman's appearance and demeanour, looking for features of general health and wellbeing. Observations of temperature, pulse, blood pressure and urinalysis are undertaken, providing a baseline for the labour. Recommendations regarding the frequency of recording the vital signs in labour are based on tradition rather than evidence. Commonly, the temperature and blood pressure are recorded 4-hourly with pulse hourly (NICE 2007).

## Abdominal examination

A detailed abdominal examination is carried out, between contractions, to determine the lie, presentation, position and level of engagement of the presenting part. This must be a gentle process, avoiding pain or discomfort and involving the couple as much as possible. The lie should be longitudinal. It is also important to determine the presentation and whether the presenting part is engaged, or will engage, in the pelvis. Auscultation of the fetal heart completes the abdominal examination; it should be strong and regular with a rate of between 110 and 160 beats per minute.

## Vaginal examination

This procedure is one of the options to help confirm the onset of labour. However, it is invasive and often very uncomfortable for the woman and also poses a potential infection risk. Women may request it in seeking reassurance about the status of labour.

## Records

When labour is established, all observations, examinations and any drug treatment are recorded on the partogram, enabling observations to be detailed on one sheet (see Fig. 36.5). The midwife's record constitutes a legal document, and throughout labour, accurate, concise and comprehensive records must be maintained in accordance with the midwives' rules and record-keeping guidance (NMC 2004, 2009). Notations must be made at the time of the event, or as near as possible, and authenticated with the midwife's full, legible signature and status.

Contemporaneous records also facilitate continuity of care in the event that care has to be transferred to another member of the team.

# GENERAL MIDWIFERY CARE IN LABOUR

## Assessment of progress

Labour progression has been the focus of extensive research over the past 40 years, though generally suffers from contextual narrowness, having been exclusively carried out in large maternity hospitals. This limits the ability to premise writing on conventional evidence sources and undermines attempts to explain the rich

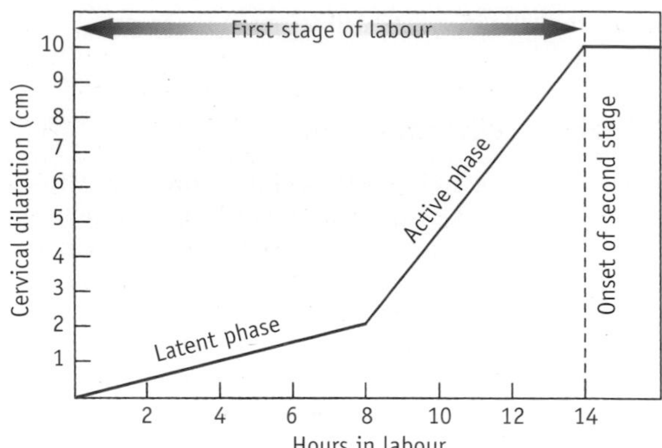


**Figure 36.6** A cervicograph.

variety of personal anecdote around individual women's labours. Research into out-of-hospital birth settings is urgently needed to explore and explain labour patterns.

### Origins of the progress paradigm

Friedman's seminal work in measuring and recording cervical dilatation over time with a cohort of women in the mid-1950s influenced understanding of average lengths of labour for primigravid and multigravid women. The resulting sigmoid-shaped Friedman curve, representing early, middle and later phases of the first stage of labour, was incorporated into obstetric and midwifery textbooks for 50 years (Friedman 1954) (Fig. 36.6).

In the early 1970s, while working in remote area of Rhodesia, concerned about the disastrous consequences of obstructed labours, Philpott & Castle (1972) added the partogram to labour records and amplified the cervicograph to give guidance regarding slow labours, with three action lines used in the active phase of the first stage of labour:

1. *Alert line* at 1 cm/hour rate – signalling the need for close monitoring.
2. *Transfer line* – 2 hours behind the alert line – need for transfer physically to a major hospital.
3. *Action line* – 2 hours behind the transfer line – rupture membranes and administer Syntocinon.

Studd (1973) measured cohorts of women admitted to UK hospitals at differing stages of labour, plotting cervical dilatation over time, raising the possibility that British women might labour at different rates to African or North American women.

### Organizational factors

This clinical imperative that long labours could indicate pathology may not have gained credence without the changes in organizational structures in how maternity care was delivered, in particular the centralizing movement of the second half of the 20th century. With more women giving birth in larger hospitals, organizational pressure increased towards processing women through delivery suites and postnatal wards. Martin (1987) railed against assembly-line childbirth in the 1980s, and Perkin's (2004) comprehensive and considered critique of US maternity care policy, likening the Henry Ford car assembly line to the organization of maternity hospital activity, highlighted the explicit adoption of an essentially business/industrial model by maternity hospitals.

A study of childbirth at a free-standing birth centre (FSBC) in the UK (Walsh 2006a) highlighted temporal differences as being the most striking factor differentiating the FSBC from maternity hospitals. Women's labours were not on a time line and there was no pressure to 'free up' rooms for new occupants. The corollary of hospitals with time restrictions on labour length is that more women can labour and birth within their space. It comes as little surprise to find that the hospitals still practising active management of labour are among the largest in Europe, with over 8000 births per year (Murphy-Lawless 1998). Midwives' anecdotes and ethnographic research point to the pressures that exist in big units to 'get through the work' (Hunt & Symonds 1995).

A backlash against the clinical imperative of labour progress began to appear in the late 1990s when Albers' research (1999) concluded that nulliparous women's labours were longer than suggested by Friedman. In a low-risk population of women cared for by midwives in nine different centres in the USA, some active phases of labour were twice the length of Friedman's cohort (17.5 hours v 8.5 hours for nulliparas, and 13.8 hours v 7 hours for multiparas) without any consequent morbidity. A later study found an average length of labour similar to that of Friedman but with a wider range of 'normal' (Cesario 2004). Primiparous women remained in the first stage for up to 26 hours, and multiparous women for 23 hours, without adverse effects. A recent RCT showed that if prescriptive action lines that limit labour length are used with primigravid women, then over 50% will require intervention, with the authors calling for a review of labour length orthodoxies (Lavender et al 2006).

One study examined patterns of cervical dilatation in 1329 nulliparous women, finding slower dilatation rates in the active phase, especially before 7 cm, where the slowest group were all below Friedman's 1 cm/hour threshold. Conclusions suggested that current diagnostic criteria for protracted or arrested labour may be too stringent, citing important contextual differences in current practice to Friedman's day (Zhang et al 2002). Improvement in the general health of the current generation of women compared with 50 years ago probably makes them less vulnerable to the effects of long labours.

These papers suggest more physiological variation between women than previously thought. Midwives have always known that many women do not fit the average of a 1 cm/hour dilatation rate and, more fundamentally, may not physiologically mimic the parameters of the 'average' cervix. Their cervix may be fully dilated at 9 or 11 cm. Given the infinite variety in women's physical appearance and psychosocial characteristics, it seems reasonable to expect subtle differences in their birth physiology.

Better understanding of the hormones regulating labour contributes to this more complex picture of physiological variation. Odent (2001) and Buckley (2004) illustrated that the 'hormonal cocktail' influencing these processes is appropriately called the 'dance of labour', the hormones' delicate interactions mediated by environmental and relational factors resembling the rhythm, beauty and harmony of skilled dancers.

## Rhythms in early labour

The division of the first stage of labour into latent and active is clinician-based and not necessarily resonant with the lived experience of labour, especially for women with a long latent phase. Traditionally, the latent phase of labour has been understood to be of varying length, culminating in a transition to the active phase at around 4 cm dilatation of the cervix (NICE 2007). Gross et al (2003) increased understanding of the phenomenon of early labour by revealing how eclectically it presents in different women and how they vary in their self-diagnosis: 60% of woman experienced contractions as the starting point of their labours and the remainder described a variety of other symptoms. Gross suggests the direction of questioning be changed from eliciting the pattern of contractions to simply enquiring *'How did you recognize the start of labour?'*.

The midwifery diagnosis of labour in hospital is not simply a unilateral clinical judgement but a complex blend of balancing the totality of the woman's situation with institutional constraints including workloads, guidelines, continuity concerns, justifying decisions to senior staff and risk management (Burvill 2002, Cheyne et al 2006). This can be contrasted with care at a home birth or in a FSBC, where the organizational and clinical parameters are secondary to women's lived experience and care is driven by the latter (Walsh 2006a).

Twenty-five years ago, Flint (1986) counselled that early labour was best experienced at home with access to a midwife, and this remains the ideal for low-risk women. Maternity services have realized that the worst place may be on a delivery suite, because, as research shows, this can result in more labour interventions (Hemminki & Simukka 1986, Rahnama et al 2006).

Recent studies demonstrate the value of triage facilities or early labour assessment centres if home assessment in early labour is not an option, as this results in fewer labour interventions (Lauzon & Hodnett 2004). The value of

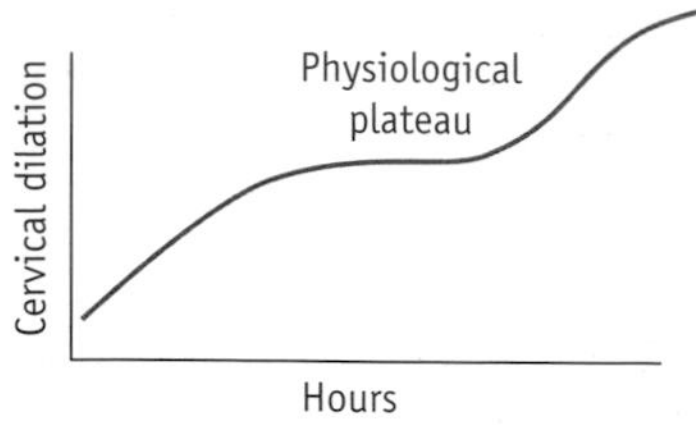


**Figure 36.7** The MANA curve. *(Davis et al 2002).*

attending an FSBC (Jackson et al 2003) and seeing a midwife rather than an obstetrician (Turnbull et al 1996) have been suggested. Individualizing care, and ongoing informational and relational continuity are all important elements of best practice for the latent phase of labour.

### Rhythms in mid labour

Midwives' understanding of the active phase of the first stage of labour has been the main focus of partogram recordings over the past 50 years. Having discussed the relaxation in timelines around this issue in recent years, the decoupling of the phenomenon of labour slowing or stopping, from the presumption that this represents pathology, can be explored. A retrospective examination of thousands of records of home birth women discovered that some had periods when the cervix stopped dilating temporarily in active labour (Davis et al 2002). This was not interpreted as pathology by birth attendants, and after variable periods of time, cervical progression began again. Apart from strong anecdotal evidence that some women experience a latent period in advanced labour, this was the first to record data on labour 'plateaus' (see Fig. 36.7).

Gaskin's (2003) description of 'pasmo' indicated that physiological delays were known about in the 19th century. Accepting the individuality of the labour experience for different women, the subtlety of hormonal interactions, and the mediating effects of environment and companions, it is entirely feasible that labour could be understood as a 'unique normality', varying from woman to woman (Downe & McCourt 2008). Midwifery skill lies in facilitating this individual expression.

Recent research into the use of differing action lines (2 hours and 4 hours behind the 1 cm/hour line) in the active phase of labour indicates that allowing for a slower rate of cervical dilatation does not result in more caesarean sections and, importantly, women are just as satisfied with longer labours (Lavender et al 2006). A cervical dilatation rate of 0.5 cm/hour in nulliparous women is now recommended (Enkin et al 2000).

## Vaginal examinations

The ubiquity of vaginal examination as a practice in labour, inextricably linked to the progress paradigm, means that the vaginal examination remains the most common procedure on labour wards. Appraisal of this common childbirth intervention is required to examine whether widespread use is justifiable. Devane's (1996) systematic literature review failed to identify the research basis for this procedure, which reveals the power of the labour progress paradigm, effectively driving adoption of the procedure on the basis of custom and practice. The literature around sexual abuse (Robohm & Buttenheim 1996) and post-traumatic stress disorder (Menage 1996) indicates that women who have experienced these find vaginal examinations very problematic. A study by Bergstrom et al (1992), based on videotaped vaginal examinations in US labour wards, revealed the ritual that has evolved around the practice in order to legitimize such an intrusion into a person's private space, showing the surgical construction of a practice undertaken by strangers, that would be totally unacceptable in any other circumstance except in an intimate sexual context between consenting adults. The adoption of a passive patient role and the marked power differential between the patient and the clinician were other taken-for-granted behaviours. In a UK-based study, similar conclusions were postulated (Stewart 2005).

Two important questions need asking before any vaginal examination is carried out (Warren 1999):

- Why do I need to know this information now?
- Is there any other way I can obtain it?

Finally, when examination is clinically justifiable, can the findings be accepted with confidence? The poor inter-observer reliability of the procedure (Clement 1994), illustrated by 'guesstimate' rather than 'estimate' scenarios of some clinical practice, may be assisted by practitioners ensuring that they undertake the examination systematically, and seek a 'second opinion' should the findings be unclear.

It is imperative that midwives approach vaginal examinations guided by negotiated and explicit consent, clear clinical justification and with sensitivity for the discomfort, embarrassment and pain that may be caused.

### Indications for vaginal examination

1. To confirm the onset of labour and establish a baseline for further progress.
2. To aid in assessing labour progress through determining the dilatation and condition of the cervix. (It is good practice to precede this with an abdominal examination to determine the fetal lie, presentation and position, the engagement or otherwise of the presentation and to auscultate the fetal heart.)
3. To diagnose the presentation when this is in doubt.
4. To rupture the membranes when necessary.

## Method

The woman is made comfortable in a semi-recumbent or lateral position with legs separated and as relaxed as possible. She can be encouraged to practice relaxation exercises. Appropriate cleansing is carried out, then the examining fingers (index and forefinger) are generously lubricated and gently inserted into the vagina.

During the examination, the midwife should note any abnormalities or deviations from normal, such as vulval varicosities, lesions (such as warts or blisters), vaginal discharge/loss, oedema and any previous scarring. She should also note the tone of the vaginal muscles and pelvic floor, and other characteristics, such as vaginal dryness or excess heat which might indicate pyrexia.

## Cervix

The cervix is assessed for consistency, effacement and dilatation (as discussed previously and in Chapter 35).

**Consistency:** The cervix is usually soft and pliable to the examining fingers. It may feel thick and is often described as having a consistency comparable to that of the lips.

**Effacement and dilatation:** The cervical canal, which usually projects into the vagina, becomes shorter, until no protrusion can be felt. This shortening, often referred to as the 'taking up' of the cervix, results from the dilatation of the internal cervical os and the gradual opening out of the cervical canal.

During and following effacement, the cervical consistency alters and it becomes progressively thinner. Complete effacement may be present in primigravidae prior to the onset of labour and prior to dilatation. In the multiparous woman, although a degree of effacement may be present prior to labour, completion of the process occurs simultaneously with cervical dilatation as labour advances.

A soft, stretchy cervix, closely in contact with the presenting part, indicates potential for normal cervical dilatation. A tight, unyielding cervix or one loosely in contact with the presenting part is less favourable and may be associated with long labour.

## Membranes

In early labour the membranes can be difficult to feel as they are usually closely applied to the head. During a contraction the increase in pressure may cause the bag of forewaters to become tense and bulge through the os uteri. The membranes may be inadvertently ruptured if pressure is applied at this time. If the head is poorly applied to the cervix, the bag of forewaters may bulge unduly early in the first stage and early rupture of membranes is likely to occur. This tends to occur with an occipitoposterior position.

## Presentation

The presentation is normally the smooth, round, hard vault of the head. Sutures and fontanelles can be felt with increasing ease as the os uteri dilates, thereby enabling confirmation of the presentation and determination of the position and attitude of the head. The degree of moulding of the fetal head can also be assessed. As labour continues, particularly if the membranes are ruptured, subsequent formation of a *caput succedaneum* may make recognition of sutures and fontanelles difficult and sometimes impossible. Rarely, a prolapsed cord may be felt as a soft loop lying in front of or alongside the fetal head. If the fetus is still alive, the cord will be felt to pulsate.

## Position

This can be determined by identification of the fontanelles and the sutures (Figs 36.8 and 36.9). An occipitoanterior position is identified by feeling the posterior fontanelle towards the anterior part of the pelvis. In an

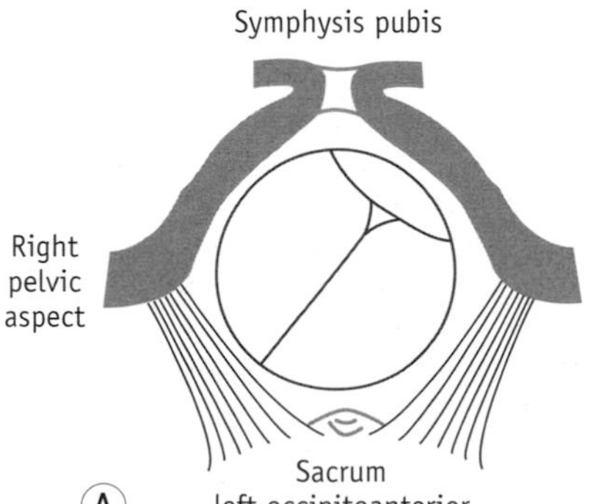


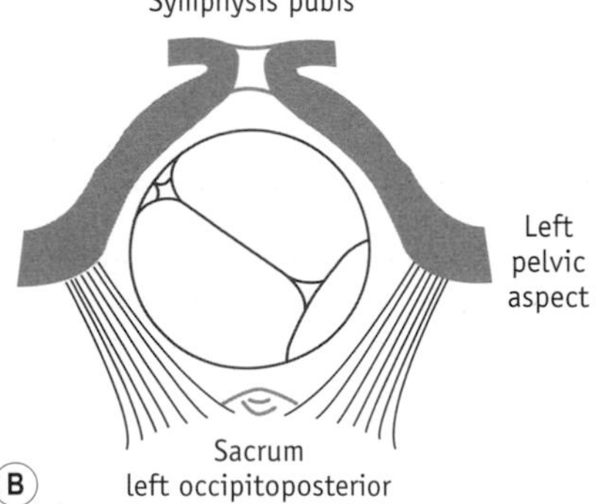


**Figure 36.8** Identifying the position of the fetus. **A.** Left occipitoanterior: the sagittal suture is in the right oblique diameter of the pelvis. **B.** Left occipitoposterior: the sagittal suture is in the left oblique diameter of the pelvis.

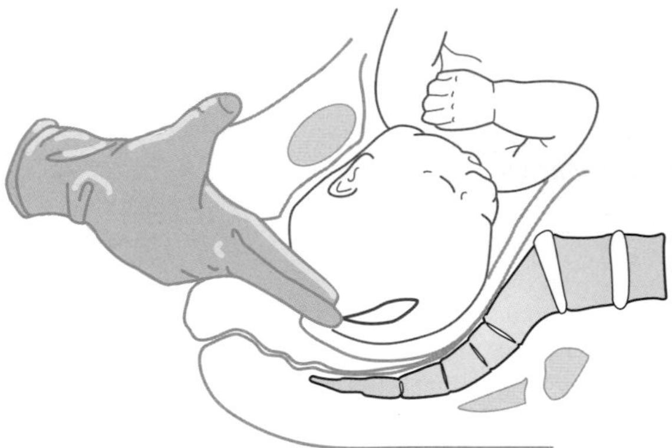

**Figure 36.9** Identifying the sagittal suture and fontanelles during vaginal examination.

**Table 36.3 Assessing the position of the fetus**

| Position of sagittal suture | Position of fontanelle | Position of fetus |
|---|---|---|
| Right oblique | Posterior fontanelle anteriorly to the left | LOA |
| | Anterior fontanelle anteriorly to the left | ROP |
| Left oblique | Posterior fontanelle anteriorly to the right | ROA |
| | Anterior fontanelle anteriorly to the right | LOP |
| Transverse diameter of the pelvis | Posterior fontanelle to the left | LOL |
| | Posterior fontanelle to the right | ROL |
| Anteroposterior diameter of the pelvis | Posterior fontanelle felt anteriorly | OA |
| | Anterior fontanelle felt anteriorly | OP |

LOA, left occipitoanterior; LOL, left occipitolateral; LOP, left occipitoposterior; OA, occipitoanterior; OP, occipitoposterior; ROA, right occipitoanterior; ROP, right occipitoposterior; ROL, right occipitolateral

occipitoposterior position, the anterior fontanelle will be felt anteriorly. The fontanelles are identified by the number of sutures which meet (see Ch. 30). See Table 36.3 and website.

Occasionally, the sagittal suture is found in the transverse diameter of the pelvis between the ischial tuberosities. It is then necessary to identify one or both fontanelles to determine the position. It may also be possible to feel an ear under the symphysis pubis and this may give an indication of the position of the fetus. Prior to delivery, when the fetal head has rotated on the pelvic floor, the sagittal suture should be in the anteroposterior diameter of the pelvis.

A summary of how to assess the position of the fetus is given in Table 36.3.

### Flexion and station

The fetal head may or may not be *flexed* at the onset of labour. In the presence of efficient uterine action and as a result of fetal axis pressure, the fetal head usually flexes, further facilitating a well-fitting presenting part. Unless the pelvis is particularly roomy or the fetal head small, deflexion of the head, and palpation of the posterior and anterior fontanelles, may be indicative of malposition of the fetal head, poor cervical stimulation and prolongation of labour.

The *station* or level of the presenting part refers to the relationship of the presenting part to the ischial spines. The maternal ischial spines are palpable as slight protuberances covered by tissue on either side of the bony pelvis. Descent in relation to the maternal ischial spines should be progressive and is expressed in centimetres as indicated in Figure 36.10.

The examination is completed by applying a vulval pad, changing any soiled linen and making the woman comfortable. The fetal heart is auscultated. All findings are recorded and the midwife analyses the findings to establish a total picture on which to make an accurate assessment of the progress of labour and to forecast how the labour is likely to advance. The midwife is able to relate to the woman and her partner the progress to date, and review with them the original birth plan for any adjustments which the woman and the midwife feel are necessary.

## Alternative skills for 'sussing out' labour

There is a dearth of any research examining alternatives to vaginal examinations for labour care, given the rich anecdotes that surround this area. Midwives have always taken into account the character of contractions, a woman's response to them and the findings from abdominal palpation. Stuart (2000) is possibly unique in relying on abdominal palpation instead of vaginal examination to ascertain progress, and most midwives weigh the results of vaginal examination above contractions and behaviour. It is the practices that are substitutional for vaginal examinations that are the most interesting. Hobbs (1998) advocated the 'purple line' method – observing a line that runs from the distal margin of the anus up between the buttocks, said to indicate full dilatation when it reaches the natal cleft. Byrne & Edmonds (1990) reported that 89% of women developed the line. In a comprehensive manual of care during normal birth, Frye (2004) identified monitoring temperature change in the lower leg. As labour

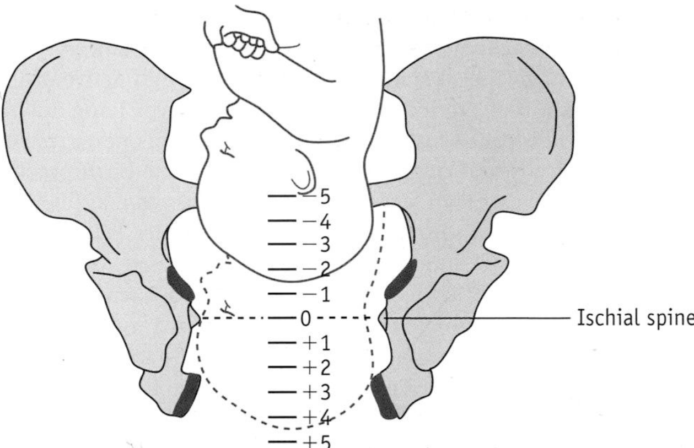


**Figure 36.10** Stations of the head in relation to the pelvis. Descent in relation to the maternal ischial spines is expressed in centimetres.

progresses, so a coldness on touch is noted to move from the ankle up the leg to the knee. Another marker may be the forehead of a woman. Possibly originating from traditional birth attendant practices in Peru, this involves feeling for the appearance of a ridge running from between the eyes up to the hairline as labour progresses.

Other wisdom comes from intuitive perceptions that many midwives may recognize but find hard to articulate, and even harder to write down, as illustrated by the story to be found on the website.

The transitional phase between the first and second stages has been studied by Baker & Kenner (1993), who noted the common vocalizations that mark it. These are just a few examples of anecdotes that abound in this area. It is an area ripe for observational research and for articles mapping the richness of midwives' experience.

Finally, there is the domain of emotional nuance reading, which may impact hugely on how labour unfolds (Kennedy et al 2004). One such episode occurred in the birth centre study by Walsh (2006b), when a teenage girl arrived in early labour, very distressed. The midwife asked her mother and sister to leave the room and gently enquired as to how she was. She burst into tears and over the next 2 hours the midwife held her in an embrace on a mattress on the floor as the girl sobbed and sobbed. Then she said she was ready and went on to have a normal, rather peaceful birth. In other settings, the girl may have been offered an epidural, but this was emotional rather than pain distress. The skill of the midwife was in her intuitive emotional nuance reading of that and how to bring comfort and support.

## 'Being with', not 'doing to', labouring women

The quest to dismantle assembly-line birth, removing women from the intrapartum timeline and rehabilitating belief in 'unique normality' of labour for individual women, challenges a radical rethink of the focus and orientation to normal labour care. Hints of a different way of midwives situating themselves with women are in the writings of midwives and they speak in paradox and metaphor. Leap (2000) tells of 'the less we do, the more we give', and Kennedy et al (2004) of 'doing nothing' in their insightful study of expert US midwives. Fahy (1998) conceptualizes the work of the midwife as 'being with' women, not 'doing to' them, and Anderson (2004) quips that good labour care requires the midwife 'to drink tea intelligently'. These writers are alluding not to a temporally regulated activity marked by task completions but to a disposition towards compassionate companionship with women that is a 'masterly inactivity' (RCM 2010). As a birth centre midwife offered during an interview: 'It's about being comfortable when there is nothing to do.'

## Loss per vaginam and rupture of the membranes

The time at which the membranes rupture should be recorded, together with the appearance of the liquor. A minor amount of blood-stained loss is consistent with a show or detachment of the membranes occurring with increasing cervical dilatation. Copious mucoid blood-stained loss may herald full cervical dilatation. A greenish colour is indicative of meconium staining, sometimes associated with fetal distress. *Frank bleeding* per vaginam is abnormal; if this occurs, the midwife must consult with the obstetrician, who will ascertain the source – whether maternal or fetal – and determine the appropriate action. Measurement of loss and monitoring of the woman's condition is vital.

## Bladder care

The woman is encouraged to empty her bladder every 2 hours. A full bladder is uncomfortable and may delay the progress of labour by inhibiting descent of the fetal head if it is above the ischial spines. This will reflexly inhibit efficient uterine contractions and cervical dilatation. Pressure on the distended bladder by the fetal head may give rise to oedema and bruising, leading to possible difficulties in micturition in the early days of the puerperium.

## Mobility and ambulation

Seven RCTs undertaken to evaluate ambulation agreed that there are no negative effects associated with mobility though there were varying conclusions as to benefit. Two studies (Flynn et al 1978, Read et al 1981) emphasized the following advantages:

- greater uterine contractility
- shorter labours
- less oxytocin augmentation
- less need for pharmacological analgesia
- fewer operative deliveries
- less fetal distress.

MacLennan et al's (1994) meta-analysis of their own trial with five others confirmed the finding of reduced analgesia requirements and noted that 46% of women in their study who declined entry to the trial did so because they did not want to lose the choice of ambulation. The most recent and largest trial (Bloom et al 1998) found that 99% of ambulant women would choose this mobility again. No other differences were noted compared with the recumbent group.

Movement appears to be a central characteristic of normal labour (Gould 2000). In an overview of trials of ambulation, Smith et al (1991) found that when given the choice, women changed position an average of seven to eight times in the course of their labours.

## Upright posture

Positive effects of gravity and lessened risk of aortocaval compression (and therefore improved fetal acid–base outcomes) were described by Bonica (1967) and Humphrey et al (1973). Mendez-Bauer et al (1975) demonstrated stronger, efficient uterine contractions. Radiological evidence from the 1950s and 1960s showed larger anteroposterior and transverse diameters of the pelvic outlet in squatting and kneeling positions (Russell 1969). Gupta & Nikodem's (2008) review of position in the second stage of labour seems to support these earlier findings. A Cochrane review of 21 studies, with a total of 3706 women, found that mobility and upright positions in the first stage of labour reduced the length of labour by about an hour (Lawrence et al 2009).

Flint (1986) discussed the idea of midwives 'fitting around women', emphasizing that nearly all common procedures, such as fetal monitoring and vaginal examinations, could be done without asking the woman to get on the bed. Props, such as beanbags and birth balls, can be used to facilitate positional and postural changes, and Robertson (1997) elaborates on these through Active Birth Workshops. Certainly, the mass trend towards lying down for childbirth, at least in western cultures, was never tested empirically and occurred largely to assist the birth practitioners to carry out technical interventions, such as forceps deliveries and administration of anaesthetics (Donnison 1988) (see Chapter 2). This will continue to be tacitly endorsed by midwives as long as the 'bed birth myth' of childbirth remains. Some independent birth centres have replaced conventional beds with sofa beds and it may be time for delivery suites across the country to follow suit. This simple, cosmetic alteration would be deeply symbolic and may have a significant impact on birth positions. Figure 36.11 illustrates a variety of positions for the first stage of labour.

**Reflective activity 36.3**

Review the records of the births you have attended, and consider the positions women adopted. Begin to include this component of the birth in your records, and evaluate the effect on the woman and on you.

## Moving and handling

Moving and handling concerns, and worries about back injuries, may preclude some midwives from assisting women who opt for an upright birth posture. If this is a real issue for practitioners, it may also have implications for assisting at recumbent births as well, as these sometimes require awkward twisting and bending. Midwives are now usually trained in 'good back care' with mandatory moving and handling sessions run by hospitals. The application of these principles should not interfere with assisting women to birth in upright postures, as these postures probably also protect women's joints and backs more than conventional bed birth.

Home birth practitioners are familiar with birth taking place in living rooms as well as bedrooms, and with the restlessness of labour, during which women move freely within the privacy of their chosen birthing space, and may choose the bed only as a prop. It is probably time to expunge the term 'confinement' from the vocabulary of childbirth once and for all, and ensure that the environment 'belongs' to the woman and her partner.

## Prevention of infection

In labour, both mother and fetus are vulnerable to infection, particularly following membrane rupture. The possibility is increased when the immune response is undermined by suboptimal health – for example, anaemia, malnourishment, chronic illness – or when the woman is

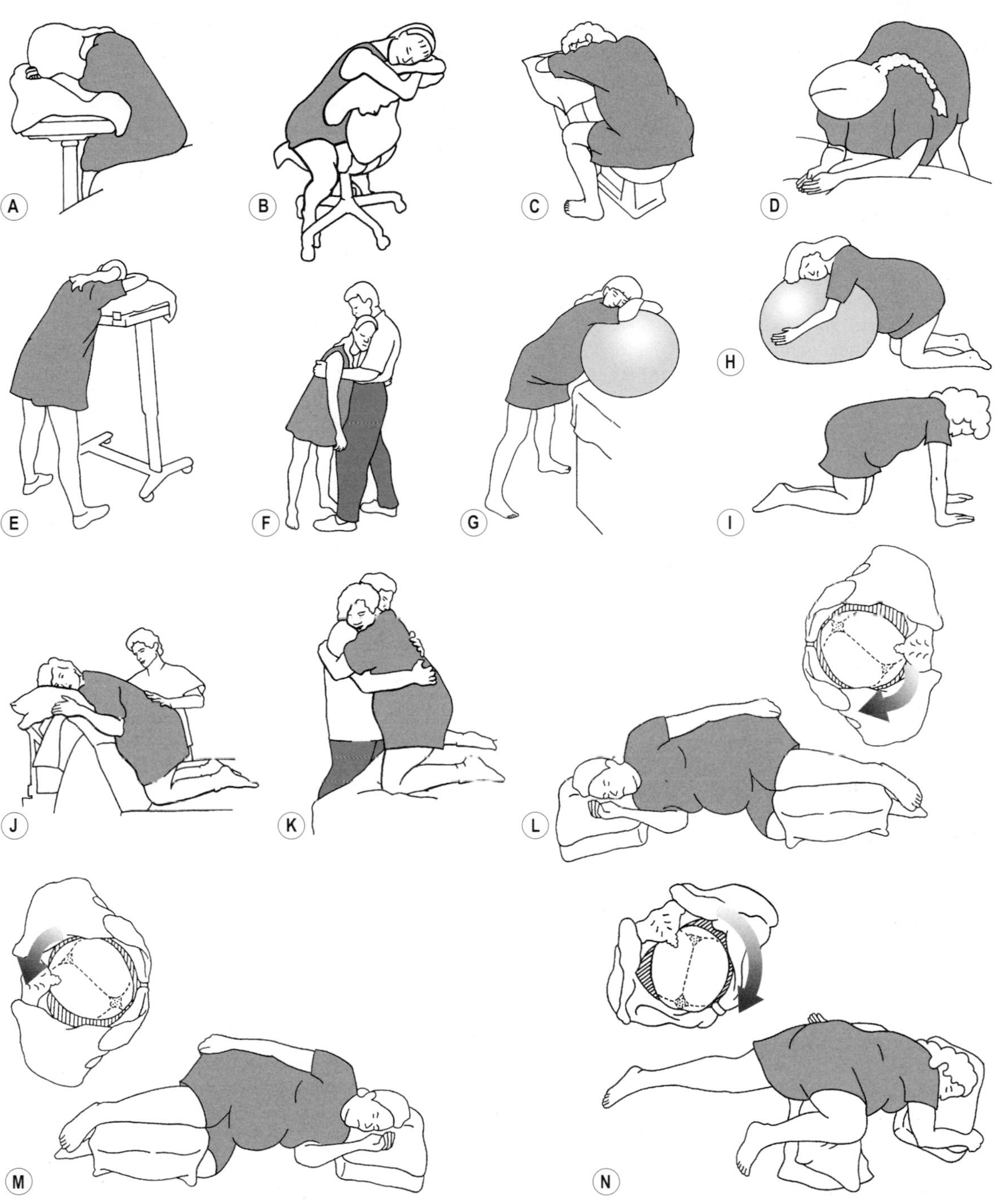


**Figure 36.11** A variety of positions for the first stage of labour. **A.** Sitting, leaning on a tray table. **B.** Straddling a chair. **C.** Straddling toilet, facing backwards. **D.** Standing, leaning on bed. **E.** Standing, leaning on a tray table. **F.** Standing, leaning forward on partner. **G.** Standing, leaning on ball. **H.** Kneeling with a ball. **I.** On hands and knees. **J.** Kneeling over bed back. **K.** Kneeling, partner support. **L.** Pure side-lying on the 'correct' side, with fetal back 'toward the bed'. If the fetus is ROP, the woman lies on her right side. Gravity pulls fetal head and trunk towards ROL. **M.** Pure side-lying on the 'wrong' (left) side for an ROP fetus. Fetal back is 'toward the ceiling'. Gravity pulls fetal occiput and trunk towards direct OP. **N.** Semi-prone on the 'correct side' – with fetal back 'toward the ceiling'. If the fetus is ROP, the semi-prone woman lies on her left side. Gravity pulls fetal occiput and trunk towards ROL, then ROA. *(From Simkin & Ancheta [2000], with permission of Blackwell Science Ltd.)*

exhausted by a long and arduous labour. The hospital environment itself may increase the woman's risk of infection as she is exposed to a variety of unfamiliar organisms and possible sources of infection.

The midwife must ensure, as far as possible, a safe environment for the woman and prevent infection and cross-infection. Such measures include good standards of hygiene and care, correct handwashing of the carers before and after attending the woman, frequent changing of vulval pads, and meticulous aseptic techniques when undertaking vaginal examination and other invasive procedures such as catheterization.

General measures, such as limiting the flow of traffic within the delivery area, scrupulous cleansing of communal equipment (for example, beds, baths, toilets and trolleys) and increasing staff awareness of the potential for, and prevention of, infection, must all be observed. A formal mechanism for infection control within hospitals must include maternity departments. One survey of surveillance of hospital-based obstetric and gynaecological infection showed a significant reduction in the incidence of infection when regular feedback to staff was implemented (Evaldon et al 1992).

## NUTRITION IN LABOUR

Controlling women's behaviours and choices in labour has traditonally included restrictions on what they can eat and drink. This was driven by concerns about aspirating stomach contents (Mendelson's sydrome) should general anaesthesia be required in an emergency. However, as regional anaesthesia has become common and anaesthetic techniques have improved, the incidence of aspiration has plummeted (Chang et al 2003). Apart from the medical risks, controlling what women eat and drink in normal labour is paternalistic and, arguably, an infringement of human rights. At home and birth centre births, the sensible approach of self-regulation has operated for decades. Women eat and drink when they feel hungry and thirsty, more commonly in early labour. Some women experience nausea as labour progresses and therefore forsake food, though they do usually continue to drink small amounts.

Odent (1998) and Anderson (1998) suggested that the smooth muscle structure of the uterus works much more efficiently than skeletal muscle, making comparatively small energy demands and utilizing fatty acids and ketones readily as an energy source. It is suggested that because the woman in physiological labour becomes withdrawn from higher cerebral activity, and as skeletal muscles are at rest, energy requirements are less than normal.

Tranmer et al (2005) tested the hypothesis that unrestricted eating and drinking during labour might reduce the incidence of labour dystocia. Though no effect was shown, it did highlight that when women self-regulate, many do choose to eat and drink, usually small amounts and often in the early stages of labour.

Imposed fasting in labour for all women is questionable in the light of evidence indicating that fasting in labour does not ensure an empty stomach or lower the acidity of stomach contents (Johnson et al 1989). Restrictions may lead to dehydration and ketosis, resulting in interventions, and this should be weighed against the alternative course of allowing women to eat and drink as desired (Johnson et al 1989).

Many maternity units require the administration of an acid inhibitor like *ranitidine* to increase the pH of the stomach contents. However, this is only appropriate in women of high risk status who might be more at risk of emergency procedures and should not be applied to women in normal labour.

## ASSESSING THE FETAL CONDITION

The midwife needs to understand the mechanisms that control fetal heart response in order to interpret the fetal response to labour. The cardioregulatory centre of the brain, situated in the medulla oblongata, is influenced by many factors. Baroreceptors situated in the arch of the aorta and carotid sinus sense alterations in blood pressure and transmit information to the cardioregulatory centre. Chemoreceptors situated in the carotid sinus and arch of the aorta will respond to changes in oxygen and carbon dioxide tensions. The cardioregulatory centre is controlled by the autonomic nervous system and, in response to varying physiological factors, either the sympathetic or parasympathetic nervous system will be stimulated. The sympathetic nervous system, via the sinoatrial node, causes an increase in heart rate, while the parasympathetic nervous system causes a rate reduction. The continuous interaction of these two systems results in minor fluctuations in the heart rate which is recognized as *variability*. Development of the sympathetic nervous system occurs early in fetal life, while the parasympathetic nervous response does not become pronounced until later in pregnancy. This accounts for the higher baseline rate of the fetal heart during early pregnancy and the lower rate at term.

### Monitoring the fetal heart

The activity of the fetal heart may be assessed intermittently using the Pinard fetal stethoscope or a Sonicaid. This provides the midwife with sample information regarding the rate and rhythm of the fetal heart. At commencement of intermittent auscultation, it is important to distinguish the maternal pulse from the fetal heart, as the former can mimic a fetal heart and, therefore, can be

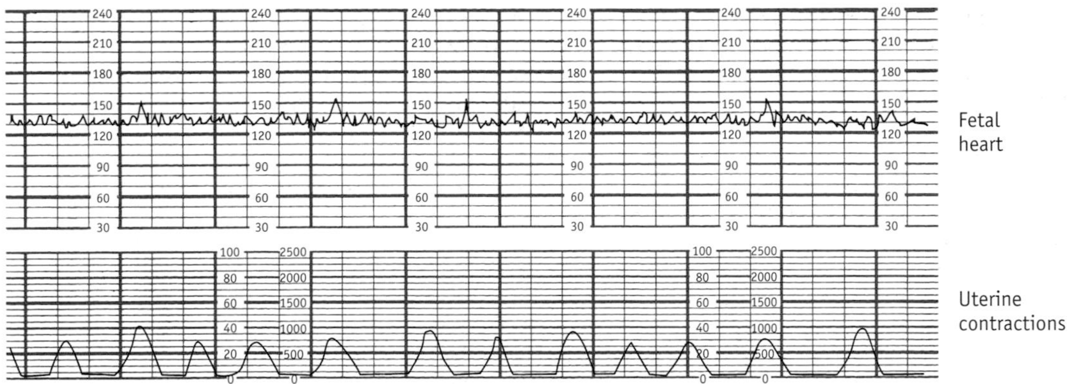


**Figure 36.12** ECG trace showing baseline variability in fetal heart rate. *(Courtesy of Sonicaid, Abingdon, Oxon.)*

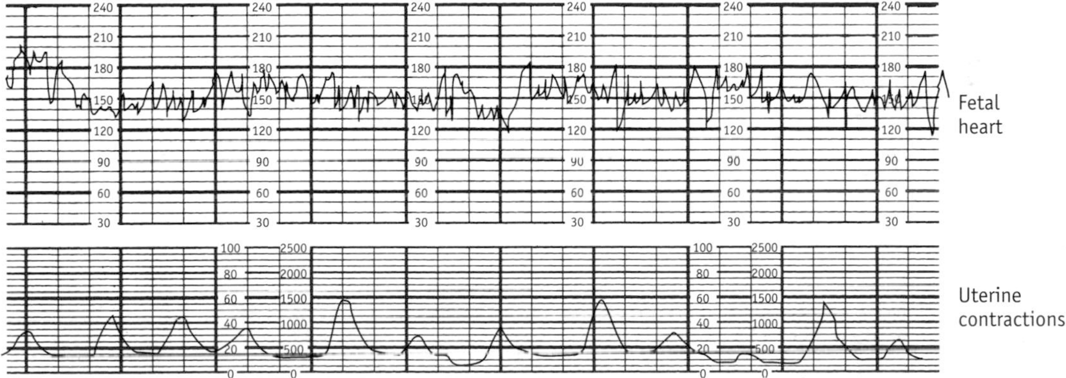


**Figure 36.13** Fetal heart rate accelerations. *(Courtesy of Sonicaid, Abingdon, Oxon.)*

falsely reassuring to the midwife. An understanding of the workings of the Sonicaid is useful, and reinforces the value of the use of the Pinard stethoscope at regular intervals even if the Sonicaid is used (Gibb & Arulkumaran 2007).

Intermittent auscultation of the fetal heart is usually undertaken every 15 minutes during the first stage of labour, though this is based on custom and practice, not research. In the second stage of labour, this increases to every 5 minutes. NICE (2007) recommends intermittent auscultation and abandonment of the 'admission trace' for women in normal labour.

## Healthy fetal heart patterns

The normal fetal heart has a baseline rate of between 110 and 160 beats per minute (bpm). The *baseline rate* refers to the heart rate present between periods of acceleration and deceleration. *Baseline variability* refers to the variation in heart rate of 5–15 bpm, occuring over a time base of 10–20 seconds. Figure 36.12 demonstrates normal baseline variability. The presence of good variability is an important sign of fetal wellbeing (NICE 2007).

Acceleration patterns of the fetal heart of 15 bpm from the baseline, as shown in Figure 36.13, are often associated with fetal activity and stimulation and are thought to be useful indicators of absence of fetal acidaemia in labour (Spencer 1993). They are not considered to be clinically significant if of short duration – that is, less than 15 seconds. When two are present within a 20-minute period, the trace is described as 'reactive' (Gibb 1988). This is considered to be a positive sign of fetal health, indicating good reflex responsiveness of the fetal circulation.

## Electronic fetal monitoring

In normal labour, continuous electronic fetal monitoring (EFM) is not required, as it results in more birth interventions without a demonstrable improvement in fetal outcome (Alfirevic et al 2006, NICE 2007). Inter- and intra-observer reliability is poor with EFM, and maternity units should regularly update all delivery suite staff in the interpretation of traces as recommended by the Confidential Enquiry into Maternal and Child Health (CEMACH) (Edwards 2004).

## CONCLUSION

Care during the first stage of labour is as much about trusting the birth process and intuitively connecting with labouring women as it is about monitoring and understanding the physiology. A social model of birth emphasizes the relational aspects of this experience and the key role of the birth environment. When these are understood and appropriately applied, physiology will be maximized and complications will occur in only a small minority of women. However, against the backdrop of increasing medicalization of childbirth, midwives may feel caught between the social and medical models and will need the support of each other if they are to facilitate empowering birth experiences for women in their care.

### KEY POINTS

- Labour is an intense, individual event, in which the midwife can play a pivotal role in supporting normality, and enabling and facilitating birth to be a positive and empowering experience.
- The midwife should be knowledgeable about the psychological, physiological and social aspects of labour in order to work in partnership with the woman, and plan care appropriately.
- The midwife must be conversant with contemporary research and evidence, and committed to sharing this knowledge with the woman and her partner.
- Continuity of care and carer provides a valued model of care and improves the outcomes of labour – where possible, this should be worked towards. Effective use of notes and records, including partograms, is a crucial part of this.
- One-to-one care during the active phase of the first stage of labour should be utilized as a means of monitoring maternal and fetal wellbeing and as an educational opportunity for the woman and birth partner.
- Models of care including birth centres, midwifery-led units and birthing suites provide an opportunity to develop women-centred care, and increase midwifery autonomy.

## REFERENCES


Adam B: *Timewatch: the social analysis of time*, Cambridge, 1995, Polity Press.

Albers L: The duration of labour in healthy women, *Journal of Perinatology* 19(2):114–119, 1999.

Alfirevic Z, Devane D, Gyte G: Continuous cardiotocography (CTG) as a form of electronic fetal monitoring (EFM) for fetal assessment during labour, *Cochrane Database of Systematic Reviews* 2006, (3):CD006066, 2006.

Anderson T: Is ketosis in labour pathological? *The Practising Midwife* 1(9):22–26, 1998.

Anderson T: The impact of the age of risk for antenatal education. *NCT conference*, Coventry 13th March, 2004.

Baker A, Kenner A: Communication of pain: vocalisation as an indicator of the stage of labour, *Australian and New Zealand Journal of Obstetrics and Gynaecology* 33(4):384–385, 1993.

Bergstrom L, Roberts J, Skillman L, et al: 'You'll feel me touching you, sweetie'. Vaginal examinations during the second stage of labour, *Birth* 19(1):10–18, 1992.

Blackburn ST: *Maternal, fetal and neonatal physiology*, ed 3, Philadelphia, 2007, WB Saunders.

Bloom S, McIntyre D, Beimer M: Lack of effect of walking on labour and delivery, *New England Journal of Medicine* 339(2):76–79, 1998.

Bonica J: *Principles and practice of obstetric analgesia and anaesthesia*, Philadelphia, 1967, FA Davis.

Buckley S: Undisturbed birth – nature's hormonal blueprint for safety, ease and ecstasy, *MIDIRS* 14(2):203–209, 2004.

Burvill S: Midwifery diagnosis of labour onset, *British Journal of Midwifery* 10(10):600–605, 2002.

Byrne D, Edmonds D: Clinical methods for evaluating progress in first stage of labour, *The Lancet* 335(1681):122, 1990.

Campbell R, McFarlane A: *Where to be born: the debate and the evidence*, ed 2, Oxford, 1994, National Perinatal Epidemiology Unit.

Cesario S: Reevaluation of Friedman's Labor Curve: a pilot study, *Journal of Obstetric, Gynecologic, and Neonatal Nursing* 33(6):713–722, 2004.

Chamberlain G, Wraight A, Crowley P: *Home births: the report of the 1994 Confidential Enquiry by the National Birthday Trust Fund*, London, 1997, Parthenon.

Chang J, Elam-Evans L, Berg C, et al: Pregnancy-related mortality surveillance – United States, 1991–1999, *MMWR Surveillance Summaries* 52(2):1–8, 2003.

Cheyne H, Dowding D, Hundley V: Making the diagnosis of labour: midwives' diagnostic judgement and management decisions, *Journal of Advanced Nursing* 53(6):625–635, 2006.

Clement S: Unwanted vaginal examinations, *British Journal of Midwifery* 2(8):368–370, 1994.

Davis B, Johnson K, Gaskin I: The MANA curve – describing plateaus in labour using the MANA database, Abstract No 30, *26th Triennial Congress ICM*, Vienna, 2002.

Department of Health (DH): *Making it better for mother and baby: clinical case for change*, London, 2007a, DH.

Department of Health (DH): *Maternity matters: choice, access and continuity of care in a safe service*, London, 2007b, DH.

Devane D: Sexuality and midwifery, *British Journal of Midwifery* 4(8):413–420, 1996.

Donnison J: *Midwives and medical men: a history of the struggle for the control of childbirth*, London, 1988, Historical Publications.

Downe S, McCourt C: *Normal birth: evidence & debate*, London, 2008, Elsevier Science.

Edwards G: *Adverse outcomes in maternity care*, Cheshire, 2004, Books for Midwives.

Enkin M, Kierse M, Neilson J. et al: *A guide to effective care in pregnancy and childbirth*, Oxford, 2000, Oxford University Press.

Evaldon GR, Frederici H, Jullig C, et al: Hospital-associated infections in obstetrics and gynaecology. Effects of surveillance, *Acta Obstetricia et Gynecologica Scandinavica* 71(1): 54–58, 1992.

Fahy K: Being a midwife or doing midwifery, *Australian Midwives College Journal* 11(2):11–16, 1998.

Fahy K: Safety of Stockholm Birth Centre Study: a critical review, *Birth* 32(2):145–150, 2005.

Flint C: *Sensitive midwifery*, London, 1986, Heinemann.

Flint C: *Midwifery teams and caseloads*, London, 1993, Butterworth Heinemann.

Flynn A, Hollins K, Lynch P: Ambulation in labour, *British Medical Journal* 2(6137):591–593, 1978.

Friedman E: The graphic analysis of labour, *American Journal of Obstetrics and Gynecology* 68:1568–1575, 1954.

Frye A: *Holistic midwifery. Volume 2: Care of the mother and baby from onset of labour through the first hours after birth*, Portland, 2004, Labry's Press.

Fullerton J, Young S: Outcomes of planned home birth: an integrative review, *Journal of Midwifery and Women's Health* 52(4):323–333, 2007.

Gagnon A, Meier K, Waghorn K: Continuity of nursing care and its link to caesarean birth rate, *Birth* 34(1):26–31, 2007.

Gaskin IM: Going backwards: the concept of 'pasmo', *The Practising Midwife* 6(8):34–36, 2003.

Gibb D: *A practical guide to labour management*, London, 1988, Blackwell Scientific.

Gibb DMF, Arulkumaran S: *Fetal monitoring in practice*, ed 3, London, 2007, Butterworth-Heinemann.

Gould D: Normal labour: a concept analysis, *Journal of Advanced Nursing* 31(2):418–427, 2000.

Green J, Coupland B, Kitzinger J: *Great expectations: a prospective study of women's expectations and experiences of childbirth*, Cambridge, 1998, Child Care and Development Group.

Gross M, Haunschild T, Stoexen T, et al: Women's recognition of the spontaneous onset of labour, *Birth* 30(4):267–271, 2003.

Gupta J, Nikodem V: Woman's position during second stage of labour (Cochrane Review), *The Cochrane Library*, Issue 2, Oxford, 2008, Update Software.

Haggerty J, Reid R, Freeman G, et al: Continuity of care: a multidisciplinary review, *British Medical Journal* 327(7425):1219–1221, 2003.

Hatem M, Sandall J, Devane D, et al: Midwife-led versus other models of care for childbearing women, *Cochrane Database of Systematic Reviews* (4):CD004667, 2008.

Healthcare Commission: *Towards better births: a review of maternity services in England*, London, 2008, Commission for Healthcare Audit and Inspection.

Hemminki E, Simukka R: The timing of hospital admission and progress of labour. *European Journal of Obstetrics, Gynaecology & Reproductive Biology* 22:85–94, 1986.

Hobbs L: Assessing cervical dilatation without VEs, *The Practising Midwife* 1(11):34–35, 1998.

Hodnett ED: Continuity of caregivers for care during pregnancy and childbirth (Cochrane Review). In *The Cochrane Library*, Issue 2, Chichester, 2008, John Wiley & Sons Ltd.

Hodnett ED, Downe S, Walsh D, Weston J: Home-like versus conventional institutional settings for birth. *The Cochrane Database of Systematic Reviews*, Issue 3, 2010.

Hodnett ED, Gates S, Hofmeyr GJ, Sakala C: Continuous support for women during childbirth. *The Cochrane Database of Systematic Reviews*, Issue 2, 2008a.

Humphrey M, Hounslow D, Morgan S: The influence of maternal posture at birth on the fetus, *Journal of Obstetrics & Gynaecology of the British Commonwealth* 80(12):1075–1080, 1973.

Hunt S, Symonds A: *The social meaning of midwifery*, Basingstoke, 1995, Macmillan.

Jackson D, Lang J, Ecker J, et al: Impact of collaborative management and early admission in labor on method of delivery, *Journal of Obstetric, Gynecologic, and Neonatal Nursing* 32(2):147–157, 2003.

Johnson C, Kierse MJNC, Enkin M, et al: Nutrition and hydration in labour. In Chalmers I, Enkin M, Kierse MJNC, editors: *Effective care in pregnancy and childbirth*, Vol. 2, Oxford, 1989, Oxford University Press.

Kennedy H, Shannon M, Chuahorm U, et al: The landscape of caring for women: a narrative study of midwifery practice, *Journal of Midwifery & Women's Health* 49(1):14–23, 2004.

Kitzinger S: *Rediscovering birth*, London, 2000, Simon & Schuster.

Lally J, Murtagh M, Macphail S, et al: More in hope than expectation: women's experience and expectations of pain relief in labour: a review, *BMC Medicine* 6:7, 2008.

Lauzon L, Hodnett ED: Labour assessment programs to delay admission to labour wards, *Cochrane Database of Systematic Reviews* (1):CD000936, 2004.

Lavender T, Alfirevic Z, Walkinshaw S: Effect of different partogram action lines on birth outcomes, *Obstetrics and Gynecology* 108(2):295–302, 2006.

Lawrence A, Lewis L, Hofmeyr GJ, et al: Maternal positions and mobility during first stage labour, *Cochrane Database of Systematic Reviews* (2):CD003934, 2009.

Leap N: The less we do, the more we give. In Kirkham M, editor: *The midwife-mother relationship*, London, 2000, Macmillan, pp 1–18.

McCoshen JA, Hoffman DR, Kredentser JV, et al: The role of fetal membranes in regulating production, transport, and metabolism of prostaglandin E2 during labor, *American Journal of Obstetrics and Gynecology* 163(5 Pt 1):1632–1640, 1990.

MacLennan A, Crowther C, Derham R: Does the option to ambulate during spontaneous labour confer any advantage or disadvantage? *Journal of Maternal and Fetal Medicine* 3(1):43–48, 1994.

Martin E: *The woman in the body: a cultural analysis of reproduction*, Milton Keynes, 1987, Open University Press.

Menage J: Post-traumatic stress disorder following obstetric/gynaecological procedures, *British Journal of Midwifery* 4(10):532–533, 1996.

Mendez-Bauer C, Arroyo J, Garcia-Ramos C: Effects of standing position on spontaneous uterine contractility and other aspects of labour, *Journal of Perinatal Medicine* 3(2):89–100, 1975.

Murphy-Lawless J: *Reading birth and death: a history of obstetric thinking*, Cork, 1998, Cork University Press.

National Institute for Health and Clinical Excellence (NICE): *Intrapartum care: care of healthy women and their babies during childbirth*, London, 2007, National Collaborating Centre for Women's and Children's Health.

North Staffordshire Changing Childbirth Research Team (NSCCRT): A randomised study of midwifery caseload care and traditional 'shared-care', *Midwifery* 16(4):295–302, 2000.

Nursing & Midwifery Council (NMC): *Midwives rules and standards*, London, 2004, NMC.

Nursing & Midwifery Council (NMC): *Record keeping: guidance for nurses and midwives*, London, 2009, NMC.

Odent M: Labouring women are not marathon runners, *The Practising Midwife* 1(9):16–18, 1998.

Odent M: New reasons and new ways to study birth physiology, *International Journal of Gynaecology & Obstetrics* 75:S39–S45, 2001.

Olsen O, Jewell D: Home versus hospital birth, *Cochrane Database of Systematic Reviews* (2):CD000352, 2006.

Page L: Putting principles into practice. In Page L, editor: *Effective group practice in midwifery: working with women*, Oxford, 1995, Blackwell Science.

Page L, McCourt C, Beake S, et al: Clinical interventions and outcomes of one-to-one midwifery practice, *Journal of Public Health Medicine* 21(3):243–248, 1999.

Pairman S: Women-centred midwifery: partnerships or professional friendships? In Kirkham M, editor: *The midwife–mother relationship*, London, 2000. Macmillan.

Perkins B: *The medical delivery business: health reform, childbirth and the economic order*, London, 2004, Rutgers University Press.

Philpott R, Castle W: Cervicographs in the management of labour on primigravidae 1. The alert line for detecting abnormal labour, *Journal of Obstetrics & Gynaecology of the British Commonwealth* 79:592–598, 1972.

Rahnama P, Ziaei S, Faghihzadeh S: Impact of early admission in labour on method of delivery, *International Journal of Gynaecology & Obstetrics* 92(3):217–220, 2006.

Read J, Miller F, Paul R: Randomised trial of ambulation versus oxytocin for labour enhancement: a preliminary report, *American Journal of Obstetrics and Gynecology* 139:669–672, 1981.

Redshaw M, Rowe R, Hockley C, et al: *Recorded delivery: a national survey of women's experience of maternity care 2006*, Oxford, 2007, NPE.

Richardson A, Mmata C: *NHS maternity statistics, England: 2005–06*, London, 2007, The Information Centre.

Robertson A: *The midwife companion*, Sydney, 1997, ACE Graphics.

Robohm J, Buttenheim M: The gynaecological care experience of adult survivors of childhood sexual abuse: a preliminary investigation, *Women and Health* 24(3):59–75, 1996.

Rosen P: Supporting women in labour: analysis of different types of caregivers, *Journal of Midwifery & Women's Health* 49:24–31, 2004.

Royal College of Midwives (RCM): Campaign for normal birth (website). http://www.rcmnormalbirth.org.uk/stories/on-the-crest-of-a-wave/masterly-inactivity/ accessed 2010.

Rudman A, El-Khouri B, Waldenstrom U: Women's satisfaction with intrapartum care – a pattern approach, *Journal of Advanced Nursing* 59(5):474–487, 2007.

Russell J: Moulding of the pelvic outlet, *Journal of Obstetrics & Gynaecology of the British Commonwealth* 76:817–820, 1969.

Schwarcz R, Diaz AG, Fescina R, et al: Latin American collaborative study on maternal posture in labour, *Birth Family Journal* 6(1):1979, 1977.

Simkin P, Ancheta R: *The labor progress handbook*, Oxford, 2000, Blackwell Science.

Smith M, Acheson L, Byrd J, et al: A critical review of labour and birth care, *Journal of Family Practice* 35:107–115, 1991.

Spencer JA: Clinical overview of cardiotocography (Review), *British Journal of Obstetrics and Gynaecology* 100(Suppl 9):4–7, 1993.

Stewart M: 'I'm just going to wash you down': sanitizing the vaginal examination, *Journal of Advanced Nursing* 51(6):587–594, 2005.

Stewart M, McCandlish R, Henderson J, et al: *Report of a structured review of birth centre outcomes 2004*, Oxford, 2005, National Perinatal Epidemiology Unit.

Stuart C: Invasive actions in labour: where have all the 'old tricks' gone? *The Practising Midwife* 3(8):30–33, 2000.

Studd J: Partograms and nomograms of cervical dilatation in management of primigravid labour, *British Medical Journal* 4(5890):451–455, 1973.

Tan BP, Hannah ME: Oxytocin for prelabour rupture of membranes at or near term (Cochrane Review) (Substantive update: 28 August 1996), *The Cochrane Library*, Issue 3, Oxford, 2002, Update Software.

Taylor S, Klein L, Lewis B, et al: Biobehavioural responses to stress in females, *Psychological Review* 107(3):411–429, 2000.

Tew M: *Safer childbirth? A critical history of maternity care*, London, 1998, Free Association Books.

Tracey S, Dahlen H, Caplice S, et al: Birth centres in Australia: a national population-based study of perinatal mortality associated with giving birth in a birth centre, *Birth* 34(3):194–201, 2007.

Tranmer J, Hodnett E, Hannah M, et al: The effect of unrestricted oral carbohydrate intake on labor progress, *Journal of Obstetric, Gynecologic, and Neonatal Nursing* 34(3):319–328, 2005.

Turnbull D, Holmes S, Cheyne H, et al: Randomised controlled trial of efficacy of midwifery-managed care, *The Lancet* 348(9022):213–218, 1996.

Walsh D: An ethnographic study of women's experience of partnership caseload midwifery practice: the professional as friend, *Midwifery* 15(3):165–176, 1999.

Walsh D: Subverting assembly-line birth: childbirth in a free-standing birth centre, *Social Science & Medicine* 62(6):1330–1340, 2006a.

Walsh D: Birth centres, community & social capital, *MIDIRS* 16(1):7–15, 2006b.

Walsh D: *Improving maternity service. Small is beautiful: lessons for maternity services from a birth centre*, Oxford, 2007a, Radcliffe Publishing.

Walsh D: *Evidence-based care for normal labour & birth: a guide for midwives*, London, 2007b, Routledge.

Walsh D, Downe S: Outcomes of free-standing, midwifery-led birth centres: a structured review of the evidence, *Birth* 31(3):222–229, 2004.

Walsh D, Newburn M: Towards a social model of childbirth. Part 1, *British Journal of Midwifery* 10(8):476–481, 2002.

Warren C: Invaders of privacy, *Midwifery Matters* 81:8–9, 1999.

Zhang J, Troendle J, Yancey M: Reassessing the labour curve, *American Journal of Obstetrics and Gynecology* 187(4):824–828, 2002.

Chapter |37|

# Care in the second stage of labour

Soo Downe

## LEARNING OUTCOMES

After reading this chapter, you will:

- understand maternal behaviours associated with transition and the expulsive stage of labour
- have enhanced your knowledge of the basic physiology of transition and the second stage
- understand some of the techniques that are currently used in childbirth
- recognize that many midwifery practices in the area of physiological birth are based on empirical but not formal evidence
- understand the importance of clear, comprehensive, accurate record-keeping.

## INTRODUCTION

The anatomical second stage of labour has been traditionally defined as the period from full dilatation of the os uteri to the birth of the baby. However, women do not experience labour and birth by its anatomical divisions, or by the dilatation of the cervix (Gross et al 2006), and labours do not usually progress at a uniform rate.

The distinctive physiological changes that occur just before or around the time the cervical os is fully dilated are traditionally defined as 'transition'. There is a paucity of formal evidence about the nature of transition, although some observational studies have been undertaken (Crawford 1983, Roberts & Hanson 2007). During or following this phase, the woman begins to feel a variable urge to bear down. Anecdotal evidence indicates that it is not uncommon for midwives to offer women pharmacological pain relief if the urge to bear down occurs when vaginal examination indicates that the anatomical second stage is still some way off. If she then progresses more quickly than expected, such pain relief may inhibit the natural urge to bear down actively. It is thus essential that midwives know how to recognize the transitional phase of labour, and how to support women effectively at this time.

## SIGNS OF PROGRESS

### Transition

Transition occurs at variable times between the late first stage and early second stage of labour. It is recognizable by a change in the behaviour of the woman, and, sometimes, by a change in the nature of the contractions she is experiencing. Any or all of the following may be noted:

- loss of control; panic
- belief that she cannot carry on
- fearfulness (sometimes of dying)
- disorientation
- nausea
- uncontrollable shivering
- demands for pain relief
- a need to shout and scream
- a slowing of contractions
- a heavy 'show' – a loss per vaginam, which is usually a mixture of blood and mucus
- a period when the woman dozes, and goes 'inside herself' (the so-called 'rest and be thankful' phase)
- a variable urge to bear down or to push.

If a vaginal examination is undertaken, the mother's cervical os will typically be found to be between 7 and 9 cm dilated, though smaller dilations have been reported (Downe et al 2008). There have been occasional reports of transition (evidenced by an early pushing urge) occurring when the cervical os is less than 7 cm dilated (Roberts et al 1987).

**Reflective activity 37.1**

Next time you are with a woman in transition and/or the expulsive phase of labour, ask yourself the following questions. If the answers conflict with local guidelines, or with the usual actions midwives are expected to take locally, consider how these guidelines or informal expectations can be examined by you and your colleagues, with a view to revision.

- Does she want/need pain relief? Could reassurance, support, and faith in her capacity to birth the baby be just as effective?
- Will firm direction be helpful for her, or will it lead her to panic?
- If her contractions are decreasing in length and strength, is this due to underlying pathology, or is it only part of a physiological transition? Does she need to rest for a short time? Is she hungry?
- Is she well hydrated?
- Does she want to be touched or not?
- Is the early pushing urge being felt because of fetal malposition, or is the head just descending very rapidly? Should she push spontaneously if you are not sure the cervical os is fully dilated?
- Is she enabled to adopt any position she wants? What would you do if she throws her arms back and brings her hips forward when she begins pushing?
- Is it difficult not to say 'hold your breath and push'?

## Expulsive phase

Initially, the strength and consistency of the pushing urge usually varies in intensity, becoming more consistent over time. The woman usually makes a characteristic grunting noise at the height of the contraction. She may feel that her bowels are emptying, which may be very embarrassing for her. The perineum bulges and is stretched thin as it is distended by the descending fetus. The anus initially pouts and then dilates with contractions. The vagina begins to gape, and finally the presenting part is visible.

Some midwives have noted the appearance of a rounded area at the level of the lower back, the so-called *rhombus of Michaelis* (Sutton & Scott 1996). Sutton & Scott note that it is caused by 'the pressure of the fetal head [which] ... lifts the sacrum and the coccyx out of the way'. They also observe that the woman's instinctive reaction to the descent of the fetus is to arch her back, push her buttocks out (or off the bed if she is semi-recumbent) and throw her arms back to grasp onto any fixed object behind her. They hypothesize that this is a physiological response, since it causes a lengthening and straightening of the curve of Carus, optimizing the fetal passage through the birth canal.

Others have noted anecdotally that women who have an epidural in situ may experience discomfort under the ribs at around about the time of full cervical dilatation. This may be a function of fetal re-alignment as the fetal head descends, causing a sensation of pressure above the level of the epidural block. The efficacy of these observations in predicting the onset of the second stage of labour for individual women remains to be researched.

If necessary, the midwife can carry out a vaginal examination to confirm full dilatation of the os uteri. If no cervix is felt, there is positive confirmation of the onset of the anatomical second stage of labour.

## PHYSIOLOGY OF THE SECOND STAGE OF LABOUR

### Contractions

On average, at this stage, studies have indicated that contractions have an amplitude of 60–80 mmHg, occur every 2–3 minutes and last for 60–70 seconds, although other patterns of second stage contractions can be effective. Marked retraction of the uterus further aids the descent of the fetus through the birth canal. There is no appreciable fall in the height of the fundus, however, because the fetal back tends to uncurl from its flexed attitude and the lower uterine segment stretches. The force of the uterine contractions and secondary powers is transmitted down the fetal spine to its head. This is *fetal axis pressure* and helps the descent of the fetus through the birth canal.

### Secondary powers

The expulsion of the fetus is further aided by the voluntary muscles of the diaphragm and abdominal wall. As the presenting part descends to approximately 1 cm above the level of the ischial spines, pressure from the fetal presentation stimulates nerve receptors in the pelvic floor, and the woman experiences the desire to bear down. This is termed the *'Ferguson reflex'* (Ferguson 1941). This sensation may occur prior to the end of the anatomical first stage of labour, or at cervical full dilatation. The voluntary muscles of the chest and abdominal wall act reflexively in concert with the uterine contractions to overcome the resistance of the vagina, pelvic floor muscles, and external parts. During this process, the diaphragm is lowered and the abdominal muscles contract.

### The pelvic floor

The advancing fetus gradually stretches the vagina and displaces the pelvic floor. Anteriorly, the pelvic floor is pushed up and the bladder is drawn up into the abdomen, where it is less likely to be damaged. Posteriorly, the pelvic floor is pushed down in front of the presenting part. The rectum is compressed; thus any faecal contents will be expelled. The perineal body becomes elongated and paper-thin as it is flattened by the advancing fetus.

## Mechanism of labour

As labour progresses, the fetus is moved through the birth canal and induced to make various twists and turns due to the forces which occur, causing it to respond to the contours and planes of the maternal pelvis. These movements are called, collectively, the *mechanism of labour*. An understanding of this mechanism enables assessment of progress in labour, and recognition of when physiological support may be required, or if a call for assistance should be made.

There is a mechanism for every fetal presentation and position. The widest diameter of the brim of the pelvis is transverse, whereas the widest diameter of the outlet is anteroposterior. To make the best use of available space, the widest presenting diameter of the fetal head usually enters the pelvis in the transverse diameter. As it descends, the fetal head and then the shoulders rotate to emerge in the anteroposterior diameter. The mechanism for the most common presentation is as follows, although it should be noted that the specific physiology of individual women and fetal pairs can alter this mechanism.

The lie is longitudinal, the presentation is cephalic and the presenting part is the area of the vertex. The attitude is one of flexion and therefore the denominator is the occiput. The engaging diameter is the suboccipitobregmatic (on average, approximately 9.5 cm). The position may be either right or left occipitoanterior.

### Descent

Descent is the process whereby the fetal head moves into the pelvis (Fig. 37.1). Engagement occurs when the widest diameter of the presenting part enters the pelvis. This is more likely to occur prior to the onset of labour in nulliparous women.

### Flexion

At the beginning of labour the fetal head is usually in an attitude of natural flexion. As labour progresses, the head meets the resistance of the pelvic floor muscles, and flexion increases. Fetal axis pressure is then transmitted through the occiput, which is pushed down lower as a consequence. The forehead is pushed upwards by the resistance of the soft parts, and so complete flexion is obtained.

### Internal rotation

When the occiput meets the resistance of the pelvic floor, it rotates forward 45° (Fig. 37.2). The slope of the pelvic floor aids this internal rotation forwards, allowing the head to emerge in the longest diameter of the pelvic outlet; that is, the anteroposterior diameter (Figs 37.3 and 37.4). The occiput then escapes under the pubic arch and the head is crowned.

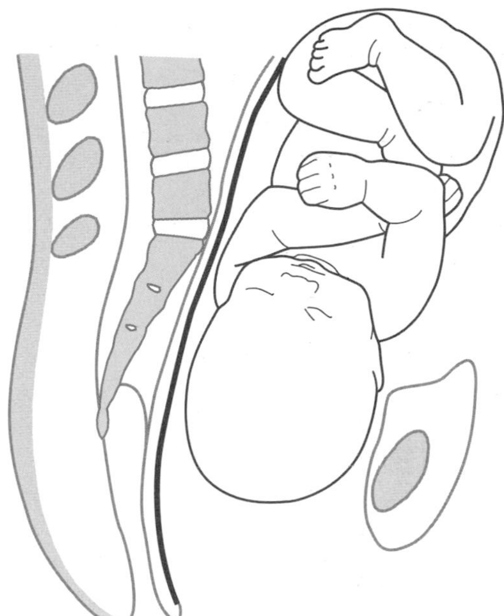

**Figure 37.1** Descent of a fetus with a well-flexed head presenting. The sagittal suture is in the transverse diameter of the pelvis. (Mother in upright position.)

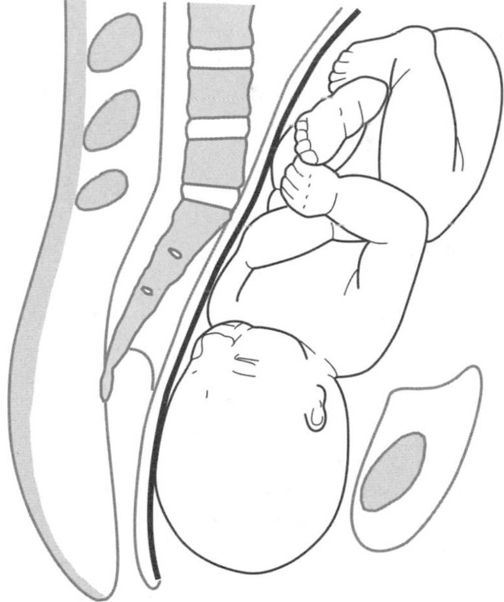

**Figure 37.2** Internal rotation occurs. The sagittal suture is in the oblique diameter of the pelvis. (Mother in upright position.)

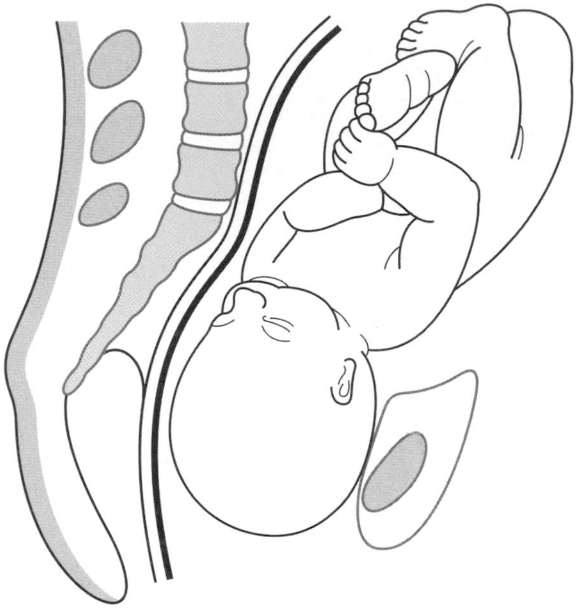

**Figure 37.3** Internal rotation complete – further descent occurs. The sagittal suture is now in the anteroposterior diameter of the pelvis. As the head deflexes slightly with descent, the sacrum and coccyx are displaced posteriorly. (Mother in upright position.)

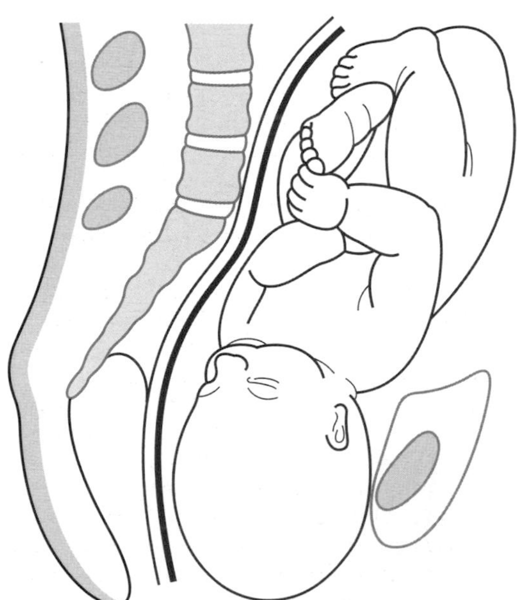

**Figure 37.4** The head descended to the vulval outlet. (Mother in upright position.)

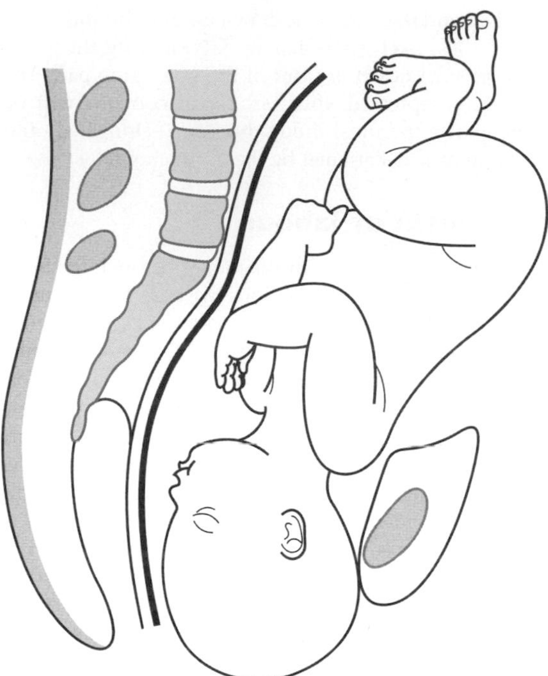

**Figure 37.5** The head is crowned. The sacrum and coccyx regain their normal position. (Mother in upright position.)

## Crowning of the head

The head is *crowned* when it has emerged under the pubic arch and no longer recedes between contractions. The widest transverse diameter of the head (the biparietal diameter) is born (Fig. 37.5).

## Extension

Once the head is crowned, extension takes place to allow the bregma, forehead, face and chin to pass over the perineum.

## Restitution

When the head is born, it rights itself with the shoulders (Fig. 37.6). During the movement of internal rotation, the head is slightly twisted because the shoulders do not rotate at that time. The baby's neck is untwisted by restitution.

## Internal rotation of the shoulders

The shoulders undergo an internal rotation similar to that of the head and then lie in the anteroposterior diameter of the outlet. The head, being free outside the birth canal, moves 45° at the same time, so internal rotation of the shoulders is accompanied by external rotation of the head. Rotation follows the direction of restitution; thus the occiput turns to the same side of the maternal pelvis as it was at the beginning of labour (Fig. 37.7).

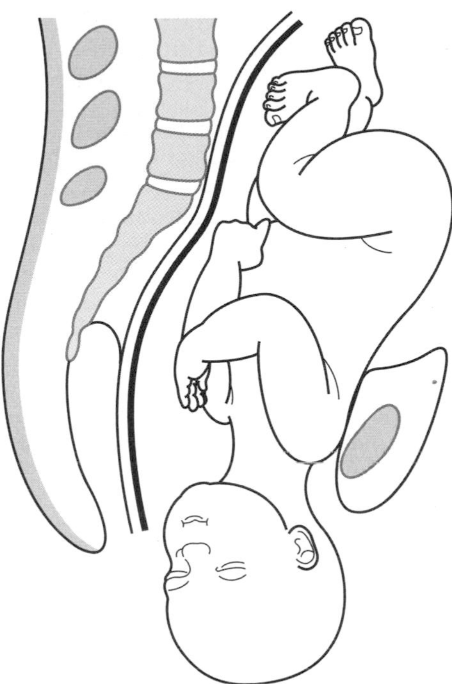

Figure 37.6 The head restitutes to the oblique, in line with the position of the shoulders. (Mother in upright position.)

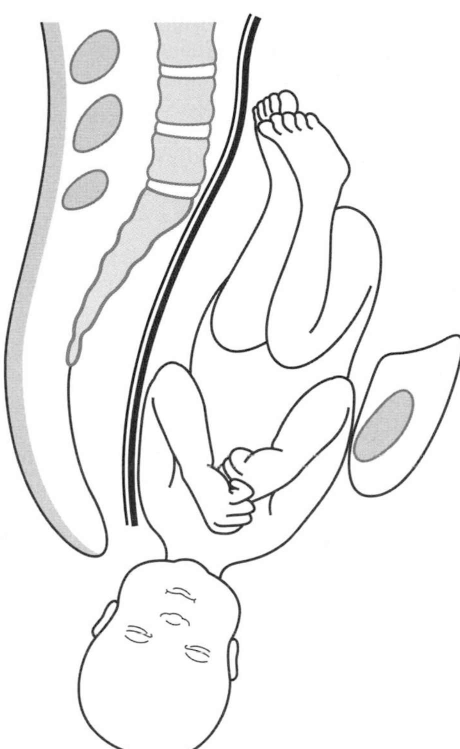

Figure 37.7 Internal rotation of the shoulders leads to external rotation of the head. (Mother in upright position.)

## Lateral flexion

In most supine or semi-recumbent maternal birthing positions, the anterior shoulder is born under the pubic arch first, then the posterior shoulder passes over the perineum. If the woman is in a position in which she is leaning forwards, the posterior shoulder may be born first because of the action of gravity and the effect of the curve of the birth canal (known as the *curve of Carus*). This curve causes the trunk of the baby to flex sideways as it is born.

## After the birth

Once the baby is born, there is a marked retraction of the uterus, which starts the process of placental separation. This is completed in the third stage of labour.

# DURATION OF THE SECOND STAGE OF LABOUR

The midwife should be aware of the rapidity with which the second stage can progress, especially for multiparous women, since their second stage sometimes lasts only a few minutes. The woman should not be left alone after the late first stage has commenced.

In the presence of effective uterine activity, where there is progressive descent of the presenting part, and the condition of the mother and fetus does not give rise for concern, time alone does not provide sufficient grounds for curtailment of the second stage. Studies in this area demonstrate increased intervention and morbidity over time, but it is not clear if this is due to actual or anticipated pathology (Altman & Lydon-Rochelle 2006). Intervention should be based on the rate of progress and the condition of the mother and baby rather than on the time which has elapsed since full dilatation of the cervix.

Many midwives take note of the pattern of progress in previous labours if the woman is multigravid; or that of labour in the sisters and mother of the labouring woman. This has not yet been tested in formal research studies.

Factors that may slow the progress of the active second stage but which can be corrected by time or by technique include a *malpositioned or deflexed fetus* (see website for Case scenario 37.1), and use of pain relief (particularly *pethidine* or *epidural analgesia*). Corrective techniques for the former include the use of optimal fetal positioning (Sutton & Scott 1996). The effect of pethidine will ameliorate with time. The use of oxytocin routinely in the second stage of labour where an epidural is in situ is not recommended (NICE 2007:122). These NICE guidelines go on to recommend that women with regional analgesia should be enabled to move around and adopt upright positions where possible; that analgesia should be continued through the second stage and until after perineal repair where this is necessary; that pushing be delayed for at least 1 hour to allow for descent and rotation of the fetal head, if all other parameters are normal; and that the second stage should ideally be completed within 4 hours in these circumstances.

## POSITIONS IN THE SECOND STAGE OF LABOUR

If left to their own devices, most women will move around during their labour and birth, as they instinctively adapt to the position of the baby and the progress of the labour. The effect of different positions on the length and outcome of labour has been the subject of much interest and investigation in recent years. Based on the latest Cochrane review in this area at the time they were developed (Gupta et al 2005), current NICE intrapartum guidelines recommend that women avoid the use of supine positions in labour (NICE 2007). The most recent Cochrane review on upright positions in labour reaches a similar conclusion (Lawrence et al 2009).

A woman who does adopt a semi-recumbent position for whatever reason should be well supported by pillows and perhaps a wedge to prevent her from sliding down and eventually adopting the dorsal position. Should this happen, the heavy gravid uterus is likely to compress the vena cava, causing subsequent hypotension, reduced placental perfusion and fetal hypoxia (Humphrey et al 1974, Johnstone et al 1987).

Whatever position the woman chooses, the midwife should be able to adapt the principles of care in labour and management of birth appropriately.

## MIDWIFERY CARE

During this period of maximum exertion, the woman should be praised for her efforts and both she and her partner should be kept fully informed of progress made. Information should be given between contractions, when the woman can relax and attend to what is being said. The midwife can help to promote confidence and allay anxiety by adopting a quiet, calm manner, and through tone of voice, tactile gestures and other non-verbal means of communication. Privacy is essential. It may help to have a 'do not disturb' sign on the door. Casual conversation between staff over the woman is never acceptable, and is particularly disrespectful at this time.

### Hygiene and comfort measures

The extreme exertion of the woman during the second stage of labour is likely to make her feel hot and sticky. She may appreciate having her face and hands sponged frequently. However, some women find this distracting as it breaks their concentration: it is very much a matter of personal choice. The woman may find drinks of iced water welcome and refreshing. If oral fluids are contraindicated, mouthwashes should be offered.

If leg cramps are experienced, these may be relieved by massage and by extending the leg and dorsiflexing the foot; that is, bending it upwards.

A full bladder may delay progressive descent of the fetus and the bladder may also be damaged by pressure as the fetus advances. Occasionally, if the fetal head has descended deeply into the pelvis and has caused upward displacement of the maternal urinary bladder, the woman may be unable to pass urine and the midwife may also find the passage of a catheter difficult. For this reason it is advisable to encourage regular micturition throughout labour, especially once the midwife recognizes that the expulsive stage of labour is imminent.

### Support during transition

This phase of labour can be difficult for the woman and for those attending and supporting her. The midwife needs to be a calm and reassuring presence, and must assess each woman carefully, since individuals react in extremely diverse ways at this time. It is important that the midwife responds to the transitional phase appropriately in each individual case. The aim is to enable the woman to regain her capacity to cope and to trust in her own ability to birth her baby, so that she can take a positive approach to the active second stage of labour. The midwife should also pay attention to the woman's other birth companions, to ensure that they are reassured that this is a normal part of labour and an indication that the birth of the baby is not far away.

### Support during the expulsive phase of labour

#### Early bearing-down efforts

Traditionally, midwives in the UK have discouraged women from bearing down until the cervical os is known to be completely dilated, particularly in the case of the primigravid woman. This has usually been advised on the assumption that active pushing prior to full cervical dilatation may cause oedema of the os uteri, which will impede or prevent the vaginal birth of the baby (Downe et al 2008). However, a few small-scale observational studies and one US survey (Bergstrom et al 1997, Petersen & Besuner 1997, Roberts et al 1987) have led to suggestions that, where the fetal head is well positioned, and the cervix is more than 8 cm dilated, spontaneous pushing may be physiological (Roberts & Hanson 2007). Given the small size and localized context of these studies to date, best practice in this area remains uncertain.

Techniques for helping women to minimize the bearing-down urge include the use of Entonox; adoption of the left lateral position; controlled breathing techniques; or, at the extremes, the administration of pain relief, including the siting of an epidural. The impact of these techniques on labour progress in this situation has not been subject to formal research.

See website for Case scenario 37.2.

## Delayed bearing-down efforts

Some women may feel little or no desire to bear down when the cervix is fully dilated, probably because the fetal head has not yet descended to compress the tissues of the pelvic floor, and therefore to stimulate muscular contractions, as in the 'Ferguson reflex' (Ferguson 1941). The role of the midwife in this situation is to ensure that the woman is well hydrated and not ketotic, and to ensure that maternal and fetal wellbeing are maintained. Assuming all is well, a watch and wait policy can be adopted until the woman begins to experience the bearing-down sensation. For some women, this can be optimized by a change to a more upright position, to encourage descent and the activation of the reflex.

## Pushing technique

Organized sustained pushing with contractions, involving breath-holding (closed glottis pushing, known as the Valsalva manoeuvre), is still practised by some midwives in the belief that it reduces the duration of the second stage of labour and therefore the period of highest risk to the fetus. This practice has been challenged intermittently since the late 1950s (Beynon 1957). The most recent authoritative statement on the subject (NICE 2007:164), based on a synthesis of the evidence to date (Bloom et al 2006, Schaffer et al 2005), concludes that *women should be informed that in the second stage they should be guided by their own urge to push. If pushing is ineffective or if requested by the woman, strategies to assist birth can be used, such as support, change of position, emptying of the bladder and encouragement.*

The observation that the woman tends to push her pelvis forward and arch herself backwards during the second stage of labour throws into question the common practice in many consultant maternity units of encouraging women who use the semi-recumbent position to abduct their legs by bending them and pushing them towards their hips, and to lean forwards as they push. This practice, and the alternatives, require more examination.

There is, as yet, no good evidence on the optimum advice for women who have an epidural in situ during the second stage of labour. However, in the absence of maternal sensation, some degree of direction from the midwife is probably necessary.

## Perineal practices

A number of practices are used by midwives in the second stage of labour in an effort to minimize trauma to the perineum. These include the use of hot or cold compresses; perineal massage as the fetal head advances; and guarding with a gentle, or, in some cases, firm pressure, to maintain fetal flexion, and to support the perineal tissues as they stretch. There is very little evidence for the benefits or risks of hot compresses or perineal massage, or for the various oils and techniques used. One large trial of the use of perineal massage found no significant differences on all parameters tested, though for the particular group studied, third degree tears were reduced (Stamp et al 2001).

One large trial assessing the effect of guarding the perineum found a small increase in mild pain at 10 days postpartum in the control group, where guarding was not employed (McCandlish et al 1998). It is not clear whether the techniques used in the study would benefit women using upright positions in labour.

## Assessing the need for episiotomy

An episiotomy is a surgical incision of the perineum to enlarge the vulval orifice. The midwife should be aware that pelvic floor and perineal trauma may have long-term implications for the woman and her partner and should not be performed as a routine, even where women have had previous third and fourth degree perineal tears (Carroli et al 2004, Hartmann et al 2005). The possibility of perineal trauma should be discussed with the woman prior to the labour. Her informed choices for this element of labour should be recorded. If an episiotomy becomes necessary, she should be informed, and the midwife must only proceed with her consent. (See Chapter 40 for more details.)

# OTHER MIDWIFERY TECHNIQUES

## Optimal fetal positioning

In recent years, the technique of optimal fetal positioning has become increasingly popular (Sutton & Scott 1996). Techniques are proposed for shifting a baby which is malpositioned or asynclitic in labour, including raising one hip, or rotating the hips, to change the angles of inclination of the pelvis. Sutton & Scott also propose that a woman's instinct to throw her hips forward and her arms back during active pushing should be respected, since this straightens the curve of Carus and optimizes maternal effort. All these observations and techniques have empirical credibility, but remain to be tested formally for their efficacy.

## Waterbirth

Therapeutic use of water in childbirth has grown in popularity. Some women may wish to spend most of their labour and birth in the water pool, others choose to spend short periods, and some women may wish to leave the water for the actual birth of the baby and birth of the placenta.

Systematic review evidence indicates that there are a number of benefits to labouring in water (Cluett et al 2004). As there is limited research evidence to guide the midwife in most aspects of waterbirth management, it is necessary to determine the benefits and risks for each woman and baby by a careful individual assessment and attention to official guidance (NICE 2007, RCOG/RCM 2006).

The essential issues to consider are as follows:

### Temperature of the water

Too high a temperature will be uncomfortable for the woman and may cause fetal tachycardia (NICE 2007). Cooler temperatures may induce respiration before the baby has been brought to the surface. Temperatures that are comfortable **for the woman** are recommended (Geissbuehler et al 2002).

### Time of entry to water

Immersion in water in the early stages of labour may inhibit uterine activity. Therefore, unless the contractions are particularly strong or painful, some midwives recommend that the woman should refrain from entering the water before the cervical os is 4–5 cm dilated. There is as yet little research to support or refute this practice.

### Infection of mother or baby

Infection risk appears to be very low, and can be minimized by using disposable bath linings, where possible, and by thorough cleaning and drying of the bath after use in accordance with current methods of prevention of cross-infection.

### Water embolism

In theory, water embolism may occur when maternal placental bed sinuses are torn in the third stage of labour. Water may then enter the circulation. For this reason it is deemed advisable for the third stage of labour to be conducted out of the water. Any oxytocic preparation, if used, should be given when the woman has left the water.

### Perineal trauma

The possibility of perineal trauma must be borne in mind. The midwife should provide verbal support to enable the woman to control her birth, allowing the head and shoulders to emerge slowly.

### Monitoring maternal and fetal health

The fetal heart can be auscultated using an underwater ultrasonic monitor, wireless electronic fetal monitoring, or Pinard's stethoscope. If pain relief is required, inhalational analgesia (Entonox) is suitable. The woman must not be left unattended while using inhalational analgesia during a waterbirth. If narcotic analgesia is required, the woman should be asked to leave the water as the drowsiness induced by the drugs compromises safety.

### The baby

The baby should be brought to the surface immediately after birth. The umbilical cord should not be clamped and cut while the baby is still under water because the sudden reduction in placental-fetal blood flow may initiate respiration, and thus water inhalation. If the umbilical cord needs to be cut prior to the birth of the baby, the woman should be asked to stand with the baby's head clear of the water so that the cord may be clamped and cut before the birth of the shoulders.

## PREPARATION FOR THE BIRTH

This is a time of great anticipation and it is now that the true value of the midwife–woman relationship, the strength of the mother, and the skills of the midwife are demonstrated. If the midwife has established a good relationship with the woman and her partner, has enabled the woman to work through her labour with confidence, and has kept the woman and her supporting companions informed of progress and what to expect in the second stage, then the woman and her companions can approach the actual birth with confidence. The atmosphere in the birth room should be calm and unhurried, so that the woman can emerge from the experience with positive memories and intact self-respect. Privacy for the mother must be ensured because it is embarrassing and stressful for her if people repeatedly enter her room.

The midwife should prepare for birth as soon as she suspects that the second stage is imminent. This is especially the case for multigravid women, who can progress very quickly, but some primigravid woman also have very short pushing phases of labour. It is essential to include the women's vocalizations and behaviour in the judgement of progress, and not to rely simply on the findings of a vaginal examination, or on stereotypes of 'typical' patterns of progress.

The room should be clean and warm for the birth of the baby. A warm cot is prepared and resuscitation equipment is checked.

## THE ACTIVITIES OF THE MIDWIFE DURING THE BIRTH

The actual methods of supporting women during birth can be learned only by experience. However, the principles remain the same and can be applied to whatever position the woman adopts for birth. She must be kept informed at all times, and her wishes must be respected.

A clean area is prepared, including a clean gown or apron and gloves for the midwife. To minimize the risk of contamination from blood or liquor splashes, and of infection with diseases such as HIV, the midwife should also wear unobtrusive eye protection, such as plain spectacles. Any other person likely to come into contact with blood or other body fluids should be similarly protected.

Local anaesthetic and syringe are made available for perineal infiltration prior to an episiotomy, should it be necessary. If the mother has consented to active management of the third stage of labour, a suitable oxytocic drug, such as, Syntometrine® 1 mL or Syntocinon 5–10 units, is checked and drawn up in readiness for use. Discussion should have taken place previously regarding active and expectant management (see Ch. 39).

If the woman is recumbent, the vulva is usually washed with warm solution, the birth area draped with clean or sterile towels, and a clean pad placed over the anus to minimize faecal contamination. Although these activities are common practice, there is no evidence that infection rates are increased if plain water is used, and the practice of draping has not been evaluated in terms of infection rates (Keane & Thornton 1998).

If the woman does not have an epidural in situ, and if the labour has progressed normally to this point, her spontaneous pushing efforts will usually be effective. The midwife will need to provide support and encouragement. If the woman is not in an upright position, and if rapid progress seems to be threatening the integrity of the perineum, the hand can be cupped over the head and the perineum to provide gentle counterpressure, or flexion maintained by placing the palm of the hand lightly on the head with fingers pointing to the sinciput. However, the head must not be held back by excessive pressure, since this risks overstretching and tearing of the deeper structures of the pelvic floor. When women are in more upright positions, a 'hands off' approach is usually adopted.

Until the head crowns, it will recede between contractions. It crowns when the widest transverse diameter, the biparietal diameter, distends the vulva, and then no longer recedes. During the birth of the head, the mother is usually asked to breathe steadily in and out to prevent the birth taking place too quickly. Inhalational analgesia can help at this point. Once crowned, the remainder of the head is born by extension. The midwife may change hand position to grasp the parietal eminences to assist in extending the head, if necessary.

When the child's head is born, most midwives will check to see if the cord is round the baby's neck. If so, it is normal practice to free the cord, or to make a loop large enough for the shoulders to pass through. A technique called the 'somersault manoeuvre' (Schorn & Blanco 1991) is widely practised in the USA (see Fig. 37.8) and has been adopted by some midwives in the UK. There is, however, no evidence that unlooping the cord as opposed to leaving it in situ improves fetal oxygenation, and some midwives report that they will not check for the cord unless the birth seems to be impeded. Rarely, if it is so tightly round the neck or shoulders as to prevent the birth of the baby, two pairs of artery forceps must be applied 2–5 cm apart, and the cord cut between them and unwound. However, this procedure should only be performed when absolutely necessary, since, once the cord is severed, the baby is no longer oxygenated, and the loss of placental blood flow may further compromise the baby if there is any subsequent delay with the shoulders.

If necessary, such as in the presence of meconium or maternal faecal matter, the baby's nose and mouth can be gently suctioned, and the eyes swabbed, from within outwards, using one swab for each eye. If the woman is in an upright position, any mucus will usually drain spontaneously as the head rests prior to *internal rotation* of the shoulders. At this stage, some mothers like to be helped into a position to see their baby's head and watch, or perhaps assist with, the birth of the trunk.

Following *restitution* and *external rotation* of the head, the shoulders will normally be in the anteroposterior diameter of the pelvis, although some babies are born with the shoulders in the oblique. If the mother is in the semi-recumbent position, and if the midwife is sure that internal rotation of the shoulders has occurred, the birth can be assisted by placing one hand each side of the baby's head. With the next contraction, gentle downward traction may be applied to the baby's head. The anterior shoulder will then come down below the symphysis pubis.

If the mother has consented to active management of the third stage of labour, an oxytocic is given as the anterior shoulder is born. The posterior shoulder is then born by guiding the head in an upward direction and the baby's trunk is carried towards the mother's abdomen, being born by lateral flexion. The baby can then be placed on the mother's abdomen, or in her arms, where she can immediately see and touch it. The time of birth is noted.

If the mother is in an upright forward-leaning position, the posterior shoulder will normally be born first, following the curve of Carus. In this circumstance, the midwife usually only needs to be in a position to receive the baby to ensure that it is brought safely to the ground, or into its mother's arms.

For most babies, nasopharyngeal suctioning is unnecessary; however, in the presence of meconium or of excessive mucus, it may be required.

Newly emerging evidence suggests that there might be benefits to delaying umbilical cord clamping for a few minutes, or until the cord has stopped pulsating (McDonald & Middleton 2008), particularly for pre-term infants. Whenever the cord is cut, prior to division, the

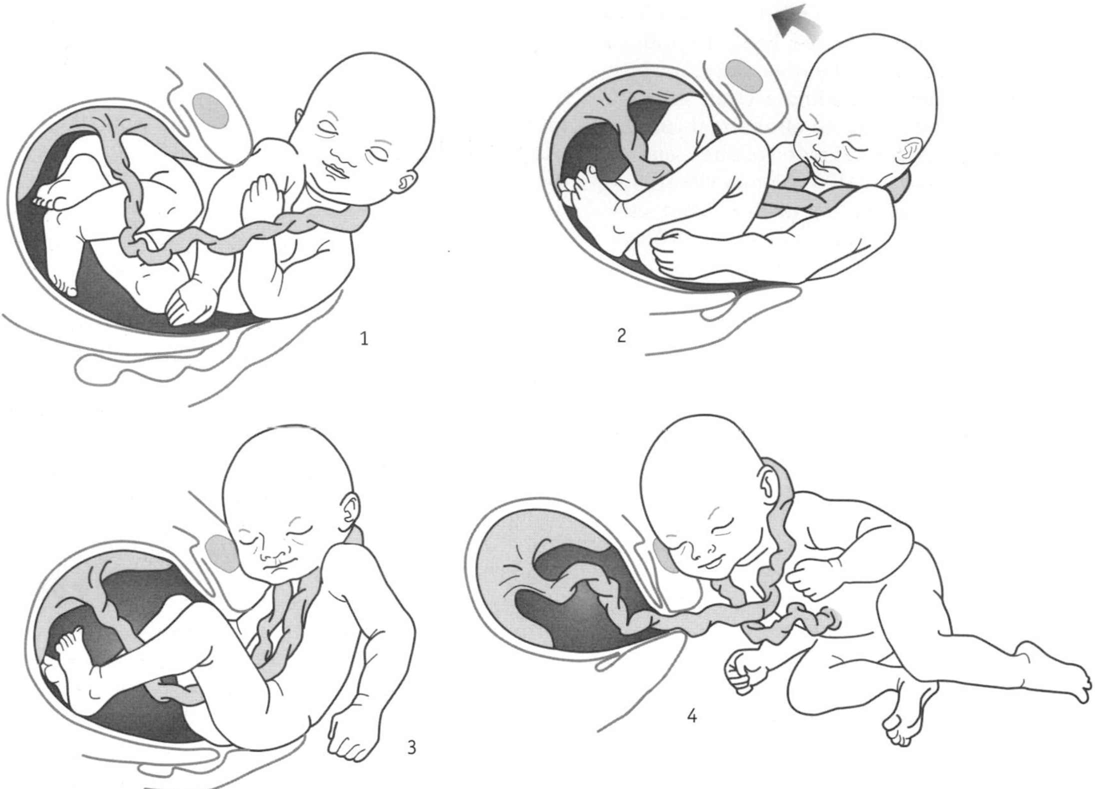


**Figure 37.8** Somersault manoeuvre: the head is delivered normally but, as the body is being born, the head is raised towards the symphysis pubis and the body is moved away from the perineum. This allows for minimum tension on the cord; the midwife can more easily unwrap it and allow the infant to reperfuse. *(From Mercer J, Skovgaard R, Peareara-Eaves J, Bowman T. Nuchal cord management and nurse-midwifery practice.* Journal of Midwifery and Women's Health, *September/October 2005. Reproduced with permission of Elsevier.)*

cord is first clamped with two artery forceps, cut between the forceps with blunt-ended scissors, and then sealed close to the umbilicus, usually with a plastic clamp. It is important to ensure that the baby is thoroughly and gently dried and covered warmly to prevent excessive heat loss, while maintaining the skin-to-skin contact with its mother which appears to be an important component of early breastfeeding success (Moore et al 2007). This is an ecstatic moment for the parents and the midwife is privileged to share their joy in the birth of their baby.

## OBSERVATIONS AND RECORDINGS

Transition and the second stage of labour are very demanding for both woman and fetus. It is a time when the capacity of the woman to birth her baby is most tested. It is also a time when the possibility of fetal hypoxia in a previously compromised baby increases as the alteration in uterine activity reduces placental-fetal oxygenation (Katz et al 1987). It is therefore important to continually assess the wellbeing of mother and fetus.

Recordings should include any discussions with the mother, and any decisions she has taken about the way the labour is conducted. The decisions and actions of the midwife must also be recorded. The woman's general condition and state of mind are noted. Her pulse is taken regularly to rule out rare acute problems, such as intrauterine infection, or a concealed intrapartum haemorrhage. Provided that the blood pressure and temperature have been within normal limits, and there is no history of hypertension or pyrexia, these measures do not need to be recorded more often than hourly. The frequency, strength and duration of uterine contractions are observed, as well as the relaxation of the uterus between contractions. Any sustained loss of uterine activity will result in delayed progress. The midwife will need to reassess the situation to establish the likely cause, and either remedy the situation or seek assistance if necessary.

NICE guidelines recommend that, in the second stage of labour, the fetal heart should be auscultated at the end of a contraction for at least 1 minute every 5 minutes (NICE 2007:161). If continuous electronic fetal heart monitoring is in progress, the cardiotocograph trace should be analysed and assessed for normality.

The amniotic fluid is observed for meconium staining. In a breech presentation, thick fresh meconium is commonly passed at this stage owing to the immense pressure exerted on the breech. While all authorities agree that thick fresh meconium in a cephalic presentation is a serious sign of fetal hypoxia, and that it poses a major risk of meconium aspiration syndrome for the neonate, the significance of thin, old meconium is subject to more controversy. Current NICE guidelines (NICE 2007) recommend continuous electronic fetal monitoring (and transfer for women who are out of hospital) for women with significant meconium-stained liquor, which is defined as either dark green or black amniotic fluid that is thick or tenacious, or any meconium-stained amniotic fluid containing lumps of meconium. NICE recommends that this approach is also considered for women with light meconium staining if a risk assessment that includes stage of labour, volume of liquor, parity, and the fetal heart rate suggests that this might be advisable (NICE 2007).

All observations, including the timing of the various stages and phases of the labour, must be recorded in locally approved labour records. Independent midwives are advised to agree their records in collaboration with their local supervisor of midwives. All actions taken by the midwife must be noted. Each entry must be dated, timed, and signed legibly. Entries made by students must always be countersigned by the attending midwife.

## FUTURE RESEARCH IN THIS AREA

Over the last few years there has been an increase in interest in the nature of normal birth and its consequences. Some of the gaps in the evidence in this area have been identified above. Examples of the areas of research relevant to midwifery that are likely to grow over the next few years include:

- physiological and biochemical outcomes of neonates and infants: comparisons between the outcomes of physiological birth and elective caesarean section
- studies of techniques in the second stage of labour
- studies of the nature of and culture around normal and optimal birth.

## CONCLUSION

For many years it has been assumed that the second stage of labour can be strictly delimited and predicted. Increasing attention to women's actual experiences has led to more formal recognition of the fluidity of the phases of labour, and to an acknowledgement of the nature of transition. Whatever the eventual findings of future research in this area, transition and the expulsive stage of labour remain times of intense hard work, profound psychological impression, and great exhilaration for the mother, her partner, and possibly her baby. The empathetic and skilled midwife is an essential companion on the journey to motherhood that is represented by this stage of labour.

### KEY POINTS

- Transition and second stage can be physically and emotionally intense and maternal behaviour is usually a good indication of progress during this time.
- It is an essential for midwives to understand the physiology and mechanisms of this phase of labour, and be able to apply this knowledge in different situations.
- A skilled midwife can offer unobtrusive support and care while ensuring the wellbeing of the mother and baby.
- Clear, comprehensive and contemporaneous record-keeping is essential.
- Empirical evidence indicates that traditional and new midwifery skills can be beneficial, but there are many gaps in the research evidence in this area, and in understanding the nature of normal and optimal birth.
- Such studies as there have been in this area generally indicate that the second stage of labour can usually be left to progress according to the pattern and activities of the individual woman.

## REFERENCES

Altman MR, Lydon-Rochelle MT: Prolonged second stage of labor and risk of adverse maternal and perinatal outcomes: a systematic review, *Birth* 33(4):315–322, 2006.

Bergstrom L, Seidel J, Skillman-Hull L, et al: 'I gotta push. Please let me push!' Social interactions during the change from first to second stage labor, *Birth* 24(3):173–180, 1997.

Beynon CL: The normal second stage of labour: a plea for reform of its conduct, *Journal of Obstetrics and Gynaecology of the British Empire* 64(6):815–820, 1957.

Bloom SL, Casey BM, Schaffer JI, et al: A randomized trial of coached versus uncoached maternal pushing during the second stage of labor, *American Journal of*

*Obstetrics and Gynecology* 194(1): 10–13, 2006.

Carroli G, Belizan J: Episiotomy for vaginal birth (Cochrane Review), *The Cochrane Library*, Issue 1, Chichester, 2004, John Wiley.

Cluett ER, Nikodem VC, McCandlish RE, et al: Immersion in water in pregnancy, labour and birth, *Cochrane Database of Systematic Reviews* (2):CD000111, 2004.

Crawford JS: The stages and phases of labour: an outworn nomenclature that invites hazard, *Lancet* 2(8344):271–272, 1983.

Downe S, Trent Midwifery Research Group, Young C, et al: Multiple midwifery discourses: the case of the early pushing urge. In Downe S, editor: *Normal birth: evidence and debate*, Oxford, 2008, Elsevier.

Ferguson JK: A study of the motility of the intact uterus of the rabbit at term, *Surgical Gynaecology and Obstetrics* 73:359–366, 1941.

Geissbuehler V, Eberhard J, Lebrecht A: Waterbirth: mother knows best! *Journal of Perinatal Medicine* 30(5):371–378, 2002.

Gross MM, Hecker H, Matterne A, et al: Does the way that women experience the onset of labour influence the duration of labour? *BJOG* 113(3):289–294, 2006.

Gupta JK, Hofmeyr GJ, Smyth RMD: Position in the second stage of labour for women without epidural anaesthesia, *Cochrane Database of Systematic Reviews* (3):CD002006, 2005.

Hartmann K, Viswanathan M, Palmieri R, et al: Outcomes of routine episiotomy: a systematic review, *Journal of the American Medical Association* 293(17):2141–2148, 2005.

Humphrey MD, Chang A, Wood EC, et al: A decrease in fetal pH during the second stage of labour when conducted in the dorsal position, *British Journal of Obstetrics and Gynaecology of the British Commonwealth* 81(8):600–602, 1974.

Johnstone FD, Aboelmagd MS, Harouny AK: Maternal posture in second stage and fetal acid-base status, *British Journal of Obstetrics and Gynaecology* 94(8):753–757, 1987.

Katz M, Lunenfeld E, Meizner I, et al: The effect of the duration of the second stage of labour on the acid-base state of the fetus, *British Journal of Obstetrics and Gynaecology* 94(5):425–430, 1987.

Keane HE, Thornton JG: A trial of cetrimide/chlorhexidine or tap water for perineal cleaning, *British Journal of Midwifery* 6(1):34–37, 1998.

Lawrence A, Lewis L, Hofmeyr GJ, et al: Maternal positions and mobility during first stage labour, *Cochrane Database of Systematic Reviews* (2):CD003934, 2009.

McCandlish R, Bowler U, van Asten H, et al: A randomised controlled trial of care of the perineum during second stage of normal labour, *British Journal of Obstetrics and Gynaecology* 105(12):1262–1272, 1998.

McDonald SJ, Middleton P: Effect of timing of umbilical cord clamping of term infants on maternal and neonatal outcomes, *Cochrane Database of Systematic Reviews* (2):CD004074, 2008.

Moore ER, Anderson GC, Bergman N: Early skin-to-skin contact for mothers and their healthy newborn infants, *Cochrane Database of Systematic Reviews* (2):CD003519, 2007.

National Institute for Health and Clinical Excellence (NICE): *Intrapartum care: care of healthy women and their babies during childbirth* (website). www.nice.org.uk/guidance/index.jsp?action=download&o=36280. 2007. Accessed October 10, 2008.

Petersen L, Besuner P: Pushing techniques during labor: issues and controversies, *Journal of Obstetric, Gynecologic, and Neonatal Nursing* 26(6):719–726, 1997.

Roberts J, Hanson L: Best practices in second stage labor care: maternal bearing down and positioning, *Journal of Midwifery & Women's Health* 52(3):238–245, 2007.

Roberts J E, Goldstein SA, Gruener JS, et al: A descriptive analysis of involuntary bearing down efforts during the expulsive phase of labour, *Journal of Obstetric, Gynecologic, and Neonatal Nursing* 16(1):48–55, 1987.

Royal College of Obstetrician and Gynaecologists (RCOG)/Royal College of Midwives (RCM): *Joint statement No.1. Immersion in water during labour and birth* (website). www.rcog.org.uk/index.asp?PageID=546. 2006. Accessed October 9, 2008.

Schaffer JI, Bloom SL, Casey BM, et al: A randomized trial of the effects of coached vs uncoached maternal pushing during the second stage of labor on postpartum pelvic floor structure and function, *American Journal of Obstetrics and Gynecology* 192(5):1692–1696, 2005.

Schorn MN, Blanco JD: Management of the nuchal cord, *Journal of Nurse Midwifery* 36(2):131–132, 1991.

Stamp G, Kruzins G, Crowther C: Perineal massage in labour and prevention of perineal trauma: randomised controlled trial, *British Medical Journal* 322(7297):1277–1280, 2001.

Sutton J, Scott P: Understanding and teaching optimal fetal positioning, ed 2, Tauranga NZ, 1996, Birth Concepts.

Chapter 38

# Pain, labour and women's choice of pain relief

*Cecelia M. Bartholomew and Margaret Yerby*

## LEARNING OUTCOMES

After reading this chapter, you will:

- understand the physiological aspect of pain processes in labour and its effect on the woman
- appreciate the impact of psychological interactions on the pain process in labour and how this impacts on the woman's perception of pain
- be aware of the effect of culture and environment on the birth process
- understand the nature of support and its relationship to women's coping mechanisms
- be familiar with the range of approaches available to the woman for the control and management of pain during labour.

## INTRODUCTION

The 9 months of pregnancy culminates in birth, an event that many women fear because the process can be painful. Some women become anxious about their ability to cope with pain and this may impact on their perceptions of control during labour and their overall satisfaction of childbirth. The challenge for midwives is in enabling women to understand the various influences upon women's interpretations and experiences of the discomforts that accompany birth. Midwives may assist women to be prepared and facilitate the optimum choices for pain relief to match women's individual needs and ensure the best outcome for both mother and fetus.

## AN EXPLORATION OF PAIN IN LABOUR

Pain is complex, personal, subjective, and a multifactorial phenomenon influenced by psychological, physiological and sociocultural factors. Though pain is universally experienced and acknowledged, it is not completely understood (Lowe 2002). Pain is *usually* associated with injury and tissue damage, thus a warning to rest and protect the area. However, in childbirth, pain is considered to be a side-effect of the process of a normal event (Simkin & Bolding 2004). Increasing pain at the end of pregnancy is often the first sign that labour has commenced (McDonald 2006).

The origins of labour pain are centred on the physiological changes which take place during labour. Pain predominates from the cervix and lower uterine segment, particularly in the first stage of labour (McDonald 2001). Effacement and dilatation of the cervix causes the stripping of membranes away from the uterine lining, hence the 'show' of early labour (McDonald 2006). This causes prostaglandin release. (See Chs 35 and 36.)

Prostaglandin aids the contractility of the myometrium, playing an important role in the initiation of labour (RPSGB & BMA 2008). Manipulation of the cervix during a vaginal examination directly stimulates the production of prostaglandins and increases pain. Nerve endings are stimulated, resulting in a form of inflammatory response in the tissues, which creates pain signals. This response produces histamine, serotonin and bradykinins, which stimulate the nociceptors in the cervix, setting up pain sequences. This stimulates an action potential in the nerve, setting up a chain reaction to the spinal cord and the higher centres in the brain (Tortora & Grabowski 2000, Yerby 2000).

## Uterine nerve supply and nerve transmission

The autonomic nervous system serves the uterus with sympathetic and parasympathetic nerve fibres (see Ch. 35). Nerve pathways supplying the uterus and cervix arise from afferent fibres of the sympathetic ganglia. Nerve endings in the uterus and cervix pass through the cervical and uterine plexuses to the pelvic plexus, the middle hypogastric plexus, the superior hypogastric plexus and then to the lumbar sympathetic nerves to eventually join the thoracic 10, 11, 12 and lumbar 1 spinal nerves (Fig. 38.1).

The nerve supply to the perineum and lower pelvis from the second and third sacral nerve roots meets the plexuses from the uterus at the Lee–Frankenhäuser plexus at the uterovaginal junction (Stjernquist & Sjöberg 1994) (see Ch. 25). These nerves transmit pain in the second stage of labour.

Nerve transmission is along fibres that conduct sensations in different strengths and at different speeds. These fibres are either *A delta,* thinly myelinated fibres, or *C* fibres, which are unmyelinated. It is the smaller C fibres which are found in the deep viscera, such as the uterus, that give rise to the deep prolonged pain of labour when stimulated by muscular contraction and chemical substances (McDonald 2006, McGann 2007).

Pain sensation is transferred by action potentials (see website) along the nerve fibres to the dorsal horn of the spinal cord, thence via upward tracts to the central nervous system (McCool et al 2004) (Fig. 38.2). Because of the release of bradykinins and histamines and other pain-inducing substances at tissue level, '*substance P*' is also released. This is a neuropeptide and is released from the afferent nerves (McGann 2007) as part of the 'signalling process' of pain on its way to the dorsal horn of the spinal cord; it could be termed a potentiator of pain sensation.

As the action potentials from the afferent neurons meet the spinal cord they enter by the posterior (dorsal) root and are transferred to the substantia gelatinosa at laminae (or layers) II and III of the grey matter of the spinal cord. These laminae decode various types of stimulus and

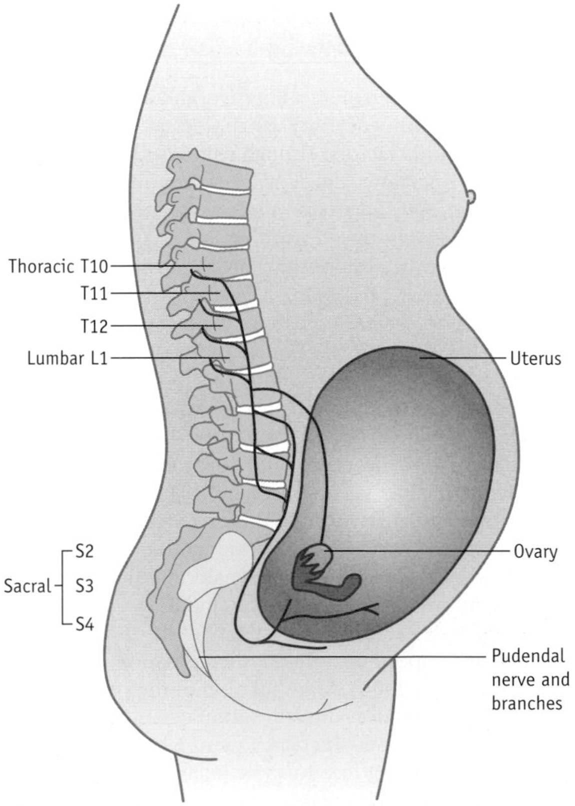

Thoracic T10
T11
T12
Lumbar L1
Uterus
Sacral S2 S3 S4
Ovary
Pudendal nerve and branches

**Figure 38.1** Pain pathways. *(Reprinted from* Pain in childbearing, *Yerby M (ed), 2000, by permission of the publisher Baillière Tindall.)*

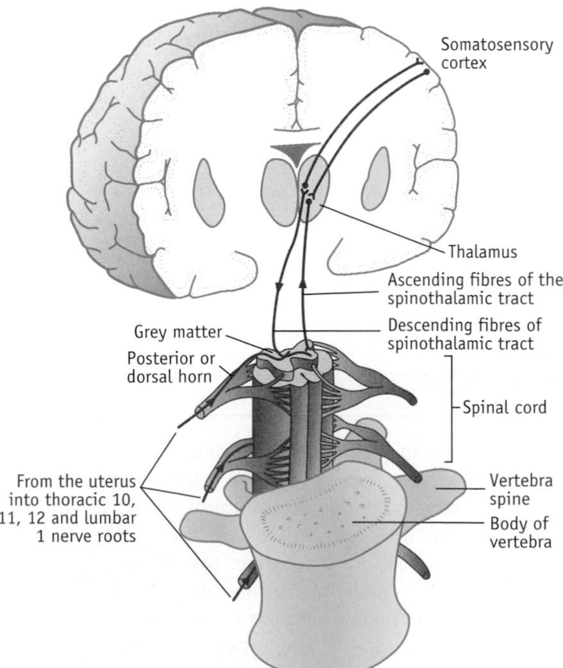


**Figure 38.2** Brain and spinal cord connections. *(Reprinted from* Pain in childbearing, *Yerby M (ed), 2000, by permission of the publisher Baillière Tindall.)*

transfer sensations to the higher centres of the brain via the anterior and lateral spinothalamic tracts, which cross to the opposite side of the cord before ascending, and are perceived as pain by the cerebral cortex (McCool et al 2004).

Descending tracts from the brain, returning to the spinal cord, may have a modulating effect on the nerve transmission of pain (Fig. 38.2). Naturally occurring endorphins at the spinal level act like exogenous opioids by modulating pain response (McGann 2007, Millan 2002).

As labour progresses, signs of the effect of pain on the woman become evident. Pain causes a boost in catecholamine secretion, thus increasing levels of adrenaline. The result is a rise in cardiac output, heart rate, and blood pressure, possibly causing hyperventilation that decreases cerebral and uterine blood flow by vasoconstriction, which may affect contractility of the uterus (McDonald 2006). Uterine contractions may be lessened by increased levels of adrenaline and cortisol and can cause uncoordinated uterine activity (McDonald & Noback 2003). Hyperventilation tends to alter oxygen balance, which may modify the acid–base status of the blood, causing maternal alkalosis, which may in turn cause fetal hypoxia (Lowe 2002).

### Pain gate theory

Melzack & Wall (1965) described a mechanism for modulating pain at spinal cord level. Opioid-like substances, namely endorphins and enkephalins, are neurotransmitters and neuromodulators. These are found principally in the sensory pathways where pain is relayed (Melzack & Wall 1965). With greater understanding of endorphins and their opiate-type properties, it was noted that they dampened the effect of substance P. They are highly effective pain-modulating substances that play a role in pleasure, learning and memory (McGann 2007).

The 'gate theory' suggests a mechanism that prevents the transfer of nerve stimuli to the higher centres of the brain where they are perceived to become conscious as a feeling of pain. At the dorsal horn root in the substantia gelatinosa of the spinal cord, substances may be blocked by a 'gating' mechanism. When the 'gate' is open, pain sensations reach the higher centres. When the 'gate' is closed, pain is blocked and does not become part of the conscious thought, and therefore pain is reduced.

## PSYCHOLOGICAL ASPECT OF PAIN

Whilst it may be easy to acknowledge physical pain, the pain in labour has a psychological component. This is a point to be appreciated by midwives and other health professionals. The psychological influences were recognized in the early theories of nociception (Eccleston 2001), which claimed that the manner in which individuals perceive and respond to pain involves more than peripheral input (Adams & Field 2001).

There exists an affective dimension of pain, which relates not only to the unpleasant feelings of discomfort but also to emotions that may be connected to memories or imagination (Price 2000a). Anxiety related to pain has a protective role that facilitates appropriate behaviours (Carleton & Asmundson 2009) which may be necessary to prepare for the impending birth. However, individuals with high levels of anxiety sensitivity tend to become fearful of the symptoms of pain, demonstrating states of hypervigilance (Thompson et al 2008). This fear may relate to the pain that is currently present but also to perceptions and concerns of what could occur (Carleton & Asmundson 2009). Individuals choose to avoid what they consider to be potentially pain-inducing situations as a result of this fear (Hirsh et al 2008). As such, this may result in what Hirsh et al (2008) describe as pain catastrophizing in reaction to childbirth – a predisposition to underestimate a personal ability to deal with pain, while exaggerating the threat of the pain anticipated. Catastrophizing has been shown to be positively associated with avoidance behaviour in labour (Flink et al 2009).

It should be noted that perceptions of pain will vary among women even when the stimuli are similar. Women react to their labour pains in different ways. This may result in a range of behaviour, such as distraction (Eccleston 2001) or feelings of anger and entrapment (Morley 2008). Maternity caregivers will need to be alert to women's expectations when dealing with their individual pain. It is important to provide clear and brief communication, repeat and explain points where necessary, and make an effort to provide consistent information and guidance (Eccleston 2001).

**Reflective activity 38.1**

Compare your experiences of caring for women during labour in different environments. Would you agree that more women rely more on pharmacological methods of pain relief in society today than in the past? Is this actually true and evidence-based?

## CULTURAL ASPECT OF PAIN

Midwives should acknowledge that the definition, understanding and manifestation of pain will be influenced by cultural experiences of both the woman and her caregivers. Culture affects attitudes toward pain in childbirth, how women cope with this and how they manage it (Callister et al 2003). While some individuals may accept intervention when in pain, others may demonstrate a more stoic approach and avoid help because of their socialization towards behaviour in such circumstances (Davidhizar & Giger 2004).

Various qualitative studies have shown how women from different backgrounds perceive and deal with the pain associated with childbirth. In their research, Johnson et al (2004) found that Dutch women felt that birth was a normal phenomenon that is accompanied by pain, which, though difficult, should not be feared, but used effectively. Somalian women in the study by Finnström & Söderhamn (2006) had been told that it was not acceptable to cry and wail when in pain. As an alternative, they felt that it was necessary to stay in control, tolerate the pain and involve a friend or a family member to help them cope with the event. In Jordan, Abushaikha (2007) found that women utilized spiritual methods to cope and were required to demonstrate patience and endurance towards the pain as a show of strong faith. The women in this study had to ensure that they were not overheard and were expected to labour silently.

Midwives' own cultural experiences of pain will affect their interpretation and attention to women in labour. A study in Scotland comparing Chinese with Scottish women, indicated through one midwifery manager's comment, that a loud coping strategy was occasionally misconstrued by health workers. They were more likely to interpret this as a sign of inability to cope and offer the women analgesia or anaesthetics. Those who remained quiet were often unnoticed (Cheung 2002).

There is a need for cultural competence when caring for women in childbirth (Brathwaite & Williams 2004). Midwives must develop their ability to interpret and understand the verbal communication of pain, and also body language, in order to address the needs of individuals from culturally diverse groups (Finnström & Söderhamn 2006). Awareness of the cultural meanings of childbirth pain, how different women cope and are expected to behave, will assist in the provision of culturally competent care (Callister et al 2003). Cultural assumptions made by midwives, as any assumptions, may prevent individualized and appropriate care.

### Impact of the environment on childbirth pains

Crafter (2000) postulated that the place of birth may have a significant impact on women's experiences of pain in labour and birth because part of a culture is expressed through its environment and organization. The Peel Report (DHSS 1970) promoted changes in the place of birth for women, who had traditionally given birth to their babies at home. Hospitalization altered women's views of birth, leading to a more medicalized birth with greater use of drugs for pain relief, which many women now accept as a normal part of the new environment. Crafter (2000) suggests that furnishings within a room may give women subliminal messages about the presiding culture. For example, an environment simulating the home may indicate behaviour of being in a home, whilst a hospital environment may promote behaviour for that environment.

If the hospital is the place of birth, a woman may adapt to this unfamiliar environment, which may distract her from identifying and adopting her own coping mechanisms during labour. Whilst individual coping strategies assist a woman's physiology of labour, these may be utilized only by women who feel comfortable within their surroundings, such as in the home or birth centre. Women in a more clinical environment may more readily opt for pharmacological preparations to relieve their pain.

## CHOICES FOR PAIN RELIEF IN LABOUR

Against this background of psychological, cultural and physical factors that influence women's experience of pain, preparation is required for individuals to feel ready to cope with their labour and to be able to make personal choices about managing the event. There are varieties of non-pharmacological and pharmacological methods from which women may choose. With an aim to make childbirth as intervention-free as possible, many women may begin by considering non-pharmacological methods, such as some of the complementary or alternative approaches.

## PREPARATION FOR PAIN IN CHILDBIRTH

The potential value of antenatal education and preparation in reducing the fear and anxiety associated with childbirth was recognized by Grantly Dick-Read (1944) and Lamaze (1958). They proposed that labour was not inherently painful. Dick-Read (1944), who appears to be the original authority in this area, endorsed the view that pain was influenced by women's socio-culturally conditioned fear and expectation of birth. They both suggested that labour pains could be controlled by psychoprophylactic techniques, such as muscle relaxation and breathing exercises. Dick-Read (1944) also postulated that providing information and encouraging women to communicate was useful in preparing women for pain in childbirth. The main goal of antenatal classes, which adopt these techniques, is based on empowering women to identify and develop their own body resources to enhance their childbirth experience (Gagnon & Sandall 2007).

The literature regarding the effectiveness of childbirth education is inconclusive (Koehn 2002). According to

Spiby et al (2003), antenatal classes have been associated with increased ability to cope, lower levels of the affective aspect of pain and less use of pharmacological pain relief in labour. However, Lothian (2003) found that only 15% of the women in her study identified childbirth education classes as their source of information about pain relief, with most women depending on their midwives or doctor for explanations. With increasing technology, women may also easily access information through other sources, including the Internet. The Cochrane review by Gagon & Sandall (2007) recognized that the benefits of antenatal education for childbirth remain ambiguous though highlighted that the main body of literature suggests that some expectant parents want antenatal classes, particularly with their first baby.

The content of antenatal classes related to pain management during labour needs to be developed. Antenatal course leaders should prepare women for their subjective experience of pain in labour (Schott 2003) by helping them to explore their own needs, attitudes and expectations of labour (Schneider 2001). Often women are not able to make choices about the management of their pain in labour because they are ignorant of their own body's resources for coping with pain (Nolan 2000). Women will need brief information on the relevant physiology of pain (Robertson 2000) and be presented with a realistic but positive approach to pain in labour (Schott 2003).

During antenatal classes, women should be helped to explore and articulate the range of coping strategies they have used in their own previous experiences of pain, so the positive methods can be enhanced and negative strategies can be replaced with an alternative (Escott et al 2004). It is not unheard of that in labour, when in a mood of panic and acute anxiety, women claim to have forgotten how to 'breathe'. Antenatally, if they have been encouraged to recall and develop their own pre-existing methods of tolerating pain, it may be easier for them to develop a greater sense of self-efficacy to deal with their labour pains (Escott et al 2005).

## CONCEPT OF SUPPORT IN LABOUR

Women need to feel supported during labour. This may take the form of informational, practical or emotional support (Hodnett et al 2007) which are all essential elements in the art of midwifery (Berg & Terstad 2006). Support in labour impacts on the sympathetic element of the autonomic nervous system, by breaking the fear–tension–pain cycle observed by Dick-Read (Mander 2000).

A correlation study in the US by Abushaikha & Sheil (2006) examined the relationship between the feeling of stress and support in labour. The findings suggested that women with greater support reported less stress compared to those who received little.

The main sources of support for some mothers are the midwife and the woman's partner. However, these sources are reliant on the society and culture to which the woman belongs. The findings of a literature review suggested that support for women varies in different countries. This support includes untrained lay women, female relatives, nurses, monitrices (midwives who were self-employed birth attendants) and doulas (Rosen 2004).

McGrath & Kennell (2008), in a randomized controlled trial, reported that women who were supported by a doula required less analgesia compared to those in the control group. A doula is an experienced woman who supports women in childbirth to enable them to achieve a rewarding birth experience (Koumouitzes-Dovia & Carr 2006). They provide care which is continuous and addresses psychological as well as the physical processes of childbirth (Pascali-Bonaro & Kroeger 2004). In the UK, doulas may be used as a supportive friend for vulnerable women who may not have access to such support from their own family.

Koumouitzes-Dovia & Carr (2006) examined women's perception of their doula support. They found that the emerging underlying themes highlighted that women felt doulas were a source of reassurance and encouragement who also provided support for their husbands. Berg & Terstad (2006), in a phenomenological study conducted in Sweden, supported these findings. They found that a doula acted as a mediator between partners, and the midwife provided stability, which made the woman calm and secure.

One of the main benefits of care by a doula is that of continuous support. In a Cochrane systematic review (Hodnett et al 2007), which consisted of 16 trials involving 13,391 women, it was demonstrated that women who had continuous support intrapartum, were more likely to have shorter labours and less likely to have analgesia. The benefit of this support was greater when the provider was not a member of the hospital staff.

## COMPLEMENTARY AND ALTERNATIVE THERAPIES FOR PAIN RELIEF

Complementary and alternative therapies (see Ch. 18) involve practices that are not categorized as conventional medicine (Smith et al 2006). The evidence regarding the efficacy of commonly used therapies in relieving pain is inconclusive (Huntley et al 2004), partly owing to a lack of relevant studies. The National Collaborating Centre for Women's and Children's Health (NCC-WCH 2007) recommended that women who want to use *acupuncture, acupressure* and *hypnosis* should not be discouraged from engaging in these practices. However, it does not encourage a standard provision of such services. There is support for other forms of coping strategies such as *music* and *massage* but more research is required in this area (Kimber et al 2008, McNabb et al 2006, NCC-WCH 2007, Nilsson 2008). Two complementary therapies that are commonly used in midwifery practice are described below.

## Hydrotherapy

Hydrotherapy is increasingly being used worldwide to provide comfort for women in labour. It is well known that a warm bath is useful for relaxation and is a simple means of reducing muscular aches and pains. There is evidence to suggest that immersion in water during the first stage of labour decreases reports of pain and the use of analgesia, without any adverse effects on the duration of labour or neonatal outcome (Cluett et al 2002). The mechanism which underpins hydrotherapy in labour is unclear (Benfield 2002) but it is thought that warm water decreases the perception of pain by stimulating the larger A delta nerve fibres blocking impulses from the smaller C fibres (Teschendorf & Evans 2000) in accordance with the gate control theory.

As women relax in the water there is a decrease in anxiety and rapid reduction in the sensation of pain (Benfield 2002). Labouring in water also enables women to move and change positions to facilitate progress in labour (Stark et al 2008), making it possible for them to play a more active part in their experience of birth (da Silva et al 2009). Women in a study by Maude & Foureur (2007) suggested that they felt protected, supported and comforted while using the water. They choose to use water to reduce their fear of pain and to cope rather than remove it.

It has been postulated that the environment in which the pool/bath is situated and the interaction with the caregivers has a significant part to play on the effect water has on women in labour (Cluett et al 2002). Therefore, the ambience created by the environment of the water pool has importance. For example, there could be a difference between the effects of labouring in a bath in a hospital setting compared with in one that is situated in a specially designed birthing unit, or located in the woman's own home.

Women relax and may become drowsy whilst in the water. The midwife must ensure the woman's safety, particularly should she require additional analgesia, such as Entonox. Women must not be left unattended in a water pool. The temperature of the woman and the water need to be monitored hourly and the water temperature should be maintained below 37.5 °C (NCC-WCH 2007). This will ensure that the woman does not become hyperthermic, as this may have adverse effects on the fetus. It remains unclear what the shape and size of the pool should be, and whether the water should be still or moving, as these aspects require further evaluation (Cluett et al 2002). However, women should have the opportunity to labour in water as a form of pain relief (NCC-WCH 2007).

**Reflective activity 38.2**

When you are next caring for a woman during labour, consider suggesting that she try different positions to cope with contractions. Which positions are the most effective? After the delivery, discuss the woman's opinion of what difference this made to her perception of pain.

## Transcutaneous electrical nerve stimulation (TENS)

TENS is the application of pulsed electrical current through surface electrodes placed on the skin parallel to and on each side of the spine (see Fig. 38.3). TENS produces small electrical sensations and is thought to assist in the prevention of the perception of pain at spinal level, stimulating naturally occurring endorphins and blocking pain (Rodriguez 2005).

The advantages of TENS are that it is a non-invasive form of pain relief that may be used effectively whether the mother is mobile or in bed, with no effect on the fetus or the woman systemically. It gives the woman a feeling of control and some responsibility for managing her own relief of pain (de Ferrer 2006). When commenced early in labour, it enables the endorphins to build up naturally as labour progresses and become more effective (Price 2000b). TENS should not be used for women in established labour as it takes about 40 minutes for the maximum endorphin level to be reached (Rodriguez 2005).

Placed in the correct position, the electrodes supply a residual voltage, which can be boosted by the woman during a contraction. This provides the woman with autonomy and helps her achieve greater emotional fulfilment from the experience of childbirth. Anecdotal evidence from women suggests that only when the electrodes are taken off in labour do they realize how useful TENS has been.

# PHARMACOLOGICAL PAIN RELIEF

Midwives should be able to give advice and explain the side-effects of pharmacological pain relief that meets the woman's needs for control and comfort without causing any harm (Green 2008). This means midwives should keep up to date with current medications and their side-effects and follow unit policies at all times (NMC 2008). An understanding of pharmacokinetics, including the changing drug absorption, metabolism, distribution and

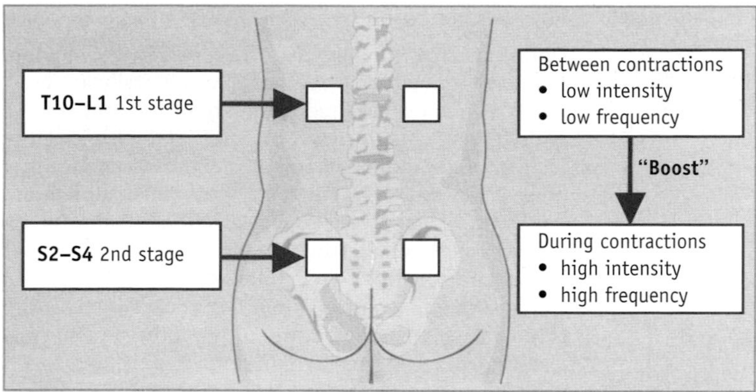


**Figure 38.3** TENS electrode positioning for use during labour *(From Johnson 1997, with permission of Mark Allen Publishing Ltd.)*

excretion in both the woman's body and that of her fetus and baby, is important in providing information and advice to the woman regarding choices of pain relief (see Ch. 10).

**Reflective activity 38.3**

When you are next on the labour ward, take an opportunity to observe the level of support a woman receives during labour and from whom.

What effect do you observe on the process of labour, and on the outcome?

Was the quality and quantity of support the same as you would observe in a home setting, or birth centre? If not, what were the key factors influencing this?

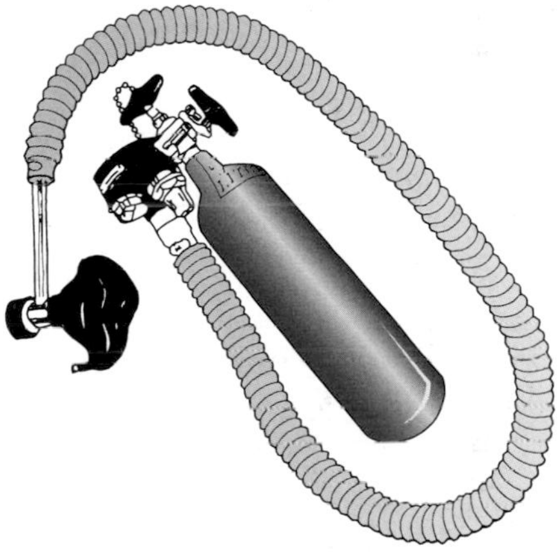

**Figure 38.4** Portable Entonox apparatus.

## Nitrous oxide

The use of inhalation analgesia for pain relief in childbirth originated from the work of Simpson of Edinburgh in 1847, who introduced chloroform for anaesthetic purposes (Crowhurst & Plaat 2001). Nitrous oxide, known as 'laughing gas', has been widely used in midwifery since the 1930s. It is used in labour in a mixture of 50% nitrous oxide and 50% oxygen as Entonox. It is supplied in small portable cylinders (Fig. 38.4) or piped directly to the delivery suite.

The two gases separate at cold temperatures, which leaves nitrous oxide at the bottom of the cylinder. Inverting the cylinder before use, warming in water or keeping at room temperature for 2 hours before use prevents the administration of 100% nitrous oxide (Anaesthesia UK 2008).

Entonox has a sedative effect in use but is not an analgesic and is self-administered by the use of a mouthpiece or mask. It is used by many women and may give them a sense of control but not total pain relief. Women should be warned about the side-effects of dry mouth or even vomiting (NCC-WCH 2007) and disorientation. The gas will only cause unconsciousness if the woman is hypoxic or if the partner is assisting in holding the apparatus. causing continuous aspiration. The effects are quite rapid, commencing 20 seconds after administration with a maximum effect at 60 seconds. It is important that deep breathing at the normal rate is encouraged. To obtain effective relief from pain at the height of the contraction, inhalation should commence immediately as the contraction begins.

Entonox is widely used in the UK and it has been suggested that respiratory depression occurs in the mother when it is combined with opioids (Yeo et al 2007). There is complete absorption through the placenta (Yentis et al 2007). The amount absorbed by the mother rapidly gains equilibrium in the fetus, but, equally so, it is rapidly cleared from the fetal system when the mother stops inhalation. Rosen's (2002) review of randomized controlled trials regarding the efficacy and safety of Entonox suggests that it does not give total pain relief but is generally safe for both mother and fetus.

## Systemic analgesia

### Pethidine

The objective of using analgesic drugs in labour is to achieve an acceptable level of pain relief without compromising the health of the mother or fetus. Opioid analgesics include the morphine-like substances derived from the opium poppy (*Papaver somniferum*) which induce 'euphoria, analgesia and sleep' (RPSGB & BMA 2008). Included in this group would be morphine, diamorphine, fentanyl, remifentanil and meptazinol (RPSGB & BMA 2008). Pethidine, a derivative, has been widely used in midwifery for women in labour since the 1950s and still continues to be used despite the effect opioids have on the mother and the fetus. Pethidine is a synthetic substance, shorter acting than morphine. It does give women some relaxant effect but occasionally causes nausea and vomiting. Its effect is rapid and lasts for approximately 3–4 hours but it is a less effective analgesic than morphine (RPSGB & BMA 2008). It may be given intramuscularly or as an intravenous injection or as an infusion, which may be self-administered. In practice, it is more often administered as a bolus intramuscular injection. The dose ranges from 50 to 200 mg, with no more than 400 mg in 24 hours (RPSGB & BMA 2008), and is dependent on the route of administration, the woman's weight, degree of pain, stage of labour and the rate of progress. A survey of UK units showed that where regional analgesia was either contraindicated or impossible to perform, pethidine or diamorphine (heroin) was used as a bolus or in the form of patient-controlled analgesia (Saravanakumar et al 2007).

#### *Physiological action on the mother*

Pethidine binds to receptor proteins to diffuse through cell membranes to exert its effect within the central nervous system. Its action at the cellular level alters potassium and calcium channels, affecting ion exchange in the neuronal membrane and calming the excitability of the nerve as it reacts to the pain-producing substances. It acts on efferent nerve pathways descending from the brain at the dorsal horn, thus playing a role in the 'gating' of pain at the spinal column level (Rang et al 2007). It is metabolized by the liver to *norpethidine* (normeperidine in America) by a process termed *n*-demethylation, which produces a substance that has half the potency of the original and has a stimulant, convulsive effect (RPSGB & BMA 2008). To prevent the side-effect of nausea and vomiting, 73.7% of UK units use a prophylactic antiemetic with pethidine (Tuckey et al 2007).

#### *Physiological effects on the fetus*

Diffusion across the placenta occurs readily, and equilibrium between maternal and fetal levels is easily achieved. This depends on the lipid solubility of the drug and its molecular weight. The lower pH levels of the fetus relative to the mother would suggest a greater transfer of the active drug (Littleford 2004). The route of administration is also important when considering fetal effects. Following an intravenous dose of pethidine, the drug has been found in the cord blood within 2 minutes; after intramuscular administration, within 30 minutes (Briggs et al 2008). Undoubtedly, pethidine passes from mother to fetus very readily, as does the metabolite norpethidine, and this is dose dependent. The fetus will also produce norpethidine and the levels in the fetal circulation may be higher than in the mother. The fetus may be more susceptible to the effects of this type of medication because of the immaturity of the blood–brain barrier and the fetal bypass of the liver, where it would normally be metabolized (Briggs et al 2008). Babies were found to be less alert, quicker to cry when disturbed, and more difficult to settle.

If the birth of the baby follows within 2–5 hours of administration, there may well be more respiratory depression in the neonate; furthermore, although this is the peak time range for neonatal effect, it may also occur if delivery occurs prior to 2 hours (Hunt 2002). Plasma half-life of pethidine in the maternal system is 3–4 hours and the substance has been found in the neonate's saliva 48 hours after birth (Briggs et al 2008).

#### *Antagonist to pethidine*

Naloxone is an antagonist, blocking the receptors to which the pethidine binds and thus blocking the action of pethidine and its consequent depressant effect on respiration. It may be given via the intramuscular route in doses of 10 mcg/kg body weight (RSPG & BMA 2008). However, it should not be given routinely as there are no studies to recommend its use in this way (Guinsburg & Wyckoff 2006, Wyllie 2008). It is contraindicated if the mother is narcotic dependent (Littleford 2004).

## The lumbar epidural

The epidural is a very effective form of pain relief. The midwife can observe the change in a woman's whole demeanour following its use. It is, however, an invasive technique that requires an anaesthetist (Bamber 2006). The risks and the benefits must be fully discussed and understood by the woman, so that she may make an informed decision. Throughout the induction procedure, the midwife should support the woman and her partner both physically and psychologically. The fetal heart rate must be monitored and record-keeping must be maintained.

An epidural is inserted in the space between the second and third lumbar vertebrae. This is made easier by

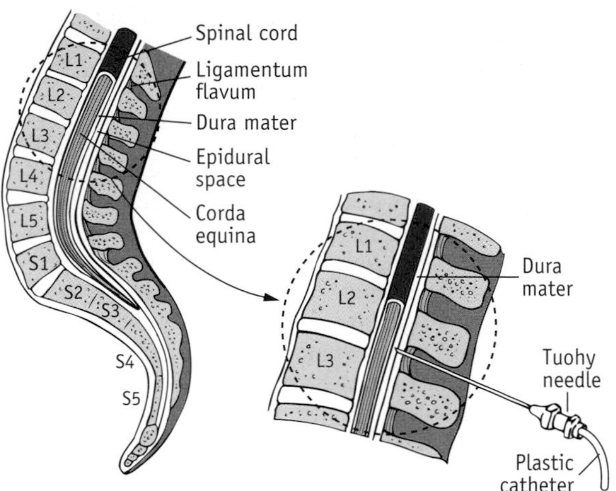


**Figure 38.5** Epidural induction: insertion of the Tuohy needle. *(Reprinted from* Pain in childbearing, *Yerby M (ed), 2000, by permission of the publisher Baillière Tindall.)*

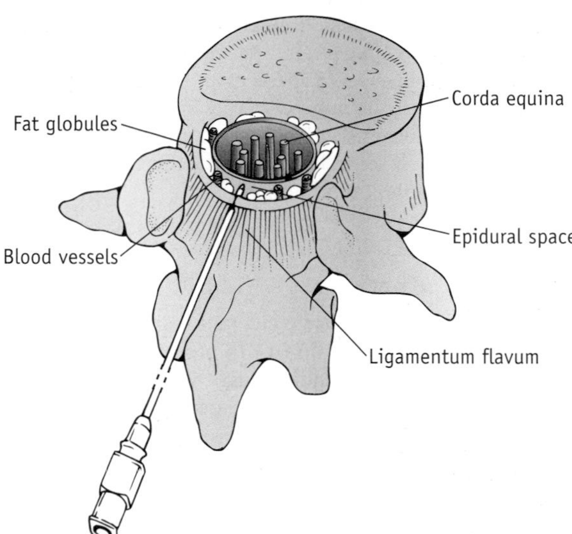


**Figure 38.6** Epidural induction: Tuohy needle positioned in the epidural space. *(Reprinted from* Pain in childbearing, *Yerby M (ed), 2000, by permission of the publisher Baillière Tindall.)*

increasing the flexion of the spine. The tough ligamentum flavum has to be overcome prior to the insertion of the needle into the 1–7-mm thick potential epidural space (Fig. 38.5) between the dura mater and arachnoid mater. The epidural space contains blood vessels, nerve roots and fat and is triangular in shape (Fernando & Price 2002). At the level of the first lumbar vertebra, the spinal cord becomes a collection of nerve fibres termed the *cauda equina*, which, as its Latin name suggests, resembles a horse's tail (Tortora & Grabowski 2000). Although anatomically the epidural space runs the length of the spinal column, occasionally the epidural injection is unsuccessful and it is believed that there may be folds in this membrane diverting the flow of analgesia away from the nerves (Russell & Reynolds 1997).

Following cleansing of the skin and application of local anaesthetic a Tuohy needle is carefully inserted into the potential space. This large-bore needle with centimetre marking and a bevelled end aids with insertion and positioning of a fine catheter (MacIntyre 2007). Smaller-gauge needles are used for spinals and could prevent dural tap (Sprigge & Harper 2008) (Fig. 38.6). The catheter is left in situ; the injection of bupivacaine into this potential space will block the autonomic nerve pathways that supply the uterus. The epidural analgesia is maintained through regular top-ups by the midwife or by the woman, using bolus doses of the anaesthetic agent (Collis 2007). The current recommendation is 0.0625–0.1% *bupivacaine* or equivalent with 2.0 mcg/mL *fentanyl* (NCC-WCH 2007).

## *Physiological effects of the epidural*

The injection of bupivacaine into the epidural space bathes the nerves of the chorda equina, blocking the autonomic nerve pathways that supply the uterus, thus changing action potentials in the nerve and preventing pain. The epidural analgesic acts on the sympathetic nervous system by altering adrenaline and noradrenaline levels in the blood (May & Leighton 2007). Lederman et al (1978) suggested that by decreasing the levels of these catecholamines, uterine activity may be improved, as high levels tend to lengthen labour.

The effect on the autonomic nervous system produces vasodilatation in the peripheral circulation, causing the extremities to feel warm, a good test that the epidural is working. However, pooling of the circulation in the periphery may cause hypotension, as there is a loss of peripheral resistance in the lower limbs. This is usually controlled by increasing intravenous fluids and repositioning the woman. If there is no sign of recovery, the anaesthetist should be informed immediately to administer a bolus dose of a vasopressor, such as ephedrine. The placental bed is unable to compensate for lowered delivery of blood to the uterus, so bradycardia in the fetus may be a problem (O'Connor 2007).

As sensation is lost, normal micturition may be affected; this does have implications on bladder care in labour to prevent postnatal urinary retention (Liang 2002). Women tend to have fewer problems with micturition when low-dose epidurals are used (Wilson et al 2009).

The pelvic floor muscles are somewhat relaxed and this may have a detrimental effect on fetal head rotation and lengthen the process of birth (Odibo 2007). In addition, the second stage could be longer because women may not feel the sensation to push. If the fetal condition is satisfactory, delayed pushing seems to decrease the need for instrumental deliveries (Roberts et al 2005) and does not appear to increase the number of caesarean sections. NCC-WCH (2007) recommend delaying pushing for 1 hour after diagnosis of second stage, with delivery of the baby before the completion of 4 hours.

### Other complications

#### *Respiratory arrest*

This may be caused by the accidental induction of a high nerve block or the injection of bupivacaine into a vein. The first sign will be a tingling tongue with a rapid deterioration; therefore, the midwife needs to be prepared for immediate resuscitation.

#### *Dural tap*

This occurs in 0.5–2% persons receiving regional anaesthetics; 70–80% of these will develop a postural headache. This is caused by a lowering of pressure of circulating cerebrospinal fluid, causing a stretching of brain tissue, in turn causing pain. Rest is important following the procedure, to prevent more spinal fluid leakage increasing headaches until the dura is healed. It can be treated with an autologous blood patch of 10–20 mL of the patient's own blood injected near the site of the epidural to seal the dura. Serious complications are rare following this procedure (O'Connor 2007).

#### *Long-term backache*

During pregnancy and labour, ligaments are altered by the hormones of pregnancy, which permits some movement, increasing pelvic size to facilitate birth. Backache is a common complaint in pregnancy and following birth. A Cochrane Update (Anim Samuah et al 2005) concluded that epidurals created more instrumental deliveries but there was no statistical evidence to suggest that epidurals caused long-term backache or increased the incidence of caesarean section.

The latest Confidential Enquiry into Maternal and Child Health (CEMACH) (Lewis 2007) states that the risk of death from regional anaesthesia is 1:100,000 parturiants.

## CONCLUSION

Pain is a multifaceted phenomenon of pregnancy, without which women would not know they were in labour. Psychological factors affect women's perceptions of pain in labour, and though education helps to decrease anxiety, it has not been proven by research to lessen women's pain. Support has been shown to be valuable, whether by partner, midwife or doula, and is valued more when care is continuous from a known midwife. Women with continuous support seem to require less pain relief, but when a labour becomes long and pain increases, women tend to require systemic pain relief. Pethidine seems to be used less often in today's delivery suites in favour of the more effective epidural analgesia, though both methods of pain relief have side-effects. Research should continue to investigate women's needs and the production of systemic analgesia that is safe in labour for both mother and fetus. Midwives should continue to develop their skills in supporting women in labour whether with or without pain relief.

### KEY POINTS

- An understanding of what pain is and how it may be experienced is influenced by women's expectations, previous experience and the effect of childbirth education on their experiences and the fear–pain–anxiety triangle.
- The midwife must take account of the physiological aspects of pain, its transmission, pain substances and the gate control theory of pain control.
- The cultural and social aspects of pain will influence the environment and coping mechanisms of women in labour, and how support may be provided by families and friends.
- There are a wide range of pain-management strategies, from the use of distractive techniques or TENS to pharmacological methods of pain relief, including Entonox, pethidine and epidural analgesia.

## REFERENCES

Abushaikha LA: Methods of coping with labor pain used by Jordanian women, *Journal of Transcultural Nursing* 18(1):35–40, 2007.

Abushaikha L, Sheil E: Labor stress and nursing support: how do they relate? *Journal of International Women's Studies* 7(4):198–208, 2006.

Adams N, Field L: Pain management 1: Psychological and social aspects of pain, *British Journal of Nursing* 10(14):903–911, 2001.

Anaesthesia UK: Commonly used drugs in obstetric anaesthesia (website). www.anaesthesiauk.com. 2008. Accessed December 2008.

Anim Samuah M, Smyth R, Howell CN: Epidural vs non epidural or no analgesia in labour, *Cochrane Database of Systematic Reviews* (4):CD000331, 2005.

Bamber J: Anaesthetist provided labour epidural analgesia, *Current Anaesthesia and Critical Care* 17(3):131–141, 2006.

Benfield RD: Hydrotherapy in labour, *Journal of Nursing Scholarship* 43(4):337–352, 2002.

Berg M, Terstad A: Swedish women's experiences of doula support during childbirth, *Midwifery* 22(4):330–338, 2006.

Brathwaite AC, Williams CC: Childbirth experiences of professional Chinese Canadian women, *Journal of Obstetric, Gynecologic, and Neonatal Nursing* 33(6):748–755, 2004.

Briggs GG, Freeman RK, Yaffe SJ, editors: *Drugs in pregnancy and lactation*, ed 8, Philadelphia, 2008, Lippincott Williams & Wilkins.

Callister LC, Khalaf I, Semenic S, et al: The pain of childbirth: perceptions of culturally diverse women, *Pain Management Nursing* 4(4):145–154, 2003.

Carleton RN, Asmundson GJ: The multidimensionality of fear of pain: construct independence for the Fear of Pain Questionnaire-Short Form and the Pain Anxiety Symptoms Scale-20, *Journal of Pain* 10(1):29–37, 2009.

Cheung NF: The cultural and social meanings of childbearing for Chinese and Scottish women in Scotland, *Midwifery* 18(4):279–295, 2002.

Cluett ER, Nikodem VC, McCandlish RE, et al: Immersion in water in pregnancy, labour and birth, *Cochrane Database of Systematic Reviews* (2):CD000111, 2002.

Collis RE: Analgesia in labour: induction and maintenance, *Anaesthesia and Intensive Care Medicine* 8(7):273–275, 2007.

Crafter H: Psychology of pain in labour. In Yerby M, editor: *Pain in childbearing*, London, 2000, Baillière Tindall.

Crowhurst JA, Plaat F: Pain relief in labour and the anaesthetist. In MacLean AB, Stones RW, Thornton S, editors: *Pain in obstetrics and gynaecology*, London, 2001, RCOG.

da Silva FMB, de Oliveira SMJ, Nobre MRC: A randomised controlled trial evaluating the effect of immersion bath on labour pain, *Midwifery* 25(3):286–294, 2009.

Davidhizar R, Giger JN: A review of the literature on care of clients in pain who are culturally diverse, *International Council of Nurses, International Nursing Review* 51(1):47–55, 2004.

de Ferrer G: TENS: non-invasive pain relief for the early stages of labour, *British Journal of Midwifery* 14(8):480–482, 2006.

Department of Health and Social Security (DHSS): *Domiciliary and maternity bed needs. Report of the Sub-committee of the Standing Midwifery and Maternity Advisory Committee (Peel Report)*, London, 1970, HMSO.

Dick-Read G: *Childbirth without fear*, New York, 1944, Harper Row.

Eccleston C: Role of psychology in pain management, *British Journal of Anesthesia* 87(1):144–152, 2001.

Escott D, Slade P, Spiby H, et al: The range of coping strategies women use to manage pain and anxiety prior to and during first experience of labour, *Midwifery* 20(2):144–156, 2004.

Escott D, Slade P, Spiby H: Preliminary evaluation of a coping strategy enhancement method of preparation for labour, *Midwifery* 21(3):278–291, 2005.

Fernando R, Price M: Regional anesthesia for labour. In Collis RE, Plaat F, Urquhart J, editors: *Textbook of obstetric anaesthesia*, Cambridge, 2002, Cambridge University Press.

Finnström B, Söderhamn O: Conceptions of pain among Somali women, *Journal of Advanced Nursing* 54(4):418–425, 2006.

Flink IK, Mroczek MZ, Sullivan MJL, et al: Pain in childbirth and postpartum recovery: the role of catastrophizing, *European Journal of Pain* 13(3):312–316, 2009.

Gagnon AJ, Sandall J: Individual or group antenatal education for childbirth or parenthood, or both, *Cochrane Database of Systematic Reviews* (3):CD002869, 2007.

Green C: Pethidine use: the ethics, *The Practising Midwife* 11(9):14–17, 2008.

Guinsburg R, Wyckoff MH: Naloxone during neonatal resuscitation: acknowledging the unknown, *Clinics in Perinatology* 33(1):121–132, 2006.

Hirsh AT, George SZ, Bialosky JE, et al: Fear of pain, pain catastrophizing, and acute pain perception: relative prediction and timing of assessment, *Journal of Pain* 9(9):806–812, 2008.

Hodnett ED, Gates S, Hofmeyr GJ, et al: Continuous support for women during childbirth, *Cochrane Database of Systematic Reviews* (3):CD003766, 2007.

Hunt S: Pethidine: love it or hate it? *MIDIRS Midwifery Digest* 12(3):363–365, 2002.

Huntley AL, Thompson JC, Ernst E: Complementary and alternative medicine for labor pain: a systematic review, *American Journal of Obstetrics and Gynecology* 191(1):36–44, 2004.

Johnson MI: Transcutaneous electrical nerve stimulation in pain management, *British Journal of Midwifery* 5(7):400–405, 1997.

Johnson TR, Clark Callister L, Freeborn DS, et al: Dutch women's perception of childbirth in the Netherlands, *American Journal of Maternal Child Nursing* 32(3):170–177, 2004.

Kimber L, McNabb M, Mc Court C, et al: Massage or music for pain relief in labour: a pilot randomised placebo controlled trial, *European Journal of Pain* 12(8):961–969, 2008.

Koehn ML: Childbirth education outcomes: an integrative review of the literature, *Journal of Perinatal Education* 11(3):10–19, 2002.

Koumouitzes-Dovia J, Carr CA: Women's perceptions of their doula support, *Journal of Perinatal Education* 15(4):34–40, 2006.

Lamaze F: *Painless childbirth* (LR Celestine Translation), London, 1958, Burke.

Lederman RP, Lederman E, Work B, et al: The relationship of maternal anxiety, plasma catecholamines, and plasma cortisol to the progression in labor, *American Journal of Obstetrics and Gynecology* 132(5):495–500, 1978.

Lewis G, editor: *The Confidential Enquiry into Maternal and Child Health (CEMACH). Saving mothers' lives: reviewing maternal deaths to make motherhood safer – 2005-2005. The seventh report on Confidential Enquiries into Maternal Deaths in the United Kingdom*, London, 2007, CEMACH.

Liang C: The effect of epidural analgesia on postpartum urinary retention in women who deliver vaginally, *International Journal of Obstetric Anaesthesia* 11(3):64–69, 2002.

Littleford J: Effects on the fetus and newborn of maternal analgesia and anesthetics: a review, *Canadian Journal of Anesthetics* 51:586–609, 2004.

Lothian JA: Listening to mothers: the first national U.S. survey of women's childbearing experiences, *Journal of Perinatal Education* 12(1):vi–viii, 2003.

Lowe NK: The nature of labor pain, *American Journal of Obstetrics and*

*Gynecology* 186(5 Suppl Nature):S16–S24, 2002.

McCool WF, Smith T, Aberg C: Pain in women's health: a multi-faceted approach toward understanding, *Journal of Midwifery and Women's Health* 49(6):473–481, 2004.

McDonald JS: Pain of childbirth. In Loeser JD, editor: *Bonica's management of pain*, ed 3, Philadelphia, 2001, Lippincott Williams & Wilkins, pp 1388–1414.

McDonald JS: Obstetric pain. In McMahon SB, Koltzenburg M, editors: *Wall and Melzack's textbook of pain*, ed 5, Edinburgh, 2006, Elsevier.

McDonald JS, Noback CP: Obstetrical pain. In Melzack R, Wall PD, editors: *Handbook of pain management*, Edinburgh, 2003, Churchill Livingstone.

McGann K: The anatomy and physiology of pain. In *Fundamental aspects of pain assessment and management*, Gateshead, 2007, Quay Books.

McGrath SK, Kennell JH: A randomized controlled trial of continuous labor support for middle-class couples: effect on cesarean delivery rates, *Birth* 35(2):92–97, 2008.

MacIntyre JWR: Regional anaesthesia safety. In Finucane BT, editor: *Complications of regional anaesthesia*, ed 2, New York, 2007, Springer.

McNabb MT, Kimber L, Haines A: Does regular massage from late pregnancy to birth decrease maternal pain perception during labour and birth? A feasibility study to investigate a programme of massage, controlled breathing and visualization, from 36 weeks of pregnancy until birth, *Complementary Therapies in Clinical Practice* 12(3):222–231, 2006.

Mander R: Does social support affect pain in labour? *British Journal of Midwifery* 8(11):667–672, 2000.

Maude RM, Foureur MJ: It's beyond water: stories of women's experience of using water for labour and birth, *Women and Birth* 20(1):17–24, 2007.

May A, Leighton R: *Epidurals for childbirth: a guide for all delivery suite staff*, ed 2, London, 2007, Cambridge University Press.

Melzack R, Wall P: Pain mechanisms: a new theory, *Science* 150(699):971–979, 1965.

Millan MJ: Descending control of pain, *Progress in Neurobiology* 66(6):355–474, 2002.

Morley S: Psychology of pain, *British Journal of Anaesthesia* 101(1):25–31, 2008.

National Collaborating Centre for Women's and Children's Health (NCC-WCH): *Intrapartum care: care of healthy women and their babies during childbirth*, London, 2007, RCOG.

Nilsson U: The anxiety- and pain-reducing effects of music interventions: a systematic review, *AORN Journal* 87(4):780–807, 2008.

Nolan M: The influence of antenatal classes on pain relief in labour, *The Practising Midwife* 3(6):26–31, 2000.

Nursing and Midwifery Council (NMC): *Standards for medicines management*, London, 2008, NMC.

O'Connor PJ: Complication of obstetric regional anaesthesia, In Finucane BT, editor: *Complications of regional anaesthesia*, ed 2, New York, 2007, Springer.

Odibo L: Does epidural analgesia affect the second stage of labour? *British Journal of Midwifery* 15(7):429–435, 2007.

Pascali-Bonaro D, Kroeger M: Continuous female companionship during childbirth: a crucial resource in times of stress or calm, *Journal of Midwifery and Women's Health* 49(4):19–27, 2004.

Price D: Psychological and neural mechanisms of the affective dimension of pain, *Science* 288(5472):1769–1772, 2000a.

Price S: Pain relief: a practical guide to obstetrics TENS machines, *British Journal of Midwifery* 8(9):550–552, 2000b.

Rang HP, Dale MM, Ritter JM: *Pharmacology*, ed 6, Edinburgh, 2007, Churchill Livingstone.

Roberts CL, Torvaldsen S, Cameron CA, et al: Delayed versus early pushing in women with epidural analgesia,: a systematic review and meta-analysis, *MIDIRS Midwifery Digest* 15(2):212–218, 2005.

Robertson A: Tell me about the pain, *The Practising Midwife* 3(7):46–47, 2000.

Rodriguez MA: Transcutaneous electrical nerve stimulation during birth, *British Journal of Midwifery* 13(8):522–526, 2005.

Rosen M: Nitrous oxide for relief of labor pain: a systematic review, *American Journal of Obstetrics and Gynecology* 186(5 Suppl Nature):S110–S126, 2002.

Rosen P: Supporting women in labor: analysis of different types of caregivers, *Journal of Midwifery and Women's Health* 49(1):24–31, 2004.

Royal Pharmaceutical Society of Great Britain (RPSBG), British Medical Association (BMA): *British National Formulary* (BNF) 56, London, 2008, Pharmaceutical Press.

Russell R, Reynolds F: Neuroscientific aspects. In: Reynolds F, editor: *Pain relief in labour*, London, 1997, BMJ Publishing.

Saravanakumar K, Garstang JS, Hasan K: Intravenous patient-controlled analgesia for labour: a survey of UK practice, *MIDIRS Midwifery Digest* 17(4):534, 2007.

Schneider Z: Antenatal education classes in Victoria: what the women said, *Australian College of Midwives Incorporated* 14(3):14–20, 2001.

Schott J: Antenatal education changes and future developments, *British Journal of Midwifery* 11(10):S15–S17, 2003.

Simkin P, Bolding A: Update on nonpharmacologic approaches to relieve labor pain and prevent suffering, *Journal of Midwifery and Women's Health* 49(6):489–504, 2004.

Smith CA, Collins CT, Cyna AM, et al: Complementary and alternative therapies for pain management, *Cochrane Database of Systematic Reviews* (4):CD003521, 2006.

Spiby H, Slade P, Escott D, et al: Coping strategies in labor: an investigation of women's experiences, *Birth* 30(3):189–194, 2003.

Sprigge JS, Harper SJ: Accidental dural puncture and post dural puncture headache in obstetric anaesthesia: presentation and management: a 23 year survey in a district general hospital, *MIDIRS Midwifery Digest* 18(3):391–396, 2008.

Stark MA, Rudell B, Haus G: Observing position and movements in hydrotherapy: a pilot study, *Journal Of Obstetric, Gynaecologic, and Neonatal Nursing* 37(1):116–122, 2008.

Stjernquist M, Sjöberg NO: Neurotransmitters in the myometrium. In Chard T, Grudzinskas JG, editors: *The uterus*, Cambridge, 1994, Cambridge University Press.

Teschendorf ME, Evans CP: Hydrotherapy during labor: an example of developing a practice policy, *MCN. The American Journal of Maternal Child Nursing* 25(4):198–203, 2000.

Thompson T, Keogh E, French C, et al: Anxiety sensitivity and pain: generalisability across noxious stimuli, *Pain* 134(1–2):187–196, 2008.

Tortora GJ, Grabowski SR: *Principles of anatomy and physiology*, ed 7, New York, 2000, Harper Collins College Publications.

Tuckey JP, Prout RE, Wee MY: Prescribing intramuscular opioids for labour analgesia in consultant-led maternity units: a survey of UK practice, *International Journal Obstetric Anaesthesia* 17(1):3–8, 2007.

Wilson MJA, MacArthur C, Shennan A: Urinary catheterization in labour with high-dose vs mobile analgesia: a randomized controlled trial, *British Journal of Anaesthesia* 102(1):97–103, 2009.

Wyllie J: Resuscitation of the term and premature baby, *Paediatrics and Child Health* 18(4):166–171, 2008.

Yentis S, May A, Malhotra S, et al: Placental transfer of drugs. In Yentis S, May A, Malhotra S, et al, editors: *Analgesia, anaesthesia and pregnancy: a practical guide*, ed 2, Cambridge, 2007, Cambridge University Press.

Yeo ST, Holdcroft A, Yentis SM, et al: Analgesia with sevflurane during labour: 11. Sevoflurane compared with Entonox for labour analgesia, *British Journal of Anaesthesia* 98(1):110–115, 2007.

Yerby M, editor: *Pain In childbearing*, Edinburgh, 2000, Baillière Tindall.

Chapter |39|

# Care in the third stage of labour

Tina Harris

## LEARNING OUTCOMES

At the end of this chapter, the reader will be able to:

- describe the physiology of the third stage of labour
- differentiate between expectant and active management
- explore the debate between expectant and active management and the implications for midwifery practice
- identify how to examine the term placenta and membranes.

## INTRODUCTION

The period from the birth of the baby until expulsion of the placenta and membranes is known as the third stage of labour. During this phase of the birthing process, the mother and child meet face to face for the first time. It is a time of great importance, when the actions of those present can have a long-term effect on developing family relationships and successful breastfeeding. It is also a time when the placenta will separate from the uterine wall, descend into the lower uterine segment and be expelled together with the membranes.

The skill and expertise of the midwife continue to be needed to support this special time between mother, baby and family whilst monitoring successful completion of the childbirth process.

Traditionally, this period of childbirth has been regarded as 'hazardous' because of the risk of excessive bleeding; haemorrhage is a major cause of maternal death in the world (Khan et al 2006). However, currently within the UK, a very small number of women die as a result of excessive bleeding (Lewis 2007). This low rate of haemorrhage has been attributed to the prophylactic or routine use of active management during the third stage of labour for all women.

Active management is a package of care which includes the administration of an oxytocic drug, early clamping and cutting of the cord, and the speedy delivery of the placenta, usually by controlled cord traction (NICE 2007).

While the benefits of active management cannot be questioned for women at risk of postpartum haemorrhage, its indiscriminate use for women at low risk experiencing normal birth has been challenged (Harris 2001, Soltani 2008). Active management is not without risk and the component of active management which reduces blood loss has still not been clearly identified. A more targeted approach for active management has therefore been suggested, rather than its indiscriminate use for all women (Harris 2001, Soltani 2008), as currently there is insufficient evidence to support a clear recommendation.

An alternative to active management is *expectant management*, also called 'passive', 'physiological', or 'natural' management. This is a package of care where there is **no** active intervention in the normal physiological processes. It is characterized by activity on the part of the woman in birthing the placenta and membranes herself; the midwife's role is one of 'watchful waiting'.

The role of the midwife during the third stage of labour is:

- to offer women a choice of care relevant to their individual needs
- to support and monitor the normal physiological, sociological and psychological processes at work
- to detect those women who deviate from the norm and offer appropriate care which may include active management of the third stage.

In achieving this, midwives need to have an understanding of the physiology of the third stage and be able to develop partnerships with women to achieve successful delivery of the placenta and membranes with the appropriate rather than indiscriminate use of intervention.

It is suggested that women often are not given information about the third stage and do not choose how it will be managed. If women are to benefit from controlling their birth experience, then this should include the third stage of labour. A discussion should ideally take place antenatally and include the benefits and limitations of both active and expectant management. Following the discussion, the woman's choice should be recorded clearly in her notes.

The midwife needs to pay careful attention to offering women clear information, which should be as value-free as possible.

Some midwives struggle in offering women this choice for a variety of reasons.

- Current evidence appears to support the continued use of prophylactic active management for all women (NICE 2007, Prendiville et al 2000).
- The majority of midwives in practice will have trained during the period when active management was regarded as appropriate for all women and to be recommended (Harris 2001).
- Some midwives may have either little or no experience of managing the third stage of labour expectantly and lack confidence in this form of care (Featherstone 1999).

If women are to have a real choice, then consideration needs to be given to educating and supporting midwives in clinical practice and in developing a reflective analytical approach to discussions about the third stage which take place between midwives and women.

**Reflective activity 39.1**

Take a few minutes to jot down notes on your feelings about the third stage of labour and how it should be managed in women experiencing normal birth. How may your personal feelings influence a woman's choice of management for the third stage?

## PHYSIOLOGY OF THE THIRD STAGE

The third stage of labour is not really a stage at all. It is an extension of what has gone before (that is, the process of giving birth) and what will happen afterwards (the control of bleeding and the return of the uterus to its non-pregnant state). During labour, the uterine muscles contract and retract under the influence of naturally produced oxytocin. These muscles continue to contract and retract during the third stage to expel the placenta and membranes. The control of bleeding is brought about by the same physiological processes.

Separation of the placenta usually begins with the contraction that delivers the baby's trunk and is completed with the next one or two contractions. As the body of the baby is delivered, there is a marked reduction in the size of the uterus because of the powerful contraction and retraction which take place. The placental site therefore greatly diminishes in size. Initially, placental separation was thought to be brought about by the bursting of decidual sinuses under pressure and the subsequent forming of a retroplacental blood clot which tore the septa of the spongiosa layer of the decidua basalis, detaching the placenta from the uterine wall (Brandt 1933). However, Dieckmann et al (1947) and more recently Herman et al (1993) suggest separation is caused by the active placental site uterine wall thickening and reducing in size, causing the placenta to 'shear off'. Krapp et al (2000, 2003) describe three phases to the third stage of labour (Fig. 39.1). These three phases have now been widely accepted as describing the process of placental detachment and expulsion.

- *Latent phase*: period of time from delivery of the infant until the beginning of placental separation. During this phase, the placenta-free uterine wall thickens under the influence of intermittent contractions, with minimal thickening of the uterine wall over the placenta (101 ± 87 seconds).
- *Detachment phase*: period of placental separation and detachment from the uterine wall, brought about by gradual thickening of the uterine wall over the site of placental attachment. The myometrium adjacent to the lower edge of the placenta contracts, thickens and reduces its surface area overall, which leads to a shearing off of the placenta in that area. This wave of placental wall thickening and placental separation continues upwards and outwards until the whole placenta is detached (56 ± 45 seconds). Separation of the placenta from the uterine wall is normally achieved within 3 minutes.
- *Expulsion phase*: period from complete separation of the placenta to vaginal expulsion. The upper uterine segment contracts strongly, forcing the placenta to fold in on itself and descend into the lower segment and from there to the vagina. Gravity, and sometimes maternal effort brought about by stimulation of the pelvic floor, leads to expulsion of the placenta and membranes (77 ± 63 seconds).

The mean length of the third stage is calculated to be approximately 6 minutes (365 ± 270 seconds) (see Fig. 39.2).

### *Cord clamping*

If the umbilical cord remains intact during the third stage, blood can pass to and from the infant until cord pulsation has ceased. The amount of blood gained or lost by the

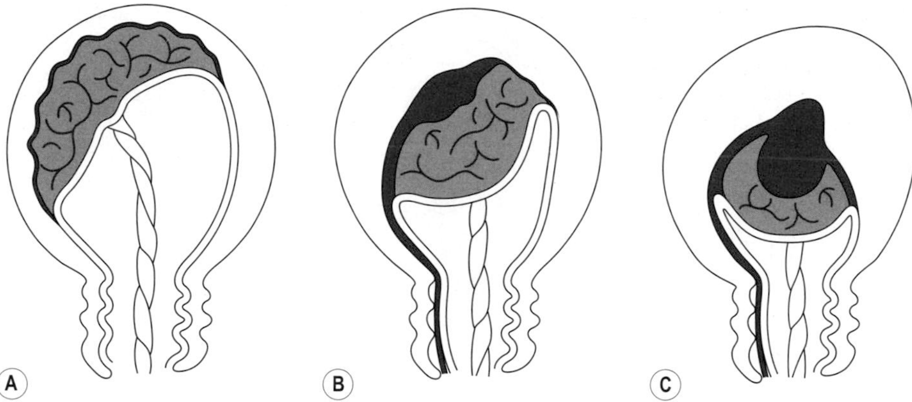


**Figure 39.1** Phases in the third stage of labour. **A.** *Latent phase*: characterized by a thick placenta-free wall and thin placental site wall. **B.** *Detachment phase*: characterized by a gradual thickening of the uterine wall over the site of placental attachment. This process can be monophasic (a constant shearing-off movement) or multiphasic (which is characterized by pauses between phases of active detachment). **C.** *Expulsion phase*: the uterine wall is uniformly thickened and drives the placenta into the lower segment for expulsion.

baby will depend on its position, with the potential for a net gain of 80 mL (Yao & Lind 1974). It is suggested that if the cord is clamped early, the resulting extra fetal blood retained in the placenta prevents it from being so tightly compressed by the uterus. As a result, contraction and retraction of the uterus may be less effective, and maternal blood loss increased, leading to a greater retroplacental blood clot being formed. Botha (1968) does not consider the formation of a retroplacental blood clot a physiological process. Rather, it occurs as a result of this intervention. Late cord clamping has also been associated with benefits for the infant (Hutton & Hassan 2007) (Box 39.1).

Detachment of the membranes begins in the first stage of labour, when separation occurs around the internal os. In the third stage, complete separation takes place assisted by the weight of the descending placenta, peeling them from the uterine wall.

During the process of separation, descent and expulsion of the placenta, a number of clinical signs may be seen.

- A small amount of blood oozes from the placental bed and tracks down between the membranes and appears as a gush of blood per vagina (sign of separation).
- Abdominally, the uterus rises up to sit on top of the descended placenta, which can resemble a full bladder as it lies in the lower uterine segment (sign of descent).
- The cord lengthens (sign of descent).

Box 39.1 **Benefits and risks associated with delayed cord clamping in the newborn**

- Increased need for phototherapy for jaundice
- Increased newborn haemoglobin up to 6 months
- Infant ferritin levels higher at 6 months
- Reduction in the risk of anaemia
- Asymptomatic polcythaemia

## Presentation of the placenta at the vulva

During the expulsive phase, the placenta may appear at the vagina in one of two ways (Fig. 39.3).

**Schultze.** The placenta appears fetal surface first, like an inverted umbrella with the membranes trailing behind. Any blood lost during the third stage will collect on the maternal surface of the placenta and be encased by the membranes. Over 80% of placentae are delivered in this way (Akiyama et al 1981).

**Matthews Duncan.** Less commonly, the placenta slips from the vagina sideways and the maternal surface appears at the vulva first. Midwives often use the term 'dirty Duncan' for this type of presentation because more bleeding is seen vaginally – blood escapes immediately from the placental site because it is not encased in the membranes. This is often associated with slower separation of the placenta and ragged membranes.

## Control of bleeding

Following placental expulsion, several mechanisms come into play to control bleeding from maternal sinuses at the site of placental attachment.

1. The empty uterus fully contracts and the uterine walls come into apposition.

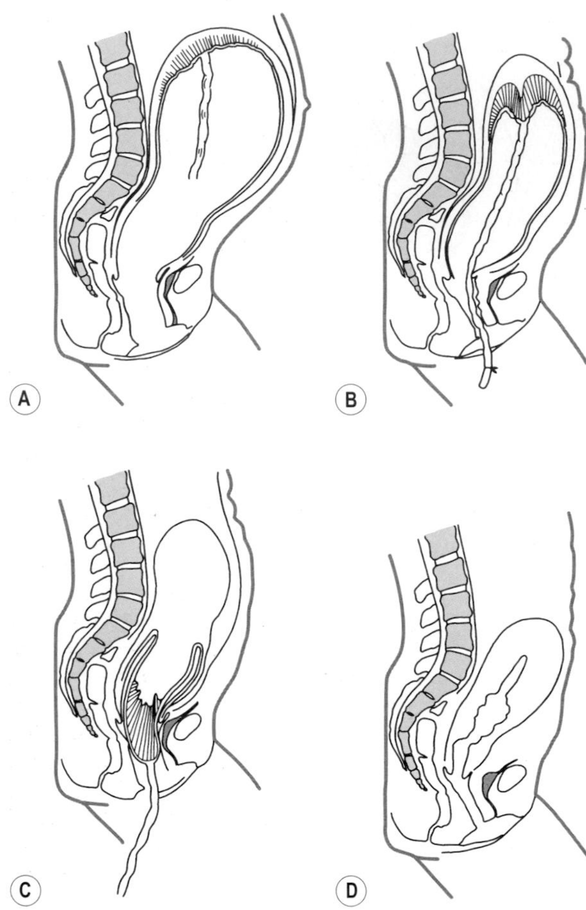


Figure 39.2 The mechanism of placental separation. **A.** The placenta before the child is born. **B.** The placenta partially separated immediately after the birth of the child. **C.** The placenta completely separated. **D.** The placenta expelled and the uterus strongly contracted and retracted.

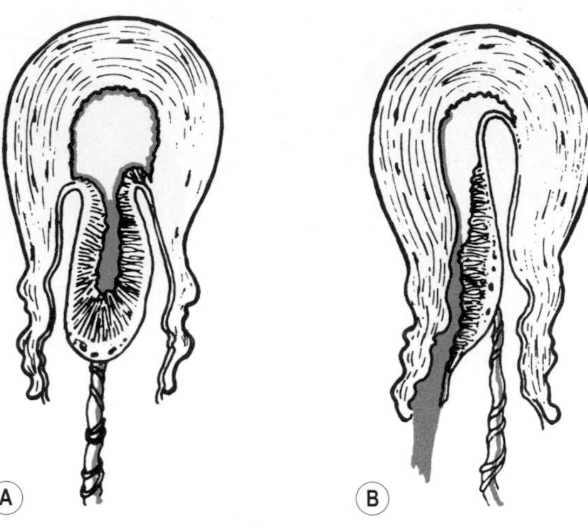


Figure 39.3 Expulsion of the placenta: **A.** Schultze method; **B.** Matthews Duncan method.

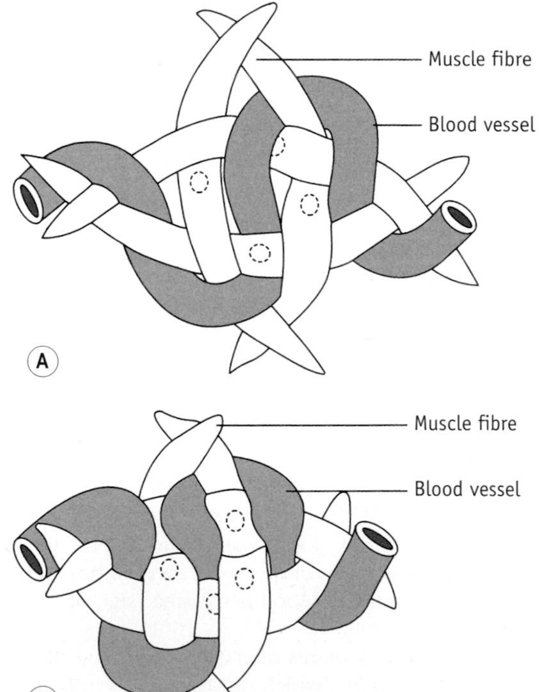


Figure 39.4 How the blood vessels run between the interlacing muscle fibres of the uterus. **A.** Muscle fibres relaxed and blood vessels not compressed. **B.** Muscle fibres contracted, blood vessels compressed and bleeding arrested.

2. The myometrium continues to contract and retract intermittently. The interlacing muscle fibres (known as living ligatures) constrict the torn blood vessels sealing them (see Fig. 39.4).
3. The process of blood clotting at the site of placental attachment is initiated and the area quickly becomes covered with a fine protective mesh.

Any factor that interferes with the normal physiological processes can influence the outcome of the third stage of labour (see Box 39.2). This includes a variety of complications of pregnancy and childbirth as well as the actions of individual midwives. Oxytocic drugs given prior to and during the third stage of labour also influence events. A woman's ability to avoid complications will also be based on her general health and by avoiding predisposing factors, such as anaemia, ketosis, exhaustion, and hypotonic uterine action.

**Box 39.2 Factors that may interfere with the physiological processes of the third stage of labour**

- Previous postpartum haemorrhage
- Anaemia
- Clotting disorders
- Pregnancy-induced hypertension
- Overdistended uterus, as in polyhydramnios, multiple pregnancy, fibroids
- Grand multiparity
- Induction/augmentation of labour
- Poor uterine action during labour and delivery
- Long first or second stage of labour
- Instrumental delivery
- Oxytocic drugs
- Dehydration during labour
- Full bladder at onset of the third stage of labour
- How the third stage of labour is managed

## MANAGEMENT OF THE THIRD STAGE OF LABOUR

Commonly, midwives describe two ways of managing the third stage: active management and expectant management. However, difficulties remain in defining what these terms mean, as midwives practise both methods in a variety of different ways (Harris 2005). The most commonly described form of each management will be outlined here with discussion about where variation may take place. The woman and her midwife will have discussed options for the third stage during the antenatal period and again during labour and made a decision over which management she would like.

### Expectant management

Expectant management is one of 'watchful anticipation' and draws upon the normal physiological processes to bring about expulsion of the placenta and membranes. The woman is active during this process and the midwife's role is a passive one involving close observation and encouragement.

#### Principles of expectant management

*Positioning the baby after birth*

Whichever position a woman chooses to give birth in, the newborn infant will be placed either on the bed/floor covering between the woman's legs or on the woman's abdomen, depending on her choice. Early skin-to-skin contact is advantageous in maintaining the infant's temperature, in promoting successful breastfeeding and in supporting development of mother–infant attachment (Moore et al 2007). The midwife then steps back to leave the woman and her family to experience undisturbed the powerful first meeting with their new baby, while continuing to observe the wellbeing of the infant and maternal vaginal blood loss.

*When to cut the cord*

There is some debate about when the umbilical cord should be clamped and cut. The potential benefits and risks to the mother and infant of delayed cord clamping (McDonald & Middleton 2008) are being considered alongside the routine use of active management which normally incorporates immediate clamping and cutting of the cord (NICE 2007, WHO 2007). In accordance with the principles of non-intervention in expectant management, Inch (1985) suggests that ideally the cord should be left intact until the placenta and membranes are completely expelled, as this enables compaction and compression of the placenta and retraction of muscle fibres to occur unhindered. There may also be beneficial effects of continued delivery of oxygenated blood to the newborn infant via the cord (Hutchon 2006), particularly in those born prematurely or asphyxiated. In a study of premature infants conducted by Kinmond et al (1993), a 30-second delay in cord clamping with the infant held 20 cm below the introitus was associated with improved outcome for the baby. A more recent study in term neonates has linked a delay in cord clamping of 2 minutes with significantly higher mean corpuscular volume, ferritin and total body iron stores in the infant up to 6 months of age (Chaparro et al 2006). Early cord clamping has also been associated with fetomaternal transfusion, of particular importance in women who are rhesus negative (Lapido 1972). Enkin et al (2000) suggest that free bleeding of the cut end of the severed umbilical cord reduces the risk of fetomaternal transfusion. Placental cord drainage has also been associated with a reduction in the length of the third stage of labour (Soltani et al 2005).

If the cord is short, this may prevent a woman from holding her baby. In these circumstances, the woman may choose to have the cord clamped and cut once it has stopped pulsating (approximately 5–10 minutes after the baby is born).

*Position of the woman during the third stage of labour*

Usually, whichever position a woman gives birth in, she will choose to sit once the baby is born. This allows her the opportunity to touch, hold and examine her baby. Skin-to-skin contact and breastfeeding should be encouraged as this aids separation and expulsion of the placenta through endogenous oxytocin release.

#### *Detection of separation and descent of the placenta*

As the uterus begins to contract again, the woman will usually indicate this and may have an urge to bear down. The midwife may also notice abdominal changes; the fundus rises up and becomes more globular. The separated placenta may be seen as a bulge, similar to a full bladder, just above the symphysis pubis, with the well-contracted uterus sitting above it. In addition, a gush of blood per vagina and cord lengthening may occur. There is no necessity to palpate the abdomen unless there is cause for concern or the midwife suspects there may be some delay. Encouraging the woman to adopt an upright position at this time will lead to rapid expulsion of the placenta and membranes. Care needs to be taken when assisting the woman to move into another position, as she will have the baby in her arms. Standing, squatting and sometimes using a toilet, bucket or bedpan can be used.

#### *Delivery of the placenta and membranes*

The placenta is delivered by maternal effort. Normally, the woman in an upright position will feel the placenta as it descends to the pelvic floor, which triggers an urge to push, or the placenta will just fall out under the influence of gravity.

The midwife's role is to let the woman know what is happening, to encourage her to adopt an upright position, and to advise her to listen to what her body is saying (to push or bear down if she wants to). A flat hand placed across the lower abdomen may assist the woman to birth the placenta, as the counterpressure compensates for poor muscle tone. The placenta and membranes are then delivered either onto the bed/floor or into a bedpan/toilet/bucket. If the membranes trail behind, they can be eased out of the vagina by turning the placenta to make a rope of the membranes, by applying gentle traction on the membranes with the fingers (usually in an up-and-down motion), or by asking the woman to cough. Once the placenta is completely expelled, the time is noted, to calculate the length of the third stage for recording later. The midwife then palpates the abdomen to ensure the uterus is well contracted and there is no excessive bleeding. The placenta and membranes can then be checked in front of the parents if they wish and any cord blood taken if the woman is rhesus negative.

It is suggested by midwives that this process normally takes between 5 and 15 minutes but can take up to an hour (Harris 2005). Whilst some authors suggest the length of the third stage is longer with expectant management than active management (Prendiville et al 1988, Rogers et al 1998), other authors looking specifically at ultrasound images suggest there is no difference (Herman et al 1993, Krapp et al 2000). If physiologically the length of the third stage is similar for both active and expectant management, perhaps time differences may be attributed to the actions of either the midwife or the woman. It has been noted that the use of an upright posture following separation appears to reduce blood loss and the length of the third stage in expectant management (Rogers et al 1998).

If there is delay in placental delivery, a number of actions can be taken. Odent (1998) suggests gently pressing upwards on the abdominal wall just above the pubic bone (with the woman lying on her back). If the cord does not move, then placental separation can be confirmed. Emptying the bladder, changing the woman's position and encouraging the woman to walk a short way may assist in placental delivery. Encouraging a woman to blow into an empty bottle has also been described (Fry 2007). According to NICE (2007), an expectant management is prolonged if not completed by 60 minutes.

## Active management

Active management is an intervention in the normal physiological processes. The administration of oxytocic drugs at the end of the second stage of labour combined with early cord clamping and controlled cord traction are used to bring about delivery of the placenta and membranes. The woman for the most part is a passive participant in this process.

### History of active management

Active intervention in the third stage of labour is not new but did not become popular until after the isolation of ergometrine (Dudley & Moir 1935) and the development of synthetic oxytocin (Syntocinon) (du Vigneaud & Tippett 1954). Initially, ergometrine was used as a treatment for postpartum haemorrhage (PPH), and it was then given following the third stage to prevent PPH. Syntometrine® (a mixture of Syntocinon and ergometrine) was marketed in the 1960s (Embrey et al 1963) as a uterotonic drug, administered at the birth of the baby's anterior shoulder and followed by cord traction. This package of care became known as active management and its popularity quickly spread. It has been so successful that it has become normal practice throughout the UK, irrespective of the degree of risk.

### Uterotonic drugs

Uterotonic drugs (drugs that make the uterus contract) are used during the third stage in three ways, as:

- *prophylaxis:* to prevent PPH irrespective of the risk status of the woman
- *a planned treatment:* when a risk of PPH has been identified, for example when a woman has a low haemoglobin level or a history of previous PPH
- *treatment in an emergency:* when uncontrolled bleeding occurs as a result of uterine atony.

While the benefits of oxytocic drugs in controlling atonic postpartum haemorrhage are recognized, their routine use in preventing the problem has been the subject of much debate and various clinical trials. A systematic review of four studies comparing active management with an expectant or physiological approach supports the prophylactic use of active management in a hospital birth situation (Prendiville et al 2000). The implications for home birth are less clear (Enkin et al 2000). The review concluded that there was an overall reduction in maternal blood loss of less than 100 mL in women having an active third stage of labour over expectant management (mean weighted difference −79.33 mL; 95% confidence interval −94.29 to −64.37) (Prendiville et al 2000). The review also highlights that certain uterotonic drugs have been associated with raised blood pressure, nausea, vomiting and headaches (Prendiville et al 2000). Higher rates of retained placenta in active management have also been reported, along with more serious complications such as postpartum eclampsia and cardiac disorders (Begley 1990, WHO 1997). It has been suggested that Syntocinon replace Syntometrine® as the drug of choice in active management as some of the complications above have been associated with the ergometrine component of Syntometrine® (McDonald et al 1993, NICE 2007).

Critics of these research studies highlight a number of factors that may have influenced the results achieved.

**Lack of skill in expectant management among midwives.** Three out of four studies were conducted in hospitals where active management was the norm (Gyte 1994). Whilst the latest study was conducted at Hinchingbrooke (Rogers et al 1998), where expectant management was said to be more common, statistics were not available as to the rate of expectant management before the trial began.

**Difficulty in defining what constitutes excessive blood loss.** It is well recognized that blood loss estimation is inaccurate, with high loss often being underestimated (Razvi et al 1996). In addition, as the reduced loss associated with active management has become the norm, midwives may interpret the slightly higher blood loss rate in expectant management as abnormal. Currently, a postpartum haemorrhage is defined as a blood loss in excess of 500 mL. In some countries this is 1000 mL, with evidence suggesting that healthy women appear to cope well with the loss of such amounts (Bais et al 2004, McDonald 2007). If this more generous definition had been used in the Hinchingbrooke study, no statistically significant difference in PPH rates would have been found between expectant and active management approaches (Rogers et al 1998). This may add weight to the growing evidence that for low-risk women an expectant management approach may not significantly increase blood loss following birth, making it a realistic option.

More recently it has been suggested that whilst oxytocics may appear to reduce blood loss at delivery in the short term, when the action wears off on the postnatal ward, the blood will be lost then (Kashanian et al 2008, Wickham 1999). Wickham (1999) observed that following active management, women often experienced a heavy blood loss when going to the bathroom for the first time, and Kashanian et al (2008) confirmed this, noting statistically significant higher blood loss in the 'fourth stage of labour' (see below) in women having active management. This may suggest that the use of uterotonics during the third stage merely delays blood loss until a time when it is less likely to be noticed. It is possible that women are supposed to lose blood at this time as they no longer require such a high circulating blood volume to supply the placental bed, and the haemodilution of pregnancy may support a woman's ability to cope with this. Further studies are required to look at what constitutes normal blood loss following childbirth and the implications of actively reducing it.

**Variation in practice.** When comparing research protocols of published trials, no consensus can be reached on a definition of what constitutes active and expectant management, which implies that there is variation in practice (Begley 1990, Prendiville et al 1988, Rogers et al 1998, Thilaganathan et al 1993). Gyte (1994) suggests that a 'piecemeal' approach, a combination of active and expectant management techniques, was used by a significant number of midwives within the Bristol trial. Inter and intra third stage practice variation among midwives has subsequently been reported (Harris 2005) as has variation in third stage policies (Winter et al 2007), intra and inter country variation in third stage care (Festin et al 2003), and variation in management between maternity care providers (Tan et al 2008). This highlights the difficulty in evaluating the results of comparative studies where variation in practice could have occurred.

Logue (1990) looked at PPH rates among doctors and midwives and found considerable variation, with some individuals having consistently much higher rates of PPH than others. She suggests that when managing the third stage, 'more conservative and patient operators show the lowest PPH rates compared with the more impatient and heavy-handed who show the highest rates' (Logue 1990:S11). This implies that the action or inaction of practitioners may have a direct impact on the outcome of the third stage and requires further exploration. This is supported in the literature by reference to the potential dangers of 'fundal fiddling' and inappropriate cord traction leading to uterine inversion (McDonald 2009).

### *Current options*

Currently, the following uterotonic drugs are available to manage the third stage of labour:

**Syntocinon.** This is a synthetically produced form of oxytocin, given either intravenously (5 IU) or intramuscularly (5–10 IU). It can be given at crowning of the head, with delivery of the anterior shoulder or shortly after the birth. Intramuscular Syntocinon acts within 2–3 minutes of administration. It is considered the oxytocic drug of choice for active management (NICE 2007). Whilst Syntometrine® remains the most effective oxytocic in reducing blood loss (McDonald et al 2004), it may cause nausea, vomiting and hypertension, making Syntocinon, which has fewer side-effects, an appropriate alternative. Syntocinon becomes inactive at high temperatures.

**Intramuscular Syntometrine® 1 mL.** This is usually given with the birth of the anterior shoulder or shortly after. Syntometrine® contains ergometrine 500 mcg and oxytocin 5 units in 1 mL. The oxytocin fraction induces strong, rhythmic contraction of the muscle fibres of the upper segment of the uterus within 2–3 minutes of administration. Its effect lasts for approximately 5–15 minutes (Baskett 1999). This rapid-acting, short-duration component is designed to initiate strong uterine action, which is sustained by the action of the ergometrine fraction, which will induce a strong, non-physiological spasm of uterine muscle within 6–8 minutes (Sorbe 1978). The effect of ergometrine is maintained for approximately 60–90 minutes (Baskett 1999). Because of the spasm-inducing properties of ergometrine there is a theoretical risk of retained placenta and therefore the midwife should aim to deliver the placenta before ergometrine takes effect. Syntometrine® becomes inactive at high temperatures.

**Intramuscular ergometrine 500 mcg.** This will cause a strong, sustained uterine contraction. If intramuscular ergometrine is administered *instead of* Syntometrine®, it is given a little earlier, at the crowning of the head, as it takes longer to act, 6–8 minutes. The World Health Organization (WHO) (1997, 2007) do not support its use for routine management in the third stage owing to its effect on blood pressure. The conclusion of a recent review of ergot alkaloids in the third stage suggests that while these drugs are effective, other drugs such as oxytocin and prostaglandins may be preferable (Liabsuetrakul et al 2007).

**Intravenous ergometrine 250–500 mcg.** This takes effect approximately 45 seconds after administration; it is usually given by a doctor but may be given by a midwife in an emergency situation, usually to control postpartum bleeding.

## Prostaglandins

There is currently some interest in exploring the use of a prostaglandin $E_1$ analogue (*misoprostol*) for management of the third stage. Misoprostol (in doses of 400–600 mg) can be given orally or rectally, needs no equipment to administer and does not become inactive at high temperatures. This makes it an ideal therapy for countries in the developing world where refrigeration and health services are limited. However, it is associated with shivering and transient pyrexia. In a systematic review of prostaglandins for preventing PPH (Gülmezoglu et al 2007), findings suggested that neither intramuscular prostaglandins nor misoprostol was as effective at preventing PPH as were injectable uterotonics.

## Nipple stimulation

A simple alternative to parenteral oxytocics for the third stage of labour is nipple stimulation, which, according to Irons et al (1994), tends to reduce the length of the third stage and the amount of blood loss. This was a small study, however, and larger trials are needed.

## Principles of active management

Currently, active management is recommended for all women, though those at low risk who request expectant management should be supported in their choice (ICM/FIGO 2003, NICE 2007, RCM 2008).

### *Positioning the baby after birth*

Where the infant is placed at birth will depend on the position that the woman chooses for birth. As discussed previously, there are significant benefits for both mother and child of early skin-to-skin contact. There is also a need to provide a safe, warm, draught-free environment.

### *When to give the uterotonic*

Traditionally, it has been recommended that during active management a uterotonic drug is administered either at the birth of the baby's anterior shoulder or shortly after the birth of the baby (if a midwife is alone). Midwives have identified that this may occur before or after the cord is clamped and cut (Harris 2005).

### *When to cut the cord*

Traditionally, midwives were advised to clamp and cut the umbilical cord as soon as possible after the birth of the baby to prevent an excess of placental blood being forced into the infant's circulation under the influence of the administered oxytocic. This was considered to have the potential to cause hypervolaemia and hyperbilirubinaemia in the neonate. Clamping occurred before or shortly after the administration of the uterotonic. However, evidence now suggests there is a benefit to delaying cord clamping for 2–3 minutes and that any subsequent polycythaemia in the neonate appears to be benign (Hutton & Hassan 2007).

### *Position of the woman during the third stage of labour*

As with expectant management, irrespective of the position in which a woman gives birth, she will usually choose to sit once the baby is born.

### Detection of separation and descent of the placenta

In active management it is normally the midwife who detects the first uterine contraction following the baby's birth by placing a hand gently on the woman's abdomen and waiting for the uterus to rise up and contract beneath it. Midwives are often warned at this time of the dangers of fundal 'fiddling', which may lead to partial separation of the placenta, with the potential for excessive bleeding to occur. Although cord traction as described by Spencer (1962) should be commenced as soon as the uterus contracts, Levy & Moore (1985) suggest waiting until signs of separation are present. This latter study found no significant difference in the incidence of postpartum haemorrhage, or the length of the third stage, between those who started controlled cord traction as soon as the uterus contracted and those who waited for signs of separation. However, the rate of postpartum haemorrhage appeared to be significantly higher when the midwife unsuccessfully used controlled cord traction without awaiting signs of separation.

### Signs of separation and descent

As the uterus contracts and the placenta separates, the fundus rises up and becomes more globular. The separated placenta may be seen as a bulge, similar to a full bladder, just above the symphysis pubis, with the well-contracted uterus sitting above it. Combined with the abdominal findings, the midwife may notice that there is a gush of blood per vagina and that the cord lengthens. The woman may experience pain at this time and also feel the urge to bear down as the placenta enters the vagina.

### Delivery of the placenta and membranes

The placenta is delivered by cord traction with the woman in a sitting/semi-recumbent position. The midwife either wraps her fingers around the cord or uses a clamp to apply downward sustained traction until the placenta appears at the vulva. When the placenta becomes visible, traction is applied upwards (following the curve of Carus) to extract the placenta from the vagina (Spencer 1962). The placenta is delivered into the midwife's hands or into a bowl placed close to the introitus. Care is taken with the membranes, which may trail behind. Some midwives ask women to cough gently, particularly if the membranes appear caught in the cervix.

Whilst applying cord traction, some midwives place a hand above the symphysis pubis and push the uterus upwards (known as 'guarding of the uterus') (Fig. 39.5). This is said to prevent uterine inversion. However, there is currently no evidence available to support this practice. Some midwives use this hand as counterpressure when applying cord traction and others suggest it provides valuable information on descent, as the placenta can be felt beneath the hand, moving down into the vagina (Harris 2005).

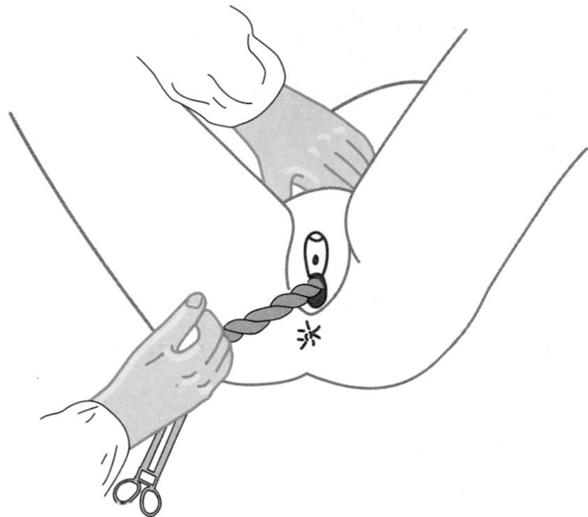

**Figure 39.5** Controlled cord traction while guarding the uterus.

In some units, women are encouraged to deliver the placenta by maternal effort (see expectant management).

Following placental delivery, the length of the third stage is noted, for recording later. The midwife palpates the abdomen to ensure the uterus is well contracted and notes vaginal blood loss.

> **Reflective activity 39.2**
>
> Consider the form of words you would choose when discussing active and expectant management of labour. What are the key points you would make, and which research and evidence would you use to explain the woman's choices?

## Examination of the placenta and membranes

Whatever management, the placenta and membranes are carefully and systematically examined as soon after delivery as possible so that, if incomplete, action can be taken immediately. The examination is to determine completeness, and to detect any abnormalities, which may suggest problems in the neonate.

Initially, the placenta is held up by the cord to view the membranes; a discrete hole, which the baby passed through, may be seen. Sometimes membranes are ragged and every attempt should be made to piece them together to ensure completeness.

The placenta is placed on a flat surface and thoroughly examined in a good light. The amnion is stripped from the chorion up to the umbilical cord to confirm that both membranes are present. The maternal surface is wiped clear of blood clots and carefully examined to ensure all the cotyledons are present. Any areas of infarction (firm

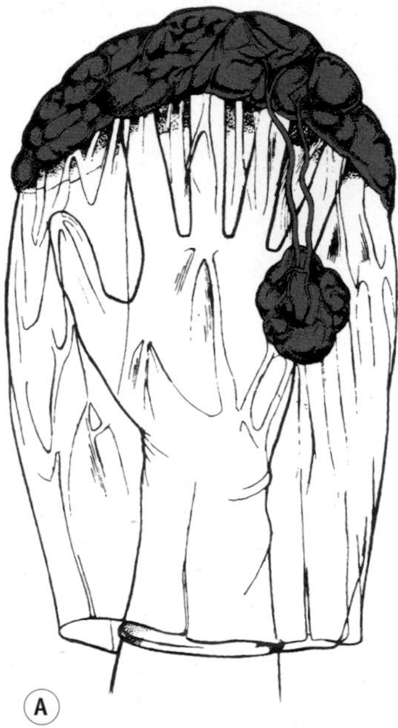


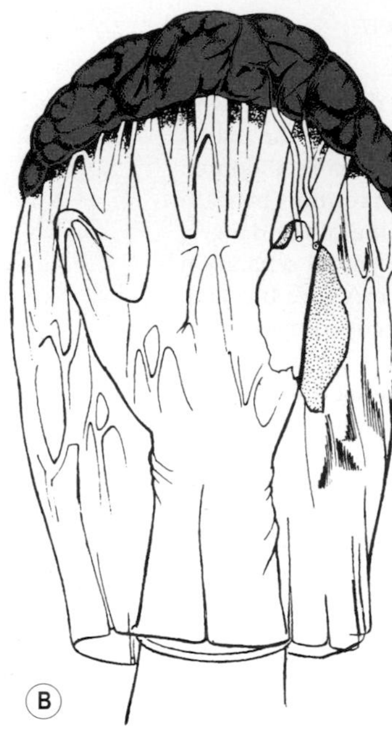


**Figure 39.6 A.** Succenturiate placenta. **B.** The torn membrane – the missing lobe is in the uterus.

whitish patches) are noted and the placental edge examined for blood vessels running into the membranes. These vessels may track back to the placenta (an erratic vessel) or go to an accessory lobe in the membranes (a succenturiate lobe). If a vessel ends at a hole in the membranes (Fig. 39.6), a succenturiate lobe may have been left behind in the uterus and the woman will need referral to an obstetrician.

The cord is examined, noting its insertion and length (though this is no longer measured) and the number of umbilical vessels. Usually the cord insertion is central and the length is approximately 50 cm. Occasionally only one umbilical artery is present; this is associated with congenital anomalies, especially renal agenesis (absence of kidneys). The paediatrician would need to be informed and a detailed examination of the newborn requested.

The placenta is usually weighed; weight at term is normally about one-sixth of the baby's birthweight. Early cord clamping increases the placental weight as it contains a greater residual blood volume.

Finally, any blood loss collected is measured and added to the estimated amount of loss which has soaked into linen and pads. Particular care is needed in estimating losses in excess of 300 mL, when amounts are often underestimated (Levy & Moore 1985), with the level of error increasing with the amount lost.

The findings are recorded in the mother's notes. Immediate referral to a doctor is made if it is thought that a piece of placental tissue has been retained.

## CARE FOLLOWING BIRTH (THE FOURTH STAGE)

Following delivery of the placenta and membranes, the midwife palpates the woman's abdomen to ensure the uterus is well contracted, assesses vaginal blood loss and examines the woman for any soft tissue damage which may require repair. The midwife makes the mother comfortable. This is an ideal time for the midwife to share the couple's delight in their baby and encourage any questions, and affords an excellent opportunity for health education to facilitate parent–baby attachment. Most women will enjoy early contact with their baby and there is evidence that this early and unhurried contact significantly affects maternal emotional wellbeing when measured 6 weeks postnatally (Ball 1994). The father, too, usually wishes to share this time with his family and should be encouraged to do so. This must be given priority over the many routine procedures (Sheridan 2010). Sensitivity is required in caring for women who appear to show little interest in their baby at birth.

Women who plan to breastfeed should be encouraged to do so soon after birth, usually within the first hour. At this time the baby usually displays a strong urge to suck and a successful feed benefits both mother and baby. Early feeding is associated with ongoing breastfeeding success and the release of endogenous oxytocin, which stimulates

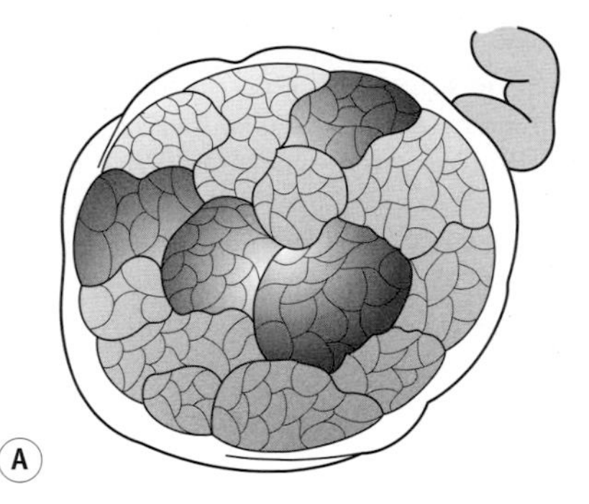


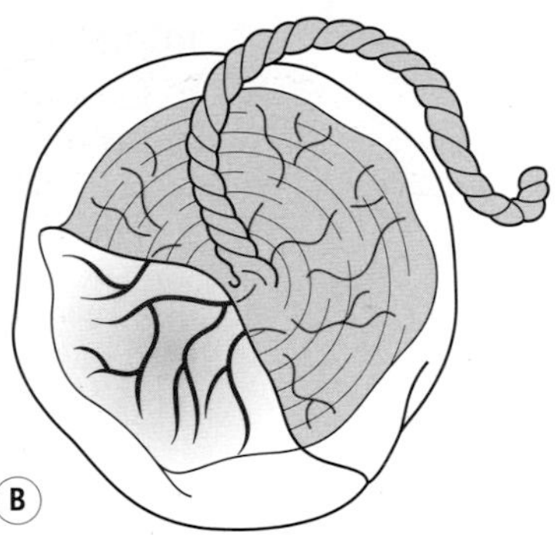


**Figure 39.7** The placenta. **A.** The maternal surface, showing the cotyledons. **B.** The fetal surface.

uterine contractions and helps to maintain haemostasis (see Ch. 43).

Ongoing care includes regular examination of the woman's abdomen to ensure the uterus remains contracted and observation of the lochia. The woman is encouraged to pass urine, as a full bladder predisposes to a relaxed uterus and heavy blood loss. If this occurs, the bladder is emptied, and then the midwife can massage the fundus of the uterus to stimulate a contraction.

Observation of the infant will include colour, respirations, and general activity. The umbilical cord is checked to ensure the cord clamp is firmly in place and that there is no bleeding. Care is taken to ensure that the baby does not become chilled; body temperature can be maintained by skin-to-skin contact or warm wrapping and cuddling by the parents. The midwife should remain in the birthing room for at least 1 hour after delivery, whether at home or in hospital.

## RECORDS

A complete and accurate account of labour must be recorded, and must be sufficiently comprehensive to enable other carers to have a clear picture of events, thus facilitating communication and avoiding discontinuity of care (NMC 2009).

Statute requires that a birth notification form be completed. This is normally undertaken by the midwife and sent, within 36 hours of the birth, to the medical officer of the district in which the birth took place (NMC 2004).

## THE PLACENTA AT TERM

At term, the placenta is flat and round or oval in shape. It is 18–20 cm in diameter and about 2.5 cm thick in the centre, becoming thinner towards the edges. Its weight is about one-sixth of the weight of the fetus and it is usually situated on the anterior or posterior wall of the uterine cavity, near the fundus. The placenta has two surfaces, maternal and fetal. The *maternal surface* is attached to the uterine decidua, is deep red in colour and divided by deep grooves or *sulci* into about 15–20 irregular lobes. These lobes (called *cotyledons*) contain masses of chorionic villi. On examination after birth, a thin greyish layer, part of the basal decidua, can be seen (Fig. 39.7). It may feel gritty due to the presence of lime salts. The *fetal surface* lies adjacent to the fetus and has a pearly white appearance as it is covered with amnion. From the insertion of the cord, which is usually situated centrally, blood vessels can be seen radiating to the periphery, like the roots of a tree. These vessels give off branches which penetrate into the substance of the placenta, each cotyledon having its own supply of fetal blood. In the centre of each cotyledon there is a main branch of the umbilical artery and vein.

## Abnormalities of the placenta

### Succenturiate lobe

A succenturiate lobe (Fig. 39.8) is a small portion or lobe of placenta which is separated from the main body. This is formed from some of the villi of the chorionic membrane which have continued to develop instead of becoming atrophied. It is attached to the main placenta by blood vessels which pass through the membrane. A succenturiate lobe may be retained in the uterus after the placenta has been expelled; and can cause postpartum haemorrhage and sepsis. When there is a small hole in the fetal membranes with placental vessels running towards it, a retained succenturiate lobe may be suspected and the woman should be referred to an obstetrician for assessment.

### Circumvallate placenta

In this type of placenta the chorion is attached not to the edge of the placenta, but to the fetal surface at some distance from the edge (Fig. 39.9). A thickened ring of membrane is seen on the fetal surface.

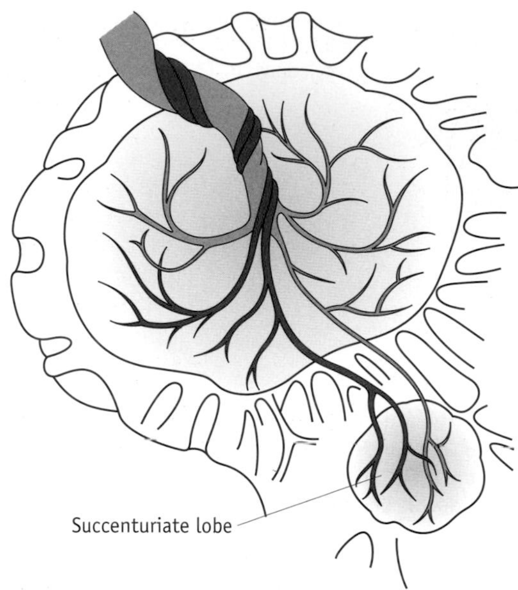


**Figure 39.8** Succenturiate placenta.

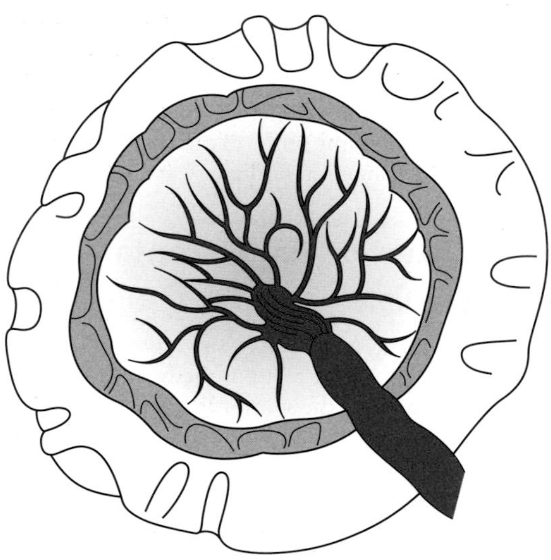

**Figure 39.9** Circumvallate placenta.

### Bipartite placenta

This is a placenta divided into two main lobes.

### Placenta accreta

This is a placenta which becomes abnormally adherent to the uterine muscle over the whole or part of its surface. It is very rare.

### Infarcts

Red or white patches are sometimes seen on the maternal surface of the placenta. These are caused by localized death of placental tissue due to interference with the blood supply.

Infarcts are red at an early stage of their development; they later become white and appear as patches of white fibrous tissue. They may be seen occasionally in any placenta, but they are often associated with pre-eclampsia.

### Calcification

On the maternal surface of the placenta, small greyish-white patches are often to be seen, particularly on the postmature placenta, owing to deposits of lime salts. They convey a gritty sensation to the fingers and are not significant.

## FETAL MEMBRANES

There are two fetal membranes: the *chorion* and *amnion*.

**The chorion.** This is the outer membrane, continuous with the edge of the placenta and derived from the trophoblast. It is opaque, thick but friable, and roughened by tiny pieces of decidua adherent to it. It lines the uterine cavity.

**The amnion.** This is the inner membrane, derived from the inner cell mass. It is smooth, transparent and the stronger membrane of the two. The two membranes lie over each other, but can be separated; the amnion may be stripped back to the insertion of the cord. The amnion secretes amniotic fluid or liquor amnii, which at term measures 1000–1500 mL.

## UMBILICAL CORD

The umbilical cord (Fig. 39.10), or *funis*, connects the placenta to the fetus. The cord is about 50 cm long and 2 cm thick. It is composed of a jelly-like substance known as Wharton's jelly; this is a primitive connective tissue, primary mesenchyme. The cord is covered externally by amnion. It supports and protects three blood vessels: one large umbilical vein carrying oxygenated blood to the fetus; and two umbilical arteries winding around the vein, carrying deoxygenated blood from the fetus to the placenta. The absence of a vessel may be associated with fetal abnormalities. The cord has a spiral twist; this torsion gives a certain amount of protection from pressure.

The function of the cord ceases as pulmonary respiration is established shortly after birth. Lacking a blood supply, the cord becomes dead tissue and quickly atrophies, as do the internal structures continuous with it. It can provide access for bacteria to enter the body, therefore care needs to be taken to keep it dry until the cord stump separates (see Ch. 41).

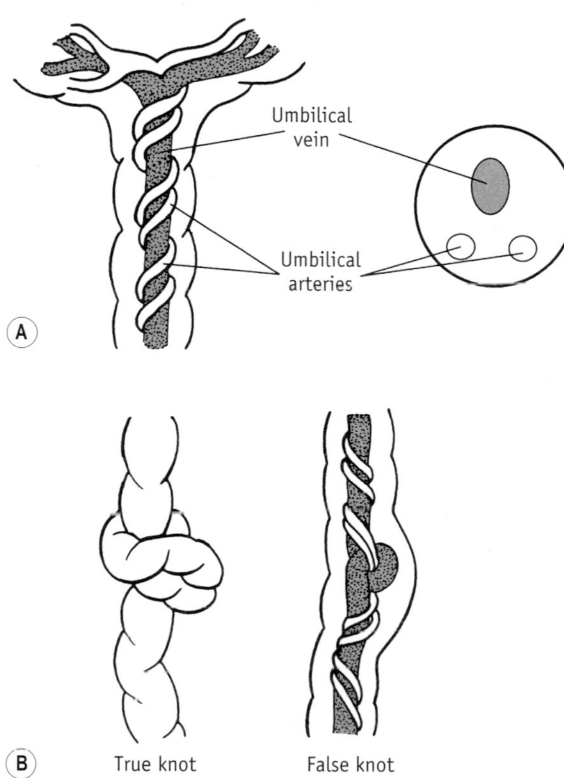


**Figure 39.10** **A.** The umbilical cord in side view and cross-section, showing the one umbilical vein with the two umbilical arteries twisting spirally around it. The vein and arteries lie in Wharton's jelly; the cord is enclosed within the amnion. **B.** True and false knots.

## Abnormalities of the umbilical cord

The cord may be too short (which may cause delay during labour), or too long, when there is a risk of cord prolapse. Occasionally it is very thick or very thin; in either case, great care is required in tying the cord and subsequently watching for haemorrhage. Rarely, a piece of fetal intestine may protrude into the cord; the possibility of this abnormality will be suspected if the cord is swollen close to the umbilicus, the size of the swelling depending on the amount of intestine which has protruded (see Ch. 48). Knots are caused by movements of the fetus before birth, the baby slipping through a loop of the cord. False knots may be due to the blood vessels being longer than the actual cord, and so doubling back upon themselves in the Wharton's jelly, or to irregularities and the formation of nodes.

### Abnormalities of insertion

The cord may be attached to one side of the placenta (an eccentric insertion) or to the margin of the placenta (a battledore insertion), or the vessels of the cord may break up and run into the membrane before reaching the placenta (a velamentous insertion) (Fig. 39.11). This is particularly dangerous if the unprotected blood vessels should lie near the internal os. This very rare condition is called vasa praevia (vessels in advance of the fetus). Should a blood vessel so situated be compressed when the membranes rupture, the fetus will suffer hypoxia. If such a vessel should actually rupture, blood will be lost from fetal vessels in the membrane. Such fetal haemorrhage is dangerous and could lead to stillbirth.

## CONCLUSION

The third stage of labour is an important period for mother and baby, when the importance of their first meeting cannot be overestimated. The midwife supports this

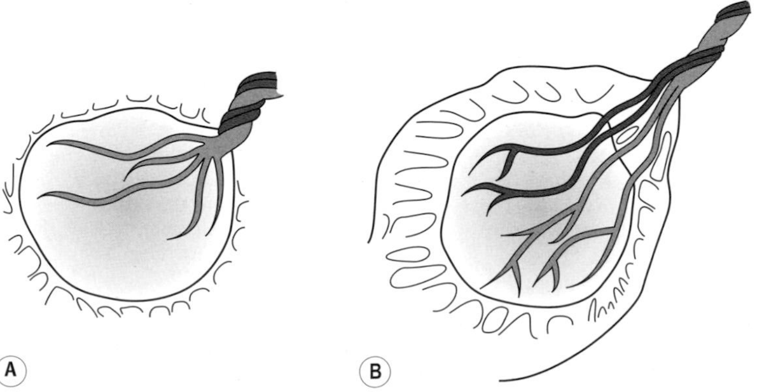


**Figure 39.11** Abnormal insertions of the cord: **A.** battledore; **B.** velamentous.

special time while monitoring successful delivery of the placenta and membranes. Currently, women appear to have little choice about how the third stage is managed, with active management being used indiscriminately. If midwives are to offer women a choice for the third stage, skills in both active and expectant management are required with a body of knowledge which enables the detection of those women who deviate from the norm, in whom active management may be the most appropriate form of care. In this way, women at low risk may be spared unnecessary intervention in the normal process of giving birth.

## KEY POINTS

- The third stage of labour is a time of great importance when mother and baby meet face to face for the first time.
- The skill and expertise of the midwife is needed to support this special time while monitoring successful completion of the childbirth process with delivery of the placenta and membranes.
- Care will be based upon knowledge of the normal physiological, sociological and psychological processes at work and the effect of interventions on that process.
- The indiscriminate use of active management for women experiencing normal birth has been challenged.
- The challenge for midwives is to change the focus for the third stage to one of normality and re-skill in expectant management techniques to include the ability to detect women deviating from the normal perspective in whom active management may be appropriate.

## REFERENCES


Akiyama H, Kohzu H, Matsuoka M: An approach to detection of placental separation and expulsion with new clinical signs: a study based on haemodynamic method and ultrasonography, *American Journal of Obstetrics and Gynecology* 140(5):505–511, 1981.

Bais JM, Eskes M, Pel M, et al: Postpartum haemorrhage in nulliparous women: incidence and risk factors in low and high risk women. A Dutch population-based cohort study on standard (>or=500 ml) and severe (>or=1000 ml) postpartum haemorrhage, *European Journal of Obstetrics Gynaecology and Reproductive Biology* 115(2):166–172, 2004.

Ball JA: *Reactions to motherhood*, Hale, 1994, Book for Midwives, pp 113–115.

Baskett TF: *Essential management of obstetric emergencies*, ed 3, Bristol, 1999, Clinical Press.

Begley C: A comparison of 'active' and 'physiological' management of the third stage of labour, *Midwifery* 6(1):3–17, 1990.

Botha MA: The management of the umbilical cord in labour, *South African Journal of Obstetrics and Gynaecology* 16(2):30–33, 1968.

Brandt M: The mechanism and management of the third stage of labour, *American Journal of Obstetrics and Gynecology* 23:662–667, 1933.

Chaparro CM, Neufeld LM, Alavez GT, et al: Effect of timing of umbilical cord clamping on iron status in Mexican infants: a randomised controlled trial, *Lancet* 367(9527):1997–2004, 2006.

Dieckmann WJ, Odell LD, Williger WM, et al: The placental stage and postpartum hemorrhage, *American Journal of Obstetrics and Gynecology* 54:415–427, 1947.

du Vigneaud VRC, Tippett S: The sequence of amino acids in oxytocin with a proposal for the structure of oxytocin, *Journal of Biological Chemistry* 205:949, 1954.

Dudley HW, Moir JC: The substance responsible for the traditional clinical effect of ergot, *British Medical Journal* 1:520–523, 1935.

Embrey MB, Barber DTC, Scudamore JH: The use of Syntometrine in prevention of post partum haemorrhage, *British Medical Journal* 1(5342):1387–1389, 1963.

Enkin M, Keirse MJNC, Neilson J, et al: The third stage of labour. In: *A guide to effective care in pregnancy and childbirth*, ed 3, Oxford, 2000, Oxford University Press.

Featherstone IE: Physiological third stage, *British Journal of Midwifery* 7(4):216–221, 1999.

Festin MP, Lumbiganon P, Tolosa JE, et al: International survey on variations in practice of the management of the third stage of labour, *Bulletin of the World Health Organization* 81(4):286–291, 2003.

Fry J: Physiological third stage of labour: support it or lose it, *British Journal of Midwifery* 15(11):693–695, 2007.

Gülmezoglu AM, Forna F, Villar J, et al: Prostaglandins for preventing postpartum haemorrhage, *Cochrane Database of Systematic Reviews* (3):CD000494, 2007.

Gyte G: Evaluation of the meta analyses on the effects, on both mother and baby, of the various components of 'active' management of the third stage of labour, *Midwifery* 10(4):183–199, 1994.

Harris T: Changing the focus for the third stage of labour, *British Journal of Midwifery* 9(1):7–12, 2001.

Harris T: *Midwifery practice in the third stage of labour*, PhD thesis, Leicester, 2005, De Montfort University.

Herman A, Weinraub Z, Bukovsky I, et al: Dynamic ultrasound imaging of the third stage of labour: new perspectives into third stage mechanisms, *American Journal of Obstetrics and Gynecology* 168(5):1496–1499, 1993.

Hutchon DJR: Delayed cord clamping may be beneficial in rich settings, *British Medical Journal* 333(7577):1073, 2006.

Hutton EK, Hassan ES: Late vs early clamping of the umbilical cord in full-term neonates, *Journal of the American Medical Association* 297(11):1241–1252, 2007.

ICM and FIGO: *Joint statement: Management of the third stage of labour to prevent postpartum haemorrhage* (website). www.pphprevention.org/files/ICM_FIGO_Joint_Statement.pdf. Accessed August 19, 2010.

Inch S: Management of the third stage of labour – another cascade of intervention, *Midwifery* 1(2):114–122, 1985.

Irons DW, Sriskandabalan P, Bullough CH: A simple alternative to parenteral oxytocics for the third stage of labour, *International Journal of Gynecology and Obstetrics* 46(1):15–18, 1994.

Kashanian M, Fekrat M, Masoomi Z, et al: Comparison of active and expectant management on the duration of the third stage of labour and the amount of blood loss during the third and fourth stages of labour: a randomised controlled trial, *Midwifery* 26(2):241–245, 2010.

Khan KS, Wojdyla D, Say L, et al: WHO analysis of causes of maternal death: a systematic review, *Lancet* 367(9516):1066–1074, 2006.

Kinmond S, Aitchison TC, Holland BM, et al: Umbilical cord clamping and preterm infants: a randomised trial, *British Medical Journal* 306(6871):172–175, 1993.

Krapp M, Baschat AA, Hankeln M, et al: Gray scale and color Doppler sonography in the third stage of labour for early detection of failed placental separation, *Ultrasound in Obstetrics and Gynecology* 15(2):138–142, 2000.

Krapp M, Katalinic A, Smrcek J, et al: Study of the third stage of labor by color Doppler sonography, *Archives of Gynecology and Obstetrics* 267(4):202–204, 2003.

Lapido OA: Management of third stage of labour with particular reference to reduction of feto-maternal transfusion, *British Medical Journal* 1(5802):721–723, 1972.

Levy V, Moore J: The midwife's management of the third stage of labour, *Nursing Times* 81(39):47–50, 1985.

Lewis G, editor: *The Confidential Enquiry into Maternal and Child Health (CEMACH). Saving mothers' lives: reviewing maternal deaths to make motherhood safer 2003-2005. The Seventh Report on Confidential Enquiries into Maternal Deaths in the UK*, London, 2007, CEMACH.

Liabsuetrakul T, Choobun T, Peeyananjarassri K, et al: Prophylactic use of ergot alkaloids in the third stage of labour, *Cochrane Databases of Systematic Reviews* (2):CD005456, 2007.

Logue M: Management of the third stage of labour: a midwife's view, *Journal of Obstetrics and Gynaecology* 10(Suppl. 2):10–12, 1990.

McDonald S: Management of the third stage of labor, *Journal of Midwifery and Women's Health* 52(3):254–261, 2007.

McDonald S: Physiology and management of the third stage of labour. In Fraser D, Cooper M, editors: *Myles textbook for midwives*, Edinburgh, 2009, Churchill Livingstone.

McDonald SJ, Middleton P: Effect of timing of umbilical cord clamping of term infants on maternal and neonatal outcomes, *Cochrane Database of Systematic Reviews* (2):CD004074, 2008.

McDonald SJ, Prendiville WJ, Blair E: Randomised controlled trial of oxytocin alone versus oxytocin and ergometrine in active management of labour, *British Medical Journal* 307(6913):1167–1171, 1993.

McDonald SJ, Abbott JM, Higgins SP: Prophylactic ergometrine-oxytocin versus oxytocin for delivery of the placenta, *Cochrane Database of Systematic Reviews* (1):CD000201, 2004.

Moore ER, Anderson GC, Bergman N: Early skin-to-skin contact for mothers and their healthy newborn infants, *Cochrane Database of Systematic Reviews* (2):CD003519, 2007.

NICE: *Intrapartum care: care of healthy women and their babies during childbirth*, London, 2007, RCOG Press.

Nursing & Midwifery Council (NMC): *Midwives Rules and Standards*, London, 2004, NMC.

Nursing & Midwifery Council (NMC): *Record keeping: guidance for nurses and midwives*, London, 2009, NMC.

Odent M: Don't manage the third stage of labour, *The Practising Midwife* 1(9):31–33, 1998.

Prendiville WJ, Harding JE, Elbourne DR, et al: The Bristol third stage trial: active versus physiological management of the third stage of labour, *British Medical Journal* 297(6659):1295–1300, 1988.

Prendiville WJ, Elbourne D, McDonald S: Active versus expectant management of the third stage of labour, *The Cochrane Library*, Issue 3, Oxford, 2000, Update Software.

Razvi K, Chua S, Arulkumaran S, et al: A comparison between visual estimation and laboratory determination of blood loss during the third stage of labour, *Australian and New Zealand Journal of Obstetrics and Gynaecology* 36(2):152–154, 1996.

Royal College of Midwives (RCM): Third stage of labour. In *Evidence-based guidelines for midwifery-led care*, London, 2008, RCM. Also available at http://www.rcm.org.uk/college/standards-and-practice/practice-guidelines/. Accessed August 2010.

Rogers J, Wood J, McCandlish R, et al: Active versus expectant management of the third stage of labour: the Hinchingbrooke randomised controlled trial, *Lancet* 351(9104):693–699, 1998.

Sheridan V: Organisational culture and routine midwifery practice on labour ward: implications for mother-baby contact, *Evidence Based Midwifery* 8(3):76–84, 2010.

Soltani H: Global implications of evidence 'biased' practice: management of the third stage of labour, *Midwifery* 24(2):138–142, 2008.

Soltani H, Dickinson F, Symonds IM: Placental cord drainage after spontaneous vaginal delivery as part of the management of the third stage of labour, *Cochrane Database of Systematic Reviews* (4):CD004665, 2005.

Sorbe B: Active pharmacologic management of the third stage of labor, *Obstetrics and Gynecology* 52(6):694–697, 1978.

Spencer PM: Controlled cord traction in management of the third stage of labour, *British Medical Journal* 1(5294):1728–1732, 1962.

Tan WM, Klein MC, Saxell L, et al: How do physicians and midwives manage the third stage of labour? *Birth* 35(3):220–229, 2008.

Thilaganathan BCA, Cutner A, Latimer J, et al: Management of the third stage of labour in women at low risk of postpartum haemorrhage, *European Journal of Obstetrics and Gynaecology and Reproductive Biology* 48(1):19–22, 1993.

Wickham S: Further thoughts on the third stage, *The Practising Midwife* 2(10):14–15, 1999.

Winter C, Macfarlane A, Deneux-Tharaux C, et al: Variation in policies for management of the third stage of labour and the immediate management of postpartum haemorrhage in Europe, *British Journal of Obstetrics and Gynaecology* 114(7):845–854, 2007.

World Health Organization (WHO): *Care in normal birth: a practical guide* (website). www.who.int/making_pregnancy_safer/documents/who_frh_msm_9624/en/. 1996. Accessed August 19, 2010.

World Health Organization (WHO): *WHO recommendations for the prevention of postpartum haemorrhage*, Geneva, 2007, WHO.

Yao AC, Lind J: Placental transfusion, *American Journal of Diseases in Children* 127(1):128–141, 1974.

Chapter 40

# The pelvic floor

Chris Kettle

## LEARNING OUTCOMES

After reading this chapter, you will:

- have enhanced your knowledge and understanding of the anatomy and function of the pelvic floor in relation to perineal trauma and repair
- understand the short- and long-term morbidity associated with perineal trauma
- be able to base practice on current research
- be aware of employing authorities' policies and guidelines and understand the legal implications associated with inadequate or incorrect repair of the perineum.

## INTRODUCTION

Perineal injury has occurred during childbirth throughout the ages and various methods and materials were used by accoucheurs in an attempt to restore the integrity of severely traumatized tissue. The earliest evidence of extensive perineal injury sustained during childbirth exists in the mummy of Henhenit, a Nubian woman aged approximately 22 years, from the harem of King Mentuhotep II of Egypt, 2050 BC (Derry 1935, Graham 1950, Magdi 1949). Despite the fact that maternity care has greatly improved over the past decade, women continue to suffer the consequences of pelvic floor damage resulting from childbirth.

## THE PELVIC FLOOR

The development of the upright posture in humans has been the dominant factor in the evolution of the pelvic floor (Benson 1992). Its main function is to provide support for the pelvic and abdominal organs and it must be strong to oppose the forces of gravity and increases in abdominal pressure. Childbirth is a known source of pelvic floor damage, causing muscle weakness, incontinence, and prolapse of the pelvic organs.

The midwife must have a sound understanding of the structure and function of the pelvic floor in order to apply this knowledge to minimize any associated morbidity during the process of childbirth.

### Structure

The ischial spines are key landmarks in understanding the location and structure of the pelvic floor. They lie laterally, in a plane which spans the pelvic cavity where many important parts of the pelvic floor are attached (Benson 1992). The soft tissues, which form the pelvic floor, fill the outlet of the bony pelvis forming a 'sling', which is higher posteriorly (Verralls 1993). In the female, the urethra, vagina, and rectum pass through its structures. It consists of the following six layers extending from the pelvic peritoneum above to the skin of the vulva, perineum, and buttocks below:

- pelvic peritoneum
- pelvic fascia
- deep muscles
- superficial muscles
- subcutaneous fat
- skin.

#### Pelvic peritoneum

This forms a smooth covering over the uterus and fallopian tubes. Anteriorly it forms the uterovesical pouch and covers the upper surface of the bladder. Posteriorly it forms the pouch of Douglas. Laterally it covers the fallopian tubes and forms the broad ligaments, which do not act as supports.

## Pelvic fascia

This connective tissue fills the space between the pelvic organs lining the pelvic cavity walls. Its function is to provide support for the organs, whilst at the same time allowing them to move within the limits of normal function (Verralls 1993). In areas where extra support is needed, it thickens to form the pelvic ligaments:

- *Transverse cervical ligaments:*
  - form the principal direct supports of the uterus
  - are known as *cardinal* or *Mackenrodt's ligaments*
  - are attached to the vaginal vault and supravaginal cervix
  - extend transversely in a fan-like way across the pelvic floor to the white line of fascia on the lateral pelvic walls.
- *Uterosacral ligaments:*
  - attach to the vaginal vault and supravaginal cervix
  - pass backwards and upwards from the cervix to the lateral border of the sacral body,
- *Round ligaments:*
  - originate just below the cornua of the uterus
  - pass through the inguinal canal and anterior abdominal wall to become inserted into each labium majus
  - assist in keeping the uterus in its normal anteverted (forward-tilted) anteflexed (bent on itself) position.
- *Pubocervical ligaments:*
  - attach to the inner part of the pubic bones
  - run posteriorly to form attachments to the bladder, vault of vagina and supravaginal cervix
  - provide support for the bladder (Verralls 1993).

## Deep muscle layer

This is formed mainly from symmetrically paired muscles, varying in thickness, collectively known as the *levator ani*. They arise at the inner circumference of the true pelvis from the white line of the obturator fascia and decussate midline between the urethra, vagina, and rectum. The muscle fibres pass downwards and backwards and are inserted medially into the upper vagina, perineal body, anal canal, anococcygeal body, coccyx, and lower borders of the sacrum.

The main function is to provide a strong sling to support the pelvic organs and to counteract any increase in the intra-abdominal pressure during coughing and laughing. When the levator ani is contracted, the pelvic floor and perineum are lifted upwards – an important mechanism to maintain continence.

The deep muscles are named after the corresponding fused bones of the innominate bone (pubis, ilium and ischium) (Fig. 40.1):

- *Pubococcygeus muscles:*
  - arise from the inner surface of the pubic bones
  - pass posteriorly below the bladder on either side of the urethra, upper vagina and anal canal to the anococcygeal body and coccyx
  - fibres cross medially and join those from the opposite sides to form U-shaped slings around the urethra, vagina, and rectum
  - the *puborectalis* muscle forms a loop around the anorectal junction and its posterior fibres communicate with the external anal sphincter
  - medial part is attached to the vagina – no direct attachment to the urethra
  - on dissection, are paler in colour, suggesting they are fast-twitch muscle capable of rapid contraction (Benson 1992)
  - function is to provide support to the urethra, vagina, and rectum to control micturition and defecation.
- *Iliococcygeus muscles:*
  - arise from the inner border of the white line of fascia on the inner aspects of the iliac bones and the ischial spines
  - join midline and are inserted posteriorly into the anococcygeal raphe and coccyx
  - on dissection, are darker in colour, suggesting they are slow-twitch muscles (Benson 1992).
- *Ischiococcygeus muscles:*
  - are triangular sheets of muscle and fibrous tissue
  - arise from the ischial spines, pass downwards and inwards to be inserted into the coccyx and lower part of the sacrum
  - are sometimes known as the coccygeus muscles
  - main function is to stabilize sacroiliac and sacrococcygeal joints.

### *Blood, lymph and nerve supply*

Blood supply is via the pudendal arteries and branches of the internal iliac artery, and the venous drainage is via corresponding veins. Lymphatic drainage is via the inguinal and external internal iliac glands and the nerve supply is via the third and fourth sacral nerves.

## Superficial perineal muscles

These are less important than the levator ani muscles; but contribute to the overall strength of the pelvic floor and likely to be damaged during vaginal delivery (Fig. 40.1):

- *Bulbospongiosus muscles (previously Bulbocavernosus in older texts):*
  - extend from central point in the perineal body, and encircle the vagina and urethra before

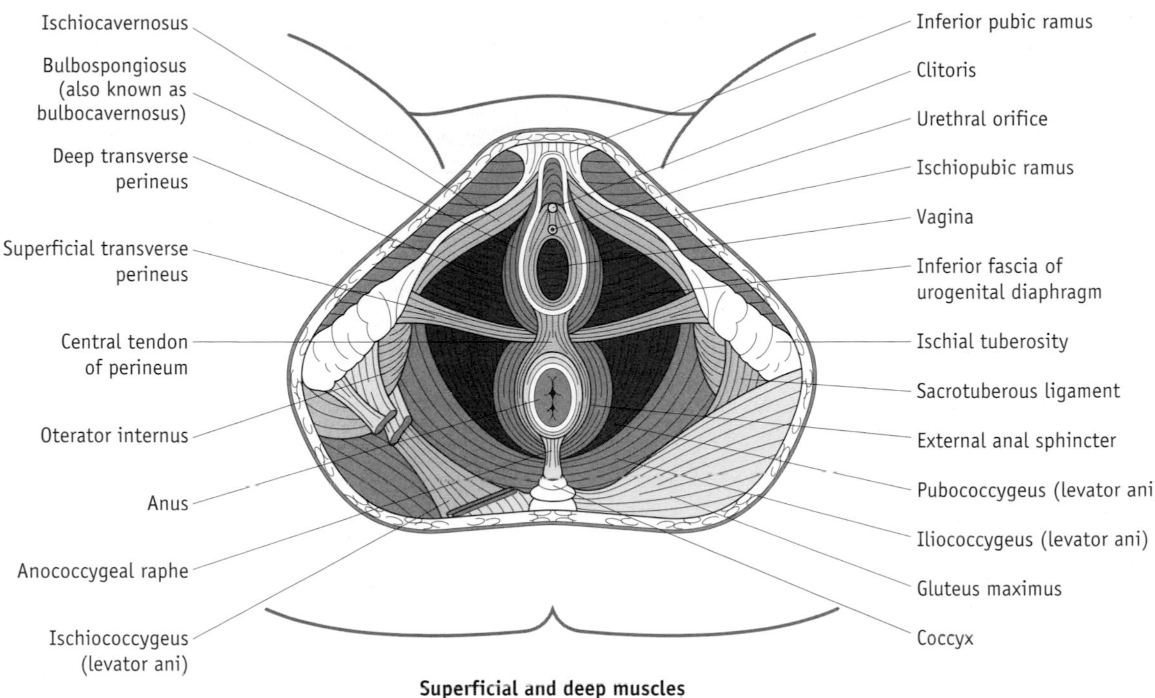


**Figure 40.1** Muscles of the pelvic floor seen in the female perineum. *(From* Principles of Anatomy and Physiology, *7th edn, by Tortora, G.J. and Grabowski, S.R. Copyright © 1993 John Wiley & Sons. Reprinted by permission of John Wiley & Sons, Inc.)*

inserting anteriorly into the corpora cavernosa of the clitoris
- posteriorly some fibres merge with the superficial transverse muscle and external anal sphincter
- situated beneath bulbocavernosus are the vestibular bulbs anteriorly and *Bartholin's glands* posteriorly
- main function is to cause erection of the clitoris and contraction of the vagina during sexual activity.

- *Ischiocavernosus muscles:*
  - arise from ischial tuberosities
  - pass upwards and inwards along the pubic arch and are inserted into the corpora cavernosa of the clitoris
  - some fibres interweave with those forming the membranous sphincter of the urethra.
- *Transverse perineal muscles:*
  - arise from ischial tuberosities
  - pass transversely to converge at central point of the perineum
  - fibres of each transverse muscle unite and interweave with the superficial tissue of the perineal body and external anal sphincter
  - provide additional support transversely across the perineal region, helping fix the position of the perineal body.

### *Sphincters*

- *Membranous sphincter of the urethra:*
  - arises from one pubic bone
  - passes above and below the urethra to the opposite pubic bone
  - not a true sphincter but capable of contracting to occlude the lumen of the urethra.
- *External anal sphincter* (EAS):
  - teardrop-shaped circle of muscle
  - surrounds the anus and is subdivided into three parts (not easily defined during dissection)
    - subcutaneous
    - superficial
    - deep
  - in females, the EAS is shorter anteriorly and fuses with the bulbocavernosus and transverse perinei in the lower part of the perineum (Sultan et al 1994a)
  - the deep EAS is inseparable from the puborectalis muscle and posteriorly is attached to the coccyx by some of its fibres
  - the circular striated (voluntary) muscle of the EAS, when dissected or torn, looks similar to 'dark red meat'
  - main function is to close the anal canal lumen and control voluntary passage of faeces and flatus.

- *Internal anal sphincter (IAS):*
  - a condensation of the circular smooth muscle of the rectum
  - approximately 3–4 cm long and 2–3 mm thick in younger women
  - not easily defined
  - on dissection, is paler in colour than the external anal sphincter
  - main function is to close the lumen of the anus and to prevent involuntary passage of faeces and flatus (very important during sleep).

**Ischiorectal fossa** is a deep wedge-shaped area, filled with fat, bounded by the *gluteus maximus, anal sphincter, transverse perinei* and *bulbocavernosus muscles*. It is a potential area for haematoma formation.

### *Blood, lymph and nerve supply*

Blood is supplied from branches of the internal iliac arteries and venous drainage is into corresponding veins. Lymphatic drainage is into the internal iliac glands. Nerve supply is from the third and fourth segments of the sacral plexus and pudendal nerve.

### Subcutaneous fat and skin

Neither has any supporting function.

## Perineal body

This is a triangular-shaped structure consisting of muscular and fibrous tissue, situated between the vagina and the anal canal, with the ischial tuberosities laterally. Each side of the triangle is approximately 3.5 cm in length: the base is the perineal skin and the apex points inwards. This is an integral part of the pelvic floor, since it is the central point where the levator ani and most of the superficial muscles unite. Blood is supplied by the pudendal arteries and venous drainage is into the corresponding veins. Lymph drains into the inguinal and external iliac glands. The nerve supply is derived from the perineal branch of the pudendal nerve.

## Midwifery implications

During pregnancy, the hormone *relaxin* softens the pelvic muscles and ligaments, allowing them to stretch during parturition to allow the passage of the term infant. After delivery, the pelvic floor is able to contract back to resume its original supporting function in a surprisingly short time, because of its remarkable elasticity.

Prolonged, repeated or extreme stretching of the pelvic floor muscles may cause permanent damage, resulting in loss of tone and elasticity. If these muscles fail to support the pelvic organs, prolapse results, though this may not manifest until later life when postmenopausal oestrogen deficiencies may predispose to muscle weakness (Haadem et al 1991). (For long term effects, please see website.)

# PERINEAL TRAUMA

*Anterior perineal trauma* is any injury to the labia, anterior vagina, urethra, or clitoris and is associated with less morbidity.

*Posterior perineal trauma* is any injury to the posterior vaginal wall, perineal muscles, or anal sphincters (external and internal) and may include disruption of the rectal mucosa.

Perineal trauma may occur spontaneously during vaginal birth or through intentional surgical incision (episiotomy) by the midwife or obstetrician to increase the diameter of the vulval outlet and facilitate delivery.

### Prevalence

Over 85% of women who have a vaginal birth will sustain some form of perineal trauma (McCandlish et al 1998) and up to 69% of these will require stitches (McCandlish et al 1998, Sleep et al 1984).

Rates will vary considerably according to individual practices and hospital policies throughout the world, illustrated by wide variations in episiotomy rates internationally from 8% in the Netherlands, 13% in England and 43% in the USA, to 99% in the Eastern European countries (Graham & Graham 1997, Graves 1995, Statistical Bulletin 2003, Wagner 1994).

Certain intrapartum interventions or alternative forms of care may also affect the rate and extent of perineal trauma; including continuous support during labour, delivery position, epidural anaesthesia, style of pushing, restricted use of episiotomy and ventouse delivery (Kettle 1999, 2001).

### Aetiology and risk factors

Perineal trauma occurs during spontaneous or assisted vaginal delivery and is usually more extensive after the first vaginal birth (Sultan et al 1996). Women who have no visible damage may be subject to transient pudendal or peripheral nerve injury due to prolonged active pushing or pressure exerted by the fetal head on the surrounding structures (Allen et al 1990).

Associated risk factors include:

- parity
- size of baby
- mode of delivery
- malpresentation and malposition of the fetus.

Other maternal factors are:

- ethnicity
- age

- tissue type
- nutritional state (Renfrew et al 1998)
- smoking – may affect perineal wound healing by causing vasoconstriction and tissue ischaemia (Mikhailidis et al 1983, Towler 2000).

### Short- and long-term effects

In the UK, approximately 23–42% of women will have perineal pain and discomfort up to 10–12 days following vaginal delivery and 7–10% of these women will continue to have long-term pain up to 18 months post partum (Glazener et al 1995, Gordon et al 1998, Grant et al 2001, McCandlish et al 1998, Mackrodt et al 1998, Sleep et al 1984).

In terms of sexual function, 62–88% of women will resume intercourse by 8–12 weeks postpartum, though 17–23% of women experience superficial dyspareunia at 3 months after delivery and 10–14% will continue to have pain at 12 months (Barrett et al 2000, Glazener 1997, Gordon et al 1998, Grant et al 2001, Kettle et al 2002, Mackrodt et al 1998).

Estimation of the extent of urinary and faecal incontinence is difficult because of under-reporting of these problems due to the sensitive nature of the complaint (Sultan et al 1996). One survey found that 15.2% of participating women (number 1782) reported stress incontinence which started for the first time within 3 months of the baby's birth, and 75% of these still had problems over a year later (MacArthur et al 1993). Sleep & Grant (1987) and MacArthur et al (1997) found that up to 4% of women reported occasional loss of bowel control.

## Antenatal preparation

The midwife can contribute to reducing the extent and rate of perineal trauma by reviewing the woman's lifestyle and giving appropriate advice regarding diet, smoking, exercise, and perineal massage. Being healthy and well nourished should ensure optimum condition of the perineal tissue prior to labour. Current evidence supports the use of antenatal perineal massage for preserving the integrity of the perineum, particularly in women having their first vaginal birth (Labrecque et al 2000, 2001). Women wishing to carry out this practice should be instructed to perform perineal massage from 34–35 weeks' gestation for 5–10 minutes daily using sweet almond oil (Labrecque et al 1999, Shipman et al 1997).

Midwives should also instruct and encourage women to carry out regular antenatal pelvic floor exercises to strengthen the muscles in preparation for childbirth and to continue these excercises into the postnatal period to reinnervate and increase the pelvic floor muscle tone in order to reduce any associated morbidity such as stress incontinence (Mason et al 2001).

## Spontaneous trauma

This can be classified as:

- **First degree**, which may involve:
  - skin and subcutaneous tissue of the anterior or posterior perineum
  - vaginal mucosa
  - a combination of the above, resulting in multiple superficial lacerations.
- **Second-degree** tears, which may involve:
  - superficial perineal muscles (bulbocavernosus, transverse perineal)
  - perineal body
  - if the trauma is very deep, possibly the pubococcygeus muscle.

Tears usually extend downwards from the posterior and/or lateral vaginal walls, through the hymenal remnants, midline downwards towards the anal margin, in the weakest part of the stretched perineum. Occasionally, they occur in a circular direction, behind the hymenal remnants, extending bilaterally upwards towards the clitoris and detaching the lower third of the vagina from the underlying structures (Sultan et al 1994a). This complex trauma causes vast disruption to the perineal body and muscles but the perineal skin may remain intact, making it difficult to repair.

- **Third-degree** tears, which involve the superficial and/or deep perineal muscles and anal sphincter(s). Recently, third-degree tears have been subclassified as:
  (**3a**) less than 50% of the external anal sphincter (EAS) torn
  (**3b**) more than 50% of the EAS torn
  (**3c**) to include internal anal sphincter (IAS) torn (Keighley et al 2000, Sultan 1999).
- **Fourth-degree** tears, involving the same structures as above, including disruption of the EAS and/or IAS and anorectal epithelium.

### Cervical tears

A cervical tear may result if an instrumental delivery (forceps or ventouse) is attempted before the cervix is fully dilated or the woman forcibly pushes the fetus through a cervix that is incompletely dilated (Oats & Abraham 2010).

Bleeding is usually very severe and will persist despite the uterus being well contracted. Postpartum haemorrhage (PPH) resulting from a cervical tear must be managed appropriately and efficiently according to guidelines (NICE 2007), as mismanagement can cause maternal mortality (see Ch. 68). Once the maternal condition has been stabilized, a skilled operator must repair the cervical tear in a theatre with good lighting, appropriate assistance, and adequate anaesthesia.

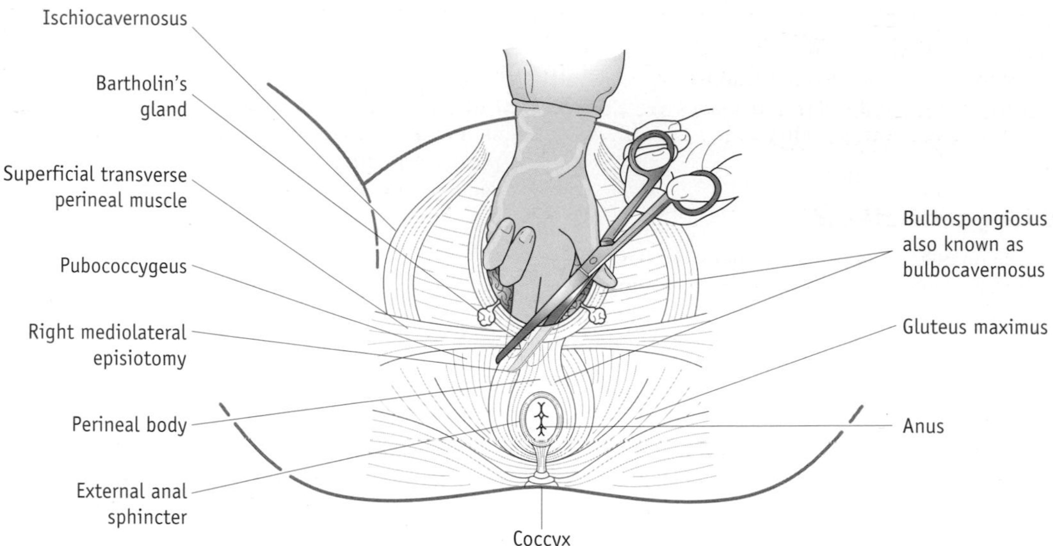


**Figure 40.2** Diagrammatic representation of a right mediolateral episiotomy showing the muscles involved when the incision is made.

## Surgical incision (episiotomy)

*Episiotomy* is a surgical incision of the perineum made to increase the diameter of the vulval outlet during childbirth.

Straight, blunt-ended Mayo episiotomy scissors are usually used because it is thought that there is less risk of accidental damage to the baby, and haemostasis of the cut tissue is promoted by the crushing action as the incision is made. Some professionals favour the scalpel and feel that it minimizes trauma to the tissues which allows better healing of the perineal wound, though no data support the validity of either of these claims (Sleep et al 1989).

An episiotomy should **not be** carried out routinely during spontaneous vaginal birth, and should only be performed if there are specific clinical needs as documented below. It should not be offered routinely following previous third- or fourth-degree trauma.

Prior to performing the incision, informed consent must always be obtained from the woman and analgesia should always be administered, except in an emergency if there is acute fetal compromise (NICE 2007).

There are two main types of incision:

*Right mediolateral:*

- Incision starts at the fourchette midline – to avoid damage to the Bartholin's gland.
- It is then directed diagonally to the right side of the posterior perineum to a point midway between the anus and ischial tuberosity, at an angle of 45–60° to the vertical axis (avoids anal sphincter complex).
- In the UK, most midwives and obstetricians perform a right mediolateral episiotomy (Fig. 40.2).

*Midline:*

- Incision starts in the midline position at the fourchette and is made vertically towards the anus.

> **Reflective activity 40.1**
>
> Find out what the episiotomy rate is for spontaneous vaginal deliveries in the maternity unit where you are working.

### Timing of the incision

An episiotomy must only be made when the presenting part is distending the perineal tissues; otherwise it will fail to accelerate delivery and excessive bleeding may occur.

### Indications

The following are not absolute, and clinical discretion must always be used:

- Rigid perineum causing delay in the second stage
- To reduce prolonged maternal 'pushing' efforts in cases of severe hypertensive or cardiac disease
- Fetal compromise
- To prevent severe perineal trauma during instrumental delivery (forceps or ventouse) or when the baby is in the direct occipitoposterior position

Table 40.1 Procedure for mediolateral episiotomy

| Action | Rationale |
|---|---|
| **1.** Explain the procedure and indications to the woman and her partner | **1.** To reassure the woman and confirm consent |
| **2.** Place the woman in a comfortable position with her legs open | **2.** To ensure that the whole perineal area is accessible |
| **3.** Cleanse the perineal area using the agreed aseptic technique | **3.** To minimize infection |
| **4.** Place the index and middle fingers into the vagina between the presenting part and perineum. Insert the needle fully into the perineal tissue starting at the centre of the fourchette and directing it midway between the ischial tuberosity and anus | **4.** To protect the baby from accidental damage |
| **5.** Draw back the plunger of the syringe prior to injecting 5–10 mL of local anaesthetic, 1% lidocaine, slowly into the tissue as the needle is withdrawn | **5.** To check that the lidocaine is not accidentally injected into a blood vessel and to provide effective anaesthesia to facilitate a pain-free incision |
| **6.** Insert the middle and index fingers into the vagina and gently pull the perineum away from the presenting fetal part | **6.** To protect the presenting fetal part from accidental damage |
| **7.** Perform the incision when the presenting part has distended the perineum | **7.** To minimize pain and blood loss |
| **8.** Insert the open scissors between the two fingers and make the incision in one single cut | **8.** To ensure a straight cut, minimize severe perineal damage and facilitate optimum anatomical realignment |
| **9.** Perform the incision – it should extend at least 3–4 cm into the perineum. The incision should start midline from the centre of the fourchette and then extend outwards in a mediolateral direction, avoiding the anal sphincter(s). Withdraw the scissors carefully | **9.** To increase the vulval outlet and facilitate delivery |
| **10.** Control delivery of the presenting part and shoulders | **10.** To prevent sudden expulsion of the presenting part and extension of the episiotomy incision |
| **11.** Apply pressure to the episiotomy incision between contractions if there is a delay in delivering the baby | **11.** To control bleeding from the wound |
| **12.** Thoroughly inspect the vagina and perineum, including a rectal examination, following completion of the third stage | **12.** To identify the extent of trauma prior to repair |

- To facilitate safe delivery in selective cases of shoulder dystocia (RCOG 2005).

*NB:* There is no scientific evidence to support the routine procedure of episiotomy to prevent intracranial haemorrhage in preterm deliveries (Woolley 1995).

## Risks

- Potentially increases the overall rate of posterior perineal trauma
- Increases intrapartum maternal blood loss
- Fourfold increased risk of anal sphincter damage (midline episiotomies) (Coats et al 1980, Thacker & Banta 1983)
- Increased postpartum pain and perineal infection
- Potential reduction in pelvic floor muscle function
- Increased vertical transmission of human immunodeficiency virus (HIV).

*NB:* The risks are clearly increased with a high episiotomy rate.

Prior to performing the episiotomy, the midwife must prepare the delivery trolley and equipment according to the practice policies and guidelines of the individual employing policies. Safety glasses and gloves must be worn during all obstetric procedures, to protect the operator against HIV and hepatitis infection. The woman's dignity and comfort must be maintained throughout the procedure (see Table 40.1). There is some debate about the incision to be used – please see website.

### Complications

- Damage to the Bartholin's gland
- Possible Batholin gland cyst formation
- Decrease in vaginal lubrication, leading to sexual difficulties
- Severe pain
- Difficulty in repair
- Possible extension of the tear if the incision is too small.

### Episiotomy rate

There seems to be no consensus as to the recommended episiotomy rate. The World Health Organization suggests that an episiotomy rate of 10%, for normal deliveries, would be 'a good goal to pursue' (WHO 1996).

### Discussion

Episiotomy has been described as the unkindest cut, but with limited evidence about use and efficacy, has been introduced into maternity care in the UK (see website).

Major variations in current national rates indicate uncertain justification for this practice (Audit Commission 1997).

Some argue that episiotomy causes more pain, weakens pelvic floor structures, interferes with breastfeeding and increases sexual problems (Greenshields & Hulme 1993, Kitzinger & Walters 1981). Others argue that episiotomy reduces the incidence of severe perineal trauma and prevents overstretching of pelvic floor muscles, so reducing the risk of stress incontinence and uterine prolapse (Donald 1979, Flood 1982). However, research carried out by Klein et al (1994) found that women who delivered with an intact perineum or spontaneous perineal tear had less pain, stronger pelvic floor muscles, and better sexual function when compared to those with an episiotomy, at 3 months postpartum.

Midwives should restrict the use of episiotomy to specific fetal and maternal indications. Previous randomized controlled trials comparing restricted to liberal use of episiotomy found that a restricted policy is associated with lower rates of posterior perineal trauma, less suturing, and reduction in pain and healing complications (Carroli & Belizan 2001). This results in a lower rate of maternal morbidity and may have significant cost-saving implications for suture materials (Carroli & Belizan 2001, Sleep et al 1984).

## Suturing the perineum

In the UK, the theory and technique of perineal repair has been included in the midwifery curriculum since 1983 (Silverton 1993). By 1986, midwives were repairing perineal trauma in over 60% of consultant units in England and Wales (Garcia et al 1986), thus achieving increased continuity of care, prompt sensitive repair, and increased job satisfaction.

### Suture materials for primary repair of perineal trauma

The ideal suture material should cause minimal tissue reaction and be absorbed once it has served its purpose of holding the tissue in apposition during the healing process (Taylor & Karran 1996). Well-aligned perineal wounds heal by primary intention with minimal complications, usually within 2 weeks of suturing. However, if the stitches remain in the tissues for longer than this period, they act as a foreign body and may impair healing, causing irritation. Local infection of the stitches will prolong the inflammatory phase and cause further tissue damage, which will delay collagen synthesis and epithelialization (Flanagan 1997).

Perineal repair using absorbable synthetic material, such as polyglactin 910 (*Vicryl*) or polyglycolic acid (*Dexon*), reduces short-term pain, though long-term effects are less clear and there are some concerns regarding the need to remove sutures up to 3 months after delivery (Kettle & Johanson 2001).

Three randomized controlled trials (RCTs) – carried out by Gemynthe et al (1996), McElhinney et al (2000) and Kettle et al (2002) – compared rapidly absorbed polyglactin 910 (*Vicryl Rapide*) to standard polyglactin 910 (*Vicryl*) and found no overall difference in short-term perineal pain between groups, but a significant reduction in the need for suture removal up to 3 months following childbirth with the rapidly absorbed material. Two of the trials (Gemynthe et al 1996, Kettle et al 2002) found a significant reduction in *'pain when walking'* at 10–14 days postpartum. One trial (McElhinney et al 2000) reported a reduction in superficial dyspareunia at 3 months postpartum. This evidence suggests that *Vicryl Rapide* is the ideal suture material for perineal repair (NICE 2007).

The arguments for recommended suture techniques for primary repair of perineal trauma are given on the website.

### Non-suturing of perineal skin

Two RCTs compared suturing the vagina and perineal muscles, leaving the perineal skin unsutured, to the conventional method of suturing the vagina, perineal muscles and skin (Gordon et al 1998, Oboro et al 2003). The UK study found no significant difference in perineal pain at

10 days postpartum between groups (Gordon et al 1998), though the Nigerian study indicated a reduction in perineal pain at 48 hours, 14 days, 6 weeks, and 3 months following birth when the skin was left unsutured (Oboro et al 2003).

### Tissue adhesive

Two small trials looked at the use of tissue adhesive for closure of perineal skin following second-degree tear or episiotomy (Adoni & Anteby 1991, Rogerson et al 2000). Both trials claim that this method is effective, but the results must be interpreted with caution owing to the poor methodological design of these studies and the small number of participants included.

### Procedure (see Table 40.2)

Perineal tears and episiotomies are repaired under aseptic conditions with a good source of light and the mother in a comfortable position so that the trauma can be easily visualized. Lithotomy poles to support the woman's legs during the repair are unnecessary and might bring back 'locked in' memories of sexual abuse, making the woman feel helpless and out of control (Walton 1994). Also, leg restraints (lithotomy poles) cause flexion and abduction of the woman's hips which results in excessive stretching of the perineum, causing the episiotomy or tear to gape (Borgatta 1989). Apart from being uncomfortable for the woman, this can make the trauma difficult for the operator to realign and suture. There is no need to use a tampon.

If the woman has a working epidural, it may be topped up to provide effective perineal area anaesthesia instead of injecting local anaesthetic. Khan & Lilford (1987) recommend that even if an epidural is used, the perineal wound should be infiltrated with normal saline or local anaesthetic to mimic tissue oedema and prevent overtight suturing.

Prior to performing the repair, the midwife must prepare the suturing trolley and check equipment according to individual employing authorities' practice guidelines. The woman's comfort and dignity must be maintained throughout the procedure.

The area should be cleaned according to the individual unit's guidelines; however, a study by Calkin (1996) found that tapwater was just as effective as chlorhexidine antiseptic.

The method of performing the repair is shown in Figure 40.3 and the rationale for each stage of the process is given in Table 40.2.

On completion of perineal repair, the woman should be given advice regarding:

- the extent of trauma
- the healing process
- methods of pain relief
- personal hygiene
- diet and rest
- pelvic floor exercise
- avoidance of constipation
- whom to contact in case of long-term perineal pain/ dyspareunia or incontinence.

## Labial lacerations

These are usually superficial but can be very painful. Some practitioners do not recommend that these are sutured; however, if the trauma is bilateral, sometimes the lacerations heal together over the urethra, causing voiding difficulties.

## Non-suturing of perineal trauma

The effects of not suturing deeper perineal trauma, such as second-degree tears or episiotomies, have not yet been robustly evaluated, though some practitioners appear to have adopted a non-suturing policy without reliable evidence to support their practice (see website).

Until robust evidence is available to support this controversial practice, midwives must be cautious about leaving trauma other than small first-degree tears unsutured unless it is the explicit wish of the woman. There is an urgent need for a large randomized controlled trial to be undertaken comparing non-suturing versus suturing of second-degree perineal trauma with long-term follow-up. Practice must be based upon scientific principles.

## Third- and fourth-degree tears

The reported incidence of clinically detectable anal sphincter injuries following childbirth ranges from 0.5% to 3% (Sultan et al 1994b, Tetzschner et al 1996), though the full extent of the problem is probably underestimated. Some third-degree tears may not be recognized following vaginal delivery (Andrews et al 2006, Groome & Paterson Brown 2000). Studies found that with increased vigilance and improvement in clinical skills, the detection of anal sphincter disruption could be vastly improved. If this type of trauma is not recognized after delivery, women can be left with long-term problems including incontinence of faeces and flatulence. Anal incontinence following anal sphincter injury varies between 7% and 59% (Goffeng et al 1998, Kamm 1994, Tetzschner et al 1996), but again may be higher due to non-reporting. In one study, only one-third of the participants with faecal incontinence had ever discussed their problem with a physician (Johanson & Lafferty 1996).

Midwives and medical staff must be aware of this type of trauma and be adequately trained to identify anal sphincter injuries when they occur (Fig. 40.4). (See website for associated risk factors.)

All perineal trauma must be thoroughly examined with the aid of a good light source and the extent of injury must be accurately documented in the hospital case notes.

**Table 40.2 Procedure for continuous method of perineal repair**

| Action | Rationale |
|---|---|
| **1.** Explain the procedure to the woman and her partner | **1.** To reassure the woman and confirm consent |
| **2.** Check maternal baseline observations and PV blood loss | **2.** To ensure that the woman's general condition is stable prior to commencing the repair |
| **3.** Assess the extent of perineal trauma | **3.** To ensure the repair is not beyond the operator's level of competence |
| **4.** Ensure that the woman is in an appropriate position | **4.** To ensure that the whole perineal area is accessible |
| **5.** Cleanse the vulva and perineal area. Drape the area with a sterile lithotomy towel | **5.** To minimize risk of infection |
| **6.** Identify anatomical landmarks. These may include hymenal remnants and tissue of different colour | **6.** To aid the operator to correctly align and approximate the traumatized tissue *NB:* Misalignment may cause long-term morbidity such as dyspareunia |
| **7.** Draw back the plunger of the syringe prior to injecting 10–20 mL of local anaesthetic, 1% lidocaine, slowly into the traumatized tissue, ensuring even distribution | **7.** To check that the lidocaine is not accidentally injected into a blood vessel and to provide effective anaesthesia to facilitate a pain-free repair |
| **8.** Identify the apex of the vaginal trauma and insert the first stitch 5–10 mm above this point | **8.** To ensure haemostasis of any bleeding vessels that may have retracted beyond the apex |
| **9.** Suture posterior vaginal trauma using a loose continuous non-locking stitch. Continue to the hymenal remnants taking care not to make the stitches too wide | **9.** To appose the edges of traumatized vaginal mucosa and muscle without causing shortening or narrowing of the vagina |
| **10.** Ensure that each stitch reaches the trough of the traumatized tissue | **10.** To close dead space, achieve haemostasis and prevent paravaginal haematoma formation |
| **11.** Visualize the needle at the trough of the trauma each time it is inserted | **11.** To prevent sutures being inserted through the rectal mucosa *NB:* A recto-vaginal fistula may form if this occurs |
| **12.** Bring the needle through the tissue underneath the hymenal ring and continue to repair the deep and superficial muscles using a loose continuous stitch | **12.** To realign the perineal muscles, close the dead space, achieve haemostasis and minimize the risk of haematoma formation |
| **13.** Reverse the stitching direction at the inferior aspect of the trauma and place the stitches loosely in the subcutaneous layer, approximately 5–10 mm apart | **13.** To appose skin edges and complete the perineal repair |
| **14.** Do not pull the stitches too tight | **14.** To prevent discomfort from overtight sutures if reactionary oedema and swelling occur |
| **15.** Complete the subcutaneous repair to the hymenal ring, swing the needle under the tissue into the vagina and complete the repair using a terminal loop knot | **15.** To secure the stitches |
| **16.** Inspect the repaired perineal trauma | **16.** To ensure the trauma has been sutured correctly and that haemostasis has been achieved<br>Check that there is no excessive bleeding from the uterus |
| **17.** Insert two fingers gently into the vagina | **17.** To confirm that the introitus and vagina have not been stitched too tightly |
| **18.** Perform a rectal examination | **18.** To confirm that no sutures have penetrated the rectal mucosa |
| **19.** Cleanse and dry the perineal area. Apply a sterile pad | **19.** To minimize infection |
| **20.** Check and record that all swabs, needles and instruments are correct | **20.** To confirm that all equipment and materials used are complete and accounted for |
| **21.** Place the woman in the position of her choice | **21.** To ensure that the woman is made comfortable following the procedure |
| **22.** Complete the appropriate documentation | **22.** To fulfil statutory requirements and to provide an accurate account of the repair |

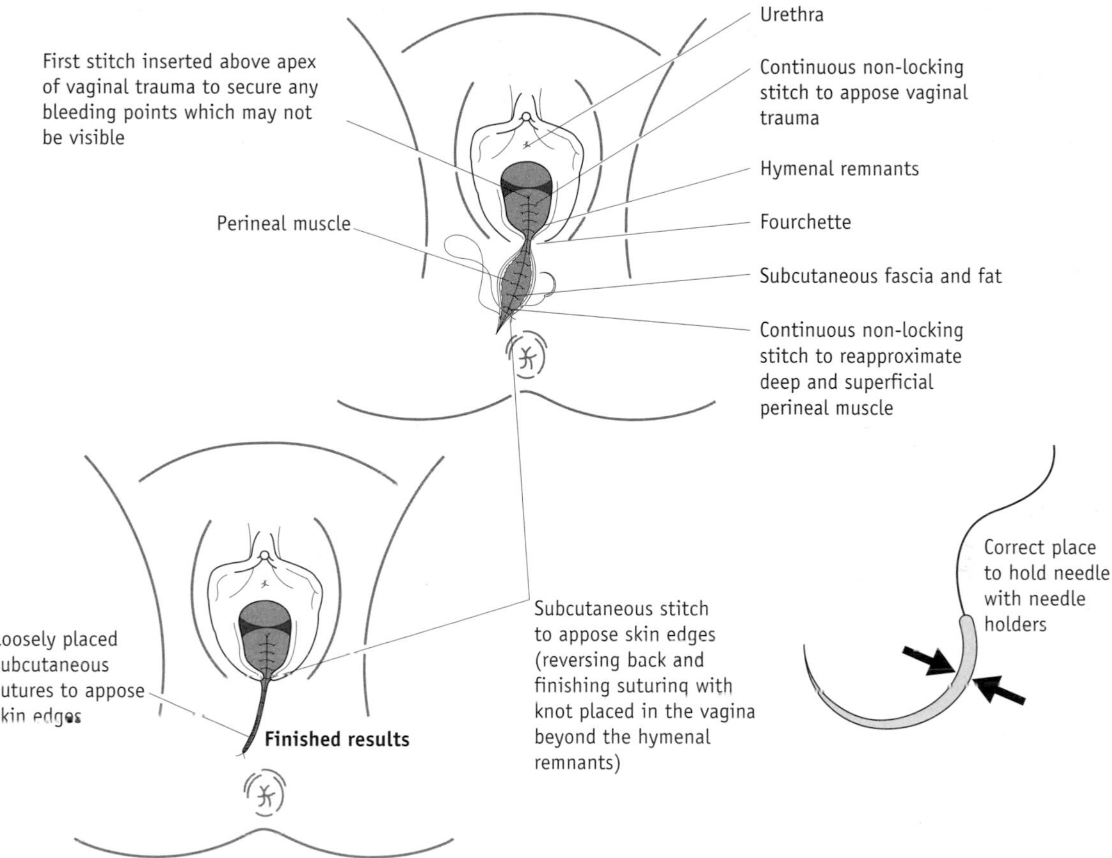


**Figure 40.3** Continuous non-locking method of perineal repair.

When assessing perineal injury after delivery, a rectal examination should be **routinely** performed to avoid missing anal sphincter trauma. If a third- or fourth-degree tear is suspected, it must be checked by an independent experienced practitioner.

## Identification of anal sphincter injury

- Look for absence of 'puckering' around the anterior section of the anus.
- Observe if the trauma extends down to the anal margin.
- Perform a digital rectal examination and ask the woman to contract the anal sphincter. If the external anal sphincter (EAS) is damaged, the torn ends will be observed retracting backwards towards the ischiorectal fossa (Fig. 40.4). *NB:* Damage to the internal anal sphincter is much more difficult to detect, as this is a less-well-defined paler muscle.

For further information on third- and fourth-degree repair, please see website.

## Professional and legal issues

Litigation is a major concern for all practitioners; however, a competent midwife has little to fear if she works within the parameters of the employing authority's policies and guidelines, and the midwives' rules (NMC 2004). In an action for damages, practitioners may be held personally liable if it can be shown that they failed to exercise appropriate skills and work within their professional boundaries.

## CONCLUSION

Mismanagement of perineal trauma has a major impact on women's health and has significant implications for health service resources. Midwives must base their practice on current research evidence and be aware of problems associated with perineal trauma and repair. Careful identification and repair of trauma by a skilled practitioner may avoid problems. It is important that prompt sensitive

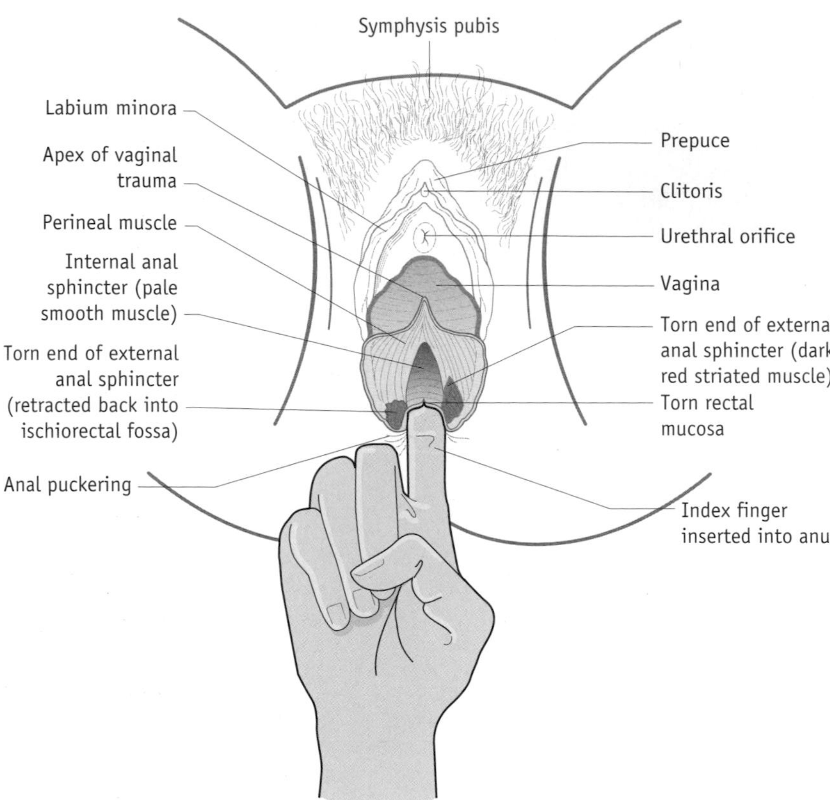


**Figure 40.4** Anal sphincter injury – fourth-degree tear. *(From Marshall & Raynor 2010.)*

treatment is provided for those women with problems in order to reduce the morbidity associated with perineal injury following childbirth.

## KEY POINTS

- A restricted episiotomy policy reduces the rates of posterior perineal trauma.
- The use of a more rapidly absorbed synthetic suture material (*Vicryl Rapide*) when compared to standard material (*Vicryl*) is associated with significantly less perineal pain when 'walking' and a reduction in the need for suture removal up to 3 months postpartum.
- The loose, continuous non-locking suturing technique for repair of vaginal tissue, perineal muscle and skin is associated with a significant reduction in pain and need for suture removal compared to the traditional interrupted method.
- It is important to recognize when anal sphincter injury has occurred and refer to the most appropriate practitioner.
- Pelvic floor exercises during pregnancy and following childbirth help to reduce morbidity.
- Women should be given clear information and advice about any trauma sustained including aftercare and reporting any deviations from normal.

## REFERENCES

Adoni A, Anteby E: The use of Histoacryl for episiotomy repair, *British Journal of Obstetrics and Gynaecology* 98(5):446–478, 1991.

Allen RE, Hosker GL, Smith ARB, et al: Pelvic floor damage and childbirth: a neurophysiological study, *British Journal of Obstetrics and Gynaecology* 97(9):770–779, 1990.

Andrews V, Sultan AH, Thakar R, et al: Occult anal sphincter injuries – myth or reality? *BJOG* 113(2):195–200, 2006.

Audit Commission: *First class delivery: improving maternity services in England and Wales*, London, 1997, Audit Commission.

Barrett G , Pendry E, Peacock J, et al: Women's sexual health after childbirth, *BJOG* 107(2):186–195, 2000.

Benson JT: *Female pelvic floor disorders: investigation and management*, London, 1992, Norton Medical Books.

Borgatta L: Association of episiotomy and delivery position with deep perineal laceration during spontaneous delivery in nulliparous women, *American Journal of Obstetrics and Gynecology* 160(2):294–297, 1989.

Calkin S: Chlorhexidine swabbing in labour, *Modern Midwife* 6(1):28–33, 1996.

Carroli G, Belizan J: Episiotomy for vaginal birth (Cochrane Review) *The Cochrane Library*, Issue 1, Oxford, 2001, Update Software.

Coats PM, Chan KK, Wilkins M, et al: A comparison between midline and mediolateral episiotomies, *British Journal of Obstetrics and Gynaecology* 87(5):408–412, 1980.

Derry DE: Notes on five pelves of women of the eleventh dynasty in Egypt, *Journal of Obstetrics and Gynaecology of the British Empire* 42(13):490–495, 1935.

Donald I: *Practical obstetric problems*, London, 1979, Lloyd-Luke.

Flanagan M: *Wound management*, New York, 1997, Churchill Livingstone.

Flood C: The real reasons for performing episiotomies, *World Medicine* 6:51, 1982.

Garcia J, Garforth S, Ayers S: Midwives confined? Labour ward policies and routines, *Research and the Midwife Conference Proceedings* 2–30, 1986.

Gemynthe A, Langhoff-Ross J, Sahl S, et al: New VICRYL formulation: an improved method of perineal repair? *British Journal of Midwifery* 4(5):230–234, 1996.

Glazener CM: Sexual function after childbirth: women's experiences, persistent morbidity and lack of professional recognition, *British Journal of Obstetrics and Gynaecology* 104(3):330–335, 1997.

Glazener CMA, Abdalla M, Stroud P, et al: Postnatal maternal morbidity: extent, causes, prevention and treatment, *British Journal of Obstetrics and Gynaecology* 102(4):286–287, 1995.

Goffeng AR, Andersch B, Andersson M, et al: Objective methods cannot predict anal incontinence after primary repair of extensive anal tears, *Acta Obstetricia et Gynecologica Scandinavica* 77(4):439–443, 1998.

Gordon B, Mackrodt C, Fern E, et al: The Ipswich Childbirth Study: 1. A randomised evaluation of two stage postpartum perineal repair leaving the skin unsutured, *British Journal of Obstetrics and Gynaecology* 105(4):435–440, 1998.

Graham H: *Eternal Eve*, London, 1950, William Heinemann Medical Books.

Graham ID, Graham DF: Episiotomy counts: trends and prevalence in Canada, 1981/1982 to 1993/1994, *Birth* 24(3):141–147, 1997.

Grant A, Gordon B, Mackrodat C, et al: The Ipswich Childbirth study: one year follow up of alternative methods of perineal repair, *Br J Obstet Gynaecol* 108(1):34–40, 2001.

Graves EJ: 1993 summary: National Hospital Discharge Survey, *Advance Data* (264):1–11, 1995.

Greenshields W, Hulme H: *The perineum in childbirth: a survey of women's experiences and midwifery practices*, London, 1993, National Childbirth Trust.

Groome KM, Paterson-Brown S: Third degree tears. are they clinically underdiagnosed? *Gastroenterology International* 13(2):76, 2000.

Haadem K, Ling L, Ferno M, et al: Estrogen receptors in the external anal sphincter, *Obstetrics and Gynecology* 164(2):609–610, 1991.

Johanson JF, Lafferty J: Epidemiology of faecal incontinence: the silent affliction, *American Journal of Gastroenterology* 91(1):33–36, 1996.

Kamm MA: Obstetric damage and faecal incontinence, *Lancet* 344(8924):730–733, 1994.

Keighley MRB, Radley S, Johanson R: Consensus on prevention and management of post-obstetric bowel incontinence and third degree tear, *Clinical Risk* 6:211–217, 2000.

Kettle C: *Perineal tears*, Nursing Times Clinical Monograph, London, 1999, Nursing Times Books.

Kettle C: Perineal care. In *BMJ clinical evidence – a compendium of the best available evidence for effective health care*, London, 2001, BMJ Publishing.

Kettle C, Johanson RB: Absorbable synthetic vs catgut suture material for perineal repair (Cochrane Review), *The Cochrane Library*, Issue 1, Oxford, 2001, Update Software.

Kettle C, Hills RK, Jones P, et al: Continuous versus interrupted perineal repair with standard or rapidly absorbed sutures after spontaneous vaginal birth: a randomised controlled trial, *The Lancet* 359(9325):2217–2223, 2002.

Khan GQ, Lilford RJ: Wound pain may be reduced by prior infiltration of the episiotomy site after delivery under spinal epidural anaesthetic, *British Journal of Obstetrics and Gynaecology* 94(4):341–344, 1987.

Kitzinger S, Walters R: *Episiotomy – physical and emotional aspects*, London, 1981, National Childbirth Trust.

Klein MC, Gauthier RJ, Robbins JM, et al: Relationship of episiotomy to perineal trauma and morbidity, sexual function, and pelvic floor relaxation, *American Journal of Obstetrics and Gynecology* 171(3):591–598, 1994.

Labrecque M, Eason E, Marcoux S, et al: Randomised controlled trial of prevention of perineal trauma by perineal massage during pregnancy, *American Journal of Obstetrics and Gynecology* 180(3 pt 1):593–600, 1999.

Labrecque M, Eason E, Marcoux S: Randomised trial of perineal massage during pregnancy: perineal symptoms three months after delivery, *American Journal of Obstetrics and Gynecology* 182(1 pt 1):76–80, 2000.

Labrecque M, Eason E, Marcoux S: Women's views on the practice of perineal massage, *British Journal of Obstetrics and Gynaecology* 108(5):499–504, 2001.

MacArthur C, Lewi M, Bick D: Stress incontinence after childbirth, *British Journal of Midwifery* 1(5):207–215, 1993.

MacArthur C, Bick D, Keighley MR: Faecal incontinence after childbirth, *British Journal of Obstetrics and Gynaecology* 104(1):46–50, 1997.

McCandlish R, Bowler U, van Asten H, et al: A randomised controlled trial of care of the perineum during second stage of normal labour, *British Journal of Obstetrics and Gynaecology* 105(12):1262–1272, 1998.

McElhinney BR, Glenn DR, Dornan G, et al: Episiotomy repair: Vicryl versus Vicryl rapide, *Ulster Medical Journal* 69(1):27–29, 2000.

Mackrodt C, Gordon B, Fern E, et al: The Ipswich Childbirth Study: 2. A randomised comparison of suture materials and suturing techniques for repair of perineal trauma, *British Journal of Obstetrics and Gynaecology* 105(4):441–445, 1998.

Magdi I: Obstetric injuries of the perineum, *Journal of Obstetrics and Gynaecology of the British Empire* 49:697–700, 1949.

Marshall JE, Raynor MD: *Advancing skills in midwifery practice*, Edinburgh, 2010, Elsevier.

Mason L, Glenn S, Walton I, et al: The instruction in pelvic floor exercises provided to women during pregnancy or following delivery, *Midwifery* 17(1):55–64, 2001.

Mikhailidis DP, Bauadas MA , Jeremy JY, et al: Cigarette smoking inhibits prostacycline formation, *The Lancet* 2(8350):627–628, 1983.

National Institute for Health and Clinical Excellence (NICE): *Intrapartum care: care of healthy women and their babies during childbirth*, Guideline No. 55, London, 2007, NICE.

Nursing and Midwifery Council (NMC): *Midwives rules and standards*, London, 2004, NMC.

Oats JK, Abraham S: *Llewellyn-Jones fundamentals of obstetrics and gynaecology*, ed 9, London, 2010, Mosby.

Oboro VO, Tabowei TO, Loto OM, et al: Multicentre evaluation of the two-layered repair of postpartum perineal trauma, *Journal of Obstetrics and Gynaecology* 23(1):5–8, 2003.

Renfrew M, Hannah W, Albers L, et al: Practices that minimize trauma to the genital tract in childbirth: a systematic review of the literature, *Birth* 25(3):143–159, 1998.

Rogerson L, Mason GC, Roberts AC: Preliminary experience with twenty perineal repairs using Indermil tissue adhesive, *European Journal of Obstetrics and Gynecology and Reproductive Biology* 88(2):139–142, 2000.

Royal College of Obstetricians and Gynaecologists (RCOG): *Shoulder dystocia*, Green-top Guideline No 42, London, 2005, RCOG.

Royal College of Obstetricians and Gynaecologists (RCOG): *Management of third and fourth degree perineal tears following vaginal delivery*, Green-top Guideline No 29 (revised version), London, 2007, RCOG.

Shipman M, Boniface D, Tefft M, et al: Antenatal perineal massage and subsequent perineal outcomes: a randomised controlled trial, *British Journal of Obstetrics and Gynaecology* 104:787–791, 1997.

Silverton L: *The art and science of midwifery*, London, 1993, Prentice Hall.

Sleep J, Grant A, Garcia J, et al: West Berkshire perineal management trial, *British Medical Journal* 298(6445):587–690, 1984.

Sleep J, Grant A: Pelvic floor exercises in postnatal care, *Midwifery* 3(4):158–164, 1987.

Sleep J, Roberts J, Chalmers I: Care during the second stage of labour. In Chalmers I, Enkin MW, Keirse MJNC, editors: *Effective care in pregnancy and childbirth*, Oxford, 1989, Oxford University Press, pp 1129–1141.

Statistical Bulletin: *NHS maternity statistics England: 2001–2002*, London, 2003, DH.

Sultan AH: Editorial: Obstetrics perineal injury and anal incontinence, *Clinical Risk* 5:193–196, 1999.

Sultan AH, Kamm MA, Bartram CI, et al: Perineal damage at delivery, *Contemporary Review of Obstetrics and Gynaecology* 6:8–24, 1994a.

Sultan AH, Kamm MA, Hudson CN, et al: Third degree anal sphincter tears: risk factors and outcome of primary repair, *British Medical Journal* 308(6933):887–891, 1994b.

Sultan AH , Monga AK, Stanton SL: The pelvic sequelae of childbirth, *British Journal of Hospital Medicine* 55(9):575–579, 1996.

Taylor I, Karran SJ, editors: *Surgical principles*, London, 1996, Oxford University Press, p. 28.

Tetzschner T, Sorenson M, Lose G, et al: Anal and urinary incontinence in women with obstetric anal sphincter rupture, *British Journal of Obstetrics and Gynaecology* 103(10):1034–1040, 1996.

Thacker SB, Banta D: Benefits and risks of episiotomy: an interpretative review of the English language literature 1860–1880, *Obstetrical & Gynecological Survey* 38(6):322–335, 1983.

Towler J: Cigarette smoking and its effects on wound healing, *Journal of Wound Care* 9(3):100–104, 2000.

Verralls S: *Anatomy and physiology applied to obstetrics*, ed 3, London, 1993, Churchill Livingstone.

Wagner M: *Pursuing the birth machine: the search for appropriate birth technology*, Camperdown, 1994, ACE Graphics, pp 165–174.

Walton I: *Sexuality and motherhood*, Hale, 1994, Books for Midwives, p. 125.

Woolley RJ: Benefits and risks of episiotomy: a review of the English-language literature since 1980. Part II, *Obstetrical & Gynecological Survey* 50(11):821–835, 1995.

World Health Organization (WHO) Maternal and Newborn Health/Safe Motherhood Unit: (1996) *Care in normal birth: a practical guide (report of a technical working group)*, Doc. No. WHO/FRH/MSM/96.24, Geneva, 1996, WHO, p. 29.

# Part 7

# The newborn baby

Chapter |41|

# Physiology, assessment and care

Stephanie Michaelides

### LEARNING OUTCOMES

At the end of this chapter, you will have:

- a clear understanding of applied physiology and the transition from fetal to neonatal life
- an understanding of the importance of providing evidence-based physiologically appropriate care and management to the neonate
- a commitment to allocating the same time and attention to the assessment and examination of the newborn as to its mother and family
- a framework for undertaking an assessment of the newborn, educating the woman about her baby's needs and how they might be met.

## INTRODUCTION

Providing the woman with support and guidance in her adjustment to motherhood is an important aspect of the midwife's role. To achieve this, the midwife works with a range of agencies and professionals to support a seamless process from the antenatal period through to early parenthood.

As well as being a screening test, examination of the newborn enables maternal/paternal–infant interaction through understanding the baby's unique development and behaviour.

### The baby as an individual

Woman-centred care has been an important development in providing choice, continuity and control to women and their families. However, it is likely that the time and attention paid to the assessment and care of the baby, even on a day-to-day basis, has been a fraction of that paid to the woman. It is crucial that babies are viewed as individuals in their own right and that midwives allocate the same attention to their assessment and care. This requires in-depth knowledge of neonatal psychological and physiological development, and complex communication and educational skills.

The baby is recognized as a person (Children Act 1989) with individual needs that require the midwife to act as an advocate and act with duty of care for those needs. Rather than relying on verbal responses, the midwife communicates with the baby via sight, touch and hearing. This must be a focused activity in order to absorb all of the information provided by the baby's responses and behaviour. Upon completion of the examination, the findings must be discussed with the parents so that the baby's management and care can be planned as a partnership. Prior to the examination, the midwife must gain consent from the legal guardian. If an unmarried woman is unable to give consent, then it has to be gained from the woman's next of kin. This should be discussed with the woman when she first attends for care, so that she can provide this information, which may be required in an emergency.

If consent is withheld, then further information, support of a peer, or medical advice may be sought. Consent needs to be obtained by the person providing the care – i.e. if the baby deviates from normal, the decision of how to proceed must be made in partnership with a senior neonatologist.

If the woman wishes the baby to be given oral (or no) vitamin K preparation, the midwife has a duty, under statute (NMC 2004), to ask the paediatrician to see the mother and ensure that the decision-making outcome is recorded in the baby's notes. If invasive treatment is required, then consent needs to be obtained by the person implementing the invasive procedure, so that the parents can be given the information they need. If the parents feel that they have not been given adequate information, then consent may not be deemed valid (DH 2001).

If the parents refuse life-saving care for the baby, the midwife needs to work with the appropriate professionals (GP or senior neonatologist) to enable the parents to understand the severity of the situation. It is crucial to record what information has been given, and any discussions that take place.

The midwife should clearly document the decisions and justification of actions and omissions, providing a clear picture of the transitional events that occurred at birth and during the first 28 days of postnatal life.

## Assessment of the newborn

This assessment is not a 'one-off' assessment but a complex, dynamic and continuous activity throughout the antenatal period, labour, at birth and in the neonatal period. Quick recognition and appropriate referral of the fetus/neonate with deviations from normal, results in an enhanced quality of life for that baby and family.

In order to achieve this, a formalized communication system between the baby and midwife is vital.

For a period of 9 months, the fetus has been in a safe, untouched and warm environment in which every need is catered for, free movement is allowed and psychological attachment to the mother is developed.

The long-term effects of the birth experience, and transition from this safe environment, are unknown, and it is imperative that birth attendants consider the baby and the environment he has recently left with equal empathy and care as that offered to the mother.

# APPLIED PHYSIOLOGY

The midwife's knowledge of the transitional events that occur at birth, and the changes to the newborn's physiology, can be applied to recognition of normal and abnormal events at birth and the difference between primary and secondary apnoea and their management. In this way, the midwife is able to provide thoughtful and reasoned practice and justify all actions.

## Respiratory system

In this section, the embryological development of lungs, role of lung fluid, fetal breathing movements, and development and function of surfactant will be explored. The respiratory system consists of:

- upper respiratory tract: the nasal cavity, pharynx and associated structures
- lower respiratory tract: the larynx, trachea, bronchi and lungs.

The transitional events that take place, in order for the baby to take the initial breath, change the lungs from passive organs filled with fluid to structures which play a vital role in aerobic metabolism.

In uterine life, the fetus obtains oxygen and excretes carbon dioxide via the placenta. Although the lungs are not used for gaseous exchange, the healthy fetus makes breathing movements 80% of the time in utero to exercise the muscles of respiration.

### Development (see also Ch. 45)

It is important to understand the growth and development of the respiratory system from its initial development at embryonic stage through to prebirth. (See website for additional information.)

A term baby who is hypothermic may exhibit expiratory grunting – where the epiglottis closes prematurely – and does not exhale all carbon dioxide. If this is not treated promptly by increasing the baby's temperature, respiratory acidosis will result, followed by metabolic acidosis and collapse.

### Lung fluid

Lung fluid, a silky clear fluid which may be seen draining from the baby's mouth at delivery, is different to surfactant. Its function appears to be mainly for cell proliferation and differentiation. At birth, the lungs must switch function from the secretion of fluid to absorption of gases. The catecholamine surge which occurs during labour is probably the final catalyst to complete this change (Milner & Vyas 1982). Some lung fluid is swallowed and then excreted via the fetal kidneys and into the amniotic fluid. At term, 10–25 mL/kg body weight of liquid remains, which is either expelled via the upper airways or absorbed via the lymphatic system of the lungs, a process commenced at the onset of labour and completed at birth (Taeusch et al 2004).

If delivered by elective lower section caesarean section (ELSCS), the burst of catecholamines provided by the onset of labour will not occur. The lungs will not have been compressed to expel lung fluid. The lung fluid is not absorbed and may be present following birth. Therefore, the midwife will need to observe the baby closely for signs and symptoms of *transient tachypnoea of the newborn* (TTN) (see Ch. 45).

### Factors affecting lung maturity

Hormones – including steroids, insulin, prolactin and thyroxine – influence lung maturity and dictate how well the baby's lung will function following birth.

**Catecholamines** are substances normally released in adults in response to stress and in the fetus may be identified around the onset of labour. These have a twofold action on the alveoli: increasing the *lecithin:sphyngomyelin ratio* to enhance synthesis of surfactant; and decreasing lung fluid production and increasing absorption of lung fluid during the labour process.

### Fetal breathing movements

Fetal breathing movements occur from 11 weeks of gestation. As the fetus grows, the strength and frequency of breathing movements increases until they are present between 40–80% of the time at a rate of 30–70 breaths per minute (Davis & Bureau 1987).

### Respiration in the neonate

**Ribcage and respiratory musculature** are immature and will continue to develop into adulthood (Harris 1988). The diaphragm and abdominal muscles are used for respiratory movement and it may be difficult to see movement of the chest when counting respiratory rate (more easily measured by observing the rise and fall of the baby's abdomen).

For the first 2–3 months of life, the baby is an obligatory nose breather and is unable to breathe through his mouth, thus it is vital that the nose is kept clear at all times of any obstacles such as eye protection pads.

**Breathing rate** is a simple guide to wellbeing but needs to be assessed alongside the baby's behaviour while validating normality. The respiratory rate is usually between 40 and 60 breaths per minute. Newborns are periodic rather than regular breathers and premature babies more so than full-term babies. They may have periods of even and uneven breathing with long gaps between breaths. A baby that has been very active or crying may have a respiratory rate above 70–80 per minute and during sleep the rate may be less than 40.

Tachypnoea (rate of >60) is a result of increased carbon dioxide and baroreceptors providing the information to the medulla; thus, an increased respiratory rate may reduce the respiratory acidosis (see Ch. 45).

**Breathing movements** should be *symmetrical*. Babies can generate spontaneous pressures above 70 cmH2O and develop a spontaneous pneumothorax; therefore, symmetrical movement of the chest confirms normality.

Babies mainly use the diaphragm to aid breathing, and so the *diaphragm* should also move symmetrically, confirming phrenic nerve integrity. Damage to the phrenic nerve can occur following shoulder dystocia and it is important to validate normality at an early stage to avoid later respiratory arrest.

#### *Abnormal signs*

*Stridor* – suggests upper airway obstruction, which could be due to oedema or abnormal growths.
*Expiratory grunting* – problem with lower airway function, such as surfactant not functioning appropriately or meconium inhalation into the alveoli.
*Nasal flaring* – the baby increases its ability to inhale oxygen by flaring the nostrils.
*Cyanosis* in room air – a late sign indicating that the baby has large amounts of unsaturated haemoglobin and is short of oxygen. Cyanosis is best observed by looking at the central circulation, such as in the gums and tongue, since they are more likely to show the level of central perfusion. A baby that is cyanosed needs to be close to resuscitation equipment, as reserves to sustain breathing are at a minimum.

### Control of respiration

The control of the respiratory system is mainly autonomic, involving the cortex, brainstem, airways, aortic/carotid chemoreceptors and central control by the medulla. The development and maturity of the central nervous system influences control of respiration, as does temperature, drugs, hypoxia, acidosis and the sleep state of the infant.

At birth, the umbilical cord is clamped and cut; this causes major circulatory changes which divert the blood to the fetal lungs rather than to the placenta for oxygenation.

## Cardiovascular system (CVS) in the embryo and fetus

The first functioning system in the embryo, the CVS, is composed of the heart and blood vessels and is a closed system that continuously circulates a given blood volume. Blood can be seen circulating in the body by the end of 3 weeks.

### Fetal circulation (see Ch. 45)

The structure of the heart provides a circulatory process different from that needed to maintain cardiovascular function after birth. There is low systemic pressure and an increased pulmonic pressure, leading to very little blood flow to the lungs, which are non-functional in utero. The fetal brain requires the highest oxygen concentration and the fetal circulation is designed to provide the vital organs such as the brain, liver and tissues with the maximum concentration of vital materials.

Within the fetal system, oxygen content varies throughout the circulation and is lower than in the neonate or adult; with a concentration of fetal haemoglobin (18–20 g/dL), fetal blood has a high affinity for oxygen.

### Changes at birth

At term, only 5–10% of the cardiac output perfuses the lungs to meet the needs of cellular nutrition, owing to pulmonary vascular resistance, the *patent ductus arteriosus* and low resistance of the placental component of the systemic circulation.

Following the birth and the taking of the first breath the right atrial pressure is lowered and the left atrial pressure is increased slightly, causing closure of the *foramen ovale*. Aeration of the lungs opens up the pulmonary capillary bed, lowering vascular resistance and increasing the pulmonary bed blood flow. The neonate can generate a pressure of up to 70 $cmH_2O$ during inspiration and 20–30 $cmH_2O$ on expiration (Strang 1977). This is thought to force fluid out of the lungs to overcome the high resistance and surface tension of the alveoli and to be necessary to establish lung volumes distributing gas through the lungs.

Oxygenation and the reduction of endogenous prostaglandins from the maternal circulation further *reduces* the vascular resistance and initiates the closure of the *ductus arteriosus*. As a result of pressure changes within the heart, the *foramen ovale* closes functionally at or soon after birth from compression of the two portions of the atrial septum. The *ductus arteriosus* is closed functionally between the fourth to seventh day, closing structurally later when fibrin is laid down – which can take several months to complete.

These physiological changes normally starts when the neonate takes the first breath. The neonatal brain must be functioning adequately in order for the baby to continue to breathe at a sufficient rate to allow homeostasis of oxygen and carbon dioxide within the body.

The vessels which in intrauterine life carried deoxygenated blood to the placenta, the umbilical and *hypogastric arteries*, and those which conveyed oxygenated blood from the placenta to the fetus, the *umbilical vein* and the *ductus venosus*, also close and later become ligaments.

These circulatory changes take place over a period of hours or even days. Respiratory and cardiac disorders accompanied by hypoxia and acidosis may delay, or even reverse, the circulatory changes in the heart and lungs.

## Changes in the blood

At birth, the baby has a high haemoglobin concentration (about 17 g/dL), mostly fetal type, HbF, which is required in utero to increase the oxygen-carrying capacity of the blood. Since oxygenated blood from the placenta is soon mixed with deoxygenated blood from the lower part of the fetus, the overall oxygen saturation of fetal blood is therefore reduced.

After birth, the high number of red blood cells is not required, so haemolysis of excess red blood cells takes place. This may result in physiological jaundice of the newborn within 2–3 days of birth (see Ch. 46). The conversion from fetal to adult haemoglobin (HbA) starts in utero and is completed during the first year or two of life. By the age of 3 months, the haemoglobin has fallen to about 12 g/dL.

At birth, the prothrombin level is low because of lack of *vitamin K*, a cofactor required for the activation of several clotting proteins in the blood. A deficiency may result; for example, following ventouse birth the baby can develop a subgaleal haemorrhage (bleeding in the potential space between the skull galea aponeurosis). Vitamin K administration can rapidly correct such a clotting problem. By the fifth or sixth day, milk feeding is usually established and the bacteria necessary for the synthesis of vitamin K are present in the intestine.

## Temperature control

Following birth, the baby must adjust to a lower and labile environmental temperature. The heat-regulating mechanism in the newborn is inefficient and the body temperature may drop unless great care is taken to avoid chilling. Heat is lost by radiation, convection, evaporation and conduction. These factors can be rectified if the baby is born into a warm environment of 26°C, dried carefully and wrapped warmly or provided with skin-to-skin contact with the mother (see Ch. 42).

## Skin

The full-term newborn's skin is well developed, opaque with few veins visible, has limited pigmentation and wrinkles around joints.

The layers of the skin include the epidermis, dermis, and subcutaneous layer. The epidermis is a thin, effective barrier preventing penetration and absorption of potential toxins and microorganisms and retaining water, heat, and other substances (see website).

The skin of full-term newborns is covered with a varying amount of vernix caseosa, a thick white, creamy substance. This forms between 17 and 20 weeks' gestation and by 40 weeks is found primarily in creases such as the axilla, neck and groins, acting as protection during uterine life (Moore & Persaud 2007). Vernix is a perfectly balanced moisturizer and any surplus should be massaged gently into the baby's skin after the birth.

## Gastrointestinal system (see website)

Normal function of the gastrointestinal (GI) system should be established prior to artificially feeding the newborn baby. This can be achieved through reviewing the woman's history and antenatal profile. Polyhydramnios, for example, may indicate disruption of the GI tract.

The midwife needs to understand glucose metabolism of the fetus and newborn in order to support the woman in her chosen method of infant feeding (de Rooy & Hawdon 2002) (see Ch. 43).

After birth, the maturation of the GI tract is stimulated by specific peptides: enteroglucagon stimulates intestinal mucosa to develop and motilin encourages gut motor activity.

Nutritive/non-nutritive sucking is the baby's main pleasure and may be satisfied by breast- or bottle-feeding alone. Babies will find solace in sucking their fingers or thumbs or suckling at the breast. Mothers need to understand why the baby is frequently feeding, so that they are reassured and not concerned that they have insufficient milk to satisfy their baby.

The knee-to-abdomen position increases abdominal pressure and may cause vomiting of newly ingested food, therefore napkin changing should be avoided soon after a feed. The supporting gastric and intestinal musculature of the newborn is relatively deficient, shown by the reduced peristaltic movement and the tendency towards distension. The use of pethidine or morphine during labour may decrease peristalsis and in some cases increase regurgitation for several days following birth.

**Meconium,** a soft, greenish black viscid substance which has gradually accumulated in the intestine from about the 16th week of intrauterine life, consists of mucus, epithelial cells, swallowed amniotic fluid, fatty acids and bile pigments.

- 0–2 days – meconium is passed – the first stool being passed within the first 48 hours. This indicates that the lower bowel is patent, though certain conditions, such as a fistula connecting the urethra and anus, may allow an apparent passage of meconium despite the absence of the anus.
- 2–4 days – as food is digested, the residue mixes with the remaining meconium and the stool changes colour to a greenish brown (*changing stool*), indicating that the GI tract is patent.
- 5th day onwards – the stools become yellow:
  - The breastfed baby passes:
    - soft, bright-yellow inoffensive stools
    - may pass stools five or more times a day as lactation is establishing
    - after 3 or 4 weeks (when lactation fully established) may only pass one soft yellow stool every 2 or 3 days as there are few waste products from breast milk.
  - The artificially fed baby passes:
    - paler, more formed stools with a slightly offensive odour
    - more regular stools when feeding is established, though constipation is more likely.

## Renal system

The fetus passes urine into the amniotic fluid during pregnancy and oligohydramnios may indicate renal abnormalities. At term, the kidneys are relatively immature, especially the renal cortex. Glomerular filtration rate and ability to concentrate urine are limited. Relatively large amounts of fluid are required to excrete solids.

The baby should pass urine, which has a low specific gravity, within 24 hours of birth. Initially, urinary output is about 20–30 mL per day, rising to 100–200 mL daily by the end of the first week as fluid intake increases.

If the baby becomes dehydrated, excretion of solids such as urea and sodium chloride is impaired. Dehydration can be recognized by a sunken fontanelle, dry mouth and skin inelasticity, and, most importantly, more than 10% loss of birth weight. It is important to note that a baby who is dehydrated will continue to pass the normal amount of urine, thus a wet nappy does not validate normality.

## Glucose metabolism

See website for fetal metabolism.

In utero, the fetus relies on the intravenous transfer of glucose and other nutrients via the umbilical vein for growth and development. Fetal metabolism is directed to anabolism under the influence of insulin, utilizing glycogen, fat and protein.

### Metabolic adjustments after birth

After birth, normoglycaemia must be maintained to protect brain function and to adapt to the intermittent delivery of milk into the gut for nutritional needs. The normal term neonate is able to adapt physiologically to episodes of starvation by utilizing ketone bodies. This is reflected in a postnatal fall in blood glucose concentration, which may be wrongly viewed as pathological and managed accordingly (de Rooy & Hawdon 2002). Following birth, the breakdown of glucose continues under the influence of insulin, but about 8 hours after birth, the baby begins to switch to glucagon metabolism.

## Musculoskeletal system

The musculoskeletal system provides stability and mobility for all physical activity and includes the bones, joints, and supporting and connecting tissue. This provides a means of protection for vital organs (brain, spinal cord), mineral storage (calcium, phosphorus) and production of red blood cells. In comparison with an adult or child's skeleton, the newborn's skeleton is flexible, the bones mainly consisting of cartilage, and joints are elastic, facilitating the passage through the birth canal.

Normal variations in shape, size, contour, or movement may be due to position in utero or genetic factors and should be distinguished from congenital anomalies and birth trauma. Early diagnosis of disorders and early intervention often prevent long-term deformity and the need for surgery.

## Central nervous system

The development of the neurological system commences 18 days post conception (see website). After birth, the brain continues to grow rapidly within the first year of life, follows a more gradual growth rate until the age of 10, and then there is minimal growth to adolescence. Physiological and psychological wellbeing are vital to the development of full neurological potential.

Babies born at term can be active participants in their environment and are capable of social interaction. It has been shown that they are able to mimic the expression of their carers and are able to some extent to self-regulate themselves.

At birth, the baby's autonomic system maintains homeostasis of all major organs, regulating temperature and cardiorespiratory function. The well newborn will have mature autonomic and motor systems which can be assessed by the ability to maintain stable cardiorespiratory function. If the baby is unwell or premature, handling will stress the autonomic system and the baby can become cyanosed and bradycardic (Roberton & Rennie 2001).

*State of consciousness* in the newborn is influenced by the reaction to stimuli, and understanding the baby's level of consciousness ensures sensitive care and management in assisting in the adaptation to the environment and advance through stages of consciousness. Providing this information to the mother assists her in caring for her baby, may assist feeding, and utilizes the baby's energy and available resources effectively (see Box 41.1).

Box 41.1 **States of consciousness in the newborn (Brazelton & Nugent 1995)**

### Sleep states

1. *Deep sleep*. Hard to waken, eyes closed, some jerky movements.
2. *Light sleep*. Eyes closed, moves from deep to light sleep, light sleep to drowsy state – may be sucking present.

### Awake states

3. *Drowsy or semi-dozing*. Eyes open or closed, reacts to source of sensory stimuli, minimal motor activity, eyes with bright look.
4. *Quiet alert*. Focuses on stimuli source, minimal motor activity in relation to stimuli, may or may not be fussing.
5. *Active alert*. Much motor activity, increased startles or activity in relation to stimuli, may or may not be fussing.
6. *Crying*. Difficult to get a response to stimuli, will need to bring infant down to state 5 to begin response to stimuli or to feed baby.

Babies are able to 'tune out' noxious stimuli and this occurs through the process of habituation. The baby stores the memory of the stimulus and with repeated episodes learns not to respond to it. Overstimulation of babies who are on system overload will cause them to suffer further stress, requiring appropriate care such as minimal handling and an environment with minimal noise and lights in order to support recovery.

The newborn baby has very poor motor development compared with other mammals but highly developed senses (sight, hearing, taste, smell); hence the importance of picking babies up, talking to them and stroking them to stimulate and evoke response. Maternal–infant interaction is facilitated by eye-to-eye contact with the mother. A 12-day-old baby is able to imitate the facial and manual gestures of adults and this may operate as a positive feedback mechanism to caregivers.

## Protection against infection

In utero, the fetus is protected from infection by the intact amniotic sac and the barrier mechanism of the placenta, although certain microorganisms do cross the placenta and may infect the fetus (see Ch. 47). During the last trimester of pregnancy, there is a transplacental transfer of IgG from the mother to the fetus, providing protection against the infectious diseases to which the mother has antibodies. These antibodies provide baby passive immunity for about 6 months (Remington & Klein 2000).

The newborn baby has no immunity to the common organisms, and when exposed to them at birth for the first time, is highly susceptible to infection. Soon after birth, the baby becomes colonized by the mother's set of microorganisms, facilitated by early and frequent contact. Clinical infection occurs when the number and virulence of the organisms overwhelm the poorly developed defence mechanisms of the baby. Breastfeeding encourages specific bacteria to multiply in the bowel and the acid conditions that result from this may help to prevent the overgrowth of potential pathogens, providing some protection from infection.

# CARE AT BIRTH

## Preparation

The midwife is obliged to support the birth of any baby showing signs of life at any gestation – in all environments, including outside hospital. It is crucial that midwives are knowledgeable about the physiology of the baby born at different gestations, and how this changes their care and management needs.

Preparations should be made prior to the baby's birth and these include identifying women whose babies are at increased risk or who will require specialist care following delivery. The midwife must be prepared to provide care for 'high-risk' and 'low-risk' women (see Box 41.2), though research indicates that the classification of risk factors remains a debatable area.

The development of complications during labour and birth is a major contributor to increased neonatal mortality and morbidity (MCHRC 2001). The midwife can identify that all is normal, detect any deviations and make appropriate referral or alter management of care accordingly.

This action plan begins antenatally to ensure that the woman is prepared and informed to self-manage her body and pregnancy so that she becomes confident and seeks appropriate support should deviations occur.

Box 41.2 **Risk factors for specialist care (Levene & Tudehope 1993)**

**High-risk pregnancy**

- Rhesus isoimmunization
- Moderate to severe pre-eclampsia
- Growth-restricted fetus
- Insulin-dependent diabetes (mother)
- Antepartum haemorrhage
- Prolonged rupture of membranes

**Abnormal labour**

- Fetal distress
- Deep transverse arrest
- Cephalopelvic disproportion

**Abnormal delivery**

- Caesarean section
- Moderate or heavy meconium staining of liquor
- Prolapsed cord
- Vacuum or high, medium forceps

**Abnormal presentation**

- Breech
- Face
- Brow
- Compound/shoulder

**Abnormal gestation**

- Pre-term delivery

**Abnormal fetus**

- Hydramnios
- Known abnormality
- Past history of abnormality
- Multiple births

At birth, the transition to independent life involves a significant physiological shift. The midwife needs to have a good insight into changes of fetal physiology, in order to evaluate the care each individual newborn baby requires.

## The Apgar score

The Apgar score, devised by Virginia Apgar in 1953 (Levene & Tudehope 1993), is a universally and commonly used quantitative measure of the neonate's wellbeing at and around birth, though criticized for its simplicity. Five indicators are used to measure this: heart rate, respiratory effort, colour, muscle tone and response to stimuli (Table 41.1).

Recording the numerical score alone provides insufficient information concerning the neonatal condition. The important factor is that the neonate's physiological condition and progress is recorded verbally and in writing until the neonate is in a good condition.

It is also advisable, if more than one practitioner is present at a delivery where resuscitation is undertaken, that the baby's Apgar score is agreed between practitioners prior to the formal record being made. Disagreements can be discussed with the supervisor of midwives and senior neonatologist. It is important for the future management of the newborn's wellbeing that an accurate assessment is given (UK Resuscitation Council 2006).

The heart and respiratory rate, the most important measures within this scoring system, will indicate the nature and timing of active resuscitation. An Apgar score of 8–9 indicates that the neonate is in good condition. The midwife should expect that most mature babies would obtain a score of about 9 as those above 38 weeks' gestation will have a mature neurological system restricting

**Table 41.1 The Apgar score**

| Sign | Score | | |
|---|---|---|---|
| | **0** | **1** | **2** |
| Heart rate | Absent | Slow < 100 | Fast > 100 |
| Respiratory effort | Absent | Slow irregular | Good/crying |
| Muscle tone | Limp | Some flexion of extremities | Active |
| Reflex irritability | No response | Grimace | Cry, cough |
| Colour | Pale blue | Body pink, extremities blue | Completely pink |

blood flow to the extremities in order to supply the brain and other major organs with extra oxygenated blood. Therefore the baby will have acrocyanosis and this continues until after 24 hours because of poor peripheral circulation (see website).

## Maternal–infant relationship

The relationship between mother and baby begins at birth. The experience of the pregnancy may act as a positive or negative foundation for this relationship. The mother's reaction to her baby will vary greatly according to her culture, experience, expectations and environment and will be affected by her physical and emotional state. In some cultures, the mother will wish to have immediate and close contact with her baby from the moment of birth. Others will want the baby cleansed before holding. So that individual needs can be appropriately met, the midwife needs to discuss the mother's wishes, expectations and fears prior to the labour.

'Bonding' is a term to be used with caution as it may imply an immediate and strong relationship at the moment of first sight. This may be very threatening and inhibiting for some mothers who will build up their relationship with their new baby in a slower and less obvious way, though the end result is as enduring and strong (see website).

Research illustrates mothers' reactions to newborn infants. The mother's first response is to touch her baby (easier if the baby is naked) with fingertips, progressing to a protective caressing movement. The mother will often then move the baby to a position to facilitate face-to-face eye contact. Throughout this time, she talks to the baby in a higher-pitched voice than usual (Klaus & Kennell 1976). Early research suggested the existence of a 'sensitive time' around the birth, at which the mother and baby should be encouraged to be together, and that women missing this time were at risk of neglecting or abusing their infants. However, Brazelton postulated that even should parent and child have to be separated, if the attendants ensure that the mother has photographs of her baby and is involved in the baby's management and care, cuddling or even just touching her child, the relationship can be effectively preserved and nurtured (Brazelton 1983).

## Warmth

The baby, accustomed to a constant intrauterine temperature of 37.8 °C, is born into a much cooler atmosphere, ideally 26 °C. At birth, the baby should be dried immediately to prevent evaporation and handed to the mother to keep warm, avoiding unnecessary exposure. Warm covers are placed over the baby, if necessary for skin-to-skin contact, and later the baby should be dressed, covered appropriately and placed in a preheated cot. Within an hour of birth, the baby's axillary temperature is taken using a low-reading thermometer (see Ch. 42).

## Identification

Two identification labels record name, date of birth and sex, using an indelible pen with clear and legible writing. These should be shown to the mother or partner and applied to the baby's ankles or wrists in the mother's presence. Should a label become detached, a replacement should be completed and placed on the baby using the same procedure. Ideally, the labels should not be removed until the baby is in his own home. During daily examination, these labels are checked by the midwife for cleanliness, comfort – neither too tight nor too loose for the baby's wrist or ankle – and number (i.e. two).

Several maternity units have developed systems to ensure that babies are properly identified and secure, including recording footprints and handprints, and these should include the names of the mother and baby.

Ideally, a resuscitaire should be situated in the delivery room, because, should the baby need resuscitation, to remove him from his parents can add significantly to their distress. If the baby has to be separated from the mother, a relative must accompany the baby to enable feedback to be given to the mother as to what events took place and to validate that the baby returned to the mother is indeed her own baby.

## Vitamin K

Following birth, free circulating vitamin K is low, decreasing during the first few days of life and gradually rising after 3–4 days. This may result in excessive bleeding if trauma occurs, for example during instrumental delivery.

It has been advised that all babies should be given vitamin K (DH) and parents should be provided with information on whether or not to give vitamin K and the route of administration as advised in the Drugs and Therapeutics Bulletin (www.dtb.org.uk/dtb/index.html).

*Vitamin K deficiency bleeding (VKDB)* (formerly known as haemorrhagic disease of the newborn) is a bleeding tendency which results from a lack of ability in the newborn to utilize vitamin K (see Ch. 44).

Signs and symptoms include bleeding from:

- the GI tract
- the intracranial space
- generalized petechiae
- mucosal surfaces
- circumcision site
- venepuncture site
- heel-prick sites
- the umbilical stump (delayed).

### Oral use of vitamin K

Absorption from the gastrointestinal tract is erratic in the newborn and there is the possibility of regurgitation, inhalation and loss of vitamin K. Additional evidence is required before firm recommendations can be made concerning the optimal dose and form of the vitamin K.

#### *Prophylaxis against late-onset haemolytic haemorrhagic disease of the newborn (HDN)*

As three babies have been reported to have developed VKDB (late onset) after being given vitamin K at birth, it cannot yet be confirmed how best to prevent this.

The blood spot (Guthrie) screening test provides a simple method for assessing VKDN. Three minutes of pressure should be applied to the site after taking the blood sample, and a note made of the time taken for the bleeding to stop. Plasters damage the baby's skin and should not be used unless absolutely necessary.

## EXAMINATION OF THE NEWBORN

The first question parents ask is whether or not their newborn baby is 'normal', as they examine him from head to toe in minute detail, equal to that of any dedicated professional. This is always an important adjunct to the midwife's assessment and, prior to any examination, parents' participation is welcomed and any concerns they have should be identified and discussed.

Three types of examination of the newborn are carried out:

- the initial post-birth examination
- the holistic examination including full assessment of eyes, heart, lungs and hips
- daily examination for general wellbeing.

Each examination has a slightly different purpose, but all should follow a systematic process, and be undertaken with the principles set over the following pages, which will provide the midwife with the best means of assessment (see Fig. 41.1).

### Initial post-birth examination

The midwife will undertake a thorough examination of the newborn soon after birth. This initial examination uses information elicited from intuitive knowledge gained from experience; the Apgar score; and physiological assessment using the senses: sound, vision and touch. It provides basic information, detects any obvious abnormalities or deviations from normal that require referral, and provides an opportunity for the midwife to support the parents in their role as carers for the new addition to their family.

Prior to this first examination, the baby should have at least 1 hour following birth to recover (NICE 2006). This allows mother and baby time to adapt to physiological changes and gives the baby time to adapt to the environment and, if breastfeeding, to feed successfully.

### The holistic examination

This examination – including heart and lung sounds, full central nervous system examination, abdominal examination and examination of the neonate's hips – is undertaken by an appropriately trained health professional. Some of these skills require postgraduate training at present. The main aim of the holistic examination is to validate normality and, where possible, detect abnormalities and communicate any action required to the parents.

Since 1994, increasingly midwives have undertaken this holistic examination rather than their medical colleagues, providing continuity of care as recommended by *Changing childbirth* (DH 1993), facilitating the midwife's self-audit and with the potential for improving interprofessional partnerships (Hall 1999).

Midwives have a vital role to recognize and validate normality and refer when deviation from the norm is detected. Any possible problems should be ascertained at the outset, providing stabilization and minimizing any future harm prior to transfer in order to ensure future wellbeing.

The United Kingdom National Screening Committee (UKNSC) of the Newborn and Infant Physical Examination (NIPE) (UKNSC 2008) advocates the first holistic examination is undertaken within 72 hours of birth, allowing the postnatal transition of major organs, such as the heart, to take place prior to examination. This is done prior to discharge and transfer to the care of a health visitor and GP. It is expected that the midwife (NICE 2006) will care for the newborn from birth to 6 to 8 weeks. It is intended that the second holistic examination is combined into a single postnatal visit at 6 weeks to validate the woman's wellbeing. In between those two examinations, the midwife will assess each baby, reviewing past and present individual history prior to deciding which criteria need assessment during physical examination and which can be validated through observation alone.

#### Examination of the newborn assessment tool

A clinical assessment tool (see website also) has been designed to assess the physiological and behavioural cues to assist the midwife to validate normality and recognize deviations (Michaelides 2010).

Using a tool enables the midwife to gather important information through assessment and analysis of the woman's oral and recorded history. A systematic framework, beginning with examination of the heart while the baby is quiet, goes through to the most intrusive testing – the Moro reflex and measuring the head circumference – at the end. The latter is undertaken last as the baby will find it uncomfortable and will require comforting upon completion.

The tool consists of 26 criteria (Fig. 41.1 A–Z), the number of which that will be fully examined at each examination being dependent on the purpose of the examination, and the experience and training of the midwife.

### Preparation

Preparation is vital to ensure a smooth and effective examination process. An area, to provide privacy and a controlled environment, needs to be set aside; an examining table with an overhead heater and light source can be utilized to examine babies at a height that will prevent practitioner back strain. It provides a safe environment for the baby (see Fig. 41.2) and a safe storage space for the required equipment (see Box 41.3). In the home environment, the midwife can use a changing mattress or table (or similar surface area) covered with a warm sheet/towel to examine the baby.

### Communication

After the examination, the midwife must explain what has been examined and why. For women who are unable to speak English, link workers or translators are essential. The midwife must demonstrate an ability to communicate with the baby, an understanding of his 'language', to observe and note physiological and behavioural wellbeing.

### Informed consent

The NIPE booklet *Screening tests for you and your baby* (see website), offered to mothers at booking, recommends midwives discuss the information with mothers at 36 weeks, and prior to the examination, enabling parents the time and information needed to give informed consent to the examination of their baby.

## Daily examination

As part of the postnatal examination, the midwife will examine the baby, including checking the eyes, skin, umbilicus and napkin area, feeding patterns, and (if in hospital) the presence of two identification labels. This examination provides an opportunity to teach the mother what to look for in monitoring her baby's wellbeing, and to learn skills in baby care.

# PHYSICAL ASSESSMENT OF THE NEWBORN

The baby enters postnatal life from a quiet, dark, warm, wet environment, with boundaries provided by the uterus, entering a whole new world. While drying the baby or, in the case of waterbirth, when the baby reaches the surface, the midwife assesses adaptation to extrauterine life by undertaking the Apgar score at 1 and 5 minutes with a brief physical assessment to exclude gross structural abnormalities.

During the first hour of life, the baby is given to the mother or father and interaction begins. As the baby is alert in this first hour, the mother should be supported to give a first breastfeed. If artificially fed, the midwife needs to undertake a fuller assessment of the gastrointestinal system. The baby who breastfeeds will take in a small, but valuable, quantity of colostrum. A baby given formula is likely to take an amount of fluid which, if the GI tract is incomplete, such as in cleft palate or imperforate anus, may cause preventable damage.

## Formal assessment of the newborn

Physical examination of the newborn baby should be performed systematically, examining each physiological system to ensure entirety (see Fig. 41.1), using the skills of observation, palpation and, where relevant, auscultation. Each system should be critically evaluated, normality validated and deviations recognized. Where deviations occur, the midwife needs to ascertain the severity in order to plan appropriate management and transfer to the care of the neonatologist as appropriate.

The midwife needs to explain that the assessment of wellbeing is a continual process and that each examination only validates normality for that moment in time. With continual observation, care and professional support through education and physical assessment, there is a growing reassurance.

## History

During the antenatal period, a full record is taken of the family, previous medical and obstetric histories of the woman and partner. The present pregnancy, labour and prenatal period should be reviewed to identify any risk factors which may affect the baby.

When obtaining a history from women, it is important that the communication process is open and interactive. Women should be given the reasons for certain questions and how this affects the care provided (see website).

Laboratory results need to be assessed by the midwife for their relevance to the assessment of the newborn. For example, a group O positive mother with a baby

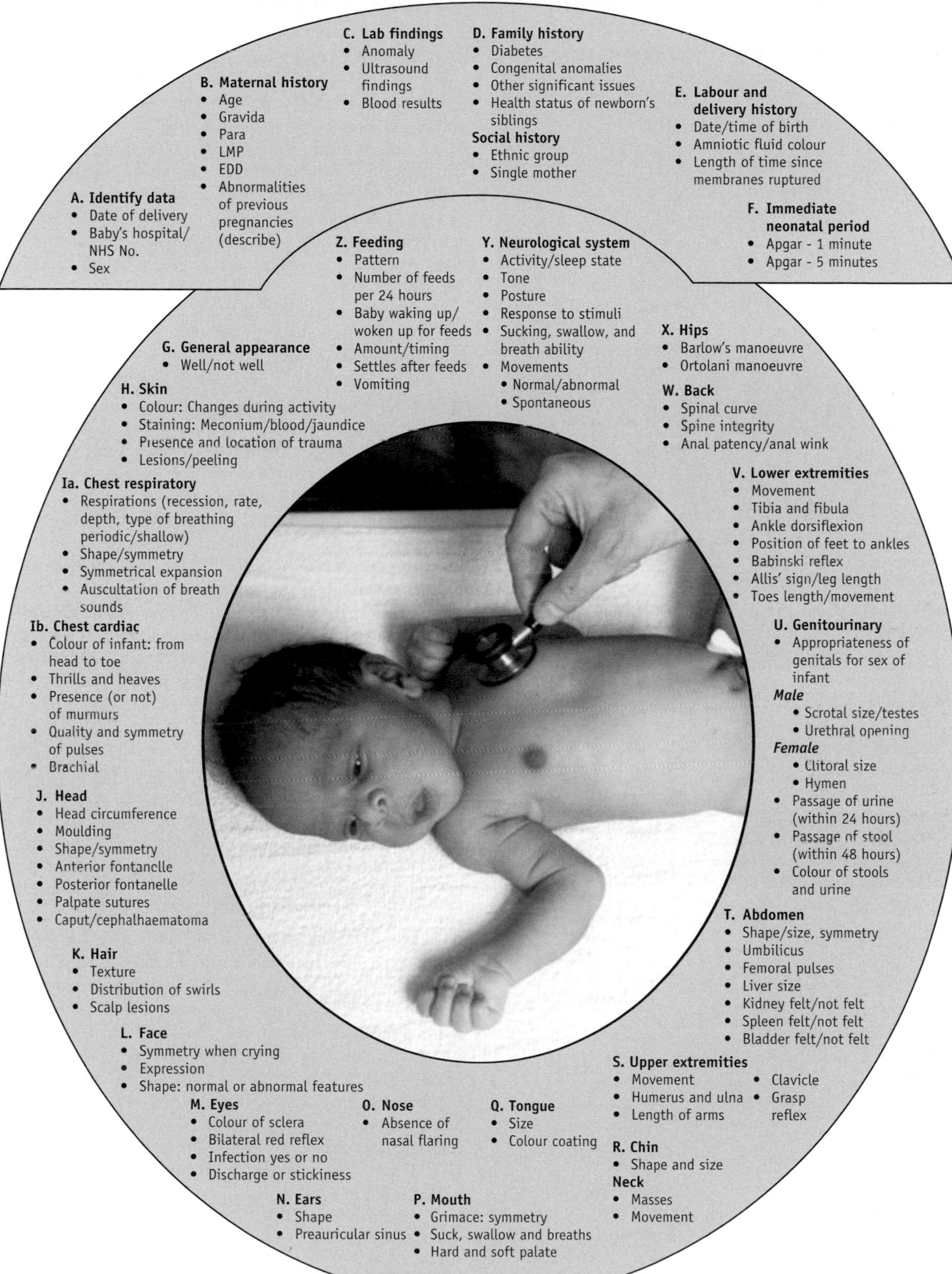
A. Identify data
• Date of delivery
• Baby's hospital/ NHS No.
• Sex
B. Maternal history
• Age
• Gravida
• Para
• LMP
• EDD
• Abnormalities of previous pregnancies (describe)
C. Lab findings
• Anomaly
• Ultrasound findings
• Blood results
D. Family history
• Diabetes
• Congenital anomalies
• Other significant issues
• Health status of newborn's siblings
Social history
• Ethnic group
• Single mother
E. Labour and delivery history
• Date/time of birth
• Amniotic fluid colour
• Length of time since membranes ruptured
F. Immediate neonatal period
• Apgar - 1 minute
• Apgar - 5 minutes
G. General appearance
• Well/not well
H. Skin
• Colour: Changes during activity
• Staining: Meconium/blood/jaundice
• Presence and location of trauma
• Lesions/peeling
Ia. Chest respiratory
• Respirations (recession, rate, depth, type of breathing periodic/shallow)
• Shape/symmetry
• Symmetrical expansion
• Auscultation of breath sounds
Ib. Chest cardiac
• Colour of infant: from head to toe
• Thrills and heaves
• Presence (or not) of murmurs
• Quality and symmetry of pulses
• Brachial
J. Head
• Head circumference
• Moulding
• Shape/symmetry
• Anterior fontanelle
• Posterior fontanelle
• Palpate sutures
• Caput/cephalhaematoma
K. Hair
• Texture
• Distribution of swirls
• Scalp lesions
L. Face
• Symmetry when crying
• Expression
• Shape: normal or abnormal features
M. Eyes
• Colour of sclera
• Bilateral red reflex
• Infection yes or no
• Discharge or stickiness
N. Ears
• Shape
• Preauricular sinus
O. Nose
• Absence of nasal flaring
P. Mouth
• Grimace: symmetry
• Suck, swallow and breaths
• Hard and soft palate
Q. Tongue
• Size
• Colour coating
R. Chin
• Shape and size
Neck
• Masses
• Movement
S. Upper extremities
• Movement
• Humerus and ulna
• Length of arms
• Clavicle
• Grasp reflex
T. Abdomen
• Shape/size, symmetry
• Umbilicus
• Femoral pulses
• Liver size
• Kidney felt/not felt
• Spleen felt/not felt
• Bladder felt/not felt
U. Genitourinary
• Appropriateness of genitals for sex of infant
Male
• Scrotal size/testes
• Urethral opening
Female
• Clitoral size
• Hymen
• Passage of urine (within 24 hours)
• Passage of stool (within 48 hours)
• Colour of stools and urine
V. Lower extremities
• Movement
• Tibia and fibula
• Ankle dorsiflexion
• Position of feet to ankles
• Babinski reflex
• Allis' sign/leg length
• Toes length/movement
W. Back
• Spinal curve
• Spine integrity
• Anal patency/anal wink
X. Hips
• Barlow's manoeuvre
• Ortolani manoeuvre
Y. Neurological system
• Activity/sleep state
• Tone
• Posture
• Response to stimuli
• Sucking, swallow, and breath ability
• Movements
• Normal/abnormal
• Spontaneous
Z. Feeding
• Pattern
• Number of feeds per 24 hours
• Baby waking up/ woken up for feeds
• Amount/timing
• Settles after feeds
• Vomiting

**Figure 41.1** The A–Z Examination of the Newborn tool, detailing the different systems.

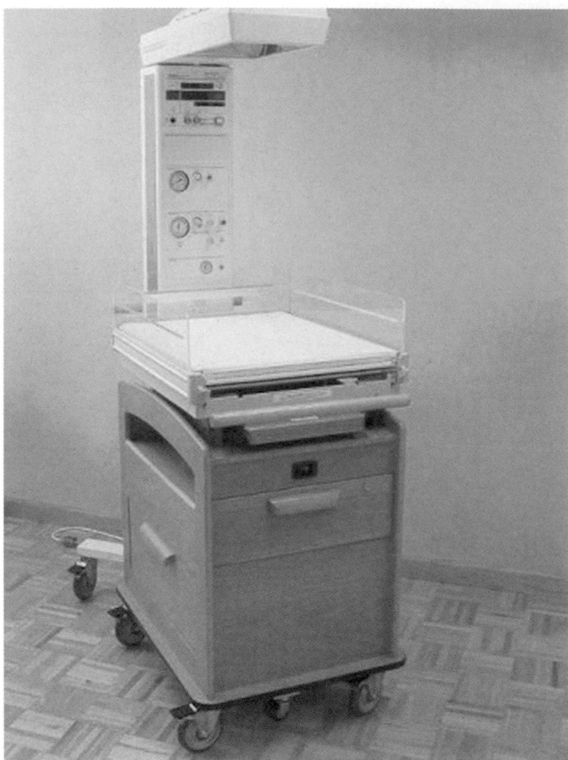

**Figure 41.2** Apparatus for examining babies.

**Box 41.3 Resources and equipment required to undertake the examination**

- Firm surface
- Sheets and blankets
- A spare nappy
- Cleaning equipment (bowl and cotton wool)
- Ophthalmoscope (cleaned and pre-set to the practitioner's eyesight)
- Stethoscope
- Small torch
- Tape measure
- Thermometer
- Mediswabs
- Gloves
- Cord clamp remover
- Bag for used nappy
- Non-stretchable tape measure
- Scales
- Supine stadiometer/roll measuring mat

who is jaundiced may trigger consideration of the possibility of *ABO incompatibility*.

*Kell antibodies* can attack the bone marrow, reduce red cell production and may result in the baby being anaemic at the time of birth. Anaemia in the newborn will render the baby hypoxic, requiring resuscitation at the time of birth and administration of fresh blood.

*Sexually transmitted diseases*, if not treated in the antenatal period, may affect the baby postnatally and thus the baby will need to be observed for signs of infection (see Ch. 47).

Health education is important though it is not always possible to reduce at-risk behaviour of women, and a non-judgemental and supportive approach is required in obtaining true and accurate information to facilitate appropriate care (see website).

Information such as the date of the first day of the last menstrual period (LMP) and the estimated date of conception (EDC) is crucial in the calculation of gestational age, an important aspect of management of care.

When undertaken correctly, fetal surveillance (see Ch. 36) can assist the midwife to have the relevant practitioners present at birth. The type of birth may affect the management of the baby – after a protracted labour, the baby may be traumatized and may require an initial superficial examination to validate wellbeing, followed by a full examination when signs of recovery are apparent. Minimal handling may assist the shocked newborn to recover. The examination should last no longer than 15 minutes.

Maternal concerns are an important guide to the focus of the examination as the majority of women will spend time examining, feeling, stroking and counting their baby's fingers and toes. In the majority of cases, they themselves will recognize if their baby deviates from normal.

## General appearance

A baby's age and gestation will influence his general appearance. Type of birth, postnatal age, and the timing of the last feed affects his behaviour. A hungry baby will be difficult to examine as many of the assessments require a quiet, calm baby, able to tolerate handling for 10–15 minutes in order to complete the physical examination.

A baby who has had a difficult birth may be very irritable or be in a deep sleep (State 1 – see Box 41.1), and the midwife uses the baby's behaviour to guide the examination. The physical examination can be delayed until the baby is able to tolerate handling and an interim observational examination undertaken.

### Observation

A 'hands-off' approach is used when observing the baby. The baby of above 38 weeks' gestation will display a flexed

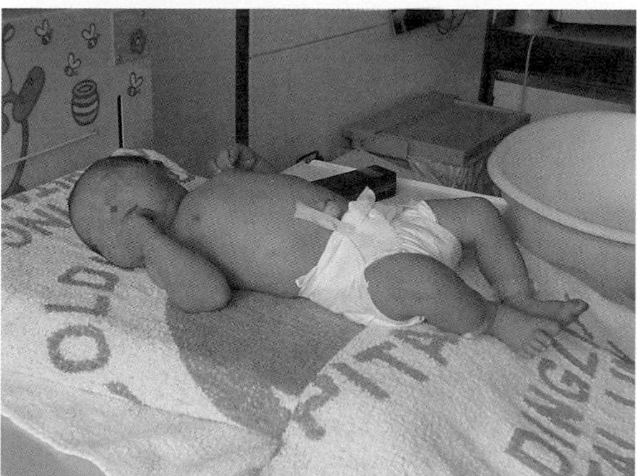

Figure 41.3 A well-flexed baby.

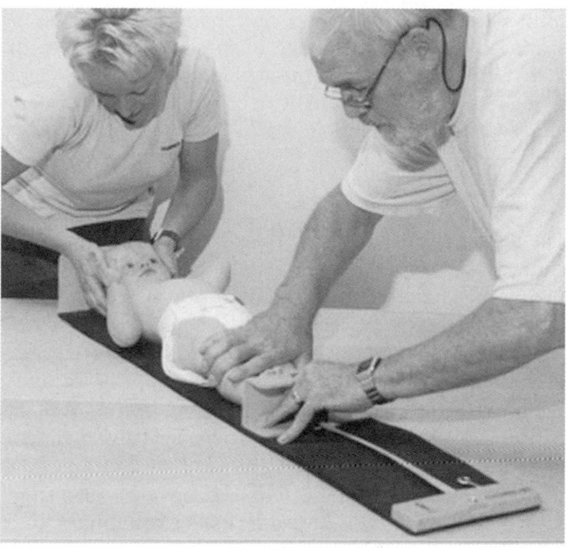

Figure 41.4 Measurement of height. *(From Jokinen 2002.)*

posture indicating good muscle tone (Fig. 41.3). General features are noted for dysmorphia.

## Gestational assessment

Previously, weight defined term and preterm babies; a baby weighing below 2500 g was deemed to be premature. Further research (Battaglia & Lubchenco 1967) showed that gestational age and whether the baby's growth is appropriate for that age is a greater predictor of outcome.

Assessment tools such as the Dubowitz scoring system (Dubowitz et al 1970) are used to assess the gestational age of the newborn using a neurological scale (see Ch. 44). This assessment is used with babies deemed to be less than 38 weeks' gestation. The main assessment of gestational age can be carried out using approximate estimates of fetal development, i.e. the LMP, the estimated date of delivery (EDD), ultrasound and physical characteristics (see website).

### *Measurements*

#### *The UK WHO growth charts*

These are based on measurements collected by the World Health Organization (WHO) (see website). Healthy breastfed babies whose mothers did not smoke and were not deprived were measured over time. Plotting the baby's weight and head circumference enables the midwife to identify the 'at risk' and validate the normal baby in order to plan future care.

#### *Weight*

Scales need to be regularly maintained for accurate measurement and recording. Care should be taken to minimize the baby's heat loss while weighing by placing him safely in the scales and ensuring that the surroundings are warm and free from draughts.

The weight can be plotted on the centile chart and babies who are small or large for gestational age identified and a plan of action developed, agreed and recorded in the baby notes. Babies below the 9th centile have reduced glycogen stores and may be more prone to hypothermia and hypoglycaemia so thermoregulation and feeding must be given extra attention.

The baby will lose 5–10% of body weight in the first week of life, then steadily gain at an average rate of 25–30 g per day until 6 months of age (Wilkinson 1997).

**Note:** A baby who has not reached his birth weight by day 10 needs to be reviewed to exclude signs of poor feeding or underlying urinary tract infection.

*Dehydration* is seen in babies who have yet to establish breastfeeding; identification is vital in order to prevent hypoglycaemia and hypernatraemia. Signs of dehydration include loss of skin turgor, dry mucous membranes, lethargy and a sunken fontanelle, and a weight loss of ≥10% is significant. Urine output is normally 1–3 mL per hour and this will continue regardless of the presence of dehydration; thus, a wet nappy does not indicate wellbeing.

#### *Length*

There is debate as to whether or not babies should be measured. Now, for accurate measurement, a supine stadiometer (Wilkinson 1997) newborn length instrument or a *rollamat* (Fig. 41.4) may be used. Both methods require the baby to be stretched, therefore two persons are required to undertake the measurement accurately.

#### *Head circumference*

This measurement is taken with a non-stretchable tape applied closely around the scalp, using the posterior fontanelle and the frontal and parietal eminences as markers. The largest estimate of three is taken. Immediately following birth, the measurement may be increased by oedema or caput, thus it needs to be repeated when any swelling has subsided.

### Vital signs

The temperature is measured while the respiratory rate is counted. If the baby is cold (less than 36.5°C), the examination may be discontinued or the baby placed under the radiant heater for the rest of the assessment.

The respiratory rate is usually between 40 and 60 breaths per minute, although the baby's behaviour prior to counting the respiratory rate needs to be taken into account. As periodic rather than regular breathers, the baby may have periods of even and very uneven breathing and long gaps between breaths. It is important to concentrate on a small area of the abdomen, and this makes counting a little easier.

**Note:** A baby that is otherwise well but has tachypnoea above **50 at rest,** may be exhibiting a sign of respiratory acidosis, and must be referred to a senior paediatrician.

## Skin

The skin protects the baby against infection and enables communication, and is sensitive to touch, pressure, temperature and pain. After birth, the baby is rubbed dry, and then touch should be gentle to minimize discomfort to the baby.

The epidermis of the skin of a newborn is thin and delicate and in postmature babies is dry and sometimes peeling (see website).

The best environment to observe the colour of the baby is in natural daylight, as artificial light can affect the depth of colour observed. Pink is the normal colour of newborns. A red/plethoric colour which, when the baby cries, becomes dusky/purple, may be due to an excessively high packed cell volume (PCV) and is deemed to be pathological as it may indicate polycythaemia (see website).

Pale skin or pallor is an indication of poor perfusion and anaemia. Infants of diabetic mothers tend to be pinker than average and 'postmature' infants are paler.

Asian and dark-skinned babies may have blue naevi scattered around any area of the body, which may be mistaken for bruises. Parents are sometimes concerned and can be reassured that this deep pigmentation of the skin will fade in a few months.

*Petechiae,* normally caused through traumatic delivery, for example a tight cord around the neck, should disappear within 24–48 hours. If this does not happen and they appear to multiply, this might be pathological and the baby needs to be referred for diagnosis.

*Jaundice* may occur physiologically after 48 hours because of extra red cell breakdown in combination with an immature liver which cannot metabolize all unconjugated bilirubin; the latter leaks under the skin and gives a jaundiced colour. The Kramer tool (see Ch. 46) enables estimation of jaundice.

Common variations of the skin include tiny milia on the nose (plugged sweat glands).

*Erythema toxicum* may be noted. These papular lesions with an erythematous base are found more on the trunk than on the extremities and fade away without treatment by 1 week of age. Occasionally their profusion is alarming.

#### Haemangiomata

- *Vascular naevi* are superficial capillary haemangiomata which may occur over the upper eyelids and the nape of the neck, sometimes hidden by the hairline. These usually diminish in size and fade by 1 year of age.
- *Capillary (strawberry) haemangioma* usually presents between birth and 2 months of age. These are most common on the face, scalp, back or chest. This haemangioma enlarges prior to diminishing by 1 year of age and disappears by the age of 5–7 years.
- *Port wine stain (naevus flammeus),* if situated on an area of skin over a nerve pathway, such as the trigeminal area on the face, may be associated with meningeal haemangioma (Sturge–Weber syndrome). Large areas of discoloration may require later laser treatment.

The skin is observed daily for soreness, rashes and septic spots.

#### Dry skin

A normal skin barrier has cells that are packed tightly together. Applying olive oil for moisturizing or massaging baby skin has been used for years. However, oleic acid, a core component of vegetable oils, disrupts the structure of skin cells, weakening the skin barrier, and either avoiding oils completely (Lavender et al 2009) or using mineral based oils may be preferable.

It has been shown that exposing a skin barrier to an oleic acid solution (10%) causes the skin to commence breakdown. However, sunflower oil is the one oil that is free of oleic acid and can safely be used on baby's skin to correct dryness (Wong 2004).

## Cardiorespiratory system

The heart and lung assessments are interlinked in order to reduce handling and ascertain how both function, to distinguish between heart and lung physiology and pathology.

### Observation

#### Colour

The infant's colour is an important index of the function of the cardiorespiratory system.

- 'Good' colour in Caucasian infants means a reddish pink hue all over, except for possible cyanosis of hands, feet, and occasionally lips (acrocyanosis)
- Mucous membranes of dark-skinned babies are more reliable indicators of cyanosis (and degree of jaundice) than the skin.
- The baby's colour should be assessed at regular intervals in the postnatal period.
- Examinations, whenever possible, should be undertaken with the baby naked in order to ascertain colour symmetry from head to toe.

### Chest

The general appearance of the chest is noted, observing the neck and collarbone area. The chest and abdomen are examined whilst observing respirations.

- Position of nipples, and presence of skin tags, accessory nipples or skin discoloration are noted.
- Chest should be rounded.
- Both sides of the chest cavity should move symmetrically, with breathing actioned by the diaphragm and abdominal muscles.
- Respiratory rate and pattern are observed for symmetrical movement of the diaphragm. [Asymmetrical movement of the diaphragm should alert the midwife to possible phrenic nerve damage. Although babies may have periodic breathing, episodes of true apnoea are deemed abnormal and may indicate neurological damage or abnormality.]
- Breathing should not draw on accessory muscles; indrawing of intercostal or subcostal muscles. Signs of accessory muscle use indicates severe respiratory distress.
- Breathing should be quiet – audible sounds are a sign of deviation from normal, and can help identify the origins of respiratory difficulty depending on the type. [For example, inspiratory grunting could indicate a problem in the upper airway, i.e. oedema or mass. An expiratory grunt suggests the cause is in the lower airways and may be due to hypothermia, surfactant deficiency or meconium aspiration.]

## Palpation

The chest is palpated gently as there may be breast enlargement due to maternal hormones and pressure can cause discomfort and pain.

- Position of the heart is checked to see whether it is on the left or right side of the chest. This is best done by auscultation (see below) but can be confirmed occasionally by palpation.
- This is followed by validation of the absence of *heaves* and *thrills* and identification of the point of maximum impulse (see website).
- *Capillary filling time* is measured using applied pressure on the chest or gently squeezing of the earlobe or toe and expecting the blood flow to return within 3 seconds.
- *Brachial and femoral pulses* are identified and palpated for strength, rhythm and volume.
- *Femoral pulses* are best palpated when the baby is quiet, and often feel quite weak in the first day or two. It is vital to validate their presence in the assessment of cardiovascular function.
- *Dorsalis pedis* pulses may be palpated in preference to femoral pulses.

## Auscultation

Normal or abnormal breath sounds may be noticed by the practitioner prior to the use of the paediatric stethoscope to identify heart and breath sounds (see website). Done after a period of observation, this can enhance the examiner's perception, knowledge of and communication with the baby. Warming the chest piece by applying friction to the stethoscope head reduces disturbance of the baby, facilitating auscultation.

Auscultation of breath sounds in the newborn is easier than in a child, as breath sounds are being established with the absence of crackles and wheezes (see Fig. 41.5).

The heart should be examined alongside other aspects such as femoral pulses. To determine whether the heart is on the right or left side, the examiner should observe precordial activity, rate, rhythm, quality of the heart sounds, and the presence or absence of murmurs.

It is difficult to examine the heart of a 'fussy' or crying baby. When the baby is peaceful, the rate, rhythm and presence of murmurs can be determined much more easily. The midwife could encourage the mother to pacify the baby by the use of her little finger or a dummy.

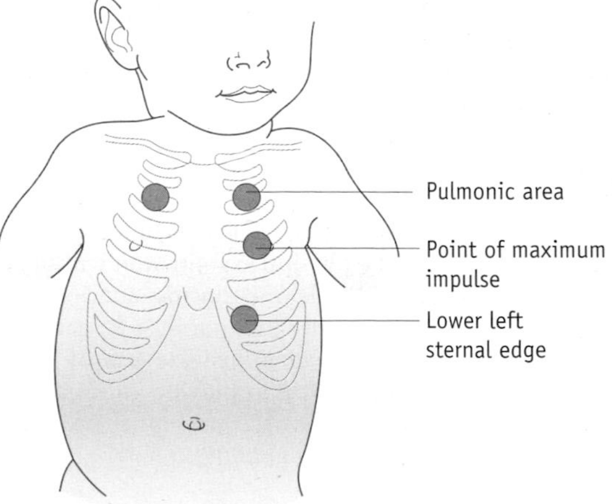


**Figure 41.5** The areas of auscultation of heart and lung sounds.

The heart rate is normally between 120 and 160 beats per minute, varying with gestational and chronological age and degree of activity.

Murmurs mean less in the newborn period than at any other time. A neonate may be found to have an extremely serious heart anomaly without any murmurs (Hall 1996). A closing ductus arteriosus may cause a murmur that, in retrospect, is only transient, but at the time is very loud, worrisome, and misleading. Gallop sounds may be an ominous finding, while the presence of a split 'S2' (i.e. *lub dub dub*) may be reassuring. If new to auscultation of heart sounds, it is difficult to ascertain SI and S2 (see website). Simultaneous palpation of the brachial pulse and auscultation of the *lub dub* makes identification of sounds easier.

The stethoscope aids assessment of the cardiovascular system. However, the best assessment is to observe or obtain an accurate history of the baby's behaviour. A baby who has been active and suddenly becomes lethargic; appears to have less tone; is not interested in feeding; or is tachypnoeic on effort, needs urgent referral and admission by ambulance to the nearest acute neonatal unit.

Major congenital abnormalities can be duct dependent, therefore most cardiac conditions will be diagnosed in the community after discharge. It is important for the parents to understand normal behaviour of the newborn in order to seek advice if their baby deviates from this.

The cardiovascular assessment is not complete until the liver is palpated and deemed to be of normal size.

### Congenital heart disease

Significant congenital heart disease (CHD) may be diagnosed at virtually any age. Some conditions are discovered in neonates; others rarely are identified during infancy. The profound haemodynamic transitions that occur at the time of birth make the clinical presentation of heart disease a challenge to practitioners to identify CHD. An understanding of the fetal circulation and transition to postnatal life can provide the clinician with the tools to anticipate and treat problems safely as they arise. For example, a baby who is suspected of having CHD and is cyanosed, is **not** given oxygen as this will encourage the ductus arteriosus to close faster.

While they cannot be prevented, there are many treatments for the defects and any related health problems. Babies in the UK have the physical examination within 72 hours following birth. While the ductus arteriosus is patent, it is difficult to identify the murmur. Research in Sweden and in the UK has identified the use of pulse oximetry as a test to be utilized to provide an improved means of identifying the at-risk newborns (de-Wahl Granelli et al 2009, Knowles et al 2005).

#### *Pulse oximetry*

Pulse oximetry is a non-invasive diagnostic test used for detecting the percentage of haemoglobin (Hb) that is saturated with oxygen. Oxygen saturation is a measure of how much oxygen the blood is carrying as a percentage of the maximum it could carry. A normal pulse reading is 98 to 100; a reading under 95 is too low and may indicate a baby at risk of CHD.

## Morphological examination

Accurate assessment of the morphological system is essential for identifying the baby who will need more thorough examination, medical/support services or family counselling. External assessment of dysmorphic features offers clues to the presence of internal anomalies. This examination requires a systematic approach to assessment, including observation and palpation.

### *The head*

Due to moulding, the shape of the head following birth can be round, bullet-shaped or an elongated oval, which may concern parents. They need to be reassured that the head will assume its natural shape, given time. This needs to be noted, as the measurement of the head circumference will differ from birth to that taken 4 or 5 days later. The average full-term head circumference, occipital–frontal diameter measurement, should be approximately 33–38 cm avoiding the ears.

The vault of the head is held in the midline while the size, shape and symmetry are assessed.

The scalp and face should be inspected for cuts, abrasions or bruises. Trauma sites such as fetal blood sample site should be identified and recorded.

The presence of caput succedaneum or cephalhaematoma should be noted (see Ch. 30).

The mobility and width of suture lines and the degree and direction of moulding of the skull bones is noted. Fontanelles are examined: large fontanelles may reflect a delay in ossification of bones and may be associated with hypothyroidism. The anterior fontanelle can provide valuable information on the wellbeing of the baby. In its normal state, it is flat and at the same level as the surrounding bones. A sunken fontanelle can be a symptom of dehydration, and a full and bulging fontanelle and wide sutures are characteristic of hydrocephalus.

### *The hair*

The condition and amount of hair is also noted, as this can be affected by certain metabolic disturbances (e.g. hypothyroidism).

### *The face*

This is examined for normal appearance and symmetry of eyes, ears and features during crying and rest.

### *The eyes*

These are checked for congenital cataracts (UKNSC 2005), and any small haemorrhages within the conjunctiva or under the eyes are noted for size and severity. The eyes may be tested for the red reflex by means of an ophthalmoscope. On examination, the retina is seen as clear and red, the amount of red pigment being dependent on race.

*Ophthalmia neonatorum* is conjunctivitis that occurs in the newborn. Conjunctivitis is an inflammation of the conjunctiva, the surface or covering of the eye, due to infectious or non-infectious causes. It is identified by an inflamed conjunctiva and watery solution or pus secreted from the eye. Simple infective conjunctivitis is often caused by *Staphylococcus aureus*, *streptococci* or *Escherichia coli*. If infection is suspected, appropriate swabs for *Chlamydia trachomatis* and *gonorrhoea* must be taken to exclude these infections which are associated with corneal ulceration and blindness (UKNSC 2008).

### *The ears*

Both are examined for symmetry and normal position on the baby. An imaginary line can be drawn from the inner canthus of the eye to the posterior fontanelle, and the helix of the ear should be above the line to validate normality. The pinna of the ear should be flexible and recoil easily. Accessory auricles, skin tags and sinuses should be noted as they may indicate further abnormalities such as renal (Roth et al 2008). The front and back of the ears should be examined closely for small spots or skin tags.

**Hearing:** Sensitivity to sounds should be noted. The ability to hear enables babies to communicate and learn about the world they live in. However, one baby will sleep through the loudest music and another will be startled by someone speaking softly. The best time to assess whether babies can hear or not is when they are fully awake. Hearing could be tested by observing the baby when a loud noise is made, but hearing can and should be tested fully at a later date.

Since March 2006, all babies in the UK have been offered a *hearing screen test* soon after birth. The screening for a hearing defect involves two painless tests – the *otoacoustic emissions test (OAE)* and the *automated auditory brainstem response test (AABR)*.

Babies are sometimes referred due to the results being affected by the baby being unsettled at the time of the test or because fluid, such as vernix or liquor, was in the ear. The test can be repeated.

### *The mouth*

This should be checked, commencing with the rooting and sucking reflexes, examining the gums for clefts and to ensure that there are no deciduous teeth present. Epstein's pearls (small white inclusion cysts clustered about the midline at the juncture of the hard and soft palate) are a normal finding. Tongue-tie, in which the frenulum restricts the movement of the tongue, should be identified. The midwife should ensure that there are neither hard nor soft palatal clefts (Bannister 2001).

The palpation and visualization of both the hard and soft palates is imperative – it may be necessary to use a torch and tongue depressor. Midwives and doctors have been shown to have missed a cleft palate (Habel et al 2006).

To examine the mouth with a tongue depressor, the baby should be swaddled and the head gently held to avoid movement during the examination. The spatula is inserted and the tongue depressed, which enables the visualization of hard and soft palates. Wood carries bacteria and multiple spatulas in one box can become contaminated when accessing individual spatulas, thus encouraging cross-infection to the newborn; consequently, spatulas require sterilization prior to use.

The mouth should be examined at regular intervals to validate normality and exclude infection, for example *Candida albicans*.

### *The nose*

This is examined for normal position and the presence of nares and possible choanal atresia which may or may not be easily identifiable.

Suctioning of babies is no longer advisable except in specific circumstances – for example, the presence of meconium or blood at birth. If a suction catheter is introduced into the nasal passages, the baby may become snuffly due to damaged epithelial lining and dissection of the mucous glands. Unless the baby has a problem with breathing, time will heal the damage and breathing should be normal within several days.

### *The neck*

This is passively examined for rotation and for anterior and lateral flexion and extension.

- Anterior flexion – the chin should touch or almost touch the chest.
- On extension, the occipital part of the head should touch or almost touch the back of the neck.

When there is asymmetrical rotation or lateral flexion or when range of motion is limited, this is recognized as abnormal. The neck should also be examined for goitre and thyroglossal or brachial arch sinus tracks, and the spaces hidden by creases, for evidence of septic spots or irritated skin.

## Sharing information with parents

If there are concerns that the baby is dysmorphic, it is important to communicate this sensitively to the parents prior to referral to a senior neonatologist, as a dysmorphic baby may be a clue to the presence of other congenital anomalies such as cardiac or gastrointestinal. One useful way to begin the discussion is to ask the parents whom the baby resembles. The parents may then feel they can disclose their concerns. Even if the baby does have a resemblance to other family members, it does not exclude genetic abnormalities and the baby should be referred to a neonatologist for follow-up. The words used to describe a dysmorphic baby need to accentuate the positive; words such as 'distinctive facial features' (Aase 1990) rather than 'abnormal' or 'deformed'.

## Musculoskeletal system

### History

Prenatal history is vital to musculoskeletal assessment because the uterine environment affects the musculoskeletal development of the fetus. Any event or condition that changes the intrauterine environment can alter fetal growth, movement or position. Factors such as oligohydramnios, breech presentation, abnormal growth patterns and exposure to teratogenic agents may adversely affect the development and maturation of the musculoskeletal system in utero. The skeletal system is interlinked with the neurological system, therefore factors such as possible birth trauma need to be considered.

The birth history, such as duration of labour, signs of fetal distress, type of birth (vaginal or caesarean), has a bearing on conditions such as cerebral palsy and brachial palsy.

In multiple gestations, the birth order is worth noting because there is a higher incidence of congenital hip dysplasia in first-born children.

An accurate gestational age assessment is necessary for assessment of the infant's posture and muscle tone.

Careful scrutiny and recording of the musculoskeletal system during the first newborn physical examination is imperative as this forms the basis for all future examinations.

### Examination

A thorough and systematic physical examination of the skeletal system, including the skull, clavicles, upper limbs, legs, spine and the hips, should be done within the first 24 hours after delivery. Then, should an abnormality of the spine be noted, the senior neonatologist will undertake the hip examination, thereby limiting stress to the newborn. As with other systems, skeletal examinations are undertaken while watching the newborn or while examining other systems.

Evaluation of the musculoskeletal system includes an appraisal of:

- posture, position, and gross anomalies
- discomfort from bone or joint movement
- range of joint motion
- muscle size, symmetry, and strength
- the configuration and mobility of the back.

**Observation** proceeds from the general to the specific and includes the ratio of extremity length to body length. General inspection includes observation for symmetry of movement as well as size, shape, general alignment, position and symmetry of different parts of the body.

Soft tissue and muscles should be observed for swelling, muscle wasting and symmetry. Asymmetry of length or circumference, constrictive bands, or length deformities of the extremities should not be present.

Palpation, along with inspection, is used on each extremity to identify component parts (for example, the two bones, radius and ulna, in the forearm), function and normal range of motion.

## Upper extremities

**Clavicles** are inspected and palpated for size, contour and crepitus (grating that can be felt or heard on movement of ends of broken bone). A fractured clavicle, one of the most common birth injuries, should be suspected when there is a history of a difficult delivery, irregularity in contour, shortening, tenderness or crepitus on palpation. It can be very uncomfortable and painful.

**Humerus** length and contour should be noted. A fractured humerus should be suspected if there is a history of difficult delivery. A mass due to haematoma formation or signs of pain during palpation may also be noted.

**Elbow, forearm, and wrist** are examined for size, shape and number of bones as well as for range of joint motion.

**Hands** should be examined for shape, size and posture, and fingers for number, shape and length. Inspection of palm creases should also be included. Although a single simian crease across the palm is usually associated with Down syndrome, it is often found in normal babies.

The fingers are usually flexed in a fist with the thumb under the fingers, The nails, usually smooth and soft and extending to the fingertips, should be examined for size and shape. The mother should be advised how to cut the nails to avoid causing infection to the nail bed, which can cause septicaemia.

Whilst dressing or undressing the newborn. the midwife should note any apparent discomfort.

## Abdomen

During fetal life, the fetus relies on the placenta for food and elimination of waste products. In order to sustain life after birth, the newborn baby must adapt to the intermittent intake of nutrients necessary for the body's metabolic requirements of growth, replacement and energy production, followed by their digestion and utilization and the excretion of waste products. The baby is able to suck and swallow but the digestion process and glucose metabolism take time to adapt to postnatal life.

Physical assessment of the gastrointestinal system therefore commences with the mouth and completes on examination of the anus to confirm normality prior to the baby being able to undertake artificial feeding as this entails a comparatively large intake volume.

The shape of the abdomen should be rounded, soft, symmetrical and slightly protruding. A flat abdomen may signify decreased tone and may herald the presence of abdominal contents in the chest cavity through a diaphragmatic hernia or abnormalities of the abdominal musculature.

Abdominal skin in the term baby is smooth and opaque with a medium-thick texture. Post-term babies have thick, parchment-like skin with superficial or sometimes deep cracking in the creases of the skin, and no vessels seen over the trunk.

*Diastasis recti* (separation of the rectus muscles) is a common finding in the newborn. Another midline malformation is an umbilical hernia, which reduces spontaneously within 2 years. If it is large, it will require surgical treatment.

**Midline defects** such as *omphalocele* or *gastroschisis* may be seen at birth. As the fetus grows during the first trimester of pregnancy, the developing intestines extend into the umbilical cord and should return to the abdomen by the 11th week of fetal development. However, if the muscles in the abdominal wall fail to close properly, the intestines may partially return to the abdominal cavity. Immediate management is to avoid fluid loss and maintain a clean environment; therefore the baby's body is placed in a special plastic bag, tied below the arms, or is wrapped in cling film from below the arms.

**Umbilical cord** is examined prior to cutting (Fig. 41.6) and applying the Hollister clamp, to exclude herniation of intestine into the cord itself and to visualize the presence of three vessels (Lissauer & Fanaroff 2008). Two vessels, one artery and a vein, sometimes indicate renal anomaly (Thummala et al 1988). The cord is a bluish white colour and gelatinous at birth. The quantity of Wharton's jelly affects the thickness of cord. Large-for-gestational-age infants have thick, gelatinous cords. Babies with congenital syphilis may also have thick cords. A thin small cord is another indication of intrauterine growth restriction.

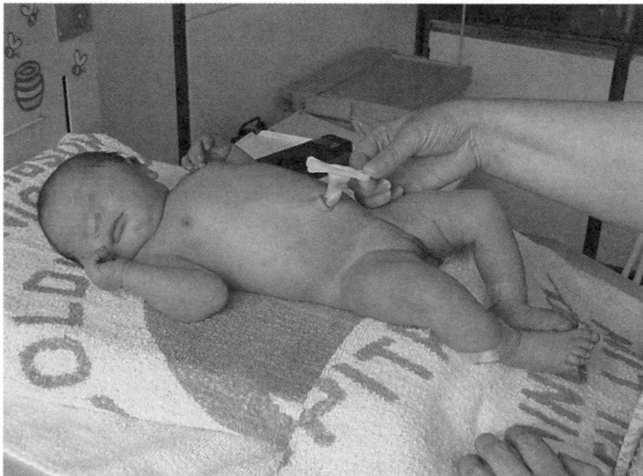

**Figure 41.6** The correct length for clamping and cutting the cord.

The cord darkens and shrivels as it dries, and separates by a process of dry gangrene, usually between the fifth and seventh day. It should be dry and without drainage of any type. Discharge of any colour before or after separation is not deemed normal; for example, clear discharge indicates a *patent urachus* or *omphalomesenteric duct* (Tappero & Honeyfield 2010).

The area around the cord is observed for any redness, which needs to be dealt with quickly to avoid serious septicaemia. The mother needs to understand the potential for infection from urine and faeces if the umbilical cord is placed inside the nappy, and the midwife can support the mother by showing her how to achieve this (Zupan et al 2004).

**Cleaning the cord:** A good handwashing technique is essential before attending to the cord, to avoid a spread of the highly dangerous *Staphylococcus aureus*. The umbilical cord is inspected daily by the midwife for signs of infection and separation. If the cord is soiled by a dirty nappy, it should be cleaned with water only and dried with cotton wool swabs.

## Peristaltic movement

The observation of movement needs to be undertaken from the side of the abdomen and at eye level. The midwife should observe for patterns and shape of movement.

Normal abdominal movements are synchronous with chest movements. After 1 hour of life, intermittent peristaltic movement is visible. Continuous peristaltic movement can imply obstruction.

It is important for the midwife to auscultate numerous neonatal bowel sounds in order to confidently validate normality.

## Palpation

Before palpating the abdomen, the midwife needs to check that the baby has not been fed a large amount prior to the examination, because such a baby will not be able to tolerate deep palpation. The midwife should stand at the side of the baby and, as with the rest of the examination, the hands must be warm and the nails short to enable palpation of the deep organs to take place without discomfort to the baby. The baby should be lying supine and be relaxed. Palpation should be light at first, progressing to deep palpation. The baby's facial expression needs to be observed for signs of discomfort or pain; and to validate that the liver and spleen are not enlarged, the baby's respirations need to be synchronized with the palpation. Flexing the baby's knee at the hip can allow the abdominal muscles to relax and aid palpation.

Light palpation of the four quadrants assesses the texture and warmth of the skin; it also reveals tenderness and guarding. Deep palpation identifies the absence of masses.

The liver is a superficial organ and palpation needs to take that into consideration. The liver edge should not be more than 2 cm inferior to the right costal margin. Babies in heart failure, where the liver acts as a sponge for fluid, will have an enlarged liver which can be palpated more than 2 cm below the costal margin. Slight oedema can sometimes also be seen around the eyelids.

The spleen is a deep organ but, if enlarged, would become a superficial organ; thus, firm but light pressure is applied in order to confirm normality. A non-palpable spleen equates to normality.

The abdominal area overlying the kidneys is also balloted, applying firm even pressure. The kidney should not be felt (RCM 2009).

### Vomiting

Most babies vomit at some time and mostly this is unimportant (Orenstein 1999). However, there are circumstances when the type of vomiting is important, the main one being green bile (Walker et al 2006). It cannot be assumed that this is meconium which was ingested at birth; and the baby should be examined by a senior neonatologist in order to exclude obstruction. Usually, the origin of blood is clear from the history, but if there is any doubt, the laboratory can perform an *Apt test* (blood mixed with sodium hydroxide), which distinguishes fetal from adult haemoglobin.

**Possets** are small, frequent vomits, particularly common in the first few days after birth, especially if the baby has swallowed any blood or meconium. 'Posseting' is also common when the milk flow is excessive. Most babies cope with these episodes quite well and either swallow the regurgitated contents or cough them out. The parents need to be informed how to manage these episodes. The baby should be left slightly on his side, while the posset is wiped away, and should not be lifted or patted on the back as both may cause overstimulation affecting the coordination of sucking, swallowing and breathing.

If the baby has inhaled a large amount of vomit, appropriate resuscitation needs to take place (Page & Jeffery 2000). Prior to any resuscitation involving mask ventilation, and when the baby has had a feed, the midwife needs to be prepared to pass a nasogastric tube to empty the contents of the stomach to avoid inhalation.

### The groin

When lying quietly, the baby's groin is flat, and if it is thin, visible pulsation of the femoral pulse may be noted. Any visible swelling on crying or on palpation must be referred urgently for diagnosis and management as this might indicate inguinal hernia or undescended testis – in the male or female – querying the sex of the baby.

## Genitourinary

### Male infant genitalia

**Scrotum:** All embryos are initially female. Under the influence of testosterone, the labia enlarge to become a scrotum, brownish in pigmentation, and should be fully rugated.

**Testes:** Normally, the testes of a full-term newborn are approximately 1.5–2 cm in length (Conner 2010). They should be palpated and have a consistency similar to that of a pea. If the scrotum appears discoloured and the testes feel solid, urgent referral is required.

The differential diagnosis for the presence of a solid scrotal mass includes testicular torsion, scrotal haematoma and testicular infarction (Diamond & Gosalbez 1998).

**Hydrocele:** The signs of a hydrocele include palpation of a cystic mass in the scrotal pouch. The whole scrotum appears swollen and firm – like a balloon filled with water – and it allows the passage of light from a torch (transillumination) (Diamond & Gosalbez 1998). Transillumination of the hydrocele excludes herniation of intestinal contents into the sac. Hydroceles are common and will disappear in time unless they are communicating types.

**Undescended testes (UDT)** is a common finding and in most cases the aetiology is unknown. There is an increased risk of infertility and testicular cancer in men with a history of UDT. The testes are very sensitive to temperature and can sometimes be seen moving up the inguinal canal. If a testis is not readily identified, a finger sweep should be performed from the anterior iliac crest along the inguinal canal. It can take up to 3 years for UDT to descend; therefore the baby will be followed up until descent. A timeline and pathway of care is provided by the NIPE standards (UKNSC 2008).

**Hypospadias:** Congenital abnormalities rarely appear singly; therefore, if the baby is noted to have UDT, extra vigilance is required to assess whether the urethral opening is central on the glans. In *hypospadias* the opening is found on the undersurface and in *epispadias* it is above the surface. Observing the baby pass urine is a good method of validating normality.

The penis shape and length are noted. *Chordee* is a lack of ventral tissue on the penis, leading to it being curved ventrally. Surgery is required to correct the condition.

## Female infant genitalia

In the female newborn, the labia majora cover the labia minora and the clitoris.

Before designating a sex to an apparently female infant, the labia majora must be parted and the clitoris observed to be an appropriate size. A discharge from the vagina will indicate that the hymen is perforated. If imperforate, the hymen appears like a tiny smooth bald head (Tappero & Honeyfield 2010). The discharge is usually creamy white at birth, occasionally being replaced after the second day by one appearing bloodstained (pseudomenses) as maternal hormones diminish.

## Ambiguous genitalia

If there is doubt as to the sex of the baby, it is important that the concerns are discussed sensitively with the parents (Ahmed & Hughes 2002). Parents will often be very distressed and continually apply pressure to be told the sex of the baby. They will take on board any terminology used, so it is important to avoid the terms 'he' or 'she' or 'it'. At the same time, the sex of the baby cannot be entered on the birth certificate until further investigations have been undertaken to confirm the sex. If the 'wrong' sex is registered, it is an extremely difficult and lengthy process to correct the mistake (Reiner 1999).

## Anus and rectum

The anus and rectum should be checked for patency and position. The practice of using a clinical thermometer to ensure anal patency is now considered outmoded. The anal sphincter is assessed by gently touching the anus and eliciting the anal 'wink' – the contraction and retraction of the muscle proving the anus is patent.

**Stools.** Record the number and character of all stools passed.

*Constipation* occurs most commonly in babies who are artificially fed. Breastfed babies may not pass a stool for 2 or 3 days once feeding is established but this is quite normal providing the stools are yellow and soft.

**Urinary output** is often less than 1 mL/kg/h during the first 12–18 hours after birth. Most healthy term babies urinate within the first 12 hours; however, a small number of healthy infants may not urinate until 24–36 hours after birth. If in doubt as to whether or not a baby has passed urine, place a piece of cotton wool at the end of the penis or urethra to elicit the passage of urine. Using bags should be avoided, as the adhesive can cause skin damage. Persistent oliguria beyond 36 hours should be evaluated in an otherwise healthy infant (Moghal & Embleton 2006).

The odour and colour of the urine are also noted. Occasionally, a red stain is found on the napkin due to urates colouring the urine.

## Lower extremities

From observation, the position of the baby's lower limbs will give a picture of the position adopted in utero. The majority of babies will lie with the legs folded on the abdomen, appearing externally rotated and bowed with everted feet. The baby delivered in a breech presentation often has flexed, abducted hips and extended knees. This positional adaptation of the lower limbs should not be confused with congenital malformations; however, a midwife who is in doubt should seek a second opinion from a peer or a neonatologist.

The midwife should examine the baby for normal appearance and for length, shape and movement of limbs, ensuring that the baby is able to move each limb fully and that the joints are functional. The legs are palpated to ascertain the presence of the femur, tibia and fibula. Femoral length can be observed by straightening both legs together and noting the length or by testing for the *Allis sign* as follows. Keeping the feet flat on the bed and the femurs aligned, flex both of the baby's knees. With the tips of the big toes in the same horizontal plane, face the feet, bend so that the baby's knees are at eye level and note the height of both knees. It will be apparent if one knee is higher than the other. This is a positive Allis sign and may indicate developmental hip displacement.

### *Ankles and feet*

Examination includes observation of resting and active movement. Passive motion of the ankle in dorsiflexion and plantar flexion varies depending on the infant's position in utero. For example, ankle and forefoot adduction, a positional deformity, can be differentiated from *congenital equinovarus* (clubfoot) malformation by passively positioning the foot in the midline and gently applying pressure to dorsiflex the foot to form a 'square window'. A clubfoot or other structurally abnormal foot and ankle will not have a full range of motion, will resist dorsiflexion and will not be able to form a square window (Bridgens & Kiely 2010).

The feet should be examined for shape, size and posture, and to check that the baby is moving both feet and adopts a normal position when at rest. The toes are examined for number, position, spacing, the presence of webbing and whether the nails are a normal shape and appearance. The soles of the feet should be inspected as part of the gestational age assessment and should therefore each be opened fully. This part of the examination is undertaken when eliciting the *Babinski reflex* (see below).

## Assessment of the back

Neural tube defects (NTD) are usually detected before birth as a result of maternal alpha-fetoprotein (AFP) measurement or ultrasound examination. Babies with NTD normally would have been born in an appropriate unit with the relevant staff, neonatologist and neonatal nurses, available at birth and afterwards. However, not all women choose antenatal screening and some may not have had antenatal care; thus, spinal neural defects could still present without warning.

On completing the examination of the lower limbs, the baby is lifted and held suspended with the examiner's hand under the chest, the back is observed to view the curvature of the spine and the baby's ability to lift the head. The spine should be straight, excluding *scoliosis, kyphosis* and *lordosis*.

The back continues to be observed with the baby lying prone. The spine is then examined from the base of the skull to the coccyx, noting any skin disruption, tufts of hair, soft or cystic masses, haemangioma, pilonidal dimple cysts or sinus tract. These deviations from normal may be signs of congenital spinal anomaly.

The position of the scapulae should also be noted while the infant is in the prone position to rule out *Sprengel's deformity*, a winged or elevated scapula.

The entire length of the spine should be gently palpated to ensure that it is complete and that there is no sign of pain.

A baby born at home found to have a meningocele (herniation of meninges) requires urgent referral and transport to hospital. Before and during transport, the lesion – especially if ruptured – should be covered with a sterile, non-adherent dressing. If that is not available, gently place sterile gauze soaked in normal saline and wrap in cling film. Pressure on the affected area must be avoided, the baby must be nursed in the prone position and gently driven into hospital.

## Hips

*Developmental dysplasia of the hip* (DDH) is the preferred term for the disease previously referred to as congenital dislocation of the hip (CDH). The new term takes into consideration that dislocation of the hip can develop after birth and although the hips can be deemed to be normal at birth, the baby can later have a positive screening for a dislocated or dislocatable hip joint.

The assessment of the baby's hips is undertaken within the first 72 hours of birth to detect conditions that may need early treatment. The UKNSC has produced standards and competencies to ensure consistency throughout the UK for improved and early detection of abnormalities to enable non-invasive treatment and avoid surgical intervention. These standards detail how the examination should be undertaken and by whom (UKNSC 2008). The assessment of the hips should be undertaken on a firm surface and one hip at a time examined by a trained professional.

The pelvic girdle of the neonate is not fully ossified and does not have the same characteristics as the adult pelvic girdle; the acetabula are shallower than in the adult. The acetabulum is still developing and it is quite possible for the femoral head to be able to move outside the acetabulum (luxation or dislocation) or through an abnormality within the acetabulum (subluxation or partial dislocation).

Early detection is vital to avoid surgical intervention. Left untreated, the hip joint develops abnormally and surgical reduction is required. Early diagnosis enables the use of splints, allowing the hip joint to develop normally.

### Examination

The ideal time to undertake examination of the hip (Fig. 41.7) is within the first 72 hours. Prior to the examination, the practitioner needs to recognize the importance of history in identifying the babies at risk. High-risk factors for DDH include (Keay & Morgan 1982):

- family history of DDH
- abnormal rotation of the developing hip during the first trimester
- neuromuscular disease, especially in the second trimester
- abnormal mechanical forces, e.g. oligohydramnios
- breech presentation in utero for a significant part of fetal life
- female infants (who are more susceptible to the maternal hormone relaxin).

The left hip is more frequently affected than the right.

Care that can prevent DDH includes postnatal application of mechanical forces associated with the baby able to fully abduct the hips, such as being allowed to lie in the prone position when awake and being carried in a sling with hips fully abducted – African babies whose

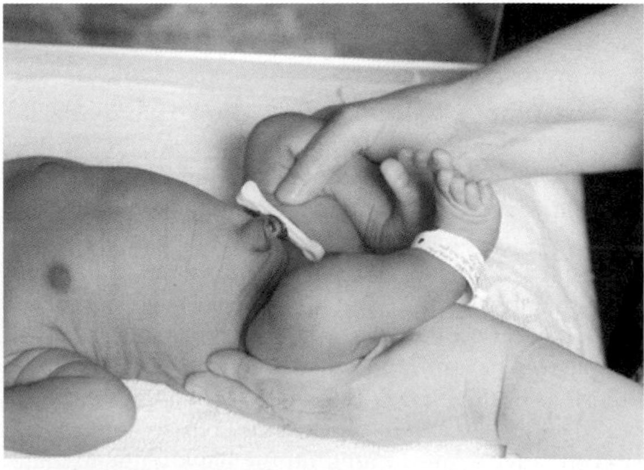

**Figure 41.7** Examination of the hips.

mothers transport them in this way have a low incidence of DDH.

The hips should be examined at regular intervals for congenital dislocation, which may be identified by the use of one of two tests:

- *Ortolani test,* which detects a dislocated hip reducing during the examination
- *Barlow test,* which detects a hip dislocating or subluxing during the examination (Sewell et al 2009).

A distinctive 'clunk' is of significance. However, 'clicks', often felt while performing these tests, are not predictive of DDH but can be confusing for an inexperienced examiner.

Ideally, examination of the hips should be the final part of the examination as it is often disruptive and uncomfortable for the baby. The midwife can utilize methods to reduce discomfort, such as sucking the mother's finger or, if bottle-feeding, the use of the pacifier.

Practitioners undertaking the examination of the hips need to have undertaken training during which they have been both taught and observed by an expert in the examination (STEPS 2004). Practice on the 'Baby Hippy' manikin is advised prior to examining a baby. An inexperienced practitioner can cause damage to the baby by failing to diagnose a false negative test, because of poor practice, or use of excessive force on a dislocated hip during abduction, causing damage to blood supply and ligaments.

## Observation

The midwife should observe the baby and note any difficulties with abduction. For example, if the baby found the procedure of examining the femoral pulses distressing or the *Allis sign* was positive, there may be an indication that the right or left hip may be dislocated.

## Ortolani and Barlow tests

The baby should be lying relaxed on a flat, firm surface in an environment warm and free from draughts. It is vital that the practitioner examines only one hip at a time with a full focus on undertaking the manoeuvre correctly.

### *Ortolani test*

- Stabilize one hip by bending the knee and hip, keeping the pelvis stable and firmly on the mattress (Fig. 41.7)
- Bend the other knee and hip
- Place two fingers over the greater trochanter (outer upper leg)
- Position the thumb on the inner trochanter
- Attempt to *abduct* (away from the midline of the body) the thigh to 90 degrees by applying pressure with the two fingers on the greater trochanter.

If the hip is dislocated, it will not be possible to abduct it and the neonate will keep the thigh at an angle less than expected. This angle is noted and recorded.

### *Barlow test*

- Continue to stabilize one hip, keeping the pelvis stable and firmly on the mattress (Fig. 41.7)
- Bend the other knee and hip
- Place two fingers over the greater trochanter (outer upper leg)
- Position the thumb on the inner trochanter
- The thigh is lifted and *adducted* (moved towards the midline of the body)
- With pressure applied with the thumb laterally, the femur is telescoped to note any movement of the head of the femur away from the acetabulum. Normality is confirmed when no movement is noted.

These two manoeuvres are then repeated with the other hip joint.

If any deviations from normal are noted, the examiner should refer the baby to a senior medical practitioner.

## Additional investigations

X-rays are unhelpful in assessment as the femoral head is cartilaginous until 6 months of age. Ultrasound examination of the hips is undertaken as part of screening for DDH; however, its effectiveness is not recognized by all.

The Ortolani and Barlow manoeuvres remain the best screening method for DDH if undertaken by a competent practitioner.

The leaflet on developmental dysplasia of the hip, congenital talipes equinovarus (clubfoot) and lower limb deficiencies (STEPS 2004) should be given to parents of affected babies. This will inform them of facts relating to deviations from normal in the lower limbs and raise awareness that although the baby's hips may be stable at the first examination, it is important to have the hips examined once again at 6 to 8 weeks to exclude the development of an abnormality.

# Neurological examination

Assessment of neurological function is important in assessing successful transition from extrauterine life and environmental factors in the perinatal period that may have caused a pathological response of the central and peripheral nervous systems. Early identification of deviations from normal can significantly reduce mortality and improve the quality of life for the newborn and family.

The Apgar score and its running commentary may indicate a baby who requires focus on the neurological system. The type of delivery, such as in shoulder dystocia, can cause brachial plexus damage, facial and Erb's palsy, paralysed vocal cords and damage to one or both of the phrenic nerves, all of which need to be excluded.

The examination of the neurological system is, in large part, undertaken by examining the other systems.

## Physical examination

Probably the most reliable information that can be obtained quickly from a neurological evaluation is through discussing the baby's behaviour with the mother and the baby's response to handling during the preceding parts of the physical examination.

**Level of consciousness:** One of the most important areas of the examination is the neonate's alertness and interaction with his mother, his overall behaviour and movement preceding and during the examination.

**Cry:** This is the baby's main method of communication to alert carers to pain, hunger, discomfort or suffering. It is important that the carers understand the types of crying in order to give appropriate care. When listening to the sound of crying, note whether it is a clear tone, without hoarseness, or nasal tone. Equally, the type of pain and whether or not pain relief is required by the baby needs to be established. Change from an uncomfortable position, a soothing bath, massage, or sucking on a finger or breast might bring relief. It takes time and skill to interpret the different sounds, and conscious effort needs to be given to listening and observing babies in order to perfect this form of communication.

**Head:** The shape and size, fontanelle and suture size are examined as stated during the morphological examination. Cranial bruit may indicate an intracranial vascular malformation.

**Face:** Facial dysmorphism may indicate a genetic syndrome such as trisomy 18, and facial features are observed during crying for facial palsy.

**Eye examination:** Pupils should be equal and react to light and the red reflex should be present and completely round in shape.

**Skin:** Cutaneous birthmarks such as café-au-lait spots may indicate the presence of a genetic disorder such as neurofibromatosis.

**Skeletal system:** The skeletal and neurological systems are interlinked and examination of the baby can indicate an abnormality; for example, a hair tuft over the spinal region may indicate a degree of spina bifida.

**Tone:** The strength and reflexes of limbs can indicate normal or abnormal movements indicating neurological damage.

## Reflexes

It is now known that babies are aware of their in-utero environment and at birth are equipped for survival. They can hear, smell, taste, see up to a distance of 30 cm (Wilkinson 1997) and favour the colours black and white. The majority of reflexes are deemed to be primitive involving the brainstem and spinal cord.

- *Rooting reflex* – a primitive survival reflex in which a touch on the baby's cheek will cause him to move his mouth to the site of touch, searching for food. When the upper lip is touched, the mouth will open. These are useful reflexes for the mother to utilize when preparing the baby for feeding, whether breast, bottle or cup feeding.
- *Sucking reflex* – can be tested by placing a clean, little finger into the baby's mouth or observing the baby feeding. The baby will tend to make sucking efforts, whether hungry or not. This confirms the baby's ability to coordinate breathe, suck and swallow – an important measure of neural integrity.
- *Grasp reflex* – can be tested by brushing the infant on the back of the hand, which will then open to grasp an offered finger. The midwife should then extend the baby's arms and lift the baby gently, observing the head and how well controlled or lax is the way in which it is held. This tests the *traction reflex*. This reflex will also need to be checked after a traumatic birth to note nerve damage that may not be obvious by observing the tone and position of the arms.
- *Moro reflex* (startle reflex) – can be observed physiologically or tested for. The baby may already have demonstrated this reflex during the examination and therefore a further demonstration is not required. If it has not been seen, the reflex can be tested by first ensuring the baby is calm and at rest. The midwife supports the baby's head with the left hand from the neck to the lower back and brings the baby's chin to his chest. The baby is then elevated several centimetres off the bed and his head allowed to drop gently to the right supporting hand. The baby will throw his arms back and then forwards towards his chest, allowing his fists to close. He may also cry. The aim of this examination is to enable the baby's head to appear to fall into an empty space; it is not to fall from a height and the head must never touch the mattress. This procedure must not be undertaken if the baby is not relaxed.
- *Asymmetrical tonic neck reflex* – the baby will extend his limbs on the side of the body his head is turned towards.
- *Stepping or walking reflex* – the baby is supported by the practitioner, with the soles of his feet flat against the mattress. This will encourage the baby to put one foot in front of the other, straighten his spine and attempt to 'walk'.
- *Babinski reflex* – the baby's foot is supported in the left hand and pressure is applied with the index finger of the other hand on the outer part of the sole

of the foot up to the small toe and across to the big toe. The normal response is for the baby to extend and fan the toes and finally to flex them. The midwife can take the opportunity to note webbing of the toes when eliciting this reflex.

The complete behavioural examination is quite dependent on infant–examiner interaction and thus the midwife should aim to examine the baby with gentleness and respect, communicating with him on both verbal and non-verbal levels.

### Cranial nerves

The 12 pairs of cranial nerves are referred to by name or roman numerals. They originate from different parts of the brain and assessment of their function confirms normality and recognizes deviations from normal (see website).

### Assessment of the autonomic nervous system

The autonomic nervous system is involved in a complex of reflex activities essential to sustain life and these are dependent on sensory input to the brain or spinal cord. Normal autonomic function in a baby at term is well developed and can be observed through the following reflex actions:

- ability to adapt temperature to the environment
- respiratory rate and heart rate changes with physical activity
- responses of the pupils to light
- contraction of the external anal sphincter (anal wink) in response to touch or when air is blown over it – the muscular opening of the anus should have a firm appearance and not be distended and lax.
- skin – harlequin sign – when the baby is lying on one side, the upper area is light and the lower area dark red.

## Identifying and managing pain and stress in the term newborn

Until the 1980s, it was thought that babies did not feel pain, therefore pain relief was rarely given.

Dummies laced with brandy and sugar were sometimes used to pacify a very distressed newborn; however, procedures which required pain relief in children or adults were undertaken on newborns without pain relief. Today, the physiology of pain pathways in babies is better understood, and it is now recognized that the baby's spinal sensory nerve cells are more excitable than those of adults. Midwives, doctors and nurses rely on patients to report their pain and its severity. The baby is unable to speak, so practitioners need to be aware of evidence of pain and obtain experience of the normal behaviour of the baby. The inability to communicate in no way negates the possibility that the baby is experiencing pain and is in need of appropriate pain relief (Lago et al 2009). Time spent observing babies is invaluable, in trying to understand how to adapt the care provided in order to minimize stress and pain to the newborn.

The physiological response to painful stimulus in the baby is greater and lasts for a longer period of time than in the adult. Adults have a sophisticated nerve pathway which can narrowly pinpoint the area of painful stimulus. In the newborn, this pathway is still developing, which means the baby is unable to localize pain but can feel pain in response not only to painful stimuli but also to touch over a wide area of the body (Anand & Scalzo 2000). Damaged skin, either from a heel prick or from ventouse or other instrumental birth, will be very sensitive to touch.

Newborns feel pain (Anand 2001) and therefore procedures that can cause pain should be kept to a minimum. Handing the baby to his mother at birth instantly provides human contact. Being stroked gently and given the opportunity to suck at the breast will reduce the newborn's pain and discomfort (Carbajal et al 2003). Bathing or washing the baby for whatever reason needs to be delayed until the baby has had time to recover and for his skin to heal prior to pressure being applied to broken or bruised skin. It is important to note that damage to the skin at birth or soon after can cause the damaged area to be oversupplied with sensory nerve terminals which will leave the area hypersensitive to touch for some weeks after the wound has heeled. This information needs to be shared with parents for them to have an insight into the baby's behaviour when that area is handled.

#### *Causes of pain*

The effect of certain procedures needs to be considered in relation to the amount of pain caused to the baby, for example:

- long or short/precipitate labour – headache
- type of labour, e.g. occipitoposterior position
- instrumental birth – bruising/trauma from ventouse cap
- heel pricks undertaken for the Guthrie test, etc.
- removal of plasters
- insertion of intravenous needles for antibiotic therapy
- delivery of fluid to the subcutaneous tissue following blockage of an intravenous cannula.

#### *Signs of pain*

One of the best indicators is vocal expression, heard in long-lasting crying. Facial expressions – brow bulge, eye squeeze, and nasolabial furrow – are also reliable indicators of pain (Stevens & Johnston 1993). Other behavioural signs of pain include pedalling movement of the legs, toes spread, legs tensed and pulled up, agitation of arms and a withdrawal reaction.

### *Sucrose administration*

The majority of research regarding non-pharmacological analgesia, performed on babies at term undergoing a heel prick procedure, recommends that prior to this procedure, if possible, the baby should:

- if breastfeeding, be held by the mother and be enabled to suckle for several minutes
- be given a dummy/finger to suck throughout the procedure (Carbajal et al 2003)
- be given 2 mL of 12–25% sucrose and allowed to suck for 2 minutes.

One study has shown that breastfeeding alone can reduce crying; however, a number of randomized controlled trials provide unequivocal evidence that babies cry less when given a combination of nutritive or non-nutritive sucking and sucrose (Carbajal et al 2003).

Many cultures recognize that the taste of sweetness reduces pain, as does massage, talking gently and obtaining eye contact with the baby.

Research on pain, undertaken on the blood spot screening and venepuncture procedures, recognizes these as being very painful for the newborn and for the parents observing a distressed newborn. There needs to be clear justification to undertake every heel-prick procedure.

### Jitteriness versus seizures

Jitteriness, although not a type of seizure, is a movement disorder characterized by movements with qualities primarily of tremulousness and occasionally of clonus. It is important to distinguish jitteriness from seizures.

If the limb that is tremulous is pressed down against the mattress and the tremors stop, seizure is excluded; if movement continues, it is a positive sign of seizure. The midwife must call for help and stay with the baby to observe the progress and length of seizures; this is also important in order to provide support if the respiratory system is involved (Silverstein & Jensen 2007).

## Assessment of feeding

The final and crucial part of the assessment to ascertain wellbeing is that of feeding. A baby who has been feeding well and who becomes tachypnoeic on feeding will require urgent further assessment.

## Bad news

Prior to undertaking the examination of the newborn, it is important for practitioners to have had training in 'giving bad news', recognizing that what they might deem good news may not produce the same reaction in the parents. A girl rather than a boy is a disaster for some parents. The smallest of deformities, such as an extra digit, can cause major concerns for parents who wished for the 'perfect' baby. For major congenital abnormalities, it is important to know specialist centres in the area and the latest management and treatment in order to have some insight when the parents start asking questions about the wellbeing of their baby.

Consequently, it is important that the examination of the newborn is undertaken where privacy is guaranteed and the parents feel that they can ask questions and that they have the professionals' full attention. If the midwife is not able to convey bad news, the examination should be delayed until the support of a senior colleague, with training and experience, is available.

## Mother–baby attachment

Parent–infant interaction is believed to play a central role in the baby's social, emotional and physiological development. The quality of the interaction between mother and baby can provide the baby with an environment for optimal development and growth. The foundation of this relationship is trust and affection. If there is failure to develop this relationship, the baby is at risk of delays in neurological developmental, child abuse, neglect and failure to thrive (Pridham et al 1999). Research has shown that educating the mother to understand her baby and his behaviour can have a positive effect on maternal–infant interaction (Anderson 1981).

Today in the UK, women stay in hospital less than 24 hours for a non-complicated birth, and therefore teaching opportunities are limited. Antenatal classes are an ideal opportunity to provide the necessary education that serves as a valuable health-promotion tool to effect positive parenting beginning at birth.

After the birth, mother and baby should be given a minimum of 1 hour of supported privacy together in the labour ward, and this should then be followed by keeping mother and baby together as much as possible during the early neonatal period when they are getting to know one another and mothering skills are developing. This is easily achieved if the birth takes place in the home but more difficult in the hospital setting. The Maternity Services Advisory Committee (MASC 1985) advocated that the baby's cot remains beside the mother's bed. Restricted contact between mother and baby in the early postnatal period is associated with less affectionate maternal behaviour and maternal feelings of incompetence and lack of confidence (Thomson & Westreich 1989). Maternal–infant attachment established from birth is strengthened by the woman getting to understand her baby, and because handling can aid this process, the mother is encouraged to care for her baby soon after birth. The use of strategies such as the shortened *Brazelton Neonatal Behavioural Assessment Scale* (see website) can assist parents to learn more about their baby's capabilities (Nugent 2004).

Unrestricted access allows the mother freedom to respond to her baby whenever he is awake. Although this aspect of initiating the relationship between mother and baby is important, the ability to enhance that relationship is dependent on the mother's physiological wellbeing.

There must be communication between mother and baby in order for interaction to take place. Mother and baby need to respond to each other's cues and the environment must be such as to facilitate that interaction. It is difficult for a woman who has had a difficult delivery to respond physically if she is unable to move and handle her baby. The midwife needs to provide the response to the cues given by the baby while allowing the mother to recover, and, in doing so, acts as a role model, educating the woman about the different cues, such as hunger, boredom, discomfort and pain, which the baby provides. A crying baby can overwhelm the woman's psychological wellbeing at this vulnerable time following birth. The father, too, should be involved in his baby's care and progress, otherwise he may feel neglected and become jealous of the close relationship developing between mother and baby.

Three stages have been described in the maternal–infant attachment process.

1. The first is when the mother and baby first become *acquainted* and involves early physical contact.
2. The next is the *care-taking relationship* when the mother learns to care for – feed, change, wash and bath – her baby.
3. The final stage, called *identity*, occurs when the child is incorporated into the family.

To reach this final stage, mother and baby grow to know and love each other as they interact. The baby may initiate interaction by crying. The mother responds by rocking the cot or picking the baby up and cuddling him. This is the expression of a mother's instinct to tend and protect her child. The baby stops crying when he is picked up and becomes alert and responsive. The mother should be encouraged to talk and establish eye-to-eye contact. In turn, the baby gazes at his mother and responds; thus mother–baby interaction is synchronized and attachment develops.

At times, mother and baby have to be separated because of maternal illness or because the baby needs intensive or special care; most mothers are likely to overcome any adverse effects of this separation (Thomson & Westreich 1989). Some consider that the degree to which a mother perceives separation as having an adverse effect on her mothering ability may be related to the outcome (Richards 1978, Ross 1980) and also the contact between mother and baby while the baby is in hospital (Moore & Nelson 2003). Women of low socioeconomic status, with low social support, may be more adversely affected by restricted contact with their baby than their more affluent counterparts (Thomson & Westreich 1989). One study demonstrated this, highlighting the benefits of early and prolonged contact following birth to women and babies with low social support (Anisfeld & Lipper 1983).

Not uncommonly, some mothers are worried that they do not feel a maternal instinct or really love their baby during the early days of motherhood. They need reassurance that their feelings are quite normal and that, as they and their baby learn to know each other, love will follow.

Each society and culture has its behavioural norms about what is accepted as normal and appropriate maternal–infant interaction and it is important to acknowledge these differences.

## Newborn behaviour

For the first 6 weeks of life, the baby does not distinguish night from day and spends 24 hours sleeping, waking, crying and feeding. Newborns have a very small stomach and require regular intake of food; they will, on the whole, feed every 3–4 hours. What parents find difficult is that the baby is awake at night and asleep during the day. Babies move from one sleep state to another, from quietly looking around, actively responding to sounds, to crying. Parents are sometimes concerned not to 'spoil' their babies and sometimes delay in answering their baby's cries. Prior to 6 months of age, the neural processes are not mature enough to enable the baby to manipulate the carer; to think 'if I cry I will get my mother to come to see to me'. If and when the baby cries, it is for a reason such as hunger, fear, discomfort, pain or boredom. Rather than spoiling the baby, if the mother/carer answers the cries immediately, the baby will develop securely, knowing his needs will be answered (Bell & Ainsworth 1972).

A baby's primary needs are for food, fluid, sleep, warmth, security and love, and the method of expressing those needs is crying. This is a signal to the carer to communicate with the baby, recognize the cry and meet the need; parents and practitioners need time to understand and interpret. Parents need to be given this information to recognize the newborn baby's needs and know what to do to help the baby calm down.

When responding to the baby's cry, the mother/carer must be 10–12 inches in front of the baby, establish eye contact and at the same time find a way to control the baby's flailing arms and legs while firmly and gently talking to him (Ludington-Hoe et al 2002). The baby can alternatively be held against the mother's body and be talked to gently.

Another method of satisfying the baby is to provide non-nutritive sucking by giving him fingers or a dummy to suck or by putting the baby to the breast. Teaching the baby the difference between night and day is also helpful. That could be accomplished by placing the baby in an environment of light and normal sounds during the day, and at night making sure the environment is dark, or the lights dimmed and sounds are gentle. Parents need to understand that they will not always succeed immediately in stopping the baby from crying; however, a variety of methods should be tried until successful. Scientifically, it is recognized that crying in the newborn can cause pathological changes to the cardiorespiratory system (Anderson 1988); therefore, listening to the baby crying without taking action to stop the crying is no longer acceptable practice.

Placing the cot near the bed will make access to the baby easier at night-time. The baby will develop an organized pattern of sleep by the age of 16 weeks (Matsuoka et al 1991). At 6 weeks the baby should begin to smile, and at 3 months take note of his surroundings.

## Sleep versus play time

Following any physical examination, the baby is dressed and given to a parent to hold. When the baby is placed in the cot, the position of the baby in the cot is informed by the 'Back to sleep' campaign to prevent sudden infant death syndrome (SIDS) (see Ch. 50). It is important to recognize that the baby is positioned on the back for sleep, but when the baby is awake, evidence recommends that he is able to play in the prone position for about 15 minutes a day. This can prevent conditions such as delays in motor skills, positional plagiocephaly (flattening of the occipital region of the head), positional torticollis (contracture of the sternocleidomastoid muscle) and shoulder retraction. None of these is life-threatening or should lead to abandoning the 'back to sleep' position (Fig. 41.8).

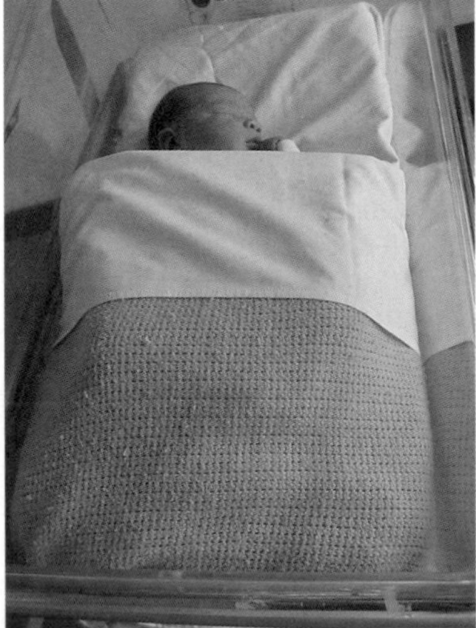

**Figure 41.8** Baby in cot in the recommended position for sleep.

# POSTNATAL CARE

Care of the newborn is based on the philosophy of a continuum of quality care that commences with antenatal and intrapartum care. This begins with getting to know the fetus both antenatally and during the intrapartum period, and that knowledge informs the management of care given to the baby from the moment of birth to 28 days.

Preparation of the parents for early detection of deviations from normal and management of the newborn is vital wherever the birth takes place. It is expected that preparation for parenthood has taken place in order to reduce the psychological stress to both the baby and family.

The UK is a multicultural society and in order for a partnership of care to be developed with parents, the cultural norms of the ethnic groups need to be understood. Many traditional practices need to be understood rather than feared. One of these practices, cup-feeding, utilized effectively today in neonatal units, was brought to the UK from Africa, where the survival of high-risk newborns was achieved by cup-feeding well before its introduction to the UK. The midwife needs to make links with women's ethnic groups and religious leaders in order to learn and understand traditional practice so that safe care can be provided to the newborn by supporting and, where necessary, sensitively changing practice.

## Follow-up of the baby

When the baby is deemed to be well and no longer requires midwifery care, the baby is transferred from the midwife to the health visitor, who usually visits the mother and baby at home. The health visitor discusses problems with the mother, gives advice on topics such as childcare and family planning, and encourages the mother to take her baby to the child health clinic or to her GP regularly. The baby's development will be followed closely by initiating the vaccination programme and developmental assessments. The GP is responsible for general medical care but some babies with medical problems are also followed up by a neonatologist/paediatrician.

### Hygiene

Because newborn infants have little resistance to microorganisms, they are highly susceptible to infection. An apparently mild infection can rapidly become a serious condition in the newborn, so every effort must be made to protect them from infection.

There are three main factors in avoiding infection:

1. Keep the baby's skin healthy and intact so bacteria have no portal of entry for invasion of tissues.
2. Limit the bacteria in the baby's surroundings.

3. Adopt a barrier-nursing technique to avoid cross-infection.

### Sources of infection

The infant may be infected in a number of ways:

**Attendants.** The nose, throat or skin of those dealing with the baby may harbour dangerous organisms (staphylococci and streptococci). This includes not only the midwife and doctor but also the parents themselves.

**Hands and clothing.** Facilities for washing the hands must be available after personal toilet and in the nursery and wards. Disposable hand towels are preferable for use. The hands must be washed before and after attending each baby. Antiseptic hand cream applied to the hands after washing is valuable. Long fingernails not only hinder many examination procedures but also can cause the baby discomfort and harbour infection.

**Dust.** The air and dust in maternity wards and nurseries contain many bacteria, one of which, *Staphylococcus aureus*, is most liable to cause infection. The ward and nursery should be adequately ventilated. Cleaning must be thorough and should minimize dust being scattered around the room. Floors are cleaned using vacuum cleaners with filters preventing bacteria passing out of the machine into the air. Damp dusting is advisable. Cots, trolleys and tables can be wiped over with dilute antiseptic and dried well.

**Fomites.** Infection may be spread by unsterilized instruments, bowls and dressings. Clothing and napkins may be the source. Before the era of pre-packed feeds and disposable bottles and teats in hospitals, inadequately sterilized bottles and teats were a source of infection. This may still be the case in some homes.

**Cross-infection.** Rooming-in, in which babies are nursed beside the mother's bed, is the usual practice nowadays. This aids the bonding process and reduces the risk of cross-infection. Overcrowding in wards and nurseries should be avoided. Individual equipment for bathing and changing should be provided, disposable articles being used whenever possible. Any baby suspected of infection should be isolated from other babies.

*The main routine care* of the baby involves changing the napkins, washing or bathing, and feeding. Soiled linen and napkins should be handled, with gloved hands, as little as possible and placed in bags and closed while carried to the waste bin.

### Bathing the baby

The issue of transmission of human immunodeficiency virus (HIV) through maternal vaginal secretions has encouraged the practice of the baby being given a bath soon after birth. Currently, there are no studies to support the reduction of HIV from this. Vernix is deemed to protect the skin, and may act as an antibacterial agent and promote healing from the trauma of birth. Bathing the baby removes this skin-protecting vernix. Work undertaken so far suggests the importance of the newborn's condition and temperature being stabilized in the normal range for 2–4 hours prior to the bath being given, in order to avoid hypothermia (see Ch. 42).

Bath time offers parents a time to get to know their baby through tactile interaction.

In order to protect the skin pH, it is important that any cleansing agents that are used have a neutral pH and minimal dyes and perfumes, and that the baby's skin is rinsed well to reduce the risk of allergic sensitization (Cetta et al 1991, NICE 2006, Crozier & Macdonald 2010).

Whilst the baby is being bathed, care must be taken to prevent abrasions of the skin which might allow entry of bacteria. Great care must also be taken with the eyes and cord, which are both sites of potential infection.

**Chafing or intertrigo**, caused by friction between two skin surfaces, is usually seen in the groin or axilla and in the folds of the neck. It indicates that the baby's skin has not been adequately dried after being washed or bathed. The energetic removal of vernix caseosa may also be the cause. After a bath, a dabbing movement with a soft towel should dry the folds in the skin. Where chafing has occurred, drying and a very light dusting with an antiseptic powder will heal the lesion.

## Dermatitis of the groin, buttocks and anus

Redness and excoriation may be produced around the groin, anus and buttocks. The development of this condition may be influenced by wetness of the skin (see website). When the skin is exposed to urine, the pH rises and changes from acid to alkaline, enabling penetration of microorganisms into the building blocks of the stratum corneum.

### Treatment and care

- Use of appropriate barrier creams containing petrolatum (soft paraffin) protects skin, maintains the acid pH, and aids healing.
- Application of zinc oxide enables skin healing.
- Exposure to air is unhelpful.
- As much urine and faeces as possible should be removed and the barrier cream reapplied to the affected areas.
- If *Candida albicans* is suspected:
  - Inspect the baby's mouth.
  - Take swabs for culture and sensitivity testing.
  - Antifungal ointment or cream should be used.
- Dermatitis is a very painful condition and great care is needed in its treatment.
- The affected area should be washed with soft absorbent cotton wool and well dried with gentle dabbing.

- Avoid use of soap or cleansing substances as they also may cause irritation to the skin.
- Maintain high standards of hygiene.

## Newborn screening tests

Various tests and examinations may be carried out in the early neonatal period to detect the presence of specific abnormal conditions. Early diagnosis and treatment may ameliorate the effects of many conditions. Thus, some inborn errors of metabolism may be managed with diet and/or drugs (see website).

### Blood spot screening test

The UK National Screening Committee recommend that all babies in the UK are offered screening for phenylketonuria (PKU), congenital hypothyroidism (CHT), sickle cell disorders (SCD), cystic fibrosis (CF) and medium-chain acyl-CoA dehydrogenase deficiency (MCADD). The test is offered to all babies in the UK at the age of 5 to 8 days.

**Phenylketonuria** is an autosomal recessive genetic condition where babies are unable to metabolize phenylalanine (an amino acid found in proteins). It affects 1 in 10,000 babies in the UK. Babies who are not treated develop serious permanent mental disability. Once diagnosed, the baby should be started on a low protein diet by day 21 of age and this will effect a good quality of life.

**Congenital hypothyroidism** affects 1 in 4000 babies in the UK. Screening is done by measuring the level of thyroxine or thyroid-stimulating hormone (TSH) in the blood sample,. Further investigations of thyroid function will be required if the test result is abnormal. If the condition is confirmed, early treatment with levothyroxine (thyroxine) sodium by the age of 21 days will prevent mental handicap and promote normal growth (Kelnar et al 1995).

**Sickle cell disorders** affect 1 in 2500 babies in the UK and the aim of screening is to identify the babies who are affected in order to commence penicillin prophylaxis. This baby is at risk of infections and severe acute anaemia in the first few years of life if left untreated.

**Deficiency of medium-chain acyl-CoA dehydrogenase** causes the accumulation of medium-chain fatty acids and impairs ketone production.

**Cystic fibrosis (CF)** affects 1 in 2500 babies across the UK. It is an autosomal recessive inherited condition which mainly affects babies' digestion and lung function. Diagnosis enables nutrition and growth to be improved and reduces chest infection.

### Hearing tests

Recent technological advances have led to improved screening methods that can identify the majority of children with impaired hearing and it is recommended that babies should be screened before leaving hospital.

The test is non-invasive and involves the measurement of otoacoustic emissions (OAE) which are low-level inaudible sounds produced by the inner ear. The screening of newborns is part of the continuum of early childhood hearing tests which screen and diagnose to improve identification of hearing impairment in young children.

The value of such a test is that children with hearing impairments can be given extra help at an early age to develop speech since the critical period for language and speech development is generally regarded as the first 2 years of life.

## Vaccinations at birth

Infants are known to be susceptible to infections in the first 2 months of life as the immune system of the newborn is immature and takes some time to develop. The UK Joint Committee for Vaccination and Immunisation (JCVI) recommends that parents give informed consent for their babies to be vaccinated against two of the most serious infections – tuberculosis (BCG) and hepatitis B – where it is necessary (DH 2009).

Vaccination is now offered in the early postnatal period to babies whose parents have emigrated from a country with high prevalence of tuberculosis or whose family members have previously been infected.

Hepatitis B vaccine is given within the first 12 hours following birth to babies whose mothers are chronic carriers of hepatitis B virus or who have had acute hepatitis B during pregnancy.

# RECORD-KEEPING

Record-keeping is an important aspect of care given to the newborn. The examination needs to be recorded along with the underpinning rationale for present and future management (NICE 2006). This commences with completing the case notes and birth notification (within the first 36 hours), which must be sent to the appropriate medical officer. Important information such as whether or not the baby has fed or has passed urine and meconium needs to be documented in the notes, in order to form a baseline for further assessments.

To midwives, the hands-on care may be seen as more important than documentation, but medico-legal experts and the NMC advise that if contemporaneous records are not kept, then legally it did not happen (NMC 2009). Good record-keeping provides evidence of actions and omissions, protects the newborn by promoting high standards of clinical care, promotes team communication, gives an accurate account of treatment, and provides the ability to detect problems at an early stage (Walton & Bedford 2007).

A common core content record is available for every child and parent and for each professional engaged in delivery, to record the progress and care given, and this record is the UK Parent-held Child Health Record (PHCHR or 'Red Book').

The new WHO growth charts are included to document and support the decisions the practitioners make in regard to the care of the newborn.

Following the first holistic physical examination, the practitioner should complete the PHCHR and give it to parents to commence the documentation of the forthcoming journey.

## CONCLUSION

The aim of this chapter has been to introduce the reader to physiology applied to the examination of the newborn and the care given to newborn babies and their families. For more detail, the reader is referred to the website for other resources and links, providing the in-depth knowledge required to undertake the examination of the newborn.

## KEY POINTS

- The transition from fetus to neonate is a complex process, and the midwife needs to be knowledgeable about fetal and neonatal physiology to recognize that the progression has been completed.
- Care of the neonate should be based upon supporting and enhancing normal transition, in early identification of deviations from normal, and appropriate management and referral.
- Midwives should allocate the same time and attention to the examination and assessment of the baby, as for the woman.
- Midwives should have a clear understanding of neonatal anatomy, physiology and behaviour in order to help women understand the behaviours, responses and care needs of their newborn baby.
- Clear, accurate and contemporaneous record-keeping is essential in ensuring continuity of care, and effective information to the parents and carers of the neonate.

## REFERENCES


Aase JM: *Diagnostic dysmorphology*, New York, 1990, Plenum Medical Book Company.

Ahmed SF, Hughes IA: The genetics of male undermasculinization, *Clinical Endocrinology* 56(1):1–18, 2002.

Anand KJ; International Evidence-Based Group for Neonatal Pain: Consensus statement for the prevention and management of pain in the newborn, *Archives of Pediatrics & Adolescent Medicine* 155:173–180, 2001.

Anand KJ, Scalzo FM: Can adverse neonatal experiences alter the brain development and subsequent behaviour? *Biology of the Neonate* 77:69–82, 2000.

Anderson CJ: Enhancing reciprocity between mother and neonate, *Nursing Research* 30:89–93, 1981.

Anderson GC: Crying, foramen ovale shunting, and cerebral volume, *Journal of Pediatrics* 113(2):411–412, 1988.

Anisfeld E, Lipper, E: Early contact, social support and mother–infant bonding, *Pediatrics* 72:79–83, 1983.

Battaglia FC, Lubchenco LO: A practical classification of newborn infants by weight and gestational age, *Journal of Pediatrics* 71(2):159–163, 1967.

Bannister P: Early feeding management. In Watson ACH, Sell DA, Grunwell P, editors: *Management of cleft lip and palate*, London, 2001, Whurr.

Bell SM, Ainsworth MD. Infant crying patterns and maternal responsiveness, *Child Development* 43(4):1171–1190, 1972.

Brazelton TB: *Infants and mothers*, New York, 1983, Delacourt Press.

Brazelton TB, Nugent JK: *Neonatal behavioral assessment scale*, Cambridge, 1995, Mac Keith Press.

Bridgens J, Kiely N: Current management of clubfoot (congenital talipes equinovarus), *British Medical Journal* 340:c355, 2010.

Carbajal R, Veerapen S, Couderc S, et al: Analgesic effect of breast feeding in term neonates: randomised controlled trial, *British Medical Journal* 326(7379):13, 2003.

Cetta F, Lambert GH, Ros SP: Newborn chemical exposure from over-the-counter skin care products, *Clinical Pediatrics* 30(5):286–289, 1991.

*Children Act*, London, 1989, HMSO.

Conner GK: Genitourinary assessment. In Tappero EP, Honeyfield ME, editors: *Physical assessment of the newborn*, Petuluma, 2010, NICU Ink.

Crozier K, Macdonald SE: Effective skin-care regimes for term newborn infants: a structured literature review, *Evidence Based Midwifery* 8(4):128–135, 2009.

Davis GM, Bureau MA: Pulmonary and chest wall mechanics in the control of respiration in the newborn, *Clinical Perinatology* 14(3):551–579, 1987.

De-Wahl Granelli A, Wennergren M, Sandberg K, Mellander M, et al: Impact of pulse oximetry screening on the detection of duct dependent congenital heart disease: a Swedish prospective screening study in 39 821 newborns, *BMJ* 338:a3037, 2009.

Department of Health (DH): *Changing childbirth. Report of the Expert Maternity Group*, London, 1993, HMSO.

Department of Health (DH): *Reference guide to consent for examination or treatment*, London, 2001, DH.

Department of Health (DH): *Birth to five*, London, 2009, DH.

De Rooy L, Hawdon J: Nutritional factors that affect the postnatal metabolic adaptation of full-term small- and large-for-gestational-age infants, *Pediatrics* 109(3):e42, 2002.

Diamond DA, Gosalbez R: Neonatal urologic emergencies. In Walsh PC, Retik AB, Vaughan ED, et al, editors: *Campbell's urology*, ed 7, Philadelphia, 1998, WB Saunders, pp 1629–1654.

Dubowitz LM, Dubowitz V, Goldberg C: Clinical assessment of gestational age in the newborn infant, *Journal of Pediatrics* 77(1):1–10, 1970.

Habel A, Elhadi N, Sommerlad B, et al: Delayed detection of cleft palate: an audit of newborn examination, *Archives of Disease in Childhood* 91:238–240, 2006.

Hall DMB: *Health for all children. Report of the Third Joint Working Party on Child Health Surveillance*, Oxford, 1996, Oxford University Press.

Hall DMB: The role of the routine neonatal examination, *British Medical Journal* 318:619–620, 1999.

Harris TR: Physiologic principles. In Goldsmith J, Karotkin E, editors: *Assisted ventilation of the neonate*, ed 2, Philadelphia, 1988, WB Saunders.

Jokinen M: Measuring newborns: does size really matter? *RCM Midwives Journal* 5(5):186–187, 2002.

Keay AJ, Morgan DM: *Craig's care of the newly born infant*, ed 7, Edinburgh, 1982, Churchill Livingstone.

Kelnar JH, Harvey D, Simpson C: *The sick newborn baby*, London, 1995, Baillière Tindall.

Klaus MH, Kennell JH: *Maternal–infant bonding*, St Louis, 1976, Mosby.

Knowles R, Griebsch I, Dezateux C, et al: Newborn screening for congenital heart defects: a systematic review and cost-effectiveness analysis, *Health Technology Assessment* 9(44):1–152, 2005.

Lago P, Garetti E, Merazzi D, et al: Guidelines for procedural pain in the newborn, *Acta Paediatrica* 98:932–939, 2009.

Lavender T, Bedwell C, Tsekiri-O'Brien E, et al: Qualitative study exploring women's and health professionals' views of newborn bathing practices, *Evidence Based Midwifery* 7(4):112–121, 2009.

Levene M, Tudehope D: *Essentials of neonatal medicine*, Oxford, 1993, Blackwell Scientific.

Lissauer T, Fanaroff A: Gatrointestinal disorders. In: *Neonatology at a glance*, Oxford, 2008, Blackwell Publishing.

Ludington-Hoe SM, Cong X, Hashemi F, Infant crying: nature, physiologic consequences and select interventions, *Neonatal Network* 21(2):29–36, 2002.

Maternal and Child Health Research Consortium (MCHRC): *Confidential enquiry into stillbirths and deaths in infancy: 8th annual report*, London, 2001, MCHRC.

Maternity Services Advisory Committee: *Maternity care in action. Part 3: Postnatal care*, London, 1985, HMSO.

Matsuoka M, Segawa M, Higurashi M: The development of sleep and wakefulness cycle in early infancy and its relationship to feeding habits, *Tohoku Journal of Experimental Medicine* 165:147–154, 1991.

Michaelides S: Clinical assessment tool. In: *Neuro-behavioural physiological assessment of the newborn*, London, 2010, Middlesex University.

Milner AD, Vyas H: Lung expansion at birth, *Pediatrics* 101(6):879–886, 1982.

Moghal NE, Embleton N: Management of acute renal failure in the newborn, *Seminars in Fetal and Neonatal Medicine* 11(3):207–213, 2006.

Moore KL, Nelson AM: Transition to motherhood, *Journal of Obstetric, Gynecologic, and Neonatal Nursing* 32:465–477, 2003.

Moore KL, Persaud TVN: *The developing human: clinically oriented embryology*, ed 8, Philadelphia, 2007, Saunders.

Motohara K, Endo F, Matsuda I: Screening for late neonatal vitamin K deficiency by acarboxyprothrombin in dried blood spots, *Archives of Disease in Childhood* 62(4):370–375, 1987.

National Institute for Health and Clinical Excellence (NICE): *Routine postnatal care of women and their babies*, London, 2006, NICE.

Nugent JK: *A relationship-building approach to family centred care* at Enriching Early Parent–Infant Relationships Conference, London, 2004, Brazelton/JJP.

Nursing and Midwifery Council (NMC): *Midwives rules and standards*, London, 2004, NMC.

Nursing and Midwifery Council (NMC): *Record keeping: guidance for nurses and midwives*, London, 2009, NMC.

Orenstein SR: Gastroesophageal reflux, *Pediatrics in Review* 20:24–28, 1999.

Page M, Jeffery H: The role of gastro-oesophageal reflux in the aetiology of SIDS, *Early Human Development* 59:127–149, 2000.

Pridham K, Kosorok MR, Greer F, et al: The effects of prescribed versus ad libitum feedings and formula caloric density on premature infant dietary intake and weight gain, *Nursing Research* 48(2):86–93, 1999.

Reiner WG: Assignment of sex in neonates with ambiguous genitalia, *Current Opinion in Pediatrics* 11(4):363–365, 1999.

Remington JS, Klein JO: *Infectious diseases of the fetus and newborn infant*, ed 5, Philadelphia, 2000, WB Saunders.

Richards MPM: Possible effect of early separation on later development. In Brimblecombe FSW, Richards MPM, Roberton NRC, editors: *Early separation and special care nurseries*, London, 1978, SIMP/Heinemann Medical Books.

Roberton NRC, Rennie J: *A manual of neonatal intensive care*, London, 2001, Hodder Arnold.

Ross GS: Parental responses to infants in intensive care: a separation issue re-evaluation, *Clinics in Perinatology* 7:47–61, 1980.

Roth DA, Hildesheimer, M, Bardenstein S, et al: Preauricular skin tags and ear pits are associated with permanent hearing impairment in newborns, *Pediatrics* 122:e884, 2008.

Royal College of Midwives (RCM): *Examination of the Newborn: Learning Resource*, London, 2009, RCM.

Sewell MD, Rosendahl, K, Eastwood DM: Developmental dysplasia of the hip, *British Medical Journal* 339:b4454, 2009.

Silverstein FS, Jensen FE: Neonatal seizures, *Annals of Neurology* 62(2):112–120, 2007.

STEPS: *Baby hip health: a guide to hip development* (website). www.steps-charity.org.uk/downloads/BHHWBaby_Hip_Health_Booklet.pdf. 2004.

Stevens B, Johnston CC: Pain in the infant: theoretical and conceptual issues, *Maternal–Child Nursing Journal* 21(1):3–14, 1993.

Strang LB: Pulmonary circulation at birth. In: *Neonatal respiration*, *physiological and clinical studies*, Oxford, 1977, Blackwell Scientific, pp 111–137.

Taeusch WH, Ballard RA, Gleason CA: *Avery's diseases of the newborn*, Philadelphia, 2004, WB Saunders.

Tappero EP, Honeyfield ME, editors: *Physical assessment of the newborn*, Petuluma, 2010, NICU Ink.

Thomson M, Westreich R: Restriction of mother–infant contact in the immediate postnatal period. In Chalmers I, Enkin M, Keirse MJNC, editors: *Effective care in pregnancy and childbirth*, Oxford, 1989, Oxford University Press, p 1324.

Thummala MR, Raju TN, Langenberg P: Isolated single umbilical artery anomaly and the risk for congenital malformations: a meta analysis, *Journal of Pediatric Surgery* 33(4):580–585, 1988.

Walker GM, Neilson A, Young D, et al: Colour of bile vomiting in intestinal obstruction in the newborn: questionnaire study, *British Medical Journal* 332(7554):1363, 2006.

Walton S, Bedford H: Parents' use and views of the national standard Personal Child Health Record: a survey in two primary care trusts, *Child: Care, Health and Development* 33(6):744–748, 2007.

Wilkinson A: Infants and children. In Epstein O, de Bono DP, Perkin GD, et al, editors: *Clinical examination*, ed 2, St. Louis, 1997, Mosby.

Wong GA, King CM: Occupational allergic contact dermatitis from olive oil in pizza making, *Contact Dermatitis* 50:102–103, 2004.

United Kingdom Resuscitation Council: *Resuscitation at birth*, Newborn Life Support Provider Course Manual, London, 2006, Resuscitation Council UK.

UK National Screening Committee (UKNSC): *Child Health Sub-Group Report on Congenital Cataract* (website). www.nelh.nhs.uk. 2005.

UK National Screening Committee (UKNSC): *Newborn and infant physical examination programme* (website). http://newbornphysical.screening.nhs.uk/. 2008.

Zupan J, Garner P, Omari AAA: Topical umbilical cord care at birth, *Cochrane Database of Systematic Reviews* (3):CD001057, 2004.

Chapter |42|

# Thermoregulation

*Stephanie Michaelides*

## LEARNING OUTCOMES

After reading this chapter, you will be able to:

- describe the mechanisms of heat loss and identify examples of each
- define the appropriate and neutral thermal environment for the newborn infant
- identify signs and symptoms of cold stress
- describe methods of preventing and correcting hypothermia and hyperthermia
- include information and advice regarding thermoregulation in antenatal and parenting education.

## INTRODUCTION

Practitioners involved in the care of the newborn need to master the art of thermoregulation to support and maintain a suitable environment for the baby's wellbeing, achieve safe and competent practice, and provide information and advice for parents and other relevant persons involved in the baby's care.

No newborn baby can afford the effects of cold stress. Those least able to tolerate hypothermia include the late preterm and/or growth-restricted and ill babies. Maintenance of an optimal thermal environment, which studies have shown to influence growth and survival, is a vital part of neonatal care. There is a rich history underpinning thermoregulation, including different infant care practices and incubator development (see website).

## PHYSIOLOGY OF THERMOREGULATION

Information from temperature receptors distributed widely in many parts of the body is transmitted to:

- the hypothalamus, where autonomic responses are coordinated
- the cerebral cortex, for behavioural responses.

When the body temperature rises, the typical adult human autonomic response is peripheral vasodilatation and sweating to cool the skin; the behavioural response is to seek a cooler environment and remove clothing. When body temperature falls, the typical responses are peripheral vasoconstriction and shivering, the need to seek warmth and put on more clothing.

Normal thermoregulatory function ensures that over a wide range of ambient temperatures, body core temperature is controlled at a relatively stable level – generally between 36.5 °C and 37.5 °C (Blackburn 2007). The ambient temperature range over which normal body temperature is achieved with minimal activation of metabolic and evaporative process is called the *thermoneutral zone*. For a naked adult, this zone is between approximately 27 °C and 33 °C.

Deviations of body temperature may take three forms:

1. Heat gain exceeds heat loss despite compensatory reactions – body temperature rises → hyperthermia
2. Heat loss exceeds heat gain – temperature falls → hypothermia
3. Control mechanisms break down and temperature alters according to environmental factors. If the

rectal temperature rises above 40.8 °C or falls lower than 35.8 °C, there is increasing malfunction and risk of tissue damage and ultimately death.

## Fetal perspective

During pregnancy, the heat generated by the mother increases by 30–35%, thus the woman can be expected to have a temperature of 37.5 °C during pregnancy. This is due to the effect of progesterone on metabolism and the basal metabolic rate (BMR), leading to the mother's perception of being more comfortable in a cool environment. In the maternal system, there is an increase of four to seven times the cutaneous blood flow and activity of sweat glands.

Fetal temperature is tightly linked to the maternal temperature regulation and cannot be autonomously controlled by the fetus (the *heat clamp*). Fetal temperature is generally about 0.3–1.0 °C above maternal body temperature (Liebeman et al 2000) – usually 37.6–37.8 °C (Blackburn 2007, Polin & Fox 2004).

The placenta is an effective heat exchanger for the fetus, and thermoregulation is influenced by:

- fetal and placental metabolic activity
- thermal diffusion capacity of heat exchange within the placenta
- rates of blood flow in the placental and intervillous spaces (Asakura 2004).

Some fetal generated heat is dissipated into the amniotic fluid via the umbilical cord (Hartman & Bung 1999, Blackburn 2007). Heat transfer is facilitated by the maternal–fetal gradient, apparent when the mother is exposed to changes in temperature, either during exercise, illness or through environmental factors such as taking a sauna.

Unstable uterine temperature, especially in the embryological state, can cause teratogenic abnormalities in the newborn (Artal & O'Toole 2003). In these cases the gradient may be reversed or reduced, which can lead to the fetal temperature rising. Changes in fetal temperature tend to be slower than maternal changes, owing to the insulatory effects of the amniotic fluid (Blackburn 2007).

## Neonatal perspective

Thermoregulation is a critical physiological function in the neonate – closely linked to survival and health status. Birth precipitates the baby into a harsh and cold environment requiring major physiological adaptations and changes, including thermoregulatory independence. Newborn babies are less efficient than adults in the ability to thermoregulate.

The ability to generate heat depends on body mass and environmental heat loss, a large surface-area-to-mass ratio (about three times higher than in the adult) leading to difficulty in maintaining body temperature in a cold environment.

Babies with a low body mass are more at risk. Although full-term babies have control over peripheral vascular circulation equal to adults, the autonomic thermoregulatory responses are not fully developed. The healthy baby can increase basal heat production by 2.5 times in response to cold within 1–2 days of birth, though less so in the first 24 hours. Newborn babies are rarely able to shiver and the increased heat comes from the noradrenergic lipolysis of the brown fat deposits characteristic of the neonate and activation of specially adapted mitochondria in the brown fat to produce heat.

The most dangerous time for the newborn to lose heat is during the first 10–20 minutes of life. If measures are not taken to halt heat loss, the baby becomes *hypothermic* (temperature <36.5 °C) soon after birth. A premature or sick baby who becomes hypothermic will be at risk of developing health problems and of dying (CESDI 2003) but the chances of survival are greatly increased if the temperature stays above 36 °C. Birth should always take place in an environmental temperature above 25 °C.

*Hyperthermia* (temperature >37.5 °C) can occur and in extreme cases can cause death within the first 24 hours after birth. Hyperthermia increases the metabolic rate, leading to increased oxygen and glucose consumption plus water loss through evaporation. This causes hypoxia, metabolic acidosis and dehydration. A core temperature above 42 °C may lead to neurological damage (WHO 1994).

Hyperthermia can be caused by infection; it is not possible to distinguish between infection and environmental factors by measuring the body temperature or by clinical signs. Therefore, a temperature above 37.7 °C in the newborn is a deviation from normal and the baby must be urgently referred to the neonatologist for assessment, diagnosis and management.

### Internal and external gradients

The external and internal gradients are interdependent. The *internal gradient* is the temperature differential between the core of the body and the skin and results in the transfer of heat from within the body to its surface. This process relies on an effective and extensive blood flow in capillaries and venous plexi influenced by tissue insulation provided by subcutaneous fat and the convective movement of heat through the blood. Heat conduction is under sympathetic control that results in changes in the skin blood flow by vasoconstriction and vasodilatation.

In the neonate, heat loss through this gradient is increased because of the thinner layer of subcutaneous fat and larger surface-to-volume ratio than in the adult (Blackburn 2007).

The *external gradient* results in heat loss from the body surface to the environment – the rate of heat loss is directly proportional to the difference between the temperature of the skin and that of the environment.

Heat transfer by the external gradient is increased in the neonate because of an increased surface area and thermal transfer coefficient. The neonate maintains temperature by means of the external gradient, that is, temperature skin changes, whereas the adult uses the internal gradient. This is especially significant for the preterm baby, for whom the control and effects of changes in the environment temperature are more profound.

## Heat loss and gain

Babies at term are *homeotherms*; meaning having the ability to produce heat to maintain body temperature within a comparatively narrow range. The newborn cannot regulate body temperature as well as an adult can, and, when the environment becomes too cold or hot, is unable to respond and maintain temperature, therefore tolerating a limited range of environmental temperatures. Thermal stability improves gradually as the baby increases in weight and age.

There are four main routes of heat loss (Hammarlund & Sedin 1986):

1. *Evaporation:* heat loss through evaporation of water from the skin and respiratory tract; highest immediately following delivery and bathing, and reduced by:
   - drying baby's head after birth and following a bath
   - using a hat
   - removing wet towels quickly following birth
   - delaying bathing until the baby's temperature is stable and above 36.8°C.
2. *Convection:* heat loss to moving air or fluid around the neonate, and dependent on the difference between skin and air or fluid temperature; the amount of body surface exposed to the environment; and the speed of air or fluid movement. Heat loss can be prevented by:
   - increasing the birthing room temperature
   - keeping room temperature above 25°C when the baby is naked
   - covering the baby with a blanket.
3. *Radiation:* heat is radiated from the skin to surrounding colder solid objects, including windows or incubator walls. This is the predominant mode of heat loss after the first week of life in babies born before 28 weeks and in all other babies throughout the neonatal period. Heat loss can be prevented by:
   - keeping the baby away from windows and draughts.
4. *Conduction:* heat loss through contact with cold objects, including cold mattress, scales and radiograph plates (Avery et al 1994). Heat loss can be prevented by:
   - warming all surfaces that the baby is likely to come in contact with (resuscitaire, scales, bedding).

(See website for more information.)

*Insensible water loss* (that is, loss through the skin, urine, faeces and respiratory tract) may lead to significant heat loss – increased in preterm and low birthweight babies (Rutter 1985) because of the large ratio of surface area to body mass; limited subcutaneous fat; immature epidermal skin layer structure; and increased body water content. Risks rise in environments where insensible water loss is increased, as 0.58 kcal of heat is lost with each gram of water lost through evaporation (Hammarlund & Sedin 1986).

The appropriate temperature of a baby depends upon the baby's age, gestation and weight. If left wet and naked, the newborn infant cannot cope with environmental temperatures of less than 32°C. If a thermometer is not available in a room, the environment must be assessed through personal comfort – what appears very warm and uncomfortable for an adult dressed in thin clothes with short sleeves is likely to be appropriate for the newborn.

## Neonatal heat production

The hypothalamus and the autonomic and sympathetic nervous systems are important aspects of maintaining the temperature within narrow set limits of 36.5–37.5°C in the newborn (see website). Constant body temperature is achieved by a functioning neurological system balancing heat gain with heat loss effector systems.

In the newborn, heat production results from metabolic processes that generate energy by oxidative metabolism of glucose, fats and proteins. The organs that generate the greatest energy are the brain, heart and liver. To maintain a constant body temperature, heat *loss* from the surface of the body must equal heat *gain*.

In the baby, though the hypothalamus will receive cold alert messages from the skin, abdomen, spinal cord and internal organs, to regulate temperature stimuli from other areas of the body, the most sensitive receptors are contained within the trigeminal area of the face (Hackman 2001).

The responses of the skin surface are determined by:

- the skin temperature
- the rate and direction of temperature change
- the size of area stimulated.

In the human newborn, cooling of the skin has been shown to increase metabolic heat production without any change in the core temperature (Polin et al 2004).

Physical mechanisms include involuntary reactions, including shivering, and voluntary reactions involving muscular activity, through crying, restlessness and hyperactivity. These responses can be affected by anaesthetics, damage to the brain, muscle relaxants or sedative drugs.

The baby may generate heat by crying and become hyperactive when cold stress is severe enough to cause jitteriness, although shivering does not appear. If cold stress is not eliminated at this point, the baby may become extremely hypothermic, hypoglycaemic, hypoxic, acidotic and lethargic, and eventually death will ensue, caused by cold injury. The full-term baby can flex the body into the 'fetal' position, which provides some protection against cold stress, but the lack of muscle tone and flaccid posture of an immature or ill baby results in a higher heat loss. Babies can also reduce shunting of internal heat to body surfaces by constricting peripheral vessels.

*Chemical* or *non-shivering thermogenesis* is the process by which the neonate generates heat through an increase in the metabolic rate and through *brown adipose tissue (BAT)* metabolism. This process can be utilized by adults and neonates – in the adult the metabolic rate can be increased by about 10–15%, whereas the neonate can increase the metabolic rate by up to 100% (Cannon & Nedergaard 2004).

## Heat production and brown adipose tissue (BAT)

A cold-stressed baby depends primarily on mechanisms that cause chemical thermogenesis. Neonatal heat production is mainly through non-shivering thermogenesis. When the baby becomes hypothermic, noradrenaline and thyroid hormones are released, inducing lipolysis in brown fat. This process can be affected by pathological events, including hypoxia, acidosis and glycaemia.

Brown adipose tissue is believed to constitute 2–7% of the newborn's weight, depending on gestation and weight. Brown fat starts to be deposited in the fetus from 28 weeks' gestation (Blackburn 2007). The brown adipocyte is uniquely suited to its role in newborn thermogenesis and differs from white adipose tissue because it is capable of rapid metabolism, heat production and heat transfer to the peripheral circulation.

The total amount of heat produced in the neonate is unknown, but may be up to 100% of its requirements (Blackburn 2007). The sympathetic nervous system stimulates the adrenal gland to release adrenaline, increasing the metabolism of brown fat and catecholamines and releasing the required glucose. The thyroid gland is also stimulated by the pituitary to release thyroid-stimulating hormone, also producing thyroxine ($T_4$) – known to enhance heat production from BAT.

Heat production within BAT is not fully understood but it is known that BAT contains high concentrations of complex mitochondria, stored triglycerides, sympathetic nerve endings, and a rich capillary network to carry heat around the body. The presence of an uncoupling protein within the mitochondria of brown fat cells supports the combustion of fatty acids to produce heat.

BAT is especially prominent in the mammalian fetus, and anatomical distribution is important to its function. The largest mass of tissue envelops the kidneys and adrenal glands; smaller masses are present around the blood vessels and muscles in the neck and there are extensions of these deposits under the clavicles and into the axillae. Further extensions accompany the great vessels entering the thoracic inlet. The proximity of BAT to large blood vessels and vital vascular organs provides the ability for rapid transfer of heat to the circulation (Okken 1995, Polk 1988). The activation of BAT metabolism *only* occurs following birth. During intrauterine life, maternal prostaglandins and adenosine do not allow non-shivering thermogenesis to take place. With the clamping of the cord, this mechanism is blocked, enabling the hypothalamus to react to hypothermia (see website).

## Feeding

From birth, the baby requires water, glucose and certain electrolytes. Calories are utilized for growth and energy in order to maintain body temperature and metabolism. The method of feeding the neonate, whether orally, by nasogastric tube or intravenously, and the frequency and volume of feeds depend on gestational age and physical condition. When gastric feeds have to be delayed for days and certainly if for more than a week, as in a case of a baby with severe respiratory distress, parenteral nutrition is required to ensure adequate calorific intake. Milk contains far more calories than dextrose given intravenously or orally (Klaus & Fanaroff 2001).

## Drugs

Medication given to pregnant women can affect thermoregulation:

- *Analgesia in labour* (such as pethidine given intramuscularly or intravenously and the use of bupivacaine for epidurals) – causes maternal vasodilatation and heat loss, rendering the fetus vulnerable to heat loss after birth.
- *Tranquillizers, antidepressants* and *hypnotics* in large doses, and *general anaesthetics* and *muscle relaxants* during caesarean section – tend to affect the neonate's muscle activity, leading to flaccidity and a resulting hypothermia.
- *Babies of women addicted to drugs* are often hyperactive with a higher metabolic rate, which can upset the thermoregulatory balance – potentially leading to hyperthermia.

# THE ROLE OF THE MIDWIFE

## During pregnancy

Advice is provided regarding maintaining a stable temperature, especially during the first trimester of pregnancy when cell division and differentiation are ocurring. There is a higher risk of congenital fetal abnormalities in women who use a sauna, especially if this is a new activity to which the mother's physiology has not adapted (Artal & O'Toole 2003, Cohen 1987, Smith et al 1988, Tikkenhan & Heinonen 1991). Care should be taken with other activities, such as hectic exercise, which significantly increase the maternal temperature.

Many women complain of heat during their pregnancy. The midwife can offer realistic and practical advice, including wearing natural fabrics, such as cotton, thin wool, silk or linen, and having cool baths/showers. The midwife should also assess the woman's health, excluding infection and/or pyrexia, taking appropriate and swift action should either be identified.

## Labour and birth

Midwives' actions prior to labour and delivery determine the wellbeing of the newborn baby. This includes controlling the neonatal environment, ensuring that the delivery room (or home) is sufficiently warm. Monitoring and recording this 4-hourly is important. Attention must also be paid to the warmth of the towels used for wrapping the baby and other factors that may affect the neonate's wellbeing, and any deviations from normal must be acted upon. A raised temperature may be an indication of infection or maternal ketosis (see Ch. 36) and may have implications for mother, fetus and neonate.

### Waterbirth

Warm water as pain relief during labour and for giving birth is increasingly being chosen by women and it is believed that warm water can improve uterine perfusion and uterine contractions, leading to a less painful birth.

The temperature of the water must be comfortable for the woman and should not rise above 37°C as this may cause hypotension in the woman and reduced blood flow to the fetus. Therefore, water temperature should be frequently measured and recorded. When the baby is delivered in warm water it is believed that breathing will not be initiated until the baby's head is lifted above the water. If the baby is asphyxiated or the water cold, then the baby may inhale some pool water (Gilbert & Tookey 1999).

### Delivery room

Whether in home or in hospital, the midwife should ensure that all professionals, and the woman and her family, understand the importance of the birthing room being warm (temperature at 25–28°C) and free from draughts caused by open windows, doors or fans. It is also helpful to discuss skin-to-skin contact for warmth after delivery, with the parents (RCM 2008, RCM 2010).

It is good practice to record the temperature of the birthing room in maternal and neonatal notes (WHO 1997).

The midwife should prepare warmed soft towels, blankets and baby clothing (including a hat) by using the radiant heater of the resuscitaire, radiator, or warming pad. If there is a clean microwave oven available, this can be used to warm clothes quickly. Blankets should be warm but not hot enough to cause any trauma to the neonate.

Prior to the birth, the cleaned resuscitaire is prepared – putting the radiant heater on pre-warmed mode, and heating sheets and blankets. Portable/transport incubators must always be fully charged and heated, with additional warmed blankets, ready to go at short notice.

### Risk factors in labour

The following aspects may lead to neonatal hypothermia or hyperthermia:

- fetal hypoxia/distress
- maternal distress – resulting in pyrexia
- maternal infection resulting in pyrexia or hypothermia
- epidural anaesthesia
- substance abuse.

If the neonate is considered to be at high risk, the midwife needs to inform the paediatrician and the special care baby nursery staff before delivery.

## Initial newborn care

A knowledge of physiology increases understanding of the implications of the neonate being exposed to heat or cold stress and directs care needs.

The neonate's head (the largest surface area) should be dried by the midwife or possibly birth partner, as it enters the cooler birthing environment. A full-term baby's temperature may drop by 1–2°C within 30 minutes of birth if heat loss is not prevented (Fanaroff & Martin 2001).

As the neonate is born, he may, according to maternal wishes, be placed on the mother's abdomen – a source of heat and comfort to the newborn baby, and an effective method of preventing heat loss whatever gestation. The midwife dries the baby, discards the damp towel, then covers the baby with a fresh warm towel. A hat may be applied, while parents provide skin-to-skin contact to reduce heat loss (RCM 2008, RCM 2010, McCall et al 2008) (see website).

When using skin-to-skin contact, the baby can be placed upright, prone on the mother's (or father's) bare chest between the breasts, head turned to the side, wearing a nappy, a hat, and covered with a warm towel. Observations are maintained to ensure that the airway is clear, and both mother and baby are comfortable (Karlsson 1996, McCall 2008). Skin-to-skin contact can maintain warmth if the baby was born by lower caesarean section under epidural, enabling the baby to stablilize its heart and respiratory rate, and maintain temperature, more effectively than if the baby remained in a cot or under radiant heat.

Babies of less than 31 weeks' gestation will have inadequate keratinization of the skin, enabling evaporation of water and heat through the skin (Avery et al 1994). Some units place the baby up to the neck in a special plastic bag after being dried. This can be useful in preventing heat and fluid loss in babies born with a congenital abnormality, such as exomphalos (see Ch. 36). It is important to note that plastic bags are only used if the baby is nursed under a radiant heater.

Care given in the first hour of life is important to the physiological wellbeing of the newborn baby and equally important is the care he receives to remove fear, discomfort and pain from the environment in which he now finds himself. Supporting the woman to breastfeed her baby within the first hour of birth can provide the same human contact that the baby has known for the previous 40 weeks of gestation and enables the development of maternal–infant interaction (Lamb 1983, Moore et al 2007 ), as well as providing a high level of nutrients to the baby to maintain brown fat metabolism (see website).

## Bathing

The timing of the first bath has depended on the hospital culture and its carers as well as the wishes of the parents. Bathing babies soon after birth should be avoided. Babies are cleaned by drying with a warm towel and bathed at least 24 hours to 5 days later, to maintain temperature and also to minimise harm to the newborn skin.

Awareness of blood as a potential risk for hepatitis B virus and human immunodeficiency virus (HIV) transmission (Hudson 1992) has led to many hospitals encouraging staff to routinely bathe babies soon after birth to reduce exposure to blood-borne pathogens for healthcare workers and family members (Varda & Behnke 2000).

Midwives owe a duty of care to the newborn and should work towards individualized care to mother and baby. Care should be driven by the needs of the neonate and the mother, avoiding routine practice and 'care by the clock'. Bathing should not be undertaken unless the baby's temperature and wellbeing are stable (Bergström et al 2005). Premature babies may be unable to tolerate the additional oxygen and glucose demands of maintaining a temperature above 36.5°C and may become cold-stressed.

Prior to a bath, the midwife needs to consider factors including the reason for bathing and the current condition of the baby, and factors that may impact on the baby's individual response (Varda & Behnke 2000):

- history of maternal pyrexia during labour and following birth
- prolonged rupture of membranes, >24 hours
- polyhydramnios
- oligohydramnios
- maternal use of medication such as aspirin to decrease body temperature, diazepam, and antihypertensives such as magnesium sulphate
- maternal diabetes
- maternal use of illicit drugs
- fetal distress
- gestational age <38 weeks
- birthweight <2500 g
- Apgar scores of below 7 at 1 and 5 minutes
- evidence of respiratory disease.

### *Where*

Bathing the baby prior to transfer to the postnatal ward exposes the baby to a greater risk of hypothermia, as differences in air temperature from one area to another may be greater than a newly bathed baby can tolerate. If mother and baby remain in the same room (as in a home birth or birth centre), this is less likely.

### *When*

Nutrition takes priority over cleanliness. The mother should be supported to breastfeed as this will facilitate successful breastfeeding. Baseline observations need to be within normal criteria (see Ch. 41). Prior to bathing, the temperature should be 36.7°C or above. The baby's temperature should be monitored and recorded in the first few hours of life (Varda & Behnke 2000).

### *How*

The ambient temperature needs to be between 25°C and 28°C, to minimize evaporative, conductive, convective and radiant heat loss. The water temperature should be 36.7°C and a radiant heater should be available to increase the environmental air temperature. After the bath, the baby should be dressed appropriately and given to parents or placed in a warmed cot.

## Resuscitation

### *Home environment*

The area prepared for resuscitation must be warm. A changing mat can be used with a nest of warmed towels in which the baby is placed after being dried and the wet towel discarded. This can be achieved by the use of heat pads.

Resuscitaires have an overhead *radiant heater* which can work from three different settings:

- *Prewarm* – used prior to birth to warm the mattress and towels.
- *Manual mode* – heat output is manually set between 50–60% (a higher output than 60% may lead the baby to become overheated).
- *Baby mode/skin probe* – the temperature is controlled by a pre-set setting, usually 36.5°C.

Thermoregulation is a life-or-death issue to the premature infant and it has been recommended that 'all labour ward and paediatric staff should be trained in the thermal care of the infants at resuscitation' (CESDI 2003).

The moment the baby is placed on the resuscitaire and under the radiant heater, the midwife needs to put the setting to either manual or servocontrol. When servo-controlled baby mode is used, the temperature is set to 36.8 °C. A small area on the left side of the baby's abdomen is cleaned of vernix using a Mediswab, the silver side of the probe placed on the abdomen, and secured with a reflective disc. This protects the probe from the infrared heat source, ensuring that it does not overheat. Overheating may result in inaccurate information going to the computerized sensor, causing the baby to become hypothermic as the radiant heat source output is reduced. The probe must be monitored regularly to ensure that it remains attached properly and keeps the baby's temperature stable.

The baby should be positioned to ensure the whole of the body is under the heat – the baby may move down the table away from the radiant heater during resuscitation. It is also important not to occlude the radiant heat source.

Poor radiant heater use can lead to hyperthermia and dehydration, or hypothermia, which causes respiratory and metabolic acidosis, increasing the risk of morbidity and mortality.

Warm gel pads can be used to provide conductive heat gain and support thermoregulation when transferring the newborn from the labour ward to the neonatal intensive care unit (NICU).

### *Oxygen therapy*

Oxygen is cold and it is important when administered facially, that a flow of 1–2 litres only is used with the mask firmly over the baby's face, avoiding the whole face/head becoming cold. In some units, resuscitaires have humidifiers attached to them which replace fluid lost and also provide warmed oxygen.

The temperature should be recorded at 30 minutes of age in order to take appropriate action if heat is being lost rapidly (CESDI 2003).

## Examination of the newborn

Once the baby is given to the parents, they will often wish to uncover and examine him carefully from head to toe. As long as the room is maintained at 25–28 °C and the baby is dry, the parents can be left to get to know their newborn baby (UKSC 2008).

The midwife usually performs an examination of the neonate soon after birth and this requires a warm and draught-free environment as the baby is usually exposed (Fanaroff & Martin 2001). The more in-depth examination requires a safe surface area and will be undertaken with the baby naked, therefore it needs to be carried out under a radiant heater and on a firm mattress at the correct height (see Ch. 41).

A superficial examination can be performed whilst the baby is in his mother's or father's arms. This keeps the baby warm through the warmth of the parent's skin and provides an opportunity for the midwife to educate the parents about what is being looked for and why. This is a time for parents to wonder at the miracle that is their baby and for the midwife to assist in this and not to rush or bustle or make it seem an everyday episode.

### *Temperature*

Within a short time, the baby's temperature begins to adjust to the extrauterine environment. If the maternal temperature is 37.8 °C immediately following the birth, the neonate could be expected to reflect that and a temperature of 38.8 °C may be acceptable.

Using the rectal route for routine temperature measurement is no longer a justifiable procedure. Historically, this was carried out to confirm the patency of the anus (now examined visually by observing whether the anus is midline and patent – see Ch. 41).

Temperature is normally measured via the axilla. If the baby becomes cold, BAT begins to metabolize, which may give rise to a normal temperature reading, and/or the area of BAT concentration being warm. The baby must be assessed carefully, and rectal temperature assessment might be required.

## Transfer

On transfer from one environment to another, there is an increased risk of temperature loss in transit. Transferring the baby from the labour ward to the postnatal ward is best done by placing the baby next to the mother, covered loosely. If transported in the cot, the baby needs to be dressed appropriately, including a hat. If the woman has not brought clothes for the baby, the neonatal unit always has clothing which can be utilized.

The best method to transport *sick and premature babies* to the neonatal unit is to place the baby in a stable environment, such as the transport incubator, facilitating warmth, observation and care.

If accompanying a woman with an in-utero transfer, the midwife must be prepared for the birth and should have towels and space blankets available to minimize heat loss while in transit.

The ideal and safe environment to transfer a baby from home to hospital is by using the portable incubator to maintain a stable warm environment. If, however, one is not available the ambulance must be sufficiently warm to allow observation of colour and respiratory effort. If the baby has no breathing problems, skin-to-skin contact can be used to support thermoregulation.

The midwife should record the temperature before and after leaving one area for another, whether in the hospital or community. Cots must be placed away from draughts and large expanses of window.

## MONITORING AND MAINTAINING TEMPERATURE

### Monitoring

Mercury devices are gradually being replaced by *infrared electronic probes* or *electronic probes* and occasionally *tympanic thermometers*. Electronic and infrared thermometers predict the temperature within 60 seconds (Leick-Rude & Bloom 1998, Dè Curtis et al 2008). Servocontrol is used to reduce handling and maintain an automatic response to temperature changes in the baby.

The *rectal temperature* is one of the most accurate measurements. The rectum bends sharply to the right and the passing of the hard thermometer may potentially cause a perforation. The probe must be well lubricated with Vaseline or soft paraffin prior to insertion, and inserted no more than **3 cm** into the rectum of the term baby and no more than **2 cm** in the preterm (Blackburn 2007, Fleming et al 1983). Stool in the rectum can influence the accuracy of readings.

Core temperature drops only when the baby's effort to produce heat has failed. A rectal temperature in the normal range does not therefore mean no cold stress; it may mean that the baby has activated brown fat metabolism and is producing chemical heat to maintain its temperature. This is achieved as the hypothalamus recognizes a temperature of less than 36.0 °C and switches on the 'central heating' in the form of non-shivering thermogenesis. The cause of the hypothermia needs to be isolated and removed prior to the baby utilizing brown fat stores and becoming cold-stressed and sick.

Temperature is now measured in the axilla, which contains a large area of brown fat tissue which, when non-shivering thermogenesis takes place, releases chemical energy, causing the area to become warmer than core temperature. Therefore, the reading will be higher than the core in a hypothermic baby (Bliss-Holtz 1991), up to 0.49 °C from the core temperature providing a false positive result, making it difficult to recognize hypothermia. Following positioning of the probe (see Fig. 42.1), the arm is brought down and held firmly against the body, which encloses the probe to avoid inaccurate results being recorded. Midwives must assess the temperature of the individual baby through behavioural and physiological signs and symptoms of cold stress. If the routine practice is to take axillary temperature, it does not preclude the midwife taking a rectal reading if the baby is assessed to be in danger of being hypothermic.

*Tactile reading/human touch* can validate the reading given by the axillary site. Comparing the abdominal temperature, which is representative of the core temperature, with the extremities, can identify a cold baby. Warm, pink feet and abdomen indicate that the baby is in thermal comfort. Cold feet and warm trunk indicates that the baby is in cold stress.

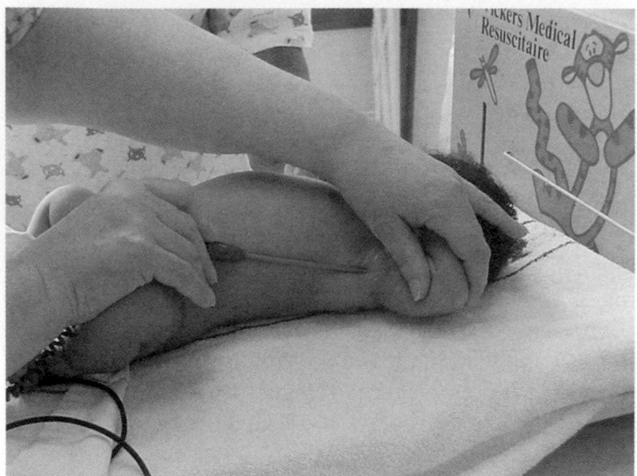


**Figure 42.1** Correct measurement of temperature via the axilla.

In *hypothermia* the feet and trunk are cold to touch (WHO 1997). If the feet are red and hot, face flushed and the baby restless, the baby could be overheated.

The use of the *inguinal site* may be useful as there is a good blood flow and no brown adipose tissue to confuse readings, but research has yet to validate it as an accurate means of monitoring temperature in the newborn.

*Tympanic temperature* appears to be an excellent and accurate way to take the temperature of children and adults but is *less accurate* for newborn babies. To obtain an accurate reading, the infrared probe must be small enough to be inserted deeply into the meatus to allow orientation of the sensor against the tympanic membrane. This may be achieved if the pinna is supported to straighten the ear canal (Craig et al 2002).

The majority of babies maintain their temperature well but there are times when parents become concerned about their baby and need to be taught a safe method to assess their baby's temperature in order to detect hypothermia or hyperthermia early. This can be done by using a thermometer or by feeling the baby's skin (touch assessment) and observing other signs.

Another non-invasive method for taking the temperature of the baby is the *Thermospot* – a 12-mm sticky black disc that changes to a 'smiley' face when the reading is complete. Parents are asked to place this high in the axilla or over the liver area in the epigastrium. This is not reliable if the temperature of the baby is below 35.5 °C (Morley & Blumenthal 2000).

### Maintaining temperature

The mother is a great source of heat for the baby when the baby is held in her arms. The midwife should encourage the mother to hold her baby close to her body to promote warmth and also engender a greater sense of intimacy. This method of maintaining temperature was investigated in a study at the Hammersmith Hospital in 1987, earning the term *kangaroo care,* also known as *skin-to-skin care,* and often used for very small neonates (Whitelaw et al 1988). A similar approach to care was used in a study in Colombia, in which very preterm and small-for-gestational-age babies were nursed inside their mothers' clothing between their breasts (Sleath 1985). There was a 95% survival rate for babies of 500–2000 g; improved rate of breastfeeding and closer maternal–baby interaction. Similar good outcomes have been found using the same approach in London.

Babies requiring surgery have particular needs which must be assessed according to the reason for and type of surgery (see website).

## MINIMIZING THE RISKS OF HYPOTHERMIA

### Wrapping and swaddling

Warm towels or blankets and clothing for the baby are essential; however, tight swaddling which restricts movement may have a detrimental effect on thermoregulation and respiration during sleep and is discouraged, especially for a baby left in a cot.

When placing the *very premature baby* under the radiant heater, the baby is usually placed into the plastic bag wet, as this minimizes water and heat loss through evaporation (Laptook & Watkinson 2008).

### Hats and clothes

The use of hats for the newborn, especially for those that are small for gestational age and preterm, and babies who are being resuscitated, has proven effective in reducing heat loss from the largest surface area of the baby.

The midwife should ensure that babies' clothing is of natural fabrics and not too close-fitting. It is better to use several layers of thin clothing rather than one or two thick layers. The midwife needs also to ensure that there are no loose threads which may become wrapped around the neonate's fingers or toes, as these can cause considerable trauma if not discovered quickly.

### Bathing

Bathing the baby cleanses and provides an opportunity to assess and validate the baby's wellbeing by observing physiological behavioural patterns, and is an excellent time for baby and family to interact (Karl 1999). This may be viewed by some midwives as a time-consuming or mundane task, better delegated to a healthcare support worker. If midwives delegate this, they must ensure that the person providing care is able to assess the wellbeing of the baby prior to the bath, provide information and advice at an appropriate level to the parents and provide a report back on the baby's wellbeing. Throughout the bath, wellbeing should be assessed following the cues the baby is providing and these should be pointed out to the mother (see Ch. 41).

### Parent education

Educating parents in the care of their babies at home includes giving advice on suitable clothing for the baby in terms of material and the number of layers required to maintain both heat and ventilation. A checklist can be useful for educating parents of small babies going home, which includes practical advice on helping babies keep warm indoors and outdoors (see website for information leaflet). This information should be translated into appropriate language for those whose first language is not English, particularly for those who have little knowledge of newborn care in the UK climate.

Social workers can be mobilized in circumstances where financial help is needed to assist with heating bills and adequate home insulation or ventilation.

## THE SICK NEONATE

### Hypothermia

Hypothermia is a temperature less than 36.5 °C. The baby is more at risk of becoming hypothermic during the first 12 hours following birth, though it can occur at other times during the neonatal period.

Signs and symptoms of cold stress initially:

- are non-specific
- may indicate other severe diseases
- may be confused with bacterial infection
- include decreased sucking ability and impaired feeding (leading to decreased heat production due to reduced energy intake).

As the body temperature continues to decrease, the baby features:

- less activity
- lethargy
- hypotonia
- increasingly weak cry
- shallow and slow respiration
- decreased heart rate.

If not addressed at this point, the baby will develop *sclerema,* which is hardening of the skin, and the face and extremities become red, giving a superficial impression of healthy rosiness.

As the baby utilizes oxygen to metabolize brown fat, it reaches its limit, and as there may already be hypoxia, this leads to impaired cardiac function and haemorrhage (especially pulmonary). Cellular function switches from

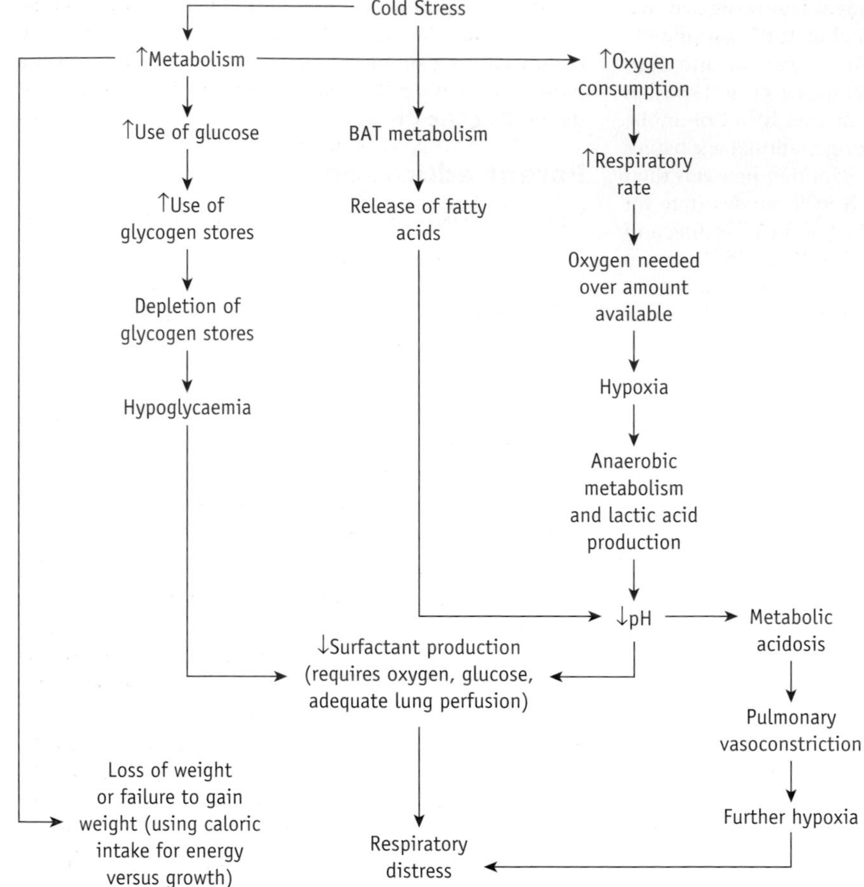


**Figure 42.2** Physiological consequences of cold stress. BAT, brown adipose tissue. *(From Blackburn 2007:718.)*

*aerobic* to *anaerobic metabolism*, leading to the production of lactic acid and metabolic acidosis (Fig. 42.2). Hypoglycaemia can also cause acidosis, and as the brain does not tolerate lack of glucose, neurological damage can occur. If severe cold stress is not treated, the baby develops kernicterus and clotting disorders and dies (Blackburn 2007, Rennie 2005).

## Management

There is no general agreement on the management of hypothermia but prevention is the best treatment. Rewarming the mildly hypothermic neonate is not problematic but debate continues about the virtues of *rapid* versus *slow* rewarming and their respective advantages and disadvantages in severe cold stress. Slow rewarming is the usual practice.

### Moderate hypothermia (temperature 32–35.9°C)

The baby is placed clothed, but not covered, under a radiant heater or in an incubator set at a temperature of 35–36°C. Alternatively, the baby can be warmed using a gel- or water-filled mattress set at 36.5°C, with the room temperature set at 32–34°C.

In the home environment, if clinically stable, skin-to-skin contact with the mother in a room with a temperature of at least 25°C can be used.

### Severe cold stress

The main aim is to maintain a thermal environment in which the baby is not required to increase his/her basal metabolic rate. The baby is rewarmed slowly to avoid hypotension due to vasodilatation of the peripheral circulation and acidosis. Rapid rewarming may induce apnoea and cardiac failure. Because oxygen consumption is minimal with gradients of less than 1.5°C, incubator temperature is set at 1.5°C higher than the baby's core temperature and adjusted every 15–30 minutes. The baby must be naked to allow the heat from the incubator or radiant warmer to warm him. The baby should preferably not be fed gastrically, as hypothermia reduces evacuation of gastric contents and reduces peristalsis. Intravenous fluids ensure adequate fluid and glucose intake but it is important to warm all fluids given to the baby prior to administration.

## Hyperthermia

Hyperthermia is a temperature of more than 37.8 °C. This is less common in newborn care. Pyrexia may be due to excessive environmental temperatures; incubator overheating (or the greenhouse effect of an incubator in the sunlight); overdressing the baby; infection; dehydration; or a change in central control by drugs or cerebral damage.

As with cold stress, hyperthermia results in increased metabolism and oxygen consumption. It is important that the baby is cooled slowly. This means removing woollens or leaving the baby with only one blanket. Extreme measures, including leaving the baby in thin clothes or restricted bedding, must be avoided.

### Reversal of heat stress

The aim in reversing hyperthermia is to reduce metabolic heat production. The baby will attempt to assume an extended position, allowing heat loss via the external gradient to the environment, and to aid this process the baby should have most of his clothes removed. Damp-sponging babies is not recommended. This encourages rapid heat loss, which may then lead to cold stress and shock (Kenner et al 1993).

Once the cause of the hyperthermia has been corrected, the temperature should return to normal within 1 hour. If improvement is not noted within that hour and the baby remains pyrexial and looks unwell, infection must be excluded and brain damage needs to be investigated (Rennie 2005).

### Effects and signs of hyperthermia

Hyperthermia increases the metabolic rate and the evaporative water loss rate, which can cause dehydration. The baby is unable to fully utilize the mechanism of sweating to reduce heat. The exception is the baby born to a mother with substance abuse, when the baby may become sweaty and wet when stressed and hyperactive. In the normal term baby, the only area of the body on which sweating takes place is the head, and, in times of shock, the palm of the hands.

Signs of hyperthermia are not easily apparent, and include restlessness and crying. As a result of metabolic rate increases, there may be tachypnoea and tachycardia. The baby's face and extremities are red because of vasodilatation. This is a serious sign of hyperthermia and must be acted upon to reverse heat gain by isolating the cause. If this does not occur and the temperature rises above 42 °C, the baby will go into shock; convulsions and coma may occur.

As with hypothermia, the main cause of hyperthermic stress in the newborn is due to misinterpreting the environmental temperature and its effect on the baby. This can happen by leaving the baby in a closed car on a hot and sunny day; overdressing the baby on a cold day whilst inside; or putting the baby too close to a heat source.

**Reflective activity 42.1**

Review your local guidelines and protocols for thermoregulation, against national guidelines and your knowledge of physiology, and consider whether these provide sufficiently up-to-date, practical information.

## EQUIPMENT

Equipment must be used appropriately and with consideration of the thermoregulatory effect.

**Incubators.** These should be used only for those babies who are ill, likely to become ill, or less than the 9th centile. Modern incubators now have double walls to stop radiant heat loss. The air temperature can be controlled manually or automatically. Incubators and radiant warmers also have an automatic servocontrol skin probe attachment.

**The transport incubator.** This is more familiar to the neonatal nurse than to the midwife, and provides the means of transferring, monitoring and supporting the small or sick neonate. The midwife should, however, gain a basic understanding of this equipment and its use (see website).

**Heated mattress.** Two types of mattress are used:

- *gel filled:* which has heat-conducting properties and is surrounded by a soft film that does not irritate the baby's skin
- *water filled:* when used in the cot, it should have holes in the base as an emergency outlet in case there is an accidental slow leak.

See website.

**Phototherapy.** This can be delivered to the baby in an incubator, cot or open bassinet with a servocontrolled overhead radiant heating source. The neonate's temperature must be monitored via the axilla, and recorded 3–4 hourly, as the baby can become hyper- or hypothermic during this treatment.

**Heat shields.** Modern incubators have reduced the need for these, but, if used, they should be checked for cracks, ease of movement and safety. Heat shields should be used when nursing a baby naked in an incubator, as well as in other situations to prevent, or help treat, hypothermia.

**Oxygen therapy.** When given in percentages greater than 30%, it should be humidified and warmed. If given via an endotracheal tube, it should be given at body temperature.

If given via a head box, it should be at the same temperature as the incubator to avoid causing physiological confusion.

## CONCLUSION

Although a homeotherm in the true sense of the word, the neonate has higher heat and water losses than those of the adult, so a thermal environment that allows a minimal resting metabolic rate must be provided. Midwives should give special attention to the maintenance of a 'normal' temperature, particularly in the 'at-risk' neonate. An understanding of the physiology of temperature control, calorific intake and application to practice is vital so as to provide a safe transition to extrauterine life.

The midwife is a key practitioner in preparing, supporting and educating the mother and her family in thermoregulation, its impact on the baby, and deviations from normal.

### KEY POINTS

- Thermoregulation is a crucial part of ensuring neonatal wellbeing, regardless of gestation and risk factors.
- The midwife requires a high level of knowledge and understanding of applied physiology of thermoregulation in order to provide safe and effective care to the woman and her baby.
- Prevention and early identification of deviations from normal can prevent long-term morbidity and mortality.
- Hypothermia and hyperthermia may be caused by sepsis, cerebral malfunction or an inadequately stable thermal environment.
- The midwife oversees and controls the environment, and ensures the provision of a neutral thermal environment, contributing to preventing hypothermia and hyperthermia.
- An important part of the midwife's role is in educating and preparing parents and other professionals regarding the thermoregulatory needs of the neonate, and integrating this into a framework of care, allowing parents to learn more about their child.
- Appropriate and effective management of hypothermia and hyperthermia, and effective use of appropriate equipment and monitoring, will reduce long-term morbidity and mortality.

## REFERENCES


Artal R, O'Toole M: Guidelines of the American College of Obstetricians and Gynecologists for exercise during pregnancy and the postpartum period, *British Journal of Sports Medicine* 37:6–12, 2003.

Asakura H: Fetal and neonatal thermoregulation, *Journal of Nippon Medical School* 71(6):360–370, 2004.

Avery G, Fletcher MA, MacDonald MG: *Neonatology: pathophysiology and management of the newborn*, Philadelphia, 1994, Lippincott Williams and Wilkins.

Bergström A, Byaruhanga R, Okong P: The impact of newborn bathing on the prevalence of neonatal hypothermia in Uganda: a randomized, controlled trial, *Acta Paediatrica* 94(10):1462–1467, 2005.

Blackburn ST: *Maternal, fetal, & neonatal physiology: a clinical perspective*, ed 3, Philadelphia, 2007, Saunders.

Bliss-Holtz J: Determining cold stress in full term newborns through temperature site comparisons, *Scholarly Inquiry for Nursing Practice* 5(2):113–123, 1991.

Cannon B, Nedergaard J: Brown adipose tissue: function and physiological significance, *Physiological Reviews* 84:277–359, 2004.

Cohen FL: Neural tube defects: epidemiology, detection and prevention, *Journal of Obstetric, Gynecologic, and Neonatal Nursing* 16(2):105–115, 1987.

Confidential Enquiries into Stillbirth and Deaths in Infancy (CESDI): *Project 27/28. An enquiry into quality of care and its effect on the survival of babies born at 27–28 weeks*, London, 2003, The Stationery Office.

Craig J, Lancaster G, Taylor S, et al: Infrared ear thermometry compared with rectal thermometry in children: a systematic review, *The Lancet* 360(9333):603–609, 2002.

De Curtis M, Calzolari F, Marciano A, et al: Comparison between rectal and infrared skin temperature in the newborn, *Archives of Disease in Childhood. Fetal and Neonatal Edition* 93(1):F55–F57, 2008.

Fanaroff AA, Martin RJ: *Neonatal–perinatal medicine: diseases of the fetus and neonate*, St Louis, 2001, Mosby.

Fleming M, Hakansson H, Svenningsen NW: A disposable temperature probe for skin measurement in the newborn nursery, *International Journal of Nursing Studies* 10(2):89–96, 1983.

Gilbert RE, Tookey PA: Perinatal mortality and morbidity among babies in water: national surveillance study, *British Medical Journal* 319(7208):483–487, 1999.

Hackman PS: Recognizing and understanding the cold-stressed term infant, *Neonatal Network* 20(8):35–41, 2001.

Hammarlund K, Sedin G: Heat loss from the skin of preterm and full term newborn infants during the first weeks after birth, *Biology of the Neonate* 50(1):1–10, 1986.

Hartman S, Bung P: Physical training during pregnancy – physiological considerations and recommendations, *J Perinat Med* 27(3):204–215, 1999.

Hudson CN: HIV infection in obstetrics and gynaecology, *Baillière's Clinical Obstetrics and Gynaecology* 6(1):137–148, 1992.

Karl D: The interactive newborn bath: using infant neurobehavior to connect parents and newborns, *MCN. The American Journal of Maternal Child Nursing* 24(6):280–286, 1999.

Karlsson H: Skin to skin care: heat balance, *Archives of Disease in Childhood* 75(2):130–132, 1996.

Kenner C, Brueggemeyer A, Gunderson LP: *Comprehensive neonatal nursing: a physiologic perspective*, Philadelphia, 1993, WB Saunders.

Klaus MH, Fanaroff AA: *Care of the high-risk neonate*, ed 5, Philadelphia, 2001, WB Saunders.

Lamb ME: Early mother–neonate contact and mother child relationship, *Journal of Child Psychology and Psychiatry* 24(3):487–494, 1983.

Laptook AR, Watkinson M: Temperature management in the delivery room, *Seminars in Fetal & Neonatal Medicine* 13(6):383–391, 2008.

Leick-Rude MK, Bloom LE: A comparison of temperature taking methods in neonates, *Neonatal Network* 17(5):21–37, 1998.

Liebeman E, Lang J, Richardson DK, et al: Intrapartum maternal fever and neonatal outcome, *Pediatrics* 105(1):8–13, 2000.

McCall EM, Alderdice F, Halliday HL, et al: Interventions to prevent hypothermia at birth in preterm and/or low birthweight infants, *Cochrane Database of Systematic Reviews* (1):CD004210, 2008.

Moore ER, Anderson GC, Bergman N: Early skin-to-skin contact for mothers and their healthy newborn infants, *Cochrane Database of Systematic Reviews* (3):CD003519, 2007.

Morley D, Blumenthal I: A neonatal hypothermia indicator, *The Lancet* 355(9204):659–660, 2000.

Okken A: The concept of thermoregulation. In Okken A, Koch J, editors: *Thermoregulation of sick and low birth weight neonates*, Berlin, 1995, Springer-Verlag.

Polin RA, Fox WW, Abman S: *Fetal and neonatal physiology*, ed 3, 2 Vol set, Philadelphia, 2004, WB Saunders.

Polk DH: Thyroid hormone effects on neonatal thermogenesis, *Clinics in Perinatology* 12:151–156, 1988.

Rennie JM: *Roberton's textbook of neonatology*, ed 4, Edinburgh, 2005, Churchill Livingstone.

Royal College of Midwives (RCM): *Midwifery Practice Guidelines, 'Immediate Care of the Newborn'*, London, 2008, RCM. http://www.rcm.org.uk/college/standards-and-practice/practice-guidelines/

Royal College of Midwives (RCM): *Revealing the evidence behind the Magic of Touch*, London, 2010, RCM. http://www.rcm.org.uk/EasySiteWeb/getresource.axd?AssetID=128609&type=full&servicetype=Attachment

Rutter N: The evaporimeter and emotional sweating in the neonate, *Clinics in Perinatology* 12:63–77, 1985.

Sleath K: Lessons from Colombia, *Nursing Mirror* 160(14):14–16, 1985.

Smith M, Upfold J, Edwards M: The dangers of heat to the newborn, *Patient Management* 3:157–165, 1988.

Tikkenhan J, Heinonen O: Maternal hyperthermia during pregnancy and cardiovascular malformations in the offspring, *European Journal of Epidemiology* 7(6):628–635, 1991.

UK National Screening Committee (UKSC): *Newborn physical examination: physical examination of the newborn and 6-8 week old* (website). http://www.screening.nhs.uk/newborninfantphysical-england.

Varda KE, Behnke R: The effect of timing of initial bath on newborn's temperature, *Journal of Obstetric, Gynecologic, and Neonatal Nursing* 29(1):27–32, 2000.

Whitelaw A, Heisterkamp G, Sleath K, et al: Skin to skin contact for very low birthweight infants and their mothers, *Archives of Disease in Childhood* 63:1377–1381, 1988.

World Health Organization (WHO) Division of Reproductive Health, Maternal and Newborn Health/Safe Motherhood: Thermal protection and/or management of neonatal hypothermia and hyperthermia. Report of a technical working group. In: *Essential newborn care*, Geneva, 1994, WHO.

World Health Organization (WHO): *Thermal protection of the newborn: a practical guide*, Geneva, 1997, WHO.

Chapter |43|

# Infant feeding

*Belinda Ackerman*

## LEARNING OUTCOMES

At the end of this chapter, you will:

- understand the nutritional requirements of the normal term neonate, and the physiology of the neonatal digestive system
- be conversant with the anatomy and physiology of lactation, and its variants
- be aware of the importance of breastfeeding, including the advantages to both the woman and baby and the impact on their long-term health, and be proficient in its promotion
- be knowledgeable about artificial feeding
- have a clear understanding of the public health role of the midwife in infant feeding.

## INTRODUCTION

This chapter will present the anatomy and physiology of infant feeding, including the maternal breast and hormonal influences, neonatal nutritional needs, and identification of public health policies for breastfeeding. Whilst human milk is the superior food for the neonate and breastfeeding is recommended by the midwife, there are some women who will choose, for a variety of reasons, not to breastfeed. It is the midwife's role to facilitate a non-judgemental environment for discussing the woman's views and expectations around infant feeding, providing factual, unbiased, evidence-based information in order that an informed decision about infant feeding can be made. It is vital that women are educated in the principles of safe preparation and administration of artificial feeds should they be unable or choose not to breastfeed.

## GOLD STANDARD

Human milk is the gold standard for nutrition of the human infant (Lawrence & Lawrence 2005, NICE 2006). It contains unique constituents valuable for brain growth, such as cholesterol, omega-3 fatty acids and the amino acid taurine, together with immune properties that cannot be matched with any substitutes. It is the standard all health professionals should endeavour to achieve for the neonate, through the information given to women and their families.

In 1989, *Protecting, promoting and supporting breastfeeding: the special role of maternity services* (WHO/UNICEF 1989) was published. This was adopted as a global initiative by policy makers at a meeting in Florence, now referred to as the *Innocenti Declaration* (Henschel & Inch 1996). In June 1991, the Baby-Friendly Hospital Initiative (BFHI) was launched at the International Paediatric Association Conference, Ankara, providing a global focus for the intent of the Innocenti Declaration. The principles of the declaration were embodied in the 'Ten steps to successful breastfeeding' (Box 43.1), designed as a set of standards that can be followed by maternity units all over the world and audited to demonstrate measurable improvements.

The *UK Baby Friendly Initiative* (UK BFI), launched in 1994, is a programme of the UK Committee for UNICEF and aims to ensure that all mothers and babies receive the health and social benefits provided by breastfeeding. The UK BFI encourages and assesses hospitals to become 'baby friendly' by implementing the 'Ten steps'.

The WHO Global Strategy for Infant and Young Child Feeding, incorporating the UNICEF recommendations, was published in 2002. This document represented 2 years of evidence and all previous initiatives and statements

**Box 43.1 The ten steps to successful breastfeeding (WHO/UNICEF 1989)**

All providers of maternity services should:

1. Have a written breastfeeding policy that is routinely communicated to all healthcare staff.
2. Train all healthcare staff in the skills necessary to implement the breastfeeding policy.
3. Inform all pregnant women about the benefits and management of breastfeeding.
4. Help mothers initiate breastfeeding soon after birth.
5. Show mothers how to breastfeed and how to maintain lactation even if they are separated from their babies.
6. Give newborn infants no food or drink other than breast milk, unless medically indicated.
7. Practise rooming in, allowing mothers and infants to remain together 24 hours a day.
8. Encourage breastfeeding on demand.
9. Give no artificial teats or dummies to breastfeeding infants.
10. Foster the establishment of breastfeeding support groups and refer mothers to them on discharge from the hospital or clinic.

Institutions which fully implement all ten steps can apply to be assessed and accredited as 'baby friendly'. A first step towards accreditation is the Certificate of Commitment, which is awarded to units which implement steps 1, 7 and 10 and adopt an action plan to meet the requirements of the remaining steps.

calling on governments to fully support breastfeeding (WHO 2002).

## PUBLIC HEALTH ISSUES

The National Service Framework for Children, Young People and Maternity Services recommends all Trusts (hospitals) have minimum standards for breastfeeding, early access to support services and specialist advice (DH 2004a).

NICE postnatal guidelines specify that a written policy for breastfeeding must be available in all healthcare settings and communicated to all staff. A lead healthcare professional must be identified to ensure this is implemented, using the Baby Friendly Initiative as a minimum standard in an environment conducive to breastfeeding (NICE 2006).

*Maternity matters* (DH 2007a) sets out the DH Policy commitment to maternity services and includes the achievement of the Public Service Agreement (PSA) targets (DH 2007b), namely *'deliver an increase of 2% points per year in breastfeeding initiation rate, focusing especially on women from disadvantaged groups'*. Breastfeeding is a key factor in reducing childhood obesity (Cross Government Obesity Unit 2008, Von Kries et al 1999) and diabetes (CEMACE 2007).

**Box 43.2 Breastfeeding Manifesto Coalition objectives 2007**

1. Implement the Global Strategy for Infant and Young Child Feeding.
2. Implement postnatal care guidance from the National Institute for Health and Clinical Excellence and the accompanying Public Health Evidence into Practice document.
3. Improve training for health professionals.
4. Work with employers to create a supportive environment for breastfeeding mothers.
5. Develop policy and practice to support breastfeeding in public places.
6. Include breastfeeding education in the curriculum.
7. Adopt the World Health Organization International Code of Marketing of Breastmilk Substitutes and subsequent relevant resolutions.

A breastfeeding manifesto was launched in May 2007 by a coalition of 33 UK membership organizations, including all the main Royal Colleges, to improve awareness of the health benefits of breastfeeding and its role in reducing health inequalities across the UK (Breastfeeding Manifesto Coalition 2007). Its guiding principles were for women to feel enabled to initiate and continue breastfeeding for as long as they wish, supported to make informed choices about feeding and ensuring awareness of the significant benefits associated with breastfeeding. See Box 43.2.

As part of the drive to promote breastfeeding, a DVD was developed by *Best Beginnings*, supported by the DH. This illustrates women discussing the practicalities and benefits of breastfeeding, and is distributed to all pregnant women in the UK (Best Beginnings 2008).

The Healthcare Commission's review of the maternity services in England recommended Trusts pay particular attention to helping women from minority ethnic groups to maintain breastfeeding (Healthcare Commission 2008).

NICE guidelines on maternal and child nutrition recommend encouraging breastfeeding during the antenatal period and ensuring that women are taught positioning and attachment and to continue breastfeeding for at least 6 months (NICE 2008a).

The strategy for children and young people's health sets out how the DH will minimize health inequalities and cement the standards set through the National Service

Framework and *Every child matters* (DH 2009a). It focuses on expanding support for women antenatally and in the immediate postnatal period within Sure Start Children's Centres and on the reduction of obesity.

Midwives should expand their public health role in educating women and their families regarding the value of breastfeeding, and in encouraging women to breastfeed. They can reduce inequalities and social deprivation by working closely with health visitors (HVs) and those specialist nurses providing the Family Nurse Partnership Programme to support women who choose to breastfeed to continue to do so (DH 1999). A multidisciplinary and longsighted approach is required, in line with governments' public health strategies, that commences preconceptually, and develops and supports women during pregnancy and through into the first few months of the baby's life.

## THE FULL-TERM NEONATE – NUTRITIONAL REQUIREMENTS

Calorific requirements were based traditionally on volumes of formula required by artificially fed babies (Riordan 2008). The calorific requirement for term infants is thought to average 440 kJ per kilogram of body weight per day (110–120 kcal/kg/day) depending on gestational age (Blackburn 2007).

Breast milk (or infant formulae) contains approximately 275 kJ (65 kcal) per 100 mL (Blackburn 2007, Riordan 2008). A baby weighing 3.5 kg requires approximately 1540 kJ in 24 hours – about 525 mL of milk per day. This amount varies depending on the gestation and age of the baby, and volume and content will vary from feed to feed. A meta-analysis of the volume of milk secreted by exclusively breastfeeding women around the world found this to be constant at around 800 mL per day. The volume of milk transferred from the breast to the baby is less than 100 mL per day for the first 24–36 hours, gradually increasing to 500 mL from 36 hours (Neville 1999).

There is no evidence to suggest that healthy term infants require larger volumes of fluid any earlier than they are made available (RCM 2009). The low volume of colostrum is important for optimal physiological adaptation of the neonate, and health professionals need to appreciate that bioavailability of breast milk's 200 known constituents identifies its superiority over formula milk.

In human milk the calorific value is derived from the carbohydrate and fat content which is absorbed easily through the gut, while cows' milk has a higher proportion of protein which is less easily digestible. The content of breast milk changes throughout a feed and during the day and night, so can never be directly compared with cows' milk or formula milk (RCM 2009).

Midwives should be conversant with the relevant DH guidelines (Statutory Instrument 77 1995), information and position statements from the Scientific Advisory Committee on Nutrition (SACN) Subgroup on Maternal and Child Nutrition, its parent body, the Food Standards Agency (FSA), and the WHO Global Strategy on Infant and Young Child Nutrition (WHO 2002).

## PHYSIOLOGY OF THE GASTROINTESTINAL TRACT

The maturation of the neonatal gut is stimulated by initiation of feeding, milk composition, hormonal regulation and genetic encoding (Blackburn 2007). Initiation of early feeding is a major stimulus for the increase of plasma concentrations of peptide hormones, for example, *enteroglucagon*, which stimulates growth of the intestinal mucosa; *gastrin*, which stimulates growth of the gastric mucosa and exocrine pancreas; and *motilin* and *neurotensin*, which stimulate gut activity. Colostrum stimulates epithelial cell turnover and maturation. Epidermal growth factor and *cortisol* also assist in the growth and development of the neonatal gastrointestinal system. None of these are available in formula milk.

Breast milk aids the passage of meconium through the gut, whereas formula milk does not. Delayed passage of meconium is associated with elevated bilirubin levels owing to reabsorption of unconjugated bilirubin and recirculation to the liver; therefore, physiological jaundice may be problematic in formula-fed infants.

Until the baby is 9 months old, intake of formula milk stimulates a greater insulin response than intake of breast milk (Blackburn 2007), thus initiating an unnecessary increase in the metabolism of glucose stores.

One of the most notable actions is that of *secretory IgA*, which has important anti-toxic and anti-allergic properties, protecting the neonatal gut from bacteria, viruses and other harmful organisms, which cannot be replicated in artificial formulae.

## NORMAL NEONATAL METABOLISM

The immature neonatal exocrine pancreatic function is a major factor in the digestion of foods in the first few weeks of life. The neonate relies on alternative/additional means for digestion of proteins, carbohydrates and fats, and compensation occurs by use of enzymes in the saliva, intestine and breast milk.

*Protein digestion* in the neonate is disadvantaged owing to the limited production of gastric pepsin (a mere trace in some) with pancreatic enterokinase output less than 10% of adults. The ratio of whey to casein proteins in breast milk is more easily digested (Hamosh 1998, Xiao-Ming 2008).

Neonatal *carbohydrate digestion* relies on amylase in breast milk, which remains high during the first 6 weeks of lactation. Neonatal salivary amylase is only one-third of adult levels, while pancreatic amylase represents only 2.5–5% of adult levels.

*Fat digestion* has been shown to be greater in breastfed versus formula-fed preterm neonates (Hamosh 1998). Though the neonate has raised gastric lipase, there is reduced pancreatic lipase for fat digestion. This is compensated by the stimulus of suckling at the breast, stimulating secretion of lingual lipase in the neonate (Blackburn 2007).

Colostrum and breast milk are uniquely tailored to assist the neonate in independent metabolism and this should be explained to the woman.

## CONSTITUENTS OF COLOSTRUM AND BREAST MILK

*Colostrum* is produced from 16 weeks' gestation and continues for the first 3–4 days postpartum, until replaced by milk. It is a yellow-orange, thick sticky fluid that assumes its colour from beta-carotene (Lawrence & Lawrence 2005), with a lower calorific value than breast milk (approx 67 kcal/100 mL versus 75 kcal/100 mL for breast milk).

The daily volume ranges from 2 to 29 mL per feed, and protein, fat-soluble vitamins and mineral percentages are higher than in breast milk, with lower levels of carbohydrate and fat. It is unique in its high concentration of protective constituents – immunoglobulins, macrophages, lymphocytes, neutrophils, and mononuclear cells – giving it a higher protein content. The concentration of growth factors is up to five times higher in colostrum than in mature milk.

*Transitional breast milk* is produced between colostrum (from 3–4 days) and mature milk and lasts for approximately 10 days to 2 weeks postpartum (Lawrence & Lawrence 2005). During this time, protein and immunoglobulin levels decrease while carbohydrate and fat levels increase. Water-soluble vitamins increase and fat-soluble vitamins decrease.

*Mature breast milk* contains approximately 90% water with 10% proteins, carbohydrate and fats with vitamins and minerals. The main solid constituent is the fatty acid component that provides 50% of the calorific requirements. Fat content varies at and during each feed according to the neonate's requirement.

### Protein

Approximately 0.9% of breast milk is protein – the more easily digested whey and casein. The ratio is reported to be 9/1 to 6/4 whey/caseins at different lactating periods (Xiao-Ming 2008). Whey is an easily digested antioxidant and can act as an antihypertensive, anticancerous, antiviral, antibacterial and chelating agent (Xiao-Ming 2008). The main components are alpha-lactalbumin, beta-lactoglobulin, serum albumin, immunoglobulins, lactoferrin and lysozyme. Casein constitutes the smaller portion of the protein. In cows' milk, the protein content is reversed, with an approximately 80% casein to 20% whey ratio (Lawrence & Lawrence 2005). Out of the 20 amino acids present, eight are essential and provide the important nitrogen content required by the neonate. Two of the most abundant amino acids are cystine and taurine. Taurine is absent from cows' milk but plays an important role in brain maturation and is thought to function as a neurotransmitter. It was originally presumed to be involved only in conjugation of bile acids. Cystine is essential for somatic growth (Riordan 2008).

### Carbohydrates

Carbohydrates comprise mainly lactose with small quantities of oligosaccharides, galactose and fructose. Lactose increases calcium absorption and is readily metabolized into galactose and glucose (assisted by the intestinal enzyme lactase), providing the necessary energy to feed the growing brain (Riordan 2008). These levels remain constant and are unaffected in malnourished women (Lawrence & Lawrence 2005).

Some oligosaccharides promote the growth of *Lactobacillus bifidus*, which increases the acidity of the neonatal gut, protecting it from pathogenic invasion (Kunz et al 1999).

### Fats

The fat content varies at different times of the day and during a feed, with higher amounts towards the end of a feed (Kunz et al 1999). Preterm fat concentrations may be 30% higher (Riordan 2008), though others did not detect any major differences in lipid composition between term and preterm breast milk apart from more medium- and intermediate-chain fatty acids (Rodriguez-Palmero et al 1999). Long-chain polyunsaturated fatty acids (LCPUFA) are important for normal visual and brain development and are absent from formula milk. Addition of LCPUFA to formula milk in one very small study was found to improve IQ at 10 months of age (Williatts et al 1998).

The majority of LCPUFA are derived from maternal body stores rather than diet. Maternal diet may directly affect the fatty acid composition of breast milk (Kunz et al 1999, SACN 2007). Vegetarian women are able to maintain a high milk content of arachidonic acid (AA) and docosahexaenoic acid (DHA). DHA is the LCPUFA associated with improved visual and neurological function (Makrides et al 1995, SACN 2007).

Approximately 98% of the fat components are triglycerides that are broken down to fatty acids and glycerol by the enzyme lipase, found in breast milk itself. The remaining fats are phospholipids (0.7%), cholesterol (0.5%) and other lipolysis products. Digestion of triglycerides is initiated in the stomach, where gastric lipase commences lipolysis, and this is continued in the intestine by pancreatic lipase. The resulting monoglycerides have potent bactericidal properties and maintain infection control in the stomach and small intestine (Rodriguez-Palmero et al 1999).

## Vitamins

Water-soluble vitamins C (ascorbic acid), $B_1$ (thiamine), $B_2$ (riboflavin and niacin), $B_6$ (pyridoxine), folate (pteroylglutamic acid), $B_{12}$ (cobalamin), pantothenic acid and biotin are all present in breast milk. Only niacin and $B_{12}$ can be increased by maternal intake if found to be deficient (Rodriguez-Palmero et al 1999).

Fat-soluble vitamins A (retinol), beta-carotene (carotenoids), D (cholecalciferol), E (alpha-tocopherol) and K (phylloquinone) are all present in breast milk.

## Minerals

These include sodium, potassium, chloride, calcium, magnesium, phosphorus, free phosphate and sulphur. Citrate binds some minerals and is soluble in water, so is important though not a mineral. Trace elements such as iron, zinc, copper, manganese, selenium, iodine and fluorine are all present in breast milk, though the latter two are absent from colostrum (Rodriguez-Palmero et al 1999).

The uptake of iron in breast milk is facilitated by the high levels of lactose and vitamin C, enabling up to 70% of absorption to take place. Absorption of exogenous iron from formula milk is limited and can adversely affect the action of lactoferrin from breast milk in the gut if the woman is mixed-feeding (see Table 43.1).

Unabsorbed iron is a contributory factor to the increased incidence of gastroenteritis in formula-fed infants.

## Defence agents

See Table 43.1.

# ADVANTAGES OF BREASTFEEDING

## The normal neonate

The recommendation of 'exclusive' breastfeeding is promoted by the DH (Kramer & Kakuma 2006, NICE 2006, Shribman & Billingham 2009) and its value to the neonate is well documented by the WHO (WHO 2007) and on the NHS website (see website) and in other publications (Britton et al 2007, Horta et al 2007, Lawrence & Lawrence 2005, NHS Centre for Reviews and Dissemination 2000, NICE 2006, Riordan 2008).

Breastfeeding has beneficial effects on the psychological and physical wellbeing of mother and baby. The action of sucking at the breast helps to initiate production of saliva that increases absorption of carbohydrate and fat. Neonatal saliva contains amylase that assists in glucose absorption and lipase that increases uptake of fatty acids (Blackburn 2007). These enzymes will be reduced if the baby is preterm and unable to suckle, as tube-feeding bypasses this process, so it is important for the midwife to assist the woman to initiate suckling as soon as the reflex is present. In addition, pancreatic secretory trypsin inhibitor is a major motogenic and protective factor in human breast milk as its presence influences gut integrity and repair (Marchbank et al 2009).

Breast milk's immune properties have been specifically highlighted (AAP 2005, Hanson 1998a, Mannick & Udall 1996, Newman 1995, Orlando 1995). It provides protection from leukaemia (Davis 1998, Shu et al 1999); rotavirus infection (Newburg et al 1998); gastrointestinal infections (Dewey et al 1995, Golding et al 1997, Mannick & Udall 1996); respiratory tract infection (Lopez-Alarcon et al 1997, Repucci 1995); *Haemophilus influenzae* meningitis (Silfverdal et al 1999); urinary tract infection (Pisacane et al 1992); otitis media (Dewey et al 1995, Duncan et al 1993); and necrotizing enterocolitis (Lucas & Cole 1990). The Millenium Cohort Study estimated that a 53% reduction of re-admisssions of children to hospital with diarrhoea and lower respiratory tract infections could have been made if women exclusively breastfed for 6 months (Quigley et al 2007).

Other benefits include: improved motor/personal and social development (Michaelsen et al 2009, Wang & Su 1996); improved IQ (Florey et al 1995, Lucas et al 1992); and protection from non-insulin-dependent diabetes mellitus (Cavallo et al 1996, Chertok et al 2009, Drash et al 1994, Pettitt et al 1997); eczema, asthma, and food allergies (Coutts 1998, Hanson 1998b, Oddy 2009, Saarinen & Kajosaari 1995); and from cardiovascular disease in later life (Horta et al 2007, Leon & Ronalds 2009, Ravelli et al 2000).

Further benefits include possible protection from schizophrenia (McCreadie 1997); juvenile rheumatoid arthritis (Mason et al 1995); inflammatory bowel disease (Mikhailov & Furner 2008); Crohn's disease and coeliac disease (Hanson 1998a, Koletzko et al 1989); development of the physiological integrity of the oral cavity, ensuring alignment of teeth and fewer problems with malocclusions (Palmer 1998); and possible protection from sudden infant death (McVea et al 2000). The action of breastfeeding has beneficial effects on dental caries, and mouth and jaw development, and reduces the risk of childhood obesity (Arenz & Von Kries 2009, Horta et al 2007, O'Tierney et al 2009).

**Table 43.1 Defence agents in breast milk (Also see RCM 2009)**

| Substance and production | Action |
|---|---|
| **1. Antimicrobial agents** | |
| Immunoglobulins | |
| Neonate produces minimal amounts of these in the first few months of life | Proteins produced by plasma cells in response to an antigen – located in the lactoglobulin fraction of breast milk |
| Secretory IgA – most abundant immunoglobulin | Important in providing passive immunity<br>More resistant to proteolytic enzymes<br>Provides resistance to a range of pathogens in gastrointestinal and respiratory tracts<br>Neutralizes viruses and toxins from microorganisms such as *Escherichia coli*, *Salmonella*, *Clostridium difficile*, rotavirus and *Vibrio cholerae* (Riordan 2008) |
| IgG, IgM, IgD and IgE | These are other immunoglobulins found in breast milk in small amounts |
| Lactoferrin – an iron-binding glycoprotein | Competes with bacteria for iron, thus depriving bacteria of nutrients for proliferation<br>Enhances iron absorption in neonate's intestinal tract<br>An essential growth factor for B and T lymphocytes (Riordan 2008) |
| Lysozyme – a whey protein | Acts with peroxide and ascorbate to destroy Gram-positive and other bacteria in the gut and respiratory system<br>Increases progressively after 6 months' lactation |
| Bifidus factor – nitrogen-containing carbohydrate | Promotes growth of anaerobic lactobacilli in the neonatal gut, providing a protective acid medium (Riordan 2008) |
| $B_{12}$-binding protein | Deprives bacteria of vitamin $B_{12}$ |
| Oligosaccharides – carbohydrates (monosaccharides) | Act by blocking antigens from attaching to the epithelium of the gastrointestinal tract<br>Prevent the attachment of pneumococci (Riordan 2008) |
| Fatty acids | Disrupt membranes surrounding certain viruses and destroy them |
| Complement (C3 and C4 components) | Has the ability to fuse bacteria bound to a specific antibody and destroy them through lysis (Lawrence & Lawrence 2005) |
| Fibronectin | Facilitates the uptake of bacteria by mononuclear phagocytic cells |
| Mucins – protein and carbohydrate molecules | Adhere to bacteria and viruses (including HIV) and prevent them from attaching to mucosal surfaces (Lawrence & Lawrence 2005) |
| **2. Anti-inflammatory factors** | |
| Secretory IgA, lactoferrin and lysozyme | Multipurpose anti-inflammatory role<br>Lactoferrin inhibits the complement system and suppresses cytokine release from macrophages that have been stimulated by bacteria (Rodriguez-Palmero et al 1999) |
| Antioxidants (alpha-tocopherol, beta-carotene cystine, ascorbic acid) | Absorbed into the circulation and have systemic anti-inflammatory effects (Rodriguez-Palmero et al 1999) |
| Epithelial growth factors | Enhance maturation of the neonatal gut and limit entry of pathogens |
| Other anti-inflammatory factors include platelet-activating factor, antiproteases (alpha-antichymotrypsin and alpha-antitrypsin) and prostaglandins | |

Table 43.1 *(continued)*

| Substance and production | Action |
|---|---|
| **3. Immunomodulators** | |
| Nucleotides, cytokines and anti-idiotypic antibodies | Appear to promote development of the neonatal immune system |
| **4. Leucocytes (white blood cells)** | |
| Approximately 90% of leucocytes in breast milk are *neutrophils* and *macrophages* | Eliminate bacteria and fungi by phagocytosis |
| 80% of the *lymphocytes* are T cells, though the cytotoxic capacity of these cells is low | |

## The preterm neonate

Breastfeeding confers all of the above advantages and, because of the reduced capability of the immune system, is vital for early protection against infection. Preterm infants are particularly vulnerable to necrotizing enterocolitis, so it is very important that women are supported to breastfeed fully (Lucas & Cole 1990). Women who give birth prematurely provide perfectly balanced breast milk for their babies – the non-protein nitrogen content is 20% higher than in those who give birth at term, providing the necessary free amino acids essential for growth (Riordan 2008). Preterm breast milk contains higher concentrations of polymeric immunoglobulin A (pIgA), lactoferrin, lysozyme and epidermal growth factor. In addition, the numbers of macrophages, neutrophils and lymphocytes are higher in the colostrum (Xanthou 1998). Lingual lipases will be reduced if the baby is preterm and unable to suckle, as tube-feeding bypasses this process (see website).

## The woman

Breastfeeeding confers significant health benefits on women, such as protection against several cancers, including premenopausal breast (Lee 2003) and ovarian cancer, improved bone density and reduction of anaemia. It can also be an effective postpartum contraceptive during 'total' breastfeeding (WHO Task Force 1999), having the added advantage of delaying menstruation and reducing anaemia (Wang & Fraser 1994). (For more information, see website.)

# CONTRAINDICATIONS TO BREASTFEEDING

There are very few absolute contraindications to breastfeeding.

## Neonatal conditions (WHO/UNICEF 2009)

### Galactosaemia

A galactose-free formula must be given.

### Maple-syrup urine disease

A special formula that is free from leucine, isoleucine and valine is required

### Phenylketonuria

A phenylalanine-free formula must be given for a period of time, with possible breastfeeding later.

## Maternal conditions

### HIV

Breastfeeding should be avoided as part of a programme of interventions to reduce the risk of mother-to-child HIV transmission (DH 2004b, RCM 1998). WHO/UNICEF advise against breastfeeding if replacement feeding is acceptable, feasible, affordable, sustainable and safe (AFASS) as is the case in the UK and developed countries (WHO/UNICEF 2009).

However, exclusive breastfeeding for the first 4–6 months continues to be advised in 'resource-constrained' settings, such as in sub-Saharan Africa, where HIV transmission has been found to be reduced by exclusive breastfeeding in comparison with mixed feeding (Coovadia et al 2007, Gray & Saloojee 2008, WHO/UNICEF 2009, WHO/UNICEF/UNAIDS/UNFPA 2007).

## Drugs – maternal medication

Certain drugs pass through breast milk and may be harmful to the neonate, and temporary or permanent avoidance of breastfeeding may be recommended, depending on the prescription of drugs currently in use by the woman (for example, antipsychotic, anticarcinogenic, iodides, anti-epileptics). Midwives can update their knowledge using the most recent *British National Formulary* (BNF) or the local pharmacy drug information service within their Trust (see website).

### Substance misuse

Substances such as nicotine, alcohol, ecstasy, amphetamines and cocaine are known to have harmful effects on the baby through breast milk. Opioids, benzodiazepines and cannabis can all cause sedation in the mother and baby. Women should be asked to abstain and cease to breastfeed while under the influence of these substances (WHO/UNICEF 2009).

## Conditions where a woman can continue to breastfeed but health problems may be of concern

### Hepatitis B

The baby should be given a hepatitis B vaccine within the first 48 hours or as soon as possible thereafter (WHO/UNICEF 2009). The woman can continue breastfeeding.

### Hepatitis C

A small study of the breast milk of seropositive women indicated a very low risk of transmitting the virus to the baby (Zimmermann et al 1995). The advice is to continue breastfeeding.

## Pollutants in breast milk

A variety of pollutants in the environment may arise in breast milk, which should not prevent breastfeeding or its promotion, as breastfeeding itself offers a degree of protection against many pollutants.

The Committee on Toxicity of Chemicals in Food, Consumer Products and the Environment examined the high quantities of polychlorinated biphenyls (PCBs) and dioxins present in breast milk and concluded that the advantages of breastfeeding still outweighed the risks (Mitchell 1997). Intake of organochlorines measured in breast milk set against the WHO acceptable daily intakes failed to demonstrate an unacceptable intake for the baby (Quinsey et al 1996). Examination of the reported levels of the pesticide DDT in breast milk fat demonstrated a decline in most areas of the world (Smith 1999), and guidance on the implications of exposure to cadmium, lead and mercury resulted in encouragement of breastfeeding under 'most circumstances' (Abadin et al 1997).

# THE ROLE OF THE MIDWIFE

## Knowledge of breastfeeding

- Midwives must be aware of their own attitudes towards and beliefs about breastfeeding prior to advising others.
- In-depth knowledge of the anatomy and physiology of lactation is crucial in order to teach women the fundamentals of 'supply and demand' and the stages of breast milk production (BFI) (Blackburn 2007, Lawrence & Lawrence 2005, NICE 2006, 2008b, Riordan 2008).
- Midwives should use the framework set out in the *Ten steps to successful breastfeeding* (BFI) (see Box 43.1). This incorporates the responsibility for training *all* healthcare staff, ensuring there is a written breastfeeding policy in each unit. The subsequent community seven-point plan (BFI) (see Box 43.3) provides guidance to healthcare professionals in the community. It sets out the gold standard for care of breastfeeding mothers in the community and should

Box 43.3 **The seven-point plan for the protection, promotion and support of breastfeeding in community healthcare settings (UNICEF UK BFI 2001)**

All providers of community healthcare should:

1. Have a written breastfeeding policy that is routinely communicated to all healthcare staff.
2. Train all staff involved in the care of mothers and babies in the skills necessary to implement the policy.
3. Inform all pregnant women about the benefits and management of breastfeeding.
4. Support mothers to initiate and maintain breastfeeding.
5. Encourage exclusive and continued breastfeeding, with appropriately timed introduction of complementary foods.
6. Provide a welcoming atmosphere for breastfeeding families.
7. Promote cooperation between healthcare staff, breastfeeding support groups and the local community.

The seven-point plan is the result of a widespread consultation procedure involving health professionals, service providers, mother support groups, professional organizations and other interested parties. It therefore reflects consensus in the UK as to what constitutes best practice in the care for and support of breastfeeding mothers and babies by the community health services.

be followed by all midwives and trusts within the UK.

- Knowledge shared with women and families must be evidence based and linked to research as far as is possible. Where there is no research, this should be made explicit in the discussion in order to ensure informed decision-making (DH). Midwives require the skills and ability to share their knowledge on breastfeeding with enthusiasm (BFI).
- Midwives should be able to confidently promote breastfeeding for its public health benefits to the woman and baby (Horta et al 2007, NICE 2006, 2008b).
- Midwives need to recognize the value and importance of breastfeeding for both mother and baby. They must be able to give practical support and advice to the woman and be sensitive to cultural issues and traditions surrounding breastfeeding (Kroeger & Smith 2004, NICE 2006, 2008a).

See website for further information.

## ANATOMY OF THE BREAST

See Figure 43.1 and material on website.

## PHYSIOLOGY OF LACTATION

### Puberty to pregnancy (mammogenesis)

Oestrogen and growth hormone stimulate the growth of the mammary ducts during puberty. In the second half of the menstrual cycle, progesterone stimulates development of the lactiferous ducts and alveoli. Proliferation of the epithelial tissue is a gradual process at each menstrual cycle.

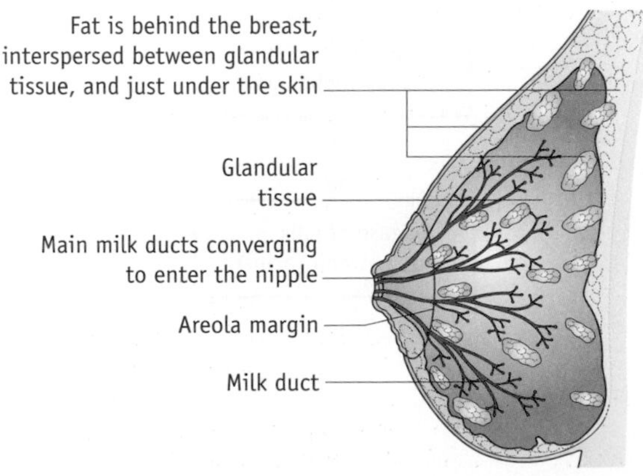


**Figure 43.1** Sagittal section of the breast.

*First trimester of pregnancy:* myoepithelial cells hypertrophy and blood vessels become more prominent under the influence of oestrogen, with a 50% increase in blood flow to the breast (Blackburn 2007).
*Second trimester:* secretion of colostrum is facilitated.
*Third trimester:* progesterone and human placental lactogen ensure that alveoli mature and milk begins to be produced. Progesterone circulates in high concentrations in pregnancy and prevents milk secretion until the birth takes place (Neville 1999).

Prolactin is a single-chain peptide hormone released from the anterior pituitary gland, and serum levels increase during pregnancy. It is thought to be essential for the development and final stages of the differentiation of the alveoli and ducts in pregnancy (Blackburn 2007, Neville 1999). Prolactin-inhibiting factor, produced by the hypothalamus, maintains low prolactin levels to prevent milk secretion in pregnancy.

Oxytocin is an octapeptide hormone produced in the hypothalamus and stored and secreted in the posterior pituitary gland (Blackburn 2007). It is produced in low levels during pregnancy (possibly due to the action of a placental enzyme). It stimulates electrical activity and muscle contractions in the myometrium during labour and is critical in the milk ejection reflex postpartum.

Other hormones, such as human placental lactogen (hPL), human chorionic gonadotrophin (hCG), growth hormone and adrenocorticotrophic hormone (ACTH), act synergistically with prolactin and progesterone to influence the growth of the glandular tissues of the alveoli to promote mammogenesis (Blackburn 2007). hPL assists in mobilization of free fatty acids and inhibition of peripheral glucose utilization and stimulates mammary growth. ACTH stimulates the adrenals to secrete corticosteroids.

### Initiation of lactation (lactogenesis)

Initiation of milk production involves a complex interaction of several hormones and factors. Following the birth, oestrogen and progesterone levels decline rapidly, allowing a rise in *prolactin* and *oxytocin* levels. Prolactin, released from the anterior pituitary gland, stimulates alveolar cells to produce milk while acting synergistically with growth hormone, insulin, cortisol, and thyrotrophin-releasing hormone (TRH) (Blackburn 2007).

Oxytocin stimulates contraction of the myoepithelial cells surrounding the alveoli, causing an ejection reflex, and milk is propelled down the lactiferous ducts to the ampulla.

The action required to stimulate both of these hormones is known as the *neurohormonal reflex* (or 'let-down' reflex). This stimulus is controlled by the effect of the neonate sucking at the breast, but may also be stimulated by the mother seeing, smelling, touching and hearing her baby.

Suckling stimulates prolactin release from the anterior pituitary gland, and therefore it is imperative that the midwife assists the woman to breastfeed as soon as possible after the birth. It is suggested that sucking movements reach a peak at 45 minutes and decline within 2–2.5 hours after the birth (Righard & Alade 1990, WHO/UNICEF 1989) in line with a physiological reduction in adrenaline levels (Widstrom et al 1990). Lack of 'priming' the alveolar prolactin receptor cells may result in shutdown and reduction of milk supply. Sensory nerve endings are activated in the nipple and areola area and this stimulates the hypothalamus via the spinal cord. As a result, oxytocin is released, prolactin-inhibiting factor is suppressed, and prolactin is released.

The levels of prolactin are increased towards the end of a feed, after approximately 20–30 minutes following a feed and at night, thus maintaining a diurnal increase (Blackburn 2007). The midwife needs to explain this to women so they understand that breastfeeding at night promotes and stimulates the production of prolactin for the next day and should be encouraged.

Prolactin release works on a *supply and demand* principle. When the baby suckles at the breast, prolactin-releasing factor is released by the hypothalamus and stimulates prolactin release from the anterior pituitary gland. When the baby stops suckling, a negative feedback *prolactin-inhibiting factor (PIF)* is released by the hypothalamus, usually by half an hour after a feed (Prentice et al 1989, Wilde et al 1995), and this inhibits prolactin supply (Fig. 43.2).

Prolactin-inhibiting factor (PIF) is a protein secreted in the breast milk itself which increases in amount as breast milk accumulates in the breast. Its function is to exert negative feedback to block future milk production when there is ineffective milk removal from the breast. Whilst prolactin and oxytocin are released systemically, therefore influencing milk production in both breasts, PIF build-up can occur in one breast, only affecting milk production in that breast. Therefore, if a baby is incorrectly attached and unable to effectively remove milk from the breast, the

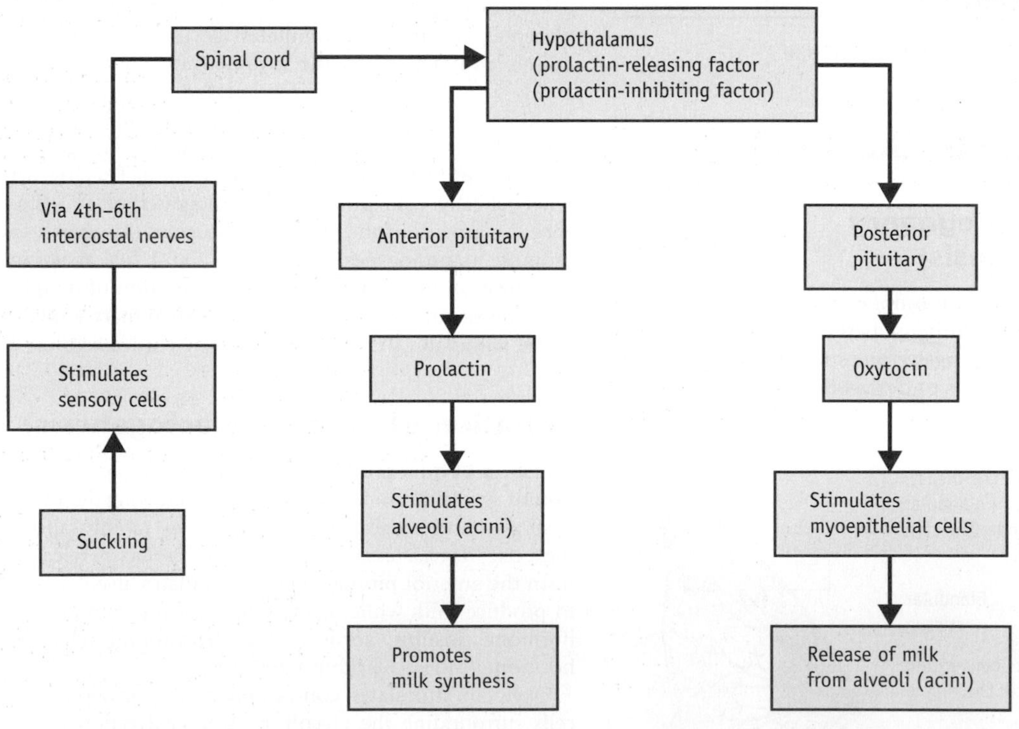


**Prolactin acts with:**
Growth hormone
Insulin
Cortisol
Thyrotrophin-releasing hormone

**Figure 43.2** Physiology of breastfeeding – overview (neurohormonal reflex).

build-up of PIF will ultimately result in a reduced milk supply. Milk production can be 'stepped up' again by effectively removing milk from the breast, thereby reducing the amount of circulating PIF in the breast milk.

Prolactin can be inhibited by oestrogen. A woman wishing to use oral contraception following the birth must be advised to take the 'progesterone-only' pill while she continues to breastfeed.

If the women 'complements' with formula milk following breastfeeds, the baby's suckling may be reduced at subsequent feeds, which ultimately interferes with the body's ability to produce the required amount of breast milk.

It is vital that the midwife discusses the physiology of lactation with the woman to dispel any fears or myths about breastfeeding.

## Maintenance of established lactation (galactopoiesis)

This phase is reliant on an intact hypothalamic–pituitary axis regulating prolactin and oxytocin levels and maintenance of frequent sucking and removal of milk by the neonate (Blackburn 2007). Growth hormone, corticosteroids, thyroxine and insulin continue to play an important part in maintaining established lactation.

The volume of milk produced commences at approximately 50 mL per day and increases to around 500 mL per day (double for twins) by 36 hours and up to 800 mL per day by 3 months (Neville 1999). Sodium and chloride levels in breast milk fall in the first few days, followed by an increase in lactose concentrations. Lactoferrin and secretory IgA rise immediately, then fall with the increase in volume in the first few days.

Regular suckling suppresses luteinizing hormone (LH) while follicle-stimulating hormone (FSH) may return to normal due to the pulsatile secretions of gonadotrophin-releasing hormone (GnRH) by 4 weeks postpartum (Neville 1999). This may have an impact on the woman's fertility.

## ASSISTING BREASTFEEDING

Midwives' contribution to the support and education of women in the antenatal and immediate postnatal period has an enormous effect on the woman's satisfaction, on breastfeeding success and on breastfeeding rates overall (NICE 2006, 2008b).

Additional support has a positive effect on the duration of breastfeeding (Britton et al 2007, Dyson et al 2005, Kramer & Kakuma 2006). This includes a range of activities, with face-to-face support in the antenatal and postnatal periods demonstrating the most positive effect 2 months postnatally.

**Early initiation of breastfeeding** It is important that skin-to-skin contact takes place in an unhurried environment for an unlimited period immediately (or as soon as possible) after delivery (Moore et al 2007, NICE 2006, WHO 2002). It increases the duration of breastfeeding, maternal–infant interaction, neonatal temperature, and glucose levels at 90 minutes, and reduces crying of the neonate (Moore et al 2007, NICE 2006). Separation of a woman and her baby within the first hour of birth for routine procedures should be avoided (NICE 2006).

The initiation of breastfeeding is increased and promoted by 'needs-based, one-to-one, informal education or support sessions, delivered either before or before and after the birth by a trained breastfeeding professional or peer counsellor' (Dyson et al 2005).

Midwives should ensure that they document and audit the timing and initiation of breastfeeding following all births.

**Positions for feeding and good attachment/latching-on** These have been cited as the key to successful breastfeeding (NICE 2006, 2008a). The midwife needs to provide the woman with simple, helpful advice on positioning and attachment. These two aspects of breastfeeding can cause major problems if they are not addressed from the birth.

Preparation of the mother is important, either sitting or lying down using cushions or pillows to support the back. Preparation of the baby so that he or she is unwrapped, with hands free (and mittens removed) enables the baby to experience touch, stimulating the neurological system and myelinization (Blackburn 2007).

*Positioning ('nose to nipple'):*

The baby is supported to face the mother, parallel to the mother's chest. The baby's neck (rather than head) should be supported enough to allow the head to extend backwards as necessary (Fig. 43.3A). The mother should then bring the baby's nose in line with her nipple and ensure the *rooting reflex* is triggered, causing the mouth to 'gape' (DH 2010a, NICE 2006, RCM 2002).

The consequences of ineffective suckling owing to poor attachment on the breast have been linked to 'failure to thrive' (Morton 1992) and early cessation of breastfeeding (Campbell 1997, Righard & Alade 1992).

Using a pacifier (dummy) can cause confusion and should be discouraged, as the baby is more likely to 'nipple-suck', leading to reduced milk production and breastfeeding (Koosha et al 2008, Neifert et al 1995, Righard & Alade 1992, UNICEF UK BFI 1998a).

**Attachment ('baby to breast')** The baby should be brought **up** to the breast quickly to ensure correct attachment, rather than the breast brought **down** to the baby, which encourages bad maternal posture and poor

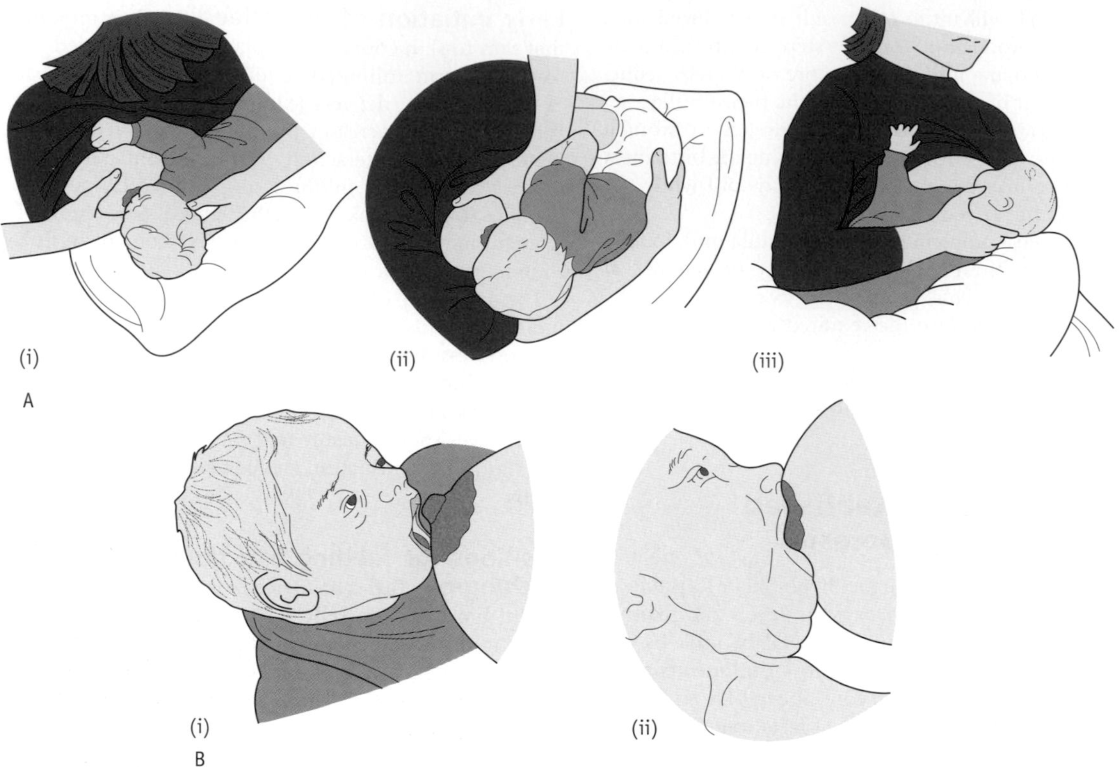


Figure 43.3 Breastfeeding. **A.** Positions. **B.** Attachment. *(From UNICEF UK BFI 1998b.)*

attachment. The baby approaches the breast leading with the chin, which enables use of the tongue and lower jaw (DH 2010a, NICE 2006).

When the baby is attached to the breast properly, 'his mouth is wide open and he has a big mouthful of breast; his chin is touching the breast; his bottom lip is curled back' (NICE 2006). The correctly attached baby will take long deep sucks with pauses, and the ear will be seen visibly moving during the process and audible swallowing is heard (Fig. 43.3B).

If the baby is attached correctly (Fig. 43.4) there should be no friction of the tongue or gum on the nipple and no movement of the breast tissue in and out of the baby's mouth (DH 2010a, RCM 2002). The midwife should share this knowledge with women and help to reduce the confusion that can occur from poor positioning, or if bottle feeds are given as a complement to breast milk.

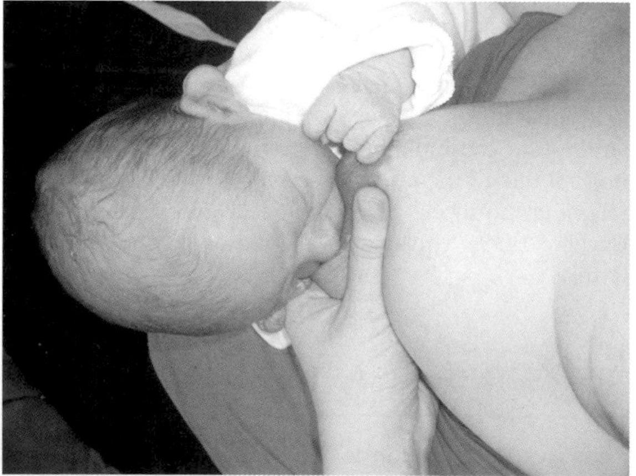

Figure 43.4 Breastfeeding.

**Expressing** Women should also be shown 'how to breastfeed and maintain lactation even if they should be separated from their infants' (NICE 2006). This includes providing information and advice on hand expression of their breast milk and storage of expressed breast milk (NICE 2006, WHO/UNICEF 1989). See Figures 43.5 and 43.6.

A Cochrane review on methods of expressing breast milk concluded there was no evidence that simultaneous pumping obtained more milk overall than sequential pumping (Becker et al 2008). However, assisting women to relax during pumping appeared to increase yield and ensuring the woman had a choice in the method of

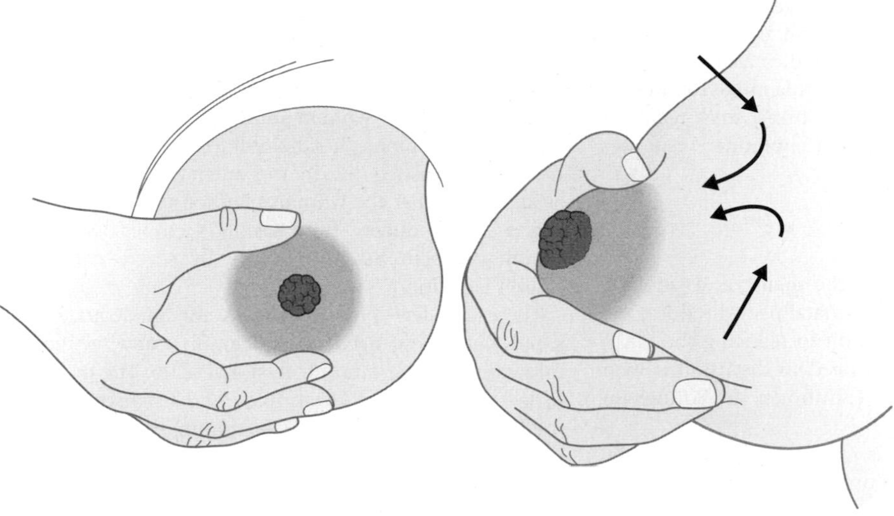

Figure 43.5 Hand-expressing breast milk. **A.** Technique 1. **B.** Technique 2. See Box 43.4 for explanatory text. *(From UNICEF UK BFI 1998b.)*

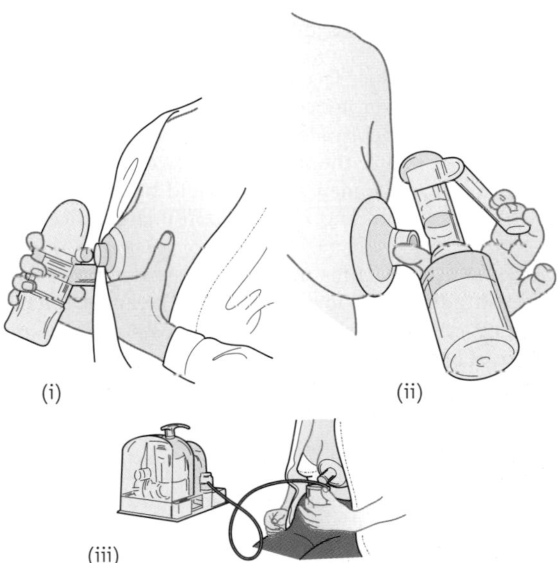


Figure 43.6 Handpumps and electric pumps. *(From UNICEF UK BFI 1998b.)*

pumping was important. The study stated that the effectiveness of the method of expressing was dependent on the reason for obtaining breast milk, for example, if the baby was in the neonatal unit (see website).

**Storage of breast milk** See website.

## Neonatal nutrition

The midwife must have adequate knowledge of the constituents of breast milk (RCM 2009). A term breastfed baby should have adequate nutrition through breastfeeding on demand. A preterm neonate (less than 37 completed weeks of gestation) or small-for-gestational-age baby will have different demands and the midwife should seek guidance from a neonatologist on frequency and volume of feeds, as this is outwith normal midwifery

Box 43.4 **Techniques for manual expression (UNICEF UK BFI 1998b)**

### Technique 1

1. Place your first finger under the breast, towards the edge of the areola, and your thumb on top of the breast opposite the first finger (Fig. 43.5A). If you have a large areola, you may need to bring your fingers in slightly. Your other fingers can be used to support the breast.
2. Gently compress the breast between the first finger and thumb.
3. Keep pressing and releasing, pressing and releasing. The milk will start to drip and then may spurt.
4. Press the areola in the same way all around the breast to make sure that the milk is expressed from all the lobes.

### Technique 2

1. Place your fingers in the same position as for technique 1.
2. Gently press your thumb and first finger back towards the chest wall as you press and release the breast tissue (Fig. 45.5B). This movement has been described as 'like easing a golf ball along a hosepipe'.

practice (NMC 2004). The advantages of breast milk for a preterm baby include protection and development of the immature gut due to antibodies and other substances that are not available in formula milk (Henderson et al 2007); and the fat content of breast milk regulates blood flow, blood clotting and immune responses (RCM 2009).

## Public health issues

*Smoking* carries higher risks for the infant, and smoking during pregnancy and in the postnatal period reduces the volume of breast milk in addition to reducing the birthweight of the baby. Midwives need to discuss this with women in early pregnancy (Shribman & Billingham 2009).

*Obesity* risk by school age is reduced by 20% if a baby is breastfed, according to the European Childhood Obesity Study Group (Koletzko et al 2009), and the Cross Government Obesity Unit Strategy recommends breastfeeding to reduce childhood obesity (Cross Government Obesity Unit 2008).

*Bed sharing* is not recommended, especially if the parents are heavy smokers, have drunk alcohol or have taken drugs that make them drowsy (DH 2009b). It is recommended that the baby is placed in its own cot after a feed and remains in the parents' room until at least 6 months of age.

*Maternal nutrition* during breastfeeding may vary according to cultural and religious differences, such as the use of 'hot' and 'cold' foods across cultures (Vincent 1999), vegetarianism and fasting.

The lactating woman should aim for a diet containing a minimum of 1800 kcal with a recommended average intake of at least 2200 kcal (Lawrence & Lawrence 2005). Women have enhanced metabolic efficiency due to hormonal influences during pregnancy and in the early postnatal period, which enables them to utilize their normal diet to produce an adequate milk supply for their baby.

Dietary restriction during lactation should be discouraged (Butte 2000) but midwives should be cautious about assuming that a poor diet will result in insufficient breast milk, which can undermine a woman's belief in her own body.

# COMMON PROBLEMS

## Insufficient milk

> *The most common cause for insufficient milk is poor attachment, ineffective milk removal and infrequent feeding*
>
> (Neifert 2004).

Women who have received continuous support are more likely to have a positive attitude to breastfeeding (Hillervik-Lindquist et al 1991). Lack of support and advice from the midwife, or immediate family and friends, can undermine the woman and lead to psychological and 'iatrogenic' problems. It is helpful for the midwife to have discussed breastfeeding in the antenatal period and be aware of whether the woman planned to breastfeed or if she is 'under duress' from family members. Stress can inhibit oxytocin but should not be severe enough to inhibit lactation (Powers 1999).

There are few physical causes for inadequate milk supply and these need to be identified and rectified by midwives and the multiprofessional team. The principles of the physiology of lactation should be discussed with the woman to ensure she is positioning the baby for adequate and frequent milk 'removal' (Powers 1999).

*Trauma* to the fetal skull during instrumental birth or difficult caesarean section can disrupt alignment of the fetal skull, cause damage to the cranial nerves and affect sucking and swallowing mechanisms (Kroeger & Smith 2004). This should gradually resolve over time with appropriate explanation, positioning advice and support.

*Certain drugs* reduce lactation (oral contraceptives containing oestrogen, bromocriptine, thiazide diuretics) and should therefore be avoided. Smoking and alcohol consumption can reduce the milk supply (Horta et al 1997, Mennella 1997). Women at risk should be identified in the antenatal period and offered appropriate advice and support.

*Anaemia* may affect the milk supply, shorten the length of breastfeeding, and lower the age of weaning (Henly et al 1995). Women who experienced postpartum haemorrhage of between 500 and 1500 mL were found to have insufficient milk supply, with infants showing failure to thrive (Willis & Livingstone 1995). Early review and treatment of such women is recommended.

*Breast surgery* may cause decreased milk production where the ducts have been severed, as in breast reduction (Neifert et al 1990). Surgery for breast enhancement involving silicone implants does not normally cause nerve and duct damage as the prosthesis is implanted beneath the pectoral muscle (Berlin 1994). The type of surgery should normally be identified by the midwife in the antenatal period and a plan of action documented.

*Nipple shields*, especially the non-silicone variety, prevent the neonate from applying the stimulus required for effective milk removal from the breast and may therefore reduce the milk supply.

*Medical disorders*, such as hyperthyroidism or hypothyroidism, can affect milk supply. Hypopituitarism (Sheehan syndrome) affects the supply of hormones from the anterior pituitary gland and therefore prevents prolactin production. All such medical conditions require prompt referral and investigation.

## Engorgement – venous/milk

Venous retention may occur because of the increase in blood and lymph circulation when the milk 'comes in', causing tenderness (Hill & Humenick 1994), but this should not be confused with 'engorgement'.

*Engorgement* of the breast is a pathological condition whereby oedema causes poor milk flow by constricting the milk ducts. This is caused by infrequent, ineffective milk removal and is preventable by good breastfeeding practices, including correct positioning and attachment. Secondary vascular and lymph stasis may occur (Hill & Humenick 1994).

Both milk and venous engorgement cause distension of the breast tissue, impeding the release of milk, and preventing the baby from 'latching on'. Engorgement may occur at any time during the first 2 weeks postpartum but is likely to peak at around the third to sixth day after delivery, or may occur following transfer home from hospital (Hill & Humenick 1994). It may last for 48 hours, during which time the woman will experience discomfort and is at risk from development of mastitis and subsequent breast abscess.

Warm flannels or a hot shower or bath may improve the milk flow by increasing the blood supply around the alveoli. Gentle hand (or pump) expression will help to release the milk flow and therefore the tension around the nipple and areola, in order to attach the baby more easily. If the baby is separated from the woman, then hand-expressing or a breast pump needs to be used regularly.

A Cochrane review reported that treatments using cold cabbage leaves or cabbage leaf extract, ultrasound versus a placebo, and oxytocin and cold packs had no demonstrable effect on the symptoms. Use of Danzen (serrapeptase – an anti-inflammatory agent) and bromelain/trypsin complex improved the overall symptoms compared to a placebo (Snowden et al 2002).

There is limited evidence surrounding the practical relief of engorgement. Midwives should be aware that it is imperative to prevent such a condition occurring in the first place, by providing advice and support with regard to correct positioning, flexible feeding arrangements, and completion of suckling on one breast at a time in order to ensure adequate milk removal (Renfrew et al 2000).

## Sore/cracked nipples

The most common cause of sore or cracked nipples is incorrect attachment – preventable by good midwifery support, education and advice (NICE 2006, RCM 2002, Renfrew et al 2000). Poor attachment and soreness are created as the neonate compresses the end of the nipple against the hard palate, causing damage, instead of taking the entire nipple in as far as the soft palate (NICE 2006).

Women with sore or cracked nipples are often prompted to wean their babies, as the pain can be unbearable. The psychological impact of nipple pain can cause high levels of emotional distress, and may affect the mother–child relationship, though both will resolve once the pain is removed (NICE 2006).

Problems in the neonate such as a short frenulum (ankyloglossia), or breast engorgement, should be identified by the midwife as these will create difficulties for the neonate in latching on (NICE 2005, 2006). See **Neonatal problems** below.

Occasionally, the woman may suffer from a condition known as *Raynaud's phenomenon* (see website).

Other conditions causing pain may present as eczema or psoriasis on the nipple or areola. Fungal infections, such as *Candida albicans* (thrush), can cause burning or shooting pain sensations, and need to be identified and treated with the appropriate medication (Amir et al 1996). Aggressive treatment with antibiotics to treat colonization of cracked nipples with *Staphyloccocus aureus* was found to improve healing and decrease the risk of developing mastitis in a randomized comparative study of 84 breastfeeding mothers in Canada (Livingstone & Stringer 1999). Midwives must be vigilant in identifying and screening for differential diagnoses rather than assuming conservative treatment is all that is required.

### Management

The midwife should assess and record the damage to the nipple for:

- location
- depth of tissue destruction
- size
- visible and non-visible characteristics of the wound
- appearance of the surrounding tissue.

Knowledge and application of current evidence-based practice reduces conflicting advice to women (Huml 1999).

Past methods including drying the nipples through exposure to air or using a hair-dryer are now known to cause scab formation and delayed healing by unnaturally drying the skin in an area that is normally moist (Inch & Fisher 2000). See website for further information.

Other suggested treatments using moisture though not demonstrating significant benefits include:

- application of teabags or warm water compresses (Lavergne 1997)
- USP-modified lanolin cream and water compresses or air (Pugh et al 1996)
- application of expressed breast milk – this uses the physiological knowledge of healing through growth and repair of skin cells but may attract yeast growth from the lactose content (Renfrew et al 2000).

The effectiveness of silicone nipple shields has been demonstrated in case studies and retrospective data following the establishment of the milk supply, but only as a last resort (Bodley & Powers 1996, Brigham 1996, Elliott 1996, Pessl 1996). They may cause a diminishing milk supply and exacerbate engorgement (Inch & Fisher 2000) so should be treated with caution and never used as a substitute for teaching correct attachment.

Treatments that have been proven to be **not** effective include chlorhexidine spray (Renfrew et al 2000) and other creams (Inch & Fisher 2000).

## Mastitis

Mastitis is an inflammatory condition of the breast which may or may not be accompanied by infection (Jones 2006).

Mastitis can be incorrectly diagnosed in the first few days but is usually caused by engorgement or milk stasis producing increased pressure in the alveoli due to non-removal of milk. The pressure builds up, forcing the milk out into the surrounding tissues.

Mastitis most commonly occurs in the second or third week postpartum (Jones 2006).

*Infective mastitis* is caused by bacterial invasion, usually via a cracked nipple. *Staphylococci* or *streptococci* are the most common organisms and these act on the milk forced outside the alveoli into the surrounding cells.

### Causes

- Most frequent is poor positioning and attachment, preventing adequate drainage of milk
- Tiredness and stress
- Initial engorgement with a blocked duct and pressure from a tight-fitting bra.

### Signs and symptoms

- 'Flu-like symptoms
- Pyrexia
- A reddened area appears around the infected breast or segment.

If left untreated, an abscess may form.

### Management

- Antibiotics
- If an abscess forms – drainage as appropriate (Jahanfar et al 2009).

The midwife's skill of preventing stasis of milk by advice on positioning, importance of emptying each breast, correct handling of the breasts and prevention of clothing restrictions will ensure good practice prevails, transmitting a positive public health message.

## Neonatal problems

### Tongue tie (ankyloglossia)

A short frenulum may present the neonate with difficulty in attaching and suckling at the breast. The tongue is unable to move forward and cup the nipple and thus stimulate release of milk from the breast. One of the first signs is sore nipples and poor weight gain due to lack of adequate milk supply, in spite of regular feeds (see website).

### Cleft lip and palate

Cleft lip and palate are congenital malformations characterized by incomplete fusing of the lip and upper jaw (Riordan 2008). This may involve the lip, or may extend to the soft and hard palate, and may be unilateral or bilateral (see website).

### Down (or Down's) syndrome

This congenital anomaly, characterized by heart defects, a protruding or large tongue and hypotonicity, can be challenging for breastfeeding. Manual expressing or pumping is often required because of inadequate stimulation of the let-down reflex by the baby.

The woman will need encouragement and advice for positioning the baby, with the emphasis on firm support of the breast and baby's head with use of pillows. Success of breastfeeding is most likely to be dictated by the severity of the cardiac abnormality, which will affect the respirations and tire the baby easily (Renfrew et al 2000).

## Breastfeeding the preterm baby

Breast milk is the optimum nutrition for the preterm infant (Henderson et al 2007). It provides additional immunity to the immature system, such as IgA, lactoferrin, lysozyme and oligosaccharides, stimulates maturation of the gastrointestinal tract and reduces necrotizing enterocolitis (RCM 2009). Different strategies, including expression and cup feeding, often need to be employed to support the development of breastfeeding. See website for more information.

## Twins and triplets

The Multiple Births Foundation produces a booklet for professionals and parents with advice and information on breastfeeding for multiples. This includes the importance of getting help and support for domestic chores as well as extra help for positioning the babies at each feed and especially at night. Cup feeding is suggested if the babies are born early (from 30 weeks' gestation) and are unable to feed at the breast initially (see Fig. 43.8).

## Going back to work

The current recommendation is for all babies to be exclusively breastfed for 6 months (WHO 2002). Many women need to return to work before this time and should be encouraged and supported by the midwife to continue breastfeeding before and after work, and to express either at work (dependent on facilities) or home and leave the expressed breast milk (EBM) with the childminder or carer. It is also useful to provide information on breastfeeding support groups and counsellors (see website).

There is no statutory right to paid breastfeeding breaks or a shorter working day in the UK but there is some legal protection under the health and safety laws – that is, the Management of Health and Safety at Work Regulations 1992 and the Employment Rights Act 1996 (Maternity Alliance 1999). If women work in the public sector, they are protected under European law. The Pregnant Workers Directive (1992) states: 'if your work affects your breastfeeding' the public sector employer must temporarily alter the working conditions and/or hours of work to protect breastfeeding or give alternative work (Maternity Alliance 1999).

## ARTIFICIAL FEEDING

The 2005 Infant Feeding Survey was the first time breastfeeding rates were provided for each separate country. Initial breastfeeding rates were 78% for England, 70% for Scotland, 67% for Wales and 63% in Northern Ireland (Bolling et al 2007). Highest incidences were found among women in the professional and managerial groups. By 6 weeks the breastfeeding rate across the UK had fallen to 48% and by 6 months only 25% were still breastfeeding.

The midwife needs to be conversant with the equipment and information for parents regarding artificial feeding (DH 2009c, 2009d, 2010b).

For information regarding constituents of artificial milk formula, see Westland & Crawley in *Infant Milks in the UK* table (RCM 2009).

### Reasons why some women may artificially feed their baby

Some women may be unable to breastfeed their baby if they have HIV or are taking certain drugs (see Contraindications to breastfeeding above). Other women may be unsupported by their families, be suffering from postnatal depression or post-traumatic stress disorder, or simply be subjected to 'peer' pressure to artificially feed their babies.

### Regulations surrounding infant formulae

Infant formulae are artificial feeds that are manufactured to take the place of human milk in providing a sole source of nutrition for the young infant. The essential composition of these formulae was set down as a Parliamentary Statute, or law, which came into force in March 1995 (Statutory Instrument 77 1995).

Midwives need to be aware of the WHO International Code of Marketing of Breastmilk Substitutes (WHO 1981), the aim of which is to ensure that infants receive safe and adequate nutrition, through the marketing and practices surrounding breast milk substitutes, advertising and donation of free samples or equipment directly to the general public.

The majority of infant formula brands can be divided into two groups: *whey* dominant and *casein* dominant. When whey is the dominant protein the whey:casein ratio is closer to that of human milk, as in 'first' milks (UNICEF UK BFI 2010). Casein-dominant formulae have a whey:casein ratio closer to that of cows' milk, as in 'follow-on' milks (RCM 2009, UNICEF UK BFI 2010).

### Types of feed available

Examples of formulae available in the UK for infant feeding are available (RCM 2009; and see website).

### Methods of artificial feeding

The most common method of feeding a term baby with formula milk is via the bottle (Fig. 43.7). There is a range of bottles to choose from and teats that mimic the shape of the nipple. The midwife needs to have a good

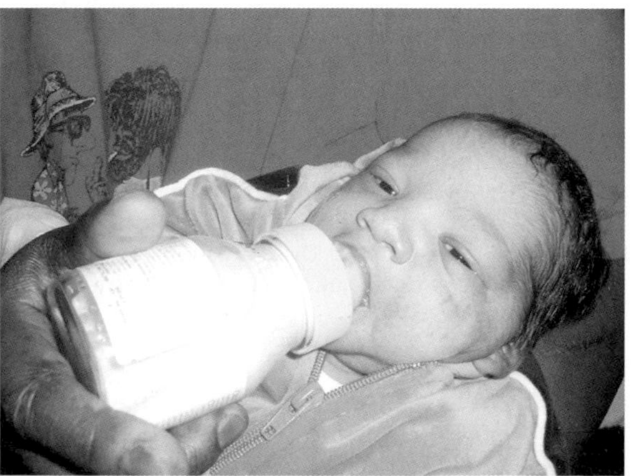

**Figure 43.7** Bottle-feeding.

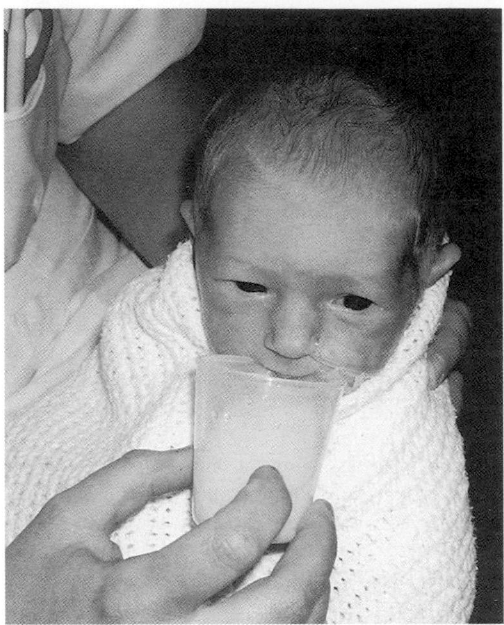

Figure 43.8 Cup-feeding. *(From Johnston et al 2003.)*

**Box 43.5 Risk factors for infections/disorders requiring hospital admission or medical treatment**

**Twice as likely**

- Respiratory infection
- Otitis media
- Atopic disease: eczema or a wheeze
- Diabetes mellitus: juvenile onset of insulin-dependent diabetes mellitus (IDDM)

**Five times more likely**

- Gastroenteritis
- Diarrhoea
- Urinary tract infection

**20 times more likely**

- Necrotizing enterocolitis (preterm babies, 30–36 weeks' gestation)

knowledge of how to teach women to make up feeds correctly (see Fig. 43.9).

### Other methods

For babies who required additional help in feeding, such as babies with feeding problems and preterm babies, there is a range of strategies, including the use of syringe feeding, cup-feeding (Fig. 43.8) and supplementary feeding. For more information, see website.

## Complementary/supplementary feeds

*Supplementary feeds* (breast milk replacements) and *complementary feeds* (breast milk substitutes) have no place in the care of a healthy term baby who is breastfeeding, as they interfere with the breastfeeding physiology (MIDIRS/NHS Centre for Reviews and Dissemination 1999). It is important that women understand the physiology of breastfeeding.

## Disadvantages of artificial feeding

Artificial feeding has been described as a risk behaviour (Minchin 2000). The scientific dangers of artificial feeding are well known amongst health professionals and the midwife should share the information with women before a decision is made to feed artificially. Babies who are artificially fed are at risk of several infections and disorders as shown in Box 43.5.

Other risks of bottle-feeding currently being researched include childhood lymphomas, inflammatory bowel disease, multiple sclerosis, dental occlusions, coronary heart disease, autoimmune thyroid disease, coeliac disease, Kawasaki disease, lower IQ, risk of sudden infant death syndrome, and obesity (MIDIRS/NHS Centre for Reviews and Dissemination 1999).

## Advantages of artificial feeding

- If the woman is HIV positive, it reduces the risk of acquired HIV infection.
- Reduction of risk of other harmful viruses, such as hepatitis B and hepatitis C, and in addition Z and T cell leukaemia (HTLV-1).
- May reduce the risk of haemorrhagic disease of the newborn as vitamin K is an additive (if pharmacological vitamin K is unavailable).
- It is the appropriate feeding method if the woman is an IV drug user or is taking medication that would be contraindicated in breastfeeding, e.g. diamorphine or anticancer drugs (MIDIRS/NHS Centre for Reviews and Dissemination 1999).
- Allows others to participate in feeding the baby.

## Preparing a bottle feed using baby milk powder

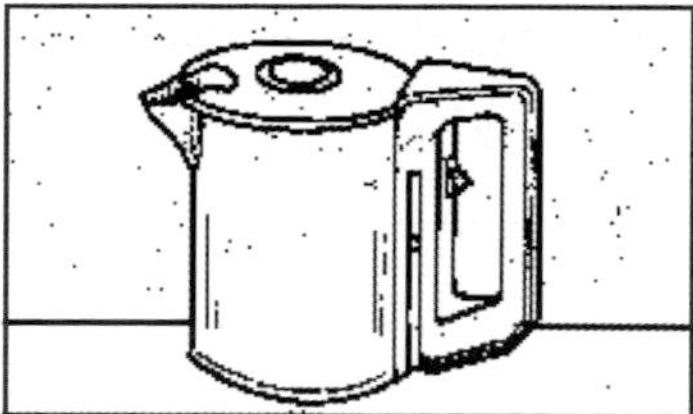

**1** Boil some fresh tap water and let it cool for a few minutes. (It should still be more than 70°C so don't leave it for more than half an hour). Do not use bottled or artificially softened water.

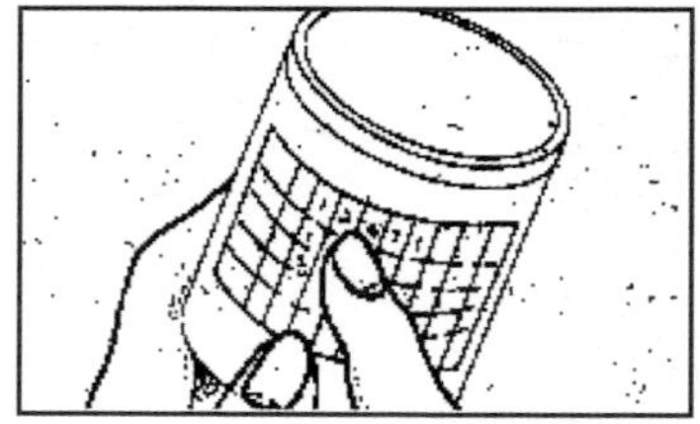

**2** Read the tin or packet to find out how much water and powder you need.
***You should make up a fresh bottle for each feed.***

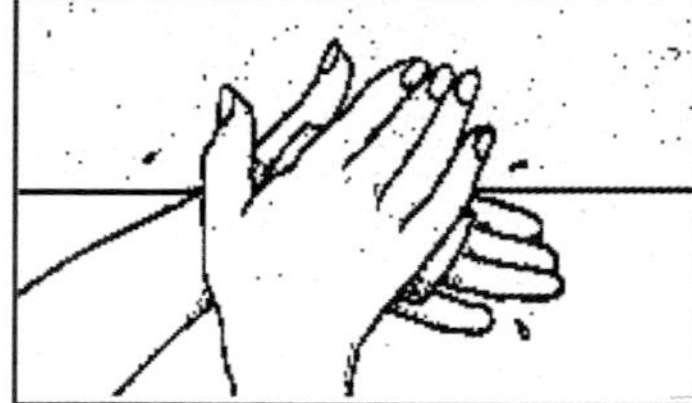

**3** Wipe clean an area on which to prepare the feed. Wash your hands very well with soap and water.

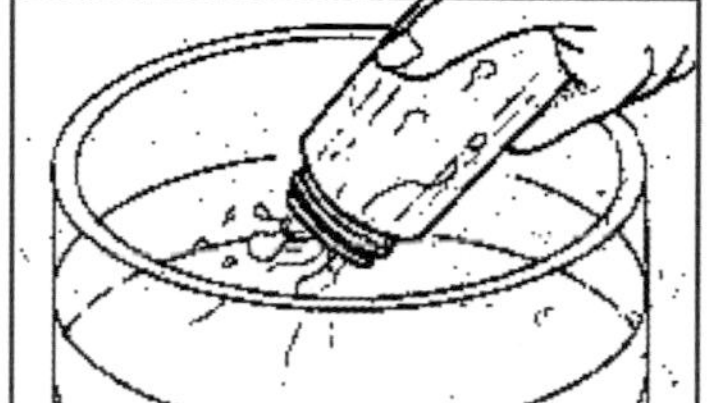

**4** If using a sterilizer, remove the lid and turn it upside down.

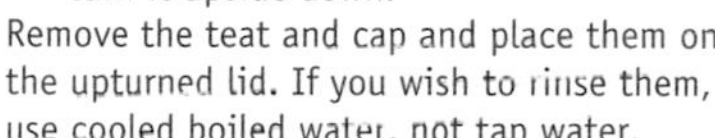

Remove the teat and cap and place them on the upturned lid. If you wish to rinse them, use cooled boiled water, not tap water.

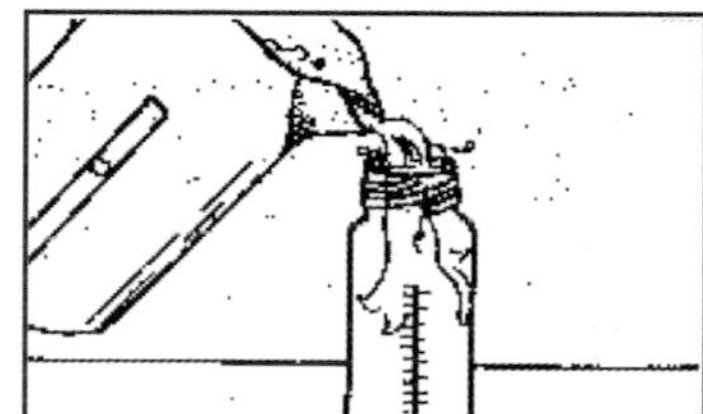

**5** Remove the bottle, rinse if wished (with the boiled water) and stand it on a clean flat surface. Pour the boiled water into the bottle up to the required mark.

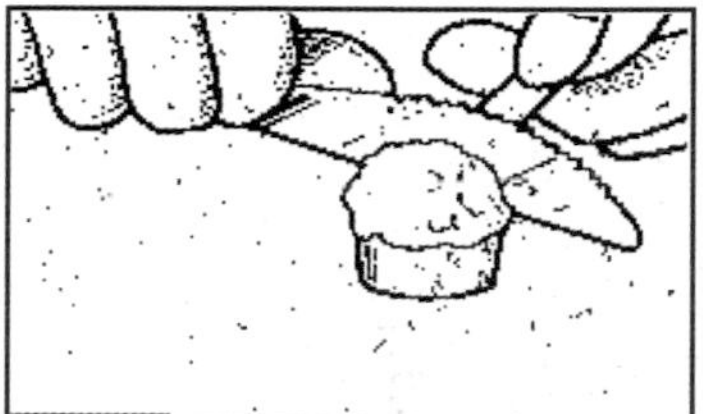

**6** Measure the exact amount of powder using the scoop provided with the milk. Level the powder in the scoop using the plastic knife or the spatula supplied with the milk powder or sterilizer.

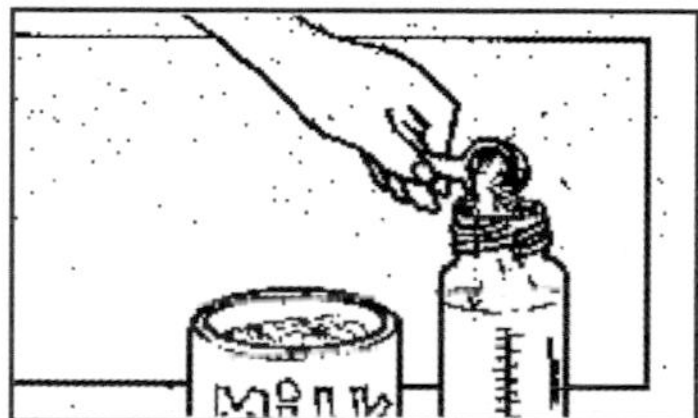


**7** **Add the powder to the water in the bottle.** All baby milks in Britain now use one scoop to 1oz (30mL) water. *Never use more than this or you will make your baby ill.* Do not add anything else to the feed.

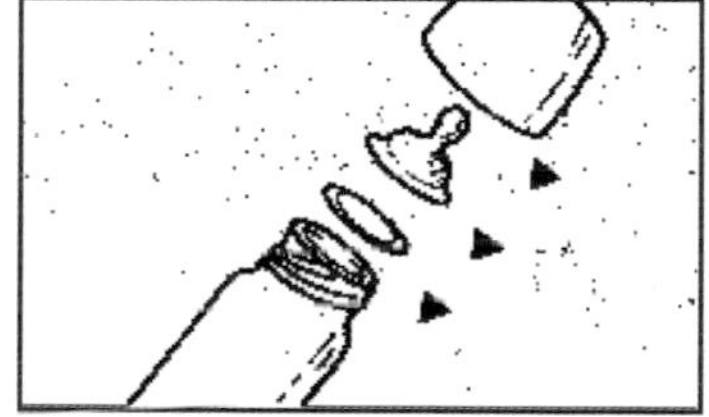

**8** Place the disc supplied on the top of the bottle, followed by the teat and cap.

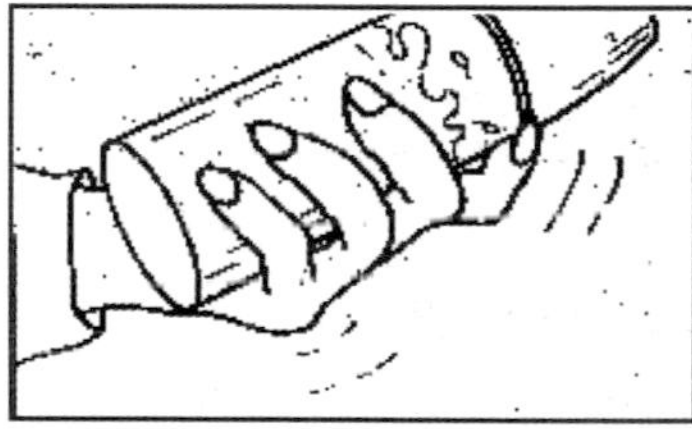

**9** Screw the cap on tightly and shake well until all the powder has dissolved.

**10** Check the temperature of the feed by dripping a little onto the inside of your wrist before giving it to your baby.

**11** After the feed, throw any unused milk away and clean the bottle. *Don't make up more than one feed at a time. Storing made-up milk increases the risk that your baby will fall ill.*

Additional tips:

- The amount of milk per feed suggested on the tin or packet is only a guide. Your baby may want more or less according to appetite.
- Use the scoop provided with the brand of milk powder you are making up - the scoop provided with another brand may be a different size.
- If your powder does not come with a spatula, you should sterilize a plastic knife and dry it on clean tissue paper. You can then keep it in the powder with the scoop.
- Powdered baby milk is not sterile. Feeds should therefore not be made in advance. If you are going to need to feed your baby while you are out it is safest to take freshly boiled water in a sealed flask and make up the feed when you need it.
- Almost all baby milk powders are made from cows' milk which has been processed to make it suitable for babies. Whey based (first) milks are more easily digested by a young baby. Casein based (second) milks take longer to digest and are not recommended for young babies.
- Ordinary cows' milk should not be given until your baby is at least a year old.
- Do not use soya or goat milk formulas without medical advice.

Reproduced by the UNICEF UK Baby Friendly Initiative, with thanks to the Women's Centre, Oxford Radcliffe Hospital NHS Trust.

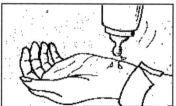

Breastfeeding is the healthiest way to feed your baby and it doesn't cost anything. If you use baby milk powder, it is very important for your baby's health that you follow all instructions carefully. It is possible, but difficult, to reverse a decision not to breastfeed or to re-start breastfeeding once you have stopped. Introducing partial bottle feeding will reduce a mother's breastmilk supply. Breastfeeding mothers do not need to eat any special foods but, just like everyone else, they are advised to follow a healthy diet. (Infant formula & follow-on formula regulations 1995)

**Figure 43.9** Preparing a bottle feed using formula milk powder. *(From UNICEF UK BFI 2001, with permission of UNICEF UK.)*

## Sterilizing baby feeding equipment

It is very important to keep any equipment used for feeding your baby either formula or breastmilk (such as bottles, teats and breastpumps) completely clean. This will help to protect your baby against infection, particularly tummy bugs (diarrhoea and vomiting). To do this you need to sterilize your equipment after you have washed it thoroughly. You will need to continue to do this until your baby is a year old. Any equipment not used straight away should be re-sterilized before use. There are several ways of sterilizing equipment. You could use:

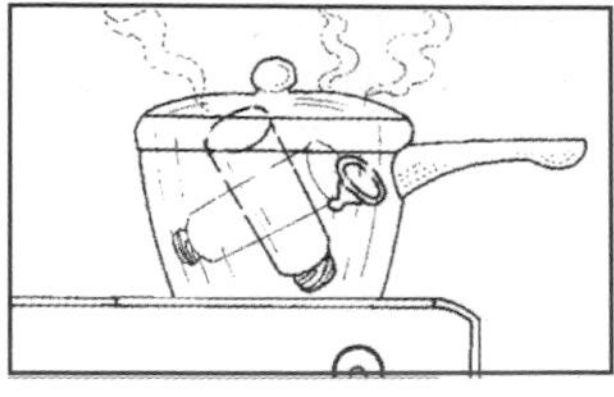

**A saucepan**

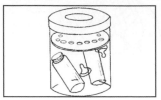

**A chemical sterilizer**
(not suitable for metal items)

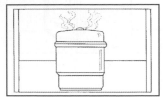

**A steam sterilizer**

You could also use a special **microwave bottle sterilizer** in a microwave oven, but this is not suitable for metal items or certain types of plastic.

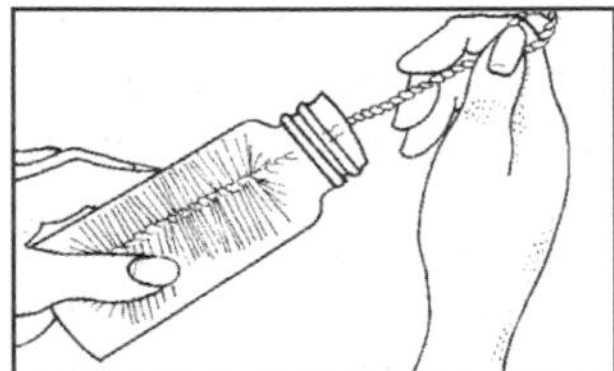

**1** Wash all bottles and other equipment thoroughly in hot soapy water using a bottle brush. Scrub the inside and outside of the bottle to remove fatty deposits. Pay particular attention to the rim.

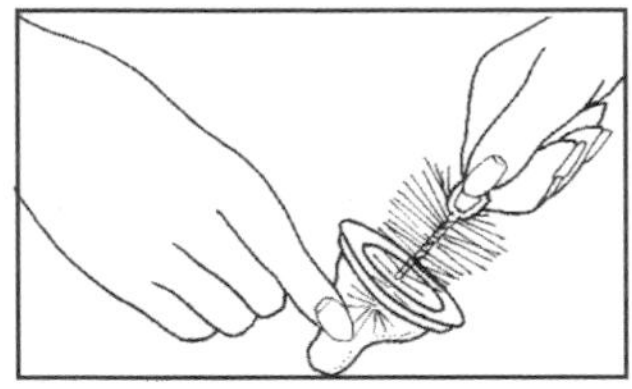

**2** Use a small teat brush to clean the inside of the teat, *or* turn it inside out and wash in hot soapy water.

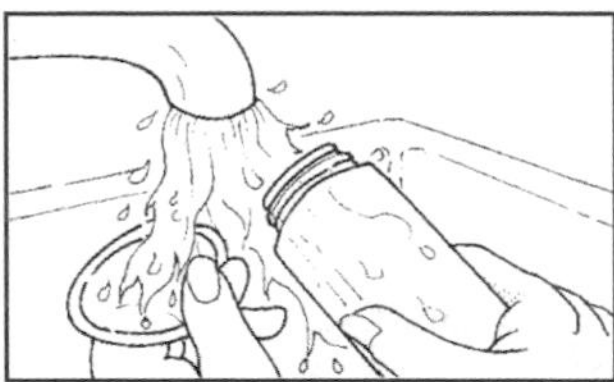

**3** Rinse all your washed equipment thoroughly before sterilizing.

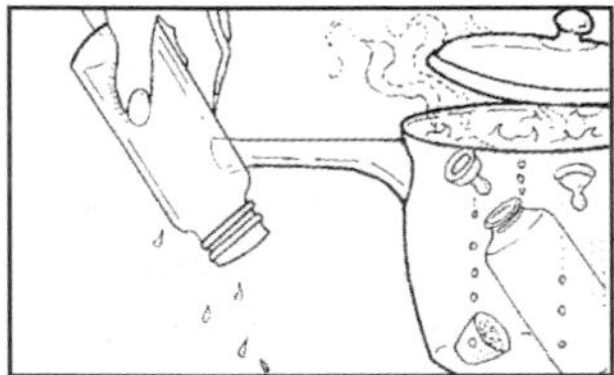

**4 To sterilize by boiling:**
Put the equipment into a large pan filled with water. Make sure there is no air trapped in the bottles or teats. Cover the pan with a lid and bring to the boil. **Boil for at least**
**10 minutes.** Make sure that the pan does not boil dry.

Keep the pan covered until the equipment is needed.

Check teats and bottles regularly for signs of deterioration. Bottles may become cloudy or cracked over time and teats get cracked or spongy. If you are unsure about a bottle of teat, it's safer to throw it away.

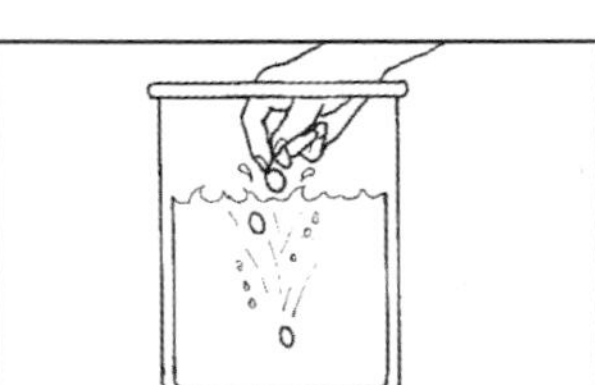

**5 To sterilize with chemicals:**
Make up the solution, using tablets or liquid, following the manufacturer's instructions. Submerge the equipment in the solution, making sure there is no air trapped
in the bottles or teats. Your sterilizing tank should have a plunger to keep all equipment under the water - or you can use a plate. **Leave in solution for at least 30 minutes.**

Make up a fresh solution every 24

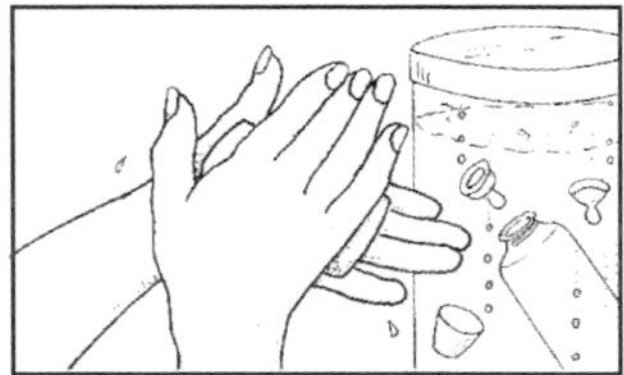

**6 To use steam or microwave sterilizers, just follow the manufacturer's instructions.**
Make sure the openings of the bottles and teats/equipment are face down in the steam sterilizer. Always wash your hands before removing equipment from your sterilizer.
If you have used a chemical sterilizer and wish to rinse your equipment prior to use, use water that has been boiled and allowed to cool.

Reproduced by the UNICEF UK Baby Friendly Initiative, with thanks to the Women's Centre, Oxford Radcliffe Hospital NHS Trust.

Breastfeeding is the healthiest way to feed your baby and it doesn't cost anything. If you use baby milk powder, it is very important for your baby's health that you follow all instructions carefully. It is possible, but difficult, to reverse a decision not to breastfeed or to re-start breastfeeding once you have stopped. Introducing partial bottle feeding will reduce a mother's breastmilk supply. Breastfeeding mothers do not need to eat any special foods but, just like everyone else, they are advised to follow a healthy diet. (Infant formula & follow-on formula regulations 1995)

**Figure 43.10** Sterilizing baby feeding equipment. *(From UNICEF UK BFI 2001, with permission of UNICEF UK.)*

## The role of the midwife in artificial feeding

The midwife needs to be:

- up to date in knowledge of the constituents of breast milk in comparison to artificial milk
- conversant with, and able to discuss with the woman, the physiology of the neonatal digestive system in relation to artificial milk
- knowledgeable about the advantages and disadvantages of artificial feeding and able to convey this information in a factual manner to facilitate a truly informed choice
- sensitive to the many factors that influence a woman's choices, such as her partner's attitude, her cultural background and her level of education
- conversant with equipment required, hygiene, and methods of sterilization of equipment (RCM 2009, UNICEF UK Baby Friendly Initiative 2001)
- able to teach the mother and family the skills of safe sterilization and making up of feeds
- expert in terms of safe storage of milk (RCM 2009, UNICEF UK Baby Friendly Initiative 2001).

## Preparation of feeds

All parents should be shown how to prepare artificial feeds and how to clean and sterilize the utensils. Ideally there should be an opportunity to practise with the midwife present so that any queries can be discussed. Women who have other children to care for may be rushed into taking shortcuts whilst making up their babies' feeds. Mistakes such as using the wrong scoop for the brand of milk, over- or underfilling the scoop, adding too little or too much water, and adding sugar or cereals to the feed are more common in parents with more than one child than in first-time parents and occur in all social classes. Hence, it is not safe to assume that multiparae or those in the higher social groups will make up feeds accurately. All parents need careful teaching and demonstrations for making up feeds by the midwife. See Figures 43.9 and 43.10.

The midwife should work in tandem with the health visitor and GP to provide a seamless service with regard to advice on infant feeding. Depending on the practice within the primary care trust, the midwife will probably 'transfer' the care of the mother and baby to the health visitor 10 days after the birth. The mother is invited to attend 'baby' clinics at the local health centre or GP surgery, where she will get advice about feeding, weaning and immunizations. The midwife may continue visiting and providing breastfeeding advice postnatally for as long as she considers neccessary (NMC 2004).

### Reflective activity 43.1

Review the advice and support you have provided for women who have experienced feeding problems. Consider whether your advice is:

- research and evidence based
- consistent with physiological principles and the advice of others
- clearly recorded in the woman's notes
- given in a way that reinforces the woman's belief in herself and her ability to breastfeed successfully.

## CONCLUSION

The mother's choice of feeding method, and her success with her chosen method, have long-term implications for the health of herself and her baby, and therefore for the health of the community as a whole. The importance of providing evidence-based, up-to-date and accurate information and sensitive support to women prior to the birth of the baby, and during the neonatal period, is fundamental to the woman's physical and psychological wellbeing and to her view of herself as a mother. Time invested by the midwife can pay huge dividends and must be seen as a priority.

### KEY POINTS

- Midwives are key professionals in providing information, education and support to the woman, her baby and family regarding infant feeding.
- Knowledge provided must be up to date, research and evidence based, and provided in an accessible, supportive and non-judgemental manner.
- Midwives need to be aware of their own biases and opinions regarding feeding choices in order to minimize the effect of both on the advice and support they provide.
- Midwives must work with professional and lay colleagues within the community to provide additional support to women and their families, whatever the feeding method.
- Women who have chosen to bottlefeed their infant should be supported, and taught the principles of correctly making up the feeds, and choosing the most appropriate milk for their baby.
- Midwives must teach all parents the principles of cleaning and sterilizing feeding equipment.

## REFERENCES


Abadin HG, Hibbs BF, Pohl HR: Breastfeeding exposure of infants to cadmium, lead and mercury: a public health viewpoint, *Toxicology and Industrial Health* 13(4):495–517, 1997.

American Academy of Pedriatrics (AAP): Policy statement, *Pediatrics* 115(2):496–506, 2005.

Amir LH, Dennerstein L, Garland SM, et al: Psychological aspects of nipple pain in lactating women, *Journal of Psychosomatic Obstetrics and Gynaecology* 17(1):53–58, 1996.

Arenz S, Von Kries R: Protective effect of breastfeeding against obesity in childhood: can a meta-analysis of published observational studies help to validate the hypothesis? *Advances in Experimental Medicine and Biology* 639:145–152, 2009.

Becker GE, McCormick FM, Renfrew MJ: Methods of milk expression for lactating women, *Cochrane Database of Systematic Reviews* (4):CD006170, 2008.

Berlin CM: Silicone breast implants and breastfeeding, *Pediatrics* 94:547–549, 1994.

Best Beginnings: From bump to breastfeeding DVD. www.bestbeginnings.info. 2008

Blackburn ST: *Maternal, fetal and neonatal physiology – a clinical perspective*, Philadelphia, 2007, WB Saunders.

Bodley V, Powers D: Long term nipple shield use – a positive perspective, *Journal of Human Lactation* 12(4):301–304, 1996.

Bolling K, Grant C, Hamlyn B, et al: *Infant feeding survey*, London, 2007, NHS Information Centre for Health & Social Care.

Breastfeeding Manifesto Coalition: *Breastfeeding manifesto*, London, 2007, UNICEF UK.

Brigham M: Mothers' reports of the outcome of nipple shield use, *Journal of Human Lactation* 12(4):291–297, 1996.

Britton C, McCormick FM, Renfrew MJ, et al: Support for breastfeeding mothers, *Cochrane Database of Systematic Reviews* (1):CD001141, 2007.

Butte NF: Dieting and exercise in overweight, lactating women, *New England Journal of Medicine* 342(7):502–503, 2000.

Cable B, Stewart M, Davis J: Nipple wound care: a new approach to an old problem, *Journal of Human Lactation* 13(4):313–318, 1997.

Campbell CMA: Early breastfeeding failure, *Update* 55(9):722, 724, 726–727, 1997.

Cavallo MG, Fava D, Monetini L, et al: Cell mediated response to beta casein in recent onset insulin dependent diabetes: implications for disease pathogenesis, *Lancet* 348(9032):926–928, 1996.

Chertok IR, Raz I, Shoham I, et al: Effects of early breastfeeding on neonatal glucose levels of term infants born to women with gestational diabetes, *Journal of Human Nutrition and Dietetics* 22(2):166–169, 2009.

Confidential Enquiry into Maternal and Child Health (CEMACE): *Diabetes in pregnancy: caring for the baby after birth*, London, 2007, CEMACH/CEMACE.

Coovadia HM, Rollins NC, Bland RM: Mother-to-child transmission of HIV-1 infection during exclusive breastfeeding in the first six months of life: an intervention cohort study, *Lancet* 369:1107–1116, 2007.

Coutts A: Pregnancy, lactation and avoidance of food allergy in the infant, *British Journal of Midwifery* 6(10):622, 1998.

Cross Government Obesity Unit: *Healthy weight, healthy lives: a cross government strategy for England*, London, 2008, DH DCSF.

Davis MK: Review of the evidence for an association between infant feeding and childhood cancer, *International Journal of Cancer* 11(Suppl):29–33, 1998.

Department of Health (DH): *Making a difference*, London, 1999, DH.

Department of Health (DH): *Maternity Standard, National Service Framework for Children, Young People and Maternity Services*, London, 2004a, DH.

Department of Health (DH): *HIV and infant feeding*, London, 2004b, DH.

Department of Health (DH): *Maternity matters*, London, 2007a, DH.

Department of Health (DH): *Review of the Health Inequalities Infant Mortality PSA Target*, London, 2007b, Health Inequalities Unit DH.

Department of Health (DH): *Reducing the risk of cot death*, London, 2009b, DH.

Department of Health (DH): *The pregnancy book*, London, 2009c, DH.

Department of Health (DH): *Birth to five*, London, 2009d, DH.

Department of Health (DH): *Off to the best start. Important information about feeding your baby (leaflet)*, London, 2010a, DH.

Department of Health (DH): *A guide to infant formula for parents who are bottle-feeding*, London, 2010b, DH.

Dewey KG, Henig J, Nommsen-Rivers LA: Differences in morbidity between breastfed and formula fed infants, *Journal of Pediatrics* 126(5):696–702, 1995.

Drash AL, Kramer MS, Swanson J, et al: Infant feeding practices and their possible relationship to the etiology of diabetes mellitus, *Pediatrics* 94(5):752–754, 1994.

Duncan B, Ey J, Holberg CJ, et al: Exclusive breast-feeding for at least 4 months protects against otitis media, *Pediatrics* 91(5):867–872, 1993.

Dyson L, McCormick FM, Renfrew MJ: Interventions for promoting the initiation of breastfeeding, *Cochrane Database of Systematic Reviews* (2):CD001688, 2005.

Elliott C: Using a silicone nipple shield to assist a baby unable to latch, *Journal of Human Lactation* 12(4):309–313, 1996.

Florey CD, Leech AM, Blackhall A: Infant feeding and mental and motor development at 18 months of age in first born singletons, *International Journal of Epidemiology* 24(3 Suppl 1):S21–S26, 1995.

Gray GE, Saloojee H: Breastfeeding, antiretroviral prophylaxis, and HIV, *New England Journal of Medicine* 359(2):189–191, 2008.

Golding J, Emmett PM, Rogers IS: Gastroenteritis, diarrhoea and breastfeeding, *Early Human Development* 49(Suppl):S83–S103, 1997.

Hamosh M: Protective function of proteins and lipids in human milk, *Biology of the Neonate* 74(2):163–176, 1998.

Hanson LA: Non breastfeeding: the most common immunodeficiency, *ALCA Galaxy* 9(3):15–18, 1998a.

Hanson LA: Breastfeeding provides passive and likely long lasting active immunity, *Annals of Allergy, Asthma & Immunology* 81(6):523–537, 1998b.

Healthcare Commission (HCC): *Towards better births: a review of the maternity services in England*, London, 2008, HCC.

Henderson G, Anthony MY, McGuire W: Formula milk versus maternal breast milk for feeding preterm or low birth weight infants, *Cochrane Database of Systematic Reviews* (4):CD002972, 2007.

Henly SJ, Anderson CM, Avery MD, et al: Anemia and insufficient milk in first-time mothers, *Birth* 22(2):87–92, 1995.

Henschel D, Inch S: *Breastfeeding. A guide for midwives*, Hale, 1996, Books for Midwives.

Hill PD, Humenick SS: The occurrence of breast engorgement, *Journal of Human Lactation* 10(2):76–86, 1994.

Hillervik-Lindquist C, Hofvander Y, Sjolin S: Studies on perceived breast milk insufficiency. III. Consequences for breast milk consumption and growth, *Acta Paediatricia Scandinavica* 80(3):297–303, 1991.

Horta BL, Victor CS, Menezes AM: Environmental tobacco smoke and the breastfeeding duration, *American Journal of Epidemiology* 146:128–133, 1997.

Horta BL, Bahl R, Martines JC, et al: *Evidence on the long-term effects on breastfeeding: Systematic reviews and meta-analyses*, Geneva, 2007, WHO.

Huml S: Sore nipples. a new look at old problems through the eyes of a dermatologist, *Practising Midwife* 2(2):28–31, 1999.

Inch S, Fisher C: Breastfeeding: early problems, *Practising Midwife* 3(1):12–15, 2000.

Jahanfar S, Ng C-J, Teng CL: Antibiotics for mastitis in breastfeeding women, *Cochrane Database of Sytematic Reviews* (1):CD005458, 2009.

Johnston PGB, Flood K, Spinks K: *The newborn child*, Edinburgh, 2003, Churchill Livingstone.

Jones W: *Breastfeeding and mastitis* (website) www.breastfeedingnetwork.org.uk. 2006.

Koletzko S, Sherman P, Corey M, et al: Role of infant feeding practices in development of Crohn's disease in childhood, *British Medical Journal* 298(6688):1617–1618, 1989.

Koletzko B, von Kries R, Monasterolo RC, et al: European Childhood Obesity Trial Study Group: Infant feeding and later obesity risk, *Advances in Experimental Medicine and Biology* 649:15–29, 2009.

Koosha A, Hashemifesharaki R, Mousavinasab N: Breastfeeding patterns and factors determining exclusive breastfeeding, *Singapore Medical Journal* 49(12):1002–1006, 2008.

Kramer MS, Kakuma R: Optimal duration of exclusive breastfeeding, *Cochrane Database of Systematic Reviews* (4):CD003517, 2006.

Kroeger M, Smith LJ: *Impact of birthing practices on breastfeeding: protecting the mother and baby continuum*, Boston, 2004, Jones & Bartlett.

Kunz C, Rodriguez-Palmero M, Koletzko B, et al: Nutritional and biochemical properties of human milk, part 1: general aspects, proteins, and carbohydrates, *Clinics in Perinatology* 26(2):307–333, 1999.

Lavergne NA: Does application of teabags provide effective relief? *Journal of Obstetric, Gynecologic and Neonatal Nursing* 26(1):53–58, 1997.

Lawrence RA, Lawrence RM: *Breastfeeding: a guide for the medical profession*, ed 6, USA, 2005, Elsevier.

Lee SY, Kim MT, Kim SW, et al: Effect of lifetime lactation on breast cancer risk: a Korean women's cohort study, *International Journal of Cancer* 105:390–393, 2003.

Leon DA, Ronalds G: Breastfeeding influences on later life – cardiovascular disease, *Advances in Experimental Medicine and Biology* 639:153–166, 2009.

Livingstone V, Stringer LJ: The treatment of Staphylococcus aureus infected sore nipples: a randomised comparative study, *Journal of Human Lactation* 15(3):241–246, 1999.

Lopez-Alarcon M, Villalpando S, Fajardo A: Breastfeeding lowers the frequency and duration of acute respiratory infection and diarrhoea in infants under six months of age, *Journal of Nutrition* 127:436–443, 1997.

Lucas A, Cole T: Breastmilk and neonatal necrotising entero-colitis, *Lancet* 336(8730):1519–1523, 1990.

Lucas A, Morley R, Cole TJ, et al: Breast milk and subsequent intelligence quotient in children born preterm, *Lancet* 339:261–264, 1992.

McCreadie RG: The Nithsdale Schizophrenia Surveys. 16. Breastfeeding and schizophrenia: preliminary results and hypotheses, *British Journal of Psychiatry* 170:334–337, 1997.

McVea KLSP, Turner PD, Peppler DK: The role of breastfeeding in sudden infant death syndrome, *Journal of Human Lactation* 16(1):13–20, 2000.

Makrides M, Neumann M, Simmer K: Are long chain polyunsaturated fatty acids essential nutrients in infancy? *Lancet* 345(8963):1463–1468, 1995.

Mannick E, Udall JN: Neonatal gastrointestinal mucosal immunity, *Clinics in Perinatology* 23(2):287–304, 1996.

Marchbank T, Weaver G, Nilsen-Hamilton M, et al: Pancreatic secretory trypsin inhibitor is a major motogenic and protective factor in human breast milk, *American Journal of Physiology. Gastrointestinal and Liver Physiology* 296:G697–G703, 2009.

Mason T, Rabinovich CE, Fredrickson DD, et al: Breastfeeding and the development of juvenile rheumatoid arthritis, *Journal of Rheumatology* 22:1166–1170, 1995.

Maternity Alliance: *Having it all – a woman's guide to combining breastfeeding and work*, London, 1999, Maternity Alliance.

Mennella JA: Infants' suckling responses to the flavor of alcohol in mothers' milk, *Alcoholism, Clinical and Experimental Research* 21:581–585, 1997.

Michaelsen KF, Lauritzen L, Mortensen EL: Effects of breastfeeding on cognitive function, *Advances in Experimental Medicine and Biology* 639:199–215, 2009.

MIDIRS/NHS *Centre for Reviews and Dissemination: Breastfeeding or bottlefeeding: helping women to choose*, ed 2, Bristol, 1999, MIDIRS.

Mikhailov TA, Furner SE: Breastfeeding and genetic factors in the etiology of inflammatory bowel disease in children, *World Journal of Gastroenterology* 15(3):270–279, 2008.

Minchin M: Artificial feeding and risk: the last taboo. *Practising Midwife* 3(3):18–20, 2000.

Mitchell P: Pollutants in breast milk cause concern, but breast is still best, *Lancet* 349(9064):1525, 1997.

Moore ER, Anderson GC, Bergman N: Early skin-to-skin contact for mothers and their healthy newborn infants, *Cochrane Database of*

*Systematic Reviews* (2):CD003519, 2007.

Morton JA: Ineffective suckling: a possible consequence of obstructive positioning, *Journal of Human Lactation* 8(2):83–85, 1992.

National Health Service (NHS) Centre for Reviews and Dissemination: Promoting the initiation of breastfeeding, *Effective Health Care Bulletin* 6(2):1–2, 2000.

National Institute for Clinical Excellence (NICE): Division of ankyloglossia (tongue-tie) for breastfeeding, *Interventional Procedure Guidance 149*, London, 2005, NICE.

National Institute for Clinical Excellence (NICE): *Postnatal care: routine postnatal care of women and their babies*, Clinical Guideline 37, London, 2006, NICE.

National Institute for Clinical Excellence (NICE): *Maternal and child nutrition*, Public Health Guidance 11, London, 2008a, NICE.

National Institute for Clinical Excellence (NICE): *Antenatal care: routine care for the healthy pregnant woman*, Clinical Guideline 62, London, 2008b, NICE.

Neifert MR: Breastmilk transfer: positioning, latch-on and screening for problems in milk transfer, *Clinical Obstetrics and Gynaecology* 47:656–675, 2004.

Neifert M, DeMarzo S, Seacat J: The influence of breast surgery, breast appearance, and pregnancy-induced breast changes on lactation sufficiency as measured by infant weight gain, *Birth* 17:31–38, 1990.

Neifert M, Lawrence R, Seacat J: Nipple confusion – towards a formal definition, *Journal of Pediatrics* 126: S125–S129, 1995.

Neville M: The physiology of lactation, *Clinics in Perinatology* 26(2):251–279, 1999.

Newburg DS, Peterson JA, Ruiz-Palacios GM, et al: Role of human-milk lactadherin in protection against symptomatic rotavirus infection, *Lancet* 351(9110):1160–1164, 1998.

Newman J: How breastmilk protects newborns, *Scientific American* Dec:58–61, 1995.

Nursing and Midwifery Council (NMC): *Midwives Rules and Standards*, London, 2004, NMC.

Oddy WH: The long term effects of breastfeeding on asthma and atopic disease, *Advances in Experimental Medicine and Biology* 639:237–251, 2009.

Orlando S: The immunologic significance of breastmilk, *Journal of Obstetric, Gynaecological and Neonatal Nursing* 24(7):678–683, 1995.

O'Tierney PF, Barker DJ, Osmond C, et al: Duration of breastfeeding and adiposity in adult life, *Journal of Nutrition* 139(2):422S–425S, 2009.

Palmer B: The influence of breastfeeding on the development of the oral cavity: a commentary, *Journal of Human Lactation* 14(2):93–98, 1998.

Pessl MM: Are we creating our own breast-feeding mythology? *Journal of Human Lactation* 12:271–272, 1996.

Pettitt DJ, Forman MR, Hanson RL, et al: Breastfeeding and incidence of non-insulin dependent diabetes mellitus in Pima Indians, *Lancet* 350(9072):166–168, 1997.

Pisacane A, Graziano L, Mazzarella G, et al: Breastfeeding and urinary tract infection, *Journal of Pediatrics* 120(1):87–89, 1992.

Powers NG: Slow weight gain and low milk supply in the breastfeeding dyad, *Clinics in Perinatology* 26(2):399–430, 1999.

Prentice A, Addey CVP, Wilde J: Evidence for local feedback control of human milk secretion, *Biochemical Society Transactions* 17:489–492, 1989.

Pugh LC, Buchko BL, Bishop BA, et al: A comparison of topical agents to relieve nipple pain and enhance breastfeeding, *Birth* 23(2):88–93, 1996.

Quigley MA, Kelly YJ, Sacker A: Breastfeeding and hospitalization for diarrheal and respiratory infection in the United Kingdom: Millennium Cohort Study, *Pediatrics* 119:e837–e842, 2007.

Quinsey PM, Donohue DC, Cumming FJ, et al: The importance of measured intake in assessing exposure of breast-fed infants to organochlorines, *European Journal of Clinical Nutrition* 50(7):438–442, 1996.

Ravelli ACJ, van der Meulen JHP, Osmond C, et al: Infant feeding and adult glucose tolerance, lipid profile, blood pressure and obesity, *Archives of Disease in Childhood* 82(3):248–252, 2000.

Renfrew M, Woolridge M, Ross McGill H: *Enabling women to breastfeed*, London, 2000, The Stationery Office.

Repucci AH: Effect of breastfeeding on hospitalization rates for lower respiratory infections, *Journal of Pediatrics* 127(4):667, 1995.

Righard L, Alade MO: Effect of delivery room routines on success of first breastfeed, *Lancet* 336(8723):1105–1107, 1990.

Righard L, Alade MO: Sucking technique and its effects on success of breastfeeding, *Birth* 19:185–189, 1992.

Riordan J: *Breastfeeding and human lactation*, ed 4 revised, Boston, 2008, Jones & Bartlett.

Rodriguez-Palmero M, Koletzko B, Kunz C, et al: Nutritional and biochemical properties of human milk: II. Lipids, micronutrients, and bioactive factors, *Clinics in Perinatology* 26(2):335–359, 1999.

Royal College of Midwives (RCM): *HIV & AIDS*, Position Paper No. 16a, London, 1998, RCM.

Royal College of Midwives (RCM): *Successful breastfeeding*, ed 3, London, 2002, Churchill Livingstone.

Royal College of Midwives (RCM): *Infant feeding*, London, 2009, RCM.

Saarinen UM, Kajosaari M: Breastfeeding as prophylaxis against atopic disease: prospective follow up study until 17 years old, *Lancet* 346(8982):1065–1069, 1995.

Scientific Advisory Committee on Nutrition (SACN): *Update on trans fatty acids and health*, Position statement, London, 2007, TSO.

Shribman S, Billingham K: *Healthy child programme – pregnancy and the first five years*, London, 2009, DH.

Shu XO, Linet MS, Steinbuch M, et al: Breastfeeding and risk of childhood acute leukaemia *Journal of the National Cancer Institute* 91(20): 1765–1772, 1999.

Silfverdal SA, Bodin L, Olc NP: Protective effect of breastfeeding: an ecologic study of Haemophilus influenzae meningitis and breastfeeding in a Swedish population, *International Journal of Epidemiology* 28(1):152–156, 1999.

Smith D: Worldwide trends in DDT levels in human breast milk, *International Journal of Epidemiology* 28(2):179–188, 1999.

Snowden HM, Renfrew MJ, Woolridge MW: Treatments for breast engorgement during lactation, *The Cochrane Library*, Issue 1, Oxford, 2002, Update Software.

Statutory Instrument No. 77: *Food. The infant formula and follow-on regulations*, London, 1995, HMSO.

UNICEF UK Baby Friendly Initiative (BFI): *Implementing the ten steps to successful breastfeeding: a guide for UK maternity service providers working towards baby friendly accreditation*, London, 1998a, UNICEF UK BFI.

UNICEF UK Baby Friendly Initiative (BFI): *Breastfeeding your baby*, London, 1998b, UNICEF UK BFI.

UNICEF UK Baby Friendly Initiative (BFI): *Implementing the baby friendly best practice standards*, London, 2001, UNICEF UK BFI.

UNICEF UK Baby Friendly Initiative (BFI): *A guide to infant formula for parents who are bottle feeding*, London, 2010, UNICEF UK BFI.

Vincent P: *Feeding our babies*, England, 1999, Hochland and Hochland.

Von Kries R, Koletzko B, Sauerwald T, et al: Breast feeding and obesity: cross sectional study, *British Medical Journal* 319:147–150, 1999.

Wang IY, Fraser IS: Reproductive function and contraception in the postpartum period, *Obstetrical & Gynecological Survey* 49(1):56–63, 1994.

Wang YS, Su SY: The effect of exclusive breastfeeding on development and incidence of infection in infants, *Journal of Human Lactation* 12(1):27–30, 1996.

Widstrom AM, Wahlberg V, Matthieson AS: Short term effects of early suckling and touch of the nipple on maternal behaviour, *Early Human Development* 21:153–163, 1990.

Wilde CJ, Addey CVP, Boddy LM, et al: Autocrine regulation of milk secretion by a protein in milk, *Biochemical Journal* 305:51–58, 1995.

Williatts P, Forsyth JS, DiModugno MK, et al: Effect of long-chain polyunsaturated fatty acids in infant formula on problem solving at 10 months of age, *Lancet* 352:688–691, 1998.

Willis CE, Livingstone V: Infant insufficient milk syndrome associated with maternal postpartum hemorrhage, *Journal of Human Lactation* 11(2):123–126, 1995.

World Health Organization (WHO): *International Code of Marketing of Breastmilk Substitutes*, Geneva, 1981, WHO.

World Health Organization (WHO): *Infant and young child nutrition – global strategy on infant and young child feeding*, Geneva, 2002, WHO.

World Health Organization (WHO): *Evidence on the long term effects on breastfeeding: systematic reviews and meta-analyses*, Geneva, 2007, WHO.

WHO Task Force on Methods for the Natural Regulation of Fertility: The World Health Organization multinational study of breastfeeding and lactational amenorrhea. III. Pregnancy during breastfeeding, *Fertility and Sterility* 72(3):431–440, 1999.

World Health Organization/United Nations Children's Fund (WHO/UNICEF): *Protecting, promoting and supporting breastfeeding: the special role of maternity services. A joint WHO/UNICEF statement*, Geneva, 1989, WHO.

WHO/UNICEF: *Acceptable medical reasons for use of breast-milk substitutes*, Geneva, 2009, WHO.

WHO/UNICEF/UNAIDS/UNFPA: *HIV and infant feeding update*, Geneva, 2007, WHO.

Xanthou M: Immune protection of human milk, *Biology of the Neonate* 74(2):121–133, 1998.

Xiao-Ming B: Nutritional management of newborn infants, *World Journal of Gastroenterology* 14(40):6133–6139, 2008.

Zimmermann R, Perucchini D, Fauchere JC: Hepatitis C virus in breastmilk, *Lancet* 345(8954):928, 1995.

Chapter |44|

# The preterm baby and the small baby

*Kathryn Eglinton*

## LEARNING OUTCOMES

At the end of this chapter, you will have:

- an understanding of classification and definitions of low-birthweight infants
- knowledge of common causes of preterm and small-for-gestational-age babies and the implications for antenatal care
- an understanding of complications relating to preterm delivery and low birthweight
- knowledge of long-term outcomes for these babies.

## INTRODUCTION

For the purpose of classification, management and research studies, newborn babies are considered according to their gestation, their birthweight relative to their gestation (centiles) and their actual birthweight. The midwife's role centres on the prevention of prematurity, on preparing parents for identifying risk factors antenatally, and, in the event of preterm birth, on working with the team to support parents in the neonatal period. Please see website for more in-depth information.

### Gestation

Low gestational age at birth is a principal factor associated with perinatal mortality. Babies born very preterm are at particular risk of sensory, cognitive and motor dysfunction (Cooke 2005, Marlowe et al 2005). Data are now available to monitor trends, and inform care for preterm births. In 2006 in England and Wales, 7.6% of live births were preterm, 88% were born at term, and 4% were born post term, with corresponding infant mortality rates of 41.0, 1.9, and 1.5 deaths per 1000 live births (ONS 2009). Almost two-thirds of all infant deaths occurred to babies born preterm. Infant mortality was highest at the very low gestational ages.

Antenatally, gestation is estimated from the date of the last menstrual period and the woman's normal cycle, clinical examination and early ultrasound scan measurements and uterine growth (see Chs 32 and 33).

Scoring systems estimate the neonatal gestation following delivery and neonatal units will use one, or an adaptation of one or two of the common ones. Improved accuracy of antenatal ultrasound scans has led to less reliance on these scales. The *Dubowitz scale* (Dubowitz et al 1970) (see Fig. 44.1) is the most widely used in the UK, and providing the baby is well and examined within a few hours of delivery, is accurate to within 2 weeks. It involves scoring the baby on neurological states as well as external criteria but may be inappropriate for use with sick or ventilated neonates.

The *Ballard score* (an adaptation of the Dubowitz score) is a newer system (Fig. 44.2).

These scoring systems require careful examination of the baby, looking at characteristics of appearance, reflexes and behaviour, providing an indication of whether the baby is small or premature.

- *Post-term:* more than 42 completed weeks of gestation.
- *Term:* 37–42 completed weeks of gestation.
- *Preterm:* fewer than 37 completed weeks of gestation.

**Reflective activity 44.1**

Examine a healthy newborn baby and assess the gestational age using the Dubowitz and Ballard scoring systems.

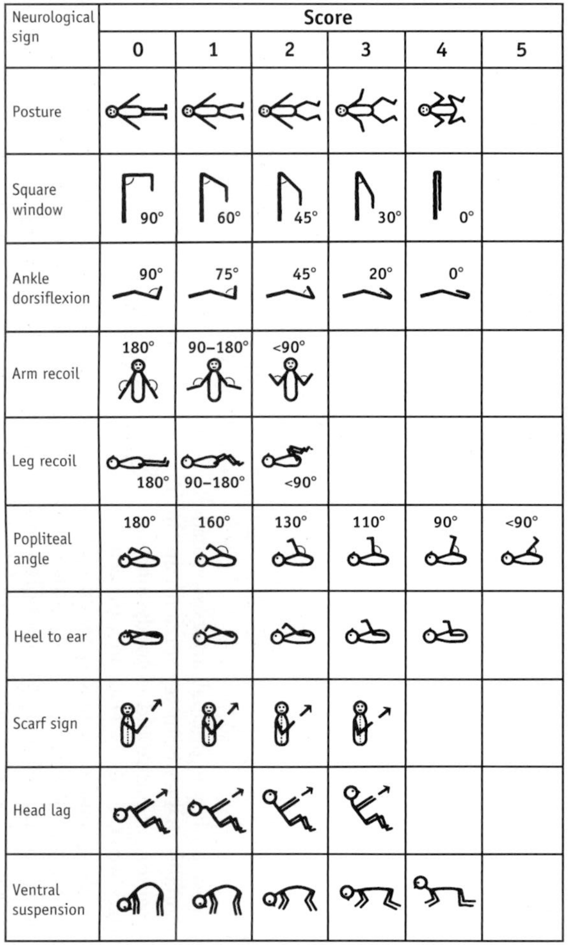

| Neurological sign | Score | | | | | |
|---|---|---|---|---|---|---|
| | 0 | 1 | 2 | 3 | 4 | 5 |
| Posture | | | | | | |
| Square window | 90° | 60° | 45° | 30° | 0° | |
| Ankle dorsiflexion | 90° | 75° | 45° | 20° | 0° | |
| Arm recoil | 180° | 90–180° | <90° | | | |
| Leg recoil | 180° | 90–180° | <90° | | | |
| Popliteal angle | 180° | 160° | 130° | 110° | 90° | <90° |
| Heel to ear | | | | | | |
| Scarf sign | | | | | | |
| Head lag | | | | | | |
| Ventral suspension | | | | | | |

Physical (external) criteria

| | Score | | | | |
|---|---|---|---|---|---|
| **External sign** | 0 | 1 | 2 | 3 | 4 |
| Oedema | Obvious oedema hands and feet; pitting over tibia | No obvious oedema hands and feet; pitting over tibia | No oedema | | |
| Skin texture | Very thin, gelatinous | Thin and smooth | Smooth, medium thickness. Rash or superficial peeling | Slight thickening. Superficial cracking and peeling, especially hands and feet | Thick and parchment-like. Superficial or deep cracking |
| Skin colour (infant not crying) | Dark red | Uniformly pink | Pale pink, variable over body | Pale. Only pink over ears, lips, palms or soles | |
| Skin opacity (trunk) | Numerous veins and venules clearly seen, especially over abdomen | Veins and tributaries seen | A few large vessels clearly seen over abdomen | A few large vessels seen indistinctly over abdomen | No blood vessels seen |
| Lanugo (over back) | No lanugo | Abundant, long and thick over whole back | Hair thinning, especially over lower back | Small amount of lanugo and bald areas | At least half of back devoid of lanugo |
| Plantar creases | No skin creases | Faint red marks over anterior half of sole | Definite red marks over more than anterior half. Indentations over more than anterior third | Indentations over more than anterior third | Definite deep indentations over more than anterior third |
| Nipple formation | Nipple barely visible, no areola | Nipple well defined, areola smooth and flat, diameter <0.75 cm | Areola stippled, edges not raised: diameter <0.75 cm | Areola stippled, edge raised: diameter >0.75 cm | |
| Breast size | No breast tissue palpable | Breast tissue on one or both sides <0.5 cm diameter | Breast tissue both sides, one or both 0.5–1.0 cm | Breast tissue both sides, one or both >1 cm | |
| Ear form | Pinna flat and shapeless, little or no incurving of edge | Incurving of part of edge of pinna | Partial incurving whole of upper pinna | Well-defined incurving whole of upper pinna | |
| Ear firmness | Pinna soft, easily folded, no recoil | Pinna soft, easily folded, slow recoil | Cartilage to edge of pinna but soft in places, ready recoil | Pinna firm, cartilage to edge, instant recoil | |
| Genitalia<br>• Male | Neither testis in scrotum | At least one testis high in scrotum | At least one testis right down | | |
| • Female (with hips half abducted) | Labia majora widely separated, labia minora protruding | Labia majora almost cover labia minora | Labia majora completely cover labia minora | | |

**Figure 44.1** The Dubowitz score: graph for reading gestational age from total score. *(From Dubowitz et al 1970 with permission.)*

Neuromuscular maturity

| | −1 | 0 | 1 | 2 | 3 | 4 | 5 |
|---|---|---|---|---|---|---|---|
| Posture | | | | | | | |
| Square window (wrist) | >90° | 90° | 60° | 45° | 30° | 0° | |
| Arm recoil | | 180° | 140–180° | 110–140° | 90–110° | <90° | |
| Popliteal angle | 180° | 160° | 140° | 120° | 100° | 90° | <90° |
| Scarf sign | | | | | | | |
| Heel to ear | | | | | | | |

Physical maturity

| | −1 | 0 | 1 | 2 | 3 | 4 | 5 |
|---|---|---|---|---|---|---|---|
| Skin | Sticky friable transparent | Gelatinous red, translucent | Smooth pink, visible veins | Superficial peeling &/or rash, few veins | Cracking pale areas rare veins | Parchment deep cracking no vessels | Leathery cracked wrinkled |
| Lanugo | none | sparse | abundant | thinning | bald areas | Mostly bald | |
| Plantar surface | heel-toe 40–50 mm: −1 <40 mm: −2 | >50 mm no crease | faint red marks | anterior transverse crease only | creases ant. 2/3 | creases over entire sole | |
| Breast | imperceptible | barely perceptible | flat areola no bud | stippled areola 1–2 mm bud | raised areola 3–4 mm bud | full areola 5–10 mm bud | |
| Eye/ear | lids fused loosely: −1 tightly: −2 | lids open pinna flat stays folded | sl. curved pinna; soft; slow recoil | well-curved pinna; soft but ready recoil | formed & firm instant recoil | thick cartilage ear stiff | |
| Genitals (male) | scrotum flat, smooth | scrotum empty faint rugae | testes in upper canal rare rugae | testes descending few rugae | testes down good rugae | testes pendulous deep rugae | |
| Genitals (female) | clitoris prominent labia flat | prominent clitoris small labia minora | prominent clitoris enlarging minora | majora & minora equally prominent | majora large minora small | majora cover clitoris & minora | |

Maturity rating

| Score | Weeks |
|---|---|
| −10 | 20 |
| −5 | 22 |
| 0 | 24 |
| 5 | 26 |
| 10 | 28 |
| 15 | 30 |
| 20 | 32 |
| 25 | 34 |
| 30 | 36 |
| 35 | 38 |
| 40 | 40 |
| 45 | 42 |
| 50 | 44 |

**Figure 44.2** The Ballard score. Each of the clinical and neurological features is assessed and scored. The gestational age is determined by comparing the total score with the maturity rating grid. *(From Johnston et al 2003.)*

## Centiles

Using an appropriate centile chart, the weight, head circumference and length of the baby is plotted against gestation and an assessment made of the growth. The centile chart forms an important part in providing a dynamic growth record and a link to the neonatal management (see Ch. 41).

The UK World Health Organization (WHO) growth charts (2009) are based on measurements collected by the WHO in six different countries (Fig. 44.3) (see website). These describe optimal rather than average growth and set breastfeeding as the norm, illustrating how all healthy children are expected to grow.

- Large for gestational age (LGA): >90$^{th}$ centile
- Appropriate for gestational age (AGA): 10$^{th}$ to 90$^{th}$ centile
- Small for gestational age (SGA): <10$^{th}$ centile.

These classifications rely on accurate assessment of gestational age at delivery.

## Birthweight

Babies may be grouped according to their birthweight – especially useful when the gestation is unknown. Many studies relate to birthweight rather than gestation as it is a better predictor of outcome. The WHO definition of low

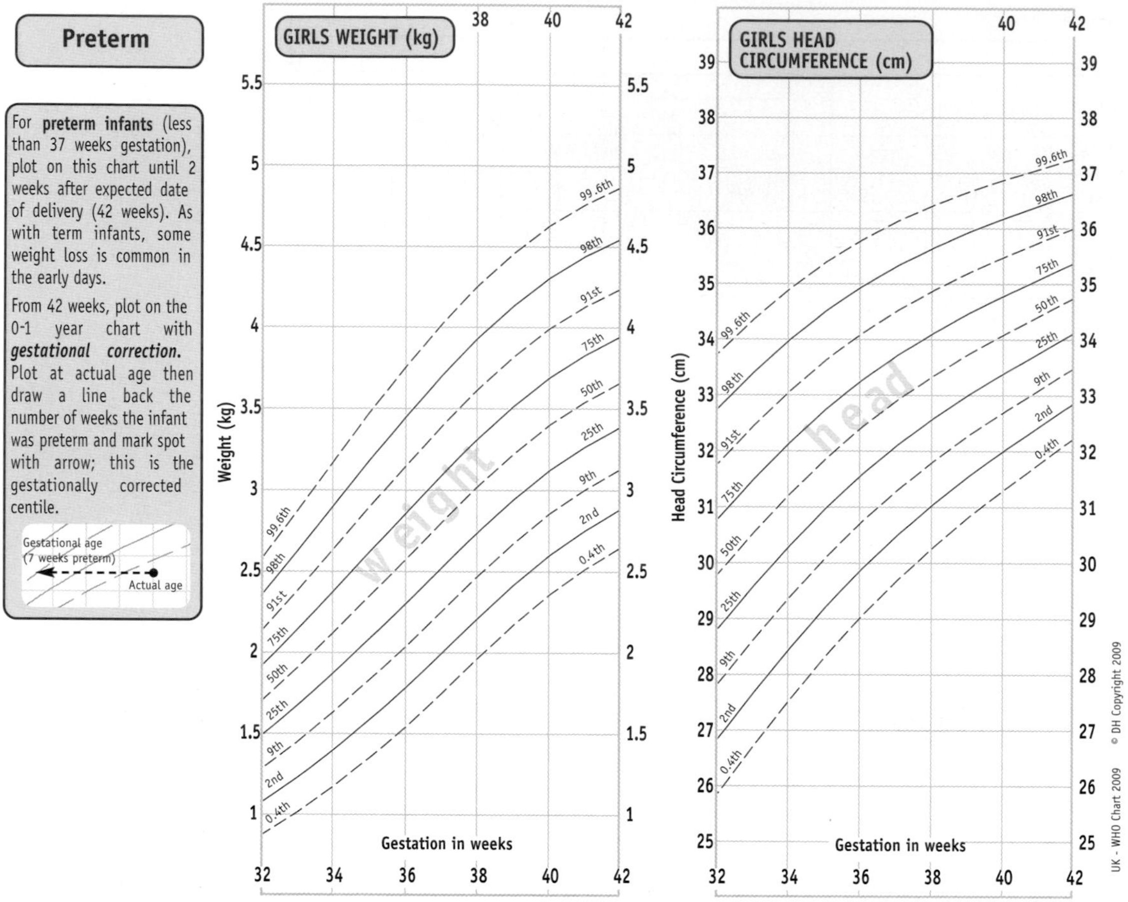

**Preterm**

For **preterm infants** (less than 37 weeks gestation), plot on this chart until 2 weeks after expected date of delivery (42 weeks). As with term infants, some weight loss is common in the early days.

From 42 weeks, plot on the 0-1 year chart with ***gestational correction.*** Plot at actual age then draw a line back the number of weeks the infant was preterm and mark spot with arrow; this is the gestationally corrected centile.

Gestational age (7 weeks preterm)

Actual age

GIRLS WEIGHT (kg)

GIRLS HEAD CIRCUMFERENCE (cm)



**Figure 44.3** WHO growth charts, preterm infants. **A.** Weight for preterm infants less than 37 weeks (female). **B.** Girls' head circumference. *(By kind permission of RCPCH/WHO/Department of Health 2009.)*

birthweight (WHO 1977) is internationally adopted, with further subdivisions as shown below:

- *Low birthweight* (LBW): lower than 2500 g at birth.
- *Very low birthweight* (VLBW): lower than 1500 g at birth.
- *Extremely low birthweight* (ELBW): lower than 1000 g at birth.

Rapid recent developments in neonatology have resulted in the survival of LBW infants above 1500 g becoming commonplace.The distribution of births by gestational age varies considerably by birthweight. This has a signifiant effect on mortality and morbidity (ONS 2009) (see website).

Preterm and SGA babies are considered separately in this chapter, although there is overlap in causes, management and complications. A baby may be preterm, SGA and LBW, and needs consideration from all perspectives.

## THE PRETERM BABY

### Causes

Infants born prematurely are at high risk of complications in the neonatal period and for later neurodevelopmental problems (Blackburn 2007). The causes of, and effective intervention strategies to prevent, preterm onset of labour have been researched. Specific events leading to onset of preterm labour and delivery are still uncertain and are likely to be a series or combination of maternal and fetal factors, or unexplained, rather than a single event, and include:

- pre-eclampsia
- placental abnormalities – antepartum haemorrhage, placenta praevia

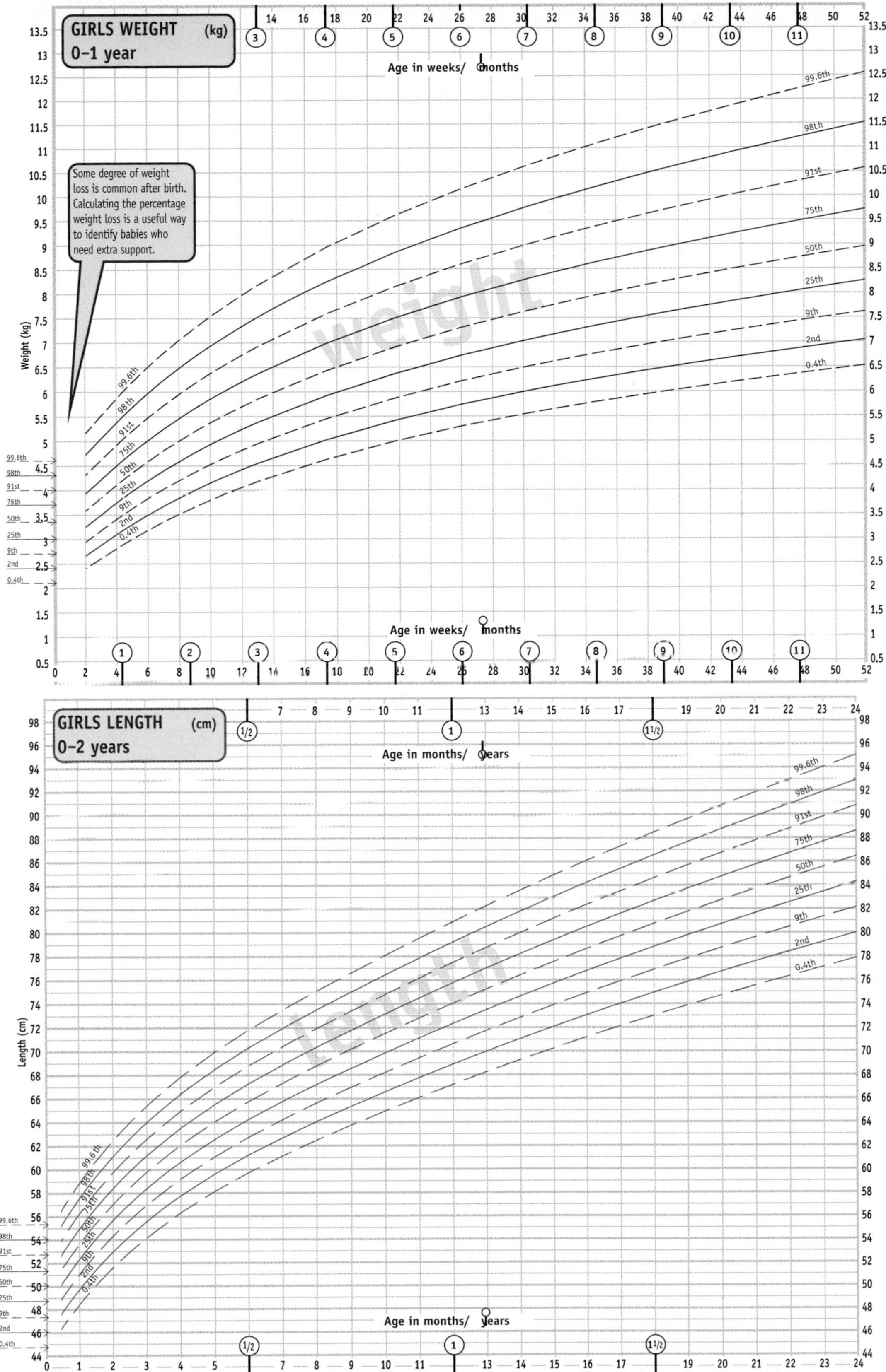


**Figure 44.3** (*continued*) **C.** Girls' weight 0–1 year. **D.** Girls' length 0–2 years. *(From http://www.rcpch.ac.uk/Research/UK-WHO-Growth-Charts, accessed 8/6/2010. Reproduced with permission.)*

- serious maternal diseases – acute or chronic, such as, pyelonephritis, chronic nephritis or essential hypertension
- premature prolonged rupture of membranes (PPROM)
- intra-amniotic infection
- cervical incompetence (history of repeated mid-trimester miscarriages)
- maternal alcohol or substance abuse – including cigarette smoking
- overdistension of the uterus – multiple pregnancies, polyhydramnios
- poor obstetric history
- maternal age <20 years or >35 years
- certain congenital abnormalities
- social class IV or V
- unexplained reasons (25–30%) (Vadillo-Ortega & Estrada-Gutierrez 2005).

Some of these problems can be addressed antenatally. A crucial part of the midwife's role is in education of women about normal pregnancy features and what should be reported to the healthcare team.

## Characteristics (Fig. 44.4)

Preterm babies are immature and not ready to adapt to extrauterine life. Their appearance depends on their maturity, but generally:

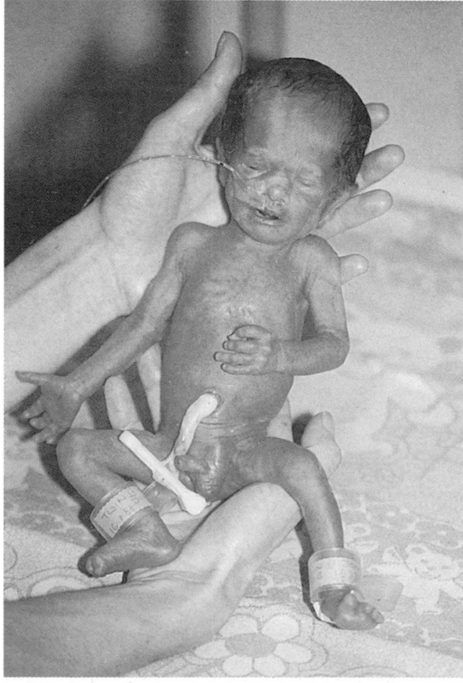

**Figure 44.4** Preterm infant. *(From Johnston et al 2003.)*

- The head is large in proportion to the body.
- Face appears small and triangular with a pointed chin.
- If very immature, the eyelids may be fused.
- Owing to poor ossification, the sutures and fontanelles are widely spaced and the skull bones soft.
- With the absence of subcutaneous fat, the skin is pinkish/red and surface veins are prominent.
- The body is covered with varying amounts of soft downy hair – *lanugo* – and often covered with protective creamy white *vernix caseosa*.
- Limbs are thin, and the more immature the baby, the greater the degree of extension of limbs.
- Poor muscle tone.
- Nails are soft.
- Chest is small and narrow with little or no breast tissue.
- Abdomen is large and umbilicus appears to be low-set.
- Genitalia are not fully developed:
  - labia majora do not cover the labia minora
  - testes may not have descended into the scrotum.
- Uncoordinated suck and swallow reflex.

## Management

The preterm baby is unable to perform many physiological functions adequately due to immaturity. Neonatal care aims to compensate for these deficiencies until the infant is able to cope unaided. Accurate assessment of the baby's condition at birth and prompt resuscitation are essential. Subsequent meticulous care and close observation are required to detect even small departures from normal physiological function, which can lead to serious complications.

## Labour and delivery

Antenatal factors that influence fetal outcome include gestational age; steroid administration; predicted fetal weight; multiple pregnancy; sex; sepsis; presence and severity of any pathology; fetal growth restriction with abnormal Doppler flow studies; and fetal anomaly.

Preterm labour often progresses rapidly. If preterm labour is anticipated, birth should be planned in a maternity unit with the appropriate level of neonatal intensive care facilities. Transfer to another hospital is increasingly likely within a managed clinical network and should be discussed if clinically appropriate. Written information, including this possibility, should be given to all parents at booking.

All resuscitation equipment must be checked and fully functional prior to the birth. An experienced paediatrician and midwife or neonatal nurse must be present at delivery to ensure immediate and expert resuscitation. Thermal care is vital at this point, as cold stress can increase mortality and morbidity in preterm infants (see Ch. 42). The radiant heater should be turned on prior to delivery. The room temperature should be increased to 26°C.

Infants over 30 weeks' gestation should be dried thoroughly and wrapped in a warm towel, and a hat applied. Infants under 30 weeks' gestation should not be dried but should have their bodies placed immediately in a plastic occlusive wrap. This should not be covered with a towel as the radiant heater needs to be directly above the baby (UK Resuscitation Council 2008). This allows visualization of the chest and ease of access whilst preventing evaporative heat loss and skin damage.

Usually, preterm infants are small and fragile and are born requiring stabilization rather than active resuscitation. Some units administer surfactant prophylactically on the resuscitaire if infants require intubation under 30 weeks' gestation. Other babies are given surfactant if they require ventilation and a diagnosis of respiratory distress syndrome is confirmed.

## Common problems

### Respiratory

The most common problems for preterm babies are respiratory disorders (discussed more fully in Chapter 45). The more preterm the baby, the more structurally and physiologically immature the respiratory system.

#### *Respiratory distress syndrome*

The incidence of *respiratory distress syndrome* (RDS) is inversely related to the gestational age of the baby. RDS is a developmental deficiency in surfactant synthesis accompanied by lung immaturity and hypoperfusion. Surfactant is usually produced in larger quantities between 32 and 35 weeks' gestation and RDS is therefore rarely seen in infants beyond this gestation. Surfactant is produced by type II pneumocytes; it assists in the reduction of the surface tension of the lung and prevents complete alveolar collapse on expiration. Surfactant synthesis is reduced with hypoxaemia and acidaemia and the asphyxiated preterm infant may make such weak respiratory effort that he cannot release what little surfactant he has from the pneumocytes. The work of breathing is increased and the baby quickly becomes exhausted. The baby tries to compensate by increasing the respiratory rate and pressures. In term or more mature preterm infants, an expiratory grunt may be audible in the baby's attempt to maintain lung volume. Intercostal and substernal recession can be quite marked – almost pulling to the backbone. There is a characteristic 'ground glass' appearance on chest X-ray with an air bronchogram as the air-filled major airways stand out.

Onset is before 4 hours, and the pattern of the disease gets worse over the first 24–36 hours, then stabilizes and gradually improves. Treatment is aimed at support and active intervention. Support includes maintaining oxygenation, ventilation, a normal pH and adequate perfusion, tissue oxygenation and hydration. Active intervention includes administration of exogenous surfactant and use of continuous positive airways pressure (CPAP) or other modes of ventilatory support if required.

#### *Apnoeas*

Many preterm babies have apnoeas associated with their prematurity and require constant monitoring (Finer et al 2006). Parents need to understand the reasons for this, appreciating they resolve with maturity. Airway position is essential when nursing preterm infants, to reduce the potential for apnoeas caused by mechanical obstruction of the airway. Apnoea monitors should be removed several days prior to discharge so that parents gain confidence and do not become reliant on them. Caffeine is given as a stimulant until these apnoeas of prematurity resolve (Darnell et al 2006).

#### *Oxygen therapy*

Oxygen has been used more than any other drug in the treatment of preterm infants in the past 60 years. Oxygen therapy should provide adequate tissue oxygenation without creating oxygen toxicity. Excessive and fluctuating quantities is one factor in the aetiology of *retinopathy of prematurity* (Campbell 1951, Tin & Gupta 2007), though clinicians are still unsure how much oxygen these babies actually need, or how much is safe to give. Further major, multi-sited research is underway in Canada (see website).

### Temperature control

Although brown fat is utilized during cold stress, VLB and preterm infants often have little or no brown fat stores to maintain the core temperature. The high surface area of preterm infants in relation to their size, and their thin, porous skin, facilitate rapid heat loss through evaporation.

Radiant heaters may exacerbate the problem by increasing the evaporative heat loss and their use is inappropriate for very small babies, who should be nursed in a humidified incubator for the first week of life.

At home, following an emergency or unexpected preterm birth, if no resuscitation is required, the midwife can place the baby on the mother's abdomen or chest for skin-to-skin contact, once dried. The baby's head should be covered with the mother and baby well wrapped in dry blankets. The aim is to maintain body temperature in the thermoneutral range, at which energy requirements are reduced to a minimum and oxygen consumption is less (see Ch. 42).

### Hypoglycaemia

This is a common problem for preterm babies in the first 48–72 hours. Stores of brown fat, white fat and glycogen are too small to maintain blood sugar level when energy requirements are particularly high. Because of the heat loss from their large surface area, increased effort of breathing that accompanies respiratory difficulties, and greater rate of growth, more energy is expended for their weight than in their term counterparts. Asphyxia, sepsis, ischaemia and hypothermia all aggravate this. Preterm infants have immature liver function, with reduced availability of liver enzymes responsible for gluconeogenesis and glycogenolysis, and are less able to produce alternative substrates, such as ketone bodies (Hume et al 2005).

Blood sugar levels should be checked every 4–6 hours during the first 48–72 hours after birth using a glucometer. Controversy still surrounds the clinical definition and significance of hypoglycaemia, but it is generally accepted that the neonatal brain can be damaged by hypoglycaemia, whether symptomatic or not (Schwarz et al 2003). Current recommendations are to maintain serum blood glucose levels above 2.6 mmol/L (Cornblath et al 2000).

## Jaundice

Physiological jaundice is exacerbated in preterm babies as the liver is immature and therefore conjugation of bilirubin is further delayed (see Ch. 46).

The severity of jaundice may be caused by the delayed passage of meconium in preterm babies, particularly if enteral feeds are not commenced for several days, or with respiratory distress syndrome. This delay can contribute to hyperbilirubinaemia as the bilirubin in meconium may be reabsorbed.

Red blood cell lifespan is related to gestational age and may be only 35–50 days in the ELBW infant who may have ongoing low-grade haemolysis. Another contributing factor is the low levels of serum albumin in ELBW infants, which may limit extracellular binding and transport of bilirubin when concentrations are high (Cashore 2000).

## Patent ductus arteriosus (PDA)

The ductus arteriosus fails to close in some very preterm and low-birthweight babies, partly because of immaturity and partly because the chemical conditions are not suitable in babies who are hypoxic and acidotic. Generally, in healthy preterm infants above 30 weeks' gestation, the ductus arteriosus has closed functionally by 4 days. Only 11% of these infants have a PDA, compared to 65% of infants less than 30 weeks' gestation with severe respiratory distress (Clyman 2004).

There are generally three physiological characteristics of a PDA in a preterm infant:

- increased flow through the lungs with diastolic volume overload
- increased flow through the left atrium, left ventricle and aorta
- left-to-right shunting to the pulmonary circulation (Blackburn 2007).

The presence of a PDA results in interstitial oedema and decreased pulmonary compliance due to pulmonary oedema. Prolonged dependence on ventilatory support increases the risk of chronic lung disease (see website).

## Nutrition

The rate of growth in preterm babies is greater than that in their mature counterparts, thus they require a greater energy intake. To achieve a rate of growth similar to that in utero, the preterm baby needs 540–600 kJ/kg/day, equating to approximately 180–200 mL/kg/day of breast milk or standard formula milk. This may be achieved by giving smaller volumes of low-birthweight formula milk, or by adding calorific supplements to breast milk. Larger babies will gain weight on smaller volumes but may also need over 200 mL/kg/day.

Wherever possible, a mother's own fresh expressed breast milk is preferred, as it will be tailor-made to her baby's requirements, whatever the gestation (Blackburn 2007) (see Ch. 43).

The mother should be encouraged to breastfeed, if possible, or start expressing milk, within a few hours of delivery, with a minimum of six times every 24 hours. The sooner this is initiated, the greater the chance of establishing breastfeeding successfully. Midwives should teach all mothers how to express milk by hand and pump and how to store breast milk safely.

Many mothers find breastfeeding a preterm baby rewarding but time-consuming and tiring, and need to be advised that stress and fatigue can adversely affect milk production. Advice should be given on ways to increase their supply should it diminish, including sufficient rest, using hand and machine expression, and an adequate diet (see Ch. 43).

*Low-birthweight formula milks* have a constitution that provides the baby with more energy, protein, vitamins and minerals per millilitre than term formula milks or breast milk. These have long-chain polyunsaturated fatty acids (LCPFA) added to them. These have been identified in human milk, term and preterm, as being important for normal development of the brain, retina and neural tissue in particular.

## Feeding methods

The method of feeding depends on the size, maturity and condition of the baby. Sucking is seen in the fetus as early as 13 weeks' gestation (Hafstrom & Kjellmer 2000), although suck and swallow coordination is not efficient until nearer term. Well babies of any size or gestation showing signs of sucking may be tried with breast, cup or bottle feeds (see Ch. 43). Careful supervision is necessary to ensure that the fluid intake is adequate and that the baby is not becoming too tired by prolonged attempts at feeding.

Immature babies have an increased risk of aspiration and must be closely monitored. They tire easily and may benefit from a regimen of mixed breast/cup/bottle and tube feeds initially, until they can cope with more. Non-nutritive sucking during gastric feeding has been shown to facilitate the development of sucking behaviour (Pinelli & Symington 2007); putting the baby to the breast at these times can be beneficial to the mother and baby and for the establishment of lactation.

### *Intravenous feeding*

Ventilated babies may be fed by the intravenous route initially, due to risks of:

- milk aspiration
- paralytic ileus and bowel obstruction.
- overexertion and increased respiratory effort
- hypotension and/or hypoxia increasing the risk of *septicaemia* or *necrotizing enterocolitis*.

If ventilation or the condition of the baby does not allow oral feeds for a prolonged period, *total parenteral nutrition* is commenced, providing the baby with individually tailored nutrients and calories based on serum electrolyte results.

### *Naso/orojejunal feeding*

Rarely, VLBW babies on long-term ventilation or those suffering from severe gastro-oesophageal reflux may be fed via a transpyloric or jejunal tube, which places milk directly into the bowel (Fig. 44.5), minimizing respiratory embarrassment by keeping the stomach empty. Once the baby's condition has improved, naso/orogastric feeding is commenced.

### *Naso/orogastric feeding*

A naso/orogastric tube is used when the baby's suck is too weak or uncoordinated to feed by breast, cup or bottle. Principles of nasogastric feeding should include:

- checking the correct position of the tube prior to feeds
- making the feed slow
- encouraging the baby to suck/positioning the baby at the breast where possible
- giving small, frequent feeds (every 1– 3 hours).

See website for further information.

## Nutritional supplements

Preterm babies have unique nutritional requirements due to inadequate stores at birth, and immaturity causing delay in developments, such as red blood cell production. They require additional supplementation of certain nutrients, including protein, vitamins, iron and minerals, to achieve optimal growth and development. Current Department of Health and NHS recommendations are that all infants should receive daily vitamin supplements, such as children's vitamin drops (vitamins A, C and D), from the age of 1 month to 5 years. These are especially important for preterm babies as they have small stores of fat-soluble vitamins and are at risk of vitamin deficiency (see website).

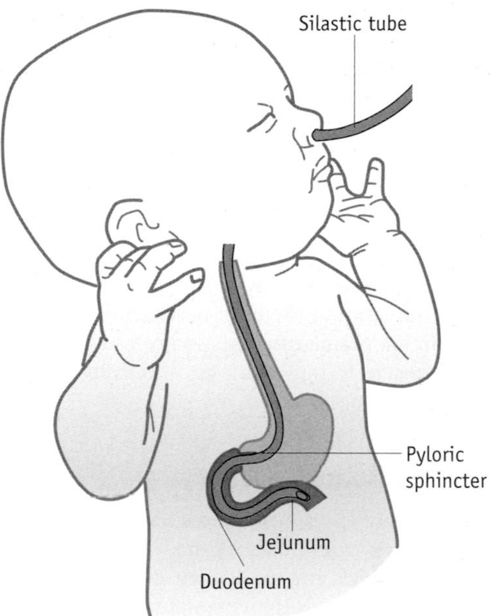


**Figure 44.5** Baby with nasojejunal tube in situ.

## Parent–baby relationship

Parents must have an opportunity to see and hold their baby, however briefly, before transfer to the neonatal unit. The paediatrician must see the parents later to provide an account of their baby's condition, care and prognosis. A mother may feel quite bereft in a postnatal ward, especially when surrounded by other mothers who have their babies beside them. It is common for parents to display signs of grief at this time, as they mourn the healthy baby they expected and fear getting attached to the small or ill baby they actually have. There must be good communication between the neonatal unit and the postnatal ward staff to ensure the family have the support they need.

Parents and siblings are encouraged to become involved in their baby's care as much as possible, from the earliest days, even if the baby is being ventilated. Very few babies are too sick to be cuddled for a short while or gently held by parents, although minimal handling techniques are generally applied to their care.

Many preterm babies are in hospital for several weeks or months before they are ready to be discharged home.

During this time, the parents participate in an increasing amount of their baby's care and will gradually gain confidence. Before discharge, it is helpful for the mother to stay in hospital to care for her baby day and night, on the neonatal unit or in a transitional care ward.

## Complications of prematurity

Several complications occur more commonly in the preterm than in the mature baby, relative to the degree of immaturity of the various systems or nerve centres controlling them. Extreme prematurity is a major cause of perinatal death, thus it is important to effectively reduce, identify and treat complications.

### Chronic lung disease (CLD)

Chronic lung disease (previously known as *bronchopulmonary dysplasia*) most commonly occurs in preterm and low-birthweight babies and is defined clinically as the sustained need for oxygen supplementation after 4 weeks of age when oxygen has been required since birth. Babies with CLD will often require long-term care and follow-up.

Features of CLD include the following:

- serious disruption of lung growth
- X-rays and lung specimens show a loss of alveoli, interstitial oedema, patches of collapse and fibrosis
- lungs are stiff and difficult to ventilate
- history of high concentrations of oxygen, need for prolonged ventilatory support and high ventilator pressures.

Rates of CLD vary considerably amongst NICUs, and with different treatment regimens (see website).

### Infection

A preterm infant is more vulnerable to infections owing to:

- low maternal IgG levels
- thin, porous skin which is an inefficient barrier to invading bacteria
- production of tears and saliva is limited with fewer antibacterial factors
- less protective stomach acid produced
- fewer and inefficient immune cells that do not respond so effectively to stress
- more invasive procedures, and multiple contacts with hospital staff.

In order to protect preterm babies as much as possible, the following guidelines should be followed:

*Handwashing* remains one of the biggest preventive measures staff and families can implement to reduce the risk of cross-infection. Parents, visitors and new staff must be taught correct handwashing techniques to perform before and after handling the baby, using an antiseptic soap, such as chlorhexidine.

Every baby should have their *own individual equipment*, including stethoscope and thermometer, which must be thoroughly cleaned between use.

*Daily cleaning of the incubator or cot* should be carried out, with cleaning and airing after discharge.

Ward areas should be *clean and well ventilated*, and soiled dressings or material placed in disposable bags and removed as soon as possible.

All staff members, family and visitors caring for a neonate must be free from any *signs of infection*, including active cold sores (herpes simplex virus), coughs and sore throats.

*Mimimal handling of preterm babies*: Parents are involved in all aspects of their care as soon as their condition permits. If sufficiently well, the baby should have the face, hands and skin folds gently washed with warm water, when necessary. The napkin area needs particular attention, as the skin is often friable and breaks down quickly when left in contact with urine or faeces.

*Oral hygiene* is necessary for babies with an endotracheal tube in situ; for those unable to suck or those receiving tube feeds.

*Antibiotic use* may render the baby susceptible to candida infection and prophylactic treatment or early identification and treatment of this is important.

*Breastfeeding is encouraged* and supported, wherever possible, and consideration should be given to the use of donor breast milk where milk bank facilities are available.

### Hypocalcaemia

Early hypocalcaemia (low serum calcium levels) may occur within the first 72 hours of life in preterm babies, infants of diabetic mothers and in those suffering from asphyxia, respiratory distress syndrome or sepsis. Asphyxia results in the excretion of high levels of calcitonin from the parathyroid glands. This reduces calcium mobilization from the bones. Vitamin D, required for parathyroid hormone action on bones and the gut, is also deficient in the preterm baby. Supplementation may be necessary.

### Hypoxic ischaemic encephalopathy (HIE) (birth asphyxia)

The preterm infant has little energy reserve should there be any interruption to the oxygen supply, and in this event the heart will not continue pumping for long. Cardiac glycogen stores allow the heart to continue in cases of asphyxia. Continued cardiac function is required to remove the accumulated lactic acid from the brain. Since glycogen stores are reduced, the capacity of the preterm baby to withstand asphyxia is reduced.

Clinical presentation of the baby with HIE varies with severity. Six aspects of clinical presentation are assessed and may be predictive of outcome:

- level of consciousness
- tone and posture – neuromuscular indicator
- primitive, complex reflexes
- presence of seizures
- autonomic functions
- duration of symptoms.

Treatment is aimed at minimizing further cerebral damage, alleviating symptoms and early detection of any complications, such as cerebral haemorrhage or hydrocephalus. Drugs are given to maintain cerebral perfusion and blood pressure, to reduce cerebral oedema and control seizures.

Investigations to assess the severity of damage include ultrasound, CT scanning, MRI scanning and EEG recording. Prognosis depends on the severity of the insult, but may result in severe neurological damage. Until recently, no treatment has shown to be effective for preventing brain damage (see website).

## Cerebral haemorrhage and associated lesions

The incidence of neonatal cerebral haemorrhages in preterm and VLBW babies has declined in the past two decades, partly due to the use of prophylactic antenatal steroids. Cranial ultrasound scanning (see Fig. 44.6) is routinely performed on all preterm babies. Small bleeds are commonly found within a few hours of birth, even after what seemed an easy delivery, and are classified depending on site and severity.

Major haemorrhages may cause ischaemic changes in the white matter around the ventricles, resulting in *periventricular cystic leucomalacia* (PVL) which is cyst formation with major neurological implications. Whilst the rate of periventricular haemorrhage (PVH) has reduced, the incidence of these ischaemic lesions appears to have increased, with implications for the morbidity of preterm and VLBW infants.

*Causes* include:

- intrapartum events
- perinatal hypoxia
- poor skull ossification
- fragile blood vessels
- episodes of hypotension, hypertension or hypoxia.

Close monitoring of fetal and neonatal wellbeing during labour and in the NNU is crucial in identifying and managing problems and maintaining stability, as is gentle handling and good pain management (see website).

*Complications* include:

- shock
- disseminated intravascular coagulation (DIC)
- pressure on parts of the brain linked with the autonomic system – influencing respiration, blood pressure and temperature control
- hydrocephalus (develops when blood in the ventricles clots and obstructs the flow of cerebrospinal fluid, or when viscosity of the cerebrospinal fluid is altered by debris from the haemorrhage)
- high incidence of cerebral palsy.

Certain drugs can reduce the rate of cerebrospinal fluid production, thereby reducing hydrocephalus. Regular lumbar punctures may be performed to relieve excess pressure, but if the problem persists, the surgical insertion of ventricular shunts may be necessary, to drain the fluid into the abdomen.

## Anaemia

Anaemia is common in preterm babies. The shorter intrauterine period prevents the accumulation of an adequate

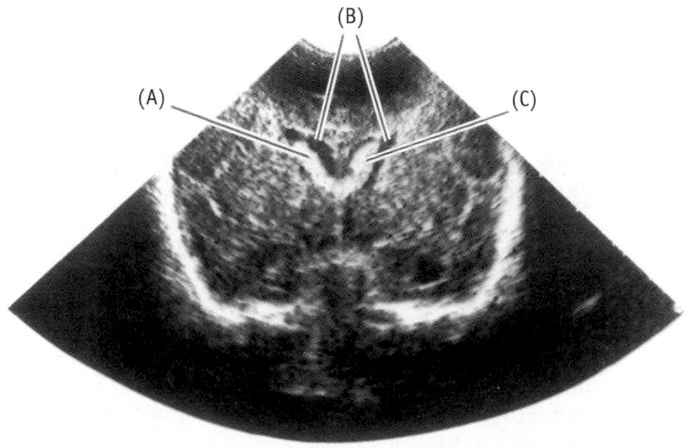


**Figure 44.6** Coronal cranial ultrasound showing intraventricular haemorrhages (B) in dilated lateral ventricles (A). *(From Kelnar et al 2007.)*

iron store and the immature gastrointestinal system does not easily digest iron supplements. The underactive bone marrow is unable to keep up sufficient red blood cell production to match the rapid rate of growth and increase in circulation. Ill babies require frequent blood tests and may have had much blood removed for sampling. Blood transfusions are often necessary, although some babies make good progress in spite of a low haemoglobin level.

### Vitamin K deficiency bleeding (VKDB)

Newborn infants have reduced levels of the vitamin K-dependent clotting factors, including prothrombin and factors VII, IX and X. This is a consequence of poor transport of vitamin K across the placenta as well as a lack of intestinal colonization by bacteria that normally synthesize vitamin K. There is substantially more vitamin K in formula milk than breast milk.

VKDB is classified according to the timing of onset:

- early: within the first 24 hours
- classic: 1–7 days
- late: 8 days–6 months.

*Early VKDB* is rare and is seen in babies of mothers taking certain drugs, such as vitamin K-antagonist anticoagulants (*warfarin*), some antituberculosis medications (*isoniazid*) and some anticonvulsants (*phenobarbital or phenytoin*). At booking, the midwife should ask about any medicines the mother is taking and refer her to the obstetrician/physician to review these. Alternative medication may reduce the neonatal risk.

*Classic VKDB* is preventable by the recommended schedule of vitamin K 0.5–1 mg intramuscularly at birth (Puckett & Offringa 2000).

*Late VKDB* occurs almost exclusively in breastfed babies and is more likely to present as intraventricular or pulmonary bleeding, rather than gastrointestinal, with an associated high morbidity rate of up to 33% (Bor et al 2000). The cause is multifactorial, often related to hepatic disease or malabsorption syndrome. Repeated transfusions of blood, plasma and/or clotting factors are given and vitamin K is administered, in an attempt to treat the condition successfully.

Babies in the high-risk group include:

- VLBW
- preterm
- hypoxic
- difficult or instrumental delivery.

Midwives need to discuss individual risk factors with parents and obtain informed consent for vitamin K administration (see website).

### Retinopathy of prematurity (ROP)

ROP is one of the few causes of childhood visual impairment that is largely preventable. Many extremely preterm babies will develop some degree of ROP, although in the majority this never progresses beyond mild disease which resolves spontaneously.

Preventive care involves reducing the incidence of preterm and low-birthweight babies and continuing with high-quality, controlled neonatal intensive care (Campbell 1951) (see website).

### Necrotizing enterocolitis (NEC)

Necrotizing enterocolitis is an inflammatory disease of the bowel normally associated with septicaemia, thought to result from the proliferation of bacteria in the bowel which then penetrate the wall at points where ischaemic damage has occured. Oedema, ulceration and haemorrhages of the bowel wall are found, which may progress to perforation or peritonitis.

The condition typically develops in preterm and low-birthweight babies who have been ill with asphyxia, respiratory distress, hypoglycaemia, hypothermia or cardiovascular disease. Predisposing factors include: variations in bowel perfusion associated with exchange transfusion; hypotension; patent ductus arteriosus; polycythaemia (when the blood is too thick to flow readily); and thrombosis or spasm of the mesenteric vessels from an umbilical catheter.

The problem usually manifests within a few days of starting milk feeds, as it is then that colonization of the intestine is more likely.

Signs and symptoms include:

- non-specific malaise
- indications of sepsis
- apnoea or septic shock
- abdominal signs such as distension, bile-stained aspirate, or the passage of blood and mucus per rectum.

The diagnosis is confirmed by the appearance of the bowel on radiography (Fig. 44.7) (see website).

Breast milk does afford some protection against NEC (Dai & Walker 1999), and midwives should promote breastfeeding for all babies, as it is particularly important for sick, low-birthweight and preterm babies.

## The neonatal intensive care unit (NICU) environment

The NICU is a busy, bright, harsh and noisy environment that could not be further from the circumstances experienced in utero. One of the aims of neonatal care is to achieve similar rates of growth and development of the baby to those that would have been attained in utero, and practitioners need to be aware of the impact of surroundings, interventions, care and treatments undertaken for the neonate's wellbeing.

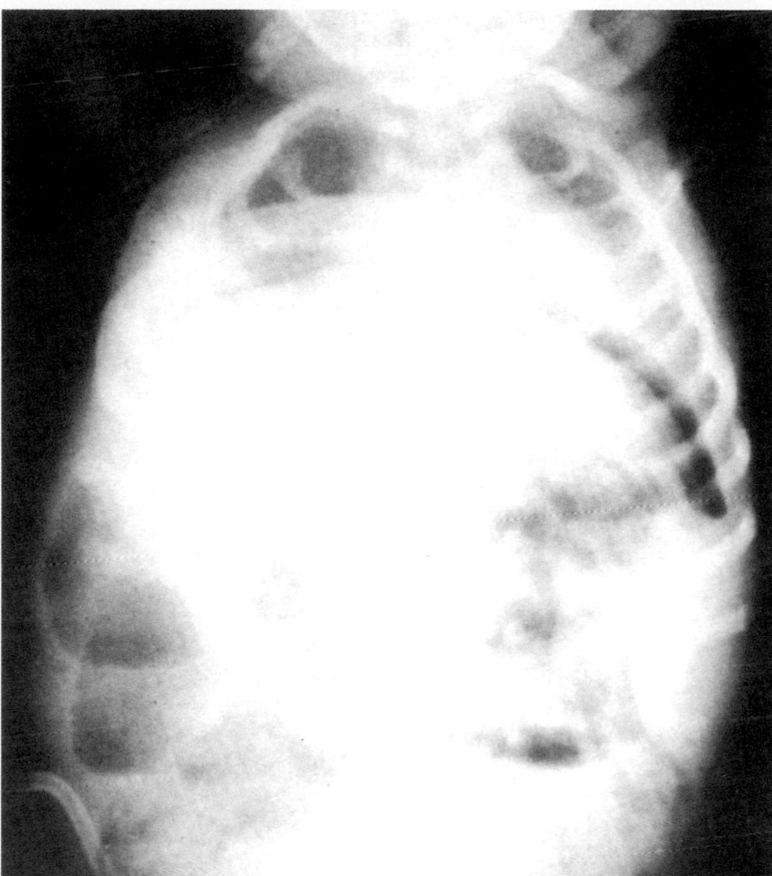

**Figure 44.7** Necrotizing enterocolitis, showing dilated loops of bowel.

Developmental care programmes are practised in many units, considering control of external stimuli, clustering of nursing activities and positioning of the neonates, particularly the preterm. Application of the synactive theory of infant development (Als et al 1994) through serial observations of the baby is helpful in identifying the baby's areas of success at coping and vulnerability. It is important to communicate these strengths and vulnerabilities to the parents and identify strategies to support the baby in the NICU.

Interventions that are used to minimize the stress encountered by these infants and individualize the care-giving according to the infant's tolerance include:

- modification of the environment
- reducing light and noise
- minimal handling
- protection of sleep states
- promoting understanding of behavioural cues
- promoting relationship-based care-giving.

These programmes appear to demonstrate some benefits to preterm babies in terms of short-term growth, decreased respiratory support, decreased length of hospital stay and improved neurological outcomes at 2 years corrected age (Symington & Pinelli 2001). However, many studies into developmental care have small sample sizes and include multiple interventions, making interpretation difficult.

## SMALL-FOR-GESTATIONAL-AGE (SGA) BABIES

### Incidence

One-third of all babies of low birthweight fall into this category and the majority of SGA babies are mature, having a gestational age of 37 weeks or more.

### Causes

It is not uncommon for preterm babies to also be SGA and many of the predisposing factors are the same in both situations:

- idiopathic – no cause identified
- placental insufficiency
- low socioeconomic groups (social classes IV and V)
- placental dysfunction (spasm of spiral arterioles reduces the intervillous blood flow and exchange of nutrients and oxygen across the placental barrier):
  - pre-eclampsia
  - essential hypertension
  - chronic renal failure
  - nephritis
- severe anaemia:
  - sickle cell disease
  - phenylketonuria
- following threatened abortion or antepartum haemorrhage
- multiple pregnancy
- viruses – rubella, toxoplasmosis, cytomegalovirus
- prescribed or abused substances: some steroids, anticonvulsants, antihypertensives, cytotoxics, nicotine, alcohol, cocaine and heroin.

## Characteristics (Fig. 44.8)

- Head appears large in relation to the wasted appearance of the body and limbs (and lack of subcutaneous fat).
- Ribs are easily visible.
- Hollowed abdomen.
- Skin often dry, loose and may be peeling.
- Skin may be meconium-stained.
- Umbilical cord is thin (may also be meconium-stained).
- Baby often appears wizened and old with an anxious, wide-awake expression.
- Muscle tone is usually good and baby is active.
- Baby will appear ravenously hungry and tends to suck a fist.
- Neurological responses usually correspond to gestational age.

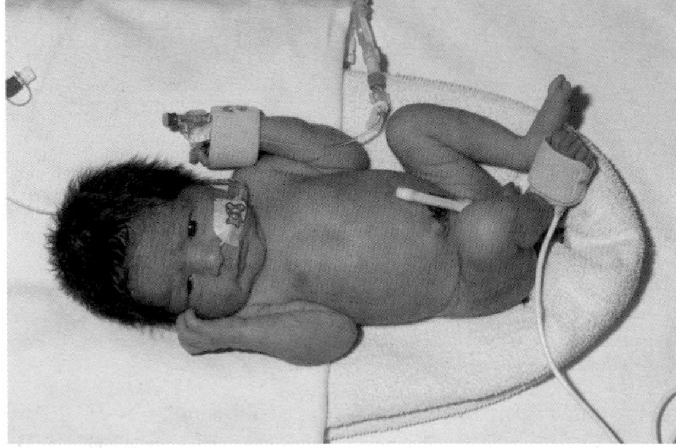

**Figure 44.8** SGA baby.

Babies who are SGA are categorized into two groups according to whether they are affected by *asymmetrical* or *symmetrical growth restriction*.

**Asymmetrical growth restriction:** Growth is normal until about the third trimester of pregnancy, when complications such as pre-eclampsia develop. This adversely affects placental function, leading to reduced growth resulting from malnutrition. This is a relatively late phenomenon and the degree of growth restriction depends on the severity of the causative condition. Head circumference and length are within normal limits for the gestational age of the baby, but birthweight is low in proportion to head circumference when plotted on a centile chart.

**Symmetrical growth restriction:** The main underlying causes are early intrauterine infections, such as *cytomegalovirus, rubella* or *toxoplasmosis*, maternal substance abuse, such as fetal alcohol syndrome, and other drugs taken early in the pregnancy. These have a toxic or teratogenic effect on the placenta, with fetal growth affected from the time these substances were introduced in the pregnancy. Some chromosomal anomalies and malformations also result in symmetrical SGA babies. The appearance of the baby is similar to that described above, but the head circumference is in proportion to the overall size and weight. The prognosis for these babies is poorer than those asymmetrically grown, since they have been compromised for a much longer period.

## Management

A detailed booking history antenatally is essential, as this may identify risk factors associated with intrauterine growth restriction (IUGR). Careful assessment of uterine size and growth is important to enable early detection of a slow or reducing rate of growth of the fetus, possibly indicating the need for a more detailed assessment of fetal wellbeing.

A great deal of the care required by SGA babies during the first 48 hours following birth, centres around prevention and early recognition of any possible complications. In most cases, these babies can be cared for in normal postnatal wards with their mothers and do not need admission to a neonatal intensive or special care unit. Transitional care wards are an ideal place to care for those babies with minor problems, such as poor temperature control.

## Labour and delivery

The growth-restricted fetus is chronically hypoxic and consequently tolerates the stresses of labour and delivery poorly, as the blood supply to the placenta is further interrupted during each contraction. The midwife should anticipate the possibility of fetal distress and perinatal asphyxia. Close fetal monitoring and observation of the liquor for meconium during labour are imperative. A paediatrician should be present at the birth if the baby is known to be significantly small or compromised. Expert and urgent resuscitation is vital, if required, particularly if there is meconium-stained liquor. This will prevent further hypoxia and respiratory complications that may result in long-term neurological damage.

SGA babies have only a thin layer of subcutaneous fat and a relatively large surface area, thus lose heat very rapidly. The room temperature must be raised prior to delivery and the baby dried and wrapped in warm blankets quickly following birth. Since 80% of heat loss occurs through the head, a hat should be placed on the baby once the head is dry.

If the baby is well enough, early feeding is important to counter hypoglycaemia resulting from insufficient energy stores in these babies.

## Complications

### Hypoxic ischaemic encephalopathy (HIE) (birth asphyxia)

This condition is mainly avoidable in countries with good antenatal care. The midwife must facilitate close and careful monitoring during labour and early intervention to expedite delivery in the event of fetal distress. Even modern methods of assessing fetal wellbeing are relatively insensitive and the midwife needs to be vigilant. SGA babies have limited reserves to cope with perinatal asphyxia and are at high risk. Mild symptoms of HIE may resolve after a few days, with little or no residual cerebral damage. More severe injuries may result in fits and cerebral palsy.

### Meconium aspiration syndrome

SGA babies tolerate perinatal stress and hypoxia poorly. Hypoxia causes relaxation of the anal sphincter, allowing meconium to be passed into the liquor. Asphyxiated fetuses gasp in utero and will inhale the liquor and meconium into the bronchial tree, and then, with the first breath at delivery, further into the trachea. This clogs the lungs and commonly leads to *pneumonitis, pneumothoraces* or a *secondary bacterial pneumonia*.

Skilled resuscitation at delivery is vital. If the baby *does not breathe*, the nares and oropharynx should be suctioned prior to bag and mask resuscitation. If examination with a laryngoscope (by a skilled practitioner) shows meconium in the larynx, the baby should be intubated and the trachea suctioned through the endotracheal tube. If the baby *does breathe* spontaneously and is vigorous, suction and intubation are unlikely to be helpful. Close observation of the baby is imperative for the first 24 hours following meconium staining of the liquor, to identify early signs of any respiratory problems or infection (see website).

### Hypothermia

Growth-restricted babies have a deficit of subcutaneous and brown fat. Hypothermia is a risk because of the relatively high surface area to bodyweight ratio. It is critical that the baby is dried and wrapped quickly following birth and the axillary temperature monitored carefully in the first 48 hours. The baby may be nursed in an incubator next to the mother in the postnatal or transitional care ward, or cared for with skin-to-skin contact with the mother to stabilize the temperature.

### Hypoglycaemia

This is a common problem for SGA babies – in most cases prevented with early and regular feeding. These babies particularly benefit from breastfeeding, as they are also at a greater risk of neonatal necrotizing enterocolitis. Low-birthweight formula milks are widely used, with the advantage of being more energy-dense than regular formula milk.

SGA babies have small livers and small glycogen stores, and their energy reserves are used during labour, particularly if prolonged or difficult. Asphyxia and hypothermia will exacerbate the problem of hypoglycaemia. Frequent recordings of the blood glucose level are important within the first 48 hours, at least 4-hourly until they are stable and maintained above 2.6 mmol/L.

### Polycythaemia

Polycythaemia occurs when the venous packed cell volume is 0.65 L/L (65%) and is a consequence of chronic intra-uterine hypoxia. To improve the oxygen-carrying capacity of the blood, the haemoglobin level may rise to more than 20 g/dL. This can result in jaundice and posibly cerebral irritation. Treatment may require exchange plasma transfusion and additional fluids (see website).

### Poor feeding

Asymmetrically growth-restricted babies tend to feed eagerly and thrive from birth. Symmetrically growth-restricted babies, however, who have been starved for a prolonged period in utero, often continue the slow rate of growth postnatally and may remain small, although a degree of catch-up growth is often evident.

### Pulmonary haemorrhage

This is a rare complication (see website).

### Substance abuse

Babies born to substance-abusing mothers are often growth restricted, particularly following the prolonged use of heroin, alcohol and nicotine (Smith et al 2006). It is often very difficult to obtain an honest and accurate history of drugs taken during pregnancy from the woman. These babies, as well as being at risk of withdrawal symptoms and future developmental problems, are often poor at withstanding labour and may suffer perinatal hypoxia, and associated complications.

The baby of a known narcotic-abusing mother is *not* given neonatal naloxone during resuscitation, as this initiates rapid withdrawal symptoms as any narcotics in the baby's circulation are rapidly broken down.

Implementing a scoring system for the frequency and severity of withdrawal symptoms, such as hyperactivity, irritability, high-pitched cry, sneezing and poor feeding, provides a framework for levels of treatment and interventions. These include nursing in quiet darkened surroundings, swaddling, and possibly medication.

## FOLLOW-UP CARE FOR SMALL AND PRETERM BABIES

The paediatrician usually follows up preterm and SGA babies after discharge from hospital to assess progress, development, and general condition. Midwives, health visitors and general practitioners see the infant more frequently and play a crucial role in monitoring for and recognizing associated complications, or deviations from normal development. Symmetrically growth-restricted and neurologically damaged babies need particularly close follow-up for several years in paediatric outpatient clinics.

Hearing must be carefully checked and most neonatal units perform hearing tests routinely for preterm, sick and SGA babies. Babies are at particular risk of hearing impairment if they have experienced hypoxia, sepsis or hyperbilirubinaemia or have received certain drugs (such as *gentamicin* or *furosemide*).

Some areas now employ specialized NICU liaison nurses or midwives to monitor these small babies in the community, offering advice and support to the parents and other health professionals. This develops continuity of advice and prevents readmission to hospital through early recognition and treatment of minor problems.

### Outcomes

Low-birthweight babies have an increased risk of:

- sudden infant death syndrome
- major disabilities
- preterm babies generally display more motor deficits: SGA babies have poorer cognitive skills
- neurological abnormalities
- long-term oxygen requirement
- ROP, PVL and/or NEC (McElrath et al 2001)
- hydrocephalus
- chronic lung disease
- perinatal mortality
- coronary heart disease and strokes in adult life (Rich-Edwards et al 1997).

With recent advances and developments in neonatal care, babies above 32 weeks' gestation and above 1500 g now have a much greater chance of intact survival than previously, and in a small study, one-third of babies born at 23 weeks' gestation survived to be discharged from hospital, but none were free from substantial morbidity (see website).

## ETHICAL ISSUES

Complex and difficult ethical issues arise in the care of very preterm and VLBW babies, especially when complications substantially increasing the risk of long-term handicap arise, or if chromosomal abnormalities or major congenital malformations are present (see website).

During the period of care, difficult decisions arise when the baby is surviving solely because of the supportive care being given, yet the risk of handicap is known to be extremely high. Professionals and parents then need time to discuss the situation openly. Space is required to reflect on the possible consequences of continuing full intensive care as long as it is required, or of withdrawing such care to allow the baby to die in peace and dignity. This is one of the most agonizing and difficult decisions both parents and professionals have to face.

Cultural factors and personal values and beliefs are deeply challenged at times like this and will influence the decisions made. Sometimes, parents appreciate the opportunity to discuss the situation with a minister of religion, or with a counsellor who is not directly involved in the care of their baby. Such help can be invaluable during this extremely stressful period (see Ch. 70).

**Reflective activity 44.2**

Review the facilities for parents and siblings of babies in your local neonatal intensive care unit.

## CONCLUSION

Many mothers feel extremely guilty when they give birth to a preterm or low-birthweight baby, often blaming themselves for actions taken or omitted during the pregnancy. Midwives must offer as much support as possible during these times.

Individuals react differently to stress and midwives and neonatal staff need to learn to recognize the signs in parents and develop appropriate skills to enable families to cope during this difficult time. They must also recognize the signs of stress in themselves and in colleagues. Opportunities to share and discuss problems can be of immense benefit to all concerned. Effective personal coping strategies are therefore essential for those working with families with preterm, sick and VLBW babies.

Midwives are a key part of the team providing care to these small babies and their parents, and need to work closely with their colleagues to ensure a seamless, sensitive and high-quality service both initially and on a long-term basis.

## KEY POINTS

- The causes of preterm labour and low birthweight are closely linked, with social factors playing a large role.
- Breastfeeding can make a significant difference to the short- and long-term health of these groups of babies, reducing the risk of complications associated with their small size or early gestation.
- Parents will require much support from the midwife, both practical and psychological, when they give birth to a very small or preterm baby. Close liaison between hospital and community staff is vital.

## REFERENCES


Als H, Lawhon G, Duffy FH, et al: Individualized developmental care for the very low birthweight preterm infant. Medical and neurofunctional effects, *Journal of the American Medical Association* 272(11):853–859, 1994.

Blackburn ST: *Maternal, fetal and neonatal physiology: a clinical perspective*, Philadelphia, 2007, WB Saunders.

Bor O, Akgun N, Yakut A, et al: Late haemorrhagic disease of the newborn, *Pediatrics International* 42(1):64–66, 2000.

Campbell K: Intensive oxygen therapy as a possible cause of retrolental fibroplasia: a clinical approach, *Medical Journal of Australia* ii:48–50, 1951.

Cashore D: Bilirubin and jaundice in the micropremie, *Clinics in Perinatology* 27:171–179, 2000.

Clyman RI: Mechanisms facilitating closure of the ductus arteriosus. In Polin RA, Fox WW, Abman SH, editors: *Fetal and neonatal physiology*, ed 3, Philadelphia, 2004, Saunders.

Cooke RWI: Perinatal and postnatal factors in very preterm infants and subsequent cognitive and motor abilities, *Archives of Disease in Childhood. Fetal and Neonatal Edition* 90(1):F60–F63, 2005.

Cornblath M, Hawdon JM, Williams AF, et al: Controversies regarding the definition of neonatal hypoglycemia: suggested operational thresholds, *Pediatrics* 105(5):1141–1145, 2000.

Dai D, Walker WA: Protective nutrients and bacterial colonization in the immature human gut, *Advances in Pediatrics* 46:353–382, 1999.

Darnell RA, Ariagno RL, Kinney HC: The late preterm infant and the control of breathing, sleep and brainstem development: a review, *Clinics In Perinatology* 33(4):883–914, 2006.

Dubowitz LMS, Dubowitz V, Goldberg C: Clinical assessment of gestational age in the newborn infant, *Journal of Pediatrics* 77(1):1–10, 1970.

Finer N, Higgins R, Kattwinkel J, et al: Summary proceedings from the Apnoea of Prematurity Group, *Pediatrics* 117(3 Pt 2):S47–S51, 2006.

Hafstrom M, Kjellmer I: Non-nutritive sucking in the healthy pre-term infant, *Early Human Development* 60(1):13–24, 2000.

Hume R, Burchell A, Williams FL, et al: Glucose homeostasis in the newborn, *Early Human Development* 81(1):95–101, 2005.

Johnston PGB, Flood K, Spinks K: *The newborn child*, ed 9, Edinburgh, 2003, Churchill Livingstone.

Kelnar CJH, Harvey D, Simpson C: *The sick newborn baby*, ed 4, London, 2007, Baillière Tindall.

McElrath TF, Robinson JN, Ecker JL, et al: Neonatal outcome of infants born at 23 weeks' gestation, *Obstetrics and Gynecology* 97(1):49–52, 2001.

Marlowe N, Wolke D, Bracewell M, et al: Neurologic and developmental disability at six years of age after extremely preterm birth, *New England Journal of Medicine* 352(1):9–19, 2005.

Office for National Statistics (ONS): *Gestation – specific infant mortality by social and biological factors, England and Wales 2006* (website). www.ons.gov.uk. 2009.

Pinelli J, Symington A: Non-nutritive sucking for promoting physiologic stability and nutrition in preterm infants, *Cochrane Database of Systematic Reviews* (4):CD001071, 2007.

Puckett RM, Offringa M: Prophylactic vitamin K for vitamin K deficiency bleeding in neonates, *Cochrane Database of Systematic Reviews* (4):CD002776, 2000.

Rich-Edwards JW, Stampfer MJ, Manson JE, et al: Birth weight and risk of cardiovascular disease in a cohort of women followed up since 1976, *British Medical Journal* 31(7105):396–400, 1997.

Royal College of Paediatrics and Child Health (RCPCH): *UK-WHO growth charts – early years*, http://www.rcpch.ac.uk/Research/UK-WHO-Growth-Charts Access Nov 2010.

Schwarz R, Cornblath M, Kalhan SC: Hypoglycaemia in the neonate. In Kendall Stevenson D, Sunshine P, Benitz W, editors: *Fetal and neonatal brain injury: mechanisms, management and the risks of practice*, Cambridge, 2003, Cambridge University Press, pp 553–570.

Smith L, LaGasse L, Derauf C, et al: The Infant Development, Environment and Lifestyle study: effects of prenatal methamphetamine exposure; polydrug exposure and poverty on intrauterine growth, *Pediatrics* 118(3):1149–1156, 2006

Symington A, Pinelli J: Developmental care for promoting development and preventing morbidity in preterm infants, *Cochrane Database of Systematic Reviews* (4):CD001814, 2001.

Tin W, Gupta S: Optimum oxygen therapy in preterm babies, *Archives of Diseases in Childhood. Fetal and Neonatal Edition* 92:F143–F147, 2007.

UK Resuscitation Council: *Resuscitation at birth*, London, 2008, Resuscitation Council UK.

Vadillo-Ortega F, Estrada-Gutierrez G: Role of matrix proteins in premature labour, *International Journal of Obstetrics and Gynaecology* 112(Suppl 1):19–22, 2005.

World Health Organization (WHO): *Manual of international statistical classification of diseases, injuries and causes of death*, Vol. I, Geneva, 1977, WHO.

Chapter 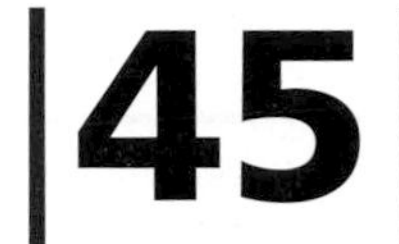

# Respiratory and cardiac disorders

Joan Cameron

### LEARNING OUTCOMES

After reading this chapter, you will be able to:

- link knowledge of fetal circulation with transitional changes at birth
- discuss the key actions in resuscitating newborn babies
- relate fetal cardiac and respiratory development to the existence of neonatal cardiac and respiratory pathology
- describe and justify the actions that a midwife should undertake to detect and treat common respiratory and cardiac disorders.

## INTRODUCTION

Developments in the organization of the maternity services means that midwives are taking on greater responsibility for the care of the newborn at birth and in the postnatal period. Midwives need to be able to respond to the challenge of resuscitating newborn babies, examining babies to confirm normality and detect abnormality, and stabilizing sick infants while awaiting transfer to tertiary facilities. This chapter provides an overview of fetal anatomy and physiology and relates this to resuscitation of the newborn (see Ch. 29). The chapter also offers an overview of some of the common respiratory and cardiac disorders midwives may encounter in practice.

## RESPIRATORY AND CARDIAC DEVELOPMENT IN THE FETUS

Midwives need to appreciate respiratory and cardiac development in utero as this facilitates understanding of normal adaptation at birth. It provides a basis for care provision in some respiratory and cardiac disorders.

### Respiratory development (Table 45.1)

Fetal lungs are filled with fluid secreted by the lungs – rather than amniotic fluid. This fluid is important in facilitating the maturation and development of the fetal lungs. Approximately 300–350 mL of fetal lung fluid is produced daily by the fetus at term. In utero, it can move up the trachea, where some is swallowed by the fetus and some escapes into the amniotic fluid. At birth, a small amount of this fluid drains from the nose but most is moved out of the alveoli into the lymphatic system with the first breaths (Greenough & Milner 2005).

*Fetal breathing movements* are rapid irregular movements, which may be seen on ultrasound as early as 10 weeks' gestation. The strength and frequency of fetal breathing movements increase with gestational age. By the third trimester, breathing movements can be detected about 30% of the time, at a rate of 30–70 breaths per minute (bpm). It is thought that fetal breathing movements are important in enhancing lung development and growth. Fetal breathing patterns can be altered during periods of hypoxia, sometimes ceasing for several hours. Monitoring fetal breathing movements by ultrasound is used as part of biophysical profiling to assess fetal wellbeing.

### Cardiac development

The cardiovascular system is the first system to develop in the embryo. The rapidly developing embryo requires an efficient and effective way of transporting oxygen and nutrients and excreting waste products (Blackburn 2007). The heart begins to develop from the neural plate at around 3 weeks post conception, at first appearing like two long strands. The cords undergo a process known as canalization to become two hollow endocardial tubes which fold back on themselves and fuse to become a

**Table 45.1 Respiratory development in the fetus**

| Post conception | |
|---|---|
| 3–6 weeks | Fetal lungs start to develop from the foregut<br>The division of the foregut and the respiratory system is complete by the end of this period.<br>Disruption at this time can lead to abnormalities such as tracheo-oesophageal fistula (Blackburn 2007) |
| 7–16 weeks | Respiratory system continues to grow and differentiate |
| 16 weeks | Tracheobronchial tree is formed<br>Cilia and mucus-producing glands are present |
| 16–26 weeks | Primitive bronchioles start to develop rich vascular network required for gaseous exchange in extrauterine life |
| 20–24 weeks | Lung is lined with epithelium composed of *Type I and Type II pneumatocytes*<br>Type II pneumatocytes start to appear<br>Type II pneumatocytes produce *surfactant*, a pulmonary lipoprotein which decreases surface tension, thus reducing the work of breathing<br>As gestational age increases, more surfactant is synthesized (Blackburn 2007) |
| 24 weeks | Vascular system proliferates<br>Leads to thinning of the vascular epithelium and the capillaries come into close contact with the developing airways – eventually becomes the *blood–gas barrier* |
| 26 weeks onwards | Terminal air sacs appear, which then develop into the alveoli<br>(Note: Despite the lack of alveoli in babies born between 24 and 26 weeks' gestation, the vascular bed is sufficient to allow some gaseous exchange and this can, with support, sustain extrauterine life [Hodson 1998]) |
| 29–35 weeks | Proliferation of alveoli starts and increases dramatically (Hodson 1998)<br>Development of alveoli continues after birth |
| 30 weeks onwards | Significant increase of total lung surface and lung volume |
| 35 weeks | Fetus has sufficient surfactant and functional alveoli to support extrauterine life |

single tube. This becomes the *endocardium*. The tissue around the outside of the endocardial tube becomes thicker and eventually becomes the *myocardium*.

The single tube is essentially upside down at this stage, with the structures that will become the atria at the lower (caudal) end and the ventricular structures at the upper (cephalic) end. By 22 days post conception, the single cardiac tube starts to beat and blood moves from the bottom of the tube to the top. As the heart enlarges, it has to fold back on itself in order to be accommodated. As the tube folds from top to bottom, it twists round so the single atrium moves to the cephalic position and the single ventricle moves to the caudal position. Between the fourth to sixth week post conception, septation occurs and divides the atrium and ventricle into two. During the septation process, the *foramen ovale* is formed, enabling movement of blood between the atria.

The process of cardiac development is complex, must take place in a specific sequence over a very short period of time and is controlled by cardiac genes. Alterations in the genetic material can lead to failure in development or altered growth patterns, giving rise to congenital cardiac malformations.

## The fetal circulation

The placenta provides the fetus with oxygen and nutrients and also disposes of waste products. In order to achieve this, the fetal circulation has a number of unique features, including temporary structures, to allow shunting of blood, allowing the mixing of oxygenated and deoxygenated blood, high pulmonary vascular resistance and a low systemic circulation (see Ch. 29 and website).

The temporary structures are:

- *ductus venosus*
- *foramen ovale*
- *ductus arteriosus*
- *hypogastric arteries*.

## TRANSITION TO EXTRAUTERINE LIFE

At birth, the newborn infant is exposed to changes in temperature and tactile stimulation, which with the hypoxic and hypercapnic changes that take place as labour progresses, stimulates the first breath. This breath inflates the lungs and forces the fetal lung fluid out into the lymphatic system (Strang 1977). Pulmonary vascular resistance decreases dramatically and the pressure in the right side of the heart falls. Because gas exchange now occurs in the lungs, alveolar oxygenation concentration levels increase.

The dramatic fall in pulmonary vascular resistance, and the increase in oxygen concentration, facilitates the closure of the ductus arteriosus. Blood flows from the lungs to the left atrium, increasing the pressure in the left side of the heart and causing the flap-like opening of the foramen ovale to close. Blood then passes from the left atrium to the left ventricle and from there into the aorta. Clamping of the umbilical cord prevents blood flowing back into the placenta and this increases the systemic circulatory pressure. The reduced blood flow through the umbilical cord vessels causes constriction of the ductus venosus.

The changes in the temporary structures may take some time to become permanent. It is recommended that auscultation of the fetal heart to elicit cardiac murmurs should be delayed until at least 6 hours after birth to allow for the closure of the ductus arteriosus and the foramen ovale (Onuzo 2006).

The changes may also be reversed in adverse conditions – hypoxia can cause the ductus arteriosus to remain patent, particularly in preterm infants. Some infants are less likely to make a successful transition to extrauterine life. Preterm infants may experience difficulty in establishing adequate lung volume or oxygenation because of poor muscle tone or lack of surfactant. Babies born at term by elective caesarean section are more likely to encounter problems clearing fetal lung fluid because of the lack of stress response associated with labour, leading to the development of *transient tachypnoea of the newborn* (Morrison et al 1995).

## RESUSCITATION OF THE NEWBORN

Although *hypoxia* is a stimulus for the onset of breathing at birth, *profound hypoxia* can depress the respiratory centre in the brain and prevent or inhibit the successful transition to extrauterine life. Neonatal hypoxia may be characterized by the absence of breathing or by the presence of profound irregular gasping movements. It has been suggested that *primary apnoea* is caused by a period of acute hypoxia. During this period, breathing ceases. Initially the heart rate remains the same, but soon falls to about 60 beats per minute (bpm). If steps are not taken to correct the hypoxia, primitive spinal centres take over and produce deep, irregular agonal gasps. Eventually the lack of oxygen causes cessation of cardiac activity and the baby enters *terminal apnoea*. At birth **it is not possible to tell** which stage the baby has reached, so the approach to newborn resuscitation is the same in all these situations.

The need for resuscitation may be anticipated in certain situations (Box 45.1), but is not always predictable; therefore, all midwives must have skills in resuscitation of the newborn. 'Fire drills' and participation at courses, including the Newborn Life Support (NLS) course, are useful ways of maintaining skills in resuscitation of the newborn.

> Box 45.1 **Anticipating the need for resuscitation**
>
> - Intrapartum hypoxia – fetal distress
> - Fetal cord accidents
> - Fetal–maternal transfusion
> - Meconium-stained liquor
> - Reduced liquor volume
> - Congenital abnormalities, e.g. diaphragmatic hernia
> - Infection
> - Drugs, such as opiates
> - Pharyngeal overstimulation – over-vigorous suctioning
> - Preterm babies – need support rather than resuscitation

### Equipment for newborn resuscitation (Box 45.2)

In an emergency, all that is required for newborn resuscitation is a flat surface and a pair of lungs to give mouth to mouth and nose breaths. However, midwives must be well prepared for resuscitation in home or the community (see website). In hospitals, community maternity units and birthing centres, a resuscitaire may be used as this provides a stable surface, warmth, and adequate lighting for effective resuscitation. The resuscitaire has suction and a source of oxygen – either piped or cylinder – and a pressure-limiting device so that the pressure used to deliver breaths can be measured and limited. Some resuscitaires incorporate a ventilator circuit so that a sick baby does not need to be moved to a separate system after being stabilized.

All equipment for neonatal resuscitation must be checked regularly and also rechecked immediately before use.

**Box 45.2 Equipment for neonatal resuscitation**

Flat, stable surface
Clock with second hand
Stethoscope
Light
Heat source
Oxygen supply
Suction and catheters
Towels or blankets (warmed)
Plastic bag for preterm births (in hospital)
500 mL self-inflating bag with a pressure-limiting device, e.g. Laerdal
Oxygen reservoir attachment for self-inflating bags
T-connector and tubing
Size 00 and 01 masks with conformable face piece
Guedel airways size 0, 00 and 000
Laryngoscope – for suction under direct vision
Endotracheal tubes 2.5, 3.0 and 3.5
Nasogastric tubes size 8 and 10 FG
2 mL, 5 mL and 10 mL syringes
21 FG and 25 FG needles

## Personnel

When the need for complex resuscitation is anticipated, a senior member of the neonatal team should be summoned. In situations where the need for resuscitation is unexpected, help should be obtained as quickly as possible. In out-of-hospital situations, this may involve calling for an ambulance, general practitioner or neonatal emergency team, depending on local circumstances. It is always best to call for help early. If the situation has resolved by the time help arrives, they are very unlikely to complain if the baby has recovered.

## Thermal control

Babies are born into an environment considerably cooler than the intrauterine environment, are wet and have a large surface area (see Chs 42, 44 and website). Prior to resuscitation, term babies should be dried and wrapped in warm towels to prevent heat loss, and their thermoregulation needs to be monitored during resuscitation.

Good practice, based on current evidence, for term babies with suspected birth asphyxia is to maintain their body temperature at 37°C.

*Induced hypothermia* as a possible method of reducing neurological damage in babies with birth asphyxia is currently under investigation, and results are awaited (Edwards & Azzopardi 2006).

## Assessment

Colour:

- Are the mucous membranes pink, blue, or pale?

Tone:

- Has the baby got good tone or is the baby floppy?

Respiratory rate:

- Is the chest moving?
- Are the movements regular or irregular gasping movements?

Heart rate:

- Listen with a stethoscope – is there a heart rate?
- Is it above 100 bpm?

A baby who is blue and floppy with a heart rate above 100 bpm is likely to respond quickly to airway opening and minimal resuscitative measures. A baby who is pale, floppy, not breathing with a slow heart rate (<60 bpm) is likely to be seriously compromised and in need of urgent resuscitation. Depending on the assessment of the baby at this stage, it may be necessary to call for additional help.

It is good practice to note the time or start the clock when the baby is born. This provides a benchmark against which treatment can be measured.

## Airway management

The baby is placed on his back on a flat surface. The prominent occiput tends to encourage the neck to flex and this can lead to airway obstruction. To correct this, the baby's head is placed in the neutral position (Fig. 45.1). To help maintain this position, a small roll may be placed under the shoulders.

If the baby has poor tone, the tongue may fall back and block the airway. To overcome this, *jaw thrust* can be employed. This involves placing the fingers under the angle of the jaw to move it forward. This can be done with one hand or two (Fig. 45.2).

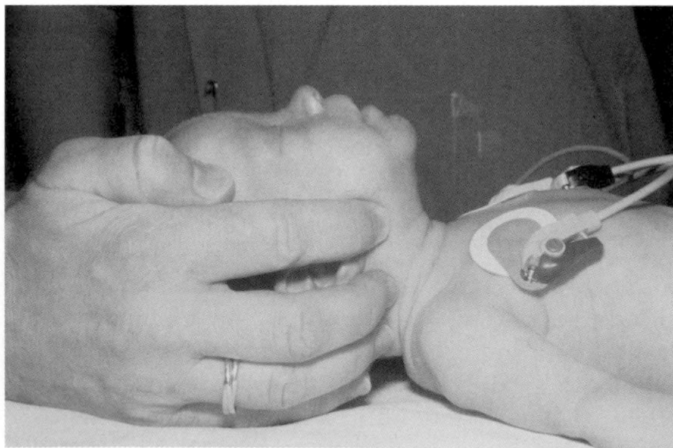

**Figure 45.1** Neutral position. *(Courtesy of UK Resuscitation Council.)*

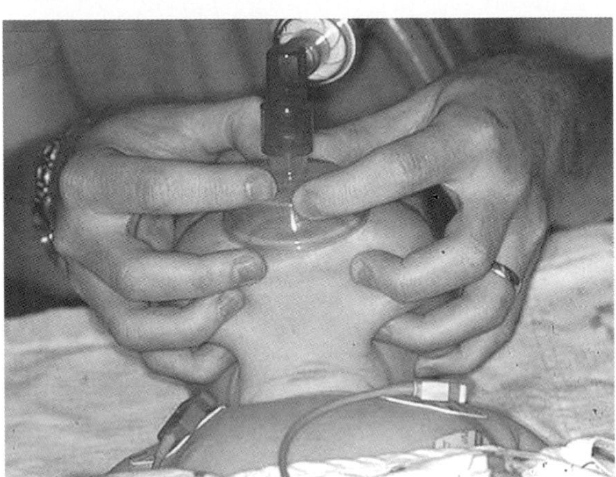

**Figure 45.2** Two-person jaw thrust. *(Courtesy of UK Resuscitation Council.)*

Alternatively, a Guedel airway can be inserted. The airway is measured from the middle of the lips to the angle of the jaw, and should be inserted with the curved surface upwards. Care must be taken to ensure that it goes over the tongue and does not force the tongue back. A laryngoscope or tongue depressor can help with this manoeuvre. At the same time, the airway can be examined for any blockages such as vernix or blood clots, which can be removed under direct vision with a large-bore suction catheter.

Once the airway is open, the situation is reassessed. If oxygen is entering the lungs, the heart rate may increase even before the chest moves. If there is no response to airway opening manoeuvres, then the next step is to provide inflation breaths.

## Breathing

A face mask which covers the nose and mouth without leaving gaps is selected and attached to either a T-piece or 500 mL self-inflating bag. If using a T-piece, the pressure setting should be checked and the blow-off valve on the self-inflating bag should be checked to ensure it works. There is debate as to whether resuscitation of the newborn requires oxygen or if air can be just as effective. Current evidence suggests that oxygen is required for preterm babies but there is a lack of good-quality information in relation to term babies (Wang et al 2008). If oxygen is available, then it should be used. If a T-piece is used, the pressure limiter should be set to a maximum of 30 $cmH_2O$ initially.

The face mask is applied to the baby's face and held firmly in place, ensuring that there are no leaks which would cause a reduction in the pressure being delivered. Five inflation breaths are then given. These 'breaths' are delivered by squeezing the self-inflating bag or occluding the T-piece for about 3 seconds. Following this, the baby is reassessed. It is very common for the heart rate to increase, even before chest movement is detected. If the chest does not move and the heart rate does not increase, then it should be assumed that the manoeuvre has been unsuccessful. The position of the baby's head should be rechecked and the inflation breaths delivered again and the situation reassessed.

Once the chest has been seen to move or the heart rate has increased, ventilation breaths are used to sustain breathing. These breaths are shorter and faster – about 30 per minute – and the pressure can be reduced to about 20 $cmH_2O$.

The baby should be reassessed every 30 seconds to ensure that resuscitation continues to be effective. If the baby has been in terminal apnoea, the first signs of spontaneous respiration may be gasping breaths. Ventilation breaths should continue to be delivered until regular breathing is sustained.

## Circulation

Once the chest has been seen to move, the heart rate will normally increase. However, in some babies, the lack of oxygenated blood in the coronary circulation means that the cardiac muscle is unable to respond to the lung inflation and the circulation of oxygenated blood. In this case, cardiac compressions may help 'bump start' the heart.

The most effective method of chest compressions is to encircle the chest with both hands, placing the thumbs just below the nipples on the sternum (David 1988). Alternatively, though less effective, a two finger technique can be used (Fig. 45.3). The chest is then compressed by about a third. Three chest compressions should be carried out for every ventilation breath. The heart rate should be assessed after 30 seconds. Once the heart rate is above 60 bpm, cardiac compressions can be stopped.

## Drugs

If the heart rate fails to respond, despite the delivery of effective ventilation breaths and cardiac compressions, it may be necessary to consider administering drugs. In newborn babies, the umbilical vein can be cannulated easily using a feeding tube. This delivers drugs and fluids directly into the inferior vena cava via the ductus venosus. There is a significant amount of dead space in the umbilical venous catheter (up to 2 mL), so each drug administration should be followed by a 2 mL flush of normal saline to ensure that the drug reaches the circulation.

*Adrenaline:* 1 : 10,000 can be used in babies who are very bradycardic. A dose of 0.1 mL/kg can be given initially. If this is unsuccessful, up to 0.3 mL/kg can be given.

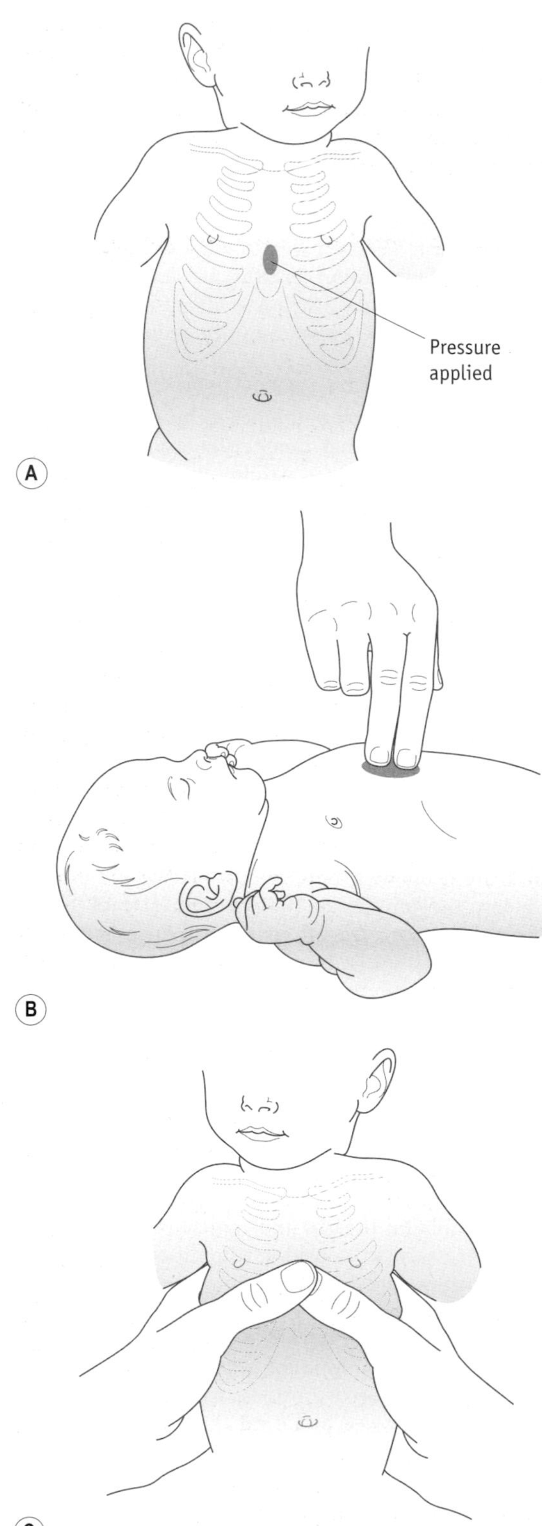


**Figure 45.3** Cardiac compression. **A.** Position for applying pressure. **B.** Using two fingers. **C.** Using two thumbs with the hands encircling the chest.

*Sodium bicarbonate:* 1–2 mmol/kg can be given to counteract acidosis. In practice this means using 2–4 mmol/ kg of 4.2% sodium bicarbonate.
*Dextrose:* can be given to correct hypoglycaemia – 2.5 mL/kg of 10%.
*Isotonic saline:* is sometimes given to correct loss of volume through either a cord accident or fetomaternal bleed. In an emergency, a bolus of 10 mL/kg of 0.9% saline can be given over 20 seconds.
*Naloxone hydrochloride* (Narcan®)*:* is not a drug of resuscitation. If a woman has been administered opiates in labour and the baby does not breathe at birth, the baby should be resuscitated first (Resuscitation Council (UK) 2008). Once effective lung inflation has been achieved, a decision may be made to administer 200 mcg of naloxone hydrochloride intramuscularly to reverse the effect of the maternal opiate. The baby's respiratory rate must be monitored closely as the effect of naloxone hydrochloride may wear off before that of the opiate. Naloxone hydrochloride should not be given to the baby of a substance-misusing woman as it can cause severe withdrawal symptoms (Suresh & Anand 1998).

## Resuscitating preterm babies

Preterm babies usually manage to breathe at birth and have a good heart rate, though face major challenges in maintaining their body temperature due to their comparatively large surface area. Hypothermia can cause hypoxia and hypoglycaemia and may interfere with surfactant production, leading to a worsening of respiratory distress syndrome (Gluck et al 1972, Stephenson et al 1970).

When a preterm birth is imminent, senior help should be available. All surfaces that the baby will touch should be warmed. At birth the baby is placed into a food-grade plastic bag up to their neck, without drying the skin, and the head should be covered with a hat. The baby should be intubated and exogenous surfactant delivered via the endotracheal tube (Verder et al 1999). Following stabilization, the baby can be transferred to the neonatal unit for ongoing care.

## Post-resuscitation care

If resuscitation is prolonged, the baby's temperature and blood glucose levels must be checked to ensure that they are within normal limits and, if not, appropriate treatment given. Most babies requiring resuscitation respond readily and can remain with the mother. If there are ongoing concerns, the baby may be transferred to a *Transitional Care Unit* or *Neonatal Unit*. The parents need accurate and up-to-date information about what is happening and care should be taken not to provide information that is unduly reassuring – especially if the baby's condition does not warrant this. Documentation should be descriptive, not opinionated, noting the condition of the baby at birth and response to any interventions.

## Discontinuing resuscitation

In some situations, the baby may not respond to resuscitation. The decision to stop resuscitation is usually taken by a senior member of the clinical team, after reviewing the situation, and in some units this might be the midwife. Protocols should be in place in community maternity units and birth centres to ensure that midwives can have access to expert advice in this situation.

## RESPIRATORY DISORDERS IN THE NEWBORN – PRINCIPLES OF CARE

A normal term neonate has a respiratory rate of between 20 and 40 bpm. Breathing is effortless and quiet. Chest movement should be equal on both sides of the chest. The mucous membranes should be pink. The expected oxygen saturation level in a newborn baby is 95–99% (Lyon 2005).

Signs of respiratory compromise may include:

- increased respiratory rate
- apnoeic episodes
- grunting – where the baby tries to exhale against a closed glottis in order to retain air in the alveoli
- nasal flaring
- sternal and intercostal recession – as the baby uses the accessory muscles of respiration to improve oxygenation
- peripheral or central cyanosis (see website).

Any baby showing signs of respiratory compromise should be carefully observed and monitored after transfer to a neonatal unit. For midwives working in community maternity units and birth centres, it may be necessary to care for the baby for several hours until specialist assistance arrives. Oxygen saturation monitoring should be used if available. The baby's respiratory rate should be monitored continuously, using either continuous monitoring or an apnoea monitor. In order to facilitate observation of the baby's respiratory function and temperature, the baby should be nursed naked in an incubator.

If the baby has a rapid respiratory rate, breastfeeding or formula feeding may be difficult and may increase the risk of aspiration. Nasogastric feeding of small volumes of milk may be possible, though a full stomach pressing on the diaphragm may cause respiratory embarrassment. If this occurs, enteral feeds are withheld and intravenous fluids given by an umbilical venous cannula to maintain glycaemic control.

The parents will be very anxious about their baby, especially if separated. It is essential that they are given accurate information and kept fully informed about the baby's condition. If the baby is to be transferred to a different hospital, the mother should be transferred to the same hospital as soon as possible.

### Meconium aspiration syndrome (MAS)

*Meconium-stained liquor* is associated with fetal hypoxia and asphyxia, and is seen primarily in term or post-term infants. It is believed that when the fetus becomes hypoxic, the anal sphincter relaxes and meconium is released into the amniotic fluid.

When meconium-stained liquor was present at birth in the past, practices such as vigorous suction of the nose and mouth and thoracic pressure during delivery were used to prevent meconium aspiration. As the pathophysiology of MAS is more complex than this, these practices are now no longer used (see website).

Meconium has been found in the alveoli of stillborn infants, which suggests that aspiration may take place in utero (Brown & Gleicher 1981). It is believed that the hypoxic fetus starts to gasp in utero and this moves meconium-stained amniotic fluid into the fetal lungs. Fetal hypoxia is associated with a rise in pulmonary artery pressure and MAS is associated with an increased incidence of *persistent pulmonary hypertension of the newborn* (PPHN). In PPHN, the pressure in the pulmonary vasculature is elevated, causing the temporary fetal structures to remain partially open after birth, causing newborn hypoxaemia. The presence of meconium in the lung may cause a chemical pneumonitis which leads to inactivation of surfactant. Meconium is a viscous substance and may also cause obstruction of the airways.

#### *Resuscitation when meconium is present in the liquor*

A multicentre randomized controlled trial compared outcomes for babies who had their nose and mouth suctioned while the head was on the perineum with those who were born without suctioning. The data concluded that prophylactic suctioning conferred no benefits (Wiswell et al 2000). This study also compared routine intubation and suctioning for all infants born through meconium-stained liquor with a selective policy where the intervention was used only for babies who were not breathing at birth. The conclusion was that babies who breathe at birth do not require routine suctioning, and therefore this intervention should be reserved for babies with no respiratory effort.

If meconium-stained liquor is present at birth – particularly if it is thick, indicating a lack of liquor – expert assistance should be called so that the baby can be intubated, if necessary. If expert help is unavailable, the baby should

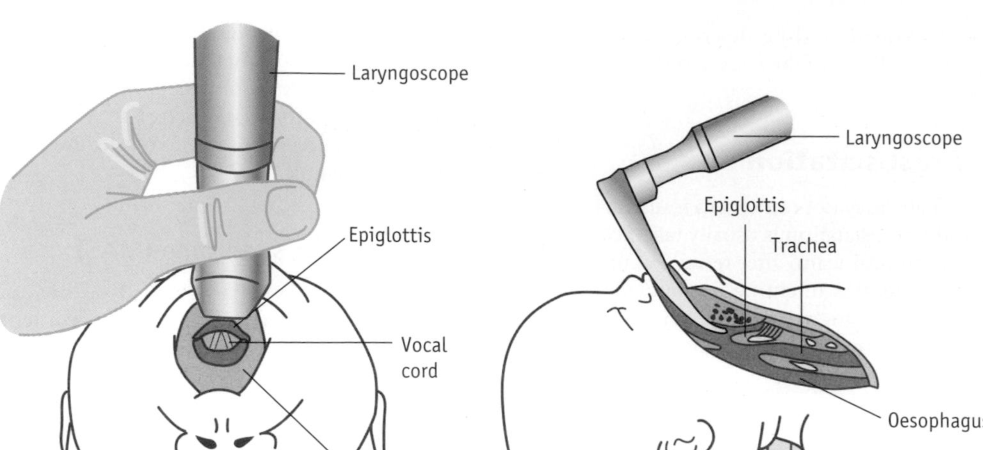


**Figure 45.4** Neonatal intubation.

be handled gently at birth, kept warm and assessed. If the baby is breathing and crying, then no further resuscitation is needed but the baby's respiratory rate must be observed over the next 4–6 hours for signs of respiratory distress (see website).

If the baby is unresponsive, a laryngoscope should be used to facilitate suction under direct vision (see Fig. 45.4). A large-bore catheter should be used to suck out particulate matter. Suctioning should stop when all visible meconium has been aspirated or the heart rate falls below 60 bpm. If the heart rate is slow, the baby's head should be placed in the *neutral position* and inflation breaths given. Once the heart rate rises above 60 bpm, any remaining meconium may be removed with suction.

**Reflective activity 45.1**

What methods of inflating the lungs are used when resuscitating babies where you practise? Are you familiar with them? If not, arrange to be updated.

### Aftercare

The majority of babies born through meconium will be well and will suffer no ill effects. It is advisable to undertake '*meconium observations*' (assessing the baby's colour, tone and respiratory rate) for up to 6 hours after birth (see website). Signs of illness in the baby include a rise in the respiratory rate (>60 bpm) and increasing cyanosis.

A baby with signs of increasing respiratory distress will need to be admitted to the neonatal unit for continuous observation. Babies with mild respiratory distress usually respond well to the administration of warmed humidified oxygen and intravenous antibiotics.

Babies with MAS who require prolonged resuscitation must be admitted to the neonatal unit for monitoring and treatment. Traditional treatments for MAS included intubation and ventilation using high concentrations of oxygen. However, the high pressures required to deliver the breaths (because of the high intrapulmonary pressures) can damage the lungs. Newer technologies for the management of MAS include the administration of *exogenous surfactant*. Because meconium inactivates surfactant, exogenous surfactant may reduce the need for more invasive treatments (Findlay et al 1996).

*Nitric oxide* is a gas which is delivered directly into the lungs via an endotracheal tube. It is a potent vasodilator and can reverse pulmonary hypertension, reducing hypoxaemia, and has been shown to be effective in treating some babies with MAS (Gupta et al 2002).

In the most severe cases of MAS, *extracorporeal membrane oxygenation* (ECMO) may be required (UK Collaborative ECMO Trial Group 1996). ECMO is a highly invasive form of treatment during which the blood is pumped out of the body, oxygenated in an oxygenator (essentially an artificial lung), and then the oxygenated blood returned to the baby (see website). Few centres in the UK provide this treatment, so a baby with MAS requiring ECMO may have to be transported many miles from the 'home' unit for treatment, resulting in separation from the parents.

Mortality and morbidity rates for babies with severe MAS are high. Mortality rates can be as high as 20% due to pulmonary complications. Some survivors of severe MAS will go on to develop chronic lung disease as a consequence of the treatment for respiratory failure. A few babies with severe MAS will have neurodevelopmental delay. It is believed that this happens as a result of cerebral damage in utero, rather than as a direct consequence of meconium inhalation (Greenough & Milner 2005).

## Transient tachypnoea of the newborn (TTN)

*Transient tachypnoea of the newborn* (also known as 'wet' lung') is believed to be due to a failure to clear fetal lung fluid during transition to extrauterine life. It almost always affects term babies and is more common in babies born by elective caesarean section. The baby presents with:

- rapid respiratory rate of 80–100 bpm soon after birth
- may be intercostal and sternal recession
- may be respiratory grunt (see website).

The clinical features of TTN are similar to those of *pneumonia* and the two conditions may coexist.

### Management

- Infection screen to exclude or confirm pneumonia
- May prescribe prophylactic antibiotics until infection is excluded
- Chest X-ray will help confirm the diagnosis of TTN
- Care in a transitional care ward with mother sharing care
- May be nursed in NNU
- Nursed in incubator to enable:
  - close observation
  - continuous monitoring of heart rate, respiratory rate and oxygen saturation levels
  - warmed humidified oxygen delivered via head box or nasal prongs.

The treatment for TTN is supportive – the condition is self-limiting and will resolve within 1–5 days, after which the baby may be discharged home to be cared for by the parents.

## Pneumonia

This may be acquired congenitally as a result of contamination with infective agents during labour or birth, or late onset – acquired after 7 days. Acquired pneumonia is most commonly seen in babies who are already intubated. The most common causative organisms are *Streptococcus A* or *Streptococcus B*, *Klebsiella* and *E. coli*.

Clinical features are similar to those for TTN:

- Rapid respiratory rate – 80–100 bpm soon after birth.
- May be intercostal and sternal recession.
- Respiratory grunt may be present (see website).
- Baby may be cyanosed.

In severe cases, the *Group B streptococcus* is associated with rapid collapse in the newborn period.

### Management

- Usually neonatal unit admission for observation
- Intravenous antibiotics usually administered
- Chest X-ray will help confirm the diagnosis of pneumonia
- Usually nursed in NNU in an incubator:
  - close observation
  - continuous monitoring of heart rate, respiratory rate and oxygen saturation levels
  - warmed humidified oxygen delivered via head box or nasal prongs
  - may require intubation and respiratory support via a ventilator.

The prognosis for term babies who contract pneumonia is good, provided the clinical features are recognized and managed promptly.

## Respiratory distress syndrome

*Respiratory distress syndrome* (RDS) is caused by a deficiency of surfactant (see Ch. 44). The severity of the condition is associated with gestational age: the lower the gestational age of the baby, the more severe the RDS. Although primarily a disease affecting the lungs, the condition impacts on all body systems as impaired oxygenation and pulmonary hypoperfusion affects blood pressure, thus inhibiting tissue oxygenation.

RDS presents soon after birth – usually within 4 hours, characterized by:

- rapidly rising respiratory rate
- marked sternal and intercostal recession
- nasal flaring
- grunting
- arterial blood gases usually show respiratory acidosis due to the trapping of carbon dioxide as the lungs are underventilated.

Administration of *corticosteroids before birth* reduces the incidence and severity of RDS (Ward 1994).

*Exogenous surfactant* is recommended following birth to stabilize the lungs (Verder et al 1999) and has been associated with:

- a dramatic fall in mortality rates from RDS (Soll 2000):
- reduced ventilator and oxygen requirements
- dramatic reduction in the risk of pneumothoraces through decreased need for ventilator support.

Surfactant is given via an endotracheal tube at birth – and further doses according to the baby's condition. Once stabilized, the baby may remain intubated with a ventilator delivering a mixture of air and oxygen directly using positive pressure to inflate the lungs. Alternatively, the baby may be extubated and placed on *continuous positive airways pressure* (CPAP) via nasal prongs. CPAP allows the baby to breathe on his own but maintains a low pressure (about 4–6 $cmH_2O$) to prevent the lungs collapsing between breaths (Greenough & Milner 2005). This facilitates gas exchange and also reduces damage to the surfactant-producing alveolar cells.

Babies with severe RDS are nursed in an incubator and have continuous monitoring of oxygenation, blood pressure, heart rate and respiratory rate. Their vulnerable state means that rapid fluctuations in blood pressure, arterial oxygen and carbon dioxide levels can affect the brain and kidneys, so care is directed at ensuring stability and detecting and correcting any abnormality.

Very preterm babies may remain in the neonatal unit for many months (see Ch. 44). Some go on to develop chronic lung disease (CLD), sometimes known as bronchopulmonary dysplasia (see website).

## Congenital abnormalities

The majority of congenital abnormalities affecting the respiratory system are usually detected antenatally. Decisions about the place of birth can be made well in advance and expert neonatal care can be available at birth. Congenital abnormalities that impact on the respiratory system include *diaphragmatic hernia, tracheo-oesophageal fistulae (TOF), oesophageal atresia,* and facial abnormalities, such as *Pierre Robin syndrome*. Depending on the severity of the condition, respiratory difficulty may present at birth or within a few hours of birth.

### Diaphragmatic hernia

Diaphragmatic hernia can range from a small hole in the muscle to complete agenesis which allows the gut contents or liver to protrude through into the thoracic cavity. This reduces the space for lung development, thus the lungs are hypoplastic and, in extreme cases, are incapable of supporting respiration. Other congenital abnormalities may be present, including cardiac and renal abnormalities. The prognosis for the baby depends largely on the extent of the diaphragmatic defect and the coexisting abnormalities. Babies diagnosed early in the antenatal period tend to have a poor prognosis (Sebire et al 1997), which may be due to the severity of the defect. Babies presenting soon after birth are more likely to have a large defect and have a significantly higher morbidity rate. Infants who present 24 hours after birth are more likely to survive.

The baby may present with increasing tachypnoea and cyanosis. Breath sounds may be reduced on the side of the hernia as the lungs are displaced by the viscera. The abdomen may have a flat appearance as the intestinal contents protrude into the thorax (Davenport 2005). Diagnosis can be confirmed by X-ray or ultrasound, which shows the presence of viscera in the thoracic cavity.

If the defect is diagnosed antenatally, arrangements should be made for the birth to take place in a maternity unit with a neonatal service capable of providing specialist care for the baby. Usually the baby will be electively intubated at birth. The extended use of a bag and mask can cause intestinal distension. A large-bore nasogastric tube should be passed and left on free drainage to decompress the bowel. The baby is then ventilated and stabilized prior to surgery to repair the defect. Delayed surgery is associated with an enhanced survival rate. The whole process is extremely worrying for the parents and intensive support from staff is required.

### Tracheo-oesophageal fistula (TOF) and oesophageal atresia

Tracheo-oesophageal atresia and fistulae are thought to occur because of abnormal separation of the primitive trachea and oesophagus in the first trimester (see Ch. 48). Oesophageal atresia may exist on its own or coexist alongside a fistula which communicates with the trachea. The defects are also associated with chromosomal abnormalities, especially trisomy 13 or 18, and may be detected antenatally on ultrasound. Oesophageal atresia is associated with maternal polyhydramnios. If diagnosed in the antenatal period, arrangements are made for the birth to take place in a maternity unit with access to a neonatal surgical unit. There may be other abnormalities present, and typically these include lower gastrointestinal abnormalities, such as duodenal atresia or anorectal abnormalities.

At birth the baby may present with frothy saliva dribbling from the mouth and may appear to choke or have frequent colour changes. In some cases, the baby may aspirate the secretions, which causes a form of respiratory distress. The initial management is to keep the airway clear. The baby should be nursed in a slightly head-up position. A *Replogle tube* (see website) has a double lumen and this is placed in the pouch at the blind end of the atresia and kept on continuous low-pressure suction. This is usually sufficient to keep the baby's airway clear. Intravenous fluids are required to maintain the baby's blood glucose level within normal limits and to maintain fluid balance prior to surgery.

If birth occurs in the birth centre or at home, the baby should be kept warm and supported in a slight head-up position. Suction can be gently applied to the mouth to keep the airway free of secretions until transfer to a neonatal unit. If there is likely to be a delay of several hours, then an umbilical venous catheter should be inserted and 10% dextrose given to maintain hydration and blood glucose levels.

Surgery is usually performed soon after birth to correct the defect. In a few cases, a wide gap between the oesophageal segments may delay surgery, to enable the two pouches to elongate. If this happens, the baby will have a gastrostomy and be fed directly into the stomach until surgery to repair the defect (Stringer et al 2005).

## CARDIAC ABNORMALITIES

The cardiovascular system is the first of the body's systems to develop and function. It is believed that the rapid development which takes place in this system makes it susceptible to teratogens. Congenital heart defects (CHD) account for about 30% of all reported congenital anomalies. Causes include the following:

- Chromosomal abnormalities – about 40% of children with Down syndrome will have a cardiac malformation.
- Genetic factors – CHD is more likely if either parent or a sibling has a history of CHD.
- Teratogens – rubella or drugs, such as phenytoin or warfarin.
- Maternal disease, specifically diabetes mellitus, significantly increases the risk of a baby having CHD.

Accurate antenatal history taking is fundamental in identifying CHD. Women who report a family history of CHD or have diabetes mellitus should be advised of the increased risk of CHD to the fetus and referred for counselling and specialized screening. General anomaly screening with a four-chamber view of the heart at 18 weeks' gestation will identify less than 50% of affected fetuses (Wyllie et al 1994). Cardiac abnormalities detected at this time are more likely to be complex and have poor outcomes. Detailed transvaginal and transabdominal ultrasound can detect cardiac abnormalities at 13–14 weeks' gestation, providing sufficient information to make accurate interpretations of the images in women with a high risk of having a fetus with CHD (Bronshtein & Zimmer 2002) (see website).

Some cardiac abnormalities may be detected in the early postnatal period when carrying out routine examinations. The family history should be reviewed and checked with the mother to ensure that nothing has been overlooked. Dysmorphic features may lead the examiner to suspect a chromosomal abnormality: in these cases, careful evaluation of the cardiovascular system should be carried out. The femoral pulses should be palpable. Absent or weak pulses are suspicious and babies in whom pulses cannot be felt should be referred for further examination.

Some babies with CHD may present with cyanosis, though this can be difficult to detect as babies may have 'dusky' episodes that pass without any ill effect. Prolonged 'duskiness' is abnormal and should be investigated. Other signs of CHD are less specific, including:

- reluctance to feed
- poor weight gain
- excessive weight gain due to fluid retention
- cold, clammy skin and persistently poor peripheral perfusion
- may have a persistent tachycardia and show signs of respiratory distress in the neonatal period.

Heart murmurs are quite common in babies as a result of the transition to extrauterine life. In the absence of any other features, the baby may be followed up after a period of 4–6 weeks to assess the possible causes of the murmur.

Many cardiac lesions present after the baby and the parents have been transferred from the care of the maternity services to the primary health care team. Parents should be advised of the importance of continuing to assess their baby's wellbeing and reporting the non-specific features of CHD to their GP or health visitor if they are concerned.

### Investigations

If CHD is suspected, *blood pressure* should be checked in the upper limbs and one leg. A difference of 20 mmHg in the systolic BP between the arms and leg is suggestive of CHD – coarctation of the aorta in particular (Archer 2005). However, the absence of a gradient does not confirm normality and babies who are unwell must continue to be observed closely and referred for further screening.

In some cases, a *hyperoxia test* can be carried out to differentiate between cyanosis that is respiratory in origin and that which is cardiac (see website).

*Chest X-rays* and *electrocardiograms* can provide information about the heart in terms of size and function. However, *transthoracic echocardiography* is more effective in diagnosing the type and extent of the cardiac defect (Archer 2005). *Doppler ultrasound* can assess blood velocity and can assist in identifying shunts and stenosis – areas of narrowing in the cardiac pathway.

### Treatment

The treatment of a baby with CHD depends on the type of defect and their general condition. Cardiac catheterization can be used for interventions such as widening stenosed vessels. Surgery may take place in stages. In the initial stage, treatment is palliative and designed to alleviate symptoms. Later, as the baby grows, corrective surgery may be carried out. In complex cases, several operations may be required.

Depending on the results of the initial investigations, the baby may be referred to a specialist centre for further investigation and treatment. In some cases, even when a defect is diagnosed, it is possible for the baby to remain in the care of the parents and be referred for treatment at a later date. Whether the baby is transferred to a specialist centre or discharged, the parents need accurate information about their baby and what the future might hold. In particular, the parents of the baby who has a delayed referral require information about the clinical features of deterioration and how they should obtain assistance if they are concerned about their baby's condition.

## Forms of congenital heart defects

Congenital heart disease is commonly divided up into two groups – *cyanotic* and *acyanotic*, which can be confusing because not all babies with cyanotic heart disease will be cyanosed initially.

### Acyanotic heart defects

These include patent ductus arteriosus, ventricular and atrial septal defects, pulmonary stenosis, aortic stenosis and coarctation of the aorta.

#### *Patent ductus arteriosus (PDA)*

The ductus arteriosus is a temporary structure which exists to divert blood away from the lungs to the aorta in the fetal circulation (see Chs 29 and 41). In term babies, the ductus arteriosus normally closes within 12–24 hours of birth in response to the circulating high partial pressure of oxygen and reduction in circulating maternal prostaglandins. Preterm babies are more likely to experience periods of hypoxia and an increase in circulating prostaglandins, which makes the ductus arteriosus more likely to remain open.

Deoxygenated blood from the pulmonary arteries shunts through the ductus arteriosus into the aorta, bypassing the lungs. Preterm babies are likely to show decreasing levels of oxygenation and worsening of RDS. Term babies may be reluctant to feed and have poor growth patterns. The baby may have tachypnoea and tachycardia. On auscultation of the heart, a murmur may be heard.

The treatment includes:

- oxygen
- preventing fluid overload
- a drug such as indometacin may be administered, which has a powerful anti-prostaglandin action which may cause duct closure
- surgical closure may be indicated if medical means fails.

#### *Atrial septal defect (ASD)*

This defect allows communication between the left and right side of the heart with mixing of oxygenated and deoxygenated blood. A simple ASD is a hole in the atrial septum and is rarely symptomatic. Closure is best performed before the onset of pulmonary hypertension. In many cases this is when the child is around 5 years of age. A complex ASD (often associated with an underlying chromosomal disorder) involves other structures, such as the mitral valve or the ventricular septum and tricuspid valve. Surgery is more complicated and there is a higher mortality rate associated with this condition.

#### *Ventricular septal defect (VSD)*

Ventricular septal defects are the most commonly occurring cardiac defect, and may occur on their own or as part of a complex heart defect. The septal defect allows mixing of blood between the two ventricles. Typically, blood from the left ventricle passes through to the right ventricle during systole. The blood is then recirculated. The flow of blood from the left to the right side of the heart can lead to elevated right ventricular pressure and pulmonary hypertension. This occurs if the defect is large. The baby may show signs of respiratory distress and cyanosis, as well as failure to thrive. Babies with a small defect may be asymptomatic. Surgical correction of the defect may be carried out. Small defects may close on their own.

#### *Coarctation of the aorta*

Coarctation of the aorta is narrowing of the aorta at the point where the ductus arteriosus joins, and may occur on its own or as part of a complex CHD. Mild forms of the defect may be undetectable and there may be no symptoms until the child is older. In more severe cases, femoral pulses may be weak or absent. Depending on the position of the coarctation, rapid collapse may follow closure of the ductus arteriosus.

Treatment options include the insertion of a *stent* or *angioplasty* to relieve the stenosis. Alternatively, surgery may be performed to remove the stenosed part of the aorta or a patch inserted to make the narrow section of the aorta wider.

#### *Pulmonary stenosis*

Pulmonary stenosis occurs when the pulmonary valve becomes narrowed. This causes an obstruction to blood leaving the right ventricle and can lead to a reduction in blood going to the lungs. The stenosis may be relieved by surgery.

#### *Aortic stenosis*

Aortic stenosis is a narrowing of the valve leading from the left ventricle into the aorta, which usually occurs alongside other heart defects. In simple cases, the baby will be asymptomatic and there may be no sign other than a cardiac murmur. In severe cases, the baby will collapse suddenly and require urgent surgery to relieve the stenosis.

### Cyanotic defects

This group of defects includes complex conditions such as *transposition of the great arteries*, *tetralogy of Fallot* and *hypoplastic left heart syndrome*.

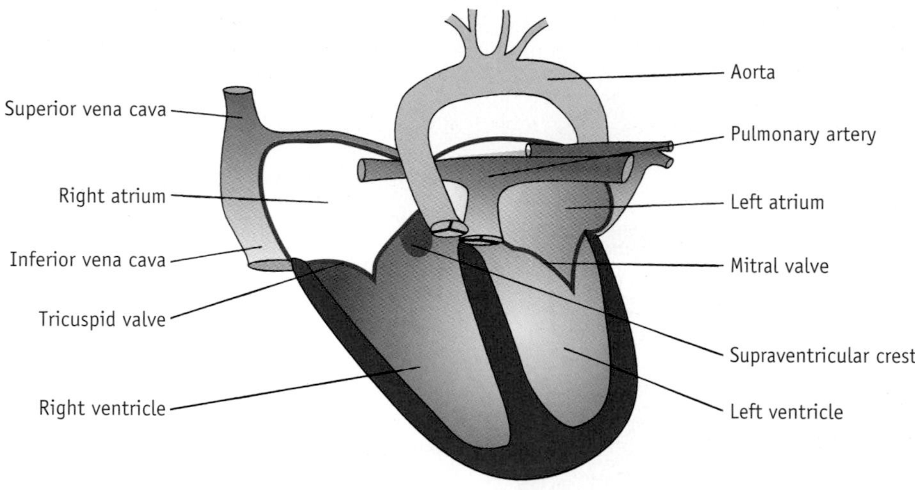


**Figure 45.5** Transposition of the great arteries.

### *Transposition of the great arteries (TGA)*

In this condition, the major heart arteries are transposed. The aorta arises from the right ventricle and the pulmonary artery arises from the left ventricle (Fig. 45.5). TGA is usually associated with other cardiac defects such as VSD. These babies usually present within the first few hours of life – especially if there is no shunt. Cyanosis may be marked and accompanied by tachypnoea and tachycardia. Initial treatment involves an infusion of prostaglandins to open the ductus arteriosus. The foramen ovale may be surgically enlarged so that well-oxygenated blood can flow from the left ventricle into the right ventricle. Surgery to correct the defect is an arterial switch procedure and is performed within 3 weeks of birth. Survival rates for surgery are around 90%.

### *Tetralogy of Fallot*

This condition comprises four abnormalities (Fig. 45.6):

- ventricular septal defect
- pulmonary stenosis
- right ventricular hypertrophy
- overriding of the aorta – the aorta is connected to the right and left ventricles and sits above the VSD.

The baby develops a right-to-left shunt. There is mixing of oxygenated and deoxygenated blood at the level of the ventricles and blood flows preferentially through the aorta, rather than the pulmonary arteries, because the pressure is lower in the larger vessel. Cyanosis may be present soon after birth or may develop in the first year of life. The baby may exhibit poor growth and failure to thrive and become breathless when engaged in any activity. The condition is treated by surgery.

### *Hypoplastic left heart syndrome*

In this condition the left side of the heart is underdeveloped (hypoplastic) (Fig. 45.7). There is atresia of the mitral and aortic valves. The left ventricle and the aorta are underdeveloped. In contrast, the right side of the heart is hypertrophied and the pulmonary artery is enlarged.

Blood passes through the ductus arteriosus into the aorta. When the ductus arteriosus closes, death follows soon afterwards. A prostaglandin infusion can be used to keep the ductus arteriosus open. Palliative surgery can be carried out so that the right ventricle is used to supply the systemic circulation. Ultimately, heart transplantation may be carried out to correct the problem.

## Parental care

Congenital cardiac defects present major challenges for families. The baby may be acutely unwell and need urgent treatment in a specialist centre located many miles away from home. Even after initial treatment, the baby may require many years of follow-up with an uncertain prognosis. Families who have babies with less complex cardiac defects may find themselves coping with feelings of uncertainty as they await treatment. Babies with CHD may be difficult to feed and may exhibit poor growth, causing further concern for the parents. Health professionals working with parents should ensure that they receive accurate, consistent information. Parents of babies with CHD may find it helpful to be given contact details of specialist support groups and voluntary organizations.

**Figure 45.6** Fallot's tetrology.

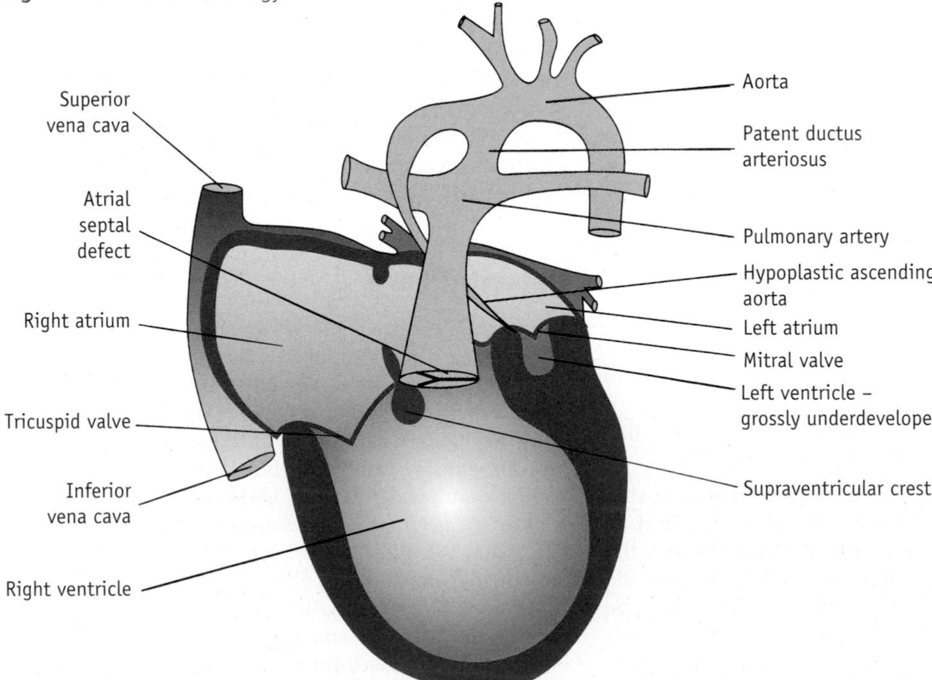


**Figure 45.7** Hypoplastic left heart syndrome.

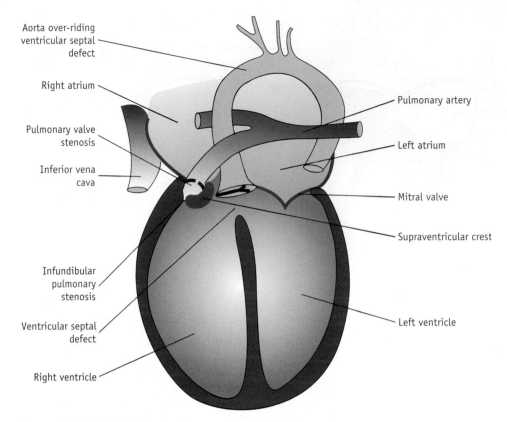

## CONCLUSION

The move towards midwife-led care means that midwives have taken on a greater responsibility for screening and detecting cardiac and respiratory disorders in the antenatal and postnatal periods. A knowledgeable and skilled midwife is able to facilitate an effective partnership with parents; the midwife should be able to provide information and support to enable them to confirm normality in their newborn infant and to have the confidence to seek support and help if they are concerned about their baby's wellbeing.

### KEY POINTS

- An understanding of normal fetal and neonatal development and physiology is crucial in recognizing the transition events at birth.
- All midwives need to be skilled in resuscitation of the newborn, and those who work in out-of-hospital settings should be able to stabilize babies with respiratory and cardiac disorders while awaiting expert help.
- Midwives need to be alert for and be able to recognize when there are deviations from normal in the neonate's cardiac or respiratory wellbeing and take the appropriate action.

## REFERENCES


Archer N: Cardiovascular disease. In Rennie J, editor: *Roberton's textbook of neonatology*, ed 4, Edinburgh, 2005, Elsevier.

Blackburn ST: *Maternal, fetal and neonatal physiology: a clinical perspective*, ed 3, St Louis, 2007, Saunders.

Bronshtein M, Zimmer EZ: The sonographic approach to the detection of fetal cardiac anomalies in early pregnancy, *Ultrasound in Obstetrics and Gynecology* 19(4): 360–365, 2002.

Brown BL, Gleicher N: Intrauterine meconium aspiration, *Obstetrics and Gynecology* 57(1):26–29, 1981.

Davenport M: Diaphragmatic hernia. In Rennie J, editor: *Roberton's textbook of neonatology*, ed 4, Edinburgh, 2005, Elsevier.

David R: Closed chest cardiac massage in the newborn infant, *Pediatrics* 81:552–554, 1988.

Edwards AD, Azzopardi DV: Therapeutic hypothermia following perinatal asphyxia, *Archives of Disease in Childhood – Fetal and Neonatal Edition* 91:F127–F131, 2006.

Findlay RD, Taeusch H, Walther FJ: Surfactant replacement therapy for meconium aspiration syndrome, *Pediatrics* 97(1):48–52, 1996.

Gluck L, Kulovich MV, Eidelman AI, et al: Biochemical development of surface activity in mammalian lung. IV. Pulmonary lecithin synthesis in the human fetus and newborn and etiology of the respiratory distress syndrome, *Pediatric Research* 6(2):81–99, 1972.

Greenough A, Milner AD: Pulmonary disease of the newborn. In Rennie J, editor: *Roberton's textbook of neonatology*, ed 4, Edinburgh, 2005, Elsevier.

Gupta AS, Rastogi S, Sahni R, et al: Inhaled nitric oxide and gentle ventilation in the treatment of pulmonary hypertension of the newborn – a single center, 5 year experience, *Journal of Perinatology* 22:435–441, 2002.

Hodson WA: Normal and abnormal structural development of the lung. In Polin RA, Fox WW, editors: *Fetal and neonatal physiology*, ed 2, Philadelphia, 1998, WB Saunders.

Lyon A: Intensive care monitoring. In Rennie J, editor: *Roberton's textbook of neonatology*, ed 4, Edinburgh, 2005, Elsevier.

Morrison JJ, Rennie JM, Milton PJ: Neonatal respiratory morbidity and mode of delivery at term: influence of timing of elective caesarean section, *British Journal of Obstetrics and Gynaecology* 102(2):101–106, 1995.

Onuzo OC: How effectively can clinical examination pick up congenital heart disease at birth? *Archives of Disease in Childhood – Fetal and Neonatal Edition* 91(4):F236–F237, 2006.

Resuscitation Council (UK): *Newborn life support manual*, ed 3, London, 2008, Resuscitation Council (UK).

Sebire NJ, Snijders RJ, Davenport M, et al: Fetal nuchal translucency thickness at 10–14 weeks' gestation and congenital diaphragmatic hernia, *Obstetrics and Gynecology* 90(6):943–946, 1997.

Soll RF: Prophylactic natural surfactant extract for preventing mortality and morbidity in preterm infants (Cochrane review), *Cochrane Database of Systematic Reviews* (2):CD000511, 2000.

Stephenson JM, Du JN, Oliver TK: The effect of cooling on blood gas tensions in newborn infants, *Journal of Pediatrics* 76:848–851, 1970.

Strang LB: *Neonatal respiration*, Oxford, 1977, Blackwell Scientific.

Stringer MD, Sugarman I, Smyth A: Congenital defects and surgical problems. In Rennie J, editor: *Roberton's textbook of neonatology*, ed 4, Edinburgh, 2005, Elsevier.

Suresh S, Anand KJ: Opioid tolerance in neonates: mechanisms, diagnosis, assessment and management, *Seminars in Perinatology* 22:425–435, 1998.

UK Collaborative ECMO Trial Group: UK Collaborative randomized trial of neonatal extracorporeal membrane oxygenation, *Lancet* 348(9020):75–82, 1996.

Verder H, Albertsen P, Ebbesen F, et al: Nasal continuous positive airway pressure and early surfactant therapy for respiratory distress syndrome in newborns of less than 30 weeks' gestation, *Pediatrics* 103:E24, 1999.

Wang CL, Anderson C, Leone T, et al: Resuscitation of preterm neonates by using room air or 100% oxygen,

*Pediatrics* 121(6):1083–1089, 2008.

Ward RM: Pharmacologic enhancement of fetal lung maturation, *Clinics in Perinatology* 21(3):523–542, 1994.

Wiswell TE, Gannon CM, Jacob J, et al: Delivery room management of the apparently vigorous meconium-stained neonate: results of the multicenter international collaborative trial, *Pediatrics* 105(1):1–7, 2000.

Wyllie J, Wren C, Hunter S: Screening for cardiac malformations, *British Heart Journal* 71(suppl):20–27, 1994.

Chapter |46|

# Neonatal jaundice

*Maggie Meeks and Stephanie Michaelides*

## LEARNING OUTCOMES

After reading this chapter, you will be able to:

- explain the normal physiology of bilirubin metabolism
- identify common causes of unconjugated hyperbilirubinaemia
- compare and contrast the principles of care of the jaundiced baby in all settings
- explain the role and risks of phototherapy and exchange transfusion
- recognize the clinical signs of conjugated hyperbilirubinaemia
- define the acute and chronic complications of kernicterus.

## INTRODUCTION

Neonatal jaundice is common and occurs physiologically in a significant number of healthy full-term babies. Midwifery practice challenges include:

- promoting and supporting successful breastfeeding to ensure adequate hydration of newly born babies
- identifying those babies who are more at risk of significant hyperbilirubinaemia (jaundice)
- identifying the jaundiced baby requiring intervention and specifically those needing referral for a paediatric opinion and phototherapy (AAP 2004).

A significant number of babies with acute bilirubin encephalopathy and subsequent kernicterus are being reported (Manning et al 2007). This may further increase as mothers and babies are discharged home earlier before feeding is established, especially if community services are not in place to support a policy of early discharge (Sellwood & Huertas-Ceballos 2008).

Understanding the normal physiology of bilirubin metabolism allows recognition of why jaundice is so common in newborn babies and explains the mechanism of jaundice in many diseases. A basic knowledge of the rare genetic diseases may also allow a greater depth of understanding of normal physiology and these will be mentioned where appropriate.

## PHYSIOLOGY

The majority of bilirubin forms from the breakdown of *heme*, an iron-containing molecule, an essential component of cytochromes, myoglobin and haemoglobin. At the end of their lifespan, red blood cells are sequestered by the spleen and the haemoglobin is broken down into component parts of *heme* and *globin*. The iron molecule is then removed from the heme to be recycled and the heme molecule is oxidized to biliverdin, which is then reduced to form unconjugated bilirubin (Dennery et al 2001). Increased red cell breakdown leads to increased levels of unconjugated bilirubin. Bilirubin is a lipid-soluble molecule that easily crosses lipid membranes, such as those within the brain. The insolubility in water means that bilirubin must be transported in the bloodstream linked to albumin. In this protein-bound state, bilirubin is not available to be filtered by the glomerulus or to enter into cell tissues (see website).

In the liver, *unconjugated bilirubin* is transported into the cells and converted into *bilirubin diglucuronide (conjugated bilirubin)* by the enzyme *UDP glucuronosyltransferase*. Conjugated bilirubin is water-soluble and actively excreted by the liver cells into the intrahepatic bile ducts with bile salts, cholesterol and phospholipids. This bile then flows down the extrahepatic ducts and into the small intestine. Within the colon some of the conjugated bilirubin is hydrolysed back to unconjugated bilirubin while the remaining is metabolized into *stercobilinogen* and *urobilinogen*. Stercobilinogen is a brown pigment that is excreted within the faeces. Urobilinogen is reabsorbed in the enterohepatic circulation to be converted back to unconjugated bilirubin. A small amount of urobilinogen is carried in the bloodstream and excreted by the kidneys.

## PHYSIOLOGICAL JAUNDICE

*Physiological jaundice* is jaundice occurring as a consequence of the changeover from intrauterine to extrauterine life. The fetus possesses a large number of red blood cells that contain fetal haemoglobin which facilitates diffusion of oxygen from placental to fetal circulation. The newborn baby begins life with 6–7 million red cells per cubic millimeter, which need to reduce to the adult level of 5 million/mm$^3$. Fetal haemoglobin needs to be replaced by adult haemoglobin, resulting in an increase in red cell breakdown and an increased bilirubin load on the immature liver. Additionally, intestinal transit is slow until enteral feeds have been established, leading to increased reabsorption of urobilinogen via the enterohepatic circulation.

### Features of physiological jaundice

- More common in breastfed babies.
- Often noted at day 3, and peaks at day 5.
- Not associated with anaemia.
- Though not as alert as normal, baby is usually well and feeding pattern is satisfactory.

Supplementing breastfeeding with water or glucose appears to have no effect on bilirubin levels in healthy newborns (Nicoll et al 1982) and should be avoided. Physiological jaundice may be exacerbated in situations that lead to increased bilirubin production (for example, polycythaemia, bruising) or decreased bilirubin excretion (poor feeding with delayed intestinal transit). In the past it was believed that physiological jaundice could **not** lead to kernicterus but unfortunately this may not be the case and vigilance is crucial.

## EVALUATION OF JAUNDICE

The practitioner needs as much information as possible to accurately assess the risk of the baby developing jaundice, its significance and management plan. The maternal blood group should be known as well as any familial predisposition to neonatal jaundice. Risk factors include infection during pregnancy and delivery, and any bruising or perinatal trauma to the baby. Babies at high risk of developing jaundice may need to remain under hospital care for longer and research continues into accurately identifying babies at risk (Sanpavat et al 2005).

It is important to assess the behaviour and feeding pattern of the baby – an alert baby feeding well is less of a concern than one who is sleepy and uninterested in feeding. Urine and bowel activity are also strong indicators of wellbeing.

Jaundice progresses from head to toe and resolves in the opposite direction, from toe to head, therefore observation of the colour of the sclera is not useful in assessing improvement. Clinical assessment of severity by experienced practitioners can be highly accurate (Riskin et al 2003), though caution is required in babies with dark skin where visual estimation alone may lead to error (AAP 2004, NICE 2010).

Clinical evaluation of jaundice requires that the baby is undressed, and cephalocaudal progression of jaundice evaluated using the five zones as in Figure 46.1. The Kramer (1969) tool facilitates assessment of the advancement of dermal icterus, and if the baby rapidly advances down the scale, swift referral to the neonatologist for diagnosis and treatment can be achieved. Jaundice becomes clinically apparent when the serum bilirubin rises above 85 µmol/L (bilirubin can be measured as a concentration recorded in µmol/L or mg/dL). Any baby with significant jaundice at 48 hours should have a further assessment by a health professional. Transcutaneous bilirubinometer devices have been developed that correlate well with serum bilirubin measurements, which may reduce the number of blood tests required (Briscoe et al 2002, NICE 2010, Rubaltelli et al 2001, Wong et al 2002) (Box 46.1; also see website). These devices should be used in infants over 35 weeks' gestation and a postnatal age of greater than 24 hours, and a reading greater than 250 µmol/L is an indication for serum bilirubin testing.

### Records

To facilitate effective management, bilirubin results should be sequentially recorded. Graphs are available for preterm

> Box 46.1 **Taking blood for serum bilirubin measurement – preparation**
>
> In order to take a heel specimen correctly, the baby's foot needs to be lower than the body and the heel needs to be warm, and this can be achieved by use of a gauze swab soaked in warm water wrapped around the heel and secured with cling film or a gel-based heel warmer. Both should be tested against the inner aspect of the practitioner's arm.
>
> For full guidance, see website.

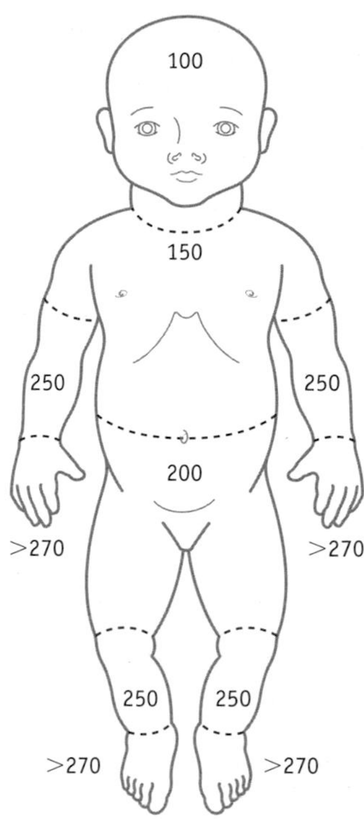


**Figure 46.1** The Kramer tool. Estimates of serum bilirubin (mmol/L) are obtained by assessing distal progression of jaundice. *(Adapted from Kramer, 1969.)*

and term babies, allowing bilirubin levels to be plotted against the time the blood sample was taken, enabling the measurement to be plotted against the baby's age in hours (AAP 2004). This helps inform the practitioner at which level phototherapy should be commenced and when exchange transfusion may be indicated. This is crucial for babies with an unconjugated hyperbilirubinaemia. In these babies, a urine dipstick will also show a positive urobilinogen (secondary to normal enterohepatic circulation of urobilinogen) and a negative bilirubin result (conjugated bilirubin will have been excreted via the liver and bowel). The National Institute for Health and Clinical Excellence (NICE) has also developed the Bili-Wheel, which measures the bilirubin level alongside the gestation to highlight interventions required (NICE 2010) (see website).

## UNCONJUGATED HYPERBILIRUBINAEMIA

Unconjugated hyperbilirubinaemia has three main causes:

- increased red cell breakdown (haemolysis)
- failure of the ability to conjugate bilirubin
- increased enterohepatic circulation.

### Increased red cell breakdown

This occurs most commonly in the neonate because of infection, bruising (for example, after ventouse or forceps delivery), polycythaemia or haemolytic disease of the newborn, or, more rarely, following localized haemorrhage or thrombosis.

### Haemolytic disease of the newborn

Haemolytic disease of the newborn is the *immune-mediated red cell breakdown* which occurs in *rhesus disease* and *ABO incompatibility* (not to be confused with *haemorrhagic disease of the newborn* – vitamin K deficiency). In haemolytic disease of the newborn, the maternal immune system has been 'immunized' against aspects of the baby's blood group (see Fig. 46.2). This 'immunization' usually occurs because of a previous pregnancy, miscarriage, or following blood transfusion when fetal blood cells have passed to the maternal circulation.

*Rhesus factor* is the rhesus C, D and E antigens expressed on red blood cells. It is the D antigen that is most likely to cause isoimmunization. An individual who is 'rhesus negative' does not express the D antigen and has the genotype dd. An individual who is 'rhesus positive' does express

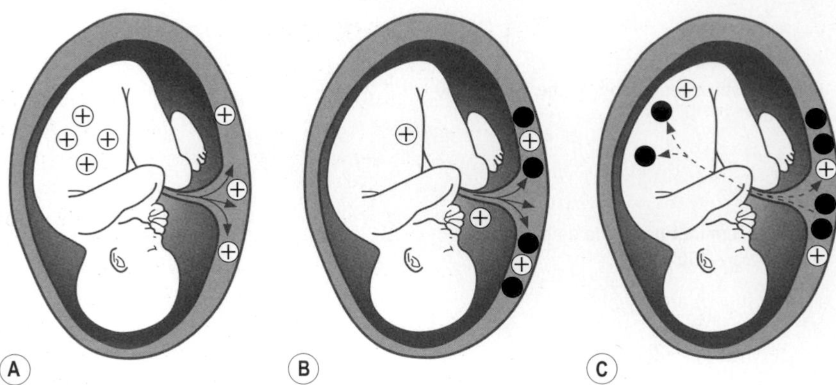


Figure 46.2 Antibody formation. **A.** The crosses represent fetal blood cells crossing over into the maternal circulation. **B.** An antibody response (black circles) is mounted by the mother. **C.** The antibodies cross into the fetal circulation where they will break down the fetal blood cells.

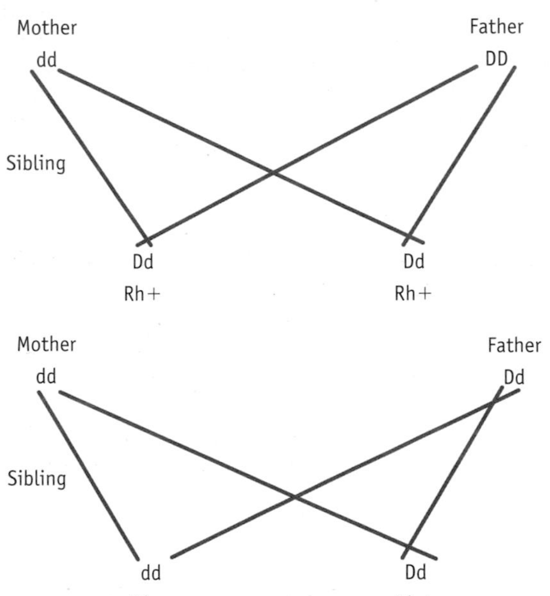


Figure 46.3 Inheritance of rhesus factor. D represents rhesus positivity, which is a dominant trait, and d represents rhesus negativity. In this instance the infant that has Dd will be rhesus positive and may result in the rhesus negative mother mounting an immune reponse.

the D antigen and can be heterozygous (Dd) or homozygous (DD) for the rhesus antigen D genes. Isoimmunization in a rhesus-negative mother can occur with a heterozygous or homozygous fetus or baby and the risk of this occurring can be predicted from a knowledge of the father's genotype as shown in Figure 46.3.

Rhesus isoimmunization can cause a severe haemolysis that may result in fetal anaemia and a need for intrauterine blood transfusions to prevent the development of *hydrops fetalis*.

In order to prevent isoimmunization, anti-D immunoglobulin is administered to women at risk, antenatally and/or postnatally forming complexes with the fetal red cells to prevent the women's immune system from mounting its own immune response. Current advice from NICE is to routinely administer anti-D prophylaxis to all rhesus-negative women antenatally at least once at 28 weeks' gestation (exact regimen depends on dose used) (NICE 2008). It can be administered at times when the women are at increased risk of isoimmunization, such as after miscarriage or after the birth of a rhesus-positive baby. Women and babies at risk can be identified by taking cord and maternal blood after delivery to determine the baby's blood group, and measure the presence of fetal blood cells and antibodies in the maternal system, as in Box 46.2.

Anti-D is a blood product; therefore, prior to administration, informed consent must be obtained. The anti-D must be prescribed on the woman's drug chart by a medical practitioner (NMC 2008).

### Box 46.2 **Coombs and Kleihauer tests**

*Direct Coombs test*: Cord blood is taken to measure the level of maternal antibodies.

*Kleihauer test:* A sample of maternal blood is taken and the number of fetal cells in the sample is estimated. A level of 50 fetal cells/50 lower-power fields is considered high.

Blood is taken from the baby (or the cord) to measure the level of maternal antibodies. One of the complications of administering prophylactic anti D to mothers is that this test may be positive secondary to the administered antibodies and not indicative of a spontaneous maternal production of antibodies.

Severe haemolysis is less common with *ABO incompatibility* than with *rhesus D incompatibility* but the principle of isoimmunization is the same. The ABO blood group refers to the pattern of expression of the A and B antigens on the red blood cells as shown below:

- blood group A – genotype heterozygous AO or homozygous AA
- blood group B – genotype heterozygous BO or homozygous BB
- blood group AB – always heterozygous AB
- blood group O – always homozygous OO.

A mother of blood group O may develop antibodies against the A and B antigens, a mother with blood group A against the B antigen, and a mother of blood group B against the A antigen. These last two examples are extremely rare and ABO incompatibility is most common in a mother who has blood group O with a fetus that has blood group A or B.

ABO incompatibility usually manifests at less than 36 hours of age, although it may not become obvious until after 48 hours. A history of mother's blood group being O positive should alert the midwife as to this possibility.

A baby diagnosed and treated for ABO incompatibility needs to be closely observed for signs of 'late' anaemia, which may occur due to ongoing haemolysis by antibodies that may persist in the baby's circulation for several weeks. Symptoms include lethargy, pallor and poor feeding history. Folate and iron may be prescribed to encourage red blood cell production in the bone marrow but it is not unusual for a baby to develop a severe anaemia requiring blood transfusion. Continuity of care by the midwife providing care up to 28 days can be very helpful.

### Genetic causes

Biochemical or structural abnormalities of red cells may lead to a shortened lifespan with increased red cell turnover and jaundice. Examples of inherited defects of red cells are:

- G6PD deficiency:
  - X-linked (males affected)
  - common in Mediterranean and Asian racial groups
  - haemolysis can be triggered by Fava (broad beans), mothballs, or a variety of drugs and infections in babies with the deficiency (see website)
- Spherocytosis:
  - autosomal dominant
  - red blood cells have a shortened lifespan due to increased sequestration within the spleen
- Pyruvate kinase deficiency:
  - autosomal recessive
  - red blood cells have a shortened lifespan due to membrane defects.

## Failure of conjugation

The ability to conjugate bilirubin varies in individuals depending on differing levels of the enzyme *UDP glucuronosyltransferase* (secondary to individual variation in gene expression) present in the liver, and immaturity of the newborn's enzyme levels.

Prolonged unconjugated hyperbilirubinaemia may occur in some breastfed babies as the enzyme may also be inhibited by breast milk, as illustrated by a study of Taiwanese babies (Huang et al 2004). There is no specific test for breast milk jaundice and diagnosis is made when all other causes have been excluded. Management is dependent on the baby's condition: usually the baby is active and feeds well but jaundice is prolonged and can take up to 6 weeks to resolve.

If the baby is well and all other causes have been excluded, the management is to encourage frequent breastfeeds as 'breastfeeding jaundice' rarely requires phototherapy treatment. Previously, practitioners have advised the discontinuation of breastfeeding in order to confirm the diagnosis, but this can provide negative feedback to the mother regarding her ability to feed and nurture her baby, so should be avoided.

### Genetic reasons

A variety of genetic conditions affect an individual's ability to conjugate bilirubin, including:

- Gilbert syndrome [autosomal recessive]
- Crigler–Najjar syndrome type II (bilirubin encephalopathy/kernicterus rare) [autosomal recessive]
- Crigler–Najjar syndrome type I (bilirubin encephalopathy/kernicterus common) [autosomal recessive].

See website for more information.

## Increased enterohepatic circulation

Delayed intestinal transit will increase the enterohepatic circulation of bilirubin and lead to an increased level of unconjugated bilirubin. In a normal newborn baby, intestinal peristalsis develops over the first few days as enteral feeds are established and a delay in establishing feeds can exacerbate jaundice. The most common medical reason for delayed intestinal transit is *congenital hypothyroidism*. Babies diagnosed with congenital hypothyroidism must be commenced on thyroxine as soon as the diagnosis has been confirmed, to minimize the complication of neurodevelopmental delay. Babies are normally screened for this by measuring thyroid-stimulating hormone (TSH) on the Guthrie card.

The enzymes in colostrum encourage the passage of meconium (see Ch. 43), and the midwife can do much to support the woman in successfully breastfeeding, thereby ensuring that the baby receives colostrum and avoids dehydration. The midwife also notes the passage of meconium as an important part of the baby's progress and wellbeing.

## Complications of unconjugated hyperbilirubinaemia

### Kernicterus

Kernicterus describes the yellow staining of the basal ganglia – usually seen on autopsy in babies who have had severe jaundice (Hachiya & Hayashi 2008). It also describes the chronic long-term clinical effects of a severe hyperbilirubinaemia (AAP 2004).

The risk of kernicterus is influenced by factors including the rate of rise of the bilirubin level as well as its maximum level. Other factors that increase an individual's susceptibility are:

- postnatal age
- prematurity
- hypoalbuminaemia (Hulzebos et al 2008)
- hypoxia/acidosis (both may reduce the effectiveness of the blood–brain barrier)
- bacterial infection (Pearlman et al 1980) – for example, Group B sepsis, urinary tract infections
- medication that interferes with bilirubin binding to albumin, such as *salicylates, sulphonamides, heparin, diazepam* and *chloramphenicol.*

There are also likely to be individual genetic factors that affect the risk of jaundice as well as sensitivity to hyperbilirubinaemia, some of which have been described above (Hansen 2000a). Kernicterus is rare in Europe and the United States (Dodd 1993, Newman & Maisels 1992) but may be increasing in incidence (Manning et al 2007). A further increase may parallel the less aggressive management of jaundice and earlier discharge into the community of newborn babies, especially those born at less than 37 weeks' gestation.

Consequences of a severe hyperbilirubinaemia can be acute or long-term complications. Acute symptoms may be reversible and without long-term complications if appropriately managed (Harris et al 2001) (Table 46.1). Up to 15% of babies who develop long-term complications may be asymptomatic in the acute stage. (See website.)

**Table 46.1 Symptoms of acute bilirubin encephalopathy**

| Age | Acute symptoms |
|---|---|
| 1–2 days | Poor suck, hypotonia, stupor, seizures |
| 3–7 days | Increased tone in extensor muscles, opisthotonos, fever |
| >1 week | Hypertonia |

## Management of unconjugated hyperbilirubinaemia

The recent trend towards home deliveries and early hospital discharge has been associated with increased readmission for jaundice and an increased reporting of babies with kernicterus. In some cases, high-risk babies can be identified (Box 46.3) and their discharge delayed. Undertaking a predischarge newborn bilirubin screening programme has been shown to reduce the rate of readmissions to hospital with significant jaundice (Eggert et al 2006). Bilitool is a web-based tool (www.bilitool.org) which facilitates this prediction of risk and allows evidence-based planning of follow-up and further bilirubin measurement (Bhutani 1999, Longhurst et al 2004). In the community there should be active breastfeeding support and careful monitoring of the jaundice by parents and community staff with early hospital review where necessary (Bhutani & Johnson 2000). Transcutaneous bilirubinometers to screen for significant hyperbilirubinaemia should also be encouraged (Briscoe et al 2002, Engle et al 2005).

Initial assessment establishes the general condition and the most appropriate investigations and management that the baby requires. Supportive measures may include the administration of antibiotics and the correction of dehydration. These may be required in the management of unconjugated hyperbilirubinaemia as meningitis and

**Box 46.3 Risk factors for developing significant unconjugated jaundice post discharge**

- Family history of neonatal jaundice:
  e.g. genetic low levels of UDP glucuronosyltransferase, G6PD deficiency
- Moderately preterm (35–37 weeks' gestation)
- Breastfeeding
- Jaundice <24 hours (haemolytic disease, e.g. rhesus/ABO)
- Asian race
- Bruising/cephalohaematoma
- Infection
- Polycythaemic babies:
  - small-for-gestational-age babies
  - large-for-gestational-age babies, e.g. baby of diabetic mother
  - babies with chromosomal abnormalities, e.g. trisomy 21
- Others:
  - e.g. hypothyroidism

septicaemia are both more common during the first month of life than at any other time during childhood, and dehydration commonly exacerbates jaundice. It may be necessary to correct acid–base defects and hypoxia since both may increase the risk of kernicterus and the administration of albumin may also reduce the amount of free bilirubin available to cross the blood–brain barrier (Ahlfors 1994).

Specific treatments for unconjugated hyperbilirubinaemia are *phototherapy* and *exchange transfusion*. The exact level of bilirubin that causes *bilirubin encephalopathy* and *kernicterus* and at what stage these treatments should be commenced remain contentious. Bilirubin encephalopathy is rare in full-term babies without underlying pathology but relaxation of treatment guidelines has led to an increase in the number of babies developing this complication (Hansen 2000b, Manning et al 2007). The aim of treatment is to identify those babies at specific risk (Bhutani & Johnson 2000) and to prevent kernicterus without exposing many more babies to unnecessary or potentially harmful treatment.

The NICE guidelines (2010) and the American Academy of Pediatrics, updating its 2001 guidelines, suggest that babies should be considered within the following groups when assessing the need for phototherapy, and the *Bilitool*™ uses these risk groups (AAP 2004, www.Bilitool.org):

- *low risk* – well infants >38 weeks
- *medium risk* – well infants 35–37+6 weeks, or infants >38 weeks with risk factors
- *higher risk* – infants 35–37+6 weeks with risk factors.

Risk factors include G6PD deficiency, evidence of hypoxia or ischaemia, haemolytic disease, infection, lethargy, and temperature instability. Table 46.2 can still be

**Table 46.2 Consensus-based bilirubin thresholds for management of babies 38 weeks or more gestational age with hyperbilirubinaemia (NICE 2010)**

| Age (hours) | Bilirubin level (µmol/l) at which the relevant action below should be taken | | | |
|---|---|---|---|---|
| 0 | | | >100 | >100 |
| 6 | >100 | >112 | >125 | >150 |
| 12 | >100 | >125 | >150 | >200 |
| 18 | >100 | >137 | >175 | >250 |
| 24 | >100 | >150 | >200 | >300 |
| 30 | >112 | >162 | >212 | >350 |
| 36 | >125 | >175 | >225 | >400 |
| 42 | >137 | >187 | >237 | >450 |
| 48 | >150 | >200 | >250 | >450 |
| 54 | >162 | >212 | >262 | >450 |
| 60 | >175 | >225 | >275 | >450 |
| 66 | >187 | >237 | >287 | >450 |
| 72 | >200 | >250 | >300 | >450 |
| 78 | | >262 | >312 | >450 |
| 84 | | >275 | >325 | >450 |
| 90 | | >287 | >337 | >450 |
| ≥96 | | >300 | >350 | >450 |
| | ↓ Repeat bilirubin measurement within 6–12 hours | ↓ Consider phototherapy (repeat bilirubin measurement within six hours) | ↓ Start phototherapy | ↓ Perform an exchange transfusion unless the bilirubin level falls below threshold while the treatment is being prepared |

considered as a guide for babies >38 weeks but local policies and recent evidence should be consulted.

## Phototherapy

The effect of light on the excretion of bilirubin has been known since the 1950s (Cremer et al 1958). Phototherapy is an artificial method that provides light of a specific wavelength to enhance bilirubin excretion. Fat-soluble unconjugated bilirubin is mainly converted into water-soluble lumirubin that can be excreted through the kidneys. The most effective light spectrum for converting the yellow bilirubin pigment to the photoisomer lumirubin is blue light and the wavelength of blue light is in the 425–475 nm range.

Other factors affecting the effectiveness of phototherapy are:

- total dose of light delivered
- energy output of light source
- number of light sources
- distance from infant
- maximum skin surface area exposed to those lights.

There are a number of ways of delivering phototherapy, including conventional phototherapy (Fig. 46.4), 360 degree units, blue light units and fibreoptic biliblanket (Figs 46.5 and 46.6) (not used as first line in term babies).

*Double phototherapy* is the combination of two phototherapy units (BiliBlanket and overhead or two overheads) placed at different positions above and/or below the infant. This can significantly increase the excretion of bilirubin (Holtrop et al 1992). There are now phototherapy units that can deliver 360° of phototherapy by completely surrounding the infant within a tunnel of light.

Overhead units have incorporated or attached UV light filters designed to protect the infant from harmful rays. Manufacturer guidelines for use of different phototherapy units (such as distance of the overhead from the infant) may vary. There have been reports of babies suffering UV burns as a direct consequence of phototherapy.

The overhead phototherapy unit requires consideration of the following aspects of care:

- May disrupt normal mother–baby interaction (BiliBlanket may be less disruptive).
- Temperature regulation – baby temperature must be regularly monitored.

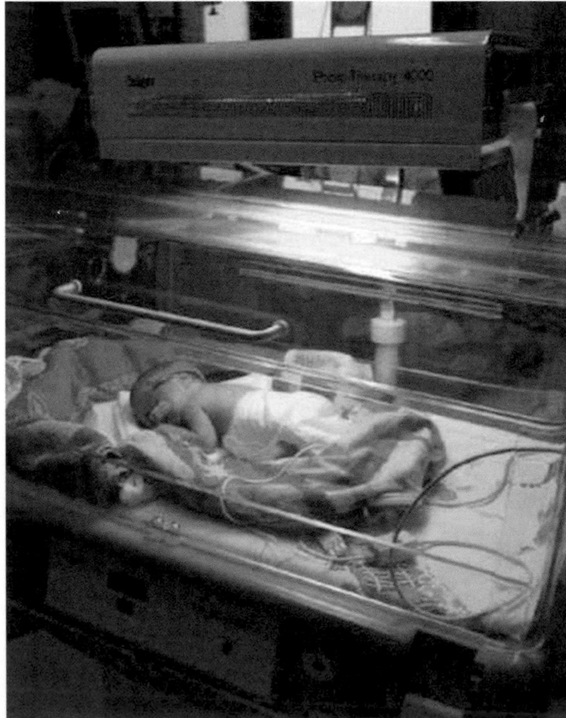

**Figure 46.4** Baby receiving phototherapy.

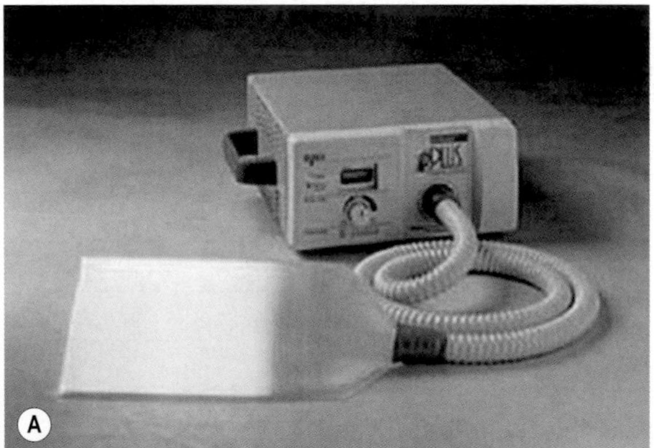


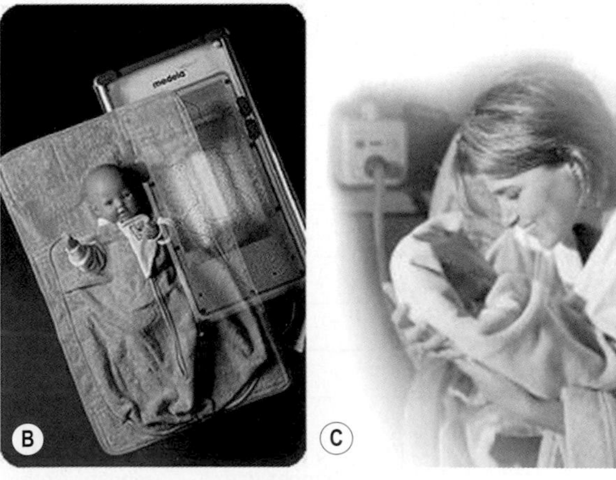


**Figure 46.5** The Ohmeda BiliBlanket. **A.** Light Source. **B.** The Biliblanket. **C.** The new Bilisoft LED phototherapy system. *(Courtesy of GE Healthcare Clinical Systems UK Ltd.)*

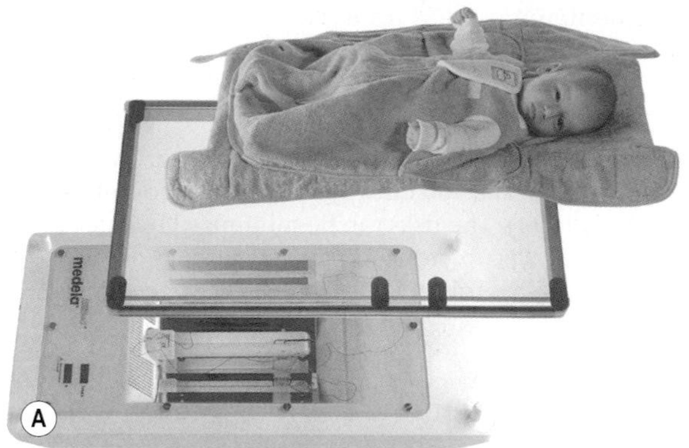


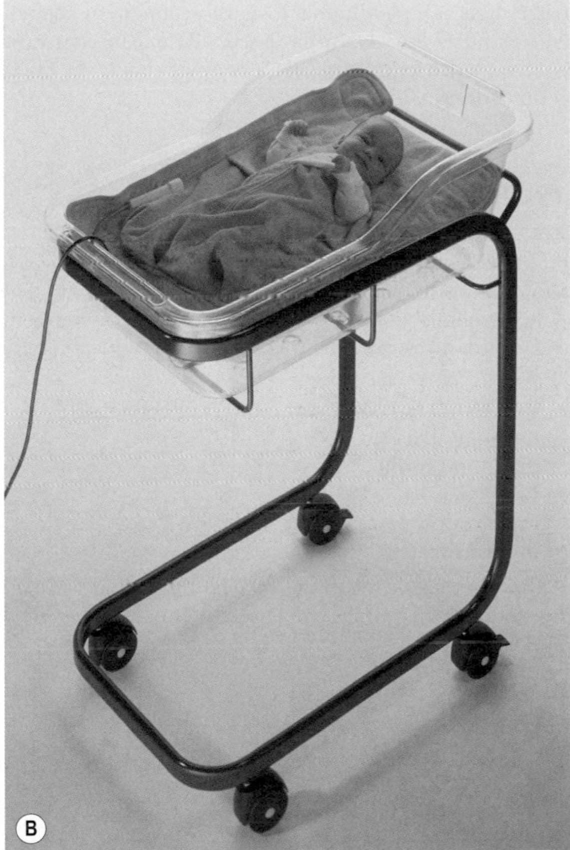


Figure 46.6 The Medela BiliBed. **A.** Phototherapy source, light-permeable support and baby in therapy blanket. **B.** Baby in crib with unit in position. *(Courtesy of Medela AG.)*

- Significant increase in fluid loss from loose stools because of an associated decreased intestinal transit time.
- Nutrition and hydration – important to continue to establish demand feeding and to prevent dehydration.

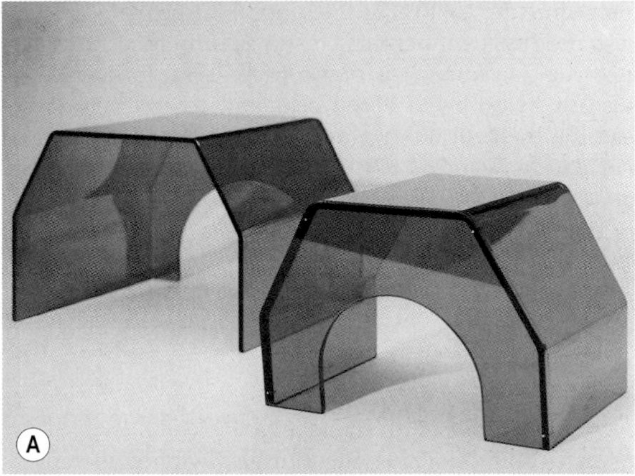


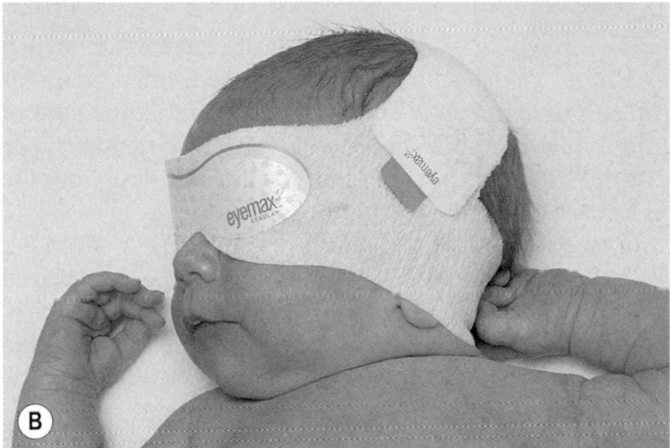


Figure 46.7 Viamed phototherapy lightshield (**A**) and eye protection (**B**). *(Courtesy of Viamed Ltd.)*

Extra fluids do not need to be routinely prescribed but the baby should be regularly assessed for signs of dehydration.

- Eye protection – the eyes must be protected as a precaution against possible damage (Fig. 46.7).
- Maternal anxiety – it is important to ensure the mother understands the reasons for her baby requiring treatment and its basic principles.

Once phototherapy has commenced, it is difficult to assess the degree of jaundice by looking at the skin, and serum bilirubin should initially be measured after 4–6 hours and then 6–12 hourly once stable or falling (NICE 2010). After stopping phototherapy, it is important to check the serum bilirubin at 12 hours (NICE) to monitor for significant rebound in hyperbilirubinaemia which may require further treatment.

## Exchange transfusion

Exchange transfusion involves removing the baby's blood, with maternal antibodies and bilirubin within it, and replacing it with fresh, rhesus-negative blood. During this procedure, up to 90% of the blood may be replaced. This was the first treatment to be successfully used for severe neonatal jaundice. It is particularly useful in haemolytic disease, as both red blood cells and red cell antibodies causing their breakdown are removed from the neonatal circulation. Removal of the antibodies prevents late-onset anaemia.

The main indications for exchange transfusion are:

- severe haemolytic disease
- hypoproteinaemia (hypoalbuminaemia)
- anaemia
- oedema
- cardiac failure
- significant hyperbilirubinaemia
- hyperbilirubinaemia uncontrolled by phototherapy
- hyperbilirubinaemia associated with polycythaemia.

The exact level of hyperbilirubinaemia at which exchange transfusion should be performed remains difficult to define. It is not recommended that the ratio of bilirubin to albumin should influence the decision (NICE 2010). Phototherapy should be continued throughout the procedure (AAP 2004, Hulzebos et al 2008).

In most cases, a two-volume exchange is performed: 160 mL/kg of the circulating blood volume is removed and replaced with transfused whole blood (commonly packed red cells and 0.9% saline or 4.5% albumin as whole blood is difficult to obtain). The procedure must be conducted slowly under strict aseptic conditions with detailed recording of the amount of blood removed and amount infused. Ideally two practitioners should undertake this in order to maintain high safety standards. There are two methods: single site or two site.

The preferred *two-site method* involves aspirating blood from a peripheral or umbilical artery at a similar rate to the infusion rate of a transfusion that is being delivered through a peripheral vein.

The *single-site method* involves cannulation of the umbilical vein with aspiration of 5–10 mL of blood through a three-way tap followed by infusion of the same quantity of donor blood. This can result in significant changes in central venous pressure and intravascular volume and is also associated with the complications of umbilical venous cannulation.

Once the transfusion is completed, the baby should continue to be monitored under phototherapy until the hyperbilirubinaemia has begun to decrease and phototherapy is no longer needed. In most cases, an exchange transfusion followed by double phototherapy is effective, however, some babies may require additional exchange transfusion.

### *Complications*

- More common than from phototherapy
- Electrolyte imbalance
- Thrombocytopenia
- Infection
- Cardiac failure
- Necrotizing enterocolitis.

An exchange transfusion should only be performed in a baby at significant risk of kernicterus in whom the benefits of transfusion outweigh the risks of complications (Ahlfors 1994). The risks can be minimized by intensively monitoring electrolytes and platelets throughout the procedure and by minimizing the changes in circulating blood volume during the procedure.

### Immunoglobulin

The use of intravenous immunoglobulin to reduce ongoing haemolysis as an additional form of treatment in haemolytic jaundice has also been described, and there is now good evidence for this (NICE 2010, Alpay et al 1999, Ergaz & Arad 1993).

## PROLONGED JAUNDICE

Prolonged jaundice is jaundice after 2 weeks of age in a term and/or in a preterm baby who remains jaundiced at 3 weeks. Both situations require paediatric assessment with some investigations. Investigation should normally include:

- split bilirubin (direct and indirect or conjugated vs unconjugated)
- full blood count
- G6PD deficiency
- urine culture (Hannam et al 2000)
- thyroid function tests.

The urgent diagnosis is to identify/exclude biliary atresia, in which case the baby may not initially be severely jaundiced but will have pale stools and dark urine (see below).

## CONJUGATED HYPERBILIRUBINAEMIA

Conjugated hyperbilirubinaemia is always pathological and refers to a situation where >15% of the total bilirubin or 25 μmol/L is in conjugated or 'direct reacting' form. This occurs as a direct consequence of interruption in the normal conjugation and hepatic excretion of bilirubin diglucuronide and results from an obstruction at any point along the pathway from the hepatocyte to the intestine. Bilirubin conjugation within the liver is often able to continue even in the presence of significant liver damage but the excretion of the conjugated bilirubin into intrahepatic bile ducts may become obstructed. Consequently, the concentration of *bilirubin diglucuronide* within the hepatocytes will continue to increase and eventually it diffuses into the bloodstream.

Conjugated jaundice can be suspected clinically in a baby with pale stools (absent stercobilinogen) and dark urine (bilirubin present). A urine dipstick test will be positive for bilirubin. These are critical clinical features as this jaundice may initially be subtle and easily missed, and always requires further assessment.

The main causes of a conjugated jaundice are as follows:

- Hepatitis with cholestasis:
  - idiopathic (unknown)
  - prolonged total parenteral nutrition (TPN)
  - congenital infection, such as CMV, toxoplasmosis, rubella
  - metabolic disease – for example, alpha-1 antitrypsin deficiency
  - galactosaemia.
- Bile duct abnormality:
  - biliary atresia
    - intrahepatic – for example, Alagille syndrome (autosomal dominant)
    - extrahepatic.

In a term baby without perinatal concerns, conjugated jaundice most commonly presents as prolonged jaundice. Any term baby who remains jaundiced at 10 days to 2 weeks of age should be investigated for conjugated jaundice by examining the stools and taking blood for a 'split' bilirubin (direct and indirect bilirubin). Infants with extrahepatic biliary atresia must be identified as early as possible, as surgery performed at 4–6 weeks improves prognosis. Short-term outcome has not been found to be improved by steroids (Vejchapipat et al 2007) and long-term outcome remains guarded with regard to long-term liver disease (Hadzic et al 2003, Hartley et al 2009).

## Complications

Complications may be general or specific complications of the underlying disease itself rather than direct complications of the jaundice.

### *General*

- Deranged clotting with bleeding concerns
- Hypoglycaemia – due to underlying hepatic dysfunction
- Reduced absorption of fat-soluble vitamins, including vitamins A, D and K – may require IV/IM vitamin K and appropriate vitamin preparations, such as Ketovite.

### *Specific*

- Septicaemia
- Cataracts in galactosaemia
- Microcephaly in congenital infection.

## Management of conjugated hyperbilirubinaemia

The main objective in the management is to establish the cause of the jaundice. Phototherapy is ineffective because conjugated bilirubin is already water-soluble and the inappropriate use of phototherapy may lead to the *'bronzed baby'* syndrome. Exchange transfusion is not indicated for a conjugated hyperbilirubinaemia because conjugated bilirubin is not lipid-soluble in the same way as unconjugated bilirubin, and will not cause kernicterus.

Signs may include the following:

- petechiae
- bruising
- bleeding
- hepatomegaly.

First-line investigations should include a blood glucose, liver function tests and clotting studies. Early advice should be sought from a paediatric hepatologist so that the most appropriate investigations and subsequent management can be arranged.

## FOLLOW-UP

All babies who have had significant unconjugated hyperbilirubineamia should be reviewed at least once following discharge. This enables results of investigations to be reviewed, further investigations to be arranged if appropriate, and the baby's clinical condition to be reassessed. Since one of the complications of hyperbilirubinaemia is sensorineural hearing loss, these babies should have formal hearing tests (see website).

Neonates who have had haemolytic jaundice require early review and regular follow-up for the first 3 months of life since the other effect of haemolysis is anaemia (especially when the treatment was phototherapy without an exchange transfusion). The baby should be seen at less than 2 weeks of age to review its clinical condition and to perform a full blood count. This investigation will provide information about the extent of the ongoing haemolysis (haemoglobin) and the baby's bone marrow response and ability to compensate (reticulocyte count). Some babies may require a later blood transfusion.

Babies that have had clinical evidence of acute bilirubin encephalopathy require continued neurodevelopmental follow-up and further investigations such as MRI to establish a guide to prognosis.

## CONCLUSION

Jaundice is a common problem of the newborn baby. An understanding of the normal physiology of bilirubin metabolism enables the midwife to predict risk factors for developing unconjugated hyperbilirubinaemia and be aware of the clinical signs suggestive of a conjugated hyperbilirubinaemia. The aim in unconjugated hyperbilirubinaemia is to prevent babies from developing severe jaundice that may lead to bilirubin encephalopathy and kernicterus. Infants with prolonged jaundice should be referred to a paediatrician to swiftly identify conjugated hyperbilirubinaemia. The midwife will often be the person who will identify the jaundice, and continue to provide care and support to the woman, baby and family. She needs to be knowledgeable about the different aspects of care and management, be able to provide accurate and evidence-based information to the family, and ensure that they feel informed and confident in the professionals providing care to the baby.

## KEY POINTS

- Jaundice is the clinical consequence of a high level of bilirubin that may be unconjugated or conjugated.
- Jaundice is common but must always be investigated when it is noted at <48 hours of age, is significant or is prolonged for more than 2 weeks.
- A baby with visible jaundice of the legs and feet requires measurement of serum bilirubin level.
- A significant unconjugated hyperbilirubinaemia must be treated with phototherapy or exchange transfusion to prevent the acute complications of kernicterus and long-term complications of deafness and athetoid cerebral palsy.
- A baby who is jaundiced with pale stools and dark urine requires urgent assessment and referral to a paediatric hepatologist.

## REFERENCES


Ahlfors CE: Criteria for exchange transfusion in jaundiced newborns, *Pediatrics* 93(3):488–494, 1994.

Alpay F, Sarici SU, Okutan V, et al: High-dose intravenous immunoglobulin therapy in neonatal immune haemolytic jaundice, *Acta Paediatrica* 88(2): 216–219, 1999.

American Academy of Pediatrics (AAP): Neonatal jaundice and kernicterus, *Pediatrics* 108(3):763–765, 2001.

American Academy of Pediatrics (AAP): Management of hyperbilirubinemia in the newborn infant 35 or more weeks of gestation, *Pediatrics* 114(1):297–316, 2004.

Bhutani VK, Johnson LH: Managing the assessment of neonatal jaundice: importance of timing, *Indian Journal of Pediatrics* 67(10):733–737, 2000.

Briscoe LS, Clark S, Yoxall CW: Can transcutaneous bilirubinometry reduce the need for blood tests in jaundiced full term babies? *Archives of Disease in Childhood – Fetal and Neonatal Edition* 86(3):F190–F192, 2002.

Cremer RJ, Perryman PW, Richards DH: Influence of light on the hyperbilirubinaemia of infants, *The Lancet*:1094–1097, 1958.

Dennery PA, Seidman DS, Stevenson DK: Neonatal hyperbilirubinaemia, *New England Journal of Medicine* 344(8):581–590, 2001.

Dodd KL: Neonatal jaundice – a lighter touch, *Archives of Disease in Childhood* 68(5 Spec No):529–532, 1993.

Eggert LD, Wiedmeier SE, Wilson J, et al: The effect of instituting a prehospital-discharge newborn bilirubin screening program in an 18-hospital health system, *Pediatrics* 117(5):e855-e862, 2006.

Engle WD, Jackson GL, Stehel EK, et al: Evaluation of a transcutaneous jaundice meter following hospital discharge in term and near-term neonates, *Journal of Perinatology* 25(7):486–490, 2005.

Ergaz Z, Arad I: (1993) Intravenous immunoglobulin therapy in neonatal immune hemolytic jaundice, *Journal of Perinatal Medicine* 21(3):183–187, 1993.

Hachiya Y, Hayashi M: Bilirubin encephalopathy: a study of neuronal subpopulations and neurodegenerative mechanisms in 12 autopsy cases, *Brain Development* 30(4):269–278, 2008.

Hadzic, N, Davenport M, Tizzard S, et al: Long-term survival following Kasai portoenterostomy: is chronic liver disease inevitable? *Journal of Pediatric Gastroenterology and Nutrition* 37(4):430–433, 2003.

Hannam S, McDonnell M, Rennie JM: Investigation of prolonged neonatal jaundice, *Acta Paediatrica* 89(6):694–697, 2000.

Hansen TW: Bilirubin oxidation in brain, *Molecular Genetics and Metabolism* 71(1–2):411–417, 2000a.

Hansen TW: Kernicterus in term and near-term infants – the specter walks again, *Acta Paediatrica* 89(10):1155–1157, 2000b.

Harris MC, Bernbaum JC, Polin JR, et al: Developmental follow-up of breastfed term and near-term infants with marked hyperbilirubinemia, *Pediatrics* 107(5):1075–1080, 2001.

Holtrop PC, Ruedisueli K, Maisels MJ: Double versus single phototherapy in low birth weight newborns, *Pediatrics* 90(5):674–677, 1992.

Hulzebos CV, van Imhoff DE, Bos AF, et al: Usefulness of the bilirubin/albumin ratio for predicting bilirubin-induced neurotoxicity in premature infants, *Archives of Disease in Childhood – Fetal and Neonatal Edition* 93(5):F384–F388, 2008.

Kramer LI: Advancement of dermal icterus in the jaundiced newborn, *American Journal of Diseases of Children* 118:454–458, 1969.

Longhurst CA, Turner S, Burgos AE: *BiliTool*, 2004; http://www.bilitool.org. Accessed November 8 2010.

Manning D, Todd P, Maxwell M, et al: Prospective surveillance study of severe hyperbilirubinaemia in the newborn in the UK and Ireland, *Archives of Disease in Childhood – Fetal and Neonatal Edition* 92(5):F342–F346, 2007.

National Institute for Health and Clinical Excellence (NICE): Pregnancy – routine anti-D prophylaxis for rhesus negative women (review of TA41), http://guidance.nice.org.uk/TA156, 2008.

National Institute for Health and Clinical Excellence (NICE): *Clinical guidelines: neonatal jaundice* (website). www.nice.org.uk/guidance/index. 2010.

Newman TB, Maisels MJ: Evaluation and treatment of jaundice in the term newborn: a kinder, gentler approach, *Pediatrics* 89(5 Pt 1): 809–818, 1992.

Nicoll A, Ginsburg R, Tripp JH: Supplementary feeding and jaundice in newborns, *Acta Paediatricia Scandinavica* 71(5):759–761, 1982.

Nursing and Midwifery Council (NMC): *Standards of medicine management*, London, 2008, NMC.

Pearlman MA, Gartner LM, Lee K, et al: The association of kernicterus with bacterial infection in the newborn, *Pediatrics* 65(1):26–29, 1980.

Riskin A, Kugelman A, Abend-Weinger M, et al: In the eye of the beholder: how accurate is clinical estimation of jaundice in newborns? *Acta Paediatrica* 92(5):574–576, 2003.

Rubaltelli FF, Gourley GR, Loskamp N, et al: Transcutaneous bilirubin measurement: a multicenter evaluation of a new device, *Pediatrics* 107(6):1264–1271, 2001.

Sanpavat S, Nuchprayoon I, Smathakanee C, et al: Nomogram for prediction of the risk of neonatal hyperbilirubinemia, using transcutaneous bilirubin, *Journal of the Medical Association of Thailand* 88(9):1187–1193, 2005.

Sellwood M, Huertas-Ceballos A: Review of NICE guidelines on routine postnatal infant care, *Archives of Disease in Childhood – Fetal and Neonatal Edition* 93(1):F10–F13, 2008.

Vejchapipat P, Passakonnirin R, Sookpotarom P, et al: High-dose steroids do not improve early outcome in biliary atresia, *Journal of Pediatric Surgery* 42(12):2102–2105, 2007.

Wong CM, van Dijk PJ, Laing IA: A comparison of transcutaneous bilirubinometers: SpectRx BiliCheck versus Minolta AirShields, *Archives of Disease in Childhood – Fetal and Neonatal Edition* 87(2):F137–F140, 2002.

Chapter |47|

# Infection

*Carol Bates*

## LEARNING OUTCOMES

After reading this chapter, you will:

- have an understanding of the neonatal immune system
- be able to apply this knowledge to practice, in order to prevent and reduce infection
- have an understanding of neonatal infections and be able to discuss when and how they occur, treatments, management and outcomes.

## INTRODUCTION

Infection is still a significant cause of abortion, fetal malformation, prematurity, infant death and long-term morbidity, especially in sick and preterm babies (Newell & Darling 2008). Normally the fetus is protected from infection during pregnancy (congenital infection) by the cervical mucus plug, intact amniotic sac and placenta, all of which act as a barrier to most bacterial conditions; but certain viruses and protozoa, because of their small molecular size, can cross the placenta, causing teratogenic (fetal malformation) effects and infections (Box 47.1).

The fetus can also acquire infection around the time of birth (perinatal infection) due to exposure to maternal infection in the birth canal or birth trauma that causes abrasion of newborn skin, giving a potential portal of entry for infection. In the neonatal period (postnatal infection) infection may be acquired from the mother, other babies, hospital equipment; inadequate handwashing by health professionals, carers and parents; and droplet infections via the respiratory route. Puncturing the skin, such as during the Guthrie blood spot test, also provides a potential portal of entry for infection, and, in certain circumstances, infection can be acquired through breastfeeding.

Bacterial infections include those caused by *group B streptococcus* (GBS) and *Listeria monocytogenes* and sexually transmitted diseases such as *chlamydia*, *gonorrhoea* and *syphilis*. Viral infections include *cytomegalovirus (CMV)*, *herpes simplex virus (HSV)*, *rubella*, *hepatitis*, *varicella–zoster* and *human immunodeficiency virus (HIV)*. *Toxoplasmosis* is a protozoal infection and *candidiasis* a fungal infection.

The effect of fetal infection depends upon the nature of the organism and the stage of gestation. For example, exposure to rubella in the first trimester of pregnancy is associated with a high risk of serious congenital defects, whereas exposure in late pregnancy poses little risk. In contrast, genital herpes infection in early pregnancy poses little risk, but if acquired at birth there is a high risk of neonatal infection. Exposure to primary CMV infection in pregnancy gives a risk of adverse neonatal outcome at any stage of pregnancy, but infection acquired during birth or in the postnatal period through breastfeeding is not associated with adverse neonatal outcome (Newell & McIntyre 2000).

Some infections have long-term sequelae which may not become apparent for months or even years. For example, the ophthalmic damage caused by chlamydia becomes apparent in the neonatal period but the pneumonia associated with chlamydia infection usually occurs months after delivery; deafness associated with congenital CMV, toxoplasmosis, syphilis and rubella infection often does not become apparent until later in childhood; and hepatitis B and C infection may result in an initial infection but chronic hepatitis develops later and after hepatitis B infection cirrhosis and carcinoma of the liver do not occur for several decades (Newell & McIntyre 2000).

**Box 47.1 TORCH**

The acronym TORCH can be used as an *aide-mémoire* for some infections that can affect the fetus in utero:

T toxoplasmosis
O other, e.g. syphilis, HIV, hepatitis
R rubella (german measles)
C cytomegalovirus
H herpes

## ANTENATAL SCREENING FOR INFECTION

Currently, all women in early pregnancy in the UK are offered screening for syphilis, HIV, hepatitis B and rubella (UKNSC/HPA 2007). Women who present in labour without having received any antenatal care should be offered screening for these four infections in labour.

At initial booking, midwives must ensure sensitive questioning reveals any risk factors for infections. Immigrants and refugees from different countries may not have had rubella vaccinations or may come from areas with a high incidence of tuberculosis or HIV. Vaccination programmes address some conditions, such as hepatitis B and rubella, and research into vaccines for other pathogens, such as HIV and GBS, continues.

## NEWBORN IMMUNITY

Both preterm and term infants are vulnerable to infection because they are naturally immunodeficient at birth. Also, because the immune system is not exposed to common organisms until birth, there is an initial delayed or diminished response to any invading organisms (Blackburn 2007).

Newborn term infants do have some degree of natural immunity at birth due to the following:

- Maternal *immunoglobulin G (IgG):* which crosses the placenta during the third trimester (it is the only immunoglobulin with a small enough molecular size to do this). Because there is no transfer of IgG until after 32 weeks' gestation, very preterm infants are even more vulnerable to infection, and they are more likely to have invasive procedures, longer hospital stays and numerous caregivers.
- *IgM:* is not passed transplacentally, but small amounts are synthesized by the fetus. It takes approximately 2 years to attain adult IgM levels; this makes babies more susceptible to Gram-negative organisms, causing gastrointestinal infections.
- *IgA:* although this is relatively deficient at birth, because IgA molecules are too big to be transferred across the placenta, serum levels rise following birth, giving some protection against respiratory and gastrointestinal infections. Breast milk, particularly colostrum, is rich in secretory IgA and *interferon,* which significantly enhances the baby's resistance to enteric infections (Kelly & Coutts 2000). Several studies show that breast milk may actively stimulate the newborn immune system (Oddy 2001).
- Breast milk also contains *IgD, lactoferrin, Lactobacillus bifidus* and *lysozyme,* an anti-infective agent. These help to ensure the gut is colonized with relatively harmless Gram-positive bifidobacteria, as opposed to coliforms and enterococci found in formula-fed infants (Dai & Walker 1999). *Lactoferrin* affects iron absorption, depleting *Escherichia coli* of the iron it needs to replicate.
- Lymphocytes are produced in the thymus gland, which is fairly large at birth. The quantity and quality of neutrophils in the neonate are relatively low compared with older babies. Breastfeeding, particularly in the early weeks, can improve these levels, as breast milk is especially rich in neutrophils and macrophages (white blood cells) (see Ch. 43).

### The complement system

The complement system is a major component of innate immunity. Complement consists of a series of plasma proteins and their fragments that, when activated, enhance other components of the immune system. For example, the effect of complement on the cell membrane of invading organisms enables their destruction by other defence mechanisms of the body (Blackburn 2007). Breast milk contains some components of the complement system but the overall action of complement is limited at birth.

## PREVENTION OF INFECTION

Midwives must be vigilant in recognizing risk factors and early symptoms of maternal and neonatal infection. To do this effectively requires multidisciplinary working to prevent, diagnose and promptly treat infection in the mother, baby and, if necessary, the midwife.

The midwife needs to educate women to be aware of sources of potential infection that may affect her and/or her child and ensure that any infection during pregnancy is managed and treated promptly. As well as maternal transmission of infection, organisms can be introduced during invasive antenatal procedures, such as amniocentesis. Intrauterine pneumonia is the commonest effect, but it depends on the pathogens introduced. Strict aseptic techniques must be assured.

Newborn infants in maternity units are at risk of cross-infection and frequent, effective handwashing remains the single most important method of preventing the spread of infection (NPSA 2010: see website). Other strategies include newborn 'rooming in' with the mother, encouraging breastfeeding to increase immune protection, using individual equipment for each baby, and, if necessary, isolation of an infected infant. Visitors should be discouraged from sitting on beds and from visiting if they have an infection or feel unwell.

To avoid exposure to bloodborne infections, such as hepatitis B and HIV, midwives must integrate into their practice the Department of Health universal precautions (DH 1998) to reduce exposure to blood and other body fluids and tissue that may contain bloodborne pathogens. Universal precautions include covering any skin cuts/lesions with a waterproof dressing, wearing rubber gloves and other protective clothing as appropriate, avoiding needlestick injuries and disposing safely of sharps (needles) and other instruments and waste, and vaccination against hepatitis B.

## SIGNS AND SYMPTOMS OF INFECTION IN THE NEWBORN

Newborn infection resulting from antenatal or intrapartum transmission of infections such as *varicella, listeriosis, HSV, GBS, rubella, syphilis, chlamydia* or *gonorrhoea* usually becomes apparent during the neonatal period. Early-onset infection occurs within the first 48 hours; late onset is after 72 hours.

The presentation of infection in the newborn is often subtle and difficult to recognize. It is important that midwives are alert to the possibility of infection so as to detect early signs and seek paediatric advice to enable prompt diagnosis and treatment.

When the membranes rupture, the fetus becomes susceptible to organisms from the birth canal; the infections most likely to be acquired in this way are pneumonia and/or meningitis due to *GBS* infection or *Listeria monocytogenes, gonococcal* and *chlamydia conjunctivitis, Candida albicans* (a fungal infection) and *herpes simplex* (Newell & Darling 2008).

The possibility of neonatal infection should always be borne in mind if labour is preterm or there is prolonged rupture of the membranes, especially if chorioamnionitis has developed. Maternal pyrexia in labour, especially if preterm, and a cardiotocogragh (CTG) showing a fetal heart rate pattern of tachycardia with reduced variability, and no acclerations, can also be indicators of the possibility of fetal infection (Gibb & Arulkumaran 2008). The midwife should seek an obstetric clinical review because maternal investigations such as blood cultures and antibiotic treatment may be required and the baby should be screened at birth.

## THE BABY AT BIRTH

Diagnosis of neonatal infection requires a high index of suspicion and if there is **any** doubt the baby should be seen by a paediatrician. A baby with infection at birth will often have an Apgar score that is within normal limits. A neonate with infection quickly becomes cold, and despite warming-up techniques being used, the temperature remains unstable. The baby appears lethargic and there is recurrent apnoea with pallor and mottling of the skin. The baby is reluctant to feed and a blood sugar, if tested, will be low.

Urgent referral to a paediatrician for further investigations is imperative as babies often deteriorate rapidly when ill. An infection screen will be carried out and includes a full blood count, blood culture, chest X-ray, and microscopy and culture of urine and cerebrospinal fluid. Treatment using broad-spectrum antibiotics will be started pending results of screening tests (Newell & Darling 2008).

## INFECTIONS ACQUIRED DURING PREGNANCY

### Listeriosis

Listeriosis is an uncommon but serious neonatal infection transmitted via the placenta. It is caused by the Gram-positive bacillus *Listeria monocytogenes*. Intrauterine infection can result in either spontaneous abortion or stillbirth; preterm labour and amnionitis are common. Listeriosis can cause a green staining of the liquor, which may be mistaken for meconium. Meconium is not normally passed prior to 34 weeks' gestation; therefore, in a labour of less than 34 weeks' gestation, green staining of the liquor should alert the midwife to the possibility of listeriosis. With listeriosis, the CTG will show a persistent tachycardia with markedly reduced variability and shallow decelerations (Fig. 47.1).

Listeriosis is usually apparent at birth or within the first few hours of life. The infant has a widespread rash with septicaemia, pneumonia and meningitis. The mortality rate is 30%. Late onset usually presents as meningitis between 1 to 8 weeks of age but has a better prognosis than early onset (Lissauer & Clayden 2007).

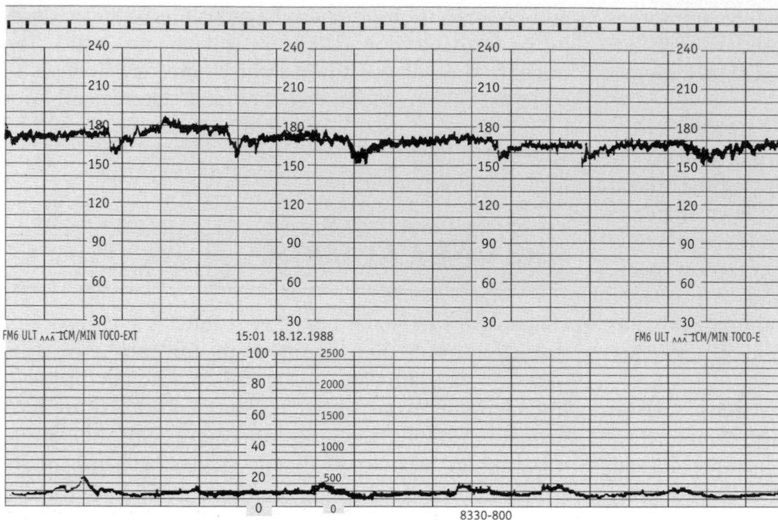


**Figure 47.1** Ominous trace: listerial infection. *(Gibb & Arulkumaran 2008:101.)*

## Syphilis

Syphilis is caused by the spirochaete *Treponema pallidum* and is acquired by direct sexual contact (see Ch. 57). Because *Treponema pallidum* crosses the placenta, all pregnant women in the UK are routinely screened for syphilis in early pregnancy. This prevents most cases of congenital syphilis because women with a confirmed positive result are referred to a sexual health clinic for assessment and treatment with parenteral penicillin which prevents mother-to-child transmission (National Collaborating Centre for Women's and Children's Health 2008). If women have a full course of treatment a month or more before birth, the infant does not require treatment and has an excellent prognosis; however, if there is any doubt about the adequacy of maternal treatment, the infant will be treated with penicillin (Lissauer & Clayden 2007).

If syphilis is not treated in pregnancy, 70% to 100% of neonates will be infected and up to one-third of these infants will be stillborn (National Collaborating Centre for Women's and Children's Health 2008). Infected infants may be asymptomatic at birth with clinical features not becoming apparent until 2 to 12 weeks after birth. Clinical features specific to congenital syphilis include a characteristic rash on the hands and soles of the feet, eye defects and microcephaly. On X-ray bone abnormalities will be seen. Congenital syphilis is very rare in the UK.

## Hepatitis B virus

Intrauterine transmission of the hepatitis B virus (HBV) is uncommon because the virus does not readily cross the placenta; transmission generally occurs in the perinatal and postnatal period. Infected infants usually become asymptomatic carriers, with approximately 30–50% developing chronic HBV liver disease, which in 10% of children may progress to cirrhosis. There is a long-term risk of hepatocellular carcinoma.

Routine antenatal testing for the hepatitis B surface antigen (HBsAg) identifies those women at risk and babies of women who are HBsAg-positive should be given hepatitis B vaccination as soon as possible after birth (within 24 hours). Hepatitis B immunoglobulin (HBIG) is given as well if the mother is also hepatitis B e antigen (HBeAg)-positive because this indicates viral activity which can persist for weeks (Newell & McIntyre 2000). Babies with a birthweight of 1500 g or less born to hepatitis B-infected mothers should receive HBIG in addition to the vaccination regardless of the antigen status of the mother (UKNSC/HPA 2007). If two injections are required, they should be given on two different sites. Further injections are required to complete the vaccination programme and are usually given at 1 month and 6 months of age although vaccination programmes can vary according to area (Newell & McIntyre 2000).

## Hepatitis C virus

Hepatitis C virus (HCV) is common amongst intravenous drug users. Mother-to-child transmission of HCV is rare unless there is co-infection with HIV. It seldom causes an acute infection but at least 50% of children will develop cirrhosis, hepatic carcinoma and eventually liver failure. Treatment is a combination of interferon and ribavirin therapy, which is successful in 50% of children (Lissauer & Clayden 2007).

## HIV

Babies are usually affected by HIV type I; the usual route of infection in the Western world is vertical transmission from mother to infant during pregnancy, labour and the postnatal period (through breastfeeding) (see Ch. 57) but the incidence of vertical transmission in Western Europe and the USA has been reduced through HIV testing in pregnancy, retroviral treatment of women and the use of infant formula feeding (HIV I DNA is present in breast milk). This has resulted in fewer than 20 of the 1000 babies born each year in the UK to HIV-positive mothers being infected with the virus (Lissauer & Clayden 2007).

Diagnosis of neonatal HIV infection is complicated by the presence of passively acquired maternal antibody, which may persist for up to 18 months of age. Prior to 18 months of age, the most sensitive test for HIV is by detection of the viral genome by HIV DNA PCR (polymerase chain reaction). Two negative HIV DNA PCRs within the first 3 months of life, at least 2 weeks after completion of postnatal antiretroviral therapy, indicate the infant is not infected, although this cannot be confirmed until after 18 months of age (Lissauer & Clayden 2007).

Infected babies appear normal at birth; however, without prophylactic treatment, nearly 25% will develop acquired immunodeficiency syndrome (AIDS) or die in the first year of life; the remaining children may not show any signs of the disease until their teenage years. Common symptoms of AIDS developing in HIV-infected infants are failure to thrive, recurrent infections, diarrhoea and severe candida (thrush) infection (Newell & Darling 2008). Infants infected with HIV are susceptible to TB but BCG vaccination should not be given because it is a live mycobacterial vaccine (Lissauer & Clayden 2007).

## Toxoplasmosis

The overall rate of fetal infection following exposure to maternal toxoplasmosis depends upon the timing of maternal infection. The rate of transmission is low (10%) during the first 2 weeks of pregnancy and increases to over 90% by the last 2 weeks of pregnancy; but the risk of adverse fetal outcome is highest following exposure to infection during the first trimester of pregnancy rather than in later pregnancy (Newell & McIntyre 2000). Clinical signs of neonatal toxoplasmosis include low birthweight, enlarged liver and spleen, hydrocephalus, jaundice and anaemia. Up to 85% of congenitally infected neonates are asymptomatic at birth, but most will develop complications, including seizures and reduced cognitive function, over time. Infected newborn infants are treated for 1 year with pyrimethamine and sulfadiazine (Lissauer & Clayden 2007). Regular blood tests are required during treatment because these drugs cause bone marrow suppression (Newell & McIntyre 2000).

## Rubella (German measles)

The extent of fetal damage following maternal rubella infection is determined by gestational age at the onset of infection. Infection before 8 weeks' gestation causes deafness, congenital heart disease and cataracts in over 80% of fetuses (Fig. 47.2). The fetus develops a viraemia which inhibits cell division and causes defects of the developing organs. Sometimes, spontaneous abortion occurs. Approximately 30% of fetuses infected between 13 and 16 weeks' gestation will have impaired hearing. Beyond 18 weeks' gestation, the risk to the fetus is minimal.

Babies with congenital rubella are very infectious and may excrete rubella virus in the urine for up to 12 months. They pose a cross-infection risk to other babies as well as to pregnant women. Isolation of mother and baby is necessary in hospital and great care required at home. Close follow-up is required, as neurological disorders, which are usually significant, may not be immediately obvious (Newell & McIntyre 2000).

## Cytomegalovirus

Cytomegalovirus (CMV) is a herpes virus. After primary infection it remains latent but may become active if immunity is compromised. Exposure to primary CMV infection at any stage of pregnancy gives a risk of adverse neonatal outcome because viraemia occurs and the virus can cross the placenta. Congenital CMV infection affects 3–4/1000

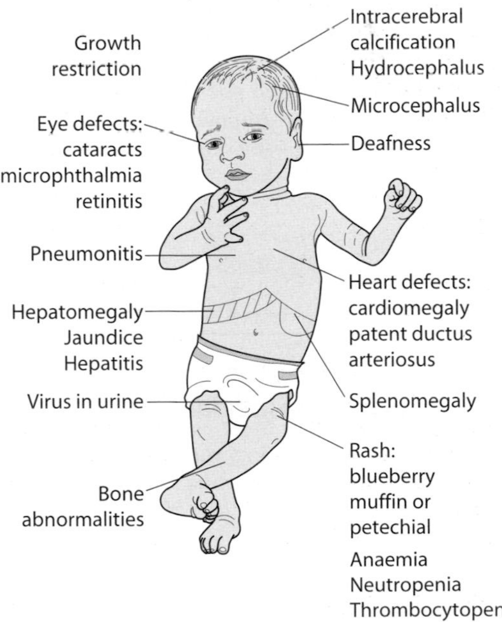


**Figure 47.2** Clinical features of congenital rubella, cytomegalovirus (CMV), toxoplasmosis and syphilis. *(Lissauer & Claydon 2007:131.)*

live births in the UK (Lissauer & Clayden 2007). It can cause intrauterine death and stillbirth but infection acquired during birth or in the postnatal period through breastfeeding is not associated with adverse neonatal outcome unless the infant is premature (Newell & McIntyre 2000).

The majority of infected infants are asymptomatic at birth and develop normally; 5% will have clinical signs and symptoms associated with congenital CMV, such as microcephaly, cerebral palsy, pneumonitis, jaundice, thrombocytopenia and virus shedding. Approximately 5% of infected infants develop problems later in life, mainly hearing problems (Lissauer & Clayden 2007). Diagnosis of CMV can be confirmed by the isolation of CMV from throat swabs and urine samples (Newell & McIntyre 2000).

## Varicella zoster

This virus is responsible for chickenpox. The effect of maternal varicella infection upon the fetus is determined by gestational age at the time of infection. Maternal varicella infection in the first 20 weeks of pregnancy results in congenital varicella syndrome in about 2% of neonates, causing chorioretinitis, skin lesions, skeletal abnormalities, encephalitis and neurological damage.

Maternal infection developing within 5 days before or 2 days after delivery has more serious implications for the neonate because the fetus is unprotected by maternal antibodies and the viral dose is high. About 25% of these infants will develop a vesicular rash. The mortality rate is 30%. These babies should be given varicella zoster immunoglobulin to reduce the risk of serious complications, including hepatic disorders and pneumonia. *Aciclovir* can also be given to the neonate prophylactically (Lissauer & Clayden 2007). Mother and baby should be isolated from other neonates.

# INFECTIONS ACQUIRED DURING BIRTH

## Group B streptococcus (*Streptococcus agalactiae*)

Group B streptococcus (GBS) is commonly found in the gastrointestinal tract and colonizes the vagina in approximately 15% to 30% of women in the UK (Feldman 2001, UKNSC/HPA 2007).

The organism possesses an enzyme which can make microscopic holes in the amniotic sac, enabling it to reach the amniotic fluid and infect the fetus through the lung epithelium (Feldman 2001).

GBS is the commonest cause of overwhelming sepsis in the newborn, including pneumonia and meningitis, with an incidence in the UK of 1:1000 live births (Feldman 2001). Eighty percent of infections are early onset, most of which are clinically apparent at or immediately after birth. The mortality rate is 18% in premature infants and 6% in the term infant (UKNSC/HPA 2007).

Late onset occurs between 7 and 90 days. The infant is not colonized with GBS at birth but acquires it at a later stage, whereupon septicaemia rapidly develops, often accompanied by meningitis (Feldman 2001).

## Diagnosis of GBS carriage in pregnancy

GBS carriage is asymptomatic but routine testing for GBS in pregnancy is not currently recommended in the UK (RCOG 2003, UKNSC/HPA 2007). Currently, a risk factor-based screening approach is used and intrapartum antibiotic prophylaxis is offered to women with recognized risk factors for early-onset GBS disease (HPA 2006a, RCOG 2003, UKNSC/HPA 2007). The risk factors are:

- maternal fever during labour (>38 °C)
- prolonged membrane rupture (>18 h)
- prematurity (<37 weeks)
- a previous infant affected by GBS disease
- being a known carrier of GBS during the current pregnancy
- incidental carriage of GBS found during pregnancy
- GBS urine infection during the current pregnancy.

A multidisciplinary GBS Working Party set up by the Health Protection Agency published *Interim 'good practice' recommendations for the prevention of early onset neonatal group B streptococcal (GBS) infection in UK* (HPA 2006a) (see Figure 47.3 and website).

### *Incidental diagnosis of GBS*

Because there is no organized approach to GBS screening in the UK, carriage is usually found incidentally either through sending a midstream specimen of urine or a HVS (high vaginal swab) for culture during pregnancy. Using a HVS is unsatisfactory because it can give false negative results, but if GBS is detected incidentally from a HVS, intrapartum antibiotic prophylaxis should be considered.

### *Specific testing for GBS*

The correct method is to take a low vaginal swab (from just inside the introitus) and then a rectal swab (the same swab or two separate swabs can be used) between 35 and 37 weeks' gestation. Swabs taken at this time are effective in predicting whether or not there will be GBS carriage during labour. A special enrichment medium is used to culture the swabs to avoid overgrowth of other organisms to increase the likelihood of GBS isolation (HPA 2006b). Vaginal GBS carriage is not treated during pregnancy but intrapartum antibiotic prophylaxis is recommended.

# INTERIM "GOOD PRACTICE" RECOMMENDATIONS FOR THE PREVENTION OF EARLY ONSET NEONATAL GROUP B STREPTOCOCCAL (GBS) INFECTION IN UK

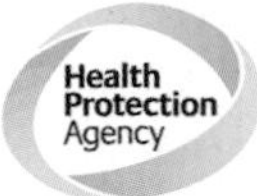


The "good practice" recommendations are not intended to be prescriptive therefore the terms fever, pre-term and prolonged have not been defined and are left to the discretion of the individual centres.

**Routine microbiological screening for antenatal GBS carriage is not recommended.**

Until it is clear that antenatal screening for GBS carriage does more good than harm and that the benefits are cost effective, there is little justification at present for recommending routine screening in the UK.

## WOMEN

*GIVE*

INTRAPARTUM ANTIBIOTIC PROPHYLAXIS (IAP) SPECIFICALLY FOR GBS TO THE FOLLOWING WOMEN:

- GBS infection in a previous baby.

*GIVE*

BROAD SPECTRUM INTRAVENOUS ANTIBIOTICS WHEN CLINICALLY INDICATED AND ENSURE THE REGIMEN INCLUDES ADEQUATE GBS COVER IN THE FOLLOWING SITUATIONS:

- Chorioamnionitis diagnosed or suspected clinically.
- Pre-term prolonged rupture of membranes.

*CONSIDER GIVING*

INTRAPARTUM ANTIBIOTIC PROPHYLAXIS (IAP) IN THE FOLLOWING SITUATIONS:

- GBS found **incidentally** in the vagina at any time during pregnancy.
- GBS found **incidentally** in the urine at any time during pregnancy.
- Labour is pre-term.
- Prolonged rupture of membranes in labour.
- Fever in labour.

## BABIES

*GIVE*

ANTIBIOTICS TO THE FOLLOWING BABIES:

- Any baby who presents at any gestation with symptoms of sepsis, eg tachypnoea, apnoea, mottling, grunting etc.
- In multiple births if one baby is diagnosed with GBS disease treat all infants.

*CONSIDER GIVING*

ANTIBIOTICS TO THE FOLLOWING BABIES:

- Babies born to mothers who should have received IAP but did not.
- Babies born to mothers who received the first dose of antibiotics less than 4 hours prior to delivery.
- Preterm babies whose mothers received IAP.

## *TREATMENT REGIMENS*

### WOMEN

Women with any of the above indications for antibiotics should be offered intravenous antibiotics during labour for at least 4 hours before delivery. However, some women prefer not to receive antibiotics if their risk is only slightly increased since it would complicate an otherwise normal birth. Also antibiotic therapy may be associated with rare but significant complications. **The risks of GBS infection in the baby must be balanced against wishes of mother and the risk of adverse reactions to antibiotics.**

- All women in whom it is recommended to GIVE antibiotics should be offered antibiotics immediately at the onset of labour.
- It is important to administer the first dose of antibiotics as soon as possible from the onset of labour because intravenous antibiotics should be given for at least 4 hours prior to delivery.

*Recommendations for specific IAP for GBS*

- Recommended doses of penicillin G are 3g (or 5mU) intravenously initially and then 1.5g (or 2.5mU) at 4-hourly intervals until delivery.
- For women allergic to penicillin, the recommended dose of clindamycin is 900mg intravenously every 8 hours until delivery.

### BABIES

Babies born to mothers in whom it is recommended to GIVE antibiotics and the mother has been given at least 1 dose at least 4 hours before should be assessed carefully by a paediatrician.

- If the indication for antibiotic administration is only the risk of GBS infection the recommended dose of penicillin G is 100mg/kg daily in 2 divided doses for neonates.
- All antimicrobial treatments used for treating unknown infections in neonates must include adequate GBS cover.

*Produced by*
Health Protection Agency GBS Working Group
August 2006

**Figure 47.3** Group B Streptococcal (GBS) guidelines *(©Health Protection Agency. Reproduced with permission.)*

### GBS urine infection

If GBS is found in the urine during pregnancy, there is a higher risk of neonatal infection. The urinary infection should be treated at the time of diagnosis and intrapartum prophylaxis should also be offered (RCOG 2003).

## GBS carriage and home birth

Women booked for a home birth may need to accept delivery in hospital if they have opted to receive intrapartum intravenous antibiotics. Routine community use of intravenous antibiotics may not be available and community midwives or GPs may be unwilling to accept the risk of anaphylaxis in the home environment.

The majority of research supporting the benefits of intrapartum prophylaxis relates to intravenous administration, but there is some evidence that the intramuscular route may be effective. If a woman fully understands that using the intramuscular route is based upon limited evidence, instead of intravenous therapy, benzyl penicillin 600 mg IM 8-hourly can be used; or erythromycin 100 mg IM 8-hourly if the woman is allergic to penicillin (UKNSC/HPA 2007).

## Ophthalmia neonatorum

Ophthalmia neonatorum is defined as a purulent discharge from the eyes of an infant within 21 days of birth. It is a notifiable condition usually acquired during birth. Causative organisms include *Staphylococcus aureus, Streptococcus pneumoniae, E. coli, Chlamydia trachomatis and Neisseria gonorrhoeae*. A paediatrician must be notified immediately and swabs taken for culture and sensitivity – differential diagnosis of the organism is essential especially for chlamydial and gonococcal infections as these two organisms can cause conjunctival scarring, corneal infiltration and blindness.

*Chlamydia trachomatis* causes a purulent discharge with swelling of the eyelids that usually occurs within 10 days of life. Treatment is with oral erythromycin. Pneumonia can affect between 1% and 22% of infants. Symptoms (coughing and cyanosis) usually appear before 2 months of age (Newell & McIntyre 2000). Treatment is a broad-spectrum antibiotic given either intravenously or orally depending upon the severity of the illness (Lissauer & Clayden 2007) (see Fig. 47.4).

*Gonococcal eye infection* also manifests as a purulent discharge and swelling of the eyelids but within 48 hours of birth. *Penicillin* is the treatment of choice or intravenous *cephalosporin* if there is the possibility of penicillin resistance. For all eye infections, the eyes must be cleaned frequently and eye drops may also be prescribed (Lissauer & Clayden 2007) (see website).

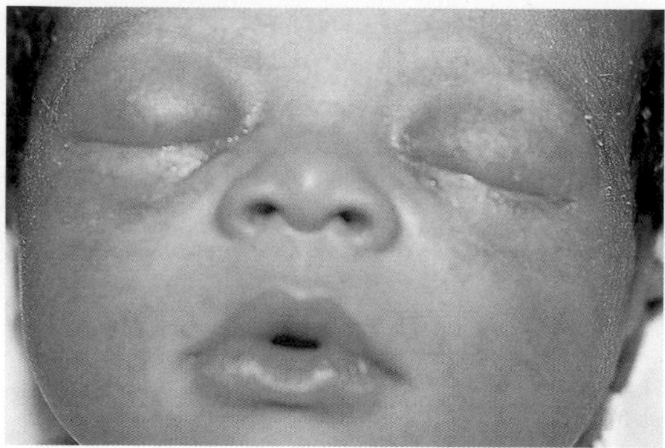

**Figure 47.4** Purulent discharge together with swollen eyelids in an 8-day-old infant. This is the characteristic presentation of conjunctivitis from *Chlamydia trachomatis. Neisseria gonorrhoeae* was absent. *(From Lissauer & Clayden 2007:165.)*

## Herpes simplex virus

Herpes simplex virus (HSV) is associated with active maternal genital herpes and is usually acquired during birth. HSV infection can be congenital and can cause a range of illnesses in the neonatal period, from skin blisters to overwhelming viraemia and encephalitis. Caesarean section may be the mode of delivery of choice when there are active herpetic lesions. Diagnosis requires culture of the virus from the affected skin, and once confirmed, treatment should be commenced as soon as the infection is identified. Infected neonates are treated with systemic *aciclovir*.

## Candida (thrush)

*Candida albicans* is the commonest cause of fungal infections in infants. It may be acquired at delivery if the mother has a vaginal infection as a result of reduced resistance during antibiotic therapy or from inadequate hygiene practices.

Oral infection appears as white patches on the tongue, gums and palate; if the patches are removed, they leave a raw red area. If the mother is breastfeeding, her nipples should also be treated to prevent reinfection. Infection in the nappy area presents with a generalized papular or vesicular rash and antifungal preparations are effective treatments.

*Disseminated candidiasis* is an overwhelming septicaemia, usually found in preterm, very low birthweight babies. There is significant associated morbidity and mortality because this serious disease can affect all the major organs. Infection of the central nervous system has a poor outcome for extremely low birthweight babies, with over

40% having severe disabilities at 2 years of age (Friedman et al 2000). Prompt treatment is essential because this is a life-threatening condition. Aggressive intravenous treatments with both antifungal and antibacterial agents are required. The treatment of choice is intravenous *fluconazole* – an antifungal agent increasingly used, instead of *amphotericin B* and *flucytosine,* and which may be given orally or intravenously in the management of neonatal *C. albicans* infection.

**Reflective activity 47.1**

Review your local policies and procedures relating to screening, detection, management and information available to women, babies and families on:

- Maternal GBS
- TORCH infections
- Hepatitis A, B and C
- Chlamydia

## POSTNATAL INFECTIONS

Mild eye infections and 'sticky eyes' are not uncommon in the newborn and in many cases no bacteria are found. It is important to teach mothers good hygiene and care of the eyes. Handwashing is essential, and cool, boiled water, or sterile saline, and sterile cotton wool swabs are used to clean the eyes from the inner aspect to the outer, discarding the swab after one sweep.

### Umbilical cord infection (Omphalitis)

Severe cord sepsis is uncommon and with good standards of hygiene can be prevented. The midwife must check the umbilicus regularly. Signs of infection include periumbilical inflammation, a moist, offensive smelling cord and delay in separation. Infection may be transported through the umbilical vein to the liver. The organism most commonly responsible is *Staph. aureus,* and, if found, antibiotics are required.

### Pemphigus neonatorum

This is a potentially fatal staphylococcal infection. Because of its highly contagious character and severe effects, the midwife should consider any skin lesion associated with the formation of a blister or pus as a possible case of pemphigus.

Blisters, which fill with pus and burst leaving a raw surface, appear on the head or trunk. This is often called the *staphylococcal scalded skin syndrome* since the appearance mimics that of a scald. As the infection spreads in the superficial tissue, large areas become involved. Complications may arise since staphylococci can also affect the lungs, gut and liver.

Treatment is with systemic antibiotics such as flucloxacillin, which are given intravenously. It is also important to monitor for dehydration and other complications caused by fluid loss.

### Gastroenteritis

This is highly infectious and carries a high risk of mortality for compromised babies. For this reason, an outbreak in a neonatal intensive care unit (NICU) or special care baby unit (SCBU) is a catastrophe. The neonate can quickly become very ill and dehydrated. Electrolyte imbalance, if not speedily treated, leads to tachycardia, hypotension and collapse. There are a number of possible causative organisms, including *Salmonella, Shigella* (a form of *E. coli*), *echovirus type II* and *rotavirus*. Isolation of infected babies is important to prevent cross-infection.

Preventive measures are of the utmost importance: high standards of hygiene must be maintained and effective handwashing practices are vital.

## PREVENTION OF NEWBORN INFECTION

A proactive approach should be taken regarding risk-identification, screening and treatment of infections in women, preconceptionally and antenatally, in order to reduce fetal and neonatal mortality and morbidity. The majority of these conditions are preventable, and midwives can do much to reduce their incidence and severity with education, awareness, early diagnosis and treatment.

**KEY POINTS**

- Midwives need to ensure they identify individual risk factors for infections for each woman, through careful history taking.
- Education and advice regarding diet, lifestyles and hygiene practices can help to prevent certain infections.
- Many maternal infections have disastrous effects on the fetus or neonate, but can be effectively treated if diagnosed antenatally.
- Early signs of infection are often subtle in neonates, and midwives must seek further advice if at all concerned.

## REFERENCES


Blackburn ST: *Maternal, fetal and neonatal physiology: a clinical perspective*, ed 3, Philadelphia, 2007, Saunders Elsevier.

Dai D, Walker WA: Protective nutrients and bacterial colonization in the immature human gut, *Advances in Pediatrics* 46:353–382, 1999.

Department of Health (DH): *Guidance for clinical health care workers: protection against infection with blood-borne viruses: recommendations of the Expert Advisory Group on AIDS and the Advisory Group on hepatitis*, London, 1998, UK Health Departments.

Feldman RG: Group B streptococcus: prevention of infection in the newborn, *The Practising Midwife* 4(3):16–18, 2001.

Friedman S, Richardson SE, Jacobs SE, et al: Systemic candida infection in extremely low birth weight infants: short term morbidity and long term neurodevelopmental outcome, *Pediatric Infectious Disease Journal* 19(6):499–504, 2000.

Gibb D, Arulkumaran S: *Fetal monitoring in practice*, ed 3, London, 2008, Churchill Livingstone.

Health Protection Agency (HPA): *Interim 'good practice' recommendations for the prevention of early onset neonatal group B streptococcal (GBS) infection in UK*, London, 2006a, London.

Health Protection Agency (HPA): *Processing swabs for group B streptococcal carriage BSOP 58*, London, 2006b, HPA.

Jones JL, Lopez A, Wilson M, et al: Congenital toxoplasmosis: a review, *Obstetrical & Gynecological Survey* 56(5):296–305, 2001.

Kelly D, Coutts AG: Early nutrition and development of immune function in the neonate, *Proceedings of the Nutrition Society* 59(2):177–185, 2000.

Lissauer T, Clayden G: *Illustrated textbook of paediatrics*, ed 3, London, 2007, Elsevier.

National Collaborating Centre for Women's and Children's Health: *Antenatal care: routine care for the healthy pregnant woman*, London, 2008, RCOG.

National Patient Safety Agency (NPSA): *Prevention of infection – correct washing hand technique* (website). www.npsa.nhs.uk/cleanyourhands/the-campaign/training-video/. 2010.

Newell SJ, Darling JC: *Paediatrics*, ed 8, Oxford, 2008, Blackwell Publishing.

Newell ML, McIntyre J: *Congenital and perinatal infections: prevention, diagnosis and treatment*, Cambridge, 2000, Cambridge University Press.

Oddy WH: Breastfeeding protects against illness and infection in infants and children: a review of the evidence, *Breastfeeding Review* 9(2):11–18, 2001.

Royal College of Obstetricians and Gynaecologists (RCOG): *Prevention of early onset neonatal group B streptococcal disease. Guideline 36*, London, 2003, RCOG.

UK National Screening Committee & Health Protection Agency (UKNSC/HPA): *Briefing paper for health professionals to support the DH UK 'screening for infectious diseases in pregnancy programme' version 4*. 2007.

Chapter |48|

# Congenital anomalies, fetal and neonatal surgery, and pain

Carol Bates

## LEARNING OUTCOMES

After reading this chapter, you will be able to:

- recognize common major congenital anomalies and syndromes
- have an understanding of the aetiology and risk factors for congenital anomalies
- appreciate the principles and problems of fetal and neonatal surgery
- have an understanding of the issues surrounding fetal and neonatal pain.

## INTRODUCTION

Congenital anomalies are defects/abnormalities present at birth, occuring in approximately 2–3% of babies (Boyd et al 2005, ONS 2010). Congenital abnormality is distinguished as:

- *malformation* – a primary defect of organ or tissue development in the embryo or fetus
- *deformation* – damage caused by external factors influencing a previously normal structure.

Congenital anomalies can affect any part of the body; and can be major, for example a congenital heart defect such as *Fallot's tetralogy*, through to minor, such as an extra digit or tongue tie. Minor anomalies are usually only registered if they are associated with other major malformations or syndromes (EUROCAT 2009). The focus of this chapter is the registered anomalies and syndromes; for more minor anomalies, see website.

## REGISTRATION OF ANOMALIES AND SYNDROMES

Ever since rubella and thalidomide were discovered as powerful teratogens, various worldwide registries have been set up to facilitate research and surveillance concerning environmental causes of congenital anomalies (Misra et al 2006). These include:

- *National Congenital Anomaly System (NCAS)* – set up in England and Wales in 1964 by the Office of National Statistics (ONS). Information is collected on anomalies associated with live and stillbirths (not termination of pregnancy or spontaneous abortion). This is a voluntary reporting system, though not all areas in England and Wales have local registers.
- *European Surveillance of Congenital Anomalies (EUROCAT)* – a register set up by the European Health Commission in 1979 to facilitate pooling and comparing of data, enabling a joint approach to European public health issues (Dolk 2005).
- *British Isles Network of Congenital Anomaly Registers (BINOCAR)* – jointly set up by the ONS and the Glasgow Register of Congenital Anomalies in 1996, collects anomaly data from terminations of pregnancy and live and stillbirths. However, in 2007, BINOCAR introduced a new classification system and the ONS was unable to fund the changes required to adapt the NCAS system to this new model. (See website.)

## ANTENATAL ANOMALY SCREENING

Ultrasound scan screening for fetal anomalies has been fully integrated into antenatal care, but ultrasound scans have their limitations and hold no guarantee that all anomalies may be identified (see Ch. 33); in a small number of cases, babies are born with abnormalities. It is vital that midwives take a detailed medical, family and obstetric history at antenatal booking in order to identify risk factors for specific diseases and facilitate genetic counselling and appropriate investigations.

It is also essential the midwife carries out a thorough initial examination of the newborn at birth because some anomalies need to be investigated and dealt with immediately (see Ch. 41).

Antenatal screening enables greater parental choice as ultrasound scanning can identify:

- anomalies incompatible with life
- anomalies associated with high morbidity and long-term disability
- fetal conditions with the potential for intrauterine therapy
- fetal conditions that will require postnatal investigation or treatment.

Midwives should ensure that women get the opportunity to discuss fully the risk factors, possible results, implications, prognosis and management options for any condition with the appropriate health professional prior to further screening to ensure informed consent is given (NICE 2008, UKNSC 2007).

## AETIOLOGY

Whilst the cause of many congenital anomalies remains unknown, there are some known factors:

### Genetic factors

Each human cell has a total of 46 chromosomes arranged in 23 pairs, one of the pair from each parent (see Ch. 26). Every chromosome carries a unique blueprint of its parent's characteristics in the form of genes. There are two sex chromosomes (X from the mother and either X or Y from the father); the remainder are called *autosomes*.

Genes may be dominant or recessive:

- *Dominant genes* will display their trait whenever they are present on just one chromosome – examples include osteogenesis imperfecta and achondroplasia.
- *Recessive genes* need to be present on both chromosomes of the pair – for example, phenylketonuria and cystic fibrosis.

The incidence of complex abnormalities is also increased with certain maternal diseases, such as unstable diabetes (Farrell et al 2002) and phenylketonuria.

### Teratogenic factors

Examples of well-documented teratogens are:

- maternal infections – including rubella, toxoplasmosis, cytomegalovirus, syphilis
- drugs – heroin, cocaine, some anticonvulsants, anticoagulants, alcohol, streptomycin, tetracycline, thalidomide
- environmental – pesticides, dioxins, radiation
- sustained hyperthermia (therefore saunas during pregnancy are discouraged)
- maternal febrile illness in the first trimester is linked to an increase in congenital heart defects (Botto et al 2001).

**Reflective activity 48.1**

Find out if your area has a high prevalence of any particular congenital anomalies and consider any known aetiological factors.

## CENTRAL NERVOUS SYSTEM ANOMALIES

### Spina bifida

Spina bifida is the commonest neural tube defect. Improved antenatal detection, therapeutic termination and routine vitamin supplementation (taking folic acid daily prior to conception and during the first 12 weeks of pregnancy) have accounted for a dramatic drop in the incidence.

There are three main types of spina bifida:

*Spina bifida meningocele* is very rare; the vertebrae develop normally but there is a protrusion of the meninges (but not neural tissue) through the vertebrae. The meningocele may or may not be covered by skin. Surgery can rectify this and no further treatment is required. There are unlikely to be any long-term health problems because neural tissue is not involved.

*Spina bifida myelomeningocele* occurs in approximately 1 : 1000 births. The vertebrae fail to fuse around the spinal cord, leaving it unprotected. This is a serious condition because it involves both the spinal cord and meninges, often accompanied by hydrocephalus. The defect can occur anywhere from the head (encephalocele) to the sacrum, but most commonly affects the lumbosacral region of the spine, with talipes, paraplegia and neurological symptoms. Cerebrospinal fluid may leak from the swelling, posing the risk of meningitis. In-utero transfer to a specialist centre for delivery should be considered because postnatal surgery will be required (see website).

*Spina bifida occulta* is the most common and usually the least serious. At birth, a dimple, depression or dark tuft of hair may be seen in the lower spine region. Because the neural tube is closed, there is no neurological impairment. An ultrasound can confirm the diagnosis. Unlike spina bifida meningocele and myelomeningocele, spina bifida occulta is not registered with EUROCAT.

## Anencephaly

The vault of the skull is absent with almost no development of the exposed brain. The baby has large protruding eyes and wide shoulders, the face presents during labour and polyhydramnios is found in about 50% of cases. Second trimester screening for abnormally elevated maternal serum alpha-fetoprotein and low oestriol concentration, has been cited as highly predictive of lethal defects, particularly anencephaly (Benn et al 2000). This condition is incompatible with life and many parents may opt for termination of pregnancy. Parents who decide to continue with the pregnancy need ongoing support, especially during labour and birth.

Whether or not parents see the baby at birth is a matter for them to decide but it has been recognized that this may assist with the grieving process and helps in understanding the nature of the abnormality; also, in reality, the baby may not look as the parents imagined (see Ch. 70) The baby should be carefully wrapped before showing the infant to the parents and the midwife should establish whether the mother wishes to hold the baby rather than just look. Not all women will initially want to hold the baby but may want to do so later and this should be accommodated. If the baby is born alive, he or she will be nursed in the Special Care Baby Unit. These babies usually do not survive more than a few days.

## Hydrocephalus

An excess of cerebrospinal fluid, caused by an obstruction or overproduction, distends the ventricles of the brain. Antenatal diagnosis is usually by ultrasound scan. The head circumference of a hydrocephalic baby is at least 2 cm larger than the 90th centile for gestational age, cranial bones are soft, fontanelles large and the sutures wide. This highlights the importance of accurate measurements at birth, which should be plotted on the appropriate centile chart.

Perinatal surgery, with the insertion of a shunt to drain fluid from the lateral ventricle into the peritoneal cavity, has proved a successful palliative treatment in more severe cases.

## Microcephaly

Microcephaly is defined as a very small vault to the skull, and may be either:

- a failure of brain growth: often caused by intrauterine infections, such as rubella, cytomegalovirus or toxoplasmosis, or by severe intrauterine hypoxia
- premature ossification of the sutures, resulting in constriction and reduction in brain growth.

These babies are usually mentally impaired and there is a high association with other abnormalities.

# ABNORMALITIES OF THE RESPIRATORY SYSTEM

## Diaphragmatic hernia

This condition develops as the result of a defect in the formation of the diaphragm, usually on the left side. The bowel and abdominal viscera herniate through the diaphragm and continue to develop in the thoracic cavity. These organs compress the developing lung and can result in pulmonary hypoplasia (Jesudason et al 2000).

This abnormality may be identified by early ultrasound scanning. Prenatal counselling should prepare parents for high mortality and morbidity rates – only approximately 50% of affected babies survive. Open fetal surgery has been carried out for this condition but carries significant risk to both mother and fetus; the development of fetoscopic surgery has improved outcomes and is considered to be the way forward (Nelson et al 2006).

Postnatal surgery involves replacing the bowel, stomach and any other herniated viscera into the abdominal cavity and repairing the diaphragmatic defect. Postoperative care centres on maintaining adequate oxygenation and respiratory support while pulmonary growth occurs.

## Choanal atresia

In this condition, the posterior nasopharynx is blocked, unilaterally or bilaterally, by a membranous or bony septum, causing acute respiratory problems from birth, as neonates breathe mainly through their nose. Dyspnoea and cyanosis relieved by crying are classic symptoms, since only in this circumstance can the baby inspire adequately. Diagnosis is confirmed by being unable to pass a nasal catheter, and immediate treatment is the insertion of an oral airway. Surgical correction is necessary.

## ABNORMALITIES OF THE ALIMENTARY SYSTEM

### Cleft lip and cleft palate

Cleft lip, with or without a cleft palate, may be unilateral or bilateral and can involve the soft palate, hard palate, or both. This is one of the most common structural birth defects, with an incidence of 1 : 700 – the incidence of cleft palate alone is 1 : 2000 births. Cleft lip is usually diagnosed on ultrasound, but cleft palate may not be; the palate should always be carefully checked during the midwife's initial examination of the neonate, as a slight deformity can easily be missed.

The cause of cleft lip and/or palate remains largely unknown. The majority are believed to have a multifactorial aetiology including genetic and environmental factors. Cleft lip and palate is also associated with other syndromes, including trisomy 13 and 18 and fetal alcohol syndrome (Hodgkinson et al 2005). There is often a family history of such abnormalities, and prenatal genetic counselling should be offered in such cases.

A cleft lip can look disfiguring, but the midwife can reassure parents that these can now be repaired extremely skilfully. Feeding problems frequently occur, often related to the baby being unable to form a seal around the nipple or teat. Breastfeeding is not impossible and should be encouraged and assisted wherever possible, with referral to a lactation specialist (see Ch. 43).

In the past, because of concern about speech function, repair would be undertaken during the neonatal period; it is now recommended that lip repair takes place at 3 months and palate repair at 8 months of age (Hodgkinson 2005).

The outcome for these babies and support for parents has improved considerably since the implementation of multidisciplinary care because many of these infants may have hearing problems and/or require ongoing speech and language therapy for many years.

### Pierre Robin syndrome

A midline cleft of the soft palate, without a cleft lip, *micrognathia* (small mandible) and abnormal tongue musculature (*glossoptosis*) are the main features of this syndrome. Until the defect is repaired, the baby must be nursed in the prone position to prevent the tongue protruding through the cleft and obstructing the airway. In severe cases, a nasal airway or dental prosthesis is kept in situ until surgical repair. There is a high incidence of aspiration pneumonia and feeding difficulties, but if the baby survives the neonatal period, the prognosis is good.

### Oesophageal atresia (OA) and tracheo-oesophageal fistula (TOF)

OA affects about 1 : 4000 neonates. In this malformation there is a blind ending to the upper end of the oesophagus, usually at the level of the third or fourth vertebra (see Fig. 48.1). Ninety per cent of babies will also have an *oesophageal fistula*, where there is a connection between one or both portions of the oesophagus and the trachea. Associated anomalies are present in 50% of cases.

Polyhydramnios should always alert the midwife to the possibility of OA/TOF, as the fetus is unable to swallow amniotic fluid, leading to its accumulation. In all cases of polyhydramnios, the midwife should pass a 10-FG nasogastric tube to assess the patency of the oesophagus before oral feeds are given. OA can sometimes be detected using ultrasound, and if this is the case, the baby should be born in a specialist unit with facilities for paediatric surgery.

OA should also be suspected at birth if copious, frothy oral secretions are present. If a fistula is present, aspiration will cause cyanotic episodes. In these circumstances, the midwife will immediately refer the infant to a paediatrican.

A 10-FG nasogatric tube will be passed to assess patency of the oesophagus. The tube should not be too soft (or small) as it may curl in the back of the throat or in the blind pouch, whilst appearing to reach the stomach. An X-ray may be taken to confirm the tube has reached the stomach. Surgery involves anastomosis of the ends of the

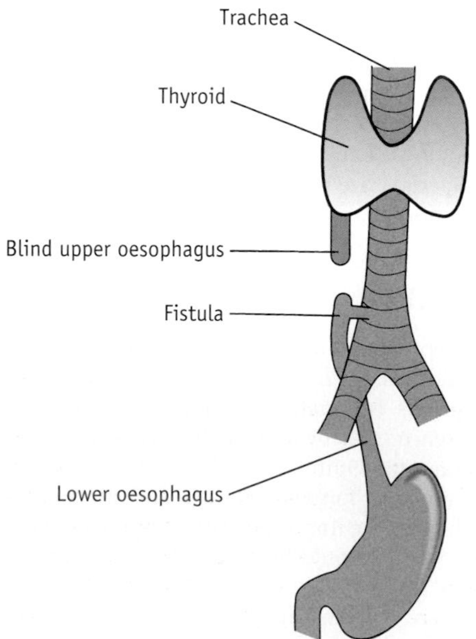


**Figure 48.1** Tracheo-oesophageal atresia with fistula.

oesophagus and division of any fistula. If the gap between the oesophageal ends is too wide, a portion of the colon or jejunum may be grafted on. Gastrostomy feeds will be necessary until repair is complete.

## Duodenal atresia

The incidence of duodenal atresia is 1 : 6000 – in one-third of cases, associated with trisomy 21. The patency of the duodenum is interrupted; projectile, bile-stained vomiting occurs within 24 hours of feeds being commenced. An abdominal X-ray shows a classic 'double bubble' appearance. Surgical correction is required.

## Imperforate anus

The incidence of imperforate anus is approximately 1–3 per 5000 births. There is a high association with other anomalies, with genitourinary abnormalities present in almost half of cases.

As part of the midwife's initial neonatal examination, the anus must be visually examined for signs of patency (see Ch. 41). No objects should be inserted, but urgent paediatric referral made if there is any doubt. It is important that the midwife notes when meconium is first passed, and referral for further investigation should be made if this does not occur within 24–36 hours. Meconium-stained liquor is not indicative of a patent anus, as a fistula may be present. In the absence of a fistula, the baby will fail to pass meconium, and will have abdominal distension and bile-stained vomiting. Surgical repair involves the formation of a temporary colostomy, which can be very distressing for parents.

## Hirschsprung's disease (aganglionosis)

This is an absence of ganglion cells in the nerve supply that controls peristalsis in the rectum and distal colon. It is an inherited disorder, involving several different genes (Martucciello et al 2000). The incidence is 1 : 5000 neonates, and four times more common in male infants.

Features include delayed passage of meconium, subsequent infrequent, offensive stools, abdominal distension and vomiting. Any baby who has not passed meconium within 24–36 hours must be referred to a paediatrician for further investigations.

A temporary colostomy may be required prior to surgery to remove the aganglionic segments of bowel. Despite apparently successful surgery, the long-term outcome may be poor for some children who can suffer severe constipation or do not gain full faecal continence until late adolescence if at all (Theocharatos & Kenny 2008). There is now greater understanding of the genetics and molecular pathology of this disease, and stem cell treatment may be used in the future, which would avoid the need for surgery and the known risk of faecal incontinence (Gershon 2007).

## Exomphalos and gastroschisis

Both anomalies occur at the end of the first trimester and involve a herniation of abdominal contents, either through the base of the umbilical cord (*exomphalos*) or through a defect in the anterior abdominal wall (*gastroschisis*). The incidence is approximately 1 per 5000–6000 neonates. There are raised maternal serum alpha-fetoprotein levels and diagnosis can be confirmed early by ultrasound scan.

*Exomphalos* has a covering of fused peritoneum and amnion, which may rupture during delivery. In up to 75% of cases there are associated chromosome or congenital abnormalities, particularly involving the alimentary tract, heart and genitourinary system.

The herniated viscera in *gastroschisis* are not protected by a covering sac and may appear oedematous or inflamed at birth. The blood supply can be disrupted to parts of the gut, resulting in necrosis, necessitating resection. If large lengths of bowel are involved, malabsorption syndrome may result. Teratogens have been implicated in its aetiology.

Babies with this condition should be delivered in a specialist centre. At birth, the defect should be covered with sterile 'cling film', or the baby's legs and abdomen placed in a special surgical plastic bag up to the armpits. The main aims are to avoid overhandling of the herniated contents, prevent infection, and reduce heat and evaporative fluid loss. Surgery will attempt to replace as much of the abdominal contents as possible, but may need to be performed in stages over subsequent months or years. Survival rates for these conditions are 90–100% in the absence of other anomalies.

# ABNORMALITIES OF THE GENITOURINARY SYSTEM

The possibility of an abnormality of the genitourinary system should be considered if only one artery is found in the umbilical cord, and the midwife must monitor the newborn to confirm that urine is passed within 24 hours of birth. If urine is not passed, or the baby is dribbling urine constantly rather than a direct stream of urine, a paediatrician should be informed immediately for further investigation.

## Posterior urethral valves (PUV)

*Anterior urethral valves* (AUV) is very rare. PUV is characterized by valves in the urethra that prevent the flow of urine from the bladder, resulting in bladder distension and back-pressure on the kidneys, leading to *hydronephrosis*. This condition is found only in male infants, occurring in 1 in 8000 births.

If undetected by antenatal ultrasound, severe renal damage may occur. Fetal surgery can alleviate the blockage, eliminating the need for elective preterm delivery. Sometimes PUV is not diagnosed until later in life.

## Hypospadias and epispadias

*Hypospadias* is a malformation in which the urethral meatus opens on the ventral surface of the penis or, in severe cases, on the perineum. The rarer condition, *epispadias*, where the meatus opens on the dorsal surface, is usually part of a *bladder exstrophy syndrome*.

Surgical correction is required in both cases, and circumcision should not be performed prior to this, as the tissue will be required for repair. The nearer the meatus is to the tip of the penis, the less severe the problem and less urgent the surgery, providing there is no urinary obstruction.

## Autosomal polycystic kidney disease (APKD)

There are two main types of *autosomal polycystic kidney disease* – recessive (ARPKD) and dominant (ADPKD).

ARPKD occurs in 1 : 20,000 live births and the fetus presents in utero with enlarged, echogenic kidneys and oligohydramnios. Approximately 30% of these neonates die following birth, from associated pulmonary hypoplasia. Survivors display a range of renal and hepatic symptoms, the severity of which dictates the course of their condition.

ADPKD is more common, occurring in 1 : 500–1000 neonates, and typically involves progressive cyst formation in many organs, particularly the kidneys and liver, and results in renal failure in late middle age.

## Renal agenesis

This is the developmental absence of one or both kidneys due to failure of the ureteral bud to develop embryologically, or regression of a dysplastic kidney. It is found in approximately 1 : 1500 antenatal ultrasound scans and if one kidney is present, is usually asymptomatic in the neonate.

There is a high association with other congenital anomalies, particularly genitourinary and musculoskeletal because they develop at the same time. Diagnosis is often incidental in the investigation of other disorders. Extra strain is placed on the solitary kidney, which commonly results in renal damage.

## Ambiguous genitalia ('disorders of sexual development')

Formerly known as *intersex disorders*, these are congenital conditions in which development of chromosomal, gonadal, or anatomical sex is atypical. Genitalia can appear ambiguous at birth; a small penis can be confused with a large clitoris, while a bifid scrotum may resemble the labia majora. True *hermaphroditism*, in which both male and female genital organs are present, is very rare. Advances in identification of molecular genetic causes of these conditions has resulted in the traditional terminology – that is, *hermaphroditism*, *pseudo-hermaphroditism* and *intersex disorders* – becoming controversial because they are confusing and can be potentially stigmatizing; the preferred term is now '*disorders of sexual development*' (Lee et al 2006).

If the genitalia are ambiguous at birth, the midwife must inform a senior paediatrician immediately. The sex of the child will usually be determined after clinical, genetic and biochemical investigations. Sometimes the sex cannot be determined, which is extremely distressing for parents. In this situation, parents should be advised to delay registering the birth until a decision is made about gender assignment (legally it is very difficult to alter a birth certificate at a later date).

Gender assignment recommendations in the newborn will depend on the diagnosis and will be based on genital appearance, surgical options, the need for lifelong replacement therapy and potential fertility. Decisions about gender assignment should also reflect family views and cultural background. Disorders of sexual development will cause parents extreme distress because it is a lifelong condition with profound pyscho-social implications at all stages of life. Specialist, multidisciplinary management is required to provide the necessary information and support, initially to parents and eventually to the child/adult (Lee et al 2006).

# ABNORMALITIES OF THE LIMBS

## Limb reduction deformities

In minor cases, these deformities are confined to one or more digits. More severe deformities may involve part or all of the limb. Teratogenic drugs taken in early pregnancy have been cited as a common cause – the best known of these being the antiemetic drug *thalidomide*. Amniotic band syndrome is another possible cause.

Some terms which may be used are:

- *amelia:* absence of one or more limbs
- *ectromelia:* absence of part of a limb
- *phocomelia:* absence of the long bones of a limb – there may be a rudimentary or well-developed hand or foot present.

## Amniotic band syndrome (ABS)

This rare condition is caused by strands of the amniotic sac separating and entangling digits, limbs, or other parts of the fetus, causing a constriction ring. The cause of the amniotic tearing is unknown and it is difficult to detect on ultrasound. The complications from ABS range from mild to severe, including syndactyly (Fig. 48.2) or amputations of fingers or toes, and clubbed feet or limb amputations (Schwarzler et al 1998).

## Chorionic villus sampling (CVS)

Early clinical trials of CVS suggested an association between CVS and a slightly increased risk for limb abnormalities (such as missing or short fingers and toes). These anomalies were only present when CVS was carried out prior to 10 weeks' gestation. The results were not considered conclusive (WHO 1992) but CVS is now only carried out after 10 weeks' gestation.

## Congenital dislocation of the hip (CDH)

In this condition, one or both hips are abnormally developed, with the head of the femur partially or wholly displaced from the acetabulum. Incidence is approximately 1:1500 births. The condition is usually of genetic origin but it may be associated with breech presentation and oligohydramnios.

*Ortolani* and *Barlow* tests assess the hips for flexion and abduction to 90 degrees, without dislocation. Eighty per cent of hips are dislocatable at birth but normalize by 2 months of age. These tests should be carried out by a practitioner trained and skilled in this examination (see Ch. 41).

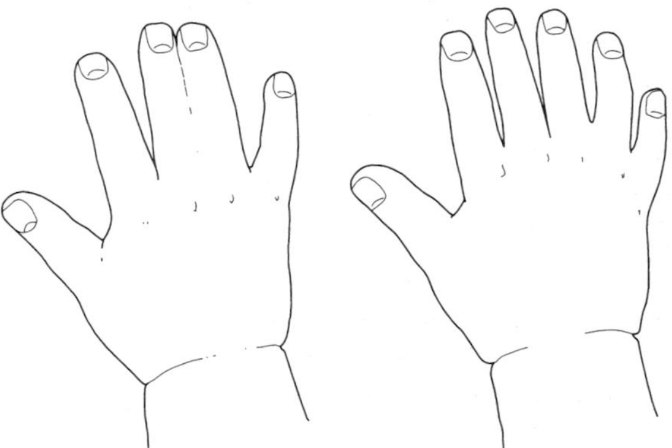

**Figure 48.2** Syndactyly (left) and polydactyly (extra digit) (right).

Early detection of CDH is essential to avoid long-term problems when the child begins to walk. Late diagnosis may necessitate 6–12 months in a hip spica, or, in the older child, long periods of traction or an open hip reduction. Ultrasound scanning of the hip joint confirms diagnosis and should routinely be performed when risk factors are present or this condition is suspected. Early orthopaedic referral is crucial, as a neonatal splint may be required.

## Achondroplasia

*Achondroplasia* (dwarfism) (Fig. 48.3) is an autosomal dominant disorder characterized by abnormal growth of cartilage and bone and occurs in approximately 1:25,000 births. The clinical features of achondroplasia are usually short stature, short limbs, and a relatively large head (*megacephaly*) which may be worsened by hydrocephalus. Neurological problems exist in 20–40% of cases, but intelligence is usually normal (Horton et al 2007).

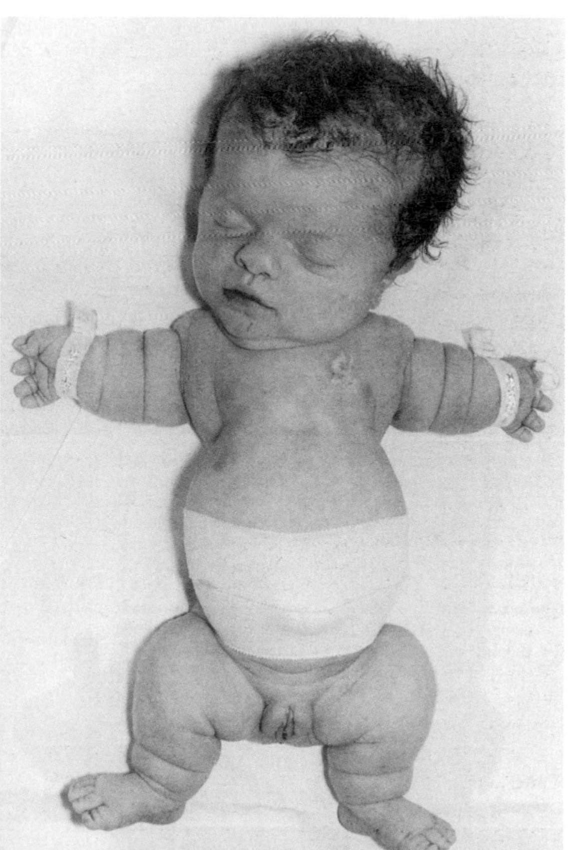

**Figure 48.3** Achondroplasia. *(From Beischer et al 1997.)*

## CHROMOSOMAL ABNORMALITIES

### Trisomy 21 (Down or Down's syndrome)

This genetic disorder results in well-recognized clinical features (see Fig. 48.4) and varying degrees of intellectual disability. The incidence of trisomy 21 is known to increase significantly with increasing maternal age and amongst very young mothers. There are three recognized forms:

1. Most commonly there is an extra chromosome 21, making 47 chromosomes in total.
2. Chromosome 21 may translocate and become attached to another chromosome pair. In these cases there are still only 46 chromosomes in total.
3. Between 1% and 2% exhibit mosaicism, where both normal and trisomic cells are present, suggesting abnormalities in the cell division processes. These individuals usually display milder intellectual disability. For further information, see website.

### Trisomy 18 (Edwards syndrome)

*Edwards syndrome* has an incidence of about 1 : 5000. It has well-recognized clinical features:

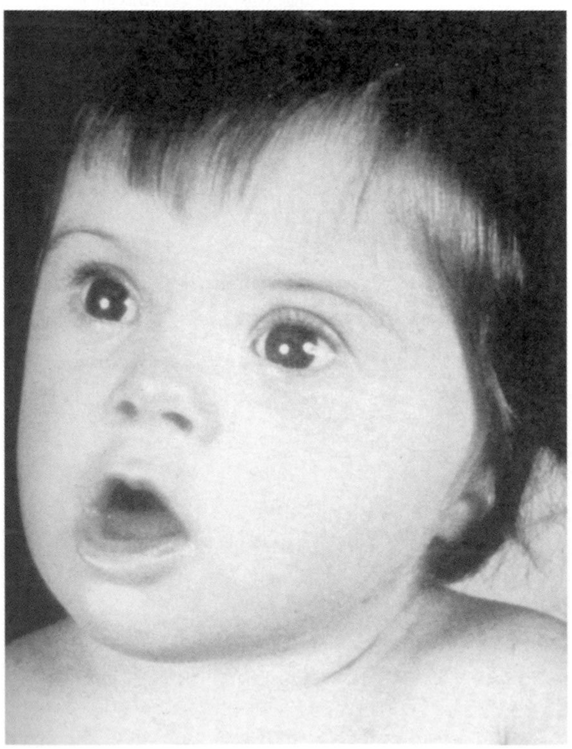

**Figure 48.4** Down syndome.

- the baby is small for gestational age
- poorly developed jaw
- often a cleft palate
- ears are malformed and low-set
- the occiput is prominent
- fingers are characteristically crossed and flexed
- prominent heels and 'rocker-bottom' feet.

Most of these children have severe congenital heart disease and gastrointestinal anomalies and die within the first year. There is often a single umbilical artery.

### Trisomy 13 (Patau syndrome)

*Patau syndrome* is relatively rare, with an incidence of about 1 : 14,000. The face is abnormal with a sloping forehead, bilateral cleft lip and/or palate, and malformed ears. Polydactyly is a common feature and the infant has prominent heels, rocker-bottom feet and a single umbilical artery. The brain is poorly developed and cardiac anomalies are common.The prognosis for these children is poor, with few living beyond 3 years.

### Potter syndrome

This condition is incompatible with sustained life. Typical features include low-set ears, furrows under the wide-set eyes, a beaked nose, and a failure to pass urine following birth owing to renal agenesis (absence of both kidneys). There are only two vessels in the umbilical cord. Associated pulmonary hypoplasia frequently manifests itself in asphyxia at birth.

### Turner syndrome

Turner syndrome – XO – only affects female infants and occurs in approximately 1 : 2500 live female births. One of the X chromosomes is missing or abnormal, manifesting itself with short stature, underdeveloped ovaries, and infertility. Many affected fetuses will spontaneously abort. Those who survive are of low birthweight, and have a webbed neck and oedema of the lower limbs. They demonstrate normal intelligence, but have a reduced life expectancy that may be related to an increased incidence of congenital heart disease, particularly coarctation of the aorta.

## ABNORMALITIES OF THE HEART AND BLOOD VESSELS

These anomalies are described fully in Chapter 45.

## FETAL SURGERY

Fetal surgery is attempted in conditions where it is considered prenatal repair or intervention will significantly reduce the mortality or morbidity of that fetus – for example, congenital diaphragmatic hernia, cystic adenomatoid malformations, and obstructive uropathy (Kumar & O'Brien 2004).

The greatest problems associated with these procedures are the high risks of precipitating preterm delivery and fetal loss (Kimber et al 1997). Open surgical procedures require a classical caesarean section and necessitate a repeat caesarean section for delivery. Open fetal surgery is relatively safe for the mother, but safety and effectiveness of the surgery for the fetus is variable and depends upon the specific procedure, gestational age and condition of the fetus. Laparoscopic techniques have been developed for many conditions and are improving fetal outcome, for example, vesico-amniotic shunt for a lower urinary tract obstruction such as posterior urethral valves (NICE 2006).

Animal experiments continue to develop techniques and technology for prenatal surgery. Long-term risks and benefits are not yet fully known for these procedures, but trials are in progress; for example, myelomeningocele reconstruction is one of the most reviewed operations and has shown some neurological benefits in survivors (NICHD 2010, Sutton et al 2001).

The physiology of wound healing in a fetus is known to be different from that in adults and results in scarless wound repair (Samuels & Tan 1999). Animal studies suggest that the advantages of this are particularly relevant in the repair of cleft lips and other disfiguring anomalies (Weinzweig et al 1999).

## NEONATAL SURGERY

Many of the major anomalies requiring surgical correction can be identified within the first or early second trimesters by ultrasound scanning. Early diagnosis enables counselling of the parents regarding the prognosis, informed choices regarding the pregnancy, and specialist perinatal care forward-planning.

To ensure optimal outcomes, in-utero transfer of the baby is recommended, if possible, to ensure that delivery takes place in a regional, specialist centre. For information about pre- and postoperative neonatal care, see website.

## NEONATAL PAIN

There has been ongoing controversy for many years over whether or not the fetus and newborn experience pain. Many of the arguments centre on what constitutes pain. Not all stimuli are painful; some may cause discomfort or a disturbance as opposed to an actual pain. Examples in the neonate would include heel pricks as painful; physical examination as a discomfort and bright lights as a disturbance. These considerations are as relevant to the midwife caring for a healthy neonate at home as to those nursing a sick infant in the neonatal intensive care unit (NICU). Babies can also manifest pain and disturbance following traumatic delivery, such as ventouse, forceps delivery or shoulder dystocia.

Since the late 1990s it has been recommended that consideration should be given to analgesia and sedation for fetuses of 24 weeks' gestation or over during fetocide and for invasive procedures, including intubation (RCOG 1997). Recent advances in neurobiology and clinical medicine have established that the fetus and newborn may experience acute, established, and chronic pain. Studies have concluded that controlling pain experience is beneficial to short-term and possibly long-term outcomes; however, despite this, pain-control measures are still used infrequently because of unresolved scientific issues (Anand et al 2006).

### Strategies for pain relief

Strategies can include:

- careful attention to the environment
- expertise at performing techniques and careful choice of equipment
- use of low noise and lighting within the NICU
- use of automated machines for heel-prick tests, as these are less painful than manual sampling
- use of interventional techniques during and following such procedures, which can be taught to parents, including:
  - comfortable positioning
  - kangaroo care
  - talking
  - gentle massage
  - cuddling
  - breastfeeding or non-nutritive sucking
  - use of sucrose (shown to be an effective analgesic agent during painful procedures (Stevens & Ohlsson 2000)
- pharmacological methods of alleviating pain – these should be considered where appropriate, and will depend on the gestation, age, weight and condition of the baby.

**Reflective activity 48.2**

What is your obstetric and neonatal unit's policy for fetal and neonatal pain awareness/relief?

## CONCLUSION

Midwives have a key role in supporting parents of a baby with a diagnosed congenital anomaly and they need to ensure that they have the necessary knowledge and skills to assist parents to reach an understanding of the short-term and long-term implications of any anomaly. In dealing with an unexpected anomaly, midwives need to draw upon their counselling and caring skills to ensure that the woman and family are provided with ongoing information and support, and that long-term services are involved at the earliest stage.

## KEY POINTS

- Midwives play a pivotal role in the provision of individualized screening, counselling and on-going support for families.
- Careful history-taking facilitates early identification of risk factors for certain anomalies.
- Antenatal identification of fetal anomalies allows preparation of the family and planned delivery in optimal conditions for specialist neonatal care.
- Fetal surgery remains experimental and investigative, but already contributes to improved mortality and morbidity rates for some serious conditions.
- Consideration should always be given to the prevention and management of pain and discomfort of neonates during examinations or procedures.

## REFERENCES


Anand KJ, Aranda JV, Berde CB, et al: Summary proceedings from the neonatal pain-control group, *Paediatrics* 11(3 part 2):S9–S22, 2006.

Beischer N, Mackay E, Colditz P: *Obstetrics and the Newborn*, London, 1997, WB Saunders.

Benn PA, Craffey A, Horne D, et al: Elevated maternal serum alpha-fetoprotein with low unconjugated estriol and the risk for lethal perinatal outcome, *Journal of Maternal-Fetal Medicine* 9(3):165–169, 2000.

Botto LD, Lynberg MC, Erickson JD: Congenital heart defects, maternal febrile illness and multivitamin use: a population-based study, *Epidemiology* 12(5):485–490, 2001.

Boyd PA, Armstrong B, Dolk H, et al: Congenital anomaly surveillance in England - ascertainment deficiencies in the national system, *British Medical Journal* 330(7481):27, 2005.

Dolk H: EUROCAT: 25 years of European surveillance of congenital anomalies, *Archives of Disease in Childhood. Fetal and Neonatal Edition* 90:F355–F358, 2005.

European Surveillance of Congenital Anomalies (EUROCAT): *Instructions for the Registration and Surveillance of Congenital Anomalies* (second revision), Northern Ireland, 2009, Eurocat Central Registry.

Farrell T, Neale L, Cundy T: Congenital anomalies in the offspring of women with type 1, type 2 and gestational diabetes, *Diabetic Medicine* 19(4):322–326, 2002.

Gershon MD: Transplanting the enteric nervous system: a step closer to treatment for aganglionosis, *Gut* 56(4):459–461, 2007.

Hodgkinson DG, Brown S, Duncan D, et al: Management of children with cleft lip and palate: a review describing the application of multidisciplinary team working in this condition based upon the experiences of a regional cleft lip and palate centre in the United Kingdom, *Fetal and Maternal Medicine Review* 16(1):1–27, 2005.

Horton WA, Hall JG, Hecht JT: Achondroplasia, *Lancet* 370(9582):162–172, 2007.

Jesudason EC, Connell MG, Fernig DG, et al: Early lung malformation in congenital diaphragmatic hernia, *Journal of Pediatric Surgery* 35(1):124–127, 2000.

Kimber C, Spitz L, Cuschierei A: Current state of antenatal in-utero surgical interventions, *Archives of Disease in Childhood* 76(2):F134–F139, 1997.

Kumar S, O'Brien A: Recent developments in fetal medicine, *British Medical Journal* 328(7446):1002–1006, 2004.

Lee PA, Houk CP, Ahmed SF, et al: Consensus statement on management of intersex disorders, *Paediatrics* 118(2):488–500, 2006.

Martucciello G, Ceccherini I, Lerone M, et al: Pathogenesis of Hirschsprung's disease, *Journal of Pediatric Surgery* 35(7):1017–1025, 2000.

Misra T, Dattani N, Majeed A: Congenital anomaly surveillance in England and Wales, *Public Health March* 120(3):256–264, 2006.

National Institute for Clinical Excellence (NICE): *Fetal vesico-amniotic shunt for lower urinary tract outflow obstruction: guidance*, 13 December 2006 (website). http://www.nice.org.uk/guidance/IPG202. Accessed Nov 2010.

National Institute for Clinical Excellence (NICE): *Antenatal care: routine care for the healthy pregnant woman*, London, 2008, NICE London.

National Institute of Child Health and Human Development (NICHD): *Management of Myelomeningocele Study (MOMS)* (website). www.spinabifidamoms.com. 2010.

Nelson SM, Cameron AD, Deprest JA: Fetoscopic surgery for in-utero management of congenital diaphragmatic hernia, *Fetal and Maternal Medicine Review* 17(1):69–104, 2006.

Office for National Statistics (ONS): *Congenital anomaly statistics England and Wales* (Series MB3) No. 23 2008, London, 2010, Office of Public Sector Information.

Royal College of Obstetricians and Gynaecologists (RCOG): *Fetal awareness. Working Party report,* London, 1997, RCOG Press.

Samuels P, Tan AK: Fetal scarless wound healing, *Journal of Otolaryngology* 28(5):296–302, 1999.

Schwarzler P, Moscoso G, Senat M-V, et al: The cobweb syndrome: first trimester sonographic diagnosis of multiple amniotic bands confirmed by fetoscopy and pathological examination, *Human Reproduction* 13(10):2966–2969, 1998.

Stevens B, Ohlsson A: Sucrose for analgesia in newborn infants undergoing painful procedures, *Cochrane Database of Systematic Reviews* (2): CD001069. Oxford, 2000, Update Software.

Sutton LN, Sun P, Adzick NS: Fetal neurosurgery, *Neurosurgery* 48(1):124–144, 2001.

Theocharatos S, Kenny SE: Hirschsprung's disease: current management and prospects for transplantation of enteric nervous system progenitor cells, *Early Human Development* 84(12):801–804, 2008.

UK National Screening Committee (UKNSC): *Consent standards for screening fetal anomalies during pregnancy: national fetal anomaly screening programmes for England NHS*, London, 2007, UKNSC.

Weinzweig J, Panter KE, Pantaloni M, et al: The fetal cleft palate: II. Scarless healing after in-utero repair of a congenital model, *Plastic and Reconstructive Surgery* 104(5):1356–1364, 1999.

World Health Organization (WHO): Chorionic villus sampling (CVS): World Health Organization European Regional Office (WHO/EURO) meeting statement on the use of CVS in prenatal diagnosis, *Journal of Assisted Reproduction and Genetics* 9(4):299–302, 1992.

Chapter 49

# Metabolic and endocrine disorders

*Carol Bates*

## LEARNING OUTCOMES

At the end of this chapter, you will have:

- developed your knowledge of newborn metabolic physiology
- an awareness of physiological metabolic disturbance and the difference between acquired and inborn metabolic disorders
- an understanding of inherited conditions, their recognition and treatment and relevance to antenatal care and screening.

## NEWBORN METABOLISM

The transition from intrauterine to extrauterine life is a complex physiological process and includes many alterations in metabolic processes. Metabolic transition to extrauterine life is characterized by a shift from anabolic to catabolic metabolism. During pregnancy, anabolic metabolism synthesizes complex molecules from simpler ones to enable *storage* of energy, whereas catabolic metabolism breaks down complex molecules into simpler ones for the *release* of energy. This is a significant shift requiring the newborn infant to begin independent provision of energy for maintenance and growth (Blackburn 2007).

During the first week of life, there is a physiological weight loss and the normal infant can lose up to 10% of its birthweight; this can lead to an electrolyte imbalance causing transient metabolic disturbances which may or may not require treatment and vigilant observation is required by the midwife. For physiology, assessment and midwifery care of the newborn see Chapter 41. For more information on metabolic and endocrine disorders see website.

Metabolic transition is influenced by genetic, environmental and endocrine factors and whilst the majority of healthy term infants successfully manage the complex adaptation to extrauterine life some infants acquire metabolic disorders and some may have inborn errors of metabolism and endocrine and exocrine disorders. There are many such conditions but this chapter will focus upon those that manifest in the first week of life and those that are subject to postnatal screening using the Guthrie test.

## ACQUIRED METABOLIC DISORDERS

Acquired metabolic disorders can occur in both term and preterm infants but are more common in preterm, growth-restricted and sick newborn infants. The most common metabolic disorder in the newborn is *hypoglycaemia* (low blood sugar levels). *Glucose homeostasis* (metabolic equilibrium) is maintained in utero by a continuous supply of maternal glucose via the placenta; from birth, newborn blood glucose levels are reliant upon already stored glycogen and fat until feeding is established.

Glucose and lactate are major carbohydrates which, along with amino acids, serve as substrates (molecules on which an enzyme acts) for metabolism and growth. In normal circumstances, endocrine changes will enable the healthy neonate to do this by breaking down already stored glycogen and glucose produced by the liver. Other sources of metabolic fuel are fatty acids released from adipose tissue and ketone bodies.

The majority of cases of hypoglycaemia are transient, occurring prior to the onset of regular feeding. Healthy term infants may have low glucose levels of 1–1.5 mmol/L but they cope with this by using alternative fuels, such as ketone bodies, lactate or fatty acids (Newell & Darling 2008).

Breastfeeding infants are particularly likely to have low blood sugar levels before feeding becomes established, but they have higher ketone body concentrations to use as an alternative metabolic fuel and therefore are unlikely to suffer any ill effects (Hawdon et al 1992, Newell & Darling 2008). An awareness of physiological hypoglycaemia is essential to ensure that infants are not unnecessarily investigated or treated unless there are other clinical indications for intervention.

Neonates with a high risk of hypoglycaemia, likely to require treatment, are preterm and growth-restricted infants (in whom there is a lack of glycogen stores), infants of diabetic mothers (where there has been excessive insulin production), sick newborn infants with a poor supply of energy, and infants with sepsis, hypothermia or following perinatal asphyxia.

## Hypoglycaemia

There has been much debate over what constitutes a normal plasma glucose value for infants of different gestation and birthweight and, therefore, what constitutes a finite biochemical definition of hypoglycaemia (Cornblath et al 2000). A generally accepted definition of hypoglycaemia since the late 1980s that continues to be used in clinical practice is a blood glucose level of <2.6 mmol/L (Koh et al 1988).

Non-specific signs of hypoglycaemia in the newborn can be vague; they include lethargy, poor feeding and a degree of jitteriness. These signs can also be due to sepsis and sometimes a healthy term infant can be sleepy and reluctant to feed. If these non-specific signs persist or worsen, the midwife should seek immediate paediatric advice and anticipate investigations for sepsis and hypoglycaemia. Specific signs of hypoglycaemia comprise increasing lethargy and irritability with a reduction in level of consciousness and eventually seizures, which are associated with the risk of cerebral damage (Newell & Darling 2008).

If a low serum glucose is confirmed using a reagent strip, then the diagnosis is definitely symptomatic hypoglycaemia and treatment is required as a matter of urgency to avoid permanent cerebral damage. The midwife should be aware that reagent strips such as BM stix can be unreliable when blood sugar readings are very low and a blood sample is needed to obtain a true (plasma) blood glucose level.

**Reflective activity 49.1**

Locate and review your local guidelines for the definition and management of hypoglycaemia in term and preterm infants – are these up to date and based on research and evidence?

## Hypocalcaemia

Hypocalcaemia is a blood calcium level less than 1.7 mmol/L (normal serum concentration is 2.2–2.7 mmol/L). There is a physiological fall in calcium levels during the first 24 hours of life, after which it rises and becomes stable in response to an increase in parathyroid hormone concentration. If this does not occur, treatment is required.

Hypocalcaemia is most likely to arise in preterm infants, infants of diabetic mothers and following birth asphyxia. It can also be caused by renal failure and hypoparathyroidism. It may cause apnoea, jitteriness or seizures. Seizures due to hypocalcaemia, unlike those due to hypoglycaemia, have a good prognosis because they are not associated with long-term brain damage (Newell & Darling 2008). Severe symptoms will be treated with intravenous calcium. Long-term treatment will depend upon the cause.

## Hyponatraemia

Hyponatraemia is a serum sodium level of less than 130 mmol/L. It is caused by either fluid overload or sodium depletion and is more common in preterm infants. It can be caused by the administration of intravenous fluids. Treatment consists of simultaneously limiting fluid intake and maintaining normal sodium intake with appropriate intravenous fluids. Chronic hyponatraemia is associated with poor neurodevelopmental outcome (Al-Dahhan et al 2002).

## Hypernatraemia

Hypernatraemia is a plasma sodium level above 143 mmol/L. This is a rare condition caused by water depletion and the loss of extracellular fluid. It can be caused by excessive intake of sodium in intravenous fluids. There is also a risk of sodium excess if parents use incorrect technique and quantities when reconstituting formula milk powder. To prevent this, the midwife should ensure parents know how to make up formula feeds correctly (see Ch. 43).

There is also a risk of hypernatraemia if breastfeeding does not establish effectively (Oddie et al 2001). This is very rare and is prevented by adequate midwifery support and supervision of breastfeeding women throughout the postnatal period.

Early signs of hypernatraemia are an increasingly fretful, thirsty baby; if left untreated, the baby will become dehydrated and pyrexial. If the mother is breastfeeding, the midwife should consider the possibility of hypernatraemia if the infant appears lethargic, is jaundiced and continues to lose rather than regain lost birthweight by the end of the first week of life.

Severe dehydration is a potentially dangerous condition which, if untreated, can lead to seizures and irreversible neurological damage. Treatment is controlled rehydration in hospital over 24–48 hours and, if a breastfed infant, assistance is given to the mother to establish breastfeeding effectively (Newell & Darling 2008).

## INBORN ERRORS OF METABOLISM

Inborn errors of metabolism are rare inherited disorders occurring in approximately 1 in 5000 births. They result primarily from enzyme deficiencies in metabolic pathways leading to an accumulation of substrate and resulting in toxicity. The error is not apparent until after birth because the placenta removes the toxic substrate during pregnancy. Inborn errors of metabolism are more common when parents are consanguineous – that is, are blood relations, such as first cousins – and accurate family history taking during the antenatal 'booking' visit is essential.

### Phenylketonuria

Phenylketonuria (PKU) occurs in about 1 : 10,000–20,000 births (Newell & Darling 2008). There is a deficiency of the enzyme *phenylalanine hydroxylase*, which converts the amino acid phenylalanine into tyrosine; once milk feeds are established, this deficiency causes a build-up of phenylpyruvic acid, which is toxic to the neonatal brain and causes irreversible neurological damage. PKU is detected using the *Guthrie test*; disability is prevented by a lifelong phenylalanine-restricted diet. This has led to excellent outcomes for children with PKU.

Pregnant women with PKU should ensure they keep to their phenylalanine-restricted diet because high phenylalanine levels cross the placenta and may lead to fetal brain damage (Newell & Darling 2008).

### Galactosaemia

Galactosaemia is a disorder of carbohydrate metabolism and occurs in about 1 : 60,000 babies. A deficiency of the enzyme *galactose-1-phosphate uridyltransferase* leads to accumulation of galactose.

Affected babies become ill almost as soon as they begin to drink milk. The clinical signs and symptoms of this disorder include vomiting, hypotonia, hypoglycaemia and jaundice. Treatment is a lactose-free diet as soon as the diagnosis is suspected.

### Glucose-6-phosphate dehydrogenase (G6PD) deficiency

G6PD deficiency is an X-linked recessive disorder (see Ch. 26) prevalent throughout tropical and subtropical regions of the world. In the UK, it is found in families of Mediterranean, African or Chinese origin, and midwives should consider ethnic origin when advising families about screening programmes.

G6PD is an enzyme necessary to maintain the integrity of the cell membrane of red blood cells. If there is a deficiency, haemolysis occurs, causing jaundice and anaemia. Common triggers for this disorder include infection, exposure to napthalane vapour (for example, moth balls) and ingestion of fava (broad) beans. G6PD deficiency manifests as jaundice that begins on the second or third day and usually subsides by the end of the first week of life. Symptoms are alleviated with phototherapy, blood transfusion, and prophylactic antioxidants such as vitamin E.

### Medium-chain acyl-CoA dehydrogenase deficiency (MCADD)

MCADD is an autosomal recessive inborn error of metabolism that occurs in 1 in 10,000–20,000 infants. It is an enzyme deficiency that prevents fatty acid oxidation, causing a build-up of medium-chain fats and toxic substances that are produced, resulting in a potentially lethal hypoglycaemia, acidosis and eventually collapse of the infant. There is a 25% mortality rate. MCADD can manifest very suddenly; emergency treatment is intravenous dextrose and glucose polymer drinks (Newell & Darling 2008).

Once diagnosis is confirmed, preventative treatment is avoidance of a metabolic crisis by ensuring the infant does not go without feeding for longer than 6 hours. In England, all infants are screened for MCADD and UK-wide screening should be in place by 2011.

## ENDOCRINE DISORDERS

Endocrine (ductless gland) disorders are relatively rare and can be serious but they are usually treatable.

### Congenital adrenal hyperplasia

Congenital adrenal hyperplasia (CAH) is due to deficiency of the enzymes responsible for hormone production in the adrenal glands. It is the commonest cause of genital ambiguity in neonates. The midwife must always carefully examine the genitalia at birth, and if the genitalia are ambiguous (Fig. 49.1), must immediately refer the baby to a senior paediatrician because chromosomal analysis will be required to determine the genetic sex, and there may be severe psychological repercussions for the baby and family should the situation not be sensitively managed.

### Thyroid disease

Normal thyroid function is necessary for healthy physical and mental growth. Congenital hypothyroidism affects approximately 1 in 4000 infants – 1 in 10 cases are

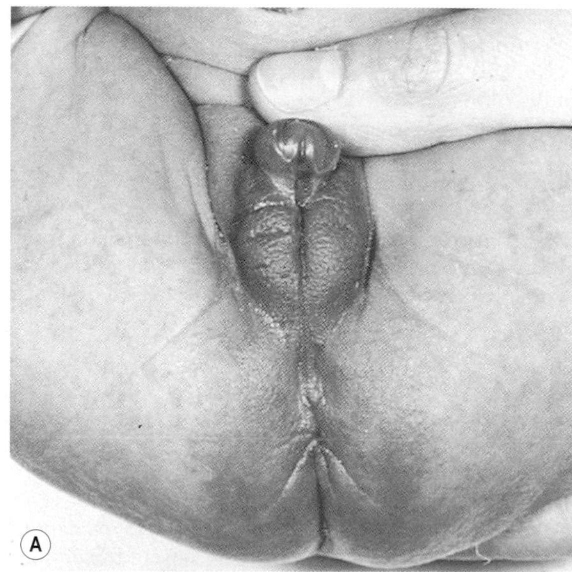

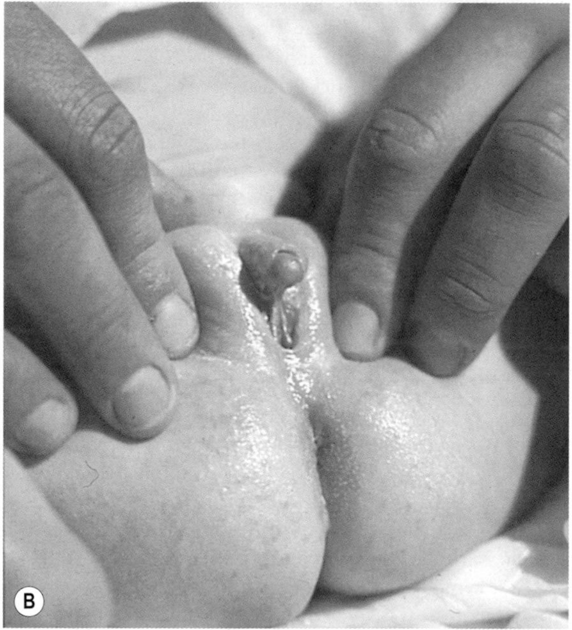

**Figure 49.1** Ambiguous genitalia. **A.** In an infant with congenital adrenal hyperplasia. **B.** In a baby with androgen insensitivity. *(From Johnston et al 2003)*

inherited. It is usually due to the absence of the thyroid gland or to metabolic problems in the gland preventing production of thyroid hormone. Untreated infants develop serious, permanent physical and mental disability. Screening for congenital hypothyroidism using the Guthrie test measures the level of thyroid-stimulating hormone (TSH), which is found to be raised. Disability is prevented by lifelong hormone replacement therapy with oral thyroxine.

## CYSTIC FIBROSIS

Cystic fibrosis (CF) is an autosomal recessive disorder caused by mutations of the *CFTR* gene on chromosome 7; it affects 1 in 2500 children in the UK and 1 in 25 of the population are asymptomatic carriers (Newell & Darling 2008).

CF affects the *exocrine* (ducted) glands. It causes production of excess secretions with abnormal electrolyte concentrations, resulting in obstruction of the ducts. This affects the pancreas, sweat glands, respiratory, intestinal and reproductive tracts. Pre-conception and antenatal testing is available for parents.

Undiagnosed CF can present in the newborn infant with a meconium ileus caused by viscid mucus making meconium so glutinous that normal peristalsis cannot move it through the bowel. In this situation, small amounts of meconium are passed but the abdomen becomes distended and vomiting develops over 24–48 hours. This highlights the need for vigilant observation of the newborn by the midwife. Meconium ileus requires urgent paediatric referrral to relieve the obstruction. Any infant who develops a meconium ileus should be tested for CF (Newell & Darling 2008).

Since 2007, CF screening of all babies has taken place in England. Guthrie samples are screened for *immunoreactive trypsinogen* levels, which are elevated in babies with CF. A sweat test to measure salt content is then carried out to confirm the diagnosis.

Treatment includes the use of synthetic proteins to break down mucus and onging physiotherapy. Heart–lung transplantations have also been carried out (Aurora et al 1999). The hope for the future is gene therapy to replace the faulty gene (Newell & Darling 2008).

## POSTNATAL SCREENING

Postnatal mass screening of neonates using the Guthrie test was introduced in 1969; intially to screen for phenylketonuria. It is now used to screen for several conditions throughout the UK, but financial, political and demographic factors will influence the range of conditions screened for in different regions. All four countries in the UK screen for phenylketonuria and congenital hypothyroidism; in England, screening also includes sickle cell disorders, cystic fibrosis and MCADD.

**Reflective activity 49.2**

Find out what disorders are routinely screened for from Guthrie cards in your area.

The Guthrie blood spots can also be used to test for other metabolic and endocrine disorders, including G6PD deficiency and congenital adrenal hyperplasia. DNA extraction from the blood spots also enables identification of Duchenne muscular dystrophy (Clague & Thomas 2002, Matern 2002).

Midwives should become familiar with the Guthrie test screening programme in their local area to enable them to give parents accurate information. Guidelines for newborn blood spot sampling (NHS National Screening Committee 2008) are available on the National Screening Committee website (www.newbornbloodspot.screening.nhs.uk). This gives information about obtaining informed consent and what to do if parents decline screening. The technique for the heel prick is clearly described and demonstrated and comfort measures are given for babies to alleviate any distress during the procedure. It recommends that the heel prick takes place on the fifth postpartum day.

In undertaking the Guthrie test, the midwife should also be alert to the possibility of conditions such as haemorrhagic disease which may be detected after the test. After taking the blood sample it is normal practice to apply pressure to the puncture wound on the heel. Prolonged bleeding should alert the midwife to potential problems. It is also useful to be aware that the use of sticking plaster should be restricted, because in removing the plaster, the first layer of epidermis may also be removed.

The Guthrie test has been a very successful mass neonatal screening programme enabling early diagnosis and treatment of metabolic disorders and conditions that untreated would result in physical and mental disability. Whilst early diagnosis of conditions such as cystic fibrosis cannot prevent the progression of the condition, it avoids delay in diagnosis and early treatment greatly improves general health and quality of life; consequently, children with the condition are living increasingly longer lives.

**Reflective activity 49.3**

List the range of conditions, including when and how screening takes place. Compile a package of information, including relevant leaflets, so that you are familiar with the information given to women and their families.

## KEY POINTS

- The transition to extrauterine life and resulting changes in neonatal metabolism can cause physiological metabolic disturbance.
- Metabolic disorders can be acquired or inherited.
- It is now possible to screen for a wide variety of neonatal metabolic conditions from Guthrie blood spots.
- Whilst most conditions are relatively rare, early diagnosis and treatment has a tremendous impact on their outcome.
- Midwives have a key role in the identification of many metabolic conditions and should be knowledgeable about their recognition, management and sequelae to effectively support and inform parents.

## REFERENCES


Al-Dahhan J, Jannoun L, Haycock GB: Effects of salt supplementation of newborn premature infants on neurodevelopmental outcome at 10–13 years of age, *Archives of Disease in Childhood. Fetal and Neonatal Edition* 86(2):F120–F123, 2002.

Aurora P, Whitehead B, Wade A, et al: Lung transplantation and life extension in children with cystic fibrosis, *The Lancet* 354(9190):1591–1593, 1999.

Blackburn ST: *Maternal fetal and neonatal physiology: a clinical perspective*, ed 3, Philadelphia, 2007, WB Saunders.

Clague A, Thomas A: Neonatal biochemical screening for disease, *Clinica Chimica Acta* 315(1–2):99–110, 2002.

Cornblath M, Hawdon JM, Williams AF, et al: Controversies regarding the definition of neonatal hypoglycaemia: suggested operational thresholds, *Pediatrics* 105(5):1141–1145, 2000.

Hawdon JM, Ward-Platt MP, Aynsley-Green A: Patterns of metabolic adaptation for preterm and term infants in the first neonatal week, *Archives of Disease in Childhood* 67(4):357–365, 1992.

Johnston PGB, Flood K, Spinks K: *The newborn child*, ed 9, London, 2003, Churchill Livingstone.

Koh THHG, Eyre JA, Ainsley-Green A: Neonatal hypoglycaemia – the controversy regarding definition, *Archives of Disease in Childhood* 63(11):1386–1388, 1988.

Matern D: Tandem mass spectrometry in newborn screening, *Endocrinology* 12(1):50–57, 2002.

Newell SJ, Darling JC: *Lecture notes. Paediatrics*, ed 8, Oxford, 2008, Blackwell.

NHS National Screening Committee: *Guidelines for newborn blood spot sampling*, London, 2008, NHS National Screening Committee.

Oddie S, Richmond S, Couthard M: Hypernatraemic dehydration and breastfeeding: a population study, *Archives of Disease in Childhood* 85(4):318–320, 2001.

Chapter |50|

# Sudden infant death syndrome

*Gail Johnson*

## LEARNING OUTCOMES

After reading this chapter, you will:

- have an understanding of the multifactorial nature of SIDS
- appreciate the risk factors associated with SIDS
- be able to advise parents on modifiable behaviours to reduce risk.

## INTRODUCTION

This chapter aims to provide an increased awareness and understanding of *sudden infant death syndrome* (SIDS) and to consider the risk factors associated with SIDS, to advise professionals and parents on minimizing risk and to enable parents to be better informed.

Sudden infant death syndrome is defined as the sudden unexpected death of a previously apparently healthy infant within the first year of life. The cause of death is frequently referred to as unexplained or unascertainable following a thorough postmortem examination. All unexpected deaths in infancy are subject to an autopsy, and where a previously undiagnosed underlying problem is found, these cases are no longer reported as SIDS (Foundation for the Study of Infant Deaths [FSID] 2009).

This chapter will address the variable terminology related to SIDS, its incidence, associated risk factors and measures to reduce the incidence, alongside national and international campaigns. In addition, the role of the midwife, health professionals and others will be considered.

## TERMINOLOGY

Sudden infant death syndrome is sometimes referred to as *sudden unexplained death in infancy* or *cot death*. Cot death is a term frequently used by parents and the media as it reflects the fact that the death usually occurs during sleep. The term sudden infant death syndrome was brought into common usage in the late 1960s to help bereaved parents and others to ascertain that the death was as a result of an unexplained or unintentional incident; to demonstrate that the parents were not considered to be blamed for the death (Gornall 2008). A diagnosis of SIDS is reached when causes of death are excluded following postmortem examination.

## INCIDENCE

The launch of the FSID 'Back to Sleep' campaign in 1991 saw a significant reduction in the number of SIDS cases reported (Fleming et al 2006, FSID 2007, Moon et al 2007). Sudden infant death syndrome was already in decline from 1989; nonetheless, the most significant reduction in the rate was in 1992, demonstrating the success of the 'Reduce the risk' campaign which encouraged parents and carers to lie babies on their back when going to sleep (FSID 2007). However, there are variations within the rates both within the UK and globally. Moon et al (2007) highlight that SIDS is the leading cause of infant mortality in the developed world. Japan and the Netherlands have the lowest rates at 0.09 and 0.1 per 1000 live births, respectively, and New Zealand has the highest rate at 0.8 per 1000 live births. Following the 'Back to Sleep' campaign, data collected and analysed for 2005 identified a decline in SIDS incidents in the UK, with a rate of 0.42 per 1000 live births (FSID 2009). There are variations in the figures across the UK, which may be due to a lack of uniformity in data collection. Whilst the figures continue to demonstrate a decline in SIDS across the UK, an estimated 300 babies a year will die.

Sudden infant death occurs most commonly within the first 4 to 8 weeks of life, and boys are more likely to die than girls, at a ratio of 60:40 (Moon et al 2007); previous data collection in the UK had put the peak of SIDS at 3 months (CEMACH 2008).

SIDS is multifactorial and a number of recommendations are made to advise parents and health professionals of the associated risk factors, to enable interventions to bring about continued decline in the rates.

## RISK FACTORS

A number of factors associated with maternal and infant health or activities have been identified as increasing the risk of SIDS.

The Department of Health, in collaboration with FSID, produced a guide on reducing the risk of 'cot death' (DH 2007a, 2009), which makes seven recommendations to reduce the risk of SIDS:

- Place your baby on the back to sleep, in a cot in a room with you.
- Cut smoking in pregnancy – fathers too!
- Do not let anyone smoke in the same room as your baby.
- Do not let your baby get too hot.
- Keep your baby's head uncovered – place your baby in the 'feet to foot position'.
- Do not share a bed with your baby if you have been drinking alcohol, take drugs or if you are a smoker.
- If your baby is unwell, seek prompt advice.

Social and health inequalities place disadvantaged families at increased risk. Poor access to healthcare and education may mean that parents are not able to seek out the appropriate advice or support. Families from black and ethnic minority groups continue to demonstrate poorer health outcomes (Bamfield 2007).

Whilst the aetiology of SIDS is not fully understood, modifying a number of behaviours is likely to reduce the incidence. The midwife and health professionals have a significant role in raising awareness of SIDS and the risk factors with parents, grandparents and carers, and supporting them to modify behaviours.

### Sleeping positions

Lying babies on their backs to sleep appears to have brought about the most significant reduction in SIDS since the 1990s. The change in sleeping positions initially caused some concern for parents and professionals as there was considered to be an increased risk of aspiration in babies lying supine. Soft bedding surfaces and blankets may make it difficult for the baby lying prone to move his head, which could be a contributory factor in cot death. Babies sleeping on their side have an increased risk of SIDS compared to babies lying in the supine position; the increased risk can be attributed in part to babies being able to roll into a prone position. Some studies have identified that gestation, age and low birthweight can lead to an increased risk for babies lying on their side (Blair et al 2006, Oyen et al 1997); however, prematurity and low birthweight are known risk factors for poorer health outcomes, making specific links or causal factors to SIDS difficult to identify. Babies nursed in special care or neonatal intensive care units are frequently laid in the prone position as it may assist the preterm or ill baby with respiration; parents observing this practice are likely to need particular advice and guidance on nursing their baby in a supine position (Esposito et al 2007).

### Sleep practices and environment

Newborn babies are less able to regulate their body temperature, and overheating has been associated with SIDS (Blair et al 2008); over-wrapping, warm centrally heated rooms and blankets can contribute to the baby becoming too hot. In addition, babies who are lying in the prone position will be less able to lose heat through their faces. Guidance from FSID and the Department of Health advises that the baby's head should not be covered by too many blankets or a hat, to prevent the baby becoming too hot. The guidance also recommends that the baby is laid with the feet at the bottom of the cot or pram, 'feet to foot' position, to prevent the baby wriggling down under the blankets (DH 2007a, 2009).

There is some evidence that indicates that where babies sleep in the same room as their parents for the first 6 months, the incidence of SIDS is reduced. This is possibly because the parents are responsive to subtle changes in the baby's breathing patterns and may react to the baby's needs more quickly (Blair et al 1999). However, *bed sharing* remains a risk factor for SIDS: there has been a rise in the number of deaths where co-sleeping was reported, with a significant increase in co-sleeping on the sofa (Fleming et al 2006, Gornall 2008, Moon et al 2007). Advice needs to reflect that the risks are increased if the parents smoke, or have taken alcohol or drugs which can cause drowsiness (James et al 2003). Extreme tiredness is an additional risk factor, one that most parents of a young baby will experience. A national audit carried out in 2003–2004 (RCM 2005) identified that women and families need clear information regarding co-sleeping, and recommended the development of multidisciplinary and evidence-based approaches to training and information for parents.

**Reflective activity 50.1**

Visit the FSID website and look at the advice and guidance for professionals and parents.

Watch the video clip 'Safe sleep for babies': www.fsid.org.uk/safe-sleep-video.html.

## Smoking

Smoking in pregnancy is known to increase the risk of preterm birth and low-birthweight babies, two factors that are associated with an increased incidence of SIDS. A number of studies reviewed by FSID suggest that the risks of SIDS and smoking in pregnancy cannot simply be attributed to prematurity and low birthweight; smoking remains a contributory factor when other confounding variables – for example, maternal age, parity, marital status and breastfeeding – are considered (FSID 2007, Moon et al 2007; Shah et al 2006). Whilst some of the evidence reviewed was undertaken in the 1990s, the conclusions were similar and suggested that the more cigarettes smoked in pregnancy the higher the risk of SIDS. The evidence highlights the benefits of encouraging women to reduce the number of cigarettes smoked in pregnancy if they are unable to stop completely.

Smoking near or in the same room as a baby continues to pose a risk of cot death – a baby who regularly spends an hour a day in a smoky environment is twice as likely to die from SIDS as a baby in a smoke-free environment. The advice not to smoke in pregnancy and around the baby applies to both the mother and father. A poll undertaken by FSID highlighted that seven in ten parents were unaware of the risk of smoking in the home and the link with cot death, despite numerous campaigns and health warnings about the risks of smoking (FSID 2008).

## Breastfeeding

Evidence indicates that breastfeeding is an important contributory factor in reducing the risk of SIDS (Fleming et al 2006, FSID 2007). The health benefits of breastfeeding are well reported and the link with a reduced risk of SIDS could be attributed to the IgA antibodies found in breast milk, which fight off bacterial toxins (Gordon et al 1999). Discouraging bed sharing may have a detrimental effect on the duration of breastfeeding. A UNICEF statement on mother–infant bed sharing advises that parents need to understand the benefits of promoting breastfeeding and that the risks of bed sharing are increased when the mother smokes (UNICEF 2005). There is some evidence that the use of dummies or pacifiers can reduce the incidence of SIDS (Mitchell et al 2006); however, the adverse effect of dummies on the duration of breastfeeding and increased risk of respiratory and gastrointestinal infections indicate that further studies need to be undertaken (Fleming et al 2000, Wickham 2006).

# THE MIDWIFE'S ROLE

Antenatal care will help to improve the wellbeing of the mother, fetus and baby through identification of risk factors, advising on modifying behaviours and seeking medical intervention where appropriate. This role will help to reduce some of the possible associated risk factors for SIDS. The midwife is in an ideal position to advise parents and the wider family on general health and raise awareness of SIDS. The midwife will also work in collaboration with general practitioners, health visitors and other practitioners to advise parents on modifying behaviours, for example, smoking cessation (DH 2007b).

**Reflective actvity 50.2**

What advice and information on SIDS or cot death is available locally to parents?

Are the risk factors associated with SIDS discussed with parents in the antenatal and postnatal period?

# AFTERMATH OF SIDS

Every unexpected death is subjected to scrutiny by the coroner, and the police are required to interview the family and may take samples of clothing and bedding away as part of the in-depth review. On top of the devastating death of a child, the parents' distress is likely to be exacerbated by the intense investigations. The investigation needs to be undertaken sensitively; the parents are likely to have many questions about the death of their baby and it is important that they are advised of any findings from the investigation.

# FUTURE PREGNANCIES

Families who have experienced the death of a baby will understandably be concerned about the health of future babies, particularly if the cause of death is not ascertained.

FSID has set up a programme of support for these families, called 'Care of Next Infant' (CONI). This uses the skills and support of the paediatrician, obstetrician, family doctor, midwife, health visitor and a local CONI coordinator. The family determines the level of support and it can include home visits to assess wellbeing and provide practical advice on room temperature and signs of ill health.

**Reflective activity 50.3**

Contact the local CONI coordinator and the midwife who is on the team to discuss their role in supporting parents.

## CONCLUSION

The death of a baby is devastating for parents, the family and health carers. Approximately 300 babies a year in the UK will succumb to SIDS. The causes are unknown but appear to be multifactorial. Advising parents on modifying behaviours, for example, the reduction or cessation of smoking, ensuring a suitable sleeping environment and encouraging breastfeeding, helps to minimize the risk factors.

**KEY POINTS**

- The aetiology of SIDS remains unclear, though a number of risk factors associated with SIDS have been identified and provide an opportunity to modify behaviours.
- Parents, grandparents and carers require advice on possible risk factors.
- Effective antenatal care may improve maternal, fetal and newborn health.
- Reducing or cessation of smoking in pregnancy and around the newborn baby reduces the risk of SIDS.
- Putting the baby on its back to sleep and avoiding overheating can reduce the risk of SIDS.

## REFERENCES


Bamfield L: Born unequal; why we need a progressive pre-birth agenda. Fabian Society Policy Report 61 (website). http://fabians.org.uk/publications/policy-reports/born-unequal-why-we-need-a-progressive-birth-agenda. 2007.

Blair PS, Fleming PJ, Smith IJ, et al: Babies sleeping with parents: case-controlled study of factors influencing the risk of the sudden infant death syndrome, *British Medical Journal* 319(7223):1457–1461, 1999.

Blair P, Platt M, Smith J, et al: Sudden infant death syndrome and sleeping positions in pre-term and low birth weight infants: an opportunity for targeted intervention, *Archives of Disease in Childhood* 91:101–106, 2006.

Blair P, Mitchell E, Heckstall-Smith E, et al: Head covering – a major modifiable risk factor for sudden infant death syndrome: a systematic review, *Archives of Disease In Childhood* 93(9):778–783, 2008.

Confidential Enquiry into Maternal and Child Health (CEMACH): *Why children die: a pilot study 2006; England (South West, North East & West Midland), Wales and Northern Ireland*, London, 2008, CEMACH.

Department of Health (DH): *Reduce the risk of cot death; an easy guide* (website). www.dh.gov.uk/cotdeath. 2007a. Accessed 2009.

Department of Health (DH): *Implementation plan for reducing health inequalities in infant mortality: a good practice guide* (website). www.dh.gov.uk/publications. 2007b. Accessed August, 2010.

Department of Health (DH): *Publications and statistics*, www.dh.gov.uk/publicationsandstatistics/index.htm. Accessed 2009.

Esposito L, Hegyi T, Ostfeld B: Educating parents about risk factors of sudden infant death syndrome; the role of Neonatal Intensive Care Unit and Well Baby Nursery Nurses, *Journal of Perinatal Neonatal Nursing* 21(2):158–164, 2007.

Fleming P, Blair P, Bacon C, et al: *The CESDI SUDI studies 1993–1996*, London, 2000, The Stationery Office.

Fleming P, Blair P, McKenna J: New knowledge, new insights, and new recommendations, *Archives of Disease in Childhood* 91(10):799–801, 2006.

Foundation for the Study of Infant Deaths (FSID): *Factfile 2* (website). www.fsid.org.uk updated November www.fsid.org.uk/editpics/612-1.pdf. 2007. Accessed July, 2010.

Foundation for the Study of Infant Deaths (FSID): Majority of parents fail to identify cot death hazards, *FSID Press Release* 21st February 2008 (website). www.fsid.org.uk/mothercare-poll-press.html. 2008. Accessed September 2008.

Gordon AE, Saadi AT, MacKenzie DA, et al: The protective effect of breast feeding in relation to sudden infant death syndrome (SIDS): III. Detection of IgA antibodies in human milk that bind to bacterial toxins implicated in SIDS, *FEMS Immunology and Medical Microbiology* 25(1–2):175–182, 1999.

Gornall J: Does cot death still exist? *British Medical Journal* 336(7639):302–304, 2008.

James C, Klenka H, Manning D: Sudden infant death syndrome: bed sharing with mothers who smoke, *Archives of Disease in Childhood* 88(2):112–113, 2003.

Mitchell E, Blair P, L'Hoir MP: Should pacifiers be recommended to prevent sudden infant death syndrome? *Paediatrics* 117(5):1755–1758, 2006.

Moon R, Horne R, Hauck F: Sudden infant death syndrome, *The Lancet* 370(9598):1578–1586, 2007.

Oyen N, Markestad T, Skaarven R, et al: Combined effects of sleeping position and prenatal risk factors in sudden infant death syndrome: the Nordic Epidemiological SIDS study, *Paediatrics* 100(4):613–621, 1997.

RCM: *A report of the findings of the RCM UK National Bed Sharing Audit*, London, 2005, RCM.

Shah T, Sullivan K, Carter J: Sudden infant death syndrome and reported maternal smoking during pregnancy, *American Journal of Public Health* 96(10):1757–1759, 2006.

UNICEF: *Sharing a bed with your baby* 2005-06_rev.qxd (website). www.babyfriendly.org.uk/pdfs/sharingbedleaflet.pdf. 2005. Modified 24/07/08. Accessed September 2008.

Wickham S: SIDS and dummies, *The Practising Midwife* 9(7):29–31, 2006.

# Part 8

# The postnatal and neonatal period

Chapter |51|

# Content and organization of postnatal care

*Pat Jackson*

## LEARNING OUTCOMES

After reading this chapter, you will be able to:

- understand the range of normal physical and psychological changes during the puerperium
- be knowledgeable about evidence-based advice and support to meet the needs of each woman
- be aware of the importance of providing culturally sensitive, individualized postnatal care for women during the puerperium
- understand the need for care provision to be undertaken in partnership with women and other care providers to ensure a seamless, high-quality service.

## INTRODUCTION

The 'puerperium' is traditionally defined as the time from immediately after the end of labour until the reproductive organs have returned as nearly as possible to their pre-gravid condition, a period estimated to be around 6–8 weeks, although the evidence base to support this duration is lacking. Recent studies suggest that, for some women, adaptation to motherhood and recovery from childbirth can take much longer than this (Bick & MacArthur 1995a, Brown & Lumley 1998).

The postnatal period is defined in the Nursing and Midwifery Council's (NMC) Midwives rules and standards (NMC 2004a) as 'the period after the end of labour during which the attendance of a midwife upon a woman and her baby is required, being not less than ten days and for such longer period as the midwife considers necessary'.

The National Service Framework (NSF) (DH 2004) describes postnatal care as professional care provided to meet the needs of women and their babies up to 6–8 weeks after birth, depending on individual need.

## AIMS OF POSTNATAL CARE

The aims of postnatal care are to:

- help the woman adapt to and confidently fulfil the role and responsibilities of motherhood
- promote and monitor the woman's and infant's physical wellbeing
- promote and monitor the woman's psychological wellbeing
- provide health promotion and educate the woman and her family in the needs and development of the infant.

## PHYSIOLOGICAL CHANGES DURING THE PUERPERIUM

During the puerperium, physiological changes take place in all women as the body returns to its pre-pregnant state (Ch. 25) and it is important that the midwife is familiar with these to ensure that appropriate care and advice is given.

### Involution of the uterus

The term *involution* describes the return of the uterus to being a pelvic organ. This includes a process of contractions, autolysis, and epithelial regeneration and proliferation. After the birth of the baby and the expulsion of the placenta, the muscles of the uterus constrict the blood vessels so that the blood circulating in the uterus is considerably reduced. This is known as *ischaemia*. There needs to be disposal of redundant *muscle, fibrous and elastic tissue*. The phagocytes of the bloodstream deal with the last two by phagocytosis, but the process is usually incomplete and some elastic tissue remains, so that the uterus never returns to its nulliparous state. Muscle fibres are digested by proteolytic enzymes, a process known as *autolysis*. The lysosomes of the cells are responsible for the removal of the waste products which pass into the bloodstream to be eliminated by the kidneys (Blackburn 2007, Coad & Dunstall 2005).

The decidual lining of the uterus is shed in the *lochia*, which also contains blood and serum. A new endometrium develops from the basal layer, beginning around the 10th postnatal day and estimated to be completed in about 6 weeks, although the evidence base for this is absent. Variations in the duration of shedding of lochia have been reported, with a range of 4 to 8 weeks (Abbott et al 1997), although duration of loss appears to be based on assumption rather than evidence. The changes in lochia have been described in three stages: *lochia rubra* (red), *lochia serosa* (pink) and *lochia alba* (white). These terms describe changes in the colour of the lochia, which together with the assumed duration of loss, have formed the basis for practice. However, they do not accurately represent the wide variability in the colour or duration of vaginal loss experienced by most women in the postnatal period (Marchant et al 1999).

The cervix and vagina lose the increased vascularity within 3 days of delivery, any oedema is reabsorbed and any bruising and tears heal rapidly (Stables & Rankin 2005). The ovaries and uterine tubes become pelvic organs again as the uterus returns to the pelvic cavity.

## Hormonal changes

Following the delivery of the placenta, the circulating levels of oestrogen and progesterone fall abruptly, but prolactin levels increase, stimulating milk secretion. (The initiation of lactation is described in full in Chapter 43.) An increase in the concentration of oxytocin occurs especially when the baby is suckling and may be experienced by the woman as a 'tingling' sensation in the breasts, as the intra-alveolar pressure is increased. There may be a cramping pain in the abdomen as a result of uterine contraction.

Eventually, negative feedback mechanisms trigger the release of the follicle-stimulating and luteinizing hormones, responsible for the resumption of the ovarian menstrual cycle. Ovulation takes place before menstruation, so that a woman may become pregnant again before she has a period; thus, all women should be advised of the need to use contraception prior to resuming sexual intercourse (Ch. 27). The re-establishment of hormonal stability in the early postnatal period will affect the emotional state of the woman (Hall 2005).

## Cardiovascular system

The diuretic effect of the removal of waste products, particularly from the uterus, via the bloodstream leads to a decrease in circulating blood volume as haemoconcentration occurs and the blood regains its former viscosity. Smooth muscle tone in the vessel walls improves as the progesterone levels fall and so the output, stroke volume and blood pressure return to pregravid levels.

## Respiratory system

Changes in the respiratory system are effected by the full ventilation of the basal lobes of the lungs which are no longer compressed by the enlarged uterus. Chest wall compliance, tidal volume and respiratory rate return to normal within 1 to 3 weeks (Coad & Dunstall 2005).

## Musculoskeletal system

The musculoskeletal system returns gradually to its pregravid state over a period of around 3 months following the birth (Wylie 2005). Ligaments of the uterus and muscles of the pelvic floor and abdomen return to their pre-pregnant state as the progesterone levels fall. This process can be aided by early ambulation and undertaking postnatal exercises (Logan 2001, NICE 2006). The rectus abdominis muscles may remain separated at the midline, a condition known as *diastasis recti*, which is most likely to occur in grande multiparous women or in those who have had a multiple pregnancy or polyhydramnios.

## Gastrointestinal system

Falling progesterone levels affect the alimentary tract so that the smooth muscle tone gradually improves and any symptoms of heartburn experienced by women should resolve. Constipation may, however, remain a common problem during the postnatal period.

## Urinary system

The *diuresis* following delivery lasts for 2–3 days and fluid and electrolyte balance returns to normal by 21 days after the birth (Coad & Dunstall 2005). Dilatation of the urinary tract, which occurs in pregnancy due to increased vascular volume and increased progesterone, resolves and the renal organs gradually return to their pregravid state.

## THE ROLE OF HEALTH PROFESSIONALS DURING THE POSTNATAL PERIOD

In the NSF (DH 2004) it states that women should receive coordinated postnatal care, delivered according to relevant guidelines with an agreed pathway of care, encompassing both medical and social needs of women and babies. Therefore the service should be delivered through the care pathway approach where linked groups of health professionals work together to ensure an equitable provision of high-quality care. All healthcare professionals caring for women and their babies should meet the relevant competences as outlined by Skills for Health (2005).

### The role of the midwife

A midwife has to provide care and monitor the progress of the mother in the postnatal period and give all necessary advice to the mother on infant care (NMC 2004a). The NICE guidelines *Routine postnatal care of women and their babies* (NICE 2006) provide guidance for midwives on the pattern and content of postnatal care with discussion of the evidence available. The midwife may delegate some appropriate aspects of care to a Maternity Care Assistant but remains the lead professional.

### The role of the GP

As part of routine postnatal care offered by the GP, a woman may receive up to five home visits and a final consultation at 6–8 weeks, following which she is discharged from the maternity services. Despite this being a routine part of care for around 50 years, the evidence of the contribution of GPs to routine community-based maternity care is hard to quantify and anecdotally there is wide variation in the extent to which GPs delegate their responsibilities to midwives (Smith & Jewell 1998).

Dowswell et al (2001) conducted a two-part study into the roles of primary care workers, in the care of childbearing women. Their survey identified that GPs had high levels of involvement in some aspects of maternity care, including postnatal visiting (76%), and the 6-week postnatal check (95%). Higher levels of GP involvement were not necessarily associated with higher levels of communication with midwives and there was some evidence of the opposite pattern. GPs within the same practice often worked and communicated with midwives in different ways.

No studies have examined the benefit to women's wellbeing of routine GP home visits and whether they are an appropriate use of GP time and skills. The few studies that have examined the 6–8-week check found that the routine content and timing may not be appropriate to meet women's health needs (Bick & MacArthur 1995b, Sharif et al 1993), although the generally high uptake suggests women value a consultation for themselves after childbirth. Discussion of contraception is routinely included as part of the 6–8-week consultation; however, one study found that more than half of postnatal women had resumed sexual intercourse within 6 weeks of the birth (Glazener 1998).

### The role of the health visitor

A health visitor will visit the woman and her infant during the postnatal period and for a number of years afterwards, until the child reaches school age. These home visits may commence whilst the midwife is still attending the woman, especially if the midwife continues to visit for up to 6 to 8 weeks or even 3 months as suggested in Standard 11 of the NSF (DH 2004).

The health visitor role, in specialist community health nursing, aims to reduce inequalities by working with individuals, families and communities, promoting health and preventing ill health, with emphasis on partnership working that cuts across disciplinary, professional and organizational boundaries (NMC 2004b). In many areas of the UK, health visitors routinely administer the Edinburgh Postnatal Depression Scale (EPDS) to postnatal women (Shakespeare et al 2003) to assist in the identification of those at risk of developing depression (Ch. 69). It is considered to be good practice to ask women who have recently given birth about their emotional wellbeing (NICE 2006); however, several studies have shown that women may not find the EPDS, or the way it is used, to be acceptable, with the consequence that they may produce ratings that do not adequately reflect their feelings (Shakespeare et al 2003).

## CONTENT OF MIDWIFERY POSTNATAL CARE

Recommendations have been identified in the NICE guidelines (2006). A documented, individualized postnatal care plan should be developed with the woman, ideally in the antenatal period or as soon as possible after birth. This should include relevant factors from the antenatal, intrapartum and immediate postnatal period. Details of the healthcare professionals involved in a woman's and her baby's care, including roles and contact details, should be provided and plans for the postnatal period should be identified. This care plan should be reviewed at each postnatal contact.

Aspects of core care and information that should be provided to maintain maternal health were also identified in the guidelines (see Box 51.1). These core observations and examinations should be performed to monitor

Box 51.1 **Routine core postnatal care and information (Adapted from the NICE guidelines 2006)**

## Within the first 24 hours after birth

1. Measure and document BP once within 6 hours after the last measurement taken soon after birth as a component of labour care.
2. Toilet facilities that are hygienic and ensure privacy should be provided in the clinical setting.
3. Document urine void within 6 hours.
4. All women should be encouraged to mobilize.

## Between 2 and 7 days (24–168 hours)

### Core information

1. The Department of Health *Birth to five* handbook should be provided to all postpartum women within the first 3 days after birth and its use discussed.
2. Women should be offered information and reassurance about:
   - perineal pain and perineal hygiene
   - urinary incontinence and micturition
   - bowel function
   - fatigue
   - headache
   - back pain
   - normal patterns of emotional changes in the postnatal period (This information should be offered by the third day)
   - contraception
   - contact details for expert contraceptive advice.
3. All women should be offered advice on diet, exercise and planning activities, including spending time with her baby.

### Core care

1. Anti-D should be offered as required according to Department of Health guideline within 72 hours of birth.
2. MMR should be offered as required according to Department of Health guideline.*
3. Enquires should be made about general wellbeing and all common health problems, including:
   - micturition and urinary incontinence
   - bowel function
   - healing of any perineal wound
   - headache
   - fatigue
   - back pain.
4. Encourage all women to use self-care techniques, such as taking gentle exercise, taking time to rest, having help to care for the baby, and talking to someone about their feelings, and ensure that they can access social support networks.
5. Ask all women about their emotional wellbeing, what family and social support they have and their usual coping strategies for dealing with day-to-day matters. All women and their families/partners should be encouraged to tell their healthcare professional about any changes in mood, emotional state and behaviour that are outside of the woman's normal pattern.
6. Observe for any risks, signs and symptoms of domestic abuse and know whom to contact for advice and management.

## Weeks 2–8 (from day 8 onward)

### Core information

1. Advise women to report any common health problems (see above).
2. Discuss initiation of sexual activity and possible dyspareunia.

### Core care

1. At any postnatal contact, enquiries should continue to be made about general wellbeing and all common health problems (see above).
2. All women should be asked about resumption of sexual intercourse and possible dyspareunia as part of an assessment of overall wellbeing 2–6 weeks after birth.
3. At 10–14 days after birth, all women should be asked about resolution of symptoms of maternal blues. If symptoms have not resolved, the woman's psychological wellbeing should continue to be assessed for postnatal depression, and if symptoms persist, evaluated.
4. Continue to observe for any indication of domestic abuse.
5. As part of the woman's individual postnatal care plan, the coordinating health professional should ensure that there is a review of the woman's physical, emotional and social wellbeing at 6–8 weeks postpartum which takes into account screening and medical history.

* MMR guidelines available on www.dh.gov.uk/en/Publicationsandstatistics/Publications/PublicationsPolicyAndGuidance/DH_074924. Section on immunization is in Chapter 6 Illness and accidents.

recovery from the birth whether in hospital or the home. Midwives should perform them as appropriate, taking into account individual women's health needs and wishes, as informed consent must always be gained before undertaking any physical examination (DH 2004, NMC 2008).

## RESEARCH UNDERPINNING CARE OF WOMEN'S PHYSICAL HEALTH DURING THE POSTNATAL PERIOD

### Uterine involution and vaginal loss

The progress of involution is usually assessed by the midwife during the postnatal period by measuring the distance between the uterine fundus and the symphysis pubis, either with a tape measure or by abdominal palpation. There is little evidence as to the accuracy or value of either method. Cluett et al (1997) found considerable variability in the pattern of uterine involution. This occurred not only in the daily rate of decline in individual women but also between women. In an earlier study by the same researchers (Cluett et al 1995), intra-observer variability was assessed and the results showed disparity, indicating that the measurement of uterine involution is unreliable. In order to ascertain if involution is associated with morbidity, other factors such as pyrexia, offensive lochia and maternal wellbeing should also be taken into account (Lewis 2007).

Recent studies have suggested that the normal duration and composition of vaginal loss is much more varied than was previously assumed (Marchant et al 1999, Visness et al 1997). Marchant et al (1999), in the Blood Loss in the Postnatal Period (BLiPP) study, described the variability of postpartum vaginal loss in relation to duration (median 21 days), amount and colour. A later study on GP consultations by women concerned about their vaginal loss, published in 2002 by the same study group, reported that 20% of the 325 women had a problem with postnatal loss between 28 days and 3 months postpartum. Visness et al (1997) reported the duration of lochia as ranging from 5 to 90 days (median 27 days). A quarter of these women reported that their blood loss stopped and recommenced.

### Pain relief

Many women experience significant pain and discomfort in the postnatal period, even if they have had a spontaneous vaginal birth with an intact perineum (Macarthur & Macarthur 2004), but as with postnatal care generally, there is little evidence regarding the most appropriate management of pain, other than some studies that have assessed pain relief for perineal trauma. In the first 3 or 4 days after delivery, pain can arise from perineal trauma, bruising, abdominal wounds, 'after pains' as a result of uterine cramps, vulval varicosities and haemorrhoids, breasts and the musculoskeletal system (Mander 1998). Many women will report pain persisting well beyond the immediate postnatal period and it is important that the midwife continues to ask about pain relief needs and ensures that these are adequately managed (NICE 2006).

**Reflective activity 51.1**

Keep a record of the rate of involution and lochial loss of primigravid and multigravid mothers for as many days as possible. Are there many differences in the pattern of involution and lochial loss between the women?

### Perineal care

The majority of women who have had a vaginal birth will experience some degree of perineal pain and will require effective pain relief (Albers et al 2005, Macarthur & Macarthur 2004). At each postpartum contact, women should be asked if they have any concerns about the healing process of any perineal wound (NICE 2006). The midwife should offer to assess the woman's perineum if she has pain or discomfort.

A combination of systemic and localized management of postpartum perineal pain (see Ch. 38) is necessary to achieve adequate pain relief (Steen et al 2006). The first line of management in most cases is oral analgesia, commonly paracetamol, unless contraindicated (Moffatt et al 2001, Steen & Marchant 2007). Combinations of paracetamol and codeine (such as *Tylex*) may be prescribed but may predispose to constipation. An alternative is the anti-inflammatory, non-steroidal *ibuprofen* (brufen) (Steen 2005).

Anti-inflammatory, non-steroidal drugs via suppository, contraindicated for women with a history of asthma and pre-eclampsia, can be effective for up to 24 hours after the birth and result in less additional pain relief being required (Hedayati et al 2003). Dodd et al (2004) concluded that the rectal route of administration was acceptable to women and provided a simple, effective and safe method of reducing the pain experienced in the first 24 hours.

In addition to analgesia, local applications can be recommended. Ice packs and cooling gel pads were the most commonly used local application in a survey of perineal care carried out by Steen et al (2006). These will provide only short-term relief but there is some evidence to suggest they promote healing. Low & Read (2000) have indicated that initial vasoconstriction is followed by vasodilatation, which improves the circulation and promotes healing. A high level of satisfaction was indicated by women who used the gel packs, as they promoted a cushioning effect as opposed to the sharp corners and firmness of ice (Steen & Marchant 2007).

Electrical therapies such as ultrasound and pulsed electromagnetic energy may also be used to relieve perineal pain, but further evidence of benefit is required. Hay-Smith (1998) reviewed the use of ultrasound for postpartum perineal pain and dyspareunia for a Cochrane review, but there was insufficient evidence to enable conclusions to be made about its use.

Bathing can relieve perineal pain and some women may find aromatherapy oils added to the bath water soothing (Steen 2003), but evidence of effectiveness is lacking. It is important that midwives acknowledge women's pain and provide appropriate advice to ensure effective relief. Perineal hygiene should be discussed with women as and when appropriate.

### Micturition and bowels

Various urinary symptoms may present in the postnatal period and it is important that the midwife is able to identify these in order to implement appropriate management and referral if necessary. In hospital, toilet facilities should be clean and privacy should be ensured. Urine voided within the first 6 hours following the birth should be documented (NICE 2006).

It could be 2–3 days after the birth before a woman has a bowel movement, especially if she has a painful perineum and/or inadequate dietary intake during labour. Constipation, defined as decreased frequency and regularity of defecation and alteration in the composition of stool (Tiran 2003), is identified by maternal self-report. Women should be asked if they have opened their bowels within 3 days of the birth and women who are constipated and uncomfortable should have their diet and fluid intake assessed. Advice on how to improve their dietary intake should be given and a gentle laxative may be recommended if dietary measures are not effective (NICE 2006). There is a dearth of research into the most effective management: dietary bran and wheat supplements were the most successful treatment in one systematic review of interventions for constipation in pregnancy (Jewell & Young 2001), but this was based on only one trial of 40 women.

Women with haemorrhoids should be advised to take dietary measures to avoid constipation (NICE 2006). Haemorrhoids can range in severity, depending upon the degree of prolapse; however, for most women, treatment with application of topical creams may be beneficial, although their use has not been proven (Alonso et al 2003).

### Breastfeeding (see Ch. 43)

Despite the benefits of breastfeeding for the woman and her infant, many women give up breastfeeding well before the end of the recommended 6-month period (WHO 2001). Baby-led feeding should be practised, with no limit on the frequency and duration of feeds (UNICEF 1992). Midwives should be available to assist women during the early days, as successful feeding is interlinked with maternal wellbeing and postnatal recovery. This aspect of the midwife's role in helping the family is underestimated, as they provide advice and support and, in particular, they promote confidence in the care of the newborn (Magill-Cuerden 2006).

## CARE OF WOMEN'S PSYCHOLOGICAL HEALTH

Pregnancy and childbirth are major life events (Clement & Elliot 1998). In addition to physical health changes, emotional and psychological changes are also experienced and midwives have an important role in monitoring them and providing support.

### Postpartum blues

This transient, self-limiting condition usually occurs between the third and tenth day after the birth and is considered a normal reaction, estimated to be experienced by around 70% of all postnatal women (Hall 2005) (see Ch. 69). Commonly reported symptoms include tearfulness, irritability and lability of mood. Although most women recover within a day or two, studies have shown a higher incidence of blues among women who suffer from postnatal depression (Beck et al 1992). Women and their family members require emotional support from the midwife and reassurance that this is a common symptom, usually of short duration. Jones & Craddock (2001) and Seyfried (2003) point out that, owing to its transient nature, professional intervention is not generally indicated, but they suggest that women with postnatal blues should be encouraged to seek further evaluation if symptoms persist beyond 7 to 10 days (Jones & Craddock 2001) or 2 weeks (Seyfried 2003).

The International Childbirth Education Association (ICEA) Position Statement and Review of Postpartum Emotional Disorders (ICEA 2003) suggests that the use of self-care techniques and good support systems will reduce the incidence of postnatal blues. These include good nutrition; regular physical activity and sleep; having realistic expectations of motherhood; taking breaks to rest; practising deep breathing; expressing and accepting negative feelings; structuring the day; nurturing a sense of humour; and postponing major life changes. NICE (2006) endorse this by including the encouragement of women to use self-care techniques as part of the core care between 2 and 7 days (see Box 51.1). There is no research evidence to underpin these suggestions.

### Postnatal debriefing and psychosocial support

There has been considerable debate as to the appropriateness of implementing postnatal debriefing to prevent post-traumatic stress disorder (PTSD). 'Debriefing' is considered to be beneficial, particularly for women who have had a traumatic labour and/or delivery, although there is limited evidence of the appropriateness of this intervention (Alexander 1999) and debate as to whether this is the correct terminology to describe the active 'listening' that midwives may implement. Two trials that evaluated the value of debriefing by midwives to prevent postnatal depression (Lavender & Walkinshaw 1998, Small et al 2000) did not show any benefit, the findings of the second study indicating that debriefing could in some cases contribute to emotional health problems. Gamble et al (2002) undertook a systematic review to assess the literature on debriefing or non-directive counselling specifically directed to prevent postpartum emotional distress and concluded that a listening visit may reduce emotional distress.

Collins (2006) undertook a review of 20 pieces of literature on the subject and provided recommendations for practice which included the suggestion that postnatal care should include *more* attention to psychological wellbeing. She proposed the facilitation of postnatal contact with the midwife present at the birth to provide answers to the woman's questions. Continuity of carer would enable this to happen. Further research is required, as in recent years there has been a growing awareness that some women's experiences of childbirth are characterized by feelings of helplessness and horror that cause severe and long-term post-traumatic stress reactions (Bailham & Joseph 2004). Midwives need to be able to recognize the signs and recommend postnatal support groups that may provide a therapeutic environment for women, although there is little research to determine their effectiveness.

All women should be asked about the level of social support available to them, to enable postnatal care to be planned to provide this if required (NICE 2006). Women should also be asked about their past or present history of mental illness and any family history of perinatal mental disorders, at the first postnatal contact with healthcare professionals. Mental disorders in the postnatal period can have serious consequences for the mother, her infant and other family members (NICE 2007). (See Chapter 69 for clinical management of mental disorders.)

## ORGANIZATION OF MIDWIFERY POSTNATAL CARE

Postnatal care commences in hospital for the majority of women, and, for those who do not experience any complications, length of stay can range from less than 6 hours to 2–3 days, with longer stays for women who have had an operative delivery. In 2006, a national survey revealed that the length of postnatal stay in hospital had fallen since 1995. A total of 63% of women had stays of less than 6 days, compared with 52% in 1995, with 24% staying between 3 and 5 days, compared with 35% in 1995 (Redshaw et al 2007).

A comparison of these 2006 data with those of 1995 for home visiting revealed a tendency for the visits to take place over a longer period. Almost all women (98%) were visited by a midwife at home, for an average of five postnatal visits. No significant differences were found in relation to parity or type of birth. Some women (19%) were also visited by a maternity support worker or maternity care assistant and this was more common for women who had not previously given birth. The last contact with the midwife was variable, but a longer duration of contact did not necessarily mean more visits, as, irrespective of the timing of the last visit, 45–56% of women had four to six visits. Where the last contact was later, there was only a slight tendency for women to have more visits. More women had home visits after 28 days in 2006 (7%) than in 1995 (2%). These changes and the variability in timing of the last contact suggest increased flexibility compared to a decade ago. Redshaw et al (2007) also found that most women thought their postnatal stay was of the right length (69%), but some would have liked a longer stay in hospital (13%) and others a shorter stay (15%). Women who had previously had a baby were more likely to say their length of stay was about right.

More than three-quarters of women were satisfied with the frequency with which midwives visited them at home for postnatal care. NICE (2006) reported that women who receive continuity of care are more likely to be satisfied with their postpartum experience. At the end of the postnatal period, the coordinating healthcare professional should ensure that the woman's physical, emotional and social wellbeing is reviewed.

## COULD POSTNATAL CARE BE MORE EFFECTIVE?

In a survey by the NCT (Singh & Newburn 2000), many women complained about the care they received in hospital, in particular inadequate support for breastfeeding and feeling left to cope alone. Baxter et al (2003) also reported how some women on postnatal wards feel a sense of abandonment. The postnatal care in hospital needs to be more responsive to the needs of the individual. Cleanliness and hygiene have been reported as causes for concern for women (Redshaw et al 2007, Wray 2006). In addition, Wray (2006) found that visiting arrangements, noise, rest, and a lack of support for infant feeding and baby care were less than satisfactory for some women, but she found that the postnatal care at home was highly regarded and valued.

**Reflective activity 51.2**

Find out the extent of postnatal visiting in your own unit. How effective do you think it is? What are the most common problems that women experience during this period?

NHS acute and primary care trusts are expected to implement the maternity standard set out in the children's NSF by the end of 2009 (DH 2007). This means that midwifery-led services should provide for the mother and her baby for at least a month after birth and up to 3 months or longer depending on individual need. NICE (2006) indicated that care from a small team of midwives may be comparable to one-to-one midwifery in terms of maternal satisfaction, continuity and clinical outcomes, and is at least as cost-effective. They suggested that the use of non-professional community support workers postpartum is unlikely to be a cost-effective use of resources. This is in contrast to Morrell et al's (2000) evaluation of the costs and benefits of community postnatal services, where they found that the cost of the support worker led to a statistically significant mean difference in total costs. They also found that women had a high level of satisfaction with the support worker service.

Following the implementation of the NSF maternity standards, postnatal services should be more flexible after transfer from hospital as women and their partners will have a choice of how and where to access care. The Department for Education and Skills (DfES) report *Every child matters* sets out proposals to reform the delivery of services for children and families (DfES 2004). Changes in the organization of care, particularly the development of Children's Centres, should lead to a more responsive service. When the mother and baby's postnatal needs have been met, responsibility for their care and support can be transferred to the health visitor (DH 2004).

A cluster randomized controlled trial implemented and evaluated a new model of midwifery-led postnatal care (the IMPaCT study). It was found that this more flexible care, tailored to individual needs, could improve women's mental health and reduce probable depression at 4 months postpartum, although the physical health assessment was the same for this group compared to the control group (MacArthur et al 2003).

## IMPLICATIONS FOR MIDWIVES

Women need to be valued as individuals and midwives must listen to them and respond to their concerns and preferences (NMC 2008). The midwife should introduce herself and explain for how long she will be providing care (NICE 2006) and must share information in a way the women and families can understand (NMC 2008). Midwives must respect and support women's rights to accept or decline treatment, or care, and work cooperatively within teams and delegate appropriately (Ch. 8).

The findings of studies described in this and the following chapter on maternal morbidity highlight the need for midwives to continuously evaluate the care they currently provide, in order to assess if this is appropriate.

### KEY POINTS

- Postnatal care must be planned, organized and delivered in partnership with women and families, tailored to their physical, emotional and cultural needs.
- Midwives should utilize available evidence and research, such as is available in the NICE postnatal guidelines, to provide high-quality care.
- Postnatal care is supported by policy initiatives such as *Maternity matters* and the National Service Framework which indicate how the postnatal care provision will change in the immediate future to provide a more flexible service to meet individual needs more effectively.

## REFERENCES


Abbott H, Bick D, MacArthur C: Health after birth. In Henderson C, Jones K, editors: *Essential midwifery*, London, 1997, Mosby.

Albers L, Sedler K, Bedrick E, et al: Midwifery care measures in the second stage of labour and reduction of genital tract trauma at birth: a randomised trial, *Journal of Midwifery and Women's Health* 50(5):365–372, 2005.

Alexander J: Can midwives reduce postpartum psychological morbidity? A randomized trial (Comments), *MIDIRS Midwifery Digest* 9:730–731, 1999.

Alonso P, Johanson J, Martinez M: Phlebotonics for haemorrhoids. *Cochrane Database of Systematic Reviews* (website). www.cochrane.org/reviews/es/info_6881021118102047 88.html. 2003. Accessed August 2008.

Bailham D, Joseph S: Traumatic childbirth: what we know and what we can do, *Midwives* 7(6):258–261, 2004.

Baxter J, McCrae A, Dorey-Irani A: Talking with women after birth, *British Journal of Midwifery* 11(5):304–309, 2003.

Beck CT, Reynolds MA, Rutowski P: Postpartum depression, *Journal of Obstetric, Gynecologic and Neonatal Nursing* 21(4):287–293, 1992.

Bick D, MacArthur C: Extent, severity and effect of health problems after childbirth, *British Journal of Midwifery* 3(1):27–31, 1995a.

Bick D, MacArthur C: Attendance, content and relevance of the 6 week postnatal examination, *Midwifery* 11(62):9–73, 1995b.

Blackburn ST: *Maternal, fetal and neonatal physiology*, ed 3, Philadelphia, 2007, WB Saunders.

Brown S, Lumley J: Maternal health after childbirth: results of an Australian population based survey, *British Journal of Obstetrics and Gynaecology* 105(2):156–161, 1998.

Clement S, Elliot S: Psychological health before, during and after childbirth. In Marsh G, Renfrew M, editors: *Community-based maternity care*, Oxford, 1998, Oxford University Press.

Cluett ER, Alexander J, Pickering RM: Is measuring postnatal symphysis–fundus distance worthwhile? *Midwifery* 11(4):174–183, 1995.

Cluett ER, Alexander J, Pickering RM: What is the normal pattern of uterine involution? An investigation of postpartum uterine involution measured by the distance between the symphysis pubis and the uterine fundus using a paper tape measure, *Midwifery* 13(1):9–16, 1997.

Coad J, Dunstall M: *Anatomy and physiology for midwives*, ed 2, Edinburgh, 2005, Churchill Livingstone.

Collins R: What is the purpose of debriefing women in the postnatal period? *Evidence Based Midwifery* 4(1):4–9, 2006.

Department for Education and Skills (DfES): *Every child matters: change for children* (website). www.everychildmatters.gov.uk/key-documents. 2004. Accessed August 2008.

Department of Health (DH): *National service framework for children, young people and maternity services* (website). www.dh.gov.uk/en/Healthcare/NationalServiceFrameworks/Children/DH_4089111. 2004. 2004. Accessed August 2008.

Department of Health (DH): *Maternity matters: choice, access and continuity of care in a safe service* (website). www.dh.gov.uk/en/Publicationsandstatistics/Publications/.../DH_073312. 2007. Accessed August 2008.

Dodd JM, Hedayati H, Pearce E, et al: Rectal analgesia for the relief of perineal pain after childbirth: a randomised controlled trial of diclofenac suppositories, *BJOG: An International Journal of Obstetrics and Gynaecology* 111(10):1059–1064, 2004.

Dowswell T, Renfrew MJ, Gregson B, et al: A review of the literature on women's views on their maternity care in the community in the UK, *Midwifery* 17(3):194–202, 2001.

Gamble J, Creedy D, Webster J, et al: A review of the literature on debriefing or non-directive counselling to prevent postpartum emotional distress, *Midwifery* 18(1):72–79, 2002.

Glazener CMA: Sexual function after childbirth: women's experiences, persistent morbidity and lack of professional recognition (Letter), *British Journal of Obstetrics and Gynaecology* 105(5):243–244, 1998.

Hall J: Postnatal emotional wellbeing, *The Practising Midwife* 8(4):35–40, 2005.

Hay-Smith E: Therapeutic ultrasound for postpartum perineal pain and dyspareunia, *Cochrane Database of Systematic Reviews* (3):CD000495, 1998.

Hedayati H, Parsons J, Crowther C: Rectal analgesia for pain from perineal trauma following childbirth, *Cochrane Database of Systematic Reviews* (3):CD003931, 2003.

International Childbirth Education Association (ICEA): *Position Statement and Review of Postpartum Emotional Disorders*, Raleigh, NC, 2003, International Childbirth Education Association.

Jewell DJ, Young G: Interventions for treating constipation in pregnancy, *Cochrane Database of Systematic Reviews* (2):CD001142, 2001.

Jones I, Craddock N: Familiality of the puerperal trigger in bipolar disorder: results of a family study, *American Journal of Psychiatry* 158(6):913–917, 2001.

Lavender T, Walkinshaw SA: Can midwives reduce postpartum psychological morbidity? A randomized trial, *Birth* 25(4):215–219, 1998.

Lewis G, editor: *The Confidential Enquiry into Maternal and Child Health (CEMACH). Saving mothers' lives: reviewing maternal deaths to make motherhood safer – 2003–2005. The Seventh Report on Confidential Enquiries into Maternal Deaths in the United Kingdom*, London, 2007, CEMACH.

Logan K: Audit on advice provided on pelvic floor exercises, *Professional Nurse* 16(9):1369–1372, 2001.

Low L, Read A: *Electrotherapy explained. Principles and practice*, ed 3, Oxford, 2000, Butterworth Heinemann.

Macarthur AJ, Macarthur C: Incidence, severity and determinants of perineal pain after vaginal delivery: a prospective cohort study, *American Journal of Obstetrics and Gynecology* 191(4):1199–1204, 2004.

MacArthur C, Winter HR, Bick D, et al: Redesigning postnatal care: a randomised controlled trial of protocol-based midwifery led care focused on individual women's physical and psychological health needs, *Health Technology Assessment* 7(37):1–98, 2003.

Magill-Cuerden J: Postnatal care in the home setting: essential support after birth, *British Journal of Midwifery* 14(1):32, 2006.

Mander R: *Pain in childbearing and its control*, Oxford, 1998, Blackwell Science.

Marchant S, Alexander J, Garcia J, et al: A survey of women's experiences of vaginal loss from 24 hours to three months of childbirth (the BLiPP study), *Midwifery* 15(2):72–81, 1999.

Moffatt H, Lavender T, Walkinshaw S: Comparing administration of paracetamol for perineal pain, *British Journal of Midwifery* 9(11):690–694, 2001.

Morrell CJ, Spiby H, Stewart P, et al: Costs and effectiveness of community postnatal support workers: randomised controlled trial, *British Medical Journal* 321(7261):593–598, 2000.

National Institute for Health and Clinical Excellence (NICE): *Routine postnatal care of women and their babies* (website). www.nice.org.uk. 2006. Accessed August 2008.

National Institute for Health and Clinical Excellence (NICE): *Antenatal and postnatal mental health* (website).

www.nice.org.uk. 2007. Accessed August 2008.

Nursing and Midwifery Council (NMC): *Midwives rules and standards*, London, 2004a, NMC.

Nursing and Midwifery Council (NMC): *Standards of proficiency for specialist community public health nurses*, London, 2004b, NMC.

Nursing and Midwifery Council (NMC): *The code: standards of conduct, performance and ethics for nurses and midwives*, London, 2008, NMC.

Redshaw M, Rowe R, Hockley C, et al: *Recorded delivery: national survey of women's experience of maternity care*, Oxford, 2007, National Perinatal Epidemiology Unit, University of Oxford.

Seyfried L: Postpartum mood disorders, *International Review of Psychiatry* 15(3):231–242, 2003.

Shakespeare J, Blake F, Garcia J: A qualitative study of the acceptability of routine screening of postnatal women using the Edinburgh Postnatal Depression Scale, *British Journal of General Practice* 53(493):614–619, 2003.

Sharif K, Clarke P, Whittle M: Routine six weeks postnatal examination: to do or not to do? *Journal of Obstetrics and Gynaecology* 4(13):251–252, 1993.

Singh D, Newburn M: *Access to maternity information and support. The experiences and needs of women before and after giving birth*, London, 2000, National Childbirth Trust (NCT).

Skills for Health. (website). www.skillsforhealth.org.uk. 2005. Accessed August 2008.

Small R, Lumley J, Donohue L, et al: Randomised controlled trial of midwife led debriefing to reduce maternal depression after operative childbirth, *British Medical Journal* 321(7268):1043–1047, 2000.

Smith L, Jewell D: General practitioners' contributions – what's really going on? In Marsh G, Renfrew M, editors: *Community based maternity care*, Oxford, 1998, Oxford University Press.

Stables D, Rankin J: *Physiology in childbearing: with anatomy and related biosciences*, ed 2, Edinburgh, 2005, Churchill Livingstone.

Steen M: Breast and perineal pain, *British Journal of Midwifery* 11(5):318–321, 2003.

Steen M: 'I can't sit down' – easing genital tract trauma, *British Journal of Midwifery* 13(5):311–314, 2005.

Steen M, Marchant P: Ice packs and cooling gel pads versus no localised treatment for relief of perineal pain: a randomised controlled trial, *Evidence Based Midwifery* 5(1):16–22, 2007.

Steen M, Briggs M, King D: Alleviating postnatal perineal trauma: to cool or not to cool? *British Journal of Midwifery* 14(5):304–306, 308, 2006.

Tiran D: Self help for constipation and haemorrhoids in pregnancy, *British Journal of Midwifery* 11(9):579–581, 2003.

UNICEF: *Baby friendly initiative: ten steps to successful breastfeeding* (website). www.babyfriendly.org.uk. 1992. Accessed August 2008.

Visness CM, Kennedy KI, Ramos R: The duration and character of postpartum bleeding among breast-feeding women, *Obstetrics and Gynecology* 89(2):159–163, 1997.

World Health Organization (WHO): *The optimal duration of exclusive breastfeeding. A systematic review*, Geneva, 2001, WHO.

Wray J: Seeking to explore what matters to women about postnatal care, *British Journal of Midwifery* 14(5):246,248,250,252,254, 2006.

Wylie L: Essential anatomy and physiology in maternity care, ed 2, Edinburgh, 2005, Churchill Livingstone.

Chapter |52|

# Morbidity following childbirth

Pat Jackson

## LEARNING OUTCOMES

After reading this chapter, you will:

- be knowledgeable about the different health problems that women can experience after childbirth
- understand the childbirth-related risk factors of the various health problems
- realize the necessity of recognizing and investigating any deviations from the expected recovery following birth
- consider the possible effects on women's physical and psychological wellbeing if postpartum problems are not identified or managed.

## INTRODUCTION

Although for most women the postnatal period is uncomplicated, core postnatal care includes recognizing any deviations from the expected recovery after birth, evaluating the situation and intervening appropriately (NICE 2006). Health problems after birth are common, may persist over time and are often under-recognized by the care providers (Leah & Albers 2000).

The NICE guidelines (2006) provide recommendations for additional postnatal care that may be needed when deviations from the expected recovery pattern occur. These recommendations have been given appropriate status levels indicating the degree of urgency required in dealing with each problem. The status levels are defined as *non-urgent, urgent* or *emergency*. If additional care is required, it should be offered so as to minimize, as much as possible, any impact on the relationship between the woman, her baby and family.

All women in the UK are offered a postnatal examination at 6–8 weeks after childbirth and this has been considered to mark the end of the puerperium and a woman's routine contact with the maternity services (NICE 2006). Although childbirth-related problems are known to occur after this time, some even requiring readmission to hospital, only recently have there been systematic investigations of longer-term postpartum morbidity. Studies, in the UK (Bick & MacArthur 1995, Glazener et al 1995) and elsewhere (Brown & Lumley 1998, Saurel-Cubizolles et al 2000), have investigated the occurrence and persistence of a range of health problems following childbirth. All these studies have identified substantial postpartum ill-health, much of which persists well past the end of the puerperium and is often not reported to health professionals, nor observed by them.

It is important to remember that not all the problems experienced following childbirth are attributable to the birth itself. Some morbidity is likely to be associated with the birth and some with pregnancy, whilst some will be due to the changes of childbirth or be unrelated to any of these events, occurring as part of a general background of morbidity present at any time in any population. Particular childbirth-related causal factors have been investigated in some of the studies and these will be referred to in the relevant sections.

## CAUSES OF POSTNATAL MORBIDITY

### Life-threatening conditions

NICE (2006) recommend that, at the first postnatal contact, women should be advised of the signs and symptoms of potentially life-threatening conditions (see Table 52.1). The incidence of these potentially life-threatening

**Table 52.1 Possible signs and symptoms of life-threatening conditions**

| Possible sign/symptom | Evaluate for | Action |
|---|---|---|
| Sudden or profuse blood loss, or blood loss and signs/symptoms of shock, including tachycardia, hypotension, hypoperfusion, change in consciousness | Postpartum haemorrhage | Emergency action |
| Offensive/excessive vaginal loss, tender abdomen or fever. If no obstetric cause, consider other causes | Postpartum haemorrhage/sepsis/ other pathology | Urgent action |
| Fever, shivering, abdominal pain and/or offensive vaginal loss. If temperature exceeds 38°C, repeat in 4–6 hours. If temperature still high or other symptoms and measurable signs, evaluate further | Infection/genital tract sepsis | Emergency action |
| Severe or persistent headache | Pre-eclampsia/eclampsia | Emergency action |
| Diastolic BP is greater than 90 mmHg and accompanied by another sign/ symptom of pre-eclampsia | Pre-eclampsia/eclampsia | Emergency action |
| Diastolic BP is greater than 90 mmHg and no other sign/symptom, repeat BP within 4 hours. If it remains above 90 mm Hg after 4 hours, evaluate | Pre-eclampsia/eclampsia | Emergency action |
| Shortness of breath or chest pain | Pulmonary embolism | Emergency action |
| Unilateral calf pain, redness or swelling | Deep vein thrombosis | Emergency action |

Adapted from NICE guideline 37 (2006)

conditions is low, but they can lead to maternal mortality and morbidity that can be avoided or reduced if appropriate action is taken. NHS Trust guidelines should be in place to enable midwives to provide women with appropriate information about the conditions and the action they should take. Details about who to contact in these circumstances should be provided.

## Common health problems

The majority of symptoms experienced after childbirth are rarely life-threatening but they can have an adverse effect on the quality of life (Bick & MacArthur 1995). Since women are often reluctant to initiate consultations about their own health, careful questioning from the midwife and other professionals is needed to enable them to discuss their symptons.

### Urinary problems

Symptoms of stress incontinence are the most common of the urinary problems that occur in association with childbirth, but some women also have retention and voiding difficulties or urinary tract infection. If urine has not been voided by 6 hours following the birth and measures, such as a warm bath or shower, are not immediately successful, the bladder should be palpated and catheterization should be considered as urgent action needs to be taken (NICE 2006). The bladder can only contain a certain amount of urine even when distended, and once that capacity is reached, the sphincter of the bladder relaxes and urine escapes. This is referred to as *retention with overflow.*

Urinary voiding difficulties and retention are generally immediate post-delivery complications. Zaki et al (2004) found that I in 60 women failed to resume normal voiding during the immediate postpartum period. Their national survey found that there was no consensus about the diagnostic criteria for retention or the optimum management for voiding dysfunction. Further research is needed, as, if it is not recognized, bladder overdistension can lead to denervation, detrusor atony and bladder dysfunction requiring, in extreme cases, self-catheterization for up to 5 weeks (Zaki et al 2004). Zaki et al reported that retention is being reported with increasing frequency, which could be due to greater awareness or an increasing use of epidural analgesia and instrumental deliveries. From day 2 onwards, pelvic floor exercises should be taught, to prevent any involuntary leakage of urine, especially if a woman reports leaking small amounts of urine. Persistent urinary incontinence should be referred for investigation and treatment (NICE 2006). A third of women are known to suffer from the problem following childbirth. Pelvic floor exercises will reduce the incidence, especially with one-to-one teaching and supervision. The exercises may be particularly beneficial for women who give birth to large babies or who have forceps deliveries (Hay-Smith et al 2008).

General population studies have shown that urinary stress incontinence among women, defined as the involuntary leakage of urine caused by pressure on the bladder from coughing, sneezing, laughing and exertion, is widely experienced (Pollock 2004). Childbirth is generally considered to be the most common cause. Viktrup & Lose (2001) reported a prevalence of stress incontinence 5 years after a first delivery of 30%, and the risk of stress incontinence at this time was related to the onset and duration of symptoms after the first pregnancy and delivery. The use of vacuum extraction or episiotomy during the first delivery also increased the risk. In their follow-up study, Glazener et al (2005) also found that about three-quarters of the women with urinary incontinence at 3 months after childbirth still had the problem 6 years later. They concluded that the moderate short-term benefits of conservative treatment may not persist. Further research is required so that appropriate management strategies can be identified. Women should be encouraged to discuss the problems of incontinence so that they can receive the advice and support that is currently available.

The risk factors in the aetiology of stress incontinence remain unclear, but it is generally considered to be linked to pelvic floor innervation damage (Allen et al 1990, Zaki et al 2004) which is more common after a longer second stage labour and the delivery of a bigger baby. Increasing maternal age, heavier infant birthweight and larger head circumference have also been identified as risk factors by Wilson et al (1996). Findings relating to the effect of forceps have been inconsistent (Brown & Lumley 1998). Delivery by caesarean section is generally associated with a lower prevalence of stress incontinence (Assassa et al 2000, Wilson et al 1996). However, Wilson et al (1996) found that a reduced occurrence only applied to women who had up to two caesarean sections.

The severity of postpartum stress incontinence and its effect on lifestyle appear to be variable. Many women practise pelvic floor exercises ineffectively and some not at all, since doing the exercises competes with all the other demands in the immediate postnatal period. A trial of treatment using pelvic floor exercise education given to women who had persistent stress incontinence at 3 months postpartum found a significant reduction in the number who still had the symptoms at 12 months (Glazener et al 2001).

There is limited information on the postpartum occurrence of urinary tract infections. Glazener et al (1995) found that 5% of women reported a urinary tract infection some time during the first postpartum year. A postpartum urinary tract infection is more common after a caesarean section and a recent Cochrane systematic review has shown that prophylactic antibiotics for women who have abdominal deliveries are effective in reducing the occurrence (Smaill & Hofmeyr 2010).

## Bowel problems

Constipation is common following delivery as the pain of perineal trauma or reduced dietary intake in labour can predispose to it. The few studies that have documented the prevalence of constipation have indicated that it occurs at some time following about 15–20% of births (Glazener et al 1995, Saurel-Cubizolles et al 2000), and is more common after instrumental delivery than after spontaneous vaginal or caesarean deliveries (Glazener et al 1995).

Haemorrhoids are also known to be common after childbirth, and faecal incontinence as well as anal fissure sometimes occur. Haemorrhoids can be extremely painful, but it has generally been considered that most cases regress within a few days of the birth (CKS 2005). However, childbirth-associated haemorrhoids can be longer lasting, with between 15% and 20% of women reporting symptoms at about 2 months after the birth (Glazener et al 1995).

Management should be as per local protocol, but severe, swollen or prolapsed haemorrhoids should be evaluated (NICE 2006). MacArthur et al (1991) found that two-thirds of the women with haemorrhoids still had them at least a year after giving birth, indicating that complete resolution of childbirth-related haemorrhoids is not common. The severity of persisting symptoms, however, is not known. Longer second stage of labour and heavier infant birthweight are associated with an increased likelihood of haemorrhoids (MacArthur et al 1991). Glazener et al (1995) found that they were more than twice as common after instrumental compared with spontaneous vaginal delivery and that women were much less likely to experience haemorrhoids after caesarean section delivery.

One study documented anal fissure, defined as a split or tear in the skin of the anal canal, as occurring in 9% of the women (Corby et al 1997). The authors noted that, without detailed investigation, many of these would have been diagnosed (if at all) as acute painful haemorrhoids, with over 90% of cases resolving without treatment. Type of delivery or perineal trauma were not associated with the occurrence of anal fissure, but postnatal constipation was much more common in the symptomatic group, which is why it is so important that midwives accurately identify and assess this problem by sensitive questioning of the woman. Midwives must also advise women on diet to ensure stools are soft and easily passed. After repair of a third or fourth degree laceration, several weeks of therapy with a stool softener, such as docusate sodium (colace), to minimize the potential for repair breakdown from straining during defecation, is recommended. Pain relief must be offered to reduce the risk of this adding to the fear of defecation (Premkumar 2005).

The occurrence of postpartum faecal incontinence, including frank incontinence, soiling and faecal urgency, is increasingly being documented. One factor associated with the development of faecal incontinence is birth injury, in particular third or fourth degree tear or disruption of the external anal sphincter muscle (Christianson et al 2003, Fenner et al 2003, Sultan et al 1999). Estimates of prevalence of faecal incontinence range from 17% to 62% if there has been severe perineal trauma at delivery, or forceps delivery. Prophylactic antibiotics can be helpful in preventing infection and breakdown of perineal wounds following third or fourth degree tears and reducing the risk of faecal incontinence (Duggal et al 2008). In addition to third or fourth degree tears, the main risk factor for postpartum faecal incontinence is instrumental delivery (Assassa et al 2000, MacArthur et al 1997, MacArthur et al 2001).

It had been considered that although obstetric injury was probably the most common cause of faecal incontinence in women, symptoms were unlikely to occur (except after a third or fourth degree tear) until later in life. Epidemiological studies of unselected obstetric populations have found that between 1% and 10% of women reported postpartum faecal incontinence. Wilson et al (1996) documented 4.9% with 'faecal incontinence' and MacArthur et al (2001) found that 9.6% reported 'losing control of bowel motions between visits to the toilet at some time since the birth'. Hay-Smith et al (2008) reported that I in 10 women leak faeces following childbirth. Studies using endosonography and manometry to image the anal sphincter muscles have obtained data on symptoms of faecal and flatus incontinence and found even higher prevalences (Sultan et al 1993). These populations, however, are smaller and include women who agree to have the anal investigative techniques, who are therefore likely to have higher symptom rates.

Pathophysiological studies have shown that childbirth-associated structural damage to the anal sphincter is more likely to be a cause of faecal incontinence than are neurological factors affecting the pelvic floor. One small study has shown that women who had symptomless anal sphincter defects after a first birth were at higher risk of developing symptoms of faecal incontinence after a second delivery (Fynes et al 1999).

Caesarean section delivery is associated with lower symptom rates but faecal incontinence has been documented after emergency procedures. First or second degree perineal laceration has not been shown to be associated with an increased risk of faecal incontinence, nor generally has episiotomy. Women with faecal incontinence must be referred for treatment (NICE 2006).

## Perineal problems

Most women who have a vaginal delivery will have a degree of perineal pain. It is probably one of the most commonly experienced immediate postpartum symptoms (Sleep 1995). Studies have shown that at least a third of women report experiencing a painful perineum soon after birth, but it can be more persistent. When women complain of perineal discomfort, the perineum should be inspected for any signs of inadequate repair, wound breakdown, delay in the healing process or infection, and appropriate advice given or referral made (NICE 2006).

Some women experience dyspareunia, defined as pain or discomfort during sexual intercourse, which can be related to perineal problems. There is little information on the prevalence of dyspareunia or any other sexual problem, possibly because of the sensitivity of the subject and the reluctance of women to seek medical consultation. If a woman expresses anxiety about resuming intercourse, reasons should be explored with her and a water-based lubricant gel may be advised to ease discomfort during sexual intercourse (NICE 2006). Further evaluation would be required if problems continue to be experienced. Brown & Lumley (1998) found that 26% of women at 6–7 months postpartum reported that they had experienced 'a sexual problem' at some time since the birth. At 8 weeks postpartum, Glazener et al (1995) showed that among the women who had attempted sexual intercourse, 28% had found this to be sore or difficult and 9% reported a lack of interest in sex. In another study it was found that 62% recalled experiencing dyspareunia some time in the first 3 months and 31% still had this at 6 months (Barrett et al 2000).

The main risk factors for perineal pain and dyspareunia relate to the type of delivery and perineal trauma. Instrumental deliveries are associated with much higher rates of perineal pain, both immediate and longer term, than are spontaneous vaginal deliveries, and caesarean sections are associated with the lowest rates (Brown & Lumley 1998, Glazener et al 1995). The pattern of association with mode of delivery is similar for dyspareunia, although the differences are less marked (Barrett et al 2000, Brown & Lumley 1998).

Descriptions from women have suggested that there is more perineal discomfort following an episiotomy than there is after a laceration and several randomized controlled trials have been undertaken to examine this issue. A Cochrane systematic review (Carroli & Mignini 2008), including eight trials on this topic, concluded that there is little evidence to justify episiotomy as a means of limiting postpartum perineal pain. The effects on perineal pain and dyspareunia of different materials used and of different suture methods are described in Chapter 40.

## Musculoskeletal system

Overall, the musculoskeletal system of the parturient woman seems to be more sensitive to various forms of injury, probably because of the laxity of ligaments resulting from the effects of progesterone and relaxin in pregnancy continuing in the postnatal period, changes in posture and positioning during the birth.

### Backache

Numerous studies undertaken in the postnatal period have documented backache with prevalences that seem to be greater than that among the general population. The range of prevalence estimates of postpartum backache is wide, from 20% to 50%, (Breen et al 1994, Brown & Lumley 1998, Glazener et al 1995, Groves et al 1994, Saurel-Cubizolles et al 2000).

In a study examining postpartum backache and its risk factors in primiparous women, Russell et al (1993) found that 29% had backache that lasted for more than 6 months after the birth, and for 15% this was new backache starting since the birth. Backache during or before pregnancy is a predisposing factor for postpartum back pain (Breen et al 1994, Östgaard & Andersson 1992, Turgut et al 1998) and some studies have found physically heavy work during pregnancy to be a risk factor (Östgaard & Andersson 1992). Epidural anaesthesia during labour has been associated with subsequent longer-term backache (Brown & Lumley 1998, Russell et al 1993) but other studies have found no association (Breen et al 1994, MacArthur et al 1995). The postulated mechanism to account for a possible association relates to stressed positions in labour, women might remain for some time in a potentially damaging position. In addition, the physical demands of childcare, lifting, bending, carrying and feeding, especially as the child increases in size, are likely to be related to the occurrence of backache.

No specific studies have examined this, but the longitudinal studies have not shown postpartum backache to reduce over time (Glazener et al 1995, Saurel-Cubizolles et al 2000). Back pain is managed as in the general population (NICE 2006). An updated Cochrane review (Roelofs et al 2008) suggested that non-steroidal anti-inflammatory drugs are effective for short-term symptomatic relief. However, the effect sizes are small and there is moderate evidence that they are not more effective than paracetamol, which has fewer side-effects (Roelofs et al 2008).

### Pelvic girdle pain

Owens et al (2003) reported an incidence of pelvic girdle pain, formally known as symphysis pubis dysfunction, of 1 in 36 in their study, which suggests the condition is more common than previously thought. An early referral should be made to the physiotherapist so that an assessment of mobility needs may be made. Regular analgesia should be provided and help with positioning for breastfeeding and babycare activities. An occupational therapist or social services advisor should be consulted about the provision of aids and equipment that may be required in order to enable the mother to cope at home.

When menstruation returns, some women may have a recurrence of symptoms. Though these may resolve within a couple of months, they may persist for longer. It is likely to recur and becomes more severe in subsequent pregnancies (Owens et al 2003). The Association of Chartered Physiotherapists in Women's Health have produced a leaflet, *Pregnancy-related pelvic girdle pain* (ACPWH 2007), to provide information and advice to women.

### Other problems

Pain and weakness in the arms and legs commencing after birth and persisting for months or even years was reported four times as often among Asian women as compared with Caucasian women in a study by MacArthur et al (1991). This could be caused by vitamin D deficiency, accentuated by the extra demands and postural stresses of pregnancy and delivery (MacArthur et al 1993a).

Paraesthesias in the legs, buttocks and lower back have been reported. MacArthur et al (1991, 1992) found that these paraesthesias, as well as those in the fingers and hands, although rare, were more common in women who had used epidural anaesthesia. Dizziness, fainting and visual disturbances, although again rare, were also more common after epidural anaesthesia and after spinal and general anaesthesia (MacArthur et al 1992).

## Headache

The occurrence of short-duration postpartum headaches, in at least a quarter of women, has been reported (Stein et al 1984) and longer-term headaches have also been documented (Glazener et al 1993, Russell et al 1993). Management of mild headache should be based on differential diagnosis of headache type and treatment as per local protocols (NICE 2006). Most postpartum headaches are probably tension-type or 'simple' headaches, but the studies that have examined headache among postnatal women have not generally specified headache type. Advice on relaxation techniques and avoidance of factors associated with the onset should be offered. Severe or persistent headache, especially associated with the other symptoms of pre-eclampsia in the early postnatal period, should be referred for treatment (NICE 2006).

MacArthur et al (1991, 1993b) found that frequent headaches in association with backache were more common in women who had had epidural anaesthesia (see Ch. 38). Headaches without backache, however, were more common in younger, lower social class women with more than one child. Headache is a common complaint, generally related to stress and fatigue.

## Fatigue

Tiredness in the early postpartum period is well recognized anecdotally, not surprisingly owing to the demands of childbirth, the additional childcare load and sleeplessness associated with night feeding. However, many women report longer-term exhaustion, which can have a significant effect on their relationships, social activities, employment and psychological health. Women rarely consult a doctor about this, possibly because they perceive it as normal at this time, or not a 'medical problem' (Bick & MacArthur 1995). Glazener et al (1993) found that 59% of the sample reported tiredness between hospital discharge and 8 weeks and 54% between then and 18 months. Brown & Lumley (1998) documented that at 6–7 months, 69% of women had experienced tiredness/exhaustion as a problem some time since the birth. In an Audit Commission study (Garcia et al 1998), women who were questioned four months postpartum said they had experienced fatigue or severe tiredness at times; 43% at 10 days, 31% at one month and 21% at 3 months. MacArthur et al (1991) asked about extreme tiredness and found that 12% of the women reported never having had such extreme tiredness before; half of these women saying it had lasted for longer than a year.

Various risk factors for postpartum fatigue shown in studies include older maternal age, being unmarried, having twins and breastfeeding (Milligan & Pugh 1994, Saurel-Cubizolles et al 2000). No significant relationship has been shown between longer-term fatigue and type of delivery, although caesarean section has been associated with increased short-term fatigue (Glazener et al 1995).

MacArthur et al (1991) found that women who had experienced postpartum haemorrhage reported more tiredness, which could plausibly be related to a low haemoglobin level. Postpartum haemorrhage still poses a risk of morbidity and mortality and estimating blood loss at birth from soaked pads and bedlinen can be challenging (NICE 2006). Postpartum anaemia is often poorly managed and Bodnar et al (2005) concluded that it warrants greater attention and higher-quality care. Haemoglobin testing is not a routine postnatal practice and it is often down to the individual women to seek treatment (Evans 2008). If women do report their tiredness and receive a prescription for iron tablets, the side-effects, most commonly constipation, may result in them taking the tablets sporadically.

One small study by Bhandal & Russell (2006) compared women having oral iron to correct postpartum anaemia with women given intravenous iron. Women treated with intravenous iron had significantly higher Hb levels on days 5 and 14 ($P < 0.01$) than those treated with oral iron, but by day 40 there was no significant difference between the two groups. More research is required to investigate the safety of this strategy. Liquid iron supplements which have higher absorption rates and reduced side-effects may be easier to continue for long-term therapy when tolerance is poor (Evans 2008). Advice about a well-balanced iron-rich diet should be provided by professionals who are knowledgeable about foods that can inhibit or enhance absorption.

Fatigue is commonly reported in association with depression and anxiety (Glazener et al 1993), although which problem arises first is not known. Brown & Lumley (2000) found that tiredness was over three times more likely to be reported by women with high scores on the Edinburgh Postnatal Depression Score (see Ch. 69).

### Depression

A study in Australia demonstrated a relationship between physical health after birth and postnatal depression and fatigue (Brown & Lumley 2000). It is important, therefore, that health professionals ensure that depression in postpartum women is identified and treated (see Ch. 69). There is accumulating evidence of the adverse effects of postpartum depression on the cognitive and emotional development of the child (Cooper & Murray 1998).

## EXTENT OF LONGER-TERM MORBIDITY

MacArthur et al (1991) found that most symptoms lasted much longer than 6 weeks: 35% of the women reported new symptoms lasting over a year and 31% still had unresolved symptoms at the time of questioning, which was between 2 and 9 years after the birth of their most recent child, indicating that many women experience childbirth-related morbidity that becomes chronic. Since the recall period in this study was lengthy for some women, it is likely that some health problems that lasted for only a few weeks or were relatively minor may not have been reported. These levels of postpartum morbidity were confirmed in a later study (Bick & MacArthur 1995).

Glazener et al (1995) also identified considerable morbidity, with the prevalence of some symptoms reducing substantially over time but not that of others. A European longitudinal study of health after birth and mothers' work, in Italy and France (Saurel-Cubizolles et al 2000), generally found very high symptom prevalences and for most symptoms these had increased at 12 months.

## MEDICAL CONSULTATION

Even though studies have shown that many women experience health problems after childbirth, it has consistently been shown that these are often not reported to a relevant health professional (Brown & Lumley 1998, Glazener et al 1995). The proportion of women in one study who said they had consulted a doctor was on average only about a third (MacArthur et al 1991). There could be many reasons for this lack of consultation. The symptom might only be mild or occur infrequently; the problem might be considered by the woman as 'normal' after having a baby; or she may have thought that there is nothing that a doctor could do. For some symptoms it may be embarrassment that accounts for a woman not seeking professional help. Whatever the reason, the effect of this lack of consultation is that the full extent of the postpartum morbidity has remained unrecognized by health professionals, and women are left with unmet health needs.

Several randomized controlled trials of revisions to current postnatal care have been undertaken to assess if improvements in maternal health outcomes could be achieved (Gunn et al 1998, MacArthur et al 2003, Morrell et al 2000). These studies differed substantially in the content of the intervention but there were no documented improvements in maternal physical health in any of the studies. Maternal satisfaction scores were higher than controls in two of the studies (Gunn et al 1998, MacArthur et al 2003) and maternal mental health scores were significantly better than controls in one study (MacArthur et al 2003).

**Reflective activity 52.1**

Use the information in this chapter to devise a symptom checklist to find out about symptoms that women may experience after childbirth.

Have a consultation with a woman in the first month after giving birth and use the checklist. Find out if she has reported any of her symptoms, if not, why, and how they might be affecting her life. Refer to the NICE guideline 37 (2006) to assess the recommendations for their management.

## IMPLICATIONS FOR MIDWIVES

Health problems after childbirth continue well past the routine discharge from maternity services and many remain unreported to the health services. This has implications for midwives and other members of the primary care team in developing strategies to identify as well as provide for women's postpartum health requirements. There will be considerable variation in the health needs of individual women and care should be tailored flexibly to take this into account. Midwives must provide a high standard of care using the best available evidence (NMC 2008) and so must ensure that their skills and knowledge are up to date and that they keep clear and accurate records to support the health and wellbeing of the women in their care. When a deviation from the norm occurs which is outside the midwife's sphere of practice, then an appropriate referral should be made to a qualified health professional who may reasonably be expected to have the necessary skills and experience to assist in providing care for the woman (NMC 2004). All relevant information must be shared with the multidisciplinary team (NMC 2008).

**KEY POINTS**

- Women can experience a range of health issues following childbirth, including physical and psychological problems.
- NICE has provided guidelines for postnatal care and highlighted potential problems with appropriate status levels indicating the degree of urgency for dealing with them.
- Some problems are associated with particular birth factors, some with postpartum, maternal or childcare characteristics.
- Many problems currently remain as unmet needs since women often do not report them and midwives and other health professionals do not always identify them.

## REFERENCES


Allen RE, Hosker GL, Smith ARB, et al: Pelvic floor damage and childbirth: a neurophysiological study, *British Journal of Obstetrics and Gynaecology* 97(9):770–779, 1990.

Assassa RP, Dallosso S, Perry C, et al and the Leicestershire MRC Incontinence Study Team: The association between obstetric factors and incontinence: a community survey, *British Journal of Obstetrics and Gynaecology* 107(6):822, 2000.

Association of Chartered Physiotherapists in Women's Health (ACPWH): *Pregnancy-related pelvic girdle pain* (website). www.acpwh.org.uk/docs/ACPWH-PGP_HP.pdf. 2007. Accessed July 2009.

Barrett G, Pendry E, Peacock J, et al: Women's sexual health after childbirth, *British Journal of Obstetrics and Gynaecology* 107(2):186–195, 2000.

Bhandal N, Russell R: Intravenous versus oral iron therapy for postpartum anaemia, *British Journal of Gynaecology* 113(11):1248–1252, 2006.

Bick DE, MacArthur C: The extent, severity and effect of health problems after childbirth, *British Journal of Midwifery* 3(i):27–31, 1995.

Bodnar LM, Cogswell ME, McDonald T: Have we forgotten the significance of postnatal iron deficiency? *American Journal of Obstetrics and Gynecology* 193(1):36–44, 2005.

Breen TW, Ransil J, Groves PA, et al: Factors associated with back pain after childbirth, *Anesthesiology* 81(6):29–34, 1994.

Brown S, Lumley J: Maternal health after childbirth: results of an Australian population based survey, *British Journal of Obstetrics and Gynaecology* 105(2):156–161, 1998.

Brown S, Lumley J: Physical health problems after childbirth and maternal depression at six to seven months postpartum, *British Journal of Obstetrics and Gynaecology* 107(10):1194–1201, 2000.

Carroli G, Mignini L: Episiotomy for vaginal birth, *Cochrane Database of Systematic Reviews* (3):CD000081, 2008.

Christianson LM, Bovbjerg VE, McDavitt E, et al: Risk factors for perineal injury during delivery, *American Journal of Obstetrics and Gynecology* 189(1):255–260, 2003.

CKS: 'Haemorrhoids' *Clinical Knowledge Summaries Service, Clinical Topic* (website). www.cks.library.nhs.uk. 2005. Accesssed June 2009.

Cooper P, Murray L: Postnatal depression, *British Medical Journal* 316(7148):1884–1886, 1998.

Corby H, Donnelly VS, O'Herlihy C, et al: Anal canal pressures are low in women with postpartum anal fissure, *British Journal of Surgery* 84(1):86–88, 1997.

Duggal N, Mercado C, Daniels K, et al: Antibiotic prophylaxis can prevent postpartum perineal wound complications, *Obstetrics and Gynecology* 111(6):1268–1273, 2008.

Evans M: Iron deficiency through the female life cycle – who needs to care? *MIDIRS Midwifery Digest* 18(3):404–408, 2008.

Fenner DE, Genberg B, Brahma P, et al: Fecal and urinary incontinence after vaginal delivery with anal sphincter disruption in an obstetrics unit in the United States, *American Journal of Obstetrics and Gynecology* 189(6):1543–1549, 2003.

Fynes M, Donnelly V, Behan M, et al: Effect of second vaginal delivery on anorectal physiology and faecal continence: a prospective study, *Lancet* 354(9183):983–986, 1999.

Garcia J, Redshaw M, Fitzsimons B, et al: *First class delivery. A national survey of women's views of maternity care*, Abingdon, 1998, Audit Commission.

Glazener CMA, Abdalla M, Russell I, et al: Postnatal care: a survey of patients' experiences, *British Journal of Midwifery* 1(2):67–74, 1993.

Glazener CMA, Abdalla M, Shroud P, et al: Postnatal maternal morbidity: extent, causes, prevention and treatment, *British Journal of Obstetrics and Gynaecology* 102(4):282–287, 1995.

Glazener CMA, Herbison GP, Wilson PD, et al: Conservative management of persistent postnatal urinary and faecal incontinence: a randomised controlled trial, *British Medical Journal* 323(7313):593–596, 2001.

Glazener CMA, Herbison GP, MacArthur C, et al: Randomised controlled trial of conservative management of postnatal urinary and faecal incontinence: six year follow up, *British Medical Journal* 330(7487):337–339, 2005.

Groves PA, Breen TW, Ransil BJ, et al: Natural history of post partum back pain and its relationship with epidural anesthesia, *Anesthesiology* 81(3A):A1167, 1994.

Gunn J, Lumley J, Chondros P, et al: Does an early postnatal check-up improve maternal health: results from a randomised controlled trial, *British Journal of Obstetrics and Gynaecology* 105(9):991–997, 1998.

Hay-Smith J, Mørkved S, Fairbrother KA, et al: Pelvic floor muscle training for prevention and treatment of urinary and faecal incontinence in antenatal and postnatal women, *Cochrane Database of Systematic Reviews* (4):CD007471, 2008.

Leah L, Albers CNM: Health problems after childbirth, *Journal of Midwifery and Women's Health* 45(1):55–57, 2000.

MacArthur C, Lewis M, Knox EG: *Health after childbirth*, London, 1991, HMSO.

MacArthur C, Lewis M, Knox EG: Investigation of long-term problems after obstetric epidural anaesthesia, *British Medical Journal* 304(6837):1279–1282, 1992.

MacArthur C, Lewis M, Knox EG: Comparison of long-term health problems following childbirth in Asian and Caucasian women, *British Journal of General Practice* 43(377):519–522, 1993a.

MacArthur C, Lewis M, Knox EG: Accidental dural puncture in obstetric patients and long-term symptoms, *British Medical Journal* 306(6882):883–885, 1993b.

MacArthur AJ, MacArthur C, Weeks S: Epidural anaesthesia and low back pain after delivery: a prospective cohort study, *British Medical Journal* 311(7016):1336–1339, 1995.

MacArthur C, Bick DE, Keighley MRB: Faecal incontinence after child birth, *British Journal of Obstetrics and Gynaecology* 104(1):46–50, 1997.

MacArthur C, Glazener CMA, Wilson PD, et al: Obstetric practice and faecal incontinence three months after delivery, *British Journal of Obstetrics and Gynaecology* 108(7):678–683, 2001.

MacArthur C, Winter HR, Bick D, et al: Redesigning postnatal care: a randomised controlled trial of protocol-based midwifery-led care focused on individual women's physical and psychological health needs, *Health Technology Assessment* 7(37):1–98, 2003.

Milligan RA, Pugh LC: Fatigue during the childbearing period, *Annual Review of Nursing Research* 12:33–49, 1994.

Morrell CJ, Spiby H, Stewart P, et al: Costs and effectiveness of community postnatal support workers: randomised controlled trial, *British Medical Journal* 321(7261):593–598, 2000.

National Institute for Health and Clinical Excellence (NICE): *Routine postnatal care of women and their babies* (website). www.nice.org.uk. 2006. Accessed August 2008.

Nursing & Midwifery Council (NMC): *Midwives rules and standards*, London, 2004, NMC.

Nursing & Midwifery Council (NMC): *The Code: standards of conduct, performance and ethics for nurses and midwives*, London, 2008, NMC.

Östgaard HC, Andersson GBJ: Postpartum low back pain, *Spine* 17(1):53–55, 1992.

Owens K, Pearson A, Mason G: Symphysis pubis dysfunction: a cause of significant obstetric morbidity, *European Journal of Obstetrics and Gynecology and Reproductive Biology* 105:143–146, 2003.

Pollock L: SUI after childbirth, *Midwives* 7(12):504, 2004.

Premkumar G: Perineal trauma: reducing associated postnatal maternal morbidity, *Midwives* 8(1):30–32, 2005.

Roelofs DDMR, Deyo RA, Koes BW, et al: Nonsteroidal anti-inflammatory drugs for low back pain: an updated Cochrane review, *Spine* 33(16):1766–1774, 2008.

Russell R, Grove P, Taub N, et al: Assessing long-term backache after childbirth, *British Medical Journal* 306(6888):1299–1303, 1993.

Saurel-Cubizolles M-J, Romito P, Lelong N, et al: Women's health after childbirth: a longitudinal study in

France and Italy, *British Journal of Obstetrics and Gynaecology* 107(10):1202–1209, 2000.

Sleep J: Postnatal perineal care revisited. In Alexander J, Levy V, Roch S, editors: *Aspects of midwifery practice: a research based approach*, London, 1995, Macmillan.

Smaill F, Gyte G: Antibiotic prophylaxis versus no prophylaxis for preventing infection after caesarean section, *Cochrane database of Systematic Reviews* (1):CD007482, 2010.

Stein GS, Morton J, Marsh A, et al: Headaches after childbirth, *Acta Neurologica Scandinavica* 69(2):74–79, 1984.

Sultan AH, Kamm MA, Hudson CN, et al: Anal sphincter disruption during vaginal delivery, *New England Journal of Medicine* 329(26):1905–1911, 1993.

Sultan AH, Monga AK, Kumar D, et al: Primary repair of obstetric anal sphincter rupture using the overlap technique, *British Journal of Obstetrics and Gynaecology* 106(3):318–323, 1999.

Turgut F, Turgut M, Cetinsahin M: A prospective study of persistent back pain after pregnancy, *European Journal of Obstetrics and Gynecology and Reproductive Biology* 80(1):45–48, 1998.

Viktrup L, Lose G: The risk of stress incontinence 5 years after first delivery, *American Journal of Obstetrics and Gynecology* 185(1):82–87, 2001.

Wilson PD, Herbison RM, Herbison GP: Obstetric practice and the prevalence of urinary incontinence three months after delivery, *British Journal of Obstetrics and Gynaecology* 103(2):154–161, 1996.

Zaki M, Pandit M, Jackson S: National survey for intrapartum and postpartum bladder care: assessing the need for guidelines, *BJOG: An International Journal of Obstetrics and Gynaecology* 111(8):874–876, 2004.

# Part | 9 |

# Problems and disorders of pregnancy, childbearing and birth and their management

Chapter |53|

# Nausea and vomiting

*Cecelia M. Bartholomew*

## LEARNING OUTCOMES

After reading this chapter, you will be able to:

- define and differentiate between physiological and pathological vomiting in pregnancy
- plan and implement appropriate midwifery action
- discuss management and possible treatments, including self help strategies
- discuss the possible consequences for mother and baby.

Nausea and vomiting are common symptoms in pregnancy, occurring in up to 90% of normal pregnancies. The dyad is often regarded as normal and a presumptive sign of pregnancy. However, the conditions may range from mild to severe, which in the latter is pathological where it can become debilitating and life-threatening to women and their fetuses. Severe vomiting is strongly associated with multiple pregnancy, hydatidiform mole and pre-eclampsia.

*Nausea* is the feeling of impending vomiting, while *vomiting* consists of retching and expulsion (Pleuvry 2006). The physiology of both reflexes is integrative and multifaceted, involving autonomic and somatic neural pathways (Palmer et al 2002). It has been postulated that they occur when the vomiting centres in the brain, situated in the lateral reticular formation of the medulla, are stimulated by the chemoreceptor trigger zones in the floor of the fourth ventricle and vagal afferents from the gut (Kumar & Clark 2001). This is despite there being no distinct anatomical vomiting centre to be located in this region of the brain (Pleuvry 2006).

There have been several theories that have been used to elucidate the function of nausea and vomiting in pregnancy. One of these suggests that through the consequential lessening of energy intake, there is a reduction of *insulin* and *insulin growth hormone-1*, which facilitates diversion of nutrients, for example, glucose from the maternal cells to the placenta and fetus in early pregnancy (Huxley 2000). Flaxman & Sherman (2008) highlight another hypothesis regarding the prophylactic benefit of nausea and vomiting to enable expulsion of foods which may contain harmful toxins and micro-organisms that trigger aversions to such foods throughout pregnancy. The specific role of nausea and vomiting remains unknown. However, Flaxman & Sherman (2008) suggest the prophylaxis hypothesis is more consistent with patterns of cravings and aversions observed in some women and societies.

The aetiology of the conditions in pregnancy is also poorly understood and the literature suggests a multiplicity of probable origins. Reviews by Davis (2004) and Verberg et al (2005) highlight factors that are predominantly promulgated as causes. These include *rising levels of hormones*, including *oestrogen, progesterone, human chorionic gonadotrophin (hCG), thyroxine* ($T_4$) and *thyroid stimulating hormone (TSH)*. This may be compounded by *physiological adaptations* to pregnancy, such as reduced gastric motility or reflux oesophagitis, and *metabolic alterations*, such as carbohydrate and vitamin B deficiency. A presumed anatomical positioning of a *right-sided corpus luteum* is also thought to cause high concentrations of sex steroids in the hepatic portal system, which induce nausea and vomiting. Female fetal sex has also been shown to be associated with the symptoms (Tan et al 2006).

While there are limited data to support the *psychogenic origins* of nausea and vomiting, 21st-century medical texts continue to suggest a link (Davis 2004). Prejudice towards women appears to have guided such concepts, which are currently being replaced by biological (Sostre et al 2008) and sociocultural theories (Munch 2002). Midwives need to be aware of the debate to ensure that they do not stereotype women and impede adequate treatment of the conditions. It is premature to advocate that there is no psychological basis for nausea and vomiting, as there appears to be an integration of various elements incorporating psychogenic, sociocultural and biological causes (Buckwalter & Simpson 2002).

## MILD AND MODERATE VOMITING IN PREGNANCY

*Mild* vomiting is an unpleasant but transient and self-limiting condition that commonly appears in the fifth week of pregnancy and peaks in severity at around 11–13 weeks. It usually resolves by 16–20 weeks (NCC-WCH 2008). The typical manifestation is that women feel nauseated on waking, and may vomit on rising from bed. Women may complain of an increased sense of smell, which initiates feelings of nausea that leads to aversion of some foods (Davis 2004). Actual vomiting recedes during the day, but nausea may persist.

*Moderate* vomiting is more serious, as the woman will vomit several times during the day, often after meals, and this may be accompanied by some weight loss and ketonuria. The fetus appears to fare well with mild and moderate vomiting (Davis 2004).

## HYPEREMESIS GRAVIDARUM

*Hyperemesis gravidarum* is a pathological condition characterized by unremitting, severe vomiting in pregnancy. It occurs in 0.3–2.0% of pregnancies and is more common in women who are younger, non-smokers and non-Caucasian (Ismail & Kenny 2007). It is diagnosed by exclusion (Kametas & Nelson-Piercy 2008) and is a leading cause of hospital admission during pregnancy (Cedergren et al 2008).

Studies have shown that a gastric infection caused by the *Helicobacter pylori* bacterium may also be linked to hyperemesis gravidarum (Golberg et al 2007). The infection responds well to antibiotic therapy, such as *erythromycin* or *clarithromycin*.

Hyperemesis gravidarum is associated with significant weight loss, ketonaemia, electrolyte imbalance and dehydration, together with hepatic, central nervous system and renal damage (Holmgren et al 2008). On examination, the woman may have sunken eyes, loss of skin elasticity, parched mouth and lips, ketonuria and/or oliguria. The woman may appear jaundiced as the condition worsens. *Oesophageal tears* (Mallory–Weiss syndrome) and *haematemesis* may occur because of the trauma produced by the persistent vomiting.

Wernicke's encephalopathy is a rare but serious complication that has been reported in women with severe hyperemesis gravidarum (Indraccolo et al 2005). It is a neuropsychiatric syndrome that is caused by severe thiamine (vitamin $B_1$) deficiency because of the persistent vomiting (Sechi & Serra 2007). It is manifest by signs of confusion, ocular abnormalities and ataxia (Chiossi et al 2006). Diagnosis may be confirmed through low red cell transketolase or an enhanced magnetic resonance imaging (MRI) scan (Kametas & Nelson-Piercy 2008). The condition responds well to thiamine (Welsh 2005).

In mild, moderate or severe cases, there appears to be a decreased risk of miscarriage, stillbirth and preterm delivery (Welsh 2005), though in very severe cases, fetal growth restriction and fetal death may also be a consequence (Turner 2007).

## CARE AND MANAGEMENT

The care and management of nausea and vomiting in pregnancy depends on the intensity of the symptoms (Davis 2004), requiring a multidisciplinary approach. The initial assessment of severity by the midwife is pivotal.

### Mild nausea and vomiting

The midwife should explain to women with *mild* nausea and vomiting that in most cases the condition will improve spontaneously within 16 to 20 weeks of gestation, with good pregnancy outcome (NCC-WCH 2008). Medication is not usually required and the woman should be advised to rest as much as possible, as tiredness and stress may exacerbate the vomiting. Frequent, small, light meals with a reduction in fatty, spicy or strong-smelling foods; a milky drink at bedtime and dry toast or a biscuit before rising; carbonated drinks, such as soda or non-alcoholic dry ginger ale, if required during the day, have been reported to alleviate the symptoms.

**Reflective activity 53.1**

Contact your local hospital dietician. What dietary modifications does he/she recommend to reduce nausea and vomiting in pregnancy?

Complementary remedies (see Ch. 18) and supplements such as vitamin $B_6$ and ginger are often useful; however, the midwife may not use any complementary therapy for her clients unless she is properly qualified in that field

(NMC 2008). Concerns about the possible toxicity of high doses of vitamin $B_6$ have not yet been resolved. Therefore, in the UK the recommended upper limit of 10 mg should not be exceeded (NCC-WCH 2008). Alternatively, ginger can be useful. It accelerates gastric emptying (Wu et al 2008) and has been found to be as effective as vitamin $B_6$ (Ensiyeh & Sakineh 2009) with no evidence of teratogenicity (Jewell & Young 2003).

Acupuncture and acupressure using the P6 point may also relieve vomiting in pregnancy. The evidence regarding its effectiveness is mixed but it appears to be more efficient than changes in diet or lifestyle (Jewell & Young 2003).

Although not clinically ill, the woman often feels miserable and her symptoms should not be regarded as trivial. Therefore, empathic support is paramount. Her partner and family will also need reassurance and guidance on how to provide assistance during this time.

## Moderate vomiting and hyperemesis

If the woman is experiencing *moderate* vomiting or suspected *hyperemesis gravidarum*, the midwife should arrange for her to be admitted to hospital without delay. She should be cared for in a single room if possible, to avoid undue disturbance. A urinalysis is conducted for ketones, bilirubin, protein and glucose, and a midstream specimen of urine is sent for culture to exclude pyelonephritis.

Antihistamines such as *promethazine hydrochloride, prochlorperazine (Stemetil) metoclopramide (Maxolon, Primperan)* (Jewell & Young 2003) or corticosteroids such as *methylprednisolone* (Ismail & Kenny 2007) are considered safe to use in pregnancy and may be utilized to control the nausea and vomiting.

Blood tests, such as aspartate aminotransferase (AST), alanine aminotransferase (ALT), urea and electrolytes, are required to assess renal and liver function. An ultrasound scan may also be useful to eliminate hydatidiform mole and multiple pregnancy as probable causes. A frequent record of the woman's weight, temperature, pulse and blood pressure is essential to monitor her wellbeing. In addition, the fetal heart rate should be appropriately auscultated (depending on the gestation) to monitor the health of the fetus.

**Reflective activity 53.2**

Locate and read your local policy for management of severe vomiting in pregnancy.

With moderate vomiting, dietary advice may help, but often the woman continues to vomit and will begin to show signs of dehydration. In cases of severe vomiting, nothing is given by mouth. Intravenous fluids with careful record of fluid balance may be essential to correct dehydration, particularly with hyperemesis gravidarum. Normal saline or Ringer's lactate (Hartmann's) solution with added potassium is commonly administered to restore the electrolyte balance. As carbohydrate increases the demand for thiamine (Sechi & Serra 2007), fluids containing dextrose should be avoided to prevent the development of Wernicke's encephalopathy (Kametas & Nelson-Piercy 2008).

In life-threatening cases of hyperemesis gravidarum, slow-drip enteral feeding may follow and total parenteral nutrition (TPN), supplemented by thiamine 100 mg daily, may be necessary (Ismail & Kenny 2007). However, such aggressive management should be a last option as both methods carry maternal risks such as life-threatening sepsis and thrombosis (Holmgren et al 2008).

Moderate vomiting usually ceases quickly and once the woman is tolerating a normal diet she may be discharged home. Most women with hyperemesis gravidarum will experience relief within 2–3 days and the vomiting is less likely to recur than when conventional antiemetics are used. Once the vomiting ceases, oral fluids and food may be gradually reintroduced and the woman may be discharged when she is taking and tolerating a normal diet and gaining weight.

In rare cases, termination of the pregnancy is considered if the vomiting is intractable and there are signs of major organ failure, such as persistent pyrexia or hypothermia, persistent tachycardia, jaundice, persistent proteinuria, polyneuritis or encephalopathy.

**Reflective activity 53.3**

Talk to women about their experiences of nausea and vomiting in pregnancy, especially their knowledge and beliefs about its causes, duration and treatment.

## EATING DISORDERS AND VOMITING IN PREGNANCY

Nausea and vomiting together with amenorrhoea are features of eating disorders such as anorexia nervosa and bulimia nervosa. One recent study found nausea and vomiting in pregnancy to be increased in women with anorexia nervosa and bulimia nervosa (Torgersen et al 2008). A pregnancy may go undetected for some time in a woman who is affected by the above. Alternatively, an existing eating disorder accompanied by such features may not become apparent as it may be mistaken for a normal aspect of a pregnancy. Fear for the health of the child may lead those affected to control and hide their symptoms. Some studies have reported that in most cases there is an apparent improvement in the eating disorder but there is regression to the pre-pregnancy state or even deterioration in the condition after giving birth (Rocco et al 2005).

Women with active eating disorders are at risk of delivering babies who are small for gestational age or with low birthweight (Koubaa et al 2005). Midwives need to be aware of suggestive signs of the eating disorders and discuss the risks of undernutrition in pregnancy (Franko & Spurrell 2000). The midwife and obstetrician need to closely monitor the pregnancy and there should be adequate support for the woman and her family to address the conditions in the postnatal period.

## CONCLUSION

Nausea and vomiting in pregnancy are common and unpleasant but the more serious and potentially life-threatening condition of hyperemesis gravidarum is fortunately rare. Some cases may be avoided if the vomiting is treated promptly and effectively. The midwife should invest time in initial assessment and identification of women who may be at risk, and ensure that support with information is available to them. The midwife should be able to differentiate between physiological and pathological vomiting and manage or refer according to severity.

### KEY POINTS

- Nausea and vomiting are common occurrences in pregnancy, but may, on rare occasions, become pathological.
- Informed and appropriate midwifery care and advice can make the discomfort tolerable for the woman.
- The midwife must be able to distinguish between physiological and pathological pregnancy vomiting and take appropriate action.
- The woman can be reassured that her baby is unlikely to come to any harm due to vomiting or medication used to control it.
- Midwives need to be aware of suggestive signs of eating disorders in women who present with nausea and vomiting.

## REFERENCES


Buckwalter JG, Simpson SW: Psychological factors in the etiology and treatment of severe nausea and vomiting in pregnancy, *American Journal of Obstetrics and Gynecology* 186(5):s210–s214, 2002.

Cedergren M, Brynhildsen J, Josefsson A, et al: Hyperemesis gravidarum that requires hospitalization and the use of antiemetic drugs in relation to maternal body composition, *American Journal of Obstetrics and Gynecology* 198(4):412.e1–412.e5, 2008.

Chiossi G, Neri I, Cavazzuti M, et al: Hyperemesis gravidarum complicated by Wernicke encephalopathy: background, case report, and review of the literature, *Obstetrics and Gynecological Survey* 61(4):255–268, 2006.

Davis M: Nausea and vomiting of pregnancy: an evidence-based review, *Journal of Perinatal and Neonatal Nursing* 18(4):312–328, 2004.

Ensiyeh J, Sakineh MAC: Comparing ginger and vitamin B6 for the treatment of nausea and vomiting in pregnancy: a randomised controlled trial, *Midwifery* 25(6):649–653, 2009.

Flaxman SM, Sherman PW: Morning sickness: adaptive cause or nonadaptive consequence of embryo viability? *The American Naturalist* 172(1):54–62, 2008.

Franko DL, Spurrell EB: Detection and management of eating disorders during pregnancy, *Obstetrics and Gynecology* 95(6 Pt 1):942–946, 2000.

Golberg D, Szilagyi A, Graves L: Hyperemesis gravidarum and Helicobacter pylori infection. A systematic review, *Obstetrics and Gynecology* 110(3):695–703, 2007.

Holmgren C, Aagaard-Tillery KM, Silver RM, et al: Hyperemesis in pregnancy: an evaluation of treatment strategies with maternal and neonatal outcomes, *American Journal of Obstetrics and Gynecology* 198(1):56.e1–56.e4, 2008.

Huxley R: Nausea and vomiting in early pregnancy: its role in placental development, *Obstetrics and Gynecology* 95(5):779–782, 2000.

Indraccolo U, Gentile G, Pomili GD, et al: Thiamine deficiency and beriberi features in a patient with hyperemesis gravidarum, *Nutrition* 21(9):967–968, 2005.

Ismail SK, Kenny L: Review on hyperemesis gravidarum, *Best Practice & Research. Clinical Gastroenterology* 21(5):755–769, 2007.

Jewell D, Young G: Interventions for nausea and vomiting in early pregnancy, *Cochrane Database of Systematic Reviews* (4):CD000145, 2003.

Kametas NA, Nelson-Piercy C: Hyperemesis gravidarum, gastrointestinal and liver disease in pregnancy, *Obstetrics, Gynaecology and Reproductive Medicine* 18(3):69–75, 2008.

Koubaa S, Hällström T, Lindholm C, et al: Pregnancy and neonatal outcomes in women with eating disorders, *Obstetrics and Gynecology* 105(2):255–260, 2005.

Kumar P, Clark M: Gastroenterology. In Kumar P, Clark M, editors: *Clinical medicine*, ed 4, Edinburgh, 2001, WB Saunders.

Munch S: Chicken or the egg? The biological-psychological controversy surrounding hyperemesis gravidarum, *Social Science and Medicine* 55(7):1267–1278, 2002.

National Collaborative Centre for Women's and Children's Health (NCC-WCH)(2008): *Antenatal care: routine care for the healthy pregnant woman*, London, 2008, RCOG Press.

Nursing and Midwifery Council (NMC): *Standards for medicines management*, London, 2008, NMC.

Palmer KR, Penman ID, Paterson-Brown S: Alimentary tract and pancreatic disease. In Haslett C, Chilvers ER, Boon NA, et al, editors: *Davidson's principles and practice of medicine*, ed 19, Edinburgh, 2002, Churchill Livingstone.

Pleuvry BJ: Physiology and pharmacology of nausea and vomiting, *Anaesthesia and Intensive Care Medicine* 7(12):473–477, 2006.

Rocco PL, Orbitello B, Perini L, et al: Effects of pregnancy on eating attitudes and disorders. A prospective study, *Journal of Psychosomatic Research* 59(3):175–179, 2005.

Sechi G, Serra A: Wernicke's encephalopathy: new clinical settings and recent advances in diagnosis and management, *Lancet Neurology* 6(5):422–455, 2007.

Sostre SO, Varma D, Sostre SS: 'Morning sickness' in pregnancy loses psychogenic stigma, *Current Psychiatry* 7(7):31–39, 2008.

Tan PC, Jacob R, Quek KF, et al: The fetal sex ratio and metabolic, biochemical, haematological and clinical indicators of severity of hyperemesis gravidarum, *BJOG: An International Journal of Obstetrics and Gynaecology* 113(6):733–737, 2006.

Torgersen L, Von Holle A, Reichborn-Kjennerud T, et al: Nausea and vomiting of pregnancy in women with bulimia nervosa and eating disorders not otherwise specified, *International Journal of Eating Disorders* 41(8):722–727, 2008.

Turner M: Hyperemesis gravidarum: providing woman-centred care, *British Journal of Midwifery* 15(9):540–544, 2007.

Verberg MFG, Gillott DJ, Al-Fardan N, et al: Hyperemesis gravidarum, a literature review, *Human Reproduction Update* 11(5):527–539, 2005.

Welsh A: Hyperemesis, gastrointestinal and liver disorders in pregnancy, *Current Obstetrics & Gynaecology* 15(2):123–131, 2005.

Wu K, Rayner CK, Chuah S, et al: Effects of ginger on gastric emptying and motility in healthy humans, *European Journal of Gastroenterology & Hepatology* 20(5):436–440, 2008.

# Chapter 54

# Bleeding in pregnancy

Amanda Hutcherson

## LEARNING OUTCOMES

After reading this chapter, you will be able to:

- identify the causes of vaginal bleeding in pregnancy
- discuss the midwife's role in bleeding in pregnancy both before and after the 24th week
- describe the possible implications for the health and wellbeing of the mother and the fetus
- discuss therapeutic termination of a pregnancy.

## INTRODUCTION

Vaginal bleeding during pregnancy is always considered to be abnormal and should always be investigated. It may be extremely frightening for the woman, so must be managed with sensitivity, ensuring that the woman is fully informed and involved in her plan of care. An important part of the management lies within the diagnosis of the cause and in the accurate assessment and reporting of the woman's previous and present history. It is also important to recognize that medical definitions and terms, such as 'abortion', will need to be explained. This term may have a different meaning for women and families.

Bleeding from the genital tract can be divided into two categories, depending on whether it occurs before or after the 24th week of pregnancy (Drife 2002).

## Bleeding before the 24th week of pregnancy

Bleeding from the genital tract in early pregnancy – that is, before the 24th week – may be caused by:

- implantation bleeding
- abortion
- hydatidiform mole
- ectopic pregnancy
- cervical lesions
- vaginitis.

## IMPLANTATION BLEEDING

There may be a little bleeding when the trophoblast embeds into the endometrial lining of the uterus. The bleeding is usually bright red and of short duration. As implantation takes place 8–12 days after fertilization, the bleeding usually occurs just before the menstrual period is due. If mistakenly thought to be a menstrual period, this may confuse the expected date of delivery. A careful menstrual history is essential to detect probable implantation bleeding, thereby avoiding miscalculation of dates.

## ABORTION

A pregnancy that ends before 24 completed weeks of gestation, and where the fetus is not alive, is termed an *abortion*. The classification is shown in Figure 54.1.

### Spontaneous abortion

Approximately 15–20% of confirmed pregnancies end in spontaneous abortion, most of these occurring before the 12th week of pregnancy. Midwives should be aware that the term 'abortion' may cause confusion. Many women who have lost a wanted pregnancy find the word offensive and it should not, therefore, be used when talking to

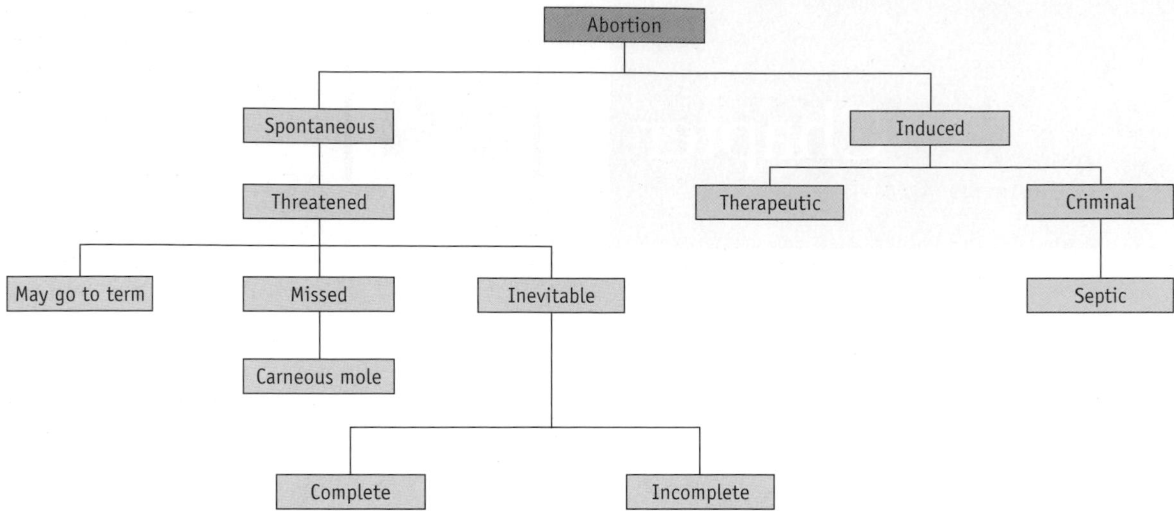


**Figure 54.1** The classification of abortion.

women about a pregnancy ending from natural causes. In these circumstances, the use of the word 'miscarriage' is more appropriate.

## Causes

- *Maldevelopment of the conceptus:* The most common cause of spontaneous abortion is a defective conceptus. Chromosomal abnormalities account for approximately 70% of defective conceptions, although spontaneous mutations may arise (Baker 2006, Beischer et al 1997).
- *Defective implantation* (Beischer et al 1997).
- *Hydatidiform mole* (Baker 2006).
- *Maternal infection:* Any acute illness, particularly a high temperature, may cause abortion. This may be due to the general metabolic effect of a high fever or the result of transplacental passage of viruses. Infections known to be associated include influenza, rubella, pneumonia, toxoplasmosis, cytomegalovirus, listeriosis, syphilis and brucellosis. Appendicitis in pregnancy may also be a cause (Silver & Branch 2007).
- *Genital tract infection*: Examples include bacterial vaginosis and vaginal mycoplasma infection (Donders et al 2000, Silver & Branch 2007).
- *Medical disorders*: These include diabetes, thyroid disease, renal disease and hypertensive disorders (Baker 2006).
- *Endocrine abnormalities*: These include poor development of the corpus luteum, inadequate secretory endometrium and low serum progesterone levels (Beischer et al 1997).
- *Uterine abnormalities*: The majority of the female genital tract arises from the two müllerian ducts, which form during embryonic life. Failure of development may cause structural abnormalities, such as double uterus, unicornuate, bicornuate, septate or subseptate uterus. Such structural uterine abnormalities are implicated in approximately 15% of early pregnancy losses. Sometimes the uterus fails to develop to the full adult size, remaining infantile. Pregnancy in such a uterus may also end in abortion (Baker 2006, Silver & Branch 2007).
- *Fibroids* (Baker 2006).
- *Retroversion of the uterus*: This does not itself cause abortion. As the uterus enlarges, it will usually rise into the abdomen. If it fails to do so, vaginal and abdominal manipulation to correct the retroversion may cause an abortion (Baker 2006).
- *Cervical weakness* ('incompetent' cervix): Laceration of the cervix or undue stretching of the internal cervical os, produced by a previous abortion or childbirth, may allow the membranes to bulge through the cervical canal and rupture. This condition is often a cause of repeated late pregnancy losses. Cervical cerclage (a nylon tape or suture inserted and tied around the cervix) at about the 14th week may prevent this. The tape must be removed before the onset of labour (Baker 2006, Beischer et al 1997).
- *Environmental factors*: External influences may be a cause. These include environmental teratogens, such as lead and radiation, and ingested teratogenic substances, such as drugs (especially cocaine) and alcohol (Carr & Coustan 2007; Silver & Branch 2007).
- *Smoking*: Exposure to tobacco smoke has been linked with spontaneous abortion but research findings remain inconclusive (Carr & Coustan 2007).

- *Maternal age*: Women in their late 30s and older have higher rates of pregnancy loss irrespective of obstetric history (Andersen et al 2000, Silver & Branch 2007).
- *Stress and anxiety*: Severe emotional upset may cause abortion by disrupting hypothalamic and pituitary functions. However, other factors may be implicated, as women experiencing adverse life events often have higher rates of smoking and alcohol use (Boyles et al 2000).
- *Paternal causes*: Poor sperm quality may be a factor. The father may also be the source of chromosomal abnormalities, particularly in cases of recurrent abortion (Beischer et al 1997, Gopalkrishnan et al 2000).
- *Immunological*: Maternal lymphocytes with natural killer cell activity may affect trophoblast development, disrupting implantation and embryonic growth. Autoimmune diseases, such as antiphospholipid syndrome, may also cause abortion (Beischer et al 1997, Silver & Branch 2007).

Despite detailed investigations, no cause can be found in the majority of cases.

## Inevitable abortion

The key feature of inevitable abortion is cervical dilatation with an outcome of unavoidable pregnancy loss. The gestation sac separates from the uterine wall and the uterus contracts to expel the conceptus. This uterine activity causes discomfort similar to that of labour contractions. Speculum examination reveals a dilating cervix, possibly with products of conception protruding through. The gestation sac may be expelled complete (*complete abortion*), or in part, usually with placental tissue retained (*incomplete abortion*).

The midwife who is called by a woman with signs of inevitable abortion should arrange immediate care. The woman's vital signs should be recorded and an estimate of blood loss made. If the fetus has been expelled and the woman is bleeding, local policies for the management of the third stage of labour and control of postpartum bleeding should be followed. Any products of conception passed should be saved for inspection. The midwife should refer the woman for medical care either by her GP or by a gynaecologist at her local hospital. If the bleeding is severe or the woman is showing signs of shock, a paramedic team from the local ambulance service should be requested. They will resuscitate the woman and stabilize her condition before transfer to hospital. In hospital, evacuation of retained products of conception (ERPC) from the uterus may be carried out and a blood transfusion may be given if blood loss has been severe.

Medical management of inevitable or incomplete abortion is possible, using prostaglandin analogues such as *misoprostol* or *gemeprost*. Once the uterus is empty, vulval hygiene is important for comfort and to reduce the likelihood of infection: the woman should be advised to change her sanitary towels frequently and keep the vulva clean, using a bidet or shower if possible. All women who have required surgical evacuation should be screened for chlamydial infection (RCOG 2006).

If the breasts begin to secrete, the woman should be advised to wear a well-fitting brassiere in order to minimize discomfort. *Cabergoline* 1 mg may be prescribed by a medical practitioner or qualified midwife prescriber to suppress lactation. If the woman is rhesus negative, anti-D gammaglobulin is given within 60 hours of abortion to prevent isoimmunization and potential rhesus problems in subsequent pregnancies. Women who are non-immune to rubella may be given rubella vaccination at this time and advised to avoid the risk of pregnancy for the next 3 months.

## Missed abortion (delayed abortion, silent abortion)

In this condition, bleeding occurs between the gestation sac and the uterine wall and the embryo dies. The uterus ceases to increase in size and as the presence of the retained fetus appears to inhibit menstruation, the woman may think that her pregnancy is continuing, although other signs of pregnancy have disappeared. The bleeding from the vagina varies from nothing, to a trickle of brownish discharge. As the signs of pregnancy gradually disappear, some women become aware that all is not well.

The diagnosis is confirmed by ultrasound. The uterus would eventually expel the fetus spontaneously, but this may not occur for some time. Treatment is usually to evacuate the uterus, either surgically or with misoprostol, either alone or in combination with methotrexate (Creinin et al 2003, Neilson et al 2006). 'Expectant' management may be offered: the woman is given the option of returning home for a few days to await spontaneous expulsion of the fetus.

If a well-formed fetus is retained in the uterus, it can become flattened and mummified as a fetus papyraceous (Fig. 54.2), rather than being reabsorbed. This is more commonly associated with a multiple pregnancy.

## Recurrent abortion

This is a term used when three or more consecutive spontaneous abortions have occurred. Careful investigation should be undertaken to find the cause. Occasionally, the causative factors are different for each, with no clear single factor associated. However, some conditions may be implicated in recurrent pregnancy loss (Backos & Regan 2006).

- *Structural abnormalities of the uterus*: These appear in up to 50% of women with recurrent abortion (for example, bicornuate uterus).

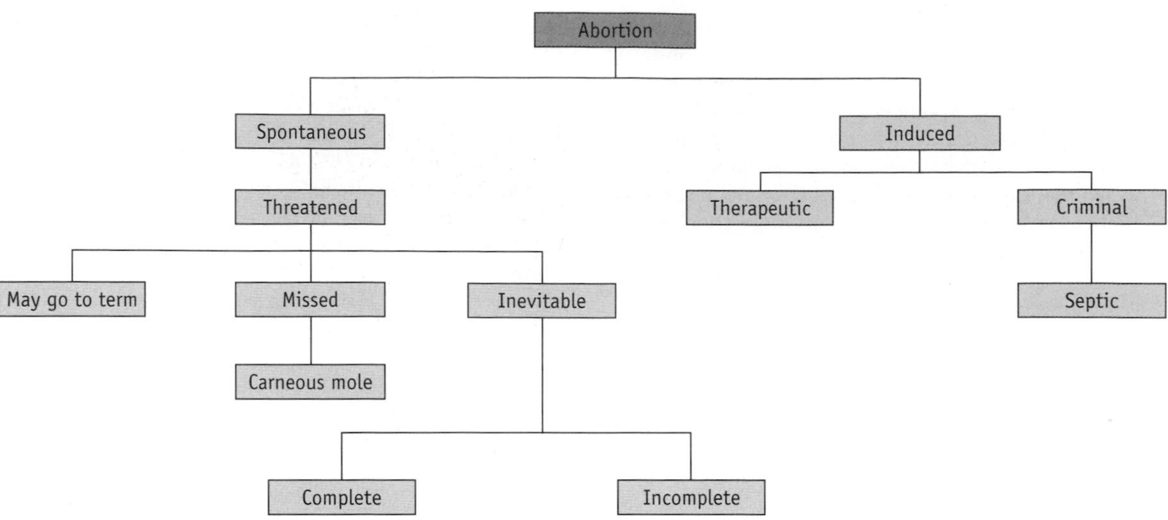


**Figure 54.2** Fetus papyraceous. *(From Beischer et al 1997.)*

- *Weak ('incompetent') cervix.*
- *Maternal systemic disease*: Diabetes and antiphospholipid antibodies.
- *Genetic causes*: The incidence of chromosome disorders is approximately 50% in first trimester abortions. The majority are balanced translocations. In cases of consanguineous or cousin marriage, a lethal recessive gene may cause recurrent losses.
- *Uterine infection*: Especially toxoplasmosis, *Mycoplasma hominis, Ureaplasma urealyticum* and chlamydia.
- *Hormonal deficiency*: Luteal phase deficits may be associated, although this theory is not universally accepted.
- *Immunological factors.*

## Psychological effects

Many women experience a marked grief reaction following abortion and may require considerable counselling and support. Psychological distress may be severe and some women become clinically depressed. The grief experienced by the partner may be as intense as that of the woman, though he is less likely to receive support (Conway & Russell 2000). Staff should treat the parents with sensitivity. The couple may wish to see their baby and staff should take account of their wishes. The guidelines written by the Stillbirth and Neonatal Death Society are useful (SANDS 2009).

After the end of the 24th week of pregnancy, the infant must be registered as a stillbirth (Home Office 2008). Many maternity hospitals offer a funeral or memorial service for pre-viable fetuses and all must offer respectful disposal. In this situation, the hospital chaplain may be a valuable source of support and advice. Antenatal Results and Choices (ARC) can provide non-directive support and counselling for parents who have received high-risk antenatal screening results or diagnosis of a fetal abnormality (ARC 2009).

**Reflective activity 54.1**

Talk to the manager of your early pregnancy unit. What are the referral criteria?

If there is no local early pregnancy unit, identify what services are available for women with early pregnancy problems and early fetal loss.

# Induced abortion

This term refers to the deliberate termination of a pregnancy. Induced abortions are classified as therapeutic or criminal.

## Therapeutic abortion

Therapeutic abortion has been legal in the UK since 1967, when the Abortion Act became law. This Act allows termination of a pregnancy if two registered medical practitioners are of the opinion that continuance of the pregnancy:

1. involves risk to the life of the pregnant woman
2. involves risk of injury to her physical or mental health
3. involves risk to any existing children of her family, greater than if the pregnancy were terminated; or
4. carries a substantial risk that if the child were born it would suffer from such physical or mental abnormalities as to be seriously handicapped.

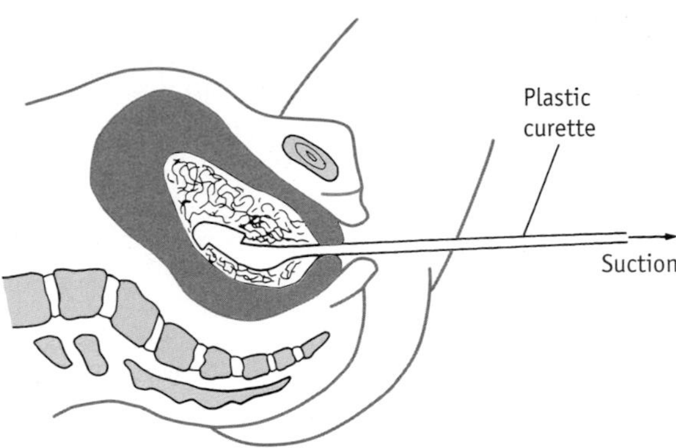


Figure 54.3 Dilatation and vacuum aspiration.

In current legislation, the upper gestation limit for legal termination is defined as the end of the 24th week (Dimond 2001, Human Fertilization and Embryology Act 1990). The only circumstances in which therapeutic abortion may be carried out after the 24th week are:

1. if there is a risk to the woman's life
2. if there is a risk of grave permanent damage to the woman's physical or mental health; or
3. if there is a substantial risk that the child would be seriously handicapped.

The law also allows for selective fetal reduction in multifetal pregnancy (see website).

Abortions after 24 weeks may only be carried out in NHS hospitals.

*Methods of surgical abortion* (Fig. 54.3)

## Criminal abortion

This is the termination of a pregnancy outside the terms of the Abortion Act, possibly by unauthorized and untrained persons, and is an offence punishable by law. The incidence has fallen sharply since the introduction of the 1967 Abortion Act. However, cases still occur: four such offences were detected in the year 2000–2001 (Home Department 2001) and seven in 2004–2005 (Home Office 2009). The abortion may be induced either by the woman herself or by some other person, by use of drugs or instruments. Whether successful or not, the action is illegal. The methods used may cause sudden death from haemorrhage, air embolus or vagal inhibition. Because of lack of asepsis, infection readily occurs and may lead to chronic ill-health or salpingitis and sterility (see website).

## Septic abortion

Uterine infection may occur after spontaneous or induced abortion. It is more likely to occur following criminal abortion or spontaneous abortion where there are retained products of conception. The incidence of septic abortion has declined in countries that allow legal termination of pregnancy but it is still a cause of maternal death: five maternal deaths from sepsis following spontaneous abortion were recorded in the UK between 1997 and 1999 (Lewis 2001), and five in the triennium 2003–2005 (Lewis 2007) (see website).

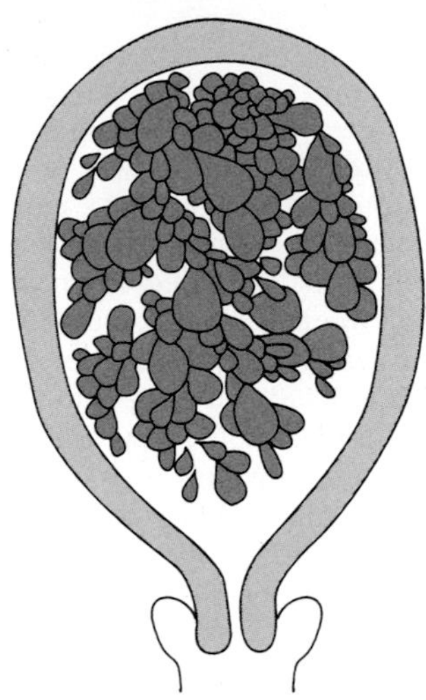

Figure 54.4 Hydatidiform mole.

**Reflective activity 54.2**

Find out what services midwives offer locally to women who have had a spontaneous abortion or second trimester termination of pregnancy.

# GESTATIONAL TROPHOBLASTIC DISEASE (HYDATIDIFORM MOLE AND CHORIOCARCINOMA)

## Hydatidiform mole

This condition occurs as a result of degeneration of the chorionic villi at an early stage of pregnancy (Fig. 54.4). Usually, the embryo is absent; occasionally, a hydatidiform mole may be found in a twin pregnancy alongside a viable fetus (Kauffman et al 1999). Molar pregnancy may be complete, with an intrauterine multivesicular mass composed of hydropic chorionic villi, or partial, where vesicular tissue is present, but less well developed, along with a fetus. Vesicle formation may occur within the placenta of an apparently normal pregnancy.

### Signs and symptoms

Often, the minor disorders of pregnancy, such as nausea and breast tenderness, are more severe. The woman may complain of intermittent bleeding per vaginam from around the 12th week of pregnancy. When the mole begins to abort, there may be profuse haemorrhage. Pre-eclampsia may develop even in the early weeks of pregnancy. Severe nausea and vomiting may occur. On abdominal examination, the uterus is usually large for the period of gestation and may feel soft and doughy to the fingers. No fetal parts are palpable and the fetal heart is absent. There may be signs of mild thyrotoxicosis due to the thyroid-stimulating hormone (TSH)-like activity of human chorionic gonadotrophin (hCG) which is secreted in large amounts by the molar vesicles. The diagnosis is suggested by the clinical findings and is confirmed by an ultrasound scan which will reveal no fetal parts but only a speckled or snowstorm appearance (Oats & Abraham 2004). Urinary or serum hCG levels wiil be high.

### Treatment

Once the diagnosis of molar pregnancy is confirmed, the uterus must be completely evacuated at once. This is achieved by careful suction curettage (see Fig. 54.3). Uterine contractions may cause molar tissue to enter the circulation via the sinuses of the placental bed. These emboli may set up metastatic disease in other sites, commonly the lungs. Medical termination should therefore be avoided. Unless the woman is haemorrhaging, oxytocic drugs are withheld until the uterus has been surgically emptied. A Syntocinon infusion may then be used to maintain uterine contraction and haemostasis. The woman should be registered at a specialist follow-up centre in London, Sheffield or Dundee (RCOG 2004a).

After treatment for hydatidiform mole, careful observation is required as approximately 3% of these women will develop malignant trophoblastic disease (choriocarcinoma). Partial moles are less likely to become malignant but still require follow-up (Seckl et al 2000). Serum beta-hCG levels are monitored fortnightly until the values fall to within the normal range. Urine samples are then normally tested every 4 weeks until 1 year after evacuation. In the second year of follow-up, urinary hCG testing is carried out every 3 months.

If any molar tissue remains in the uterus, it will continue to grow and may invade the myometrium. Perforation of the uterine wall is then likely and this will cause major internal haemorrhage. Signs that the mole is continuing to grow are indicated by the persistence of high hCG levels 24 hours after uterine evacuation and high levels 1 month after treatment. If the serum or urinary hCG fails to return to normal levels within 6 months or begins to rise again, the woman is at risk of malignant trophoblastic disease.

The woman must avoid another pregnancy until she has been discharged from the follow-up programme. Use of the oral contraceptive pill increases the risk of the development of invasive disease and should therefore be avoided until hCG levels have been normal for three successive months.

## Choriocarcinoma

Choriocarcinoma is a malignant disease of trophoblastic tissue. It occurs following approximately 3% of complete moles (Seckl et al 2000). hCG levels will rise and the pregnancy test will become strongly positive again. Choriocarcinoma may occur in the next normal pregnancy following an evacuation of a mole.

As the growth infiltrates the uterus and vagina, the affected woman will experience increasingly severe pain. The condition will be rapidly fatal unless treated. The disease spreads by local invasion and via the bloodstream; metastases may occur in the lungs, liver and brain. Transplacental fetal metastases may occur during a pregnancy but this is very rare.

Choriocarcinoma responds extremely well to chemotherapy. Cytotoxic drugs, such as *methotrexate, etoposide* and *actinomycin-D,* are used singly or as combination therapy, and are nearly always completely successful. The woman should avoid another pregnancy for at least 1 year after the completion of treatment and will require hCG monitoring after any future pregnancy, as there is a risk of disease recurrence (Oats & Abraham 2004).

# ECTOPIC OR EXTRAUTERINE GESTATION

Ectopic pregnancy occurs when the fertilized ovum implants outside the uterine cavity. In 95% of cases the site of implantation is the uterine tube and these are known as tubal pregnancies. Occasionally, the site may be the ovary, the abdominal cavity or the cervical canal, but these are rare. The incidence of ectopic pregnancy is 1 : 150 pregnancies (Baker 2006). Ectopic pregnancy is the major cause of maternal death before 20 weeks' gestation in the industrialized world (Benrubi 2005, Lewis 2007).

## Tubal pregnancy

This is the commonest type of ectopic pregnancy and the incidence has increased two- to threefold in the last 30 years (Wiznitzer & Shener 2007). Tubal pregnancy occurs when there is a delay in the transport of the zygote along the fallopian tube. This may be due to a congenital malformation of the uterine tubes or more commonly to tubal scarring following pelvic infection. The ovum implants

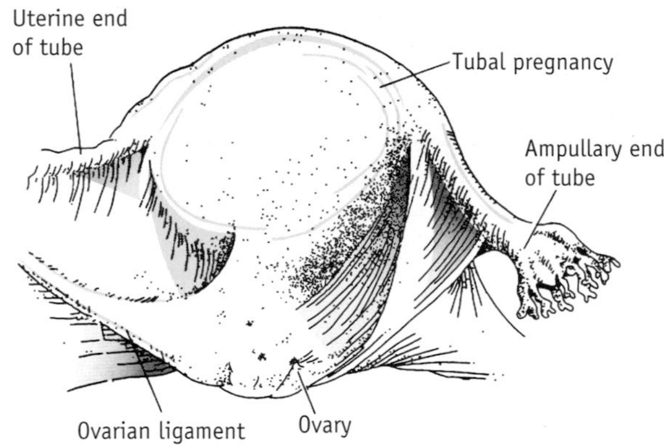


Figure 54.5 Tubal pregnancy.

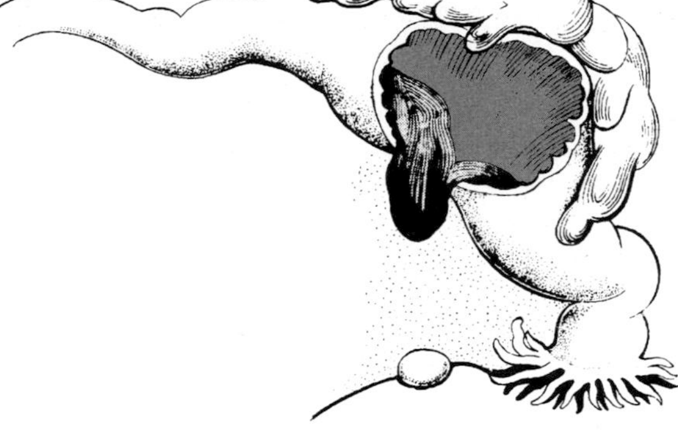

Figure 54.6 Rupture of the uterine tube.

and begins to develop in the lining of the tube. The ampulla is the most common site (Fig. 54.5).

Although tubal pregnancy may occur in the absence of any significant history, there are certain risk factors (Lemus 2000, Wiznitzer & Shener 2007):

- *History of previous tubal pregnancy.*
- *Tubal surgery.*
- *Hormonal ovulation induction* – drugs such as clomifene may interfere with tubal motility.
- *Progesterone-releasing intrauterine contraceptive devices* (this is related to higher-dose devices).
- *Tubal endometriosis.*
- *Pelvic inflammatory disease.*
- *Appendicectomy, pelvic or abdominal surgery* which may cause adhesion formation.
- *Postcoital contraception using diethylstilbestrol.*
- *Contraceptive methods* – the intrauterine contraceptive device and the progesterone-only pill may increase the relative risk because they protect against intrauterine pregnancy but do not prevent ovulation and fertilization. This may make tubal pregnancy more likely in a woman who conceives while using these methods.
- *IVF pregnancy.*

## Diagnosis

Diagnosis based on clinical signs alone may be difficult because the clinical picture may appear similar to pelvic inflammatory disease or threatened abortion. Delay in diagnosis and treatment may contribute to maternal mortality and morbidity. The most accurate method currently available is a combination of serum hCG levels and transvaginal ultrasound scanning. hCG levels rise steadily in early pregnancy. Levels lower than normal or falling below the doubling time (the time in which serum levels can be expected to double) are indicative of ectopic gestation (Tin-Chiu et al 1999). The ultrasound scan may reveal a

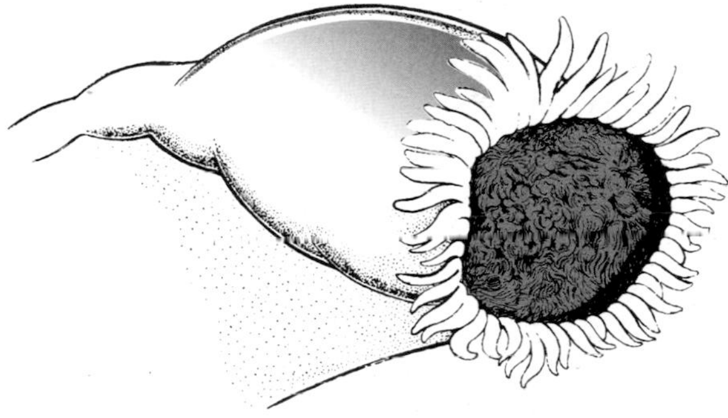

Figure 54.7 Tubal abortion.

tubal mass or a fluid collection in the pelvis but is most useful for confirming the *absence* of an intrauterine sac. As the conceptus develops and grows, the tube distends to accommodate it.

Initially, the woman will experience the usual signs of pregnancy, such as nausea and breast changes, although amenorrhoea is not always present. The uterus will soften and enlarge under the influence of the pregnancy hormones. As the tube becomes further distended, the woman will experience abdominal pain and some vaginal bleeding. The blood loss is uterine in origin and signifies endometrial degeneration. Gastrointestinal disturbance such as diarrhoea and pain on defecation are also common signs (Baker 2006, Lewis 2007).

If the site of implantation is the narrower proximal end of the tube, tubal rupture is likely to occur between the 5th and 7th weeks of pregnancy (Fig. 54.6).

If the pregnancy is located in the wider ampullary section, the gestation may continue until the 10th week. Occasionally, the gestation sac is expelled from the fimbriated end (Fig. 54.7).

As the ovum separates from its attachment to the ampullary part of the tube, layers of blood clot may be deposited around the dead ovum to form a mass of blood clot which may remain in the uterine tube or be expelled from the fimbriated end of the tube. When the tube ruptures, there will be severe intraperitoneal haemorrhage and the woman will experience intense abdominal pain. There may also be referred shoulder-tip pain on lying down as blood tracks up towards the diaphragm. The woman will appear pale, shocked and nauseated and may collapse. The abdomen is tender and may be distended. Pelvic examination is usually exquisitely tender, especially on movement of the cervix. Ruptured ectopic pregnancy is an acute surgical emergency requiring immediate treatment.

### Management

If ectopic pregnancy is suspected, a large-bore intravenous cannula (size 16 gauge) should be inserted and blood taken for cross-matching. The woman must be transferred to theatre as soon as possible. Laparoscopic salpingotomy may be performed unless the woman is suffering from haemorrhagic shock, when laparotomy is preferable.

If the condition is detected in the early stages, non-surgical management may be attempted with injections of prostaglandin $F_{2a}$ or systemic prostaglandin $E_2$. Methotrexate may also be given, either intramuscularly or directly into the gestation sac (RCOG 2004b, Reis et al 2008).

## Heterotopic or combined pregnancy

Heterotopic pregnancy occurs when a blastocyst from a multiple gestation implants outside the uterine cavity. It is associated with dizygotic twinning, and the extrauterine pregnancy is nearly always tubal. It may follow in vitro fertilization and embryo transfer. The incidence is thought to be approximately 1 : 15000 and is likely to rise as the incidence of both multiple gestation and ectopic pregnancy rises. Diagnosis can be difficult and management options are limited by the presence of the intrauterine pregnancy. The ectopic sac must be removed but the uterus should be disturbed as little as possible and methotrexate must be avoided if the intrauterine pregnancy is to survive (Wiznitzer & Shener 2007).

## Secondary abdominal pregnancy

Very rarely, when rupture of a tubal pregnancy occurs, there may be partial extrusion of the ovum into the peritoneal cavity but with enough chorionic villi remaining attached to the tube to ensure that the embryo does not die. Chorionic villi on the surface of the ovum then become attached to the neighbouring abdominal organs and the pregnancy continues with the fetus developing free within the abdominal cavity (see website). The fetus is at risk of severe growth restriction because of the relatively poor placentation and may also suffer pressure deformities as there is no protective uterine wall.

This condition is usually detected by ultrasound scanning but may be suggested by a persistently abnormal fetal lie and the fact that fetal parts are unusually easy to palpate. Delivery is by laparotomy. The placenta is usually left in situ to be absorbed, as an attempt to detach it may cause uncontrollable haemorrhage.

Ectopic pregnancy is a significant cause of maternal death and the incidence is rising. There were 10 reported deaths in the UK from this cause between 2003 and 2005 (Lewis 2007). The midwife must be aware of the associated risk factors and seek an obstetric opinion for any woman with signs or symptoms suggestive of extrauterine gestation without delay.

## BLEEDING FROM ASSOCIATED CONDITIONS

The following conditions may cause bleeding, although, strictly speaking, they are not bleeding of early pregnancy since the bleeding is not from the site of the pregnancy.

### Cervical polyp

This is a small red gelatinous growth attached by a pedicle to the cervix, close to the external os. It may give rise to slight irregular bleeding.

### Ectropion of the cervix

A cervical erosion is formed when the columnar epithelium lining the cervical canal proliferates owing to the action of the pregnancy hormones. The ectropion forms a reddish area on the cervix, extending outwards from the external os. It may give rise to a blood-stained discharge from the vagina. No treatment is necessary and the ectropion will recede during the puerperium.

### Carcinoma of the cervix

Invasive cervical carcinoma is rarely seen in pregnancy, although cervical intraepithelial neoplasia (CIN) may occasionally be discovered if a cervical smear is taken. If the cervical cytology report suggests precancerous changes, colposcopy is performed to identify the affected areas and a small cervical biopsy may be carried out. Treatment is deferred until after delivery if the condition is not invasive.

Invasive cervical cancer is very serious as the disease may progress quickly. On vaginal examination, the cervix is hard and irregular and bleeds when touched. There may also be a purulent vaginal discharge. If the condition is discovered in the first trimester, the pregnancy may be terminated and treatment initiated. In the third trimester, the fetus is viable and may be delivered by caesarean section. Once the infant is born, the obstetrician may carry out a radical hysterectomy (Wertheim's hysterectomy). Vaginal delivery is associated with a poorer prognosis for the mother as cervical dilatation may cause dissemination of tumour cells and metastases have been reported in episiotomy sites (Sood et al 2000).

A dilemma arises if the condition is discovered in the second trimester, because the fetus is unlikely to survive if delivered. The woman may choose to postpone treatment for a time to allow further fetal growth; however, the delay should be no longer than 4 weeks.

Bleeding in early pregnancy may occur for a variety of reasons. It is a serious sign and the underlying condition may be life-threatening. Any woman who reports vaginal bleeding during pregnancy must be referred to an obstetrician without delay.

## Bleeding after the 24th week – antepartum haemorrhage

Antepartum haemorrhage is defined as bleeding from the genital tract after the 24th week of pregnancy and before the birth of the baby. Bleeding that occurs during labour is sometimes referred to as intrapartum haemorrhage.

Antepartum haemorrhage is a serious complication which may result in the death of the mother or the baby.

There are two main varieties of haemorrhage:

- *Placenta praevia* (unavoidable or inevitable haemorrhage) is bleeding from separation of an abnormally situated placenta. (The placenta lies partly or wholly in the lower uterine segment and bleeding is inevitable when labour begins.)
- *Abruptio placentae* (placental abruption) is bleeding from separation of a normally situated placenta.

However, extraplacental bleeding may sometimes occur. This is vaginal bleeding from some other part of the birth canal, for example, a cervical polyp, as described above.

## PLACENTA PRAEVIA

The incidence of placenta praevia at term ranges from 0.5% to 1%. It is usually detected on ultrasound scanning in early pregnancy and may be seen in as many as one-quarter of all pregnancies in the second trimester. As the lower segment grows and stretches, the placental site appears to rise up the uterine wall, away from the internal os uteri, until at term in the majority of cases the placenta no longer occupies the lower segment. Those cases where the placenta overlies the internal os in early pregnancy, are at highest risk of haemorrhage. The classification of placenta praevia is shown in Table 54.1. The types are illustrated in Figure 54.8.

**Table 54.1 Classification of placenta praevia**

| | |
|---|---|
| Low-lying placenta | Placenta mainly in the upper segment but encroaching on the lower segment |
| Marginal | Placenta reaches to, but does not cover, the internal os |
| Partial | Placenta covers the internal os when closed but not completely when it is dilated |
| Total | Placenta completely covers the internal os |

### Causes

The cause of placenta praevia is unknown but the following factors are known to be associated (Baker 2006, Benrubi 2005, Handler et al 1994):

- *Multiparity*: The increased size of the uterine cavity following repeated childbearing may predispose to placenta praevia.
- *Multiple pregnancy*: The larger placental site is more likely to encroach on the lower segment of the uterus.
- *Age*: Risk rises with maternal age.
- *Scarred uterus*: One previous caesarean section doubles the risk of placenta praevia.
- *Previous myomectomy or hysterotomy*.
- *Smoking*: The exact mechanism is unclear but the relative hypoxia induced by smoking may cause enlargement of the placenta in order to compensate for the reduced oxygen supply.
- *Placental abnormality*: Bipartite and succenturiate placentae may cause placenta praevia. Placenta membranacea (placenta diffusa) may also be a cause. This is a rare developmental abnormality of the placenta where all the chorion is covered with functioning villi. The placenta develops as a thin membranous structure, covering an unusually large surface of the uterus. The condition may be diagnosed on ultrasound. It may cause severe haemorrhage possibly requiring hysterectomy. It may not separate readily in the third stage of labour. Fetal nutrition appears to be relatively undisturbed in cases of placenta membranacea.
- *Fetal sex*: There may be an association between male fetal sex and placenta praevia (Wen et al 2000).

### Associated conditions

A low-lying placenta puts the woman and her fetus at risk of other complications. The most serious of these is

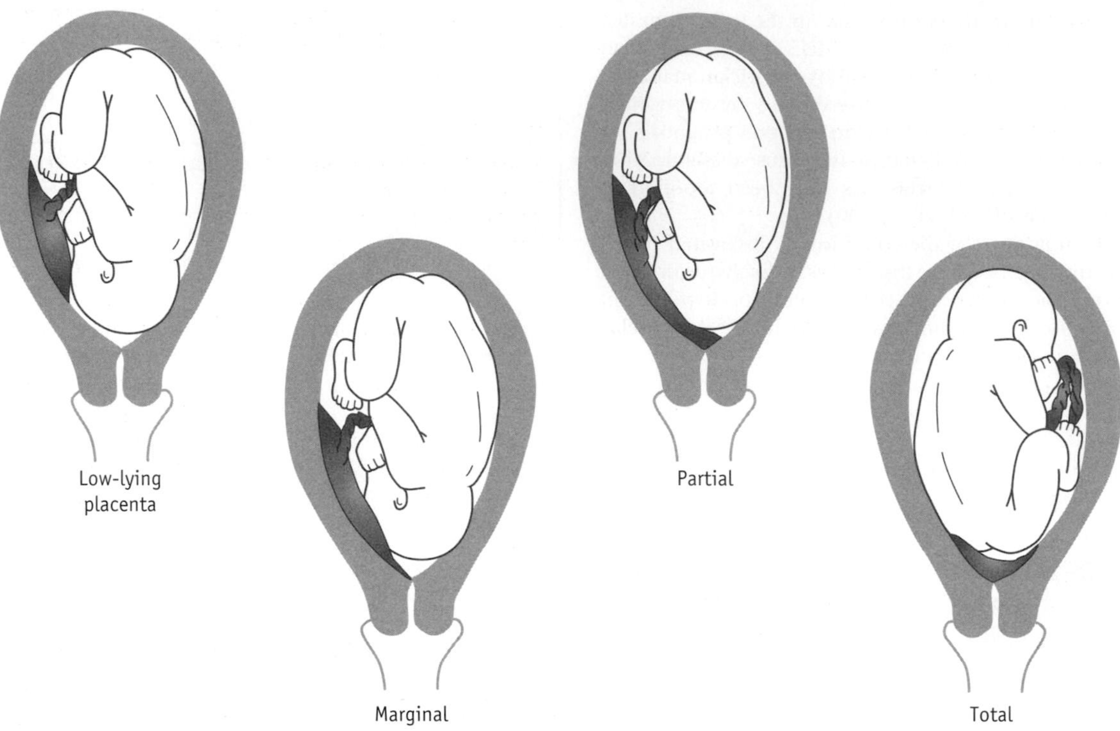


**Figure 54.8** Placenta praevia.

placenta accreta. This usually occurs where the previous delivery was by caesarean section (Yang et al 2007). The combination of the relatively thin decidua in the lower segment and the presence of scar tissue increases the likelihood of trophoblastic invasion of the myometrium.

Intrauterine growth restriction may occur, possibly as a result of repeated small haemorrhages (Drife 2002).

## Signs and symptoms

As placenta praevia is normally diagnosed on ultrasound scanning in early pregnancy (Baulies et al 2007), midwives will usually be aware of any woman in their care who has a low-lying placenta. However, there are women who will not have had an ultrasound scan during pregnancy, including women who choose not to do so, women who have concealed their pregnancy, women who have not accessed care, or women who may have spent their antenatal period in a country where ultrasound scans are not readily available. Therefore the midwife must be aware of the signs that indicate a possible placenta praevia:

- *Malpresentation of the fetus*: Although the presentation may be cephalic, often it is not. The placenta occupies space in the pelvis and the midwife may find that the breech presents, as there is more room for the head in the fundus, or that the lie is oblique and the fetal shoulder presents.
- *Non-engagement of the presenting part*: This is especially likely with a partial or total placenta praevia.
- *Difficulty in identifying fetal parts on palpation*: An anterior placenta praevia lies between the fetus and the midwife's hand like a cushion. This makes the fetal parts relatively difficult to identify.
- *Loud maternal pulse below the umbilicus:* An anterior placenta praevia may often be detected by the presence of loud maternal arterial sounds from the placental bed. This is more easily heard with an electronic fetal heart monitor (Doppler). The fetal heart sounds may be difficult to detect as they are muffled by the placenta, especially in a cephalic presentation.

  An anterior placenta praevia will cushion some of the fetal movements and the woman may mention that she only feels fetal movement above the umbilicus.
- *Bleeding after sexual intercourse:* Stimulation of the cervix during intercourse may provoke bleeding.

When bleeding occurs, it usually begins after the 24th–28th week of pregnancy, although it may occur earlier. In the third trimester of pregnancy, the lower segment is completing its development, Braxton Hicks contractions are increasing, and towards the end of pregnancy, the cervix is becoming effaced. Bleeding is caused by detachment of the placenta which cannot stretch to adapt to these changes in uterine structure. As the placenta is in the lower pole of the uterus, the blood escapes easily, thus giving rise to the classical unprovoked, fresh, painless bleeding of placenta praevia. 'Warning haemorrhages' are associated with placenta praevia. These are small, recurrent, fresh and painless haemorrhages occurring during the third trimester. Each episode of bleeding indicates further placental detachment. If the placenta is torn, some fetal bleeding will occur and this will further compromise the condition of the fetus. Torrential maternal haemorrhage may occur at any time but is more likely once labour begins as the cervix begins to dilate.

It is impossible to predict the course of events in a case of placenta praevia and even in the absence of bleeding the condition is regarded as a major and life-threatening complication of pregnancy.

## Management

If no serious haemorrhage has made it imperative to act, the woman will be delivered at about 38 weeks' gestation, which should avoid problems of prematurity for the infant.

If the placental location is unclear, an examination may be carried out in theatre, by a senior obstetrician, with the woman suitably anaesthetized and the theatre set up in readiness for a caesarean section. An intravenous infusion is commenced and four units of cross-matched blood is immediately available. With the woman in the lithotomy position, the obstetrician makes a very gentle and cautious vaginal examination, passing a finger through the cervix into the lower pole of the uterus. If the placenta is palpable, the obstetrician will immediately perform a caesarean section. If the placenta is not palpable in the lower segment, the membranes may be ruptured and the woman allowed to labour. This procedure avoids unnecessary caesarean section for women in whom placenta praevia is not confirmed.

However, nearly all women have access to ultrasound scanning and the diagnosis is usually clear. Vaginal delivery is usually possible in cases of a low lying placenta, if the fetal head is engaged. However, the presence of placental tissue within 2 cm of the internal os is a contraindication to vaginal birth (RCOG 2005).

### *Active treatment*

In cases where bleeding first occurs at 38 weeks or later, conservative treatment is not appropriate, as the fetus is mature. Active treatment is also necessary in cases where labour has started, if bleeding is severe or there are signs of fetal distress. An intravenous infusion is commenced and the woman's condition is stabilized if necessary. A senior obstetrician performs an emergency caesarean section under general anaesthesia. A paediatrician should be present to attend to the baby, who may be asphyxiated at birth. Preterm infants of mothers with placenta praevia have an increased risk of developing respiratory distress syndrome (Lin et al 2001).

### *Third stage*

Postpartum haemorrhage may complicate the third stage of labour since there are few oblique muscle fibres to control bleeding from the placental site in the lower uterine segment.

Placenta accreta may occur in women who have had a previous caesarean section and torrential haemorrhage may result from attempts to separate the placenta. Surgical treatments, such as ligation of the internal iliac arteries and interventional radiology, may be required in order to control the haemorrhage (RCOG 2007). Hysterectomy is undertaken as a last resort to save the woman's life. The midwife must be familiar with local guidelines for management of massive obstetric haemorrhage (see Box 54.1) and adequate supplies of cross-matched blood should be available before surgery commences.

Box 54.1 **Key points from guidelines for the management of massive obstetric haemorrhage (DH 1994, Lewis 2007)**

- Dealing with ill, bleeding women requires skilled teamwork between obstetric and anaesthetic teams, with appropriate help from other specialists, including haematologists, vascular surgeons and radiologists
- Immediate involvement of all key staff, including senior obstetrician, anaesthetist, haematologist, blood transfusion service and portering staff
- Minimum 20 mL sample of blood for cross-matching and coagulation studies
- Minimum 6 units of cross-matched blood, with use of plasma expanders as necessary (not dextrans)
- Blood of the patient's own group to be used for transfusion; uncross-matched O-negative blood to be used only if immediate transfusion is required
- Minimum of two peripheral intravenous lines, using 16-gauge cannulae
- Immediate commencement of CVP monitoring
- Facilities for monitoring central venous and intra-arterial pressure, ECG, blood gases and acid–base status should be available in consultant units
- Rapid administration of blood and fluids (blood filtration is not necessary)
- Use of blood-warming equipment
- Repeated estimation of haemoglobin and coagulation studies
- Use of an early warning scoring system such as the Modified Early Warning Scoring System (MEWSS)

*It cannot be emphasized too strongly that vaginal examination in placenta praevia is an extremely dangerous procedure and should not be attempted, except with the precautions described above.*

Current interventions for suspected placenta praevia are reviewed by Neilson et al (2003), a summary of which can be found on the website.

## ABRUPTIO PLACENTAE

Abruptio placentae is bleeding due to the separation of a normally situated placenta (Fig. 54.9). It is sometimes referred to as placental abruption or 'accidental' bleeding. Placental abruption may occur at any stage of pregnancy, or during labour, and may complicate approximately 1% of pregnancies.

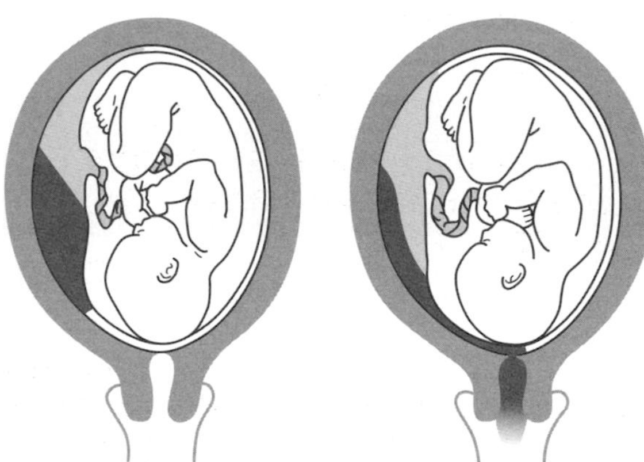

**Figure 54.9** Abruptio placentae.

### Causes

The cause of the placental separation cannot always be satisfactorily explained and in 40% of cases no cause can be found (Rana et al 1999). The following risk factors have been associated with the condition (Carr & Coustan 2007, Ray & Laskin 1999, Reis et al 2000)

- *Hypertensive disease*: essential hypertension, pregnancy-induced hypertension (PIH) or pre-eclampsia.
- *Sudden decompression of the uterus*: such as may follow spontaneous rupture of the membranes in cases of polyhydramnios.
- *Preterm prelabour*: rupture of the membranes.
- *Previous history*: placental abruption.
- *Trauma*: for example, following external cephalic version, road traffic accident, a fall or a blow.
- *Smoking*.
- *Drug abuse*: for example, cocaine, crack or marijuana.
- *Folate and vitamin $B_{12}$ deficiency*: although the evidence for this association is not conclusive.

Maternal hypertension is the most consistent finding in cases of placental abruption.

### Types

The bleeding may be revealed, concealed or partially revealed (Fig. 54.10).

**Revealed bleeding:** This occurs when the site of detachment is at the placental margin. The blood thus dissects between the membranes and the decidua and escapes through the os uteri. With revealed placental abruption the degree of shock is in proportion to the visible vaginal blood loss.

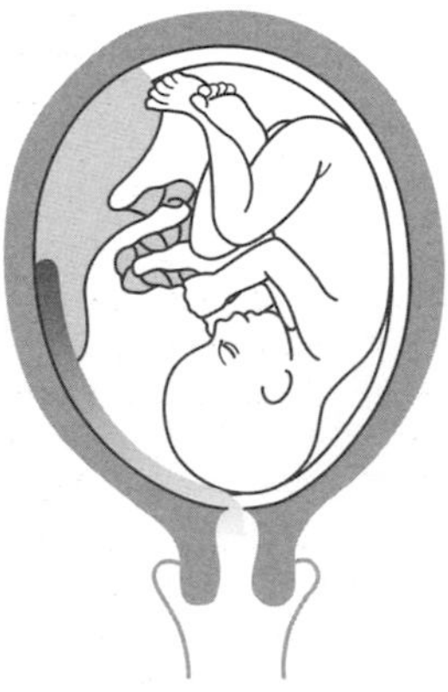



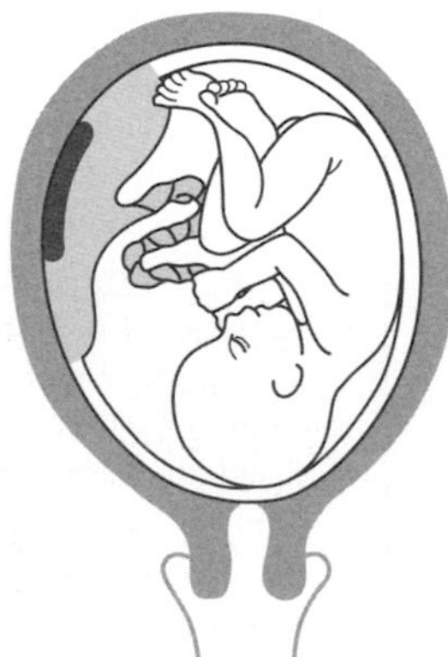



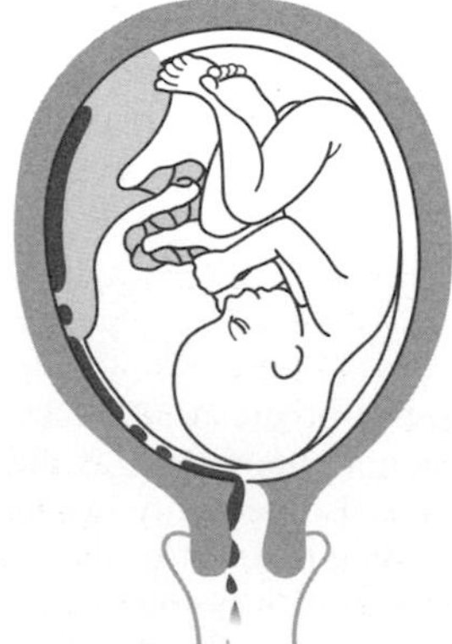



**Figure 54.10** Types of abruptio placentae.

**Concealed bleeding:** This occurs when the site of detachment is close to the centre of the placenta. The blood cannot escape and a large retroplacental clot forms. The blood may infiltrate the myometrium, sometimes as far as the peritoneal covering, causing a marbled, petechial pattern of bleeding. This is called a *Couvelaire uterus*. There is no visible blood loss but the pain and shock may be severe as the intrauterine tension rises. Increasing abdominal girth or rising fundal height are suspicious signs of concealed haemorrhage. Backache may accompany abruption in a posteriorly sited placenta.

**Partially revealed bleeding:** This occurs when some of the blood trickles between the membranes and the decidua to become visible as vaginal bleeding. Not all the blood escapes and a variable amount remains concealed. In this situation the bleeding and thus the degree of shock will be much more severe than the visible loss suggests.

The severity of placental abruption may be classified as mild, moderate or severe.

**Mild abruptio placentae:** The loss is usually slight and the bleeding may be entirely concealed, although often there is a slight trickle per vaginam. The woman may experience no more than mild abdominal pain, the uterus is not tender and the fetus is alive. There is no sign of maternal shock.

**Moderate abruptio placentae:** The blood loss is heavier, the abdominal pain more severe and, on palpation, the uterus may be tender and firm. The mother may be hypotensive and have a tachycardia and usually there are signs of fetal distress.

**Severe abruptio placentae:** This is an obstetric emergency. More than half the placenta will have separated, the blood loss will exceed 1 litre and the mother will be very shocked. Abdominal pain will be severe. On palpation, the uterus may be hard and tender, and on auscultation, fetal heart sounds will not be heard. There is an increased risk of coagulation disorders. It is essential to remember that the amount of bleeding per vaginam is **no guide** to the degree of placental separation.

## Outcome

If there is only minor detachment of the placenta and the mother and fetus are in good condition, the woman will be advised to stay in hospital for observation. If the bleeding ceases and all appears well, she may be discharged. The pregnancy will be closely monitored with ultrasound scans and regular cardiotocography to assess fetal growth and wellbeing. There is an increased risk of poor fetal growth and preterm birth following an episode of placental abruption (Rasmussen et al 2000).

In a case of moderate or severe abruptio placentae, the most important treatment is to empty the uterus. If fetal condition permits, labour is induced by rupturing the membranes and an oxytocic infusion is commenced. Vaginal delivery may be possible.

If the fetus is in poor condition, delivery will be by caesarean section unless the woman is already in the second stage of labour, when a forceps delivery will be performed. Ergometrine 500 mcg is given intravenously at delivery to control haemorrhage in the third stage of labour. It is usual to continue the Syntocinon infusion for some hours after delivery in order to maintain uterine contraction.

The most effective treatment for severe haemorrhage and defective coagulation is the transfusion of fresh blood. If fresh blood is not available, fresh frozen plasma should be given as this contains fibrinogen, platelets and clotting factors III, V and VIII.

**Reflective activity 54.3**

Locate and read your Unit policy for management of bleeding in later pregnancy.

## MANAGEMENT OF ANTEPARTUM HAEMORRHAGE AND THE MIDWIFE'S ROLE

### At home

If called by a woman with bleeding, the midwife must ascertain the amount of bleeding and organize immediate care. If the reported bleeding is heavy, the midwife should ask a paramedic team from the local ambulance service to attend in order to avoid delay in transfer to hospital.

The woman should lie on her side or with a pillow or towel wedged under the right hip to achieve a slight pelvic tilt and avoid supine hypotensive syndrome. Blood pressure, pulse rate and temperature should be recorded, blood loss noted and a sanitary pad applied. The presence of pain is suggestive of abruptio placentae, while painless bright bleeding may indicate placenta praevia. Soiled pads and clothing should be saved to allow accurate estimation of blood lost. An obstetrician from the local hospital must be contacted, as the woman will need to be admitted. The midwife should inform the obstetrician of the severity of the bleeding, colour of the blood (fresh or dark), nature and location of pain, if present, and the woman's general condition. If the initial loss is small, the woman's blood pressure and pulse rate will be normal and she will appear well. The assessment of blood pressure should be treated with caution, with reference to the woman's medical record if possible. A normal blood pressure may falsely represent a low blood pressure in women with a history of hypertension. In these cases, the pulse and respiration rate may be more indicative of bleeding. Should the loss be severe, she will present the typical picture of a woman who has had a haemorrhage: pale, sweating, restless, thirsty, with a rising pulse rate, rising respiration rate and falling blood pressure. In this case, emergency assistance is needed and a paramedic team from the ambulance service should be called. An intravenous infusion is started and group O rhesus-negative blood may be given if necessary. Plasma expanders, such as *Haemaccel, Gelofusine* or *hetastarch* (*Hespan*) preparations, may be used.

When attending to a woman who is bleeding, *no vaginal examination should be made*. If this is a case of placenta praevia, a vaginal examination could precipitate a disastrous haemorrhage. Rectal examinations are similarly dangerous. Abdominal examination should be avoided if possible as this may provoke Braxton Hicks contractions, which may accelerate bleeding.

## In hospital

The woman is admitted to the delivery suite and the attendance of a senior obstetrician is requested. If there are signs of severe haemorrhage, a senior anaesthetist and haematologist should also be in attendance.

Until the diagnosis is clear, she must be treated as having a potential placenta praevia, although there may be some features which help in making a diagnosis (see Table 54.2). Often the distinction is not clear; it is particularly difficult if the mother has had a small revealed abruption but no pain, no apparent cause for the bleeding and no signs of pre-eclampsia.

If bleeding has been severe, the treatment must be swift, as the woman's condition may deteriorate rapidly. The aim is to restore normal blood volume and thus improve the mother's general condition, deliver the baby if necessary, and avoid the dangerous complications of renal failure and blood coagulation disorders. Two intravenous cannulae (16 guage) are inserted, blood is taken for grouping and cross-matching, and the duty haematologist and blood bank must be informed if large quantities of blood are likely to be needed. Other blood tests include full blood count (essential for haemoglobin estimation and platelet count), urea and electrolytes, clotting studies and fibrin degradation products.

Temperature, pulse, blood pressure, fetal heart and vaginal loss should be observed. The pulse and blood pressure are recorded as frequently as the woman's condition dictates: quarter-hourly if the bleeding is continuing. Maternal oxygen saturation should be observed using a pulse oximeter. Oxygen may be given by facemask if required. The fetal heart should be continuously monitored by external cardiotocography whilst bleeding persists. Gentle pressure should be used so as not to stimulate further bleeding or uterine activity. Placing a mark on the abdomen durng the first assessment of the fetal heart may reduce excessive palpation. A Foley urinary catheter is inserted and the urinary output is closely monitored, a marked decrease being a grave sign. The urine is tested for protein. The midwife records an estimate of blood loss, observing for the appearance of blood clotting: blood with normal clotting factors will clot in room air; if this fails to

**Table 54.2 Differential diagnosis with placenta praevia**

| Clinical sign | Placenta praevia | Abruptio placentae |
|---|---|---|
| Pain | No pain | Uterine pain, may be severe; backache if placenta is posterior |
| Colour of blood loss | Bright, fresh | May be darker |
| 'Warning' haemorrhages | Yes | No |
| Onset of bleeding | Possibly following coitus, otherwise unexpected | May follow trauma, exertion |
| Degree of shock | In proportion to visible loss | May be more severe than visible loss suggests |
| Consistency of uterus | Soft, non-tender | Increased uterine tone, may be tense, rigid, 'woody' |
| Palpation | Fetus usually fairly easy to palpate | Tense uterus makes palpation difficult |
| Presentation | May be a malpresentation | Probably cephalic |
| Engagement | Not engaged | May be engaged |
| Fetal heartbeat | Probably present | May be absent |
| Abdominal girth | Equivalent to gestation | May increase due to concealed haemorrhage |

happen, deranged clotting should be suspected. Analgesia, such as morphine, may be required if the woman is in pain. An intravenous infusion of normal saline 0.9% or Hartmann's solution (Ringer's lactate) will be commenced. Blood transfusion may be required and several units of blood or packed cells may be needed if the haemorrhage has been substantial. In such cases, central venous pressure should be monitored to avoid the dangers of over- or undertransfusion.

The abdominal girth is sometimes measured and recorded. Meticulous observation and recording of vital signs, blood loss and fluid balance are essential in order to assess the woman's condition and plan her care. Ongoing management of the situation is governed by the condition of the mother and fetus. The midwife may need to involve the social worker if there are other children at home for whom care arrangements need to be made. The needs of the partner should also be addressed, which include support and information.

If the haemorrhage is not severe and urgent delivery is not indicated, the woman may be transferred to the antenatal ward once the bleeding settles and her condition is stable. In the absence of pain or active bleeding, the woman should not be confined to her bed and can be encouraged to wear her usual clothes during the day. In cases of placenta praevia, at least two units of cross-matched blood should always be available; local policy will dictate the regularity of sample update, usually weekly. This enables cross-match of fresh blood and ensures ready availability of blood should haemorrhage occur. If the bleeding is due to placenta praevia, the woman may be advised to remain in hospital until delivery. The midwife must ensure that the woman and her partner are fully informed about her condition and the likely management.

Following antepartum haemorrhage, tests to assess fetal wellbeing will be carried out because premature separation of the placenta may result in impaired placental function. Fetal growth will be assessed by ultrasound, and periodic continuous fetal heart monitoring will be performed. Women who have a rhesus-negative blood group should be given anti-D gammaglobulin in line with local policy, after each episode of bleeding.

## COMPLICATIONS

**Blood coagulation disorders (see Ch. 68):** When tissue damage occurs, there is a release of thromboplastin from the local cells. Thromboplastin activates the clotting mechanism and this results in the conversion of fibrinogen into fibrin. The sticky web of fibrin traps the cellular components of the blood and a clot forms, sealing off the bleeding point. The clot is later dispersed by plasmin, which is the active product of the fibrinolytic system. When a clot is broken down, fibrin degradation products (FDPs) are formed. Clot dispersal is a protective mechanism to prevent capillary blockage.

The system of initial clot formation followed by fibrinolysis is normally delicately balanced. If the coagulation system fails, bleeding will persist, while if the fibrinolytic system fails, clotting will persist.

Occasionally, tissue damage is so severe or widespread that there is a massive release of thromboplastin into the general circulation. Widespread clotting will then occur throughout the body. This condition is known as *disseminated intravascular coagulation* (DIC). This is extremely dangerous as the microthrombi generated by the thromboplastin will occlude small blood vessels. This results in ischaemic tissue damage within the body organs: the damaged tissue releases thromboplastin, which stimulates further clotting. Thus a vicious circle of tissue damage and uncontrolled clotting occurs. Any body organ may be affected: renal damage will result in oliguria or anuria; liver damage will lead to jaundice. If the lungs are affected, dyspnoea and cyanosis will occur; convulsions or coma indicate cerebral involvement. Microthrombi in the retina may cause blindness; if the pituitary gland is affected, Sheehan's syndrome, a condition that may have serious long-term effects on the mother's health and her future fertility, may occur (see website). Eventually, the available circulating platelets are depleted. Clotting factors, such as prothrombin (factor II), thromboplastin (factor III), proaccelerin (factor V), antihaemophilic factor (factor VIII) and fibrinogen (factor I), are exhausted. No further coagulation can take place: bleeding becomes apparent. This may take the form of oozing from venepuncture sites, mucous membrane bleeding, petechiae and uncontrollable uterine haemorrhage.

DIC is always a secondary event, occurring as a result of massive tissue damage and thromboplastin release. It may complicate conditions such as severe pre-eclampsia, septicaemia or amniotic fluid embolism. It may also occur following abruptio placentae when thromboplastin is released from the damaged placental, decidual and myometrial tissue. Unless DIC is recognized and treated promptly, the condition may become uncontrollable with death an inevitable outcome. The midwife must be aware of any woman who is at risk of DIC and be alert for the signs of coagulation failure. All maternity units should have an emergency protocol for dealing with such cases. Any woman with an abruptio placentae should have screening tests for coagulation defects. These tests include:

- partial thromboplastin time (normally 35–45 seconds)
- prothrombin time (normally 10–14 seconds)
- thrombin time (normally 10–15 seconds)
- fibrinogen levels (2.5–4 g/L)
- fibrin degradation products
- whole blood film and platelet count.

Fresh frozen plasma, packed cells and platelets are used in the treatment of DIC. Heparin is rarely used as it may exacerbate the haemorrhage, especially if the uterus is not empty.

**Acute renal failure:** This may occur following severe shock in cases of antepartum haemorrhage.

**Postpartum haemorrhage:** Following severe abruptio placentae, postpartum haemorrhage is most likely to be caused by a blood coagulation disorder, whereas following placenta praevia it is due to the inability of the lower uterine segment to contract effectively. Aortic compression may be necessary to control cases of intractable haemorrhage.

**Infection:** Sepsis is likely owing to the woman's lowered resistance following a state of severe shock, a large blood transfusion, increased intervention in labour and anaemia.

**Anaemia:** The haemoglobin must be checked and anaemia corrected in the puerperium.

**Psychological disturbances/psychoses:** Psychological disorders after childbirth are more likely following complications of pregnancy and labour, and may be due to the ensuing anaemia or post-traumatic stress (PTS) syndrome (Ch. 69).

## VASA PRAEVIA

This unusual condition may result in vaginal bleeding. It is associated with velamentous insertion of the cord. One of the fetal vessels traverses the membranes in the region of the internal os, in front of the presenting part. Occlusion of the vessel may occur as the presenting part compresses the membranes. When the membranes rupture, the vessel can be torn and severe fetal bleeding occurs. The perinatal mortality associated with this condition is high (Suzuki & Igarash 2008). Diagnosis is difficult but a pulsating vessel may be felt on vaginal examination. Velamentous insertion can often be detected on routine ultrasound examination from the second trimester of pregnancy and vasa praevia can be confirmed by transvaginal colour Doppler scanning (Nomiyama et al 1998).

If vasa praevia is suspected, the midwife should leave the membranes intact and inform the obstetrician.

The midwife should be aware that there is a higher risk of vasa praevia in placenta praevia, where there is a succenturiate lobe and in IVF pregnancies (Olayinka et al 1999).

## CONCLUSION

Bleeding in pregnancy remains a major cause of maternal morbidity and mortality. The midwife must be familiar with local policy for management of bleeding in pregnancy and regular emergency drills should be held in maternity units to ensure that the obstetric team can respond to haemorrhage quickly and appropriately (Lewis 2007). Midwives should be familiar with the recommended guidelines for the management of massive obstetric haemorrhage, to be found in Lewis (2007).

Midwives also need to be able to identify women who might be at risk, and refer appropriately, also ensuring that the woman and her family are informed and supported throughout. Often the midwife will be the person providing continuity during the woman's pregnancy, facilitating holistic, sensitive and appropriate care to the woman, her baby and family.

### KEY POINTS

- Vaginal bleeding at any stage of pregnancy is always abnormal and may be indicative of a serious complication.
- Midwives need to educate the woman and her family regarding deviations from normal, and ensure that they are aware of what action should be taken and with whom they should communicate.
- Midwives must be aware of the possible causes of bleeding in pregnancy.
- A prompt and appropriate response may prevent the loss of the fetus and may save the mother's life.
- Midwives must be aware of the possible emotional, social and psychological impact of bleeding or pregnancy loss for the woman and her partner.

## REFERENCES

*Abortion Act*, London, 1967, HMSO.

Andersen N, Wohlfahrt J, Christens P, et al: Maternal age and fetal loss: population based register linkage study, *British Medical Journal* 320(7251):1708–1712, 2000.

ARC (Antenatal Results and Choices) (website). www.arc-org.uk 2009. Accessed January 27, 2009.

Backos M, Regan L: *High risk pregnancy: management options*, Edinburgh, 2006, Saunders.

Baker PN: *Obstetrics by Ten Teachers*, London, 2006, Arnold.

Baulies S, Maize N, Munoz A, et al: Prenatal ultrasound diagnosis of placenta previa and analysis of risk factors, *Prenatal Diagnosis* 27(7):595–599, 2007.

Beischer N, Mackay E, Colditz P: *Obstetrics and the newborn*, London, 1997, WB Saunders.

Benrubi GI: *Handbook of obstetric emergencies*, Philadelphia, 2005, Lippincott Williams & Wilkins.

Boyles S, Ness R, Grisso J, et al: Life event stress and the association with spontaneous abortion in gravid women at an urban emergency department, *Health Psychology* 19(6):510–514, 2000.

Carr R, Coustan D: Nonprescription drugs and alcohol: abuse and effects in pregnancy. In Reece EA, Hobbins JC, editors: *Clinical obstetrics: the fetus & mother*, ed 3, Oxford, 2007, Blackwell.

Conway K, Russell G: Couples' grief and experience of support in the aftermath of miscarriage, *British Journal of Medical Psychology* 73(4):531–545, 2000.

Creinin MD, Potter C, Holovanisin M, et al: Mifepristone and misoprostol and methotrexate/misoprostol in clinical practice for abortion, *American Journal of Obstetrics and Gynecology* 188(3):664–669, 2003.

Department of Health (DH): *Report on Confidential Enquiries into Maternal Deaths in the United Kingdom 1988–1990*, London, 1994, HMSO.

Dimond B: Termination of pregnancy, *British Journal of Midwifery* 9(2):108, 2001.

Donders G, Van Bulck B, Caudron J, et al: Relationship of bacterial vaginosis and mycoplasmas to the risk of spontaneous abortion, *American Journal of Obstetrics and Gynecology* 183(2):431–437, 2000.

Drife J: Bleeding in pregnancy. In Chamberlain G, editor: *Turnbull's obstetrics*, Edinburgh, 2002, Churchill Livingstone.

Gopalkrishnan K, Padwal V, Meherji P, et al: Poor quality sperm as it affects repeated early pregnancy loss, *Archives of Andrology* 45(2):111–117, 2000.

Handler A, Mason E, Rosenberg D, et al: The relationship between exposure during pregnancy to cigarette smoking and cocaine use and placenta praevia, *American Journal of Obstetrics and Gynecology* 170(3):884–889, 1994.

Home Department: *Criminal statistics England and Wales 2000*, London, 2001, The Stationery Office.

Home Office: Identity and Passport Service, General Registrar Office, official information on births, deaths and marriages (website). www.gro.gov.uk/gro/content. 2008. Accessed January 26, 2009.

Home Office: Crime statistics (website). www.homeoffice.gov.uk/rds/recordedcrime1.html. 2009. Accessed February 12, 2009.

Human Fertilization and Embryology Act, London, 1990, Office of Public Sector Information.

Kauffman D, Sutkin G, Heine R, et al: Metastatic complete hydatidiform mole with a surviving co-existent twin. A case report, *Journal of Reproductive Medicine* 44(2):131–134, 1999.

Lemus J: Ectopic pregnancy: an update, *Current Opinion in Obstetrics and Gynecology* 12(5):369–375, 2000.

Lewis G, editor: *Why mothers die 1997–1999: the fifth report of the Confidential Enquiries into Maternal Deaths in the United Kingdom*, London, 2001, RCOG.

Lewis G, editor: *Saving mothers' lives: reviewing maternal deaths to make motherhood safer – 2003–2005. The Seventh Report on Confidential Enquiries into Maternal Deaths in the United Kingdom*, London, 2007, CEMACH.

Lin C, Wang S, Hsu Y, et al: Risk for respiratory distress syndrome in preterm infants born to mothers complicated by placenta previa, *Early Human Development* 60(3):215–224, 2001.

Neilson JP: Interventions for suspected placenta praevia, *Cochrane Database of Systematic Reviews (Online)* (2):CD001998, 2003.

Neilson JP, Hickey M, Vazquez J: Medical treatment for early fetal death (less than 24 weeks) *Cochrane Database of Systematic Reviews (Online)* (3):CD002253, 2006.

Nomiyama M, Toyota Y, Kawano H: Antenatal diagnosis of velamentous umbilical cord insertion and vasa previa with color Doppler imaging, *Ultrasound in Obstetrics and Gynecology* 12(6):426–429, 1998.

Oats JN, Abraham S: *Llewellyn-Jones fundamentals of obstetrics and gynaecology*, ed 8, London, 2004, Elsevier.

Olayinka K, Turner M, Lees C, et al: Vasa previa: an avoidable obstetric tragedy, *Obstetrical and Gynecological Survey* 54(2):138–145, 1999.

Rana A, Sawhney H, Gopolan S, et al: Abruptio placentae and chorioamnionitis – microbiological and histological correlation, *Acta Obstetricia et Gynecologica Scandinavica* 78(5):363–366, 1999.

Rasmussen S, Irgens L, Dalaker K: Outcome of pregnancies subsequent to placental abruption: a risk assessment, *Acta Obstetricia et Gynecologica Scandinavica* 79(6):496–501, 2000.

Ray J, Laskin C: Folic acid and homocystine metabolic defects and the risk of placental abruption, pre-eclampsia and spontaneous pregnancy loss: a systematic review, *Placenta* 20(7):519–529, 1999.

Reis P, Sander C, Pearlman M: Abruptio placentae after auto accidents. A case control study, *Journal of Reproductive Medicine* 45(1):6–10, 2000.

Reis JL, Condeco P, Ventura P, et al: Conservative management of a cervical pregnancy with methotrexate, *Female Patient* 33(3):36–38, 2008.

Royal College of Obstetricians and Gynaecologists (RCOG): *The management of gestational trophoblastic neoplasia. Green top guideline 38*, London, 2004a, RCOG.

Royal College of Obstetricians and Gynaecologists. *The management of tubal pregnancies. Green top guideline 21*, London, 2004b, RCOG.

Royal College of Obstetricians and Gynaecologists (RCOG): *Placenta praevia and placenta praevia acreta: diagnosis and management. Green top guideline 27*, London, 2005, RCOG.

Royal College of Obstetricians and Gynaecologists (RCOG): (2006) *Management of early pregnancy loss. Green top guideline 25*, London, 2006, RCOG.

Royal College of Obstetricians and Gynaecologists (RCOG): *The role of emergency and elective interventional radiology in postpartum haemorrhage. Practice guideline 6*, London, 2007, RCOG.

Seckl M, Fisher R, Salwerno G, et al: Choriocarcinoma and partial hydatidiform moles, *Lancet* 356(9223):36–39, 2000.

Silver R, Branch D: Sporadic and recurrent pregnancy loss. In Reece EA, Hobbins JC, editors: *Clinical obstetrics: the fetus & mother*, ed 3, Oxford, 2007, Blackwell.

Sood A, Sorosky J, Mayr N, et al: Cervical cancer diagnosed shortly after pregnancy: prognostic variables and delivery routes, *Obstetrics and Gynecology* 95(6 Pt 1):832–838, 2000.

Stillbirth and Neonatal Death Society (SANDS): www.uk-sands.org. 2009. Stillbirth and neonatal death charity supporting anyone affected by the death of a baby and promoting research to reduce the loss of babies' lives. Accessed July 13, 2010.

Suzuki S, Igarash M: Clinical significance of pregnancies with succenturiate lobes of the placenta, *Archives of Gynecology and Obstetrics* 227(4):299–301, 2008.

Tin-Chiu L, Bates S, Pearce M: Biochemical tests in complications in early pregnancy. In O'Brien P, editor: The yearbook of obstetrics and gynaecology vol 7, London, 1999, RCOG.

Wen S, Demissie K, Liu S, et al: Placenta praevia and male sex at birth: results from a population-based study, *Paediatric and Perinatal Epidemiology* 14(4):300–304, 2000.

Wiznitzer A, Shener E: Ectopic and heterotopic pregnancies. In Reece EA, Hobbins JC, editors: *Clinical obstetrics: the fetus & mother*, Oxford, 2007, Blackwell.

Yang Q, Wen SW, Oppeheimer I, et al: Association of caesarean delivery for first birth with placenta previa and placental abruption in second pregnancy, *British Journal of Obstetrics and Gynaecology* 114(5):609–613, 2007.

Chapter 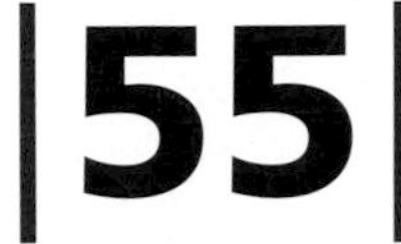

# Medical disorders of pregnancy

Chris Bewley

## LEARNING OUTCOMES

After reading this chapter, you will be able to:

- have an overview of some pre-existing medical and other disorders which affect or are affected by pregnancy
- recognize the signs and symptoms which require immediate referral for appropriate medical help
- build on knowledge of normal physiology to gain insight into the underlying pathophysiology of some conditions
- be familiar with some of the drugs used in various medical conditions
- realize the importance of the midwife's role in the multidisciplinary team supporting women whose pregnancy is complicated by a medical disorder.

## INTRODUCTION

Midwives are mainly concerned with normal pregnancy; however, they must be aware of pre-existing conditions which make a woman unsuitable for booking in a low-risk environment and be able to recognize signs of deterioration in a woman's condition, and know what action to take (Lewis 2007, NMC 2008). With modern treatment, many women with medical conditions who previously would not have reached childbearing age, now do so. Trends in childbearing also show that women are having children at a later age, by which time they may have developed medical conditions such as heart disease, hypertension and diabetes which are associated with unhealthy lifestyles and obesity (Lewis 2008). Lewis also suggests that while health professionals have given effective attention to the 'big obstetric killers' such as haemorrhage, sepsis and pre-eclampsia, more women now die from indirect causes relating to their medical conditions (Lewis 2008).

Women with pre-existing medical conditions have often received lifelong treatment and are experts in their own care and treatment. They will often be familiar with a medical team, and may have received pre-conception advice prior to planning the pregnancy. More rarely, they may have received advice against becoming pregnant and may be considering a termination, or have deliberately decided to embark on a pregnancy regardless of personal risk. Whether or not the pregnancy continues, women with complicated pregnancies report that they feel 'out of control' and experience high levels of anxiety. They feel the focus of pregnancy is on the fetus and once the baby is born, care is not so intense, so they feel isolated in the postnatal period (Spencer 2007, Thomas 1999).

An in-depth approach to all medical conditions is beyond the scope of this chapter; however, a range of medical conditions is considered, all of which, if disclosed at the antenatal booking interview, require a multidisciplinary approach (NICE 2008a). It cannot be overemphasized that some of the signs and symptoms associated with severe maternal illness, such as breathlessness and heartburn, are common towards term in a normal pregnancy, which is why they can be easily overlooked or disregarded (Lewis 2007).

Some conditions are discussed in further detail in the chapter, outlining the effects on mother and fetus/neonate, treatment, and specific midwifery care. Recommendations are given on the website for further reading, and include some of the excellent new publications, specifically written for midwives.

## ANAEMIA

Anaemia is a deficiency in the quality or quantity of red blood cells, resulting in reduced oxygen-carrying capacity of the blood. In the UK, NICE guidelines for antenatal care indicate that routine iron supplementation during pregnancy is unnecessary, suggesting that investigations and/or supplementation are warranted only when haemoglobin levels are lower than 11 g/dL at first contact, and 10.5 g/dL at 28 weeks (NICE 2008a). However, Evans (2008) suggests that iron deficiency anaemia (IDA) has a profound impact on women's lives throughout the lifespan, and that postnatal anaemia contributes to poor health and low mood which is frequently overlooked. Work from the World Health Organization (WHO) also highlights the risks of anaemia to pregnant and non-pregnant women (WHO 1992), and this was illustrated by data gathered by McLean et al (2007) which plotted the prevalence of anaemia in children and women of reproductive age throughout the world, indicating the highest rates in the African and Indian continents.

### Types of anaemia

Anaemias can be classified according to their causes:

1. Iron deficiency anaemia
2. Folic acid deficiency anaemia
3. Haemoglobinopathies, which include sickle cell disease and thalassaemia
4. Anaemia as a result of blood loss or secondary to infection
5. Aplastic varieties (rare in pregnancy).

### Effects on pregnancy and childbirth

Anaemia will have the following effects:

- Undermining of the woman's general health
- Lowering of resistance to infection
- Exacerbation of the minor disorders of pregnancy, such as digestive problems
- In severe cases – may cause intrauterine hypoxia
- Perinatal mortality is increased in severe anaemia
- Antepartum and postpartum haemorrhage are more serious
- Higher risk of thromboembolic disorders
- Increased risk of postnatal depression
- Risk of maternal mortality is increased.

### Signs and symptoms

- Pallor of mucous membranes
- Tiredness, dizziness and fainting
- Dyspnoea on exertion
- Palpitations
- Oedema
- Digestive upsets and loss of appetite commonly occur and tend to exacerbate the condition.

**Reflective activity 55.1**

When are blood tests carried out in your unit to determine women's haemoglobin levels, and what tests are done? At what point is action taken? How does this relate to the information given above?

## Iron deficiency anaemia

Iron deficiency is the commonest cause of anaemia in women. Anaemia may predate pregnancy, arising from poor diet, menorrhagia, or repeated pregnancies, especially if close together. Bleeding from haemorrhoids or antepartum haemorrhage may also cause anaemia, as may hookworm or parasitic infestation.

### Investigations

After taking a detailed history about general health, diet, infection, blood loss and other relevant information, further investigations such as haemoglobin level, mean corpuscular volume (MCV), packed cell volume (PCV), total iron binding capacity, and serum ferritin will give a full picture (McKay 2000, NICE 2008a) (see Ch. 33).

### Management

Where iron deficiency anaemia has been diagnosed, oral iron 120–140 mg daily may be given as:

- *ferrous sulphate* – 200 mg tablet twice daily, giving 120 mg iron; or
- *ferrous gluconate* – two 300 mg tablets twice daily, giving 140 mg iron.

Women need to know that iron absorption is enhanced by vitamin C and inhibited by tannin in tea, and that there might be some side-effects, such as blackness of stools, nausea, epigastric pain, diarrhoea and constipation. Side-effects may be reduced by taking the iron after meals, although this decreases iron absorption. It may be better tolerated at bedtime, and by leaving 6 to 8 hours between doses. However, the type and dose may need to be changed if symptoms persist (Jordan 2002). This is also a good opportunity for the midwife to provide dietary advice (see Ch. 17).

In more severe cases of anaemia, the woman may be given intramuscular injections of iron. Special precautions should be taken when administering this, to avoid permanent staining of the skin (Jordan 2002).

**Table 55.1 Haemoglobin combination in sickle cell disorders**

| | |
|---|---|
| HbSS | Homozygous sickle cell disease (sickle cell anaemia) |
| HbSC | Heterozygous sickle cell disease (sickle cell C disease) |
| HbCC | Homozygous CC disease (*not* a sickling disorder) |
| HbS beta/thal | Sickle/beta thalassaemia |
| HbAS | Sickle cell trait |

## Folic acid deficiency anaemia

Folic acid is necessary for formation of nuclei in all body cells. In pregnancy, when there is proliferation of cells, a deficiency may occur unless the intake is increased.

### Management

Dietary sources of folic acid are lightly cooked green leafy vegetables, such as broccoli and spinach (see Ch. 17). Following the demonstrated link between neural tube defects and intake of folic acid, all pregnant women, and those intending to become pregnant, are advised to take 0.4–4 mg folic acid daily (NICE 2006).

## Haemoglobinopathies

Haemoglobinopathies are inherited conditions in which one or more abnormal types wholly or partly replace normal adult haemoglobin HbA. The main haemoglobinopathies which complicate pregnancy are sickle cell disease and thalassaemia. These conditions are genetically complex and are presented here in a simplified form, with patterns of inheritance illustrated in Tables 55.1. and 55.2.

### Sickle cell trait and sickle cell disease

In sickle cell disease, erythrocytes containing HbS have a short lifespan of 5–10 days (rather than the normal span of 120 days). '*Sickling*' occurs when cells become sickle shaped under conditions of low oxygen tension, including hypoxia, dehydration, infection, acidosis and cold (Dike 2007, Nelson-Piercy 2006). Cells are easily haemolysed and cause extremely painful vaso-occlusive symptoms in joints, in the abdomen and in the extremities during acute exacerbations, known as a *crisis*. This leads to chronic haemolytic anaemia, and an increase in the rate of haemoglobin synthesis in the bone marrow, which may lead to folic acid deficiency. Other complications are thromboembolic disorders, retinopathy, renal papillary necrosis, leg ulcers, and increased risk of infection because of disorders in the function of the spleen (Dike 2007, Nelson-Piercy 2006). Acute chest syndrome may occur, in which there is pyrexia, tachypnoea, leucocytosis and pleuritic chest pain.

**Table 55.2 Patterns of inheritance in sickle cell anaemia**

| | Mother | | Father | |
|---|---|---|---|---|
| | Sickle cell anaemia (HbSS) | | Normal haemoglobin (HbAA) | |
| Infants | HbAS | HbAS | HbAS | HbAS |
| | (All infants will have sickle cell trait) | | | |
| | Sickle cell anaemia (HbSS) | | Sickle cell trait (HbAS) | |
| Infants | HbAS | HbAS | HbSS | HbSS |
| | Sickle cell trait (HbAS) | | Sickle cell trait (HbAS) | |
| Infants | HbAA | HbAS | HbAS | HbSS |

*Effect on pregnancy*

The diagnosis is usually made in childhood, once most fetal haemoglobin (HbF) has been replaced, and all women at risk should be tested. Nelson-Piercy (2006) observes that 35% of pregnancies will be complicated by crises, and perinatal mortality is increased four- to sixfold. Pregnancy may be complicated by increased risk of miscarriage, intrauterine growth restriction (IUGR), preterm labour, and pre-eclampsia.

### Management

#### *Pregnancy*

All women at risk, together with their partners, should be screened for haemoglobinopathies in early pregnancy. Iron therapy should be avoided but folic acid given routinely throughout pregnancy. Blood transfusions may be required to treat severe anaemia, and exchange transfusions carried out to remove abnormal HbS and replace it with normal HbA, although the advantages of this are debatable.

Women with sickle cell disease may have poor appetites and need to have regular small meals including meat, fish, eggs, cheese, fruit and wholemeal bread. They should be aware of the symptoms of infection, and who to contact if they feel unwell. In the case of a crisis, the woman will be admitted to hospital, where she should be kept warm, and given pain relief, usually morphine (Nelson-Piercy 2006). Oxygen levels are monitored by pulse oximetry or arterial blood gases.

#### *Labour*

Dehydration, acidosis and infection all lead to *sickling*, and must be avoided, whilst avoiding fluid overload.

Unless there are obstetric indications, caesarean section is not indicated, and general anaesthesia should be avoided. Management must involve the haematology department, and colleagues knowledgeable in the care and management of women with sickle cell disease, and the woman should be encouraged to report any problems.

### *Postnatally*

Specialist help is available to women and their partners and screening tests may be offered during pregnancy and postnatally, to detect abnormal haemoglobins in the baby.

### Thalassaemia

Thalassaemia is a condition in which there is an abnormal amount of $HbA_2$. It is most common in people of Mediterranean and Asian origin. The condition arises from defects in the alpha or beta globin chains resulting in thin, shortly lived red cells, often misshapen and deficient in haemoglobin, causing profound anaemia. As with sickle cell trait, thalassaemia in its mild forms confers some protection against malaria.

### Management

As iron stores are likely to be overloaded, rather than depleted, iron supplements are not usually given. Folic acid is given throughout pregnancy, however, because the bone marrow is active in replacing the short-lived red blood cells.

## Other causes of anaemia

### Glucose-6-phosphate dehydrogenase (G-6-PD) deficiency

This rare, X-linked inherited enzyme deficiency typically affects people of African, Asian and Mediterranean origin. Haemolytic crises occur if the affected person takes certain drugs, including antimalarial preparations, sulphonamides and antibiotics (nitrofurantoin, nalidixic acid and possibly chloramphenicol) or eats broad (fava) beans. It may be implicated in cases of prolonged neonatal jaundice.

**Reflective activity 55.2**

Where is your nearest specialist centre for haemoglobinopathies? Does this reflect the ethnic mix of your community?

## HEART DISEASE

Heart disease is the leading non-obstetric cause of maternal death in the UK, with 48 maternal deaths reported in the triennium 2003–2005 (Lewis 2007). Myocardial infarction is the most common cardiac cause of maternal death. The total incidence of cardiac disease in pregnancy is 0.5–2% (McLean et al 2008).

Signs and symptoms of cardiac disease are:

- dyspnoea
- chest pain
- limitation of activity
- palpitations/arrhythmias/dysrhythmias
- cyanosis
- heart sound changes.

During pregnancy, women with pre-existing heart disease may experience a worsening of symptoms, due to physiological changes of pregnancy (see Ch. 31). There is an increase in circulating blood volume, increased resting oxygen consumption, decreased peripheral vascular resistance, an increase in stroke volume and a slight increase in resting heart rate (Adamson et al 2007). These changes influence haemodynamics, increasing strain on the heart, which is further compromised during labour. A wide range of conditions affect the heart in a mild, moderate or severe way, and conditions may be congenital or acquired, as outlined below.

### Congenital heart disease

Congenital defects relate to the structure of the heart, and the most common are atrial septal defects, patent ductus arteriosus, and ventricular septal defects. Other more serious lesions include *Fallot's tetralogy* (ventricular septal defect, pulmonary stenosis, overriding aorta and right ventricular hypertrophy) and *Eisenmenger's syndrome* (ventricular septal defect, overriding aorta and right ventricular hypertrophy). Most lesions are corrected by surgery in childhood. *Marfan's syndrome* is a genetic condition in which cardiac anomalies occur. Pregnancy outcome is worst where there is pulmonary hypertension in Eisenmenger's syndrome and in Marfan's syndrome where there is aortic involvement (Adamson et al 2007). Many pre-existing cardiac disorders are complex, and pre-pregnancy counselling is essential, so that women know their own health status in relation to likely outcome. Some women, particularly those with cyanotic heart disease and pulmonary hypertension, may be advised to avoid pregnancy, or, if pregnant, may be advised to have termination of pregnancy (Adamson et al 2007). However, the woman's choice must be respected.

### Acquired heart disease

This usually involves damage to heart valves, such as stenosis, where the valve is constricted, or incompetence, where the valve fails to close completely. Valvular problems are often subsequent to infection or rheumatic heart disease, now rare in the UK but prevalent in developing countries, and a problem for immigrant mothers (Lewis 2007). Women who have had valve replacements will be on anticoagulant therapy, and choices need to be made to balance the need for anticoagulants against the risks they pose for the fetus. *Warfarin* is teratogenic in early pregnancy and may lead to fetal haemorrhage at any time. There is considerable debate about appropriate combinations of *warfarin* and *heparin* and whether fetal risks may be reduced by changing to self-administered subcutaneous or intravenous heparin, which does not cross the placenta, after the first trimester (Adamson et al 2007). The effects of heparin are reversed by *protamine sulphate.*

Peripartum cardiomyopathy is a rare, functional, cardiac complication, with sudden cardiac failure, arising in the last month of pregnancy or in the first 5 months postpartum, where there has been no evidence of heart disease pre-pregnancy. It is more common in women of black race, multiparity, and higher maternal age, and is a significant cause of maternal mortality (Adamson et al 2007, Lewis 2007, McLean et al 2008).

### Effects on the fetus in maternal cardiac disease

- Increased risk of congenital cardiac defects
- Intrauterine hypoxia
- Intrauterine death
- Effects of maternal medication.

### Antenatal care

Pre-pregnancy counselling and then care in a dedicated antenatal cardiac clinic are required, with input from obstetrician, cardiologist, anaesthetist and midwife (Adamson et al 2007).

Aims of antenatal care are to detect heart failure and disturbances of cardiac rhythm. Women and their partners need help and support during what may be a particularly anxious time. Practical help may be needed with housework, transport to clinics and childcare.

A high-protein, low-carbohydrate, low-salt diet is recommended. Weight control is important, as excessive weight gain places extra strain on the heart. Infection is treated with antibiotics to reduce the risk of bacterial endocarditis; dental work, which may be a potential source of infection, should be carried out early in pregnancy.

Major antenatal complications are acute pulmonary oedema and congestive cardiac failure. Women and partners should be aware of symptoms which indicate worsening of the condition, such as dyspnoea, cough or chest pain, which will need hospital admission immediately for stabilization.

### Labour

Depending on the type of cardiac disorder and the progress of the pregnancy, labour may be spontaneous or induced or an elective caesarean section may be carried out. Prophylactic antibiotics may be given to reduce the risk of bacterial endocarditis (Adamson et al 2007). Epidural analgesia is recommended, but with caution in regard to hypotension, and it is contraindicated in women on anticoagulant therapy. The optimum position for the woman is the 'cardiac position' supported left lateral, or semi-upright, with the legs lower than the abdomen (Adamson et al 2007). In addition to usual midwifery observations in labour, the following are important:

- colour in case of cyanosis
- respiratory rate – should remain below 24 per minute
- degree of dyspnoea
- radial and apical pulses – should remain below 110 per minute
- ECG may be continuous throughout labour
- fluid balance to prevent overload
- continuous electronic fetal monitoring.

In the absence of obstetric complications, vaginal delivery causes less haemodynamic fluctuation than caesarean section (Adamson et al 2007).

There is no reason for elective instrumental delivery if birth is proceeding well; however, excessive pushing should be avoided since it alters haemodynamics and may compromise cardiac activity. If the woman feels the urge to push, short pushes with the mouth open should be encouraged. Sudden strong uterine contraction in the third stage may direct so much of the uterine circulation of blood to the systemic circulation that the impaired heart may become seriously compromised, therefore ergometrine and syntometrine are not used. Syntocinon should be used with caution, and is contraindicated in cases of heart failure (Adamson et al 2007).

### Postnatal care

Continuing close observation of vital signs is necessary as heart failure or peripartum cardiomyopathy may occur in the first few days postnatally. Women require rest, but not complete immobilization. Physiotherapy helps to reduce the risk of thromboembolic disorders. There is usually no contraindication to breastfeeding. The risk of congenital heart disease in the baby is increased and, therefore, careful examination of the baby is essential.

Careful plans should be made for transfer to the community. Women need practical help to enable them to rest, and cope with the demands of the baby. An appointment should be made with the cardiologist 4–6 weeks postnatally, to assess cardiac function. Advice should be given on appropriate contraception postnatally, and pre-conception counselling for future pregnancies.

## THYROID DISORDERS

Physiological changes in pregnancy lead to alterations in thyroid function and iodine uptake, and can adversely affect women who have pre-existing thyroid disorders, as described below.

## Thyrotoxicosis (hyperthyroidism, *Graves' disease*)

Thyrotoxicosis occurs in about 1:500 pregnancies, with 95% of these associated with an autoimmune disorder in which thyroid-stimulating hormone (TSH) receptor antibodies are produced. When untreated, the condition is associated with infertility,, but conception occurs commonly in women who are treated. The condition does not appear to be made worse by pregnancy (Nelson-Piercy 2006).

Women with thyrotoxicosis experience sensitivity to heat, tachycardia, palpitations, vomiting, palmar erythema and emotional lability. Whilst all of these are also features of normal pregnancy, women with thyrotoxicosis also experience weight loss, tremor, persistent tachycardia, eyelid lag and prominent eyes. The disease usually predates pregnancy, but may arise for the first time in the first or early second trimester (Nelson-Piercy 2006) and may be mistaken for hyperemesis gravidarum.

If untreated, there is an increased risk of miscarriage, IUGR, preterm labour, and perinatal mortality. In women who are poorly controlled, there is a risk of a thyroid crisis, or 'storm', with hyperpyrexia, palpitations and tachycardia, which may lead to heart failure, especially in labour (Nelson-Piercy 2006).

### Treatment

Treatment is by *carbimazole* or *propylthiouracil* (PTU), either for 12–18 months following diagnosis, or over a longer period. Both drugs cross the placenta (PTU less so) and may cause fetal hypothyroidism and/or goitre (Nelson-Piercy 2006), but they are unlikely to cause teratogenic problems at therapeutic levels. In the early management of the disease, beta-blockers may be given for the first month to control palpitations, tachycardia and tremor.

Fetal effects are unlikely with good control, but outcomes are unpredictable. There may be fetal tachycardia, IUGR, fetal goitre, and a 50% increase in mortality if the disease is untreated. After delivery, the baby may develop thyrotoxicosis, with weight loss, tachycardia, jitteriness, and poor feeding. Treatment is by antithyroid drugs. The neonatal condition will resolve once maternal thyroid-stimulating antibodies have cleared from the neonatal system.

During the antenatal period, assessment of maternal heart rate, weight gain, and experience of nausea and vomiting should be carried out. Clinical assessment of fetal condition includes monitoring for IUGR; listening to the fetal heart; and may include serial ultrasound scans to assess growth and to detect goitre. During labour, observation of temperature, heart rate and rhythm are necessary, in addition to usual midwifery care. Minimal amounts of antithyroid drugs are excreted in breast milk, so breastfeeding is not contraindicated (Nelson-Piercy 2006).

## Hypothyroidism

This occurs in about 1% of pregnancies and there is usually a family history. It is characterized by weight gain, lethargy, hair loss, dry skin, constipation, fluid retention, carpal tunnel syndrome and possibly goitre. There is also intolerance of cold and a low pulse rate. Like hyperthyroidism, it is thought to be an autoimmune disorder.

Untreated, it may lead to infertility, increased risk of miscarriage and fetal loss. Treatment is by thyroxine supplementation, and when well controlled there are no adverse effects on pregnancy. Little thyroxine crosses the placenta, and neonatal hypothyroidism is very rare (Nelson-Piercy 2006).

# RENAL CONDITIONS

Three common forms of urinary tract infection occur during pregnancy: *asymptomatic bacteriuria*, *cystitis* and *pyelonephritis*. Infection may arise in pregnancy because of physiological changes, as the ureters and pelvis of the kidney become dilated and urinary stasis may occur. Dilatation of the ureters is further accentuated when the enlarging uterus presses on the ureters at the pelvic brim, particularly on the right side since the uterus inclines to the right. Other predisposing factors are vesicoureteric reflux of urine containing bacteria, urinary catheterization (even with impeccable technique), and abnormalities of the renal tract (Gilbert & Harmon 2002).

### Causative organisms

The main causative organism is *Escherichia coli*, a normal inhabitant of the intestines, which may increase in virulence during pregnancy under the influence of oestrogen. Occasionally, other organisms, such as *Proteus vulgaris*, *Streptococcus faecalis* or *Pseudomonas aeruginosa*, are involved.

## Asymptomatic bacteriuria

Between 2% and 10% of all women have asymptomatic bacteriuria, that is, the presence of more than 100,000 colony-forming units of a single organism per millilitre of urine (Nelson-Piercy 2006). Untreated, it leads to urinary tract infection in 30–40% of women, in the form of cystitis and/or pyelonephritis. NICE guidelines recommend that women are offered screening for asymptomatic bacteruria (NICE 2008a).

## Cystitis

Cystitis, or infection of the urinary bladder, occurs in up to 1.5% of pregnancies. Women may experience:

- dysuria
- haematuria
- frequency/urgency
- suprapubic pain
- backache.

Diagnosis is by culture from a midstream specimen of urine, and treatment is by antibiotics, typically *ampicillin*. Follow-up testing of urine should be carried out as the condition may recur. Women should be advised to drink plenty of fluids, preferably not acidic or carbonated, to wipe the perineum from front to back, and to empty the bladder immediately before and following sexual intercourse. Cranberry juice or capsules may help in the treatment and prevention of urinary tract infection, particularly that associated with *E. coli* (Lavender 2000). It is thought that tannins in cranberries prevent P-fimbriated *E. coli* from attaching themselves to uroepithelial cells, thereby inhibiting infection. Low-sugar versions are suitable for women with diabetes.

Women also need to know the signs and symptoms of further infection and be encouraged to report these to the midwife or GP (Gilbert & Harmon 2002), as ascending infection may lead to the more serious condition of pyelonephritis.

## Pyelonephritis

Pyelonephritis occurs in 1–2% of all pregnancies and is more common in women who exhibit bacteriuria (Nelson-Piercy 2006). Renal tubules become inflamed, and their ability to reabsorb sodium is adversely affected. Normally, sodium and water are excreted in the urine, but where reabsorption is affected, they remain in the body, causing oedema and increased pressure on the cardiovascular system. There is a consequent decrease in urine output. Additionally, buffer production of potassium and ammonia is affected, causing accumulation of free hydrogen ions and acidaemia.

When glomerular damage occurs, nitrogenous waste cannot be removed from the blood, causing an increase in serum creatinine, urea and uric acid, and a decrease in urinary creatinine, urea and uric acid. Glomerular damage also causes loss of plasma proteins into the urine, changing osmotic pressure and leading to further oedema (Marieb 2006).

Thus, infections need to be treated quickly and effectively, and the woman's wellbeing and response to treatment carefully monitored.

### Signs and symptoms

- Pain from the loin to the groin, often on the right side
- Headache
- Nausea and vomiting
- Dysuria
- Frequency
- Pyrexia, sometimes accompanied by rigors
- Tachycardia
- The woman may be anaemic and urinary output may be diminished.

### Diagnosis

Diagnosis is confirmed by microscopic examination of a midstream specimen of urine. This will reveal pus cells and more than 100,000 bacteria per millilitre. The urine is acid, smells offensive and contains red blood cells and protein. Blood cultures may also be taken.

### Management

The woman may be admitted to hospital for rest, observation and treatment. A broad-spectrum antibiotic such as *ampicillin* (500 mg every 6–8 hours) is usually prescribed but may be changed once sensitivity of the causative organism is established. Initially, intravenous administration is more effective. The woman should drink plenty of fluids to avoid urinary stasis. Fluid balance is monitored.

Lying on the unaffected side will help to relieve the pain and assist drainage. Analgesics are prescribed as necessary. Temperature, pulse and respirations are recorded 4-hourly. Midstream specimens of urine are tested until urine is free of pus. The haemoglobin is checked due to risk of anaemia.

Recurrence of the infection may occur during pregnancy or postnatally, necessitating follow-up. Antibiotic therapy is continued for a month, and sometimes throughout pregnancy. Three months following delivery when the renal tract has returned to normal, further renal investigations may be carried out (Gilbert & Harmon 2002).

### Effects on the fetus

Risk of miscarriage and preterm labour is increased, and maternal hyperpyrexia may result in intrauterine fetal death. Preterm labour may not be recognized if the woman is already in severe pain from the illness, and labour may only be detected by cardiotocography. Maternal plasma volume may be reduced, leading to poor placental perfusion. This can result in IUGR. There may also be fetal hypoxia. If the mother has a urinary tract infection at the time of delivery, the infant is at substantial risk of congenital infection.

## Chronic renal disease

Chronic renal disease may arise as a result of any of the following:

- glomerulonephritis (acute or chronic)
- polycystic renal disease
- chronic pyelonephritis
- diabetic nephropathy
- systemic lupus erythematosus
- scleroderma
- renal calculi
- congenital abnormality of the lower urinary tract
- solitary kidney
- nephrotic syndrome.

The underlying pathophysiology described for pyelonephritis leads to the same maternal and fetal consequences in chronic renal disease. However, chronic renal disease is further complicated when damage to renal tissue results in reduced blood supply to the kidney. When this occurs, renin is produced to increase blood supply (see Ch. 56), with a consequent rise in blood pressure.

Chronic renal disease is usually classified as mild, moderate or severe, depending on levels of plasma creatinine (Nelson-Piercy 2006). Women with severe disease may be advised against pregnancy, since 85% of them are likely to experience problems.

The outcome of pregnancy depends on the nature and severity of the disease. Outcome is best where renal function is only moderately compromised, with little or no hypertension, and worse where renal function is less than 50% (Nelson-Piercy 2006). The woman is at risk of deterioration of renal function, proteinuria, and worsening of hypertension. There is also an increased risk of miscarriage, superimposed pre-eclampsia, IUGR, preterm delivery and fetal death.

The aim of care is to avoid further deterioration in renal function. More frequent antenatal visits are required for maternal and fetal monitoring by the multidisciplinary team. The woman may need extra rest and help with childcare and household work. She may need to be admitted to hospital for rest and observation. Labour and delivery may be spontaneous or induced, or elective caesarean section may be performed, depending on maternal and fetal condition.

## Renal transplant

Following successful renal transplantation, pregnancy occurs in 1 in 20 female transplant patients of childbearing age (Robson 1999).

Pre-pregnancy counselling is essential for these women, and, generally, the following advice is given:

- The woman must have been in good health for 2 years after transplantation.
- There should be no proteinuria and no significant hypertension.
- There should be no sign of rejection of the transplanted kidney.
- There should be no sign of distension of the renal pelvis or calyces.
- Plasma creatinine should be 200 mmol/L or less.
- Immunosuppressive drug dosages should be at maintenance levels.

The woman should be cared for by a nephrologist and an obstetrician; however, she still requires midwifery care and support. Regular monitoring of blood pressure, renal function and fetal condition, including ultrasound assessment of growth and Doppler studies of umbilical and placental circulation, must be carried out.

Predisposition to urinary tract infection in pregnancy and immunosuppressive drugs taken by transplant patients make the woman prone to infection. Hypertension and anaemia can also occur.

Labour may occur spontaneously unless there is an obstetric indication for intervention. Steroid therapy is increased and antibiotics must be given prophylactically for any surgical intervention, including episiotomy (Nelson-Piercy 2006).

Neonatal problems include preterm delivery, IUGR, respiratory distress syndrome, adrenocortical insufficiency, thrombocytopenia, leucopenia, cytomegalovirus and other infections. Theoretically, breastfeeding is possible, but so many uncertainties surround the effects of some of the drugs used that it is not advised (Joint Formulary Committee 2008).

## Acute renal failure

A fall in urinary output is the first sign of acute renal failure. An output of less than 500 mL in 24 hours is considered a sign of renal failure.

### Causes

Acute renal failure in pregnancy is rare (0.005%), but mild to moderate renal impairment may occur (Billington & Heptinstall 2007). It may occur in association with severe haemorrhage, pre-eclampsia and eclampsia and infection, including septic abortion. It is rarely associated with pyelonephritis (Nelson-Piercy 2006). The kidneys are unable to excrete creatinine and urea, with rising serum levels leading to acidosis. Though rare, it is serious and its course is unpredictable. Women with renal failure should be transferred to a unit where renal dialysis is available.

### Management

Management depends on the cause, which may be prerenal (e.g. hypovolaemia) or renal (tubular or cortical necrosis). It is important to be aware that acute renal failure can occur and to prevent its onset by adequate fluid replacement, while avoiding fluid overload, which particularly in cases of pre-eclampsia, can lead to pulmonary oedema (Nelson-Piercy, 2006). Emphasis is on avoiding and/or treating uraemia, acidosis, hyperkalaemia and fluid overload. Renal dialysis may be needed.

Women and their families need support from the multidisciplinary team, since not only is the woman extremely ill but also she will be concerned for her baby. Postnatal care should include full information about the nature of her illness, effects on future pregnancies and information about appropriate contraception.

**Reflective activity 55.3**

This section and others in this chapter have highlighted the need for women to have practical help with daily activities. How could this be accomplished?

## DIABETES MELLITUS

Diabetes is a disorder of the endocrine system that affects the metabolism of carbohydrates, fats and protein. Glucose is essential to cell function, and, in a complex metabolic process, insulin enables glucose to enter cells. It is important to remember that in diabetes there is no shortage of glucose, rather there is a lack of insulin. Diabetes affects many body systems, although the principal signs and symptoms of diabetes arise as the body tries to metabolize fat and protein to provide energy.

The main signs and symptoms are hyperglycaemia, thirst, polydipsia, fatigue and blurred vision. Some 2–4% of pregnancies involve women who have diabetes, and there are associated risks for the woman and her baby, with generally poorer outcomes than for women who do not have diabetes (NICE 2008b). Understanding of the condition and how it affects and is affected by pregnancy is, therefore, essential for midwives. Diabetes arises for a number of reasons and is classified as follows.

#### *Type 1: insulin-dependent diabetes (IDD) mellitus*

This is most common in young people and there is an almost complete lack of insulin, because of an absence of, or destruction of, beta cells in the pancreatic islets of Langerhans. This type of diabetes is insulin dependent. It is a genetically mediated autoimmune disorder involving human leucocyte antigens (HLA) on chromosome 6 (de Swiet 2001). Hyperglycaemia, polyuria and ketosis are present and there is usually significant weight loss. Untreated, or poorly controlled, this can lead to metabolic acidosis, coma and death. Type 1 diabetes causes multisystem, microvascular complications, relating to high levels of blood glucose. Complications include retinopathy, causing problems with vision; nephropathy, causing deterioration in renal function and associated hypertension; and neuropathy, mostly affecting the feet and legs which may lead to ulceration and gangrene. Those with type 1 diabetes are also more likely to develop cataracts.

#### *Type 2: non-insulin-dependent diabetes (NIDD) mellitus*

This condition can exist without any symptoms. There is resistance in the tissues to the action of insulin; it is often diagnosed later in life, and frequently affects those who are overweight. It is not dependent on insulin, and may be controlled by weight loss and diet, or by oral hypoglycaemic agents.

#### *Gestational diabetes mellitus*

The glucose tolerance test is normal except in times of stress, when there may be signs of diabetes. When this occurs in pregnancy, it is known as *gestational diabetes mellitus* (GDM). NICE guidelines do not support routine screening for GDM (NICE 2008b), but deem it appropriate if the woman has any of the following risk markers at the first antenatal booking interview:

- family origin with a high prevalence of diabetes (South Asian, Black Caribbean, Middle Eastern)
- history of diabetes in first-degree relatives
- previous gestational diabetes
- previous baby weighing more than 4.5 kg
- BMI above 30kg/m$^2$.

In these cases, screening should be offered. Where the woman has previously had GDM, she can monitor blood glucose herself in early pregnancy, or a 2-hour 75 g oral glucose tolerance test can be offered at 16–18 weeks. If abnormal, treatment would be started; if normal, it can be repeated at 28 weeks (NICE 2008b).

Midwives need to be aware that women with gestational diabetes and those with pre-existing diabetes mellitus require knowledgeable and skilled care with a recognition of them as women in their own right rather than a reflection of a medical condition.

### Pregnancy and diabetes

A number of hormonal and metabolic changes occur naturally as a result of pregnancy, and these changes, together with their accepted physiological norms, have been well documented (see Ch. 17).

Type 1 and type 2 diabetes mellitus are complicated by the physiological changes which take place in glucose metabolism during pregnancy and, as previously stated, diabetes may develop during the pregnancy.

## Care of women with diabetes

### Pre-conception care

Although more complications occur in the pregnancies of diabetic mothers, the maternal mortality rate is no higher than 0.5% (Nelson-Piercy 2006). Good glycaemic control pre-pregnancy can help reduce the risks of miscarriage, congenital malformation, stillbirth and neonatal death, as can folic acid supplements (5 mg/day, taken pre-conception and up to 12 weeks' gestation). Weight control is important and women with a BMI over 27 kg/m$^2$ should be encouraged to lose weight. Retinal and renal assessment should be offered. Women should be advised about local and national support systems (NICE 2008b). Maternal and fetal risks and complications affecting women with pre-existing diabetes are:

- unstable diabetic control
- fetal macrosomia + risk of consequent shoulder dystocia
- birth trauma (mother and baby)
- pre-eclampsia
- miscarriage
- preterm labour
- induction of labour or caesarean section
- congenital malformation
- intrauterine death
- stillbirth
- transient neonatal morbidity (neonatal hypoglycaemia, hypocalcaemia, jaundice, polycythaemia, respiratory distress syndrome)
- neonatal death
- obesity and/or diabetes developing later in the baby.

## Care during pregnancy

Care is from the multidisciplinary team, and women will need individualized care according to their own particular health needs. The place of birth should be discussed and should be in a hospital with advanced neonatal resuscitation facilities available 24 hours per day (NICE 2008b). In pregnancy, insulin requirements will be increased to cope with the relative fasting hypoglycaemia, and insulin requirements should be reviewed. Women with type 2 diabetes may also require insulin at this stage. Rapid-acting insulin (*aspart* and *lispro*) are considered safe in pregnancy, and of the long-acting insulins, *isophane* is recommended (NICE 2008b). Oral hypoglycaemics other than *metformin* are not considered safe in pregnancy. Women should perform their own blood glucose monitoring at home and aim for fasting blood glucose values between 3.5 and 5.9 mmol/L. They should aim to keep 1-hour postprandial (after food) levels below 7.8 mmol/L. Some women find an insulin pump gives better control than multiple injections (NICE 2008b). They should also have ketone testing strips for urinalysis because of the risk of ketoacidosis.

If not already carried out, renal and retinal assessment should be offered. Retinal assessment can be offered again at 28 weeks, or earlier if there are signs of retinopathy. Renal assessment can be followed up by referral to a nephrologist if serum creatinine is raised (120 micromol/L or more), or there is proteinuria >5 g/day (NICE 2008b).

### *Diet*

The carbohydrate energy content of the diet should be related to the energy requirements of the individual. In most cases it does not exceed 40%, but it can be higher without adverse effects. Fat intake should be restricted because of the increased risk of arterial disease in diabetics. A high fibre intake is recommended because the slower gastric emptying delays the absorption of sugar into the bloodstream. Hypoglycaemia may exacerbate the effects of morning sickness; glucose and sugary foods should be avoided, and hypoglycaemia prevented by taking milk and a light snack. Concentrated oral glucose should be available for all women taking insulin, and glucagon for women with type 1 diabetes, in case of hypoglycaemia. Family members should also know when and how to give it.

Diabetes is particularly common in British women of Asian origin. Dietary considerations for such women should avoid sweets, such as gulab juman, halwa and jelabi, and, where the woman is also overweight, foods fried in ghee or oil should be avoided.

### *Glycosylated haemoglobin ($HbA_{1C}$)*

Glycosylated haemoglobin ($HbA_{1C}$) can also be measured every 2–4 weeks, and helps to assess diabetic control. It is a type of adult haemoglobin where one part of the beta chain has been combined with glucose. $HbA_{1C}$ has been found to increase in diabetes, especially when the blood glucose control is poor, although its levels are not indicators of present diabetic status but of blood glucose levels during the preceding 1–3 months. Levels of 10% or lower are considered a sign of good control, while levels of more than 10% indicate poor control (Nelson-Piercy 2006). Women should be offered monthly estimations of $HbA_{1c}$ (NICE 2008b).

## Fetal wellbeing

Women should be offered cardiac screening for the fetus at 18–20 weeks, as well as all other usual antenatal screening tests that would be offered at that time. At 28, 32 and 36 weeks, further scans for fetal growth assessment and amniotic fluid volume should be offered (NICE 2008b).

## Care during labour

The midwife cares for the woman in conjunction with medical and obstetric colleagues; labour onset may be spontaneous or induced, or delivery may be by elective caesarean section if there are obstetric indications.

In addition to usual care in labour, blood glucose is checked hourly, and the aim is to keep blood glucose levels between 4 and 7 mmol/L. Where this is not possible, or in cases of type 1 diabetes, dextrose/insulin regimens may be used (NICE 2008b).

Electronic fetal monitoring should be continuous because of the increased risks of fetal hypoxia during labour.

### Postnatal care

Maternal insulin requirements fall sharply after the birth of the baby and placenta, so frequent blood glucose estimations are made to detect hypoglycaemia. The insulin dosage is reduced and the woman is gradually restabilized.

Breastfeeding should be encouraged, and women may need additional carbohydrate to facilitate this. They may be advised to have a snack before and during feeding, in case they become hypoglycaemic. Infection is an increased risk, so education about good hygiene is important. When women are transferred into the community, they should resume attendance at their regular specialist clinic with routine diabetes care.

Women with type 2 diabetes can resume oral hypoglycaemics, but only *metformin* and *glibenclamide*, if they are breastfeeding.

Women with gestational diabetes should stop medication after the birth, and receive information about weight control, exercise, diet, and how to recognize hyperglycaemia. They may also be offered a blood glucose test before transfer into the community, and offered a fasting plasma glucose test at 6 weeks, and then yearly.

### Care of the baby

Mother and baby should not be separated unless the baby is ill, and babies should not go home until they are 24 hours old, feeding well, and have stable blood glucose levels (NICE 2008b). These babies are particularly prone to respiratory distress syndrome and hypoglycaemia, so require close observation. In intrauterine life, the hypertrophic islets of Langerhans produce more insulin in response to the high maternal blood sugar levels. After birth, the pancreas continues to produce excess insulin initially, so the baby becomes hypoglycaemic. To prevent this, early feeding within 30 minutes of birth, then 2 to 3 hourly, is essential and the baby's blood glucose levels are measured 2–4 hours after birth, or earlier if there are signs of hypoglycaemia (NICE 2008b).

Other neonatal complications include skin infections, hyperbilirubinaemia and bleeding from a very thick cord, and the incidence of congenital malformations is increased.

> **Reflective activity 55.4**
>
> Does your unit have a policy for routine screening for diabetes? How does it compare with the NICE guidelines?

## RESPIRATORY PROBLEMS

### Tuberculosis

Pulmonary tuberculosis (TB) is responsible for 6% of all deaths worldwide, and up to half the world's population is infected with the disease in its latent or active form (Mays 1993, Nelson-Piercy 2006). In the UK, TB is becoming more prevalent, particularly among the homeless, where there is overcrowding, and exposure through contact with people from countries where the disease is widespread. All new UK entrant pregnant women and children younger than 11 years should have a *Mantoux test* (NICE 2006). Women may become pregnant whilst being treated for TB, or may develop the disease during pregnancy.

Classic symptoms are chronic cough and blood-streaked sputum, with fever, weight loss and night sweats occurring late in the disease. The onset is insidious and there is also a feeling of general malaise.

#### Diagnosis

Diagnosis is made when the causative organism (*Mycobacterium tuberculosis* or the tubercle bacillus) is found in sputum and by chest X-ray.

#### Pregnancy care

Care in pregnancy should include input by an obstetrician, respiratory physician, GP and midwife, and possibly a social worker if social and economic factors are involved. Help is needed with housework and childcare during and after pregnancy, since the woman will be tired. Liaison with other healthcare workers may be necessary, since family members may need to be screened and educated as to the nature of the disease and the steps needed to prevent its spread.

Infection is spread by airborne transmission of droplet nuclei from a person with active TB, so if the woman is infectious, she needs a single room in hospital.

Drugs used to treat TB have side-effects for both mother and fetus; however, treatment in pregancy is safe (Robson & Waugh 2008) (see Table 55.3). Courses of treatment are long – 6 to 9 months or longer – but the symptoms of the disease resolve after only 3 weeks, and the woman will be non-infectious after 2 (Nelson-Piercy 2006). Women must

**Table 55.3 Drugs used for the treatment of active TB in pregnancy**

| Drug | Dose | Possible side-effects | |
|---|---|---|---|
| | | **Maternal** | **Fetal** |
| Isoniazid | 5 mg/kg/day<br>Max. 300 mg | Hepatitis<br>Peripheral neuropathy<br>Agranulocytosis | None |
| Rifampicin | 10 mg/kg/day<br>Max. 600 mg | Hepatitis<br>Decreased effectiveness of oral contraceptive | Increase in neural tube defects |
| Ethambutol | 15–25 mg/kg/day<br>Max. 2.5 g | Optic neuritis<br>Visual problems | None |
| Pyrazinamide | 15–30 mg/kg/day | Hepatitis<br>Arthralgias | None |

*Note:* Streptomycin is not given in pregnancy since it causes damage to fetal auditory and vestibular nerves.

be encouraged to continue treatment, otherwise drug-resistant strains of TB may develop.

In the absence of obstetric indications, labour onset is spontaneous and care is as for normal labour. After birth, the woman should continue treatment. There are no contraindications to breastfeeding. The baby should have BCG vaccination and may have *syrup of isoniazid* prophylactically. There should be a paediatric review before discharge (NICE 2006). Unless the disease is active, the mother and baby are not separated (Nelson-Piercy 2006).

Advice about family-spacing methods will be needed, as women with active TB should avoid pregnancy until there are no further signs of the disease, usually for a period of 2 years.

## Asthma

Asthma is an obstructive disease of the respiratory system characterized by episodic breathlessness, wheezing, cough, thick sputum and feelings of tightness in the chest. It affects 5–10% of the general population and 3–12% of pregnant women (Rey & Boulet 2007). Acute attacks are caused by inflammation, narrowing of the airways, and contraction of the smooth muscle of the airway walls, and are characterized by any one of the following:

- increased respiratory rate (>25 breaths/minute)
- increased heart rate (>110 beats/min) and wheezing
- inability to speak in complete sentences
- use of accessory muscles of respiration.

An acute attack can be life-threatening, leading to bradycardia, dysryhthmia or hypotension, with exhaustion, confusion, coma and death (BTS/SIGN 2008).

Known factors in asthma attacks are:

- allergens, such as pollen, animals, house dust mites
- certain foods/medicines, such as dairy products, orange juice
- environmental factors, such as dust, chemicals, cigarette smoke, perfumes
- exercise
- cold or dry air
- emotional responses, such as laughing or crying
- upper respiratory tract infections.

There is a complex link between pregnancy and asthma. Some pregnant women experience fewer asthmatic attacks, possibly owing to the increased production of corticosteroids in pregnancy, some may stay the same, but a few may have more, particularly those who have severe asthma. Links have been shown between asthma and poor pregnancy outcomes, including pre-eclampsia, placenta praevia, miscarriage, haemorrhage, and poor placental function, leading to low birthweight. Studies suggest that female gender of the fetus causes a worsening of symptoms in the mother. Causes are unknown but the conditions are less likely to arise where asthma is controlled well (Nelson-Piercy 2006, Rey & Boulet 2007) so it is important to encourage women to maintain their drug therapy.

Drug therapy is often by inhaled anti-inflammatory agents, beta-agonists or steroids. These are safe during pregnancy and midwives should assure women of this. As Nelson-Piercy (2006) points out, poorly controlled asthma carries greater risks for the fetus than do the drugs used to treat it. Women should be advised to use spacers when inhaling steroids to avoid oral thrush, and if they smoke, should be offered help in stopping.

Oral steroids such as *prednisolone* may be used to control exacerbations; however, these are diabetogenic and women will therefore need regular estimation of blood glucose. Women on oral steroids will need hydrocortisone during labour (Nelson-Piercy 2006). Entonox, epidural and other forms of pain relief can be used in labour; however, opiates are respiratory depressants, and would not be used if the woman had an attack during labour. Epidural anaesthesia is safer for caesarean section, as it avoids the problems of chest infection and atelectasis associated with general anaesthesia.

Breastfeeding is not contraindicated, and may protect the baby from developing atopic asthma (BTS/SIGN 2008, Nelson-Piercy 2006).

## EPILEPSY

Epilepsy is a condition of abnormal cerebral function causing convulsive seizures. One in 200 people are affected, with an incidence in pregnancy of 0.6–1% (Nelson-Piercy 2006). Seizures may be partial, arising in the frontal or temporal lobe of the brain, or generalized (petit mal and grand mal). Petit mal or 'absence' seizures are short (< 20 seconds), while grand mal seizures typically follow a pattern with four phases:

1. *Premonitory stage* or aura/warning.
2. *Tonic stage*: Muscles go into spasm. Fists are clenched and arms and legs rigid for up to a minute.
3. *Clonic stage*: The spasm ceases; violent, jerky muscular movements begin, while frothy, often blood-stained saliva appears at the lips and mucus or blood may be inhaled. This restless phase lasts up to 2 minutes.
4. *Comatose stage*: There may be a period of unconsciousness or confusion lasting only a few minutes, or much longer.

Risks during a seizure are trauma, including biting of the tongue, inhalation of mucus or blood, and cerebral hypoxia. In pregnancy, the fetus is also subject to hypoxia and there may be IUGR. A phenomenon known as sudden unexpected death in epilepsy (SUDEP) can also occur, but may be unrelated to a seizure. In many cases the cause is unknown (idiopathic), but it may follow cerebral trauma, congenital abnormality, space-occupying lesions in the brain, vascular disorders, degenerative disorders, infection, metabolic disorders such as hypoglycaemia, or withdrawal from drugs or alcohol. Seizures may be triggered when women are stressed, tired, in pain, or in hot and steamy environments, and women should be advised about this (Billington & Stevenson 2007).

*Status epilepticus* is a rare but serious condition in which myoclonic seizures occur in rapid succession. It is controlled by increasing antiepileptic drugs (AEDs), administering *diazepam* and by intravenous dextrose to prevent hypoglycaemia. CEMACH (Lewis 2007) records 11 deaths related to epilepsy in the 2003–2005 triennium. Six of these deaths were sudden unexpected death in epilepsy (SUDEP). Previous deaths have been due to accident, drowning in the bath, and aspiration of vomit during seizures. A list of safety measures which may help avoid such accidents is given at the end of this section.

Epilepsy may be controlled, but not cured, by antiepileptic drugs (AEDs), such as *phenytoin sodium, phenobarbital, carbamezapine* and *sodium valproate*. All cross the placenta and are teratogenic, and may lead to some major congenital malformations, including neural tube and cardiac defects, with *sodium valproate* carrying the greatest risk and *carbamezapine* the least. Abnormalities occur more often in women who receive combinations of AEDs (polytherapy), so, during pregnancy, monotherapy is recommended. However, about 96% of women will have a normal baby (Morrow et al 2006). Pregnancy has a variable effect on seizures: some women will have fewer seizures and about a third will have more (Epilepsy Action 2006). The aim is to be as seizure-free as possible. Physiological changes in pregnancy result in lower concentrations of AEDs, which may need to be increased. These drugs alter the absorption of folic acid and 5 mg/day should be given as a prophylactic precaution preconception and during the first trimester, and throughout pregnancy for women taking sodium valproate. For the same reason, clotting factors may be inhibited in both mother and baby. Women may be given 10–20 mg/day vitamin K orally for 4 weeks from 36 weeks, and babies should receive 1 mg vitamin K intramuscularly post delivery (Epilepsy Action 2006, Nelson-Piercy 2006).

In the absence of obstetric complications, labour and delivery will be spontaneous, and midwifery care as for any woman in labour. Pain relief can include TENS, Entonox or epidural, and overbreathing should be avoided as this can trigger seizures, as can pethidine. It is important to make sure women continue to take their AEDs.

All AEDs are secreted in breast milk, but there is no contraindication to breastfeeding.

Individualized parenting programmes can help women and their families keep healthy and safe during pregnancy and after the birth. Advice for the woman may include the following:

- Make sure the family knows how to put the woman in the recovery position following a seizure.
- Avoid becoming overtired, hypoglycaemic or stressed.
- Avoid having a bath or shower when alone in the house.
- Share care of the baby to avoid becoming overtired.
- Sit on the floor when feeding the baby.
- Use gates at the top and bottom of stairs.

More information can be found on the Epilepsy Action website (www.epilepsy.org.uk).

## OBSTETRIC CHOLESTASIS

Obstetric cholestasis (formerly known as intrahepatic cholestasis of pregnancy) is a disease arising in the third trimester which is characterized by intense pruritus (itching) without a rash, abnormal liver function tests (LFTs), dark-coloured urine, anorexia, malabsorption of fat and elevated maternal bile acid levels. It is thought to arise from a genetic hypersensitivity to oestrogen and is associated with increased rates of fetal mortality and morbidity, and with maternal coagulation defects, due to inability to absorb vitamin K, which is fat-soluble (Nelson-Piercy 2006). It occurs in 0.7% of pregnancies in multi-ethnic populations, with a higher incidence (1.2–1.5%) in women of Indian-Asian or Pakistani-Asian origin (RCOG 2006). The condition was once thought to be benign, but it is now recognized that it may be a factor in 'unexplained' fetal deaths, some of which are sudden, and are almost impossible to predict. It is thought that bile acids cause placental vasoconstriction, resulting in fetal hypoxia. In up to 40% of pregnancies complicated by obstetric cholestasis, there will be meconium in the amniotic fluid, with the risk of meconium aspiration (Redfearn & Chambers 1996).

Any woman complaining of severe itching, which often begins on the palms of the hands, should be referred for liver function tests. If obstetric cholestasis is diagnosed, careful monitoring is required to detect and prevent coagulation defects by giving vitamin K. Fetal wellbeing is monitored, checking growth, liquor volume and blood flow, using Doppler studies. Early delivery has not been shown to decrease the risk of perinatal mortality (RCOG 2006).

The most distressing aspect of the condition for women is the interruption of sleep because of itching. Antihistamines such as *promethazine (Phenergan)* may be given to alleviate itching, and women should be encouraged to wear loose cotton clothing. Topical applications of calamine lotion or aqueous cream may also help.

Although symptoms will disappear following delivery, the risk of recurrence in subsequent pregnancies is as high as 50%. Since the condition is related to oestrogen, women should avoid oral contraceptives containing oestrogen (Nelson-Piercy 2006).

## CONCLUSION

This chapter has reviewed some of the medical disorders midwives may encounter when working with pregnant women. Whilst pathophysiology and practical care are important, emphasis must also be placed on the need to treat women as individuals, and not merely a reflection of their condition. The midwife has an important role in identifying women with pre-existing medical conditions, and women who may be at risk of developing such conditions, and in monitoring the wellbeing of the woman and her baby throughout. The need to educate and support women and involve them in planning and participating in their care will ensure that even should intervention be required, complications and problems should be minimized and the women will feel empowered during the process.

### KEY POINTS

- Women with pre-existing medical disorders may be well informed about their condition and its management and be aware of risks associated with pregnancy.
- The midwife needs to be knowledgeable about medical disorders and contemporary management and care in order that she can interpret and explain this information to women and their families, working towards a partnership model of care.
- Women who develop medical disorders during pregnancy need education and support in relation to their condition.
- Strategies for reducing risk and preventing problems that medical disorders may present need to be explored with women and their families.
- Women and their families need to be aware of signs and symptoms of deterioration and how to deal with them.
- Women and families may need antenatal education specifically tailored to their needs.
- Collaborative, multidisciplinary care is essential.

## REFERENCES


Adamson DL, Dhanjal MK, Nelson-Piercy C, et al: Cardiac disease in pregnancy. In Greer I, Nelson-Piercy C, Walters B, editors: *Maternal medicine: medical problems in pregnancy*, Edinburgh, 2007, Churchill Livingstone.

Billington M, Heptinstall T: Medical disorders and critical care. In Billington M, Stevenson M, editors: *Critical care in childbearing for midwives*, Oxford, 2007, Blackwell.

Billington M, Stevenson M, editors: *Critical care in childbearing for midwives*, Oxford, 2007, Blackwell.

British Thoracic Society (BTS)/Scottish Intercollegiate Guidelines Network (SIGN): *British guideline on the management of asthma: a national clinical guideline*, London, 2008, BTS/SIGN.

de Swiet M: Medical disorders in pregnancy. In Chamberlain G, editor: *Turnbull's obstetrics*, ed 3, Edinburgh, 2001, Churchill Livingstone.

Dike P: Haematological disorders and the critically ill woman. In Billington M, Stevenson M, editors: *Critical care in childbearing for midwives*, Oxford, 2007, Blackwell.

Epilepsy Action: Epilepsy and pregnancy (website). www.epilepsy.org.uk. 2006. Accessed May, 2009.

Evans M: Iron deficiency anaemia throughout the female life cycle – who needs to care, *MIDIRS Midwifery Digest* 18(3):404–408, 2008.

Gilbert E, Harmon J: *Manual of high risk pregnancy and delivery*, ed 3, St Louis, 2002, Mosby.

Joint Formulary Committee: *British National Formulary*, ed 56, London, 2008, British Medical Association and Royal Pharmaceutical Society of Great Britain.

Jordan S: *Pharmacology for midwives: the evidence base for safe practice*, Basingstoke, 2002, Palgrave.

Lavender R: Cranberry juice: the facts, *Nursing Times Plus* 96(40):11–12, 2000.

Lewis G, editor: *The Confidential Enquiry into Maternal and Child Health (CEMACH). Saving mothers' lives: reviewing maternal deaths to make motherhood safer – 2003–2005. The Seventh Report on Confidential Enquiries into Maternal Deaths in the United Kingdom*, London, 2007, CEMACH.

Lewis G: Foreword. In Robson SE, Waugh J, editors: *Medical disorders in pregnancy: a manual for midwives*, Oxford, 2008, Blackwell.

McKay K: Blood tests in pregnancy (2) Iron deficiency anaemia, *The Practising Midwife* 3(4):25–27, 2000.

McLean E, Cogswell M, Egli I, et al: Worldwide prevalence of anaemia in preschool aged children, pregnant women and non-pregnant women of reproductive age. In Kraemer K, Zimmermann MB, editors: *Nutritional anaemia*, Basel, 2007, Sight and Life.

McLean M, Bu'Lock F, Robson SE: Heart disease. In Robson SE, Waugh J, editors: *Medical disorders in pregnancy: a manual for midwives*, Oxford, 2008, Blackwell.

Marieb E: *Human anatomy and physiology*, ed 8, California, 2006, Benjamin Cummings.

Mays M: Tuberculosis: a comprehensive review for the certified nurse-midwife, *Journal of Nurse-Midwifery* 38(3):132–139, 1993.

Morrow JI, Russell A, Guthrie E, et al: Malformation risks of anti-epileptic drugs in pregnancy: A prospective study from the UK Epilepsy and Pregnancy Register, *Journal of Neurology, Neurosurgery and Psychiatry* 77(2):193–198, 2006.

National Institute for Health and Clinical Excellence (NICE): Guideline CG033. Clinical diagnosis and management of tuberculosis, and measurements for its prevention and control (website). www.nice.org.uk. 2006. Available online. Accessed August, 2010.

National Institute for Health and Clinical Excellence (NICE): Guideline 62. Antenatal care (website). www.nice.org.uk. 2008a. Available online. Accessed August, 2010.

National Institute for Health and Clinical Excellence (NICE): Guideline 63. Diabetes in pregnancy (website). www.nice.org.uk. 2008b. Available online. Accessed August, 2010.

Nelson-Piercy C: *Handbook of obstetric medicine*, ed 3, Oxford, 2006, Informa Healthcare.

Nursing and Midwifery Council (NMC): *Standards for pre-registration midwifery education*, London, 2008, NMC.

Redfearn J, Chambers J: Obstetric cholestasis. Itching in pregnancy? Midwives must be alert, *Midwives* 109(1297):36–37, 1996.

Rey E, Boulet LP: Asthma in pregnancy, *British Medical Journal* 31(334):582–585, 2007.

Robson SC: Hypertension and renal disease in pregnancy. In Edmonds DK, editor: *Dewhurst's textbook of obstetrics and gynaecology for postgraduates*, Oxford, 1999, Blackwell Science.

Robson SE, Waugh J, editors: *Medical disorders in pregnancy: a manual for midwives*, Oxford, 2008, Blackwell.

Royal College of Ostetricians and Gynaecologists (RCOG): Greentop guideline no 43: Obstetric cholestasis (website). www.rcog.org.uk. 2006. Accessed August, 2010.

Spencer L: Psychological care. In Billington M, Stevenson M, editors: *Critical care in childbearing for midwives*, Oxford, 2007, Blackwell.

Thomas H: Women's experiences of major illness during pregnancy, *MIDIRS Midwifery Digest* 9(3):312–316, 1999.

World Health Organization (WHO): The prevalence of anaemia in women, Geneva, 1992, WHO.

Chapter |56|

# Hypertensive disorders of pregnancy

Chris Bewley

## LEARNING OUTCOMES

After reading this chapter, you will:

- understand the role of the midwife in the multidisciplinary approach to care
- be aware that hypertension may be associated with pre-eclampsia, chronic or essential hypertension, or renal disease
- understand the pathophysiology of pre-eclampsia
- recognize the outward signs of pre-eclampsia and relate them to pathophysiology
- be aware of the psychological support needed for women who are diagnosed with pre-eclampsia.

## INTRODUCTION

This chapter draws on the most recent guidelines for health professionals, and on other significant literature on hypertensive disorders in pregnancy, to provide an overview of the nature, prevalence, diagnosis and outcomes in women and their babies. A midwifery approach to collaborative care is proposed, which maximizes recognition and minimizes adverse pregnancy outcomes for mother and baby, yet retains maternal choice, input and understanding. Definitions of pregnancy-induced hypertension (PIH), pre-eclampsia, eclampsia and HELLP (*h*aemolysis, *e*levated *l*iver enzymes, *l*ow *p*latelets) syndrome are provided, and recommendations are given for further, more in-depth reading.

The incidence of hypertensive disorders in the UK is difficult to gauge, owing to the variety of ways in which they present; however, approximately 12% of all pregnancies will be affected by pregnancy-induced hypertension and 3–5% by pre-eclampsia (Duley et al 2006, Walker 2000). Hypertensive disorders in pregnancy accounted for 18 maternal deaths in the UK between 2003 and 2005 (Lewis 2007); of these, six women developed eclamptic seizures (five in the antenatal period), and eight were diagnosed with HELLP syndrome.

Effects on maternal systems and effects on the fetus/neonate are as follows:

**Central nervous system**
- Cerebral haemorrhage
- Eclampsia (seizures)
- Cerebral oedema
- Retinal oedema/retinal blindness

**Pulmonary system**
- Pulmonary oedema
- Laryngeal oedema

**Renal system**
- Cortical necrosis
- Tubular necrosis

**Liver**
- HELLP syndrome
- Hepatic rupture
- Jaundice

**Haematological (specifically coagulation)**
- Disseminated intravascular coagulation (DIC)
- Haemolysis

**Placenta**
- Placental abruption
- Placenta ischaemia/infarction

**Fetus/Neonate**
- Intrauterine growth restriction (IUGR)
- Prematurity
- Low birthweight
- Intrauterine hypoxia leading to neurological complications
- Perinatal death

(Duley et al 2006, Stevenson & Billington 2007).

## TERMINOLOGY

Various terms have been applied to a condition arising in pregnancy characterized by hypertension, proteinuria, and a combination of other signs and symptoms including seizures (sometimes called convulsions, or fits) (Salas 1999). Box 56.1 shows the range of terms in use, together with the signs and symptoms relating to each. However, for midwives, more important than terminology, is the ability to recognize that a woman is unwell, and to refer swiftly and appropriately (Lewis 2007).

### Definition

Most authorities agree that a blood pressure of 140/90 mmHg or more and/or an increase in diastolic pressure of 20 mmHg or more from the booking blood pressure, after the 20th week of pregnancy constitute grounds for further monitoring. A further recommendation is that women whose systolic blood pressure is above 160 on two separate occasions should be referred and treated for hypertension (Lewis 2007, PRECOG Development Group 2004, RCOG 2006).

**Box 56.1 Features of hypertensive disorders in pregnancy**

**Pregnancy-induced hypertension (PIH)/ Gestational hypertension (GH)**

Blood pressure of ≥140/90 mmHg or a rise of 15–20 mmHg in the diastolic blood pressure after 20 weeks' gestation

Systolic blood pressure of <160 mmHg on more than one occasion

**Gestational proteinuric hypertension (GPH)**

As PIH and GPH, with the addition of proteinuria

**Pre-eclampsia**

As PIH and GPH, plus any one of the following:

- General malaise or complaints of feeling unwell
- Severe persistent frontal headache, probably associated with cerebral oedema
- Visual disturbances, resulting from oedema of the retina. Vision may be dim or blurred, difficulty reading, spots or flashes of light
- Vomiting, which may be related to cerebral oedema or associated with abdominal pain
- Epigastric pain or tenderness, possibly caused by haemorrhages under the liver capsule; this can be a warning that eclampsia is imminent. Pain may also be associated with placental abruption
- Hyper-reflexia
- Sudden severe swelling of the hands, feet, or face
- Oliguria (>30 mL urine/hour) may indicate the onset of eclampsia or renal involvement

Note: Not all women with severe pre-eclampsia present with all these symptoms and signs. Indeed any one symptom, with or without hypertension and proteinuria, is sufficient to indicate that the condition is worsening and that eclampsia may be imminent.

**Reflective activity 56.1**

What does your unit protocol indicate about levels of blood pressure and referral?

What definition of 'hypertensive' is used, and are the protocols evidence-based?

## PRE-ECLAMPSIA

Pre-eclampsia is the term used when hypertension is accompanied by one or more other signs and symptoms in the mother (see Box 56.1).

### Pathophysiology

Despite much research, the cause of pre-eclampsia and HELLP syndrome is uncertain, and it remains a 'disease of theories' (Duley et al 2006, Redman & Walker 1996). There are some indications that low dietary calcium may be a factor and that antioxidant vitamins may help prevent the disease, but these areas remain under examination. Although it is associated with implantation of the placenta, there is a generalized response in the maternal endothelial system which leads to widespread platelet aggregation and vasoconstriction. It is thought that initial underperfusion of the placenta triggers a maternal circulatory response, leading to a generalized condition of hypovolaemia and vasospasm.

In normal pregnancy, physiological dilatation of the spiral arterioles in the placental bed occurs, by the stripping away of their muscle coating. This allows pooling of maternal blood in the intervillous spaces of the placental bed, creating a shunt, which lowers maternal blood pressure. This occurs around 16–18 weeks of pregnancy, and leads to the physiological fall in blood pressure commonly observed in the second trimester of normal pregnancy. In pre-eclampsia and HELLP syndrome, dilatation fails to occur and the blood pressure is raised as the blood is forced through constricted arterioles. There is generalized abnormal vascular tone and vasospasm, which leads to endothelial dysfunction and disturbances of maternal microcirculation. There is consequent hypoperfusion and vasoconstriction in the maternal brain, kidneys and liver, and in the placenta (Walker 2000). Similar circumstances arise in conditions where the placenta is large, such as diabetes and multiple pregnancy, and in hydatidiform mole, where the embryo dies, and only placental tissue remains (Roberts 2000).

## Predisposing factors

Pre-eclampsia is more common in first pregnancies; even if the first pregnancy results in miscarriage, and more so after termination of pregnancy. There is a reduced incidence of pre-eclampsia in the second pregnancy, suggesting some immunological factors (Eras et al 2000). Li & Wi (2000) suggest that changing paternity also affects the woman's likelihood of developing pre-eclampsia, while Smith et al (1997) suggest some partner-specific maternal immune response.

The Pre-eclampsia Community Guideline (PRECOG Development Group 2004) and National Institute for Health and Clinical Excellence guidelines (NICE 2008) suggest that women with any of the following are predisposed to the development of pre-eclampsia:

- first pregnancy
- pre-eclampsia in a previous pregnancy
- 10 years since a previous pregnancy
- age 40 years or more
- body mass index (BMI) 35 or more
- family history of pre-eclampsia (in mother or sister)
- booking diastolic blood pressure of 80 mmHg or more
- booking proteinuria of 1+ or more, on more than one occasion, or quantified at >0.3 g/24 hours in the absence of infection
- multiple pregnancy
- underlying pre-existing medical conditions such as diabetes, hypertension, renal disease, antiphospholipid antibodies.

## Diagnosis

Clearly, accurate history taking at antenatal booking will determine future care, and provides a good baseline. The major areas for consideration when screening for pre-eclampsia, at booking and at follow-up antenatal visits, are previous history, noting any of the above, blood pressure and urinalysis, as discussed below.

### *Blood pressure*

A reading of 140/90 mmHg is regarded as the upper limit of normal, but a rise in diastolic blood pressure of 15–20 mmHg or more above the level recorded prior to 20 weeks' gestation is significant (Moran & Davison 1999). The diastolic pressure is no longer considered more significant than the systolic, and the Confidential Enquiry into Maternal and Child Health (CEMACH) suggests a systolic pressure of 160 mmHg on more than one occasion warrants investigation and treatment (Lewis 2007).

Accurate measurement of blood pressure is essential. The diastolic measurement is taken at stage V (five) of the Korotkov sounds (absence of sound) (PRECOG Development Group 2004, RCOG 2006). However, where there is no complete disappearance of sound (in about 15% of women), both 'muffling' and disappearance levels should be recorded (PRECOG Development Group 2004). The woman should be in a sitting or semi-reclining position, so that her arm and the sphygmomanometer cuff are at the same level as the left atrium. Large-size cuffs should be available for women weighing more than 85 kg (NICE 2008, PRECOG Development Group 2004, RCOG 2006). Although automated blood pressure devices are useful, they may underestimate blood pressure by as much as 30 mmHg (Natarajan et al 1999, RCOG 2006).

**Reflective activity 56.2**

How does your technique of taking blood pressure compare with the above?

Does your unit have a clear policy for the standard of measuring blood pressure?

### *Urinalysis*

Proteinuria of 1+ or more on dipstick, on two occasions more than 4 hours apart, in an uncontaminated specimen, and once infection has been excluded, is always serious in conjunction with hypertension (NICE 2008). It indicates damage to endothelial tissue, with leakage of albumin, the smallest plasma protein, from the blood into the urine. Protein loss changes osmotic pressure within the capillaries and may lead to pathological oedema. Hypertension and proteinuria occurring prior to 33 weeks' gestation often has a poor prognosis (Mattar & Sibbai 1999).

Volume and concentration of urine affect random readings, and can result in false positives or negatives. Also, protein excretion is variable according to the time of day. A 24-hour urine collection remains the 'gold standard' for quantification of protein, and significant proteinuria is said to exist where protein exceeds 300 mg/24 hours (NICE 2008, RCOG 2006).

### *Oedema*

Although 85% of women with pre-eclampsia develop oedema, it is no longer considered a cardinal sign, because it is a feature of normotensive as well as hypertensive pregnancies (see Ch. 31).

Pathological oedema associated with pre-eclampsia occurs in the pretibial area, hands, face and abdomen, and does not resolve with rest. Excessive weight gain may be due to occult oedema. During the latter half of pregnancy, normal weight gain should be approximately 0.5 kg per week. Weight gain significantly in excess of this, sometimes defined as exceeding 2 kg in a 1 week period, accompanied by hypertension and proteinuria is likely to be associated with pre-eclampsia (Duley et al 2006).

### Diagnostic tests

Hypertension and proteinuria are not the only signs of pre-eclampsia, or necessarily the most important; they constitute evidence of significant organ damage within an ongoing process. Diagnosis is usually made on physical signs rather than symptoms. This is important, since a woman may have severe pre-eclampsia and yet feel well.

Diagnostic tests to assess renal function, cardiovascular changes and liver enzymes are necessary to diagnose the extent to which the maternal system is affected (Lewis 2007, PRECOG Development Group 2004, RCOG 2006).

## The midwife's responsibility

It has been customary to describe pre-eclampsia as mild, moderate or severe, but it may also be helpful for midwives to consider 'red flag' signs and symptoms (Lewis 2007), as discussed below, which warrant immediate referral (see Ch. 55).

Early diagnosis is essential; so midwives must begin with an accurate recording of the woman's history to identify risk factors and establish a baseline blood pressure using a standardized technique (Moran & Davison 1999). Thereafter, in addition to assessing general wellbeing, regular antenatal screening involves blood pressure readings, testing urine for protein at each visit, and assessing for significant non-dependent oedema.

Although hypertension and proteinuria, with or without oedema, occur in pre-eclampsia, the severity of these signs varies considerably. A small number of women present with symptoms such as headache, visual disturbances, epigastric pain or generally feeling unwell, which may be indicative of serious systemic complications, and may be followed by eclampsia (Lewis 2007). If a woman complains of these symptoms, the midwife must take her blood pressure, test the urine for protein, and then refer her to an obstetrician immediately, even if her blood pressure is not significantly raised. It is now known that convulsions may precede hypertension or proteinuria (Lewis 2007). Lewis (2007) suggests that same-day referral to an obstetrician is required for women who have hypertension >160 mmHg systolic and/or >90 mmHg diastolic or proteinuria >1+ on dipstick.

Following referral, women need follow-up care in a multidisciplinary team setting. With the changes in general practitioner (GP) involvement with antenatal care, and the arrangements for out-of-hours referral, midwives, in common with all health professionals, should make sure that GPs receive details of referrals and results of tests for their records (Lewis 2007).

Day assessment units (DAUs) or maternity day units (MDUs) offer facilities for ongoing assessment on an outpatient basis, with mothers actively involved in their own screening programmes (Moran & Davison 1999). All of the following tests can be carried out in this setting.

### Assessment of renal functions

- *Uric acid levels* indicate progress and severity of pre-eclampsia, with increased levels in cases of hypertension, usually before the development of proteinuria.
- *Blood urea and creatinine levels* may be raised, and a high level (>110 micromol/L) indicates a late stage of renal involvement.
- *24-hour urinary protein excretion* of ≥0.3 g/24 hours indicates renal involvement.

### Assessment of liver functions

Serial measurements of *liver enzymes*, particularly alanine amino transferase (ALT) or aspartate amino transferase (AST), are performed, and where these rise above 70 IU/L, liver function tests may be carried out (RCOG 2006).

### Assessment of coagulation complications

Repeated investigations to detect the development of coagulation complications should also be performed. These investigations include:

- *blood film*
- *platelet count*, which often decreases to below 100 × $10^6$/L in pre-eclampsia
- *coagulation studies*: coagulation levels are usually unchanged in pre-eclampsia, unless *disseminated intravascular coagulation (DIC)* is present, when thrombin time will be prolonged in the presence of fibrin degradation, heparin or reduced fibrinogen.

The multisystem nature of the condition is reflected in changes which take place in the blood and may give rise to HELLP syndrome, characterized by *h*aemolysis, *e*levated *l*iver enzymes and *l*ow *p*latelets (RCOG 2006).

### Assessment of fetal wellbeing

The following investigations may be used to assess fetal condition, where there is a possibility of IUGR or intrauterine hypoxia:

- *Cardiotocography:* although this can be unreliable at under 30 weeks' gestation, a reactive and variable trace is generally indicative of satisfactory fetal condition. Loss of variability or decelerations suggest deterioration. Walker (2000) suggests that the tracings can be reassuring for the mother.
- *Measurement of symphyseal–fundal height.*
- *A record of fetal movements.*
- *Ultrasound scanning* for:
  - amniotic fluid index
  - fetal growth – as fetal growth restriction may occur prior to any other signs of pre-eclampsia (Lewis 2007)
  - umbilical artery Doppler analysis.

In case of abnormality in any of the above, Moran & Davison (1999) suggest a biophysical profile of the fetus is performed, which includes:

- record of fetal breathing movements
- tone
- gross body movements
- heart rate activity
- liquor volume.

Women attending the DAU/MDU will need to be kept fully informed of their situation, and may need considerable support from the midwife. Women who have experienced pre-eclampsia speak of how frightened they were and how they feared for their baby (Duley et al 2006, Fallon & Engel 2008, Redman & Walker 1996) and reported that compassionate care from the midwife was appreciated.

**Reflective activity 56.3**

Visit a maternity day assessment unit and find out what tests are carried out to assess the progress of pre-eclampsia. List what the normal test results should be, and keep these in your personal record/resource book.

## Severe pre-eclampsia

Depending on the severity of pre-eclampsia and the gestation, conservative treatment may 'buy time' to bring the fetus to the optimal time of delivery, without endangering the mother. Moran & Davison (1999) suggest that, apart from women with diabetes, renal disease, thrombocytopenia and IUGR, pregnancy may be prolonged by up to 15 days without maternal compromise. Antihypertensive drugs control the blood pressure, reducing the risk of cerebral haemorrhage and eclampsia, and therefore the risk of maternal death (Moran & Davison 1999), although they do not improve the underlying effects of the disease. Mattar & Sibai (1999) suggest that outcome is poorest for women who develop pre-eclampsia at or before 32 weeks.

The dangers to mother and baby are:

- *Maternal*: eclampsia, placental abruption, disseminated intravascular coagulation, pulmonary oedema, cerebral oedema, cerebrovascular haemorrhage, renal or hepatic failure, and death.
- *Fetal*: IUGR, fetal hypoxia, intrauterine death, preterm delivery.

### Management

The midwife is part of the multidisciplinary team approach which aims to deliver the baby before life-threatening complications occur. In addition to ongoing monitoring of blood pressure and urine, the following are significant:

**Bedrest:** This is traditionally advised for women with severe pre-eclampsia, although Norwitz et al (1999) suggest that the course of the disease and perinatal outcome is unchanged even for women at high risk. Bedrest itself carries the risk of thromboembolism (Moran & Davison 1999).

**Fluid balance:** Accurate monitoring of fluid intake and urinary output is essential, as overtransfusion has caused pulmonary oedema in the past. However, it is now disputed that aiming for a specific urinary output, usually 30 mL per hour, will prevent renal involvement, which nowadays is rare in the UK (RCOG 2006). Lewis (2007) suggests that there are now fewer complications relating to overtransfusion, probably due to better fluid monitoring, and the restriction of fluids to 80 mL or 1 mL/kg per hour (RCOG 2006). However, this regimen would be inappropriate in the case of maternal haemorrhage.

**Emotional care:** The woman must be kept informed and involved in all aspects of care, using information that is accessible and evidence-based. It is also important to ensure that she has antenatal and parenting education, including a visit to the neonatal intensive care unit (NICU), and opportunity to talk to staff there. Women and their families may be extremely anxious, and information and full involvement in decision making is crucial for them (Crafter 2000, Fallon & Engel 2008, Hartley 1998).

**Antihypertensive drugs:** There is considerable discussion about the levels of hypertension at which drugs should be given, the efficacy and suitability of the various drugs, and the evidence on which their use is based (RCOG 2006). Women taking antihypertensives may experience feelings of sedation, and dizziness on standing. Jordan (2002) advises that women taking oral antihypertensives assume 'the sick role'. They should take time off work and should rest.

Box 56.2 shows the range, dosage, mode of action and side-effects of commonly used drugs.

## ECLAMPSIA

Eclampsia is the onset of seizures (fits) in pregnancy, usually, but not always, complicated by pre-eclampsia. The incidence of eclampsia in the UK is 26.8 per 100,000 maternities (Lewis 2007). One in 200 women who have pre-eclampsia will develop eclampsia (Walker 2000). It is not unusual for women to die after only one seizure (Lewis 2007).

In severe pre-eclampsia there is likely to be cerebral hypoxia due to intense vasospasm and oedema. Cerebral hypoxia leads to increased cerebral dysrhythmia and this may be the cause of the convulsions. Some women have an underlying cerebral dysrhythmia and therefore

### Box 56.2 Antihypertensive drugs

#### Methyldopa

- Proven as safe long term (RCOG 2006)
- Can be used antenatally and during labour
- 1–3 mg daily in divided doses, or at night, by mouth
- Can also be given intravenously
- Acts centrally by inhibiting sympathetic outflow, causing decreased peripheral resistance and bradycardia, leading to reduced blood pressure
- Reduces the risk of developing severe hypertension (Collins & Wallenburg 1989)

*Side-effects:* include postural hypertension, maternal sedation and depression. Not suitable for women with history of depression. Also passes into breast milk, causing neonatal sedation, therefore not suitable for postnatal use (Moran & Davison 1999).

#### Labetolol

- Can be used antenatally, during labour and postnatally
- Dose – up to 2.5 g daily orally
- May also be given intravenously (as a second choice to hydralazine)
- A combined α- and β-antagonist, it reduces peripheral resistance and cardiac output, thereby reducing blood pressure
- In common with β-adrenoceptor antagonists such as propanolol and atenolol, may result in severe fetal and neonatal bradycardia
- Thought to be generally as safe and effective as methyldopa, with an antihypertensive action that may be more controlled than that of hydralazine
- Prevents relaxation of bronchioles, therefore not suitable for women with asthma
- Prevents normal responses to hypoglycaemia, so not suitable for women with diabetes
- Present in breast milk in small amounts, but advice is to monitor the baby

#### Hydralazine

- Can be used at any time during pregnancy or postnatally
- Usually the intravenous drug of choice
- Dose 5–10 mg diluted with 10 mL 0.9% normal saline given intravenously as a bolus over 1–2 minutes
- Is effective in approximately 15 minutes and can be repeated at 20-minute intervals until blood pressure is stabilized
- Can cause sudden, profound maternal hypotension with fetal consequences due to poor placental perfusion, therefore needs constant monitoring of blood pressure
- Present in breast milk but not known to be harmful; however, advice is to monitor the baby

#### Nifedipine

- Can be given orally in 1-mg doses
- Is a *calcium antagonist*
- Lowers blood pressure by inhibiting calcium ion activity in smooth muscles of blood vessels, resulting in decreased peripheral vascular resistance
- Present in breast milk in amounts too small to be harmful, but manufacturers advise avoiding

#### ACE inhibitors

These act by blocking the action of angiotensin-converting enzyme, preventing the production of angiotensin II, which causes vasoconstriction and the production of aldosterone and vasopressin. However, ACE inhibitors are considered unsuitable for use during pregnancy as they have adverse fetal and neonatal effects.

(Joint Formulary Committee 2008, Jordan 2002)

convulsions may occur following less severe forms of pre-eclampsia.

The seizures may occur before, during or after labour. Even if antenatal care and care in labour are of a high standard, postpartum convulsions may still occur. Monitoring of blood pressure and urine for proteinuria must therefore continue during the postpartum period.

There is one sign of eclampsia, namely, the eclamptic convulsion. This is similar to an epileptic seizure (see Ch. 55), and to aid medical differential diagnosis, it is important to observe carefully the duration and nature of the seizure. There are four main phases:

1. *Premonitory stage*: There may be rolling of eyes and facial and hand muscle twitching.
2. *Tonic stage*: Muscles go into violent spasm, with fists clenched and leg rigidity. The jaw is rigid and clenched, and the tongue may be bitten. Breathing is suspended, and the woman may become cyanosed. This lasts for about 30 seconds.
3. *Clonic stage*: The spasm ceases, and there are jerky muscular movements, which increase in intensity, moving the body sometimes violently. Breathing is harsh and noisy, and there may be frothy, blood-stained saliva. This stage lasts for around 2 minutes
4. *Comatose stage*: The woman is unconscious, often breathing is noisy. Cyanosis resolves, though the face may remain swollen and congested. This stage may last a few minutes, or hours.

During a seizure there are dangers for both mother and fetus.

**Maternal** If maternal blood pressure is high, there may be cerebral haemorrhage; inhalation of blood or mucus may lead to asphyxia or pneumonia. Any of these complications may be fatal.

**Fetal** The fetus may already be affected by placental insufficiency. This leads to IUGR and hypoxia. During the seizure when the mother stops breathing, the fetal oxygen supply, already impaired, is further reduced. Intrapartum convulsions are hazardous to the fetus because intrauterine hypoxia is already increased owing to uterine contractions.

## Management

During a seizure, the basic principles of resuscitation must be followed:

- Remain with the woman
- Call for appropriate help; depending on where the woman is, this may be an anaesthetist, senior obstetrician, or, at home, an ambulance paramedic
- Clear the airway of mucus and blood and maintain a clear airway, using the recovery position
- Turn the woman onto her left side
- Protect her from injury
- Administer oxygen (RCOG 2006).

*Anticonvulsant* and *antihypertensive* drugs are given immediately to try to stabilize eclampsia and to lower the blood pressure. Unless there is an immediate problem with the fetus, such as bradycardia, plans for induction of labour or caesarean section can be made once the maternal condition is stabilized. The risks of eclampsia, placental insufficiency and abruption, and intrauterine fetal death must be considered against those of prematurity (Lewis 2007, RCOG 2006).

*Magnesium sulphate* ($MgSO_4$) is the anticonvulsant drug of choice (WHO 1995, 2002). *Diazepam* and *phenytoin* are no longer used in the first instance, although diazepam may be used in single doses in persistent seizures (RCOG 2006). Magnesium sulphate is effective and acts rapidly. An example of how this may be given is as an initial intravenous loading dose of 4 g given as 10% $MgSO_4$, injected over 5–10 minutes via syringe driver, followed by an infusion of 1–2 g/hour. This should be continued for 24 hours after the last seizure (Lewis 2007). It is believed to inhibit presynaptic activity but does not have antihypertensive or sedative properties. Blood levels must be monitored regularly to ensure that these remain within the therapeutic range (2–4 mmol/L).

Toxicity leads to loss of maternal reflexes and eventually muscle paralysis, respiratory arrest and cardiac arrest. Signs of toxicity are loss of patellar reflexes, weakness, nausea, flushes, sleepiness, double vision, and slurred speech. The antidote is intravenous *calcium gluconate* 10 mL of 10% solution (Moran & Davison 1999). There are no known long-term adverse fetal or neonatal effects, but a study by Riaz et al (1998) of 26 infants whose mothers received magnesium sulphate suggests they were hypotonic and had lower Apgar scores immediately after delivery than did the control group of 26.

*Blood pressure* is controlled by the use of antihypertensive drugs (see Box 56.2).

### Midwifery care

The scope of midwifery care is dependent on the severity of illness, and is similar in severe pre-eclampsia and eclampsia. Women may be extremely ill and may be cared for in a high-dependency unit (HDU) by a multidisciplinary team. A specialized chart, like those used in ICUs or HDUs, should be used to record observations.

Any stimulus may precipitate convulsions, so external stimuli such as noise, bright lights and handling are reduced to a minimum. The woman is kept in a quiet, single room and, until her condition is stabilized, she must never be left alone. Suction and oxygen equipment must be available. Although bright sunshine should be excluded, the room should be light enough for the midwife to be able to assess the woman's condition without switching lights on and off. Only essential procedures such as turning 2-hourly to avoid hypostatic pneumonia, treatment of pressure areas and mouth care are carried out initially.

### Observations

1. Restlessness or twitching may indicate a seizure.
2. Continuous oxygen saturation should be measured. Cyanosis is an important sign of cardiorespiratory failure, and therefore the midwife needs to monitor this visually as well as electronically. Cyanosis is an indication for the administration of oxygen.
3. The temperature is recorded hourly. If there is no obvious sign of infection, a rise in temperature could indicate anoxic damage to the temperature-regulating centres in the midbrain.
4. Pulse and respirations may be recorded as often as every 15 minutes.
5. Blood pressure is recorded frequently, usually every 15 minutes. If automatic sphygmomanometers are used, there should be an initial check using a manual machine to monitor any difference between the two (Lewis 2007, RCOG 2006).
6. An accurate record of fluid intake and output is essential. A self-retaining catheter is inserted into the bladder and released hourly; thus, urinary output can be measured accurately and the woman will not have to be disturbed to pass urine. Urinary output of less than 30 mL/hour suggests renal involvement. Urine is tested for protein.
7. The fetal heart is continuously monitored.
8. Monitor for signs of labour, as this may start spontaneously. Any loss per vaginam is noted and the fundus should be gently palpated if the woman appears to be restless at regular intervals because she could be being disturbed by uterine contractions. A

comatose woman could progress to an advanced stage of labour unless the signs are recognized.

9. Blood should be taken every 12–24 hours for full blood count, urea and electrolytes, creatinine and liver function tests.
10. Information and support should be provided to the woman, and to her family, in clear terms that they will understand. This may require the use of a translator if English is not their first language.

## CARE DURING LABOUR AND POSTNATALLY

### Mode of delivery

Pre-eclampsia will resolve only after delivery, but not immediately. Moran & Davison (1999) contend that fetal maturity can be assumed at 36 weeks, and that if the woman has reached that far she is likely to have a vaginal delivery. The disease usually resolves within 48–72 hours of delivery.

As soon as the woman's condition is stabilized, arrangements are made for delivery. Walker (2000) suggests that rushing the delivery contributes to postpartum risks, but there should be no unnecessary delay. The woman should be transferred to a unit with specialized facilities, especially those for neonatal intensive care, and discussion between senior medical staff at each institution must occur (Walker 2000). Dexamethasone or betamethasone may be given intramuscularly or orally to the woman to aid fetal lung maturity as their effects are beneficial even before 24 hours have elapsed. Walker (2000) suggests that prior to 32 weeks, caesarean section is appropriate, but that after 34 weeks, vaginal delivery should be aimed for.

### Care in labour for women with pre-eclampsia or eclampsia

In addition to the midwifery care already described, and the continuation of observations, effective analgesia is essential and can best be achieved by epidural anaesthesia. This has the advantage of lowering the blood pressure, although it is more advantageous in preventing the rise in blood pressure associated with pain in labour. Continuous monitoring of the fetal heart and uterine contractions should be carried out. As long as the woman's condition remains stable, there is no need for routine instrumental delivery (Walker 2000).

Syntocinon should be given for third stage delivery, since ergometrine causes a rise in blood pressure. CEMACH (Lewis 2007) advice is that syntocinon is also used for women who have not had their blood pressure taken in labour, for example, those who present in an advanced stage of labour and give birth quickly.

A paediatrician, or practitioner skilled in neonatal resuscitation must be present at the birth.

### Management after delivery

Following an initial improvement after delivery, 60% of women will worsen within 48 hours, and most maternal deaths occur in the postpartum period (Moran & Davison 1999, Walker 2000). Antihypertensive drugs are usually continued for a further 48 hours, as there is still a risk of postpartum seizures.

The special midwifery care and observations previously described are continued. Unsatisfactory postpartum care accounts for a significant proportion of the mortality from pre-eclampsia and eclampsia (Lewis 2007). Depending on the gestational age, the baby may be cared for in the NICU unit or in a postnatal area with the mother. Parents must be appropriately supported to care for their baby, and, given the connection between sudden infant death syndrome (SIDS) and pre-eclampsia, they should be particularly encouraged to follow the protocols for preventing SIDS (Li & Wi 2000).

### Psychological and follow-up care

Problems resulting from hypertensive disorders may be minor, and be a matter of the woman needing medication to control her blood pressure; or may be major, and result in her having instrumental delivery, and even requiring high-dependency or intensive care. This may be considerably different from the woman's birth expectations (Duley et al 2006). It can also cause post-traumatic stress syndrome, with debilitating symptoms such as flashbacks, nightmares and depression (Hammett 1992).

The midwife needs to provide space and an opportunity for the woman, and often her partner, to review and debrief, if they wish. This will often clarify issues of confusion for the woman, assisting her to begin to understand and accept events. It also allows the midwife to identify a woman who may require additional support or counselling (Fallon & Engel 2008).

**Reflective activity 56.4**

Review the literature and the level of information available locally to women.

Follow-up investigations of blood pressure or assessment of renal function may be necessary for women who have suffered serious hypertensive disease in pregnancy, although persistent renal problems are now rare in the UK (RCOG 2006). Women may also be advised to obtain preconception advice and counselling before embarking on a future pregnancy. Eclampsia rarely occurs in a subsequent pregnancy, but pre-eclampsia recurs in up to 1:20 cases where severe pre-eclampsia was present in a first pregnancy, and in up to 1:3 where it occurred in a second pregnancy (Redman & Walker 1996). It is not associated with a higher incidence of essential hypertension in later life.

The charity Action on Pre-eclampsia (APEC) seeks to inform all pregnant women of the risks of pregnancy-induced hypertension, emphasizing the fact that the disorder is largely asymptomatic and must be diagnosed by active screening. Whilst the charity welcomes the demedicalization of childbirth, it emphasizes the importance of informing women and securing their cooperation in all aspects of antenatal care (APEC 2008). This is congruent with the midwifery concept of health promotion (Crafter 2000), and the participation of women in their own antenatal care, by regular antenatal checks, by providing a urine specimen, and by being aware of the significance of headaches, visual disturbances and abdominal pain. It could be argued that some women will be inappropriately stressed by unnecessary tests and investigations, and some will develop pre-eclampsia despite regular antenatal care. However, monitoring of blood pressure and urinalysis remain relatively cheap and easy methods of detecting pre-eclampsia (Stevenson & Billington 2007).

**Reflective activity 56.5**

Check your unit protocol, how is the development of any of the above assessed and dealt with?

## ESSENTIAL/CHRONIC HYPERTENSION

Essential hypertension is a condition of permanently raised blood pressure, often with no apparent cause. It may also be associated with renal disease (see Ch. 55), phaeochromocytoma or coarctation of the aorta. It is familial and complicates 2–5% of all pregnancies (Roberts & Redman 1993) with 15–20% of women developing a superimposed pre-eclampsia (Sibai 1991). A woman attending the antenatal clinic is said to have essential hypertension if her blood pressure in early pregnancy is 140/90 mmHg or more, or her 6-week postpartum blood pressure remains high following hypertension in pregnancy. It is distinguished from pre-eclampsia by the fact that it is present in the early weeks of pregnancy, long before pre-eclampsia normally arises, and, in the absence of renal disease, there is no oedema or proteinuria.

Mid trimester, the blood pressure often falls to a normal level, which may mask hypertension if the woman begins antenatal care after the 18th week of pregnancy.

### Management

The woman will require antenatal care from a consultant obstetrician, physician and midwife. She is likely to have a normal pregnancy and labour but is advised to avoid excessive weight gain. She should be advised not to smoke, as this contributes to hypertension. Fetal wellbeing is monitored closely to detect growth restriction. Antihypertensive drugs may be prescribed if the diastolic blood pressure exceeds 100 mmHg (RCOG 2006, Sibai 1991). Investigations are carried out as described for pre-eclampsia. In addition, *urinary catecholamines* or *vanillylmandelic acid* (VMA) are usually measured, because severe hypertension may be caused by phaeochromocytoma, a tumour of the adrenals.

Renal failure, heart failure and cerebral haemorrhage are potential complications if the blood pressure is exceptionally high. The fetus is at risk, because the placental circulation is poor; hence, IUGR and hypoxia may occur.

If the blood pressure cannot be controlled or there are signs of fetal growth restriction or hypoxia, labour is induced or, if the danger is more acute or arises earlier, caesarean section may be performed. Women with essential or chronic hypertension require the same midwifery input as women with pre-eclampsia; however, from a psychological point of view, their disease is ongoing and progressive.

**Reflective activity 56.6**

Is there a copy of the latest Confidential Enquiry into Maternal Deaths available on the maternity unit?

Review the chapter on hypertensive disorders of pregnancy.

Consider:

- Do you think any of these case studies could happen in your unit/locality?
- Does your unit management mirror the recommendations – if not, why not?

## CONCLUSION

Hypertension complicates a significant number of pregnancies, and midwives play a key role in the detection of pre-eclampsia, and in the care of women who experience hypertensive disorders during pregnancy. The midwife works with the woman and her family in a partnership role, ensuring that the woman is sufficiently informed and prepared, so she can report problems and unusual symptoms early. Within the multidisciplinary team, the midwife can provide the crucial element of continuity, during and following the pregnancy. This can help to ensure holistic care to provide as positive and safe an experience as is possible to mother and baby (Crafter 2000).

**KEY POINTS**

- Hypertensive disorders of pregnancy include pre-existing essential or chronic hypertension,

hypertension associated with renal disease, pre-eclampsia and eclampsia.

- Pre-eclampsia and eclampsia are major contributors to maternal and perinatal morbidity and mortality.
- Involvement of senior midwifery and medical personnel at an early stage, and throughout the care, is essential.
- Women and their partners need information about pre-eclampsia and its effects, given in a sensitive way.
- Effective assessment, monitoring and referral by the midwife will ensure that care is tailored to the woman's needs and that complications are speedily dealt with.
- Follow-up investigations may be necessary to safeguard women's physical and psychological wellbeing.

## REFERENCES


Action on Pre-eclampsia (APEC): How to reduce errors in blood pressure measurement and improving the reliability of proteinuria estimate using dipstick testing (website). www.apec.org.uk. 2008. Accessed October 23, 2008.

Collins R, Wallenburg HCS: Pharmacological prevention and treatment of pregnancy. In Chamberlain I, Enkin M, Keirse MJNC, editors: *Effective care in pregnancy and childbirth*, Oxford, 1989, Oxford University Press.

Crafter H: Working with Action on Pre-eclampsia: the role of a childbirth charity advisor and trustee, *MIDIRS Midwifery Digest* 10(2):184–186, 2000.

Duley L, Meher S, Abalos E: Management of pre eclampsia, *British Medical Journal* 332(7539):463–468, 2006.

Eras JL, Saftlas AF, Triche E: Abortion and its effect on risk of pre-eclampsia and transient hypertension, *Epidemiology* 11(1):36–43, 2000.

Fallon A, Engel C: Midwifery basics: caring for women with medical conditions (1) Hypertensive disorders of pregnancy, *The Practising Midwife* 11(9):32–37, 2008.

Hammett PL: Midwives and debriefing. In Abbott P, Sapsford R, editors: *Research into practice*, Buckingham, 1992, Open University Press, pp 135–159.

Hartley J: Diagnosis, treatment and care of the pre eclamptic woman, *RCM Midwives Journal* 1(1):17–20, 1998.

Joint Formulary Committee: *British National Formulary*, ed 56, London, 2008, British Medical Association and Royal Pharmaceutical Society of Great Britain.

Jordan S: *Pharmacology for midwives: the evidence base for safe practice*, Basingstoke, 2002, Palgrave.

Lewis G, editor: *The Confidential Enquiry into Maternal and Child Health (CEMACH). Saving mothers' lives: reviewing maternal deaths to make motherhood safer – 2003–2005 The Seventh Report on Confidential Enquiries into Maternal Deaths in the United Kingdom*, London, 2007, CEMACH.

Li D, Wi S: Maternal pre-eclampsia/eclampsia and the risk of sudden infant death in offspring, *Paediatric and Perinatal Epidemiology* 14(2):141–144, 2000.

Mattar F, Sibai BM: Eclampsia VIII Risk factors for maternal morbidity, *American Journal of Obstetrics and Gynecology* 182(2):307–312, 1999.

Moran P, Davison JM: Clinical management of established pre-eclampsia, *Baillière's Best Practice: Clinical Obstetrics and Gynaecology* 13(1):77–93, 1999.

Natarajan P, Shennan AH, Penny J: Comparison of auscaltatory and oscillometric automated blood pressure monitors in the setting of pre-eclampsia, *American Journal of Obstetrics and Gynecology* 181(5 Pt 1):1203–1210, 1999.

National Institute for Health and Clinical Excellence (NICE): *NICE clinical guideline 62. Antenatal care: routine care for the healthy pregnant woman*, London, 2008, NICE.

Norwitz ER, Robinson JN, Repke JT: Prevention of pre-eclampsia: is it possible? *Clinical Obstetrics and Gynecology* 42(3):436–454, 1999.

PRECOG Development Group: Pre-Eclampsia Community Guideline (PRECOG) (website). www.apec.org.uk. 2004. Accessed October 24, 2008.

Redman C, Walker I: *Pre-eclampsia: the facts*, Harrow, 1996, Action on Pre-eclampsia.

Riaz M, Porat B, Brodsky NL, et al: The effects of maternal magnesium sulfate treatment on newborns: a prospective controlled study, *Journal of Perinatology* 18(6 Pt 1):449–454, 1998.

Roberts JM: Pre-eclampsia: what we know and what we do not know, *Seminars in Perinatology* 24(1):24–28, 2000.

Roberts JM, Redman C: Pre-eclampsia: more than pregnancy induced hypertension, *Lancet* 341(8858): 1447–1451, 1993.

Royal College of Obstetricians and Gynaecologists (RCOG): Clinical greentop guidelines. Management of severe pre eclampsia/eclampsia (website). www.rcog.org.uk. 2006. Accessed August, 2010.

Salas SP: What causes pre-eclampsia? *Baillière's Best Practice: Clinical Obstetrics and Gynaecology* 13(1):41–57, 1999.

Sibai BM: Diagnosis and management of chronic hypertension in pregnancy, *Obstetrics and Gynecology* 78(3 Pt 1):451–461, 1991.

Smith GN, Walker M, Tessier JL, et al: Increased incidence of pre-eclampsia in women conceiving by intrauterine insemination with donor versus partner sperm for treatment of primary infertility, *American Journal of Obstetrics and Gynecology* 177(2):455–458, 1997.

Stevenson M, Billington M: Hypertensive disorders and the critically ill woman. In Billington M,

Stevenson M, editors: *Critical care in childbearing for midwives*, Oxford, 2007, Blackwell.

Walker J: Severe pre-eclampsia and eclampsia, *Baillière's Best Practice: Clinical Obstetrics and Gynaecology* 14(1):57–71, 2000.

World Health Organization (WHO): Magnesium sulphate is the drug of choice for eclampsia, *Safe Motherhood – A Newsletter Of Worldwide Activity* 18(2):3, 13, 1995.

World Health Organization (WHO): The selection and use of essential medicines. Report of the WHO Expert Committee, 2002 (including the 12th Model List of Essential Medicines), WHO Technical Report Series, No. 920, Geneva, 2003, WHO.

Chapter |57|

# Sexually transmitted infections

Jane Susan Bott

## LEARNING OUTCOMES

This chapter aims to enable the reader to:

- understand the midwife's role in offering and recommending screening for human immunodeficiency virus (HIV), syphilis, and hepatitis B virus (HBV) infection during pregnancy
- be aware of the ethical principles which underpin midwifery practice
- discuss the clinical presentation, pregnancy implications and management of common sexually transmitted infections (STIs).

## INTRODUCTION

Most STIs are transmitted during sexual intercourse, non-penetrative genital contact, sex toys shared between partners or oral sex (BUPA 2007). Twenty-five types of STIs have been identified, although some – for example, vaginal candidiasis, pubic lice and scabies – can be acquired without sexual contact (Brook Advisory Centres 2008). Chlamydia, gonorrhoea, genital herpes simplex virus (HSV), genital human papillomavirus (HPV), non-specific infections, HIV, syphilis, HBV and trichomoniasis are the most common STIs.

Adverse trends in STIs in the UK are mainly attributable to rates of new HIV diagnoses and STIs in men who have sex with men. Although levels are relatively low, there has also been a steady increase in heterosexual HIV transmission, especially in the black ethnic minority. Most of the partners of infected black African and Caribbean people had probably been infected abroad (UK Collaborative Group for HIV and STI Surveillance 2007). Young adults (16–24 years of age) also appear to present a challenge as:

- 66% of genital chlamydia, 55% of genital warts, and 48% of gonorrhoea infections that were diagnosed at genitourinary medicine clinics during 2006 were in young adults
- 75% of the women diagnosed with genital chlamydia were under 25 years of age
- there was a 16% rise in diagnoses of genital HSV among teenage women between 2005 and 2006.

Controlling the transmission of HIV and STIs is a major public health challenge and midwifery practice involves responding to the challenge. Midwives are required to promote routine screening for HIV, HBV, and syphilis (DH 2003) to all pregnant women. Midwives encouraging sexual health and education during the booking visit may reduce transmission of infection, including mother-to-infant transmission, as well as facilitate early diagnosis and treatment of infected persons, which reduces associated morbidity and mortality. Midwives should ensure that women receive information about these screening tests, and advice about reducing the risk of STIs by reducing the number of partners and frequency of partner change, and using condoms correctly and consistently during sexual intercourse (HPA 2008a).

Most STIs, if detected early, are treatable and can be cured with antibiotics, for example, gonorrhoea and syphilis. However, patients with viral infection, such as HSV, experience recurrences, as the virus remains in the body and reactivates on occasions. HIV is more serious as currently no cure is available and the effects may be more devastating for a pregnant woman and her family.

This chapter will examine the midwife's role and underpinning ethical principles in relation to HIV screening, including the complex issues involved in decision making for the woman (Box 57.1). These principles, including accurate information based upon evidence, may also be applied to the midwife's role when offering and recommending screening for HBV and syphilis. These STIs, in addition to other common STIs, will be discussed, with reference to clinical presentation, pregnancy implications and management. An understanding of the clinical presentation and management of STIs will enable midwives to effectively meet women's sexual health needs.

## HUMAN IMMUNODEFICIENCY VIRUS (HIV)

Unlinked anonymous surveillance of newborn infant dried blood spots shows that HIV prevalence in women giving birth varies widely nationally (Fig. 57.1) and is highest in urban areas, particularly London, where the prevalence has increased from 0.19% (200/106,407) in 1997 to 0.42% (502/119,614) in 2006 (UK Collaborative Group for HIV and STI Surveillance 2007). Women born abroad, especially in areas with generalized HIV epidemics, have a higher HIV prevalence than those born in the UK. One in every 2013 UK-born women giving birth in England was HIV-infected, compared with 1 in 138 non-UK-born women.

| Box 57.1 **Ethical principles** |
|---|
| Beneficence |
| Non-maleficence |
| Informed consent |
| Autonomy |
| Confidentiality |

### Disease progression

Sexual exposure is the primary method of spread of HIV infection worldwide. If left untreated, HIV damages the immune system, causing chronic and progressive illness as the infected person becomes vulnerable to a variety of infections (Bradley Hare 2006). Different stages of the disease have been identified (Pratt 2003):

- *Primary infection:* During the first few months, some people are asymptomatic; others develop an acute illness (acute retroviral seroconversion syndrome), experiencing symptoms including fatigue, headache, fever, joint and muscle pains, lymphadenopathy, diarrhoea, nausea and vomiting, skin rash and neurological illness, such as meningitis. Others develop persistent generalized lymphadenopathy. Seroconversion takes place during this phase as HIV-1 antibodies and p24 antigen (website) become positive within the first few weeks or months or in most cases.
- *Clinical latency:* Even without antiretroviral therapy, most people remain asymptomatic for many years. However, there is slow progressive loss of CD4 T-lymphocytes (website) with a corresponding increase in viral load.
- *Symptomatic disease:* People with 'early symptomatic disease' are affected by conditions: cervical dysplasia and cervical carcinoma, listeriosis and pelvic inflammatory disease. Progression to acquired immunodeficiency syndrome (AIDS)-defining conditions, referred to as 'late symptomatic disease', is when people are affected by a range of life-threatening opportunistic cancers and infections, for example, pneumocystis carinii pneumonia (PCP), candidiasis of the oesophagus, trachea and lungs, toxoplasmosis of the brain, pulmonary tuberculosis, herpes simplex virus infection, invasive cervical cancer, cryptosporidiosis with diarrhoea lasting more than 1 month and cytomegalovirus.

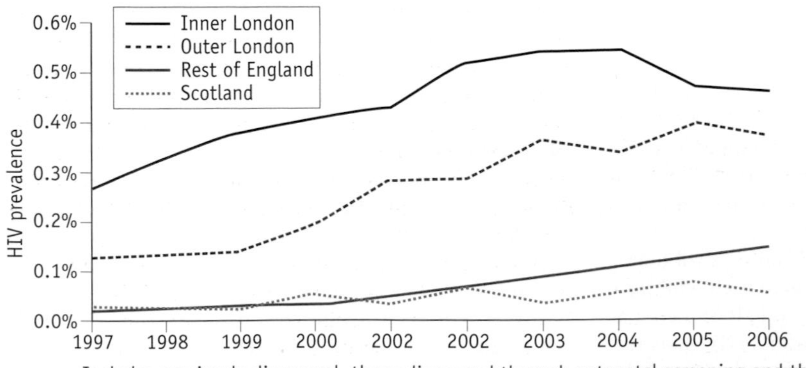


**Figure 57.1** HIV prevalence among pregnant women by area of residence, England & Scotland (UK Collaborative Group for HIV and STI Surveillance 2007).

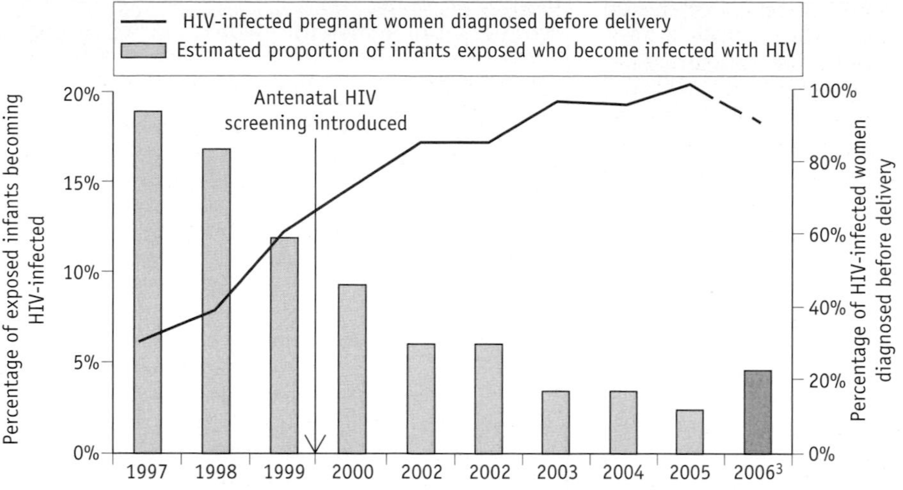


**Figure 57.2** Estimated proportion of HIV-infected pregnant women diagnosed before delivery[1] and of exposed infants becoming infected with HIV[2], England and Scotland (UK Collaborative Group for HIV and STI Surveillance 2007).

## HIV screening during pregnancy

Since the implementation of routine screening during pregnancy, improved diagnostic rates for HIV have enabled infected women to make informed choices regarding interventions, reducing risks of mother-to-child-transmission (MTCT) of HIV infection from 25–30% to less than 2% (RCOG 2004). By 2006, more than 90% of pregnant women were aware of their HIV infection, resulting in a MTCT rate of less than 5% in the UK, compared with about 20% in 1997 (Fig. 57.2) (UK Collaborative Group for HIV and STI Surveillance 2007).

## Beneficence

When applying ethical principles of beneficence (Ch. 8), the midwife should ensure outcomes of care result in 'good' being done to the woman and her baby. This entails informing women of the advantages of HIV testing during pregnancy, the benefits of which are listed below.

### *Preventing mother-to-child-transmission*

Several well-conducted studies have shown that MTCT can be reduced by use of antiretroviral therapy, elective caesarean section (CS) and exclusively formula feeding the baby (Bott 2005). The HIV physician is responsible for determining treatment for individual women, taking into consideration maternal and fetal factors. For example, women with a low plasma viral load and a well-preserved CD4 T-lymphocyte count (website) can be treated either with single therapy (zidovudine) or with a combination of drugs referred to as HAART (highly active antiretroviral therapy) following a consideration of the benefits (British HIV Association & Children's HIV Association 2008, RCOG 2004) (Box 57.2). Women with advanced HIV (website) are likely to have symptomatic infection and falling CD4 T-lymphocyte counts and should be treated with a HAART regimen to improve maternal morbidity and mortality and prevent MTCT (RCOG 2004).

Further research to evaluate the effect on MTCT and maternal health of planned CS for women who are taking HAART or who have very low viral loads is indicated in British guidelines. However, delivery by CS is recommended for other women. Women choosing vaginal birth benefit from discussing a birth plan with their midwife, including guidelines for vaginal and CS births, to ensure maximum benefit and minimum harm (British HIV Association & Children's HIV Association 2008, RCOG 2004) (Box 57.3).

Several studies have confirmed a 10–24% increase in MTCT of HIV when women breastfeed their babies (British HIV Association & Children's HIV Association 2008). Transmission may occur throughout the period of breastfeeding, though the risk is influenced by breast milk virus load, which is highest early after delivery. Breastfeeding women have significantly higher median virus load in

**Box 57.2 Therapeutic options for women with a low plasma viral load and a well preserved CD4 T-lymphocyte count**

**Option 1: Single-agent zidovudine regimen**

- Zidovudine is given orally twice a day during pregnancy, commencing at 28 weeks gestation
- Zidovudine is given intravenously intrapartum
- Zidovudine is usually discontinued immediately after delivery
- Delivery should be by elective CS

**Benefits**

- Exposure of the mother and fetus to larger numbers of potentially toxic drugs is avoided

**Option 2: Short-term antiretroviral therapy regimen (START)**

- HAART is given during pregnancy, commencing at 20–28 weeks gestation
- HAART may be discontinued shortly after delivery, provided that the maternal viral load is undetectable

**Benefits**

- Maternal plasma viraemia is more likely to be suppressed to undetectable levels
- Fewer mother to infant transmissions are therefore envisaged
- Risk of the mother developing resistant virus may be lower

- Zidovudine is usually administered orally to the neonate for 4–6 weeks, commencing as soon as possible after the birth
- Antiretroviral therapy for invasive genetic diagnostic tests

British HIV Association & Children's HIV Association 2008, RCOG 2004

colostrum/early milk, compared with the mature breast milk collected 14 days after the birth of the baby (Rousseau et al 2003), and women with more advanced HIV are also more at risk of breast milk transmission (British HIV Association & Children's HIV Association 2008). In the UK, midwives should advise all women who are HIV-positive to bottle-feed their babies to prevent MTCT (RCOG 2004). The Department of Health has issued guidance for healthcare professionals involved in supporting HIV-infected women to breastfeed their babies (see below).

To further reduce MTCT, HIV-infected women should be screened for other genital infections as early as possible in pregnancy and again at 28 weeks' gestation (RCOG 2004).

Results from a comprehensive national surveillance study in England and Ireland conducted during 2002–2006 show that current options and treatment offered to pregnant women according to British guidelines appear to be effective in reducing MTCT. The overall MTCT was 1.2%, and it was 0.8% for women who received at least 14 days of antiretroviral therapy. Transmission rates were 0.7% for HAART with planned CS, 0.7% for HAART with planned vaginal delivery, and 0% for zidovudine monotherapy with planned CS (Townsend et al 2008). The transmissions that occurred despite woman taking HAART were mainly attributable to adherence problems and short duration of treatment.

**Box 57.3 Guidelines for vaginal and CS births**

**Elective CS**

- Elective CS should be performed at 38–39 weeks
- Commence zidovudine infusion 4 hours before CS and continue until cord has been clamped

**Planned vaginal delivery**

- Amniotomy should be avoided unless there is slowing of progress during second stage of labour
- Avoid use of fetal scalp electrode and fetal blood sampling
- Continue HAART regime throughout labour
- If an intravenous infusion of zidovudine is required, start it at beginning of labour and continue until cord has been clamped

- Clamp the cord as soon as possible after birth of baby
- Test maternal blood at delivery for plasma viral load
- Bath baby immediately after birth

British HIV Association & Children's HIV Association 2008, RCOG 2004

### *Benefits for the mother*

Early diagnosis of HIV improves maternal health and life expectancy as affected women benefit from being monitored and treated. The use of HAART has dramatically cut the number of deaths from AIDS-related illnesses and women benefit from PCP prophylaxis with co-trimoxazole, which is usually administered when the CD4 T-lymphocyte count is below $200 \times 10^6$/L. With appropriate treatment, affected people now have a near-normal life expectancy (BUPA 2008, RCOG 2004).

### *Benefits for the baby*

Babies benefit from being followed up, and receiving appropriate treatment as necessary. Virologic testing of babies to diagnose HIV infection is recommended at 1 day, 6 weeks and 12 weeks of age (British HIV Association & Children's HIV Association 2008). If the test results show a baby is HIV-infected, urgent referral to a specialist clinic enables early commencement of combination antiretroviral therapy. If the test results are negative, parents can be reassured that their baby is not infected with HIV, providing breastfeeding has been avoided. PCP prophylaxis is recommended for babies born to mothers at high risk of MTCT (British HIV Association & Children's HIV Association 2008). A negative HIV antibody test result at 18 months of age will confirm that the child is uninfected (RCOG 2004).

Mortality, AIDS, and hospital admission rates have declined substantially in perinatally HIV-infected children in the UK and Ireland, paralleling the increased use of combination antiretroviral therapy. Mortality decreased by 80% between 1997 and 2001–02, AIDS progression decreased by 50% and hospital admission rates decreased by 80% (Gibb et al 2003).

### *Benefits for the family*

Informed decisions regarding the current pregnancy in terms of effective interventions to prevent MTCT and planning future pregnancies may be made by women, possibly in consultations with their partners, or they may make informed choices to terminate the pregnancy if in their best interests. Preventing the spread of HIV infection may be through testing other family members for HIV and giving advice.

## Non-maleficence

When applying the ethical principle of non-maleficence, the midwife should ensure that any act or omission does not result in harm. Being aware of the potential 'harm' (Box 57.4) facilitates discussion of individual concerns with women, who themselves must decide whether screening is in their best interests. Knowledge regarding potential effects of different treatments and interventions assists provision of optimum care.

Some women may be inclined to regard a negative test result as justification for an unhealthy lifestyle, described as the 'certificate of health effect' (Tymstra & Bieleman 1987). Screening may have adverse consequences should it lead to denial of the need to change 'risky' behaviour.

Box 57.4 **Potential 'harm'**

- Possible adverse consequences of a negative result
- Psychological impact
- Social sequelae – impact on work/family/relationships
- Stigma/discrimination
- Insurance/mortgage issues (if positive)
- Unnecessary treatment of about 85% of mothers and their uninfected babies
- Side-effects of antiretroviral therapy
- Avoidance of breastfeeding

McIntyre (2005) argues that women need to be informed that their risk of HIV acquisition during pregnancy is doubled, probably owing to biological changes, and messages to prevent infections should be reinforced. Midwives can therefore reduce 'harm' when discussing the implications of a negative test result. Also, women should understand that screening detects HIV antibodies present in the blood. The possibility of recent exposure or suspected exposure to HIV and re-testing later in pregnancy should be discussed, as a negative test result does not guarantee against newly acquired infection. It has been argued that further testing for HIV later in pregnancy, especially for women in an ethnically diverse area such as London, should be considered (Moses et al 2008).

Awaiting the results of HIV testing and receiving a positive result can be considerably stressful and midwives need to be sensitive to individual needs for support. Receiving an HIV diagnosis is a traumatic experience, resulting in reactions of shock, fear and anguish (Stevens & Tighe 1997). Women often experience unrelenting misery, escalating drug use and transmission risks, and destabilization of relationships, income and shelter. Other examples of harm include risk of rejection, isolation, domestic violence (Lester et al 1995) and suicide (Campbell 1995). Therefore, it is important that midwives are able to refer women to specialist counsellors and social workers as appropriate, to reduce the potential social and psychological 'harm'. Details of HIV support groups may also be given (website).

Informing women of the 15–20% risk of vertical transmission is the same as telling them that 80–85% of babies will not be infected, and therefore the majority of mothers who accept interventions on offer will be exposing themselves and their babies to unnecessary treatment (RCOG 1997). Midwives can give women *A guide to HIV, pregnancy & women's health*, which is freely available in different languages, to help them understand the different treatments, including different drug combinations, and the possible effects on the baby (i-base 2007).

Olivero et al (1997) warn of the potential toxicity of antiretroviral drugs and the need for long-term follow-up of children born to HIV-infected women. Monitoring the effects of perinatal exposure is particularly important in cases where these drugs have been administered during the period of embryogenesis, when teratogenicity is more likely to be a problem. Increasing numbers of women have been diagnosed with HIV before pregnancy and have been taking HAART prior to conception and throughout pregnancy. Long-term side-effects fall into four categories: teratogenic, carcinogenic, developmental and mitochondrial. The Antiretroviral Pregnancy Registry, which detects major teratogenic effects for each licensed antiretroviral drug, has found no increased risk of birth defects so far among the overall population exposed to antiretroviral drugs throughout pregnancy, or among those exposed during the second and third trimesters, when compared with the general population. However, there was an increased frequency of birth defects when didanosine only was used and a significantly elevated rate of hypospadias after first-trimester exposure to zidovudine (Antiretroviral Pregnancy Registry 2008). (See website for explanation of HAART.)

Short-term effects of mitochondrial (see website for relevant web-link) toxicity are rare, resulting in severe lactic acidosis, multisystem failure and anaemia. With appropriate care, affected babies are able to make a good recovery (Giaquinto et al 2001). Zidovudine has been associated with a higher incidence of neonatal haemoglobin concentration of less than 9 g/dL, although by 12 weeks of age this effect was no longer apparent (Connor et al 1994). However, a more recent study has reported a significant negative effect on haematopoiesis up to the age of 18 months (Le Chenadec et al 2003).

Some studies have shown a significant association between HAART and preterm delivery, especially before 34 weeks, and an increased risk of pre-eclampsia (British HIV Association & Children's HIV Association 2008). Lactic acidosis, a recognized complication of HAART, may mimic the signs of pre-eclampsia. Signs of lactic acidosis include gastrointestinal disturbances, fatigue, fever and breathlessness. Other antiretroviral toxicities include hepatoxicity, rashes, glucose intolerance and diabetes (RCOG 2004).

Many HIV-infected women in the UK would prefer to breastfeed their babies if it was safe. Randomized controlled studies are currently being conducted in Africa to determine the safety of breastfeeding when mothers are on combination antiretroviral therapy (British HIV Association & Children's HIV Association 2008).

When HIV-infected mothers choose to breastfeed, under the Children Act 1989, courts have a statutory duty to treat the welfare of the baby as paramount. If the midwife's duty of care to the mother conflicts with the needs of the baby, it is vital to ensure, with an interpreter if necessary, that the mother understands why bottle-feeding is recommended and explore reasons why a mother might feel unable to avoid breastfeeding. In exceptional circumstances, when a midwife is required to support an HIV-infected mother who persists in wanting to breastfeed her baby, the social worker, paediatrician and supervisor of midwives should all be informed. Accurate records of care should be kept. The UK Chief Medical Officers' Expert Advisory Group on AIDS (2004) advises the following strategies to protect the infant from possible MTCT of HIV:

- antiretroviral drug therapy for mother and baby
- exclusive breastfeeding
- early discontinuation of breastfeeding, substituting infant formula milk for breast milk before 6 months or solid foods after 6 months
- ensure correct positioning and attachment of baby to the breast to prevent cracked nipples and mastitis (Pillay et al 2000)
- examine the baby's mouth for signs of oral candidiasis, and treat promptly if appropriate.

### Informed consent

Women need to be aware of the implications of receiving an HIV diagnosis in order to decide whether to be tested, and, if necessary, make informed decisions regarding treatment and interventions (Ch. 8). Midwives must ensure that women are provided with relevant up-to-date information 'in a way they can understand' (NMC 2008). Leaflets, available in different languages, are helpful in facilitating this process (DH 2000).

### Autonomy

Autonomy (Ch. 8) is inextricably linked with consent and entails facilitating a woman's ability to formulate and carry out her own plans so that she is in control of her life and can act freely within the context of rational decision making (Downie & Calman 1987). Midwives must 'respect and support people's rights to accept or decline treatment and care' (NMC 2008). Lack of feelings of autonomy and control may discourage some women from seeking antenatal care.

### Confidentiality

A breach of confidentiality (Ch. 8) is particularly serious for women who are HIV-positive, because of the risk of discrimination. The Nursing and Midwifery Council (NMC 2008) requires midwives to disclose information if they believe someone may be at risk of harm, in line with the law of the country in which they are practising.

**Reflective activity 57.1**

Refer to your local trust protocol for midwives offering and recommending HIV screening during pregnancy. What guidelines have been included in relation to ensuring that confidentiality is maintained? Are these adequate? If not, what improvements could be made?

## HEPATITIS B VIRUS (HBV)

Routine screening for HBV during pregnancy was introduced in 1998 and the estimated uptake was 93% in 2005 (UK Collaborative Group for HIV and STI Surveillance 2007). Standards for screening aim to ensure immunization of babies born to infected mothers to reduce the perinatal transmission of this infection. Partners and children of infected women are offered screening and follow-up, with hepatitis B immunization as appropriate (DH 2003). Leaflets in different languages can be given to women to facilitate the process of informed consent (DH 2007) (see website).

Many people infected with HBV are unaware of their infection. Those who do experience symptoms commonly have a 'flu-like' illness and jaundice (DH & RCM 2000). Approximately 10% of infected people become carriers of the virus (Sira 1998) and 20% of carriers develop serious liver disease, such as cirrhosis or hepatocellular carcinoma (Wright & Lau 1993). Vertical transmission may occur at or around the time of birth (DH & RCM 2000), and up to 90% of infected infants become chronic carriers (Grosheide & Van Damme 1996). These infants are at risk of premature death from chronic liver disease. Immunization can prevent 95% of cases of such infants developing carrier status (Hadler & Margolis 1992).

Screening involves testing a blood specimen for HBV surface antigen (HBsAg). If the screening test is positive, confirmatory testing is undertaken. If infection is confirmed, tests for hepatitis B e-markers are carried out to determine whether the newborn baby should be given hepatitis B specific immunoglobulin (HBIg), in addition to hepatitis B vaccine.

Babies born to carrier mothers should be immunized with hepatitis B vaccine within 24 hours of birth. If the mother carries the hepatitis B e-antigen or has had acute HBV infection during pregnancy, the baby should also receive HBIg. Further vaccinations are given at 1 and 2 months of age. At 12 months, a booster dose is given, and follow-up testing should also be carried out (DH & RCM 2000). Breastfeeding is not contraindicated, therefore this should be encouraged and supported. Also, mothers should be referred to a specialist with expertise in liver disease.

**Reflective activity 57.2**

Find the local trust protocol for midwives offering and recommending HBV screening. What written information is given to infected mothers regarding when injections should be given to their babies, and who is responsible for administering each dose and follow-up appointments?

## SYPHILIS

Syphilis is caused by *Treponema pallidum*, a spirochaete, which enters the body through tiny breaks in the skin of the external genitalia during sexual intercourse.

If untreated, the disease progresses through four consecutive stages:

- *Primary stage*: Small painless papules, known as chancres, develop around the external genitalia, healing spontaneously after 1–2 months.
- *Secondary stage*: Bloodborne spirochaetes disseminate throughout the body, causing a widespread rash over the trunk and extremities. Fever, myalgia, lymphadenopathy, headache and sore throat are common. The kidneys and joints may also be affected, causing arthritis, glomerulonephritis and nephrotic syndrome. Symptoms resolve over 4–12 weeks.
- *Latent period*: lasts for months or years.
- *Tertiary syphilis*: About 25% of people will develop complications as multiple organs are affected, including the cardiovascular and nervous systems. About 50% of these people will die, usually from cardiovascular complications.

During the primary or secondary stage of syphilis, MTCT will inevitably occur at any stage of pregnancy. Complications include miscarriage, stillbirth, premature delivery, and congenital syphilis, and 50% of babies born to these infected women will die within 4 weeks (Heffner & Schust 2006) .

UK pregnant women have been screened routinely for syphilis for many years, with an estimated uptake in 2005 of 95%. Increasing numbers of women have been diagnosed in recent years (from 268 in 2002 to 553 in 2006) and high screening uptake rates must be maintained to prevent future cases of congenital syphilis (UK Collaborative Group for HIV and STI Surveillance 2007). Penicillin is the treatment of choice in all but highly allergic patients.

Syphilis is not transmitted during breastfeeding, unless an infectious lesion is present on the breast (Genc & Ledger 2000). Midwives should ensure that women are given this information.

## GONORRHOEA

Gonorrhoea is caused by the bacterium *Neisseria gonorrhoeae* (HPA 2008a).

Affected men commonly develop urethritis, with dysuria and/or a purulent urethral discharge. Many women are asymptomatic. Others present with dysuria and vaginal discharge from cervicitis or purulent drainage from the Bartolin's glands (Heffner & Schust 2006). If untreated, it can cause chronic pelvic pain, pelvic inflammatory disease, ectopic pregnancy and infertility (UK Collaborative Group for HIV and STI Surveillance 2007).

During pregnancy, gonorrhoea has been associated with low birthweight, premature delivery, preterm rupture of the membranes, chorioamnionitis and postpartum sepsis. Without treatment with antibiotics, MTCT can occur and 30–50% of babies will develop ophthalmia neonatorum within 3–14 days of life, which may cause blindness. Otitis media and nasopharyngitis may also occur (Heffner & Schust 2006, Mitchell 2004).

## GENITAL HERPES SIMPLEX VIRUS (HSV)

Genital herpes is a lifelong disease, as HSV establishes a latent infection in the sacral dorsal root ganglia which can be reactivated when exposed to certain conditions, including fever, sun exposure and hormonal changes. There are two types of HSV (HPA 2010):

- Type 2 is almost exclusively associated with genital infections
- Type 1 causes oral herpes but has increasingly been implicated in genital infections.

About 55% of people with genital HSV are asymptomatic and may be unaware that viral shedding, which commonly persists for at least 8–10 years, may contribute significantly to genital HSV transmission (UK Collaborative Group for HIV and STI Surveillance 2007).

Of those who do experience symptoms after initial infection (*primary episode*), over 80% present with symptoms of mucocutaneous infection around the infection site, including painful penile or vulval lesions or blisters, dysuria, urethral or vaginal discharge, and painful inguinal adenopathy. Other symptoms include fever, headache, malaise, urinary retention and proctitis. Aseptic meningitis occurs in about 12–30% of patients. No HSV antibodies are detectable in a patient's serum during this acute phase, demonstrating that there has been no prior HSV infection. Others will present initially with symptoms suggesting the occurrence of genital HSV infection, which tends to be milder than a primary first episode, and HSV antibodies will be detectable in the patient's serum. This is referred to as a *non-primary episode*.

Following the primary episode, HSV virions travel to the dorsal root ganglia of the sacral plexus, where they remain in a non-replicative state until reactivation. *Recurrent episodes* of genital HSV-2 disease occur when the virus is reactivated. There is a dramatic increase in viral DNA synthesis and the virus spreads back down the sensory neurons to the skin. Affected people experience painful breakouts of penile or vulval and cervical lesions. The duration of symptoms and viral shedding is much shorter with recurrences.

Maternal primary HSV has been associated with spontaneous abortion, low birthweight, premature delivery and stillbirth (Mitchell 2004). Life-threatening neonatal herpectic infections may also occur as the baby becomes infected from the genital tract of the mother at delivery. The risk of MTCT varies and is dependent upon the likelihood of the virus being shed from the cervix (Heffner & Schust 2006) (Table 57.1). There is also an increased risk of MTCT among immunocompromised women, such as those infected with HIV (Chen et al 2005, Hitti et al 1997).

Women with a primary episode of genital herpes during pregnancy are offered treatment with aciclovir, and delivery by caesarean section is recommended for women with primary episode genital herpes lesions at the time of delivery, or within 6 weeks of the expected date of delivery, to prevent neonatal herpectic infection (RCOG 2007).

**Table 57.1 Risk of neonatal HSV infection**

| Clinical scenario | MTCT | Risk of cervical shedding among women |
|---|---|---|
| Primary episode of HSV-2 | 50% | 90% |
| Primary episode of HSV-1 | 50% | 70% |
| Non-primary episode of HSV-2 | | 70% |
| Recurrent episodes | 5% | 12–20% |

Heffner & Schust 2006

Babies with localized or disseminated neonatal infection are treated with intravenous antiviral therapy. However, even with effective treatment, 70% of babies with disseminated infection will die. Survivors have a high risk of neurological complications (Mitchell 2004).

## CHLAMYDIA

There is a high prevalence of genital chlamydia infection among young heterosexuals in the UK (UK Collaborative Group for HIV and STI Surveillance 2007). Infection with the bacterium, *Chlamydia trachomatis*, can cause mucopurulent vaginal discharge, bleeding between periods, painful micturition and lower abdominal pain in women. Untreated infection, which is likely because 70% of women are asymptomatic, may cause chronic pain, pelvic inflammatory disease, ectopic pregnancy and infertility (HPA 2008b).

Symptoms in men include discharge from the penis, burning and itching in the genital area, and painful micturition. Complications, which are rarer than in women, include epididymitis and Reiter's syndrome. As 50% of infected men are asymptomatic, they may unknowingly transmit infection to a female partner. Early diagnosis is beneficial in preventing complications and reducing the spread of infection. England's National Chlamydia Screening Programme enables many young people to access screening for chlamydia in a wide choice of settings, including general practice, contraception clinics and young people's sexual health clinics. Infected people are treated with antibiotics such as azithromycin or doxycycline (HPA 2008b).

MTCT of infection can occur as the fetus passes through the birth canal of a woman who has not received appropriate antibiotic treatment (doxycycline is contraindicated in pregnancy) prior to delivery, causing the baby to be born with conjunctivitis or pneumonia. However, both are treatable.

## TRICHOMONIASIS

Trichomoniasis, a very common STI, is caused by *Trichomonas vaginalis*, a flagellated protozoan. Infected women commonly experience vulval itching, dysuria and vaginal discharge, which may be frothy yellow and have an offensive odour; occasionally, women complain of low abdominal discomfort; however, 10–50% are asymptomatic. Men commonly present with urethral discharge and/or dysuria, urethral irritation and frequency of micturition, although 15–50% are asymptomatic (BASHH 2007).

It is unclear whether pregnant women with trichomoniasis are more likely to give birth prematurely, or have other pregnancy complications. Metronidazole, given as a single dose, is likely to cure trichomoniasis, but it is not known whether this treatment will have any effect on pregnancy outcomes (Gülmezoglu 2002).

## HUMAN PAPILLOMAVIRUS (HPV)

Genital HPV infections are extremely common, particularly in the first few years after onset of sexual activity. There are 40 types of HPV. Many types cause infections which are asymptomatic and resolve without causing disease. Others are oncogenic or 'high-risk' types that cause cervical cancer. High-risk HPV infections are also associated with cancer of the penis, vulva, vagina, anus, mouth and oropharynx. Those that do not cause cancer are termed 'low-risk' types. Two of the 'low-risk' types cause genital warts (HPA 2008c).

The National Health Service (NHS) Cervical Screening Programme aims to detect pre-cancerous lesions and cervical cancers at early asymptomatic stages when they can be successfully treated (Table 57.2).

To protect girls aged 12–13 years against infection with HPV 16 and 18 (associated with 70% of cervical cancers), HPV vaccination was introduced into the national immunization programme from September 2008, with a 2-year catch-up campaign offering vaccination to girls aged between 16 and 18 from autumn 2009, and to girls aged between 15 and 17 from autumn 2010 (HPA 2008c, NHS Screening Programmes 2008).

**Table 57.2 The NHS Cervical Screening Programme**

| Age group (years) | Frequency of screening |
|---|---|
| 25 | First invitation |
| 25–49 | 3-yearly |
| 50–64 | 5-yearly |
| 65+ | Only screen those who have not been screened since age 50 or have had recent abnormal tests |

## VAGINAL CANDIDIASIS

Vaginal candidiasis is caused by a yeast, *Candida albicans*, which often inhabits warm moist areas of the body such as the mouth, vagina, perineum and groin. More common in pregnancy or after the use of broad-spectrum antibiotics, infected women often have no symptoms, although some experience vaginal soreness and itching, a white curdy vaginal discharge and reddening of the labia. Midwives can reassure pregnant women that there is no evidence that this infection, commonly known as 'thrush', harms the unborn child.

Although candida may be sexually transmitted, recurrent infection is more likely to be a result of reinfection from the bowel. Women should be informed of preventive measures, including wiping from front to back and avoiding tight underwear (especially synthetics). In addition, women should be advised to avoid excessive washing, and use of bubble baths and perfumed soaps that may damage the vaginal natural protective flora (Young & Jewell 2001).

Topical imidazoles should be used for treating symptomatic vaginal candidiasis in pregnancy. A 4-day course will cure just over half of infections, whereas a 7-day course cures over 90% (Young & Jewell 2001).

## CONCLUSION

Significant increases in HIV prevalence in UK-born women giving birth between 2000 and 2006 occurred. Routine screening for HIV, introduced throughout the UK between 2000 and 2003, continues to be a highly successful public health intervention. Midwives have a key role in offering and recommending screening for HIV, HBV and syphilis during pregnancy, enabling infected women to benefit from interventions. This improves health outcomes for women and their families, reducing further spread of infection. Women should receive relevant information regarding issues surrounding testing to make an informed choice. Specially designed leaflets are useful, and midwives' roles are to ensure these are easily understood and different languages meet individual needs. Details of support groups may also benefit women who are diagnosed during pregnancy.

Midwives require appropriate knowledge, skills and attitudes when providing care in relation to sexually transmitted diseases in pregnancy. Effectively working within a multidisciplinary context ensures maximum benefit and minimum harm for all women and families.

**Reflective activity 57.3**

Design an information leaflet to be given to women for one STI. Include details of transmission, clinical presentation, pregnancy implications, management/advice and contact details of useful support groups/sources of further information.

**KEY POINTS**

- Midwives have an important role in screening and eliciting appropriate information and providing education.
- Midwives should respect women's autonomy by facilitating their ability to make important decisions, and ensure standards of confidentiality are maintained.

## REFERENCES


Antiretroviral Pregnancy Registry: Antiretroviral Pregnancy Registry International Interim Report for 1 January 1989–1931 January 2008 (website). www.apregistry.com/forms/exec-summary.pdf. 2008. Accessed July 14, 2008.

Bott JS: *HIV and midwifery practice*, London, 2005, MA Healthcare.

Bradley Hare C: Clinical overview of HIV disease (website). hivinsite.ucsf.edu/InSite?page=kb-03-01-01#S5X. 2006. Accessed July 9, 2008.

British Association of Sexual Health and HIV (BASHH): *United Kingdom national guideline on the management of Trichomonas vaginalis*, London, 2007, BASHH.

British HIV Association & Children's HIV Association: BHIVA and CHIVA guidelines for the management of HIV infection in pregnant women (website). www.bhiva.org/cms1221368.asp. 2008. Accessed July 14, 2008.

Brook Advisory Centres: Sexually transmitted infections (STIs) (website). www.brook.org.uk/content/M2_4_sti.asp. 2008. Accessed July 8, 2008.

BUPA (health information team): Sexually transmitted infections (website). hcd2.bupa.co.uk/fact_sheets/html/Sexually_transmitted_diseases.html. 2007. Accessed July 8, 2008.

BUPA (health information team): HIV/AIDS (website). hcd2.bupa.co.uk/fact_sheets/html/aids.html#5. 2008. Accessed July 12, 2008.

Campbell J: HIV and suicide: is there a relationship? *AIDS Care* 7(Suppl 2):S107–S108, 1995.

Chen KT, Segú M, Lumey LH, et al: New York City Perinatal AIDS Collaborative Transmission Study (PACTS) Group. Genital herpes simplex virus infection and perinatal transmission of human immunodeficiency virus, *Obstetrics and Gynaecology* 106(6):1341–1348, 2005.

Connor EM, Sperling RS, Gelber R, et al: Reduction of maternal–infant transmission of human immunodeficiency virus type 1 with zidovudine treatment, *New England Journal of Medicine* 331(18):1173–1180, 1994.

Department of Health (DH): HIV testing as part of your antenatal care: better for your baby (website). www.dh.gov.uk/en/Publicationsandstatistics/Publications/PublicationsPolicyAndGuidance/DH_4131234. 2000. Accessed November 27, 2008.

Department of Health (DH): *Screening for infectious diseases in pregnancy: standards to support the UK antenatal screening programme*, London, 2003, DH.

Department of Health (DH): *Hepatitis B: how to protect your baby*, London, 2007, DH.

Department of Health (DH) & Royal College of Midwives (RCM): *Information for midwives – hepatitis B testing in pregnancy. Helping women choose*, London, 2000, DH.

Downie RS, Calman KC: *Health respect – ethics in health care*, London, 1987, Faber & Faber.

Genc M, Ledger WJ: Syphilis in pregnancy, *Sexually Transmitted Infections* 76(2):73–79, 2000.

Giaquinto C, De Romeo A, Giacomet V, et al: Lactic acid levels in children perinatally treated with antiretroviral agents to prevent HIV transmission, *AIDS* 15(8):1074–1075, 2001.

Gibb DM, Duong T, Tookey PA, et al: Decline in mortality, AIDS, and hospital admissions in perinatally HIV-1 infected children in the United Kingdom and Ireland, *British Medical Journal* 327(7422):1019–1025, 2003.

Grosheide PM, Van Damme P: *Prevention and control of hepatitis B in the community*. Communicable Diseases Series 1:1–60. Antwerp, 1996, Viral Hepatitis Prevention Board Secretariat.

Gülmezoglu AM: Interventions for trichomoniasis in pregnancy, *Cochrane Database of Systematic Reviews* (3):CD000220, 2002.

Hadler S, Margolis H: Hepatitis B immunization: vaccine types, efficacy, and indications for immunization. In Remington J, Swart M, editors: *Current Clinical Topics in Infectious Diseases*, Boston, 1992, Blackwell Scientific.

Health Protection Agency (HPA): Gonorrhoea (website). www.hpa.org.uk/webw/HPAweb&Page&HPAwebAutoListName/Page/1191942171519?p=1191942171519#what. 2008a. Accessed September 10, 2008.

Health Protection Agency (HPA): Genital chlamydia (website). www.hpa.org.uk/webw/HPAweb&Page&HPAwebAutoListName/Page/1191942172070?p=1191942172070. 2008b. Accessed September 12, 2008.

Health Protection Agency (HPA): Human papillomavirus (HPV) – cervical cancer and genital warts (website). www.hpa.org.uk/webw/HPAweb&Page&HPAwebAutoListName/Page/1191942128136?p=1191942128136. 2008c. Accessed September 16, 2008.

Health Protection Agency (HPA): Genital herpes (website). www.hpa.org.uk/Topics/InfectiousDiseases/InfectionsAZ/GenitalHerpes/GeneralInformation/#what. Accessed July 21, 2010.

Heffner LJ, Schust DJ: *The reproductive system at a glance*, Oxford, 2006, Blackwell.

Hitti J, Watts DH, Burchett SK, et al: Herpes simplex virus seropositivity and reactivation at delivery among pregnant women infected with human immunodeficiency virus-1, *American Journal of Obstetrics and Gynecology* 177(2):450–454, 1997.

i-base: A guide to HIV, pregnancy & women's health (website). www.i-base.info/guides/pregnancy/Introduction.html#changes. 2007. Accessed July 14, 2008.

Le Chenadec J, Mayaux MJ, Guihenneuc-Jouyaux C, et al: Perinatal antiretroviral treatment and hematopoiesis in HIV uninfected infants, *AIDS* 17(14):2053–2061, 2003.

Lester P, Partridge JC, Chesney MA, et al: The consequences of a positive prenatal HIV antibody test for women, *Journal of Acquired Immunodeficiency Syndrome* 10(3):341–349, 1995.

McIntyre JA: Sex, pregnancy, hormones and HIV, *The Lancet* 366(9492):1141–1142, 2005.

Mitchell H: Sexually transmitted infections in pregnancy. In Adler M, Cowan F, French P, et al, editors: *ABC of sexually transmitted infections*, London, 2004, BMJ Books, pp 34–38.

Moses SE, Tosswill J, Sudhanva M, et al: HIV-1 seroconversion during pregnancy resulting in vertical transmission, *Journal of Clinical Virology* 41(2):152–153, 2008.

NHS Screening Programmes: NHS Cervical Screening Programme (website). www.cancerscreening.nhs.uk/cervical/#future. 2008. Accessed September 16, 2008.

Nursing and Midwifery Council (NMC): The code. Standards of conduct, performance and ethics for nurses and midwives (website). www.nmc-uk.org/aFrameDisplay.aspx?DocumentID=3954. 2008. Accessed November 27, 2008.

Olivero OA, Anderson LM, Diwan BA, et al: Transplacental effects of 39-azido-29, 39-dideoxythymidine (AZT): tumorigenicity in mice and genotoxicity in mice and monkeys, *Journal of the National Cancer Institute* 89(21):1602–1608, 1997.

Pillay K, Coutsoudis A, York D, et al: Cell-free virus in breast milk of HIV-1-seropositive women, *Journal of Acquired Immune Deficiency Syndromes* 24:330–336, 2000.

Pratt RJ: *HIV and AIDS: a foundation for nursing and healthcare practice*, ed 5, London, 2003, Arnold.

Rousseau CM, Nduati RW, Richardson BA, et al: Longitudinal analysis of human immunodeficiency virus type 1 RNA in breast milk and of its relationship to infant infection and maternal disease, *Journal of Infectious Diseases* 87(5):741–747, 2003.

Royal College of Obstetrics and Gynaecology (RCOG): *HIV infection in maternity care. Working Party report*, London, 1997, RCOG.

Royal College of Obstetrics and Gynaecology (RCOG): Management of HIV in pregnancy. RCOG Guideline No. 39 (website). www.rcog.org.uk/resources/Public/pdf/RCOG_Guideline_39_low.pdf. 2004. Accessed July 9, 2008.

Royal College of Obstetrics and Gynaecology (RCOG): Green-top Guideline No. 30. *Management of genital herpes in pregnancy* (website). www.rcog.org.uk/resources/Public/pdf/greentop30_genital_herpes0907.pdf. 2007. Accessed September 12, 2008.

Sira J: Hepatitis: exploding the myths, *Primary Health Care* 8(3):31–38, 1998.

Stevens PE, Tighe DB: Trauma of discovery: women's narratives of being informed they are HIV infected, *Aids Care* 9(5):523–538, 1997.

Townsend CL, Cortina-Borja M, Peckham KS, et al: Low rates of mother-to-child transmission of HIV following effective pregnancy interventions in the United Kingdom and Ireland, 2002–2006, *AIDS* 22(8):973–981, 2008.

Tymstra T, Bieleman B: The psychological impact of mass screening for cardiovascular risk factors, *Family Practice* 4(4):287–290, 1987.

UK Chief Medical Officers' Expert Advisory Group on AIDS: *HIV and infant feeding: guidance from the UK Chief Medical Officers' Expert Advisory Group on AIDS*, London, 2004, DH.

UK Collaborative Group for HIV and STI Surveillance: *Testing times. HIV and other sexually transmitted infections in the United Kingdom: 2007*, London, 2007, Health Protection Agency, Centre for Infections.

Wright TL, Lau JYN: Clinical aspects of hepatitis B virus infection, *The Lancet* 342(8883):1340–1344, 1993.

Young GL, Jewell D: Topical treatment for vaginal candidiasis (thrush) in pregnancy, *Cochrane Database of Systematic Reviews* (4):CD000225, 2001.

Chapter |58|

# Abnormalities of the genital tract

*Patricia Lindsay*

## LEARNING OUTCOMES

After reading this chapter, you will be able to:

- identify the major anomalies of the female genital tract and discuss their origin
- discuss their impact on fertility, pregnancy, labour and the puerperium
- discuss three main types of uterine displacement and their impact on labour
- discuss the implications of female genital mutilation
- identify the role of the midwife in the care of a woman with a genital tract anomaly.

## INTRODUCTION

The true incidence of reproductive tract anomalies is uncertain and their role in reproductive difficulties is unclear (Saravelos et al 2008, Shulman 2008). While structural abnormalities of the uterus are particularly likely to cause problems, pregnancy and labour may also be affected by other conditions such as fibroids or uterine displacements. Female genital mutilation (also known as female circumcision) presents clear health risks for mother and baby. The midwife must be able to give appropriate and safe care for any woman presenting with a genital tract anomaly.

## DEVELOPMENTAL ANOMALIES

Most of the female genital tract arises from the müllerian ducts (see Ch. 29), which form during embryonic life and which fuse by the 12th week after fertilization. The median septum then breaks down, thus forming a single uterus (Laufer et al 2005). Should this process fail, abnormalities such as *double uterus* (with or without a double cervix and vagina), *bicornuate uterus* or *subseptate uterus* will occur (Fig. 58.1). As the müllerian ducts and wolffian ducts (see Ch. 29) develop close together, genital tract anomalies may be accompanied by malformations of the kidney and ureters. Care should include assessment of the urinary system (Laufer et al 2005).

### Diethylstilbestrol (DES)

This synthetic non-steroidal oestrogen was used for approximately 30 years to treat conditions such as recurrent pregnancy loss and threatened abortion. It is still sometimes used as a form of postcoital contraception (Mackay Hart & Norman 2008). Girls who have been exposed to DES in utero have an unusually high incidence of uncommon anomalies. These include an increased incidence of:

- cervical anomalies
- uterine malformations such as hypoplastic and T-shaped uteri
- cervical cancer.

Reproductive function is impaired. Conception may be difficult; ectopic pregnancy and preterm birth are commoner (RCOG 2002).

### Unicornuate uterus

This uncommon abnormality arises from failure of development of one of the müllerian ducts. There is a higher rate of spontaneous abortion, breech presentation, fetal growth restriction and preterm labour, possibly due to the limited space in the uterine cavity (Akar et al 2005).

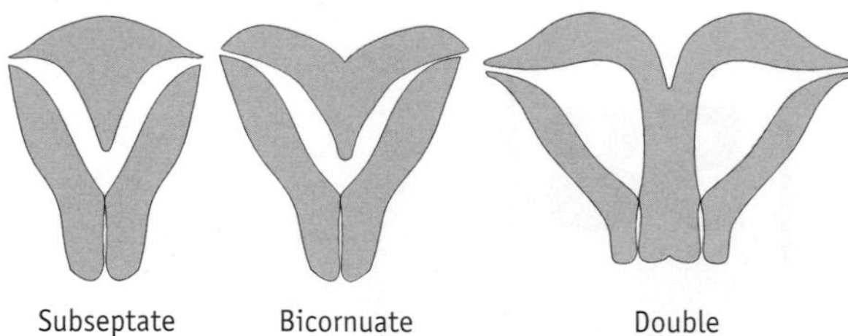

**Figure 58.1** Uterine malformations.

Caesarean delivery is therefore more likely. If the pregnancy develops in a rudimentary horn, the outcome is usually spontaneous abortion or occasionally rupture of the rudimentary horn, as the myometrium becomes rapidly stretched.

## Double uterus (uterus didelphys)

This may be accompanied by a double vagina or a longitudinal vaginal septum. As the pregnancy progresses, the midwife will notice that the fundus is abnormal in shape and may feel unusually wide. Breech presentation is common. As the pregnancy continues, the non-pregnant uterus will enlarge under the influence of the pregnancy hormones and may occupy space in the pelvis, thus obstructing labour. Twin pregnancy (one fetus in each horn) has been recorded (Ahmad et al 2000).

## Subseptate and bicornuate uterus

This occurs when complete obliteration of the müllerian septum fails. A subseptate uterus is outwardly normal, but the midwife may recognize a bicornuate uterus, which has a wide, heart-shaped fundus. This can be detected on abdominal examination and may be visible under the abdominal wall in a slim woman, especially after the third stage of labour. These anomalies do not usually cause difficulties in conception or in early pregnancy. However, they are associated with transverse lie and breech presentation, as the abnormal uterine structure hinders the normal process of spontaneous version between 30 and 34 weeks' gestation. Attempts at external cephalic version of the fetus will be unsuccessful.

The midwife should consider the possibility of structural abnormality of the uterus in any woman with a history of recurrent malpresentation. The progress of the first and second stage of labour is usually normal where there is a subseptate or bicornuate uterus. However, retained placenta may occur in the third stage.

## Vaginal septum

A vaginal septum (Fig. 58.2) may be longitudinal or transverse, complete or partial. It may be detected on vaginal examination, but, as the tissue is usually soft and is easily deflected by the examining fingers, the diagnosis is often overlooked. A vaginal septum may obstruct fetal descent during labour (Heinonen 2000).

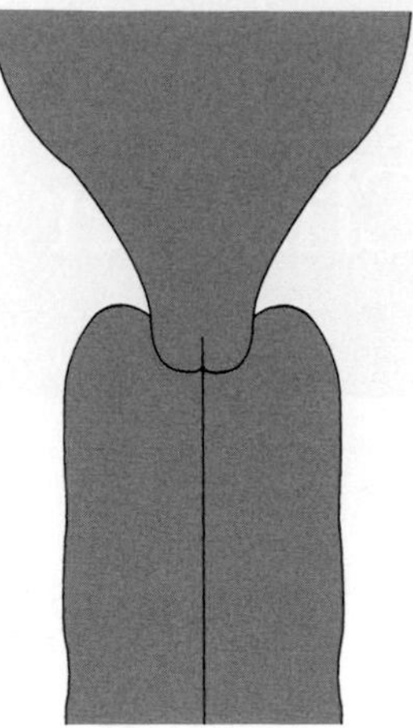
**Figure 58.2** Longitudinal vaginal septum.

## Associated problems

The presence of a uterine malformation is associated with an increased risk of recurrent spontaneous miscarriage and preterm birth (Mackay Hart & Norman 2008, Woelfer et al 2001).

The midwife should refer the woman to an obstetrician so that appropriate care may be planned as there is a higher likelihood of the need for intervention during labour.

**Reflective activity 58.1**

Think about the potential needs of a woman with a double uterus. What factors would you discuss with her? What would you include in her care plan?

# DISPLACEMENTS OF THE UTERUS

## Retroversion of the gravid uterus

Retroversion of the uterus, where the pregnant uterus falls back into the hollow of the sacrum (Fig. 58.3), is normally of little clinical significance (Mackay Hart & Norman 2008). During pregnancy, the condition usually resolves spontaneously as the uterus grows and rises into the abdomen around the 12th week (Mukhopadhyay & Arulkumaran 2004).

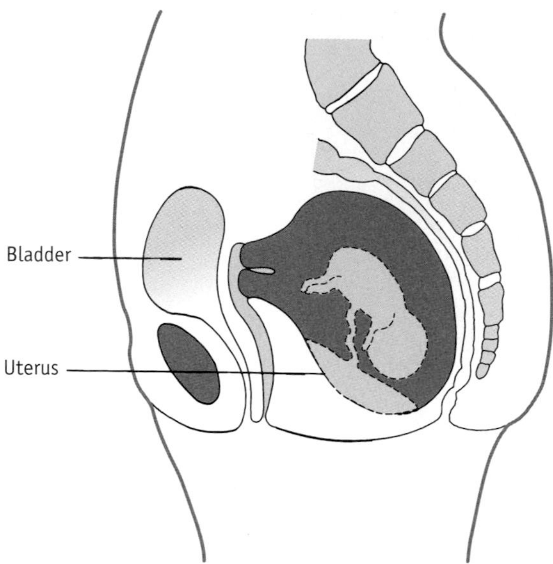


Figure 58.3 Incarceration of the gravid uterus.

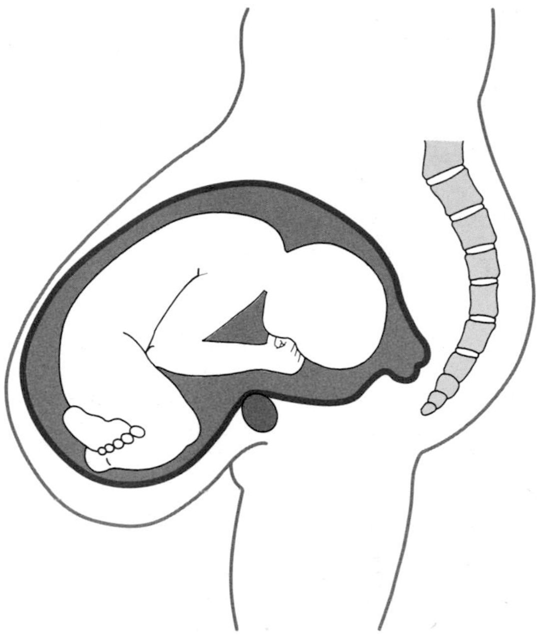

Figure 58.4 Pendulous abdomen.

However, rarely, the retroversion fails to resolve and the uterus becomes fixed or incarcerated in the pelvis. Between the 12th and 16th week of pregnancy the retroverted pregnant uterus fills the pelvis and the cervix is drawn up towards the pelvic brim. The anterior vaginal wall and the urethra become stretched, the urethra narrows and the mother is unable to pass urine.

## Diagnosis

The woman will initially complain of pelvic pressure and difficulty in micturition and later of complete inability to pass urine. The bladder becomes more distended and, if unrelieved, overflow incontinence will occur.

The woman will experience severe abdominal pain. On abdominal examination there is a soft swelling (the bladder) above the pubes, which may extend to the umbilicus and may be mistaken for the uterus. The fundus is not palpable at the brim of the pelvis. A pelvic ultrasound scan will assist the diagnosis (Mukhopadhyay & Arulkumaran 2004).

## Treatment

The bladder is emptied with an indwelling catheter and is then kept empty until bladder tone returns. Once the bladder is empty, the uterus usually corrects its malposition spontaneously. This may be assisted if the mother lies in the semi-prone or Sims position (see Ch. 61). The retroversion will not recur, since the uterus will, in a few days, be too big to fall back into the pelvis. Persistent retroversion has been reported but is rare (Hamoda et al 2002).

## Dangers

- *Urinary tract infection,* owing to stasis of urine in the overdistended bladder. A catheter specimen of urine should be sent for microscopy, and any infection must be treated promptly.
- *Sloughing of the bladder* and rupture may occur.
- *Spontaneous abortion.*
- *Persistent incarceration,* which may cause sacculation of the anterior uterine wall. The pregnancy will then enlarge into the abdomen and this may confuse the diagnosis. Delivery will be by caesarean section.

# Anteversion of the gravid uterus (pendulous abdomen)

This rare condition (Fig. 58.4) may occur in multiparous women whose abdominal muscles have been weakened by repeated pregnancies or those who have a midline abdominal wall hernia, possibly associated with an old scar (Saha et al 2006). Separation of the rectus abdominis muscle allows the uterus to fall forward and in extreme cases the fundus may lie below the symphysis pubis. As the uterus becomes heavier, the woman experiences backache and abdominal pain. The presenting part will not engage and dystocia is likely because the long axis of the uterus is at an angle to the pelvic brim. An abdominal binder may bring relief (Saha et al 2006). This should be worn during labour to facilitate engagement and descent of the fetus. The 'all-fours' delivery position should be avoided.

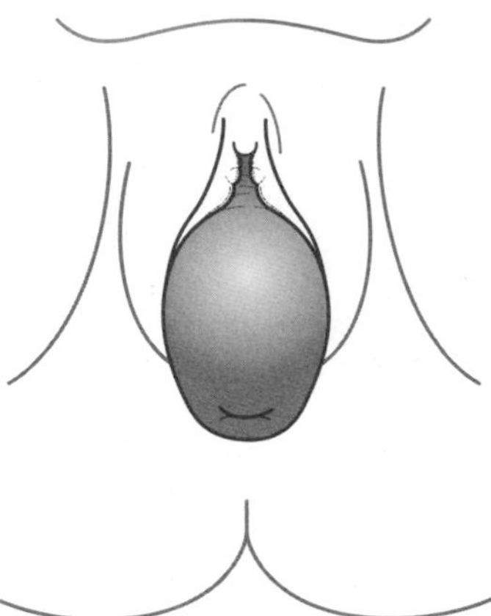

Figure 58.5 Complete uterine prolapse (uterine procidentia), non-pregnant uterus.

## Prolapse of the gravid uterus

Uterine prolapse is rare in pregnancy (Fig. 58.5). Laxness of the uterovaginal supports allows the uterus to descend so that the cervix is found at or just behind the vaginal introitus. The condition is most troublesome in the first trimester of pregnancy as the uterus increases in size and weight and the ligaments soften and relax. A ring pessary may relieve the prolapse. As the uterus grows into the abdomen, the condition improves, although it may recur in late pregnancy. Caesarean section may be recommended to prevent further damage to the uterovaginal supports (Mukhopadhyay & Arulkumaran 2004).

**Reflective activity 58.2**

What information and advice would you give a woman who (at 8 weeks' gestation) has been told that she has a retroverted uterus?

# PELVIC MASSES

## Fibromyomata (fibroids)

Fibroids are the commonest pelvic tumours, occurring in up to 30% of women of childbearing age (Cooper & Okolo 2005). They are commoner in older women and in young West Indian and West African women. The presence of fibroids (leiomyomas) increases the risk of complications such as threatened abortion, antepartum haemorrhage, breech presentation and caesarean birth (Mukhopadhyay & Arulkumaran 2004).

On uterine palpation, one or more swellings may be felt, continuous with the uterine wall (Fig. 58.6). A large fibroid may be mistaken for the fetal head. In pregnancy, hypertrophy of the myometrial fibres and increased vascularity and oedema cause the fibroid to enlarge and soften.

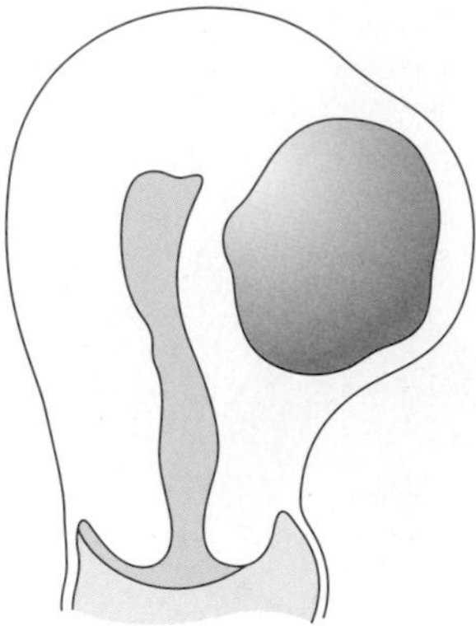

Figure 58.6 Uterine fibroid.

*Red degeneration of a fibroid* (see website) may cause acute pain and vomiting in pregnancy and torsion of a pedunculated fibroid (see website) may require myomectomy (Cunningham et al 2005). Most fibroids are found in the body of the uterus and do not affect the course of labour. Rarely, one may occur in the lower segment beneath the presenting part. This will prevent fetal descent into the pelvis and may obstruct labour. During the third stage of labour, postpartum haemorrhage may occur (Mukhopadhyay & Arulkumaran 2004).

Pregnancy complicated by fibroids is considered high risk and the labour and birth should take place in hospital in case difficulty should arise. During the puerperium, fibroids regress and become smaller as autolysis reduces the myometrial mass (Mukhopadhyay & Arulkumaran 2004).

The midwife should be aware of any woman who has a history of treatment for fibroids prior to pregnancy. Myomectomy involves incisions on the uterus and this may pose a risk of scar rupture in future pregnancy (Hockstein 2000). Selective embolization of fibroids is often the preferred treatment and the risks to future fertility are believed to be small (McLucas et al 2001).

## Ovarian cyst

Sonographically detectable adnexal masses occur in up to 6% of fertile women (Bayar et al 2005). Corpus luteum cysts are common in the first trimester and usually regress spontaneously. A 12-year retrospective study found a 13% malignancy rate in ovarian cysts (Sherard et al 2003).

The cyst may be in the abdomen or in the pelvis (Fig. 58.7). There is a risk of malignancy or torsion, the risk of malignancy rising with increasing age. Torsion is most likely during the second trimester or in the puerperium (Mukhopadhyay & Arulkumaran 2004). Simple non-malignant cysts can be successfully aspirated during pregnancy, although conservative management is also an option (Caspi et al 2000, Zanetta et al 2003).

## FEMALE GENITAL MUTILATION (FEMALE GENITAL CUTTING, FEMALE CIRCUMCISION)

Female genital mutilation (FGM) is the removal of all or part of the external female genitalia for non-medical reasons (WHO 2008). The custom still persists among some groups, particularly those from Nigeria, Ethiopia, the Sudan and Egypt. It is a cultural requirement and may be a rite of passage into adult status within the community. It is usually performed before the age of 15 (WHO 2008).

The World Health Organization (2008) classifies FGM as follows:

- *type 1: clitoridectomy* – partial or total removal of the clitoris and/or the prepuce (Fig. 58.8)
- *type 2: partial or total excision of the clitoris and labia minora* with or without excision of the labia majora (Fig. 58.8)
- *type 3: infibulation* – narrowing of the vaginal opening, excision of part or all of the external genitalia and stitching/narrowing of the vaginal opening (*also called pharaonic circumcision*) (Figs 58.8 and 58.9)
- *type 4: any other harmful procedure carried out for non-medical reasons*. This includes pricking, piercing, scraping, incising or cautery of the female genitalia.

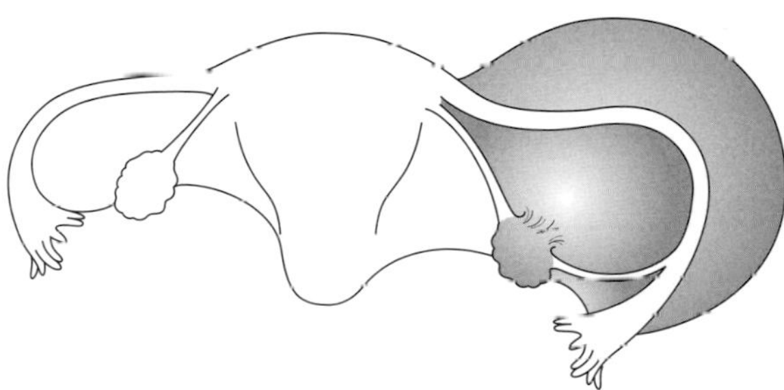

Figure 58.7 A uterus with a simple serous cyst.

Female genital mutilation is illegal in the UK and many other countries and is considered to be a violation of human rights (WHO 2008). It carries a significant immediate mortality from haemorrhage and sepsis. Lifelong morbidity from urinary infection, pelvic inflammatory disease, endometriosis and renal damage may follow.

Infibulation presents particular problems in childbearing. In pregnancy, urinary tract infection is more likely. The rates of caesarean section, postpartum haemorrhage and perinatal death are increased in women who have undergone FGM (WHO 2006). When attending the woman in childbirth, the midwife must be prepared to perform an anterior episiotomy, separating the labial remnants (Fig. 58.10), and the perineum must be meticulously repaired. Repair of the labia in such a way as to restore the infibulated state is illegal (RCOG 2003).

If the infant is a girl, the midwife must be aware that the family may wish to have the child circumcised. Under the terms of the Female Genital Mutilation Act 2004 it is now illegal to have this carried out abroad under the principle of 'extra-territoriality' (see website) (Kwateng-Kluvitse 2005). Midwives should initiate their local Child Protection process if they feel that a female child is at risk.

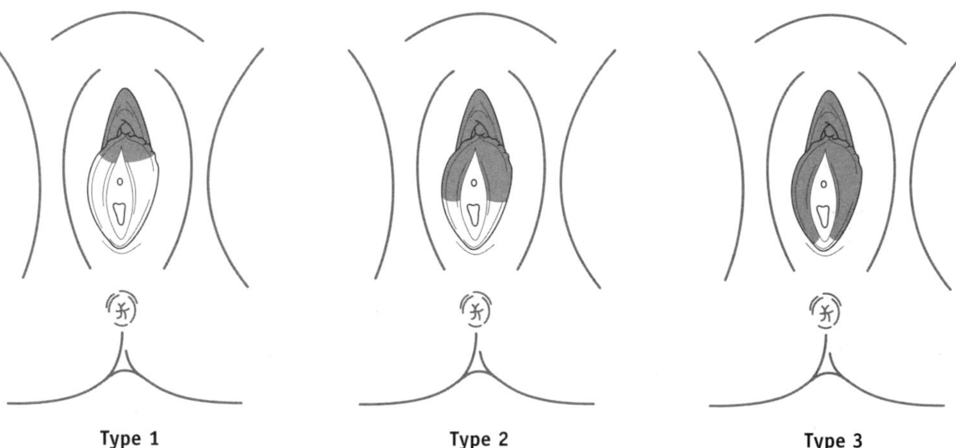


Figure 58.8 Types of surgery.

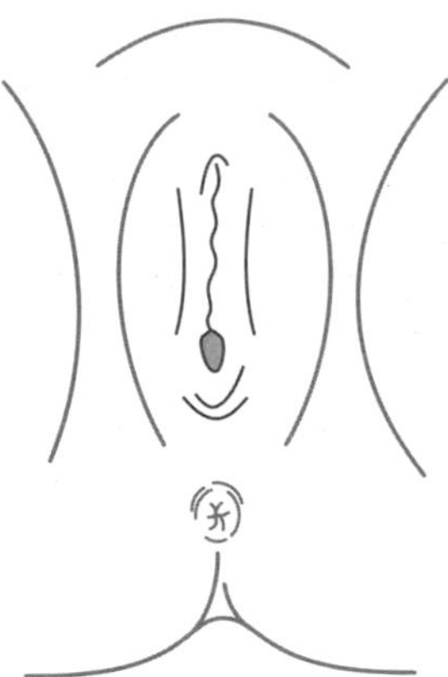

**Figure 58.9** Appearance after healing of type 3 (infibulation).

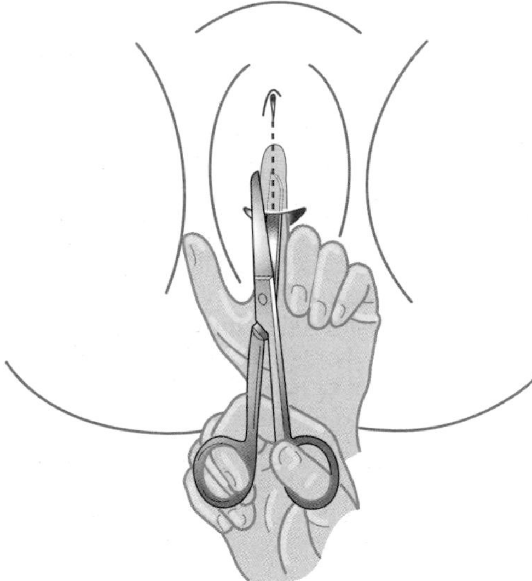

**Figure 58.10** Direction of anterior episiotomy for type 3 (infibulation).

At booking, the midwife should ascertain whether the woman has undergone genital mutilation. The words used should reflect the midwife's attitude and approach, which must be well informed, non-judgmental and sensitive. Good communication is essential. If the woman and the midwife do not speak the same language, an interpreter must be found – this should *not* be a family member. A careful history must be taken; details of any previous births must be recorded, including any surgical interventions required, the condition of the infant and the woman's health since the birth. A physical examination should be carried out, with consent. Minor degrees of genital mutilation will probably require no special attention, apart from ascertaining the woman's wishes regarding her labour and delivery care.

Infibulation, however, may present problems. Detailed information about previous pregnancies and births will help to inform the current management. The woman's beliefs and knowledge about the impact of her surgery on childbirth must be assessed. Her wishes for this pregnancy and birth should be discussed, but the midwife must make it clear that re-infibulation following the birth is not permitted by law. The possibility of the need for episiotomy should be raised. Advice regarding hygiene in pregnancy is essential, especially the need to reduce the risk of urinary tract infection.

De-infibulation services should be available to women who request it. Ideally, this procedure should be performed before pregnancy, or around 20 weeks' gestation (RCOG 2003). The midwife should refer the woman to an obstetrician. In all her communication, the midwife must be aware of the social implications of her advice and actions.

The Foundation for Women's Health, Research and Development (FORWARD) website contains information on FGM, including potential sequelae such as obstetric fistula formation.

**Reflective activity 58.3**

Find and read your unit policy for the care of a woman with type 3 genital mutilation. If there is no policy, how would you get one written? What issues would you include?

## CONCLUSION: IMPLICATIONS OF GENITAL TRACT ANOMALIES FOR MIDWIFERY PRACTICE

The true incidence of genital tract anomaly is unknown. The diagnosis may be made only following investigations for reproductive problems, such as recurrent pregnancy loss, pain or infertility.

A thorough but tactful history must be taken, with attention to privacy during the consultation. The midwife should assess the woman's general health and enquire about the information and advice which may have been given by other health professionals. Lower abdominal or periumbilical scars suggest gynaecological surgery and the midwife should enquire about the procedure. If there is a history of reproductive problems or gynaecological surgery, the woman should be referred to an obstetrician for an opinion on management of the pregnancy and labour.

Psychological support is essential. The midwife must be sensitive in ascertaining the history and giving advice and care during pregnancy. Working in partnership with the woman may ameliorate some of the psychological impact by focusing on normality, as far as is compatible with safety. Anxiety may be reduced and feelings of control and satisfaction enhanced if the woman is an informed and equal partner.

The midwife may be the first healthcare practitioner that the woman comes into contact with, and may pave the way not just for this pregnancy, but for interactions with other practitioners within the health services. A sensitive, respectful and caring approach ensures that the woman's experience of healthcare is positive, and will also contribute to the health of the woman, her baby and family.

## KEY POINTS

- The true incidence of anomalies is unknown but may have significant implications for fertility and childbearing.
- Midwives must be able to identify women at risk of related problems and implement appropriate care.
- Midwives should be aware of different cultural practices in their own practice areas, and be knowledgeable about the impact of such practices on the reproductive health of the woman and on her baby.
- The legal and ethical difficulties which may present in this area must be considered, whilst maintaining respect and sensitivity for the views and beliefs of others.

## REFERENCES


Ahmad F, Sherman S, Hagglund K: Twin gestation in a woman with a uterus didelphys. A case report, *Journal Of Reproductive Medicine* 45(4):357–359, 2000.

Akar M, Bayar D, Yildiz S, et al: Reproductive outcome of women with a unicornuate uterus, *Australian and New Zealand Journal of Obstetrics and Gynaecology* 45(2):148–150, 2005.

Bayar Ü, Barat A, Ayoğlu F: Diagnosis and management of simple ovarian cysts, *International Journal of Gynecology & Obstetrics* 91(2):187–188, 2005.

Caspi B, Ben-Arie A, Appelman Z, et al: Aspiration of simple pelvic cysts during pregnancy, *Gynecological and Obstetric Investigations* 49(2):102–105, 2000.

Cooper N, Okolo S: Fibroids in pregnancy – common but poorly understood, *Obstetrical & Gynecological Survey* 60(2):132–138, 2005.

Cunningham F, Leveno K, Bloom S, et al: *Williams obstetrics*, ed 22, London, 2005, McGraw-Hill.

Foundation for Women's Health, Research and Development (FORWARD): Female genital mutilation (website). www.forwarduk.org.uk/key-issues/fgm. Accessed January 19, 2009.

Hamoda H, Chamberlain P, Moore N, et al: Conservative treatment of incarcerated gravid uterus, *British Journal of Obstetrics & Gynaecology* 109(9):1074–1075, 2002.

Heinonen P: Clinical implications of the didelphic uterus: long term follow up of 49 cases, *European Journal of Obstetrics & Gynecology* 91(2):183–190, 2000.

Hockstein S: Spontaneous uterine rupture in the early third trimester after laparoscopically assisted myomectomy, *Journal of Reproductive Medicine* 45(2):139–141, 2000.

Kwateng-Kluvitse A: Female genital mutilation and child protection In Momoh C, editor: *Female genital mutilation*, Oxford, 2005, Radcliffe.

Laufer M, Goldstein D, Hendren W: Structural abnormalities of the female reproductive tract. In Emans S, Laufer M, Goldstein D, editors: *Pediatric and adolescent gynecology*, ed 5, London, 2005, Lippincott, Williams & Wilkins.

Mackay Hart D, Norman J: *Gynaecology illustrated*, ed 5, London, 2008, Churchill Livingstone.

McLucas B, Adler L , Perrella R: Uterine fibroid embolization: non-surgical treatment for symptomatic fibroids, *Journal of the American College of Surgeons* 192(1):95–105, 2001.

Mukhopadhyay S, Arulkumaran S: Gynecological disorders in pregnancy. In Arulkumaran S, Sivanesaratnam V, Chatterjee A, et al, editors: *Essentials of obstetrics*, Tunbridge Wells, 2004, Anshan.

Royal College of Obstetricians and Gynaecologists (RCOG): *Fetal and maternal risks of diethylstilboestrol exposure in pregnancy*, London, 2002, RCOG.

Royal College of Obstetricians and Gynaecologists (RCOG): *Female genital mutilation*, London, 2003, RCOG.

Saha P, Rohilla M, Prasad GR, et al: Herniation of gravid uterus: report of 2 cases and review of literature, *MedGenMed. Medscape General Medicine* 8(4):14, 2006.

Saravelos S, Cocksedge K, Li T-C: Prevalence and diagnosis of congenital uterine anomalies in women with reproductive failure: a critical appraisal, *Human Reproduction Update* 14(5):415–429, 2008.

Sherard G, Hodson C, Williams H, et al: Adnexal masses and pregnancy: a 12-year experience, *American Journal of Obstetrics & Gynecology* 189(2):358–362, 2003.

Shulman L: Müllerian anomalies, *Clinical Obstetrics and Gynecology* 51(1):214–222, 2008.

Woelfer B, Salim R, Banerjee S, et al: Reproductive outcomes in women with congenital uterine anomalies detected by three-dimensional ultrasound screening, *Obstetrics and Gynecology* 98(6):1099–1103, 2001.

World Health Organization (WHO): Female genital mutilation and obstetric outcome: WHO collaborative prospective study in six African countries, *The Lancet* 367(9525):1835–1841, 2006.

World Health Organization (WHO): *Eliminating female genital mutilation: an inter-agency statement*, Geneva, 2008, WHO.

Zanetta G, Mariani E, Lissoni A, et al: A prospective study of the role of ultrasound in the management of adnexal masses in pregnancy, *British Journal of Obstetrics and Gynaecology* 110(6):578–583, 2003.

Chapter |59|

# Multiple pregnancy

*Jane Denton and Margie Davies*

## LEARNING OUTCOMES

After reading this chapter, you will be aware of the following:

- the incidence of multiple births
- how twins arise and the importance of determination of chorionicity and zygosity
- additional information and support required to prepare women to care for two or more babies
- risks and complications associated with twin births
- how to support and care for bereaved parents.

## THE INCIDENCE OF MULTIPLE BIRTHS

The incidence of multiple births continues to rise, mainly because of the increased availability of treatments for infertility (Kurinczuk 2006). A decline in the 1970s was followed by a rise from the early 1980s onwards (Fig. 59.1) (MacFarlane & Mugford 2000). In the UK, the multiple birth rate in 2008 was 15.48 per thousand maternities (Fig. 59.2). A total of 11,573 sets of twins and 149 sets of triplets were born (Fig. 59.3).

Multiple pregnancies carry higher risks for the mothers and babies, and can impose a greater burden practically, financially and emotionally on the parents (Botting et al 1990) and also on neonatal services (Collins & Graves 2000).

The rate of conception of multiple pregnancies is almost certainly higher than the recorded data suggest. Early ultrasound scans have shown that although there may be two or more fetal sacs in the first few weeks, some fetuses may die during the first trimester. This is described as 'the vanishing twin syndrome' (Landy & Nies 1995). If a multiple birth occurs before 24 weeks' gestation and includes both live births and dead fetuses, the fetal deaths are not registerable.

If a dead fetus is delivered with a live birth after 24 weeks' gestation, it should be registered as a stillbirth even if death occurred much earlier in the pregnancy (MacFarlane & Mugford 2000).

## FACTS ABOUT MULTIPLES

### How twins arise

There are two types of twins: monozygotic and dizygotic.

- *Monozygotic* ('identical', MZ, monozygous, uniovular) twins arise when a fertilized egg (zygote) divides into two identical halves during the first 14 days after fertilization. They will have the same genetic make-up and will therefore be of the same sex, apart from the rare case of an XO/XY chromosomal anomaly (Perlman et al 1990).
- *Dizygotic* ('non-identical', DZ, dizygous, fraternal or binovular) twins result from the fertilization of two separate ova (eggs) by two separate sperm. They may be of the same or of different sex and are no more genetically alike than any other siblings.

### Causes of twinning

The cause of monozygotic twinning is unknown, but recent reports suggest that slightly more are born after the use of drugs to stimulate ovulation and assisted conception procedures. The incidence of MZ twins throughout

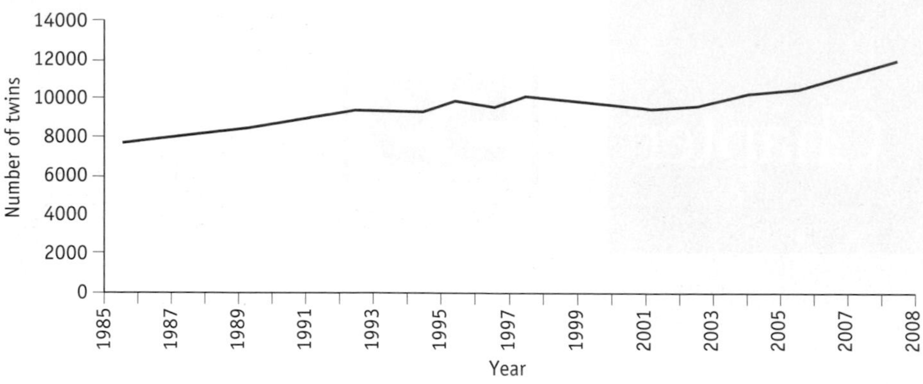


**Figure 59.1** Twinning rate in UK 1985–2008. *(Source: ONS London, GRO Northern Ireland and GRO Scotland.)*

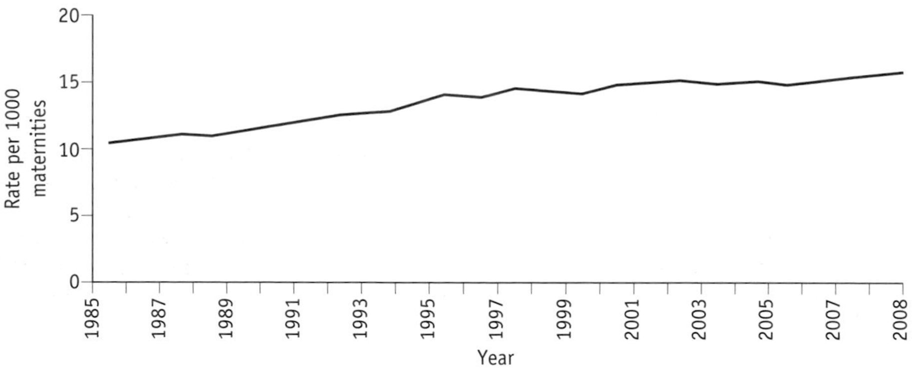


**Figure 59.2** Multiple births in England and Wales, 1985–2008. *(Source: ONS, Birth Statistics, Series FM1.)*

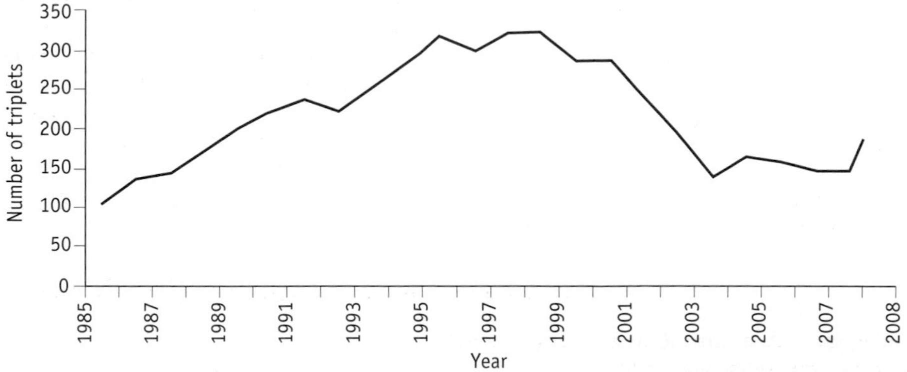


**Figure 59.3** Triplet and higher-order births in England and Wales, 1985–2008. *(Source: ONS.)*

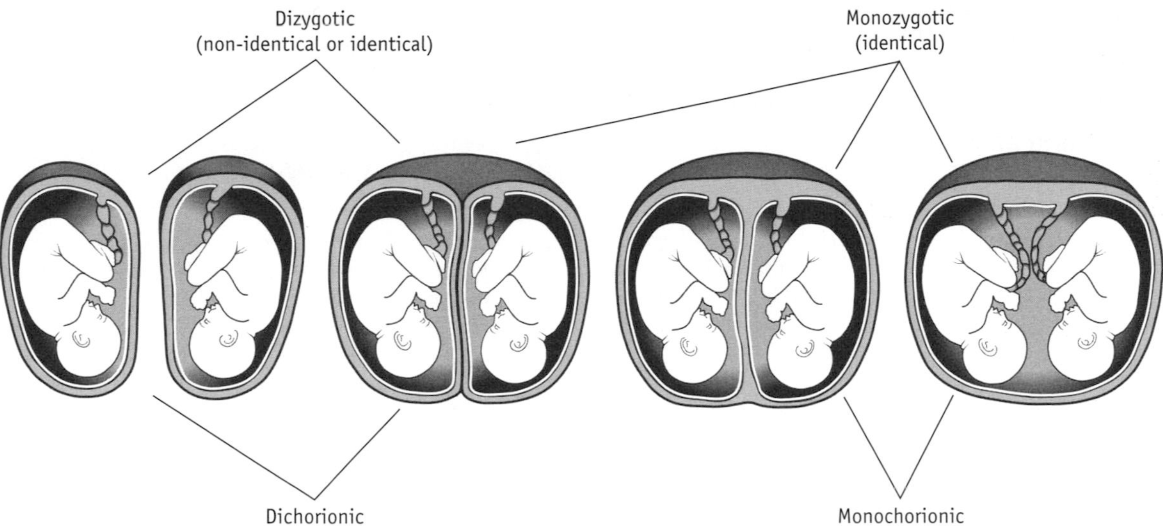


**Figure 59.4** The relationship between zygosity and chorionicity.

the world was approximately 3.5–4 per 1000 until the recent slight rise which may be associated with fertility treatments (Derom et al 2001).

Dizygotic twinning is different as there are several known associated factors (Chitayat & Hall 2006): maternal age, parity, race, maternal height and weight, and infertility treatments.

## DETERMINATION OF ZYGOSITY

Zygosity determination means finding out whether or not twins, triplets or more are monozygotic (identical). Midwives should understand the importance of this for the clinical care of the mothers and babies, so that it is not incorrectly assumed that, if the babies are the same sex and dichoronic, they are necessarily dizygotic (non-identical) (see placentation above). Accurate information about zygosity and how it can be determined should be provided as soon as a multiple pregnancy is diagnosed.

### Placentation

There can be two separate placentas (dichorionic) or a single placenta (monochorionic), which can sometimes be fused (dichorionic) (Fig. 59.4). All dizygous twins have dichorionic (two chorions) and diamniotic (two amnions) placentas (DCDA).

About one-third of monozygous twins also have DCDA placentas; this arises if the embryo divides within the first 3 or 4 days after fertilization, before implanting in the uterus. In about two-thirds of cases, the division occurs between 4 and 8 days and this placenta will be monochorionic diamniotic (MCDA). Monoamniotic twins (MCMA) occur in about 1% of cases and arise when the embryo divides later, between 9 and 12 days.

Despite the now well-established facts about placentation and zygosity, many parents are still told incorrectly that if same-sex twins are dichorionic they must be non-identical.

### Importance of chorionicity

When a twin pregnancy is diagnosed on ultrasound scan, an assessment of the chorionicity should be made (preferably during the first trimester) by measuring the thickness of the dividing membranes (Fisk & Bryan 1993). Nearly all monochorionic placentas have blood vessels linking the placenta together. As long as the bloodflow can pass in both directions, there will not be a problem; however, if anastomoses occur between an artery and a vein, causing the blood to flow in one direction only, *twin-to-twin transfusion syndrome* is likely to occur. This happens in approximately 15% of MCDA twins.

## Zygosity determination after birth

### DNA testing

The most accurate method of zygosity determination currently is to compare DNA (see The Multiple Births Foundation website: www.multiplebirths.org.uk).

**Reflective activity 59.1**

Find out what information is available in your unit about zygosity determination and DNA tests.

## DIAGNOSIS OF A MULTIPLE PREGNANCY

### Ultrasound examination

Ultrasound screening may be carried out as early as 6 weeks into the pregnancy and most women are aware of the multiple conception by 20 weeks. When the diagnosis is made in the first trimester, the risk of the 'vanishing twin syndrome' should be explained (Landy & Nies 1995). Chorionicity should be determined in the first trimester.

### Inspection

A midwife must always be alert to the possibility of twins if, on inspection, the uterus looks larger than expected for the gestation, especially after 20 weeks, and fetal movements are seen over a wide area, although the diagnosis need not always be of twins. A history of twins in the family should also be taken into account.

### Palpation

On abdominal palpation, the fundal height may be greater than expected for the period of gestation.

If two fetal poles (head or breech) are felt in the fundus of the uterus and multiple fetal limbs are palpable, this may be indicative of a multiple pregnancy. A smaller-than-expected head for the size of the uterus may suggest that the fetus is small and there may be more than one present. Location of three poles is diagnostic of at least two fetuses.

### Auscultation

Hearing two fetal heart rates is not diagnostic of a twin pregnancy, as one heart rate can be heard over a wide area. The use of 'Sonicaid' machines in monitoring fetal heartbeats has improved detection of more than one fetal heart rate, but heartbeats must be listened to simultaneously for at least 1 minute. If the two heartbeats have a variation of more than 10 beats per minute, almost certainly twin infants are present.

## ANTENATAL SCREENING

The UK National Screening Committee standard for screening in multiple pregnancy is by measurement of nuchal translucency (NT), preferably in combination with biochemistry. Biochemical screening alone should not be used.

Chorionic villus sampling (CVS) can be performed from the 11th week and has a 3–4% risk of miscarriage in a multiple pregnancy. Amniocentesis can also be performed in twin pregnancies, usually between 15 and 20 weeks. The risk of miscarriage is 2.5%. Both tests should be performed in a specialist fetal medicine centre.

## ANTENATAL PREPARATION

Early diagnosis of multiple pregnancy and chorionicity is extremely important so that parents have the additional specialist support and advice they need.

At whatever stage parents are told, it is essential that whoever shares the news is aware of the effect the revelation may have. Although some mothers and fathers are delighted to know that more than one baby is expected, in many cases there are reactions of shock and disbelief (Spillman 1986). It is important that an obstetrician or midwife is available to answer questions and give appropriate counselling at this time. It is helpful if the mother can be put in touch with other parents of twins who can understand and provide reassurance. Contact numbers for local twins groups and information about other relevant support organizations can be a great source of reassurance (see website).

### Parent education

As soon as a multiple pregnancy is diagnosed, written information should be given containing contact numbers of the local twins club, the parent education department at the local hospital, and national twin organizations, such as The Multiple Births Foundation (MBF) and The Twins and Multiple Births Association (Tamba). The news that two babies are expected can come as a considerable shock to some families, and the midwife should give them every opportunity to discuss any concerns they have.

Routine parentcraft classes need to be booked as early as possible; ideally, the mother should commence these at 24 weeks' gestation, which is earlier than for a singleton pregnancy, or specialist multiple pregnancy classes at 28 weeks (Davies 1995). When planning classes, contact with the local twins club can provide a very useful source of practical information. Mothers from twins clubs are usually delighted to participate and offer practical information, such as on equipment, clothes and breastfeeding (Denton & Bryan 1995).

The aim, as for all pregnant women, should be for continuity of care throughout the pregnancy. Multiples are considered high-risk pregnancies; if dedicated 'twin clinics' are held, these midwives specialize in the care of women expecting twins or more and offer the specific care, continuity and support needed.

Midwives must be aware of the enhanced role of fathers in the care of multiples and their cooperation in the mother's care should be sought from the start.

**Reflective activity 59.2**

Find out what information and education is provided for parents specific to multiple births in your local area.

### Preparation for breastfeeding

Mothers expecting twins or triplets will inevitably give a lot of thought to how they are going to feed their babies, not only from the nutritional aspect but also from the practical one because feeding will take a large part of the first months. Mothers should be encouraged that breastfeeding not only is possible for two babies and in some cases three (Fuducia 1995), but can be a very rewarding experience for all. Breast milk is ideal for all babies and especially important because twins, and more so triplets, tend to be born prematurely and of low birthweight.

Early in the pregnancy the mother should be given as much information about breastfeeding as possible, with contact numbers of local breastfeeding organizations. Both parents should have the chance to talk through any issues; a good idea is to suggest they meet with another mother who is successfully breastfeeding twins (see Davies & Denton 1999).

## COMPLICATIONS ASSOCIATED WITH A MULTIPLE PREGNANCY

When the pregnancy is multiple, minor disturbances are likely to be exaggerated. Morning sickness is often severe and prolonged. Heartburn can be persistent. Increased pressure may cause oedema of the ankles and varicose veins in the legs and vulva. As the pregnancy progresses, dyspnoea, backache and exhaustion are common.

### More serious complications

- *Pre-eclampsia* is reported to be more frequent in multiple pregnancies (Bryan et al 1997). The woman who has pre-eclampsia in her first pregnancy is usually less likely to experience this in subsequent pregnancies, unless she has changed her partner; then the risk is the same as in the first pregnancy, but the midwife must be aware of confidentiality in dealing with this (Salha et al 1999).
- *Anaemia:* Two or more fetuses make greater demands on the mother's stores of iron and folic acid. The literature on nutrition in pregnancy is focused on singletons and so is difficult to apply to multiple pregnancies. Practice varies – some units suggest supplements only if iron deficiency is detected, whereas others offer iron combined with folic acid routinely (Carlin & Neilson 2006).
- *Acute polyhydramnios* can occur as early as 16 weeks. It may be associated with fetal abnormalities, but with monochorionic twin pregnancies it is more likely to be due to twin-to-twin transfusion syndrome (TTTS) (see below) (Steinberg et al 1990). The midwife should always be alert for the mother who complains of a rapid increase in her abdominal girth in the second trimester, as well as a uterus that is continuously hard. This is due to the rapid increase in amniotic fluid (polyhydramnios). Urgent obstetric intervention is required to prevent premature labour and possible fetal demise.
- *Twin-to-twin transfusion syndrome* (TTTS) can be acute or chronic and occurs in approximately 15% of monochorionic diamniotic twin pregnancies (Fisk 1995). It arises because of unequal bloodflow through placental anastomoses from one fetus to the other. The donor twin transfuses blood via arteriovenous anastomoses of the placenta to the recipient twin. This results in growth restriction, oligohydramnios and anaemia in the donor twin ('stuck twin') and polycythaemia with circulatory overload in the recipient twin (hydrops). The fetal and neonatal mortality is high; early intervention with serial amnioreduction, laser coagulation of connecting placental vessels or amniotic septostomy may prolong the pregnancy until the fetuses are viable.
- *Preterm labour* is a major risk with multiple pregnancy.
- *Antepartum haemorrhage* is significantly increased (MacGillivray & Campbell 1988). Placenta praevia is also more common, because of the large placental site encroaching on the lower uterine segment, and placental abruption may occur following rupture of the membranes and subsequent diminution in uterine size, or be associated with pregnancy-induced hypertension.

## FETAL ABNORMALITIES ASSOCIATED WITH MONOZYGOTIC TWINS

**Conjoined twins:** This results from the incomplete monozygotic division of the fertilized ovum. It is extremely rare, occurring in approximately 1.3 per 100,000 births. Delivery has to be by caesarean section; separation of the babies is sometimes possible, depending on which internal organs are involved.

**Acardiac twins (twin reversed arterial perfusion, TRAP):** In acardia, one twin presents without a well-defined cardiac structure and is only kept alive through placental anastomoses to the circulatory system of the healthy co-twin (Moore et al 1990).

**Fetus-in-fetu (endoparasite):** In fetus-in-fetu, parts of a fetus become lodged within the other, usually healthy, twin. This can only happen in monozygotic twins and is seen equally in both sexes (Baldwin 1994).

## INTRAPARTUM CARE

It is advisable that all mothers expecting a multiple birth be booked for delivery in a consultant unit. Ideally, in the case of triplets and higher-order births, this should be a hospital that can offer intensive neonatal care facilities, such as a regional referral unit.

### Complications

The risks during labour to mother and babies is much greater in a multiple pregnancy. As well as preterm delivery, other complications are more common.

**Malpresentation:** Although malpresentations can occur more frequently than with singleton births, in about half of twin pregnancies both babies are cephalic presentations and in three-quarters of cases the first baby presents by the vertex.

**Cord prolapse:** This is a particular risk in cases of premature rupture of the membranes, malpresentation, polyhydramnios and in the interval between the births of the first and second twin.

**Prolonged labour:** The length of the first stage of labour is usually similar to that of a singleton birth. However, because of the overdistension of the uterus and abdominal muscles, there may be uterine inertia in some mothers.

**Monoamniotic twins:** As monoamniotic twins share the same sac, there is the risk of cord entanglement. Delivery is recommended around 32–34 weeks' gestation and by caesarean section (Pasquini et al 2006).

**Locking of twins:** This is an extremely rare phenomenon (Khunda 1972).

**Deferred delivery of the second twin:** In the last few years there have been cases reported where the first twin has been born, often very prematurely, and then labour has stopped. Labour in some instances has not recommenced again for a period of time; pregnancies have been recorded with a gap of 30 days or more. This can be beneficial to the second twin, as *betamethasone* can be administered to help mature the lungs. Throughout this period, the mother will need an enormous amount of support from midwives. She will be concerned about the twin who has been born as well as still being pregnant and concerned for that baby. She will need close monitoring for signs of infection.

### Onset of labour

The average gestational duration of multiple pregnancies with two, three and four babies are as follows:

- twins: 37 weeks
- triplets: 34 weeks
- quadruplets: 32 weeks.

Approximately 30% of twins and 80–95% of triplets are born spontaneously before 37 weeks (Clarke & Roman 1994). If labour does begin prematurely when the chances of survival are not good, the mother may be given drugs to inhibit uterine activity. Intravenous *salbutamol* and *sulindac* tablets are the drugs most commonly used. The cause of the premature labour must be determined quickly, so that it can be treated if possible; for example, a urinary tract infection should be treated with antibiotics. Most twin pregnancies are induced by 38 weeks.

### Care in labour

When a mother expecting a multiple birth is admitted in labour, the team who will be present at the delivery should be informed. As well as midwives and obstetric medical staff, an anaesthetist and paediatricians should be available (Bryan et al 1997). All those in attendance should be introduced to the parents, and their presence and role explained. If students and other observers are included, the mother's permission must be sought; ideally this should be prior to labour commencement.

#### First stage

The first stage of labour is conducted as for a singleton labour, though a multiple pregnancy is considered high risk. Regular monitoring of each baby must be observed – two external transducers can achieve this, or once the membranes are ruptured, a scalp electrode on the presenting twin and the external monitor on the second twin. Uterine activity should also be monitored. Epidural anaesthesia is now the pain relief of choice offered to mothers giving birth to multiples. This form of pain relief has the added advantage that if manoeuvres, such as internal version, forceps delivery, ventouse extraction and emergency caesarean section, are needed, adequate pain relief is in situ. The use of analgesia, such as pethidine, is usually avoided as this may cause respiratory depression, particularly in the case of the second baby, who may already be experiencing reduced oxygen levels (Bryan et al 1997). It is widely accepted that the risk to the second-born infant is significantly higher (MacGillivray & Campbell 1988). Thompson et al (1983), in a Scottish study, report a death rate for first twins of 47.6 per 1000 compared with 64.6 for second twins.

If there are any signs of fetal distress at any time during the first stage of labour to either baby, then an emergency caesarean section must be performed.

## Second stage

The obstetrician, anaesthetist and paediatrician should be present together with the midwife because of the risk of complications. Continuous monitoring of contractions and both infants' heartbeats should be in progress.

The delivery room should be suitable for an emergency caesarean section or in close proximity to an operating theatre. Two sets of resuscitation equipment and incubators should be prepared. The delivery trolley should include the requirements for episiotomy, amniotomy, instrumental delivery and extra cord clamps. Equipment for local and general anaesthesia should be available if epidural anaesthetic is not already established and effective.

The second stage is conducted as usual for the birth of the first baby. When the labour is preterm, forceps may be used to protect the infant's head during delivery. The cord should be firmly clamped in two places and cut between the clamps. Extra cord clamps may be needed if blood gases have to be taken; local unit policy should be followed for this. If the maternal side is not secure, the second baby, in the case of monochorionic twins, may suffer exsanguination. When the first twin is born, the time of delivery must be noted. The first infant and the cord should be clearly labelled 'Twin 1' or with the parents' chosen name, if known. The baby should be shown to the mother if the condition is satisfactory, or the parents constantly informed of progress if resuscitation is required. When the condition is satisfactory, the suckling of the baby breastfeeding will stimulate uterine activity.

The lie, presentation and position of the second baby must be ascertained by abdominal palpation and confirmed by vaginal examination. If transverse or oblique, this must be corrected by external version to longitudinal. If this is not possible, an emergency caesarean section is performed. The fetal heart rate and the mother's blood pressure and pulse rate must be checked after each procedure.

When it has been confirmed that there is no cord presentation, the second sac of membranes is ruptured and a scalp electrode applied. Once again, a check is made to make sure that the cord has not prolapsed. If contractions do not resume very soon after delivery of the first twin, then a Syntocinon infusion may be needed. The delivery is conducted in the normal way, taking care to note the time and label the baby 'Twin 2', and the same for the cord. The interval between the births varies considerably. It has been suggested that 30 minutes should be the maximum time (Barrett 2006). Depending upon gestation and individual circumstances, delayed delivery may be considered, but this is not usual practice.

If more than two babies are expected, the delivery is usually by caesarean section (see below).

### *Undiagnosed twins*

It is unusual nowadays for a multiple pregnancy to remain undiagnosed at the time of delivery. However, where ultrasonography is not available or not used routinely for all expectant mothers, or in the case of an unbooked woman, this can still occur. In this situation, *ergometrine* or *Syntometrine* should not be administered until after the birth of the baby, so there is no risk to a possible twin of severe anoxia, which may lead to death, or precipitate delivery of a possibly brain-damaged infant. Rupture of the uterus is also a risk. If drugs have been administered, the second baby requires immediate delivery. A general anaesthetic may be required and a muscle relaxant given. Caesarean section may be indicated.

It should be appreciated that both parents in this situation are likely to be in a state of shock (Theroux 1989). Suddenly there are two babies to whom they must relate. They may already have formed a bond with the first infant and find it difficult to accept the unexpected baby (Bryan et al 1997). Midwives, if aware of the possible problem, can give extra support to allow expression of negative feelings and help acceptance of the new situation.

## Third stage

Management may vary in different hospitals. It is usual to give an injection of *ergometrine maleate* 250–500 mcg intravenously or *Syntometrine* 1 ml intramuscularly with the birth of the anterior shoulder of the last baby. When the uterus is felt to contract, controlled cord traction is applied to both/all cords at the same time.

Following delivery, there is an increased risk of haemorrhage from the large placental site and overdistended uterine muscles, which may also contribute, as the abdominal muscles are more relaxed.

## Examination of placenta and membranes

The midwife must make the usual examination to ensure completeness and detect any deviation from normal. If the babies are of different sex, then they must be dizygotic twins, with either two separate placentas or one that has fused together, but each will have its own set of membranes, that is, amnion and chorion. When the babies are of the same sex, they may be monozygotic or dizygotic. It used to be thought that there was only a single chorion in the case of all monozygotic twins. However, research has revealed that one-third of monozygotic twins have dichorionic placentas. DNA testing is advisable to confirm zygosity.

## Delivery of triplets and higher-order births

The greatest problem for triplet and higher-order births is preterm delivery.

The recommended method of delivery is by caesarean section and in many series of data this rate is greater than 90% for triplets (Lipitz et al 1994). The higher the order, the more likely this becomes (Pons et al 1988).

The delivery of triplets or more is a major event for all staff as well as parents. As much information as possible should be given to the parents about the procedure, and the roles of the many personnel in the delivery room should be explained (Bryan et al 1997). It is crucial that the resuscitation teams are briefed well in advance of the delivery and that each baby has its own paediatric team.

However many infants are involved, the parents should be shown their babies as soon as possible after delivery.

If it is necessary to transfer some or all of the infants to the neonatal unit, photographs should be taken and brought to the mother as soon as possible. Ideally, the babies should be photographed together so that the realities of the multiple birth are established. However, if this is not possible, the pictures should be clearly labelled with the birth order of the babies.

# POSTNATAL CARE

The immediate postnatal care for a mother who has given birth to twins or more is the same as for a singleton mother, but with special attention to her blood loss and the involution of the uterus. As the babies are likely to be smaller and preterm, it is more difficult for them to maintain their body temperature, so they must be kept warm.

Following delivery, the mother is likely to be very tired. She has probably suffered from a sleep deficit over several months, and a more complicated delivery or caesarean section may compound her exhaustion. The lochia in the first few days is often heavier than after a singleton delivery and the mother is more likely to complain of afterpains.

In addition, the mother has two or more babies for whom she must care and relate. Her anxieties may be increased if her babies are preterm. One, both, or, in the case of triplets or more, all, may be nursed in the neonatal unit. The mother will need additional support and help if she has one baby on the postnatal ward with her and one in the NICU. She may feel more inclined to stay with the healthy baby on the ward rather than the one in NICU, though if the long-term outcome is uncertain she should be encouraged to spend as much time as possible with the sick baby.

Some units have established transitional care wards where small, well babies can remain with their mothers with the aid of specially trained midwives or nurses who are available to support, assist and advise them on the care and specialized feeding the babies need.

Sadly, it is not uncommon for very sick babies to be transferred, sometimes without their mother, from the delivery hospital to a regional referral unit where intensive neonatal nursing care can be offered. The distances involved can be great and extremely costly to the parents and the neonatal services (Papiernik 1991). This situation is traumatic for all the family. Midwifery staff must strive to reunite the family as soon as the condition of the babies allows. Regular communication during the separation is vital. The splitting up of the family group is often avoided if the babies are transferred to the regional referral unit in utero. Bowman et al (1988) demonstrated that such babies had a better prognosis than those who needed to be transferred after birth.

## Feeding multiples

During the first few weeks, the mother is going to need a lot of extra support and advice to help her establish breastfeeding. She should allow 4–6 weeks to get into a routine and achieve this. Twins can breastfeed separately or together; if fed together, the feeds will only take a little longer than with a single baby. The mother will have more quality time with her babies, as she has no bottles to sterilize or feeds to make up (see Ch. 43).

Whilst in hospital, help should be available at every feed until the mother feels confident. It is advisable in the first few days for her to feed her babies separately; this gives her a chance to get to know each baby as an individual and to feel confident handling and putting the baby to the breast. It can be overwhelming for the mother with a first baby to try to perfect feeding two babies together right from the start. Once breastfeeding is established, some mothers prefer to feed both infants together, thus saving time; others prefer to feed separately but wake the second to feed immediately after the first so the routine is maintained. There is no one right way (Davies & Denton 1999); it has to be the mother's preference and what fits in with her family, developing the mother's confidence and ability to cope. One of the main causes of nipple soreness and backache is incorrect positioning of both babies at the breast and the mother's sitting position whilst feeding. It is very important for mothers to be taught right from the start to use plenty of pillows to support their backs and also to take the weight of the babies for feeding. The pillows should bring the babies up to nipple level so the mother can sit with her back straight and not lean forwards over the babies. As the weight of the babies is taken by the pillows, the mother's hands are free to reposition a baby should either of them come off the breast and to lift one baby up for winding purposes. There are a variety of positions in which the mother can hold her babies for

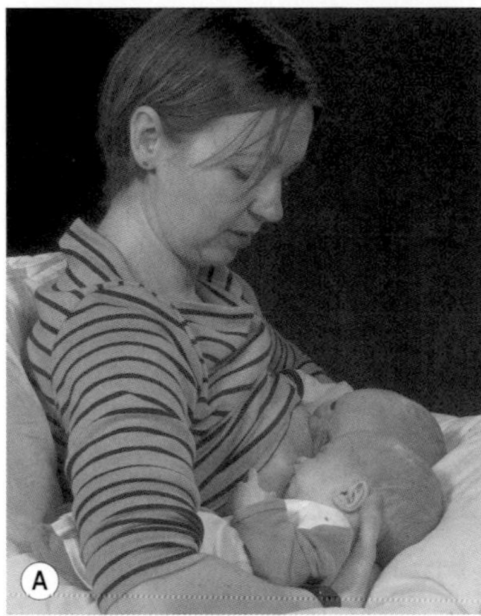
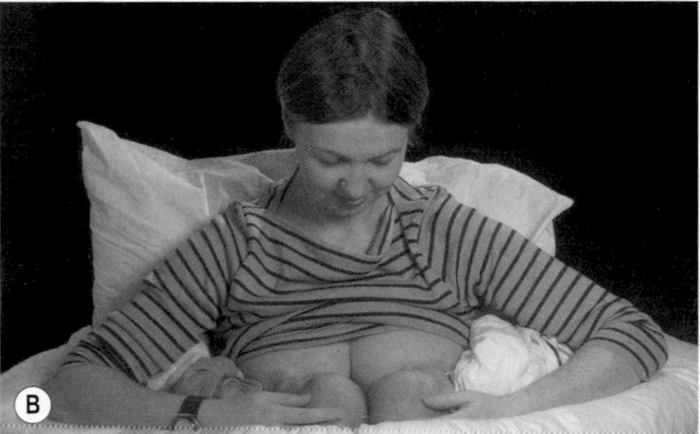

**Figure 59.5** A mother well positioned successfully breastfeeding twins using the underarm hold.

feeding. The most usual one for newborns is the underarm hold (Fig. 59.5).

Some mothers will choose to wholly or partially bottle feed their babies. Partners, family and friends are then able to share in feeding routines.

Whatever the mother's choice of feeding method, the midwife should support her in that choice.

## Coming home

If the babies have been born preterm, the mother may go home several days or weeks before her babies. It is unusual for babies to be discharged home at different times, but there are occasions when this happens. This will put added strain on the parents, who have to care for one baby at home whilst finding time to visit the sick one in hospital. Criticism of parents who do not visit frequently should be avoided. It may be necessary to arrange for a room on the NICU for the mother to room-in so she gains confidence in caring for the babies before discharge. This transition will be smoother if the mother has adequate help at home for the first few weeks after discharge.

### Sources of help

There is no statutory help routinely available for mothers of twins, triplets or more in the UK. If there are concerns about the family circumstances and the parents' ability to cope, then social services should be contacted before the babies are born. Further Education Colleges running the Diploma in Child Care and Education often welcome the opportunity to place their students with families for work experience. *Home Start* is another organization which may be able to assist (see website). Local Sure Start centres may have details of other help available.

## Family relationships

A mother may find it more difficult to relate to both/all of her babies at the beginning. This is very common and she should be reassured that these feelings will pass and she will bond with all her babies.

A strong preference may develop for one of the babies in the early days. Research has shown that this is usually for the baby who was heavier at birth (Spillman 1984). The mother should be reassured that this is normal and in time her relationship with the other baby or babies will improve.

Becoming overtired and feeling overwhelmed with the immensity of their task is also a risk for both parents. There may also be problems with other children in the family, especially toddlers. It is hard enough for a 2-year-old child to accept one new baby. When two or more arrive simultaneously, there may be real difficulties. Single older children may see their parents as a pair and the twins as a pair and themselves on their own, so it is helpful for the parents to arrange for a special friend to spend time with the older child. It is usual for the new babies to give a present to their older sibling; it is a good idea for the older child to choose a small different gift for each twin. Cuddly toys are a good idea. Being the first gifts the twins receive can make the sibling feel very special.

## Individuality and identity

Most parents of twins appreciate the importance of their children developing their own identities. This, ideally, should be discussed in the antenatal period. Parents of twins are encouraged to treat their children as individuals, giving them the same opportunities as a single-born child. Ways in which they can emphasize their individuality should be discussed in parent education classes. These include choosing names that do not sound the same or rhyme and commence with a different first letter, and dressing the children in different-coloured clothes (Bryan & Hallett 2001).

## Postnatal depression

In view of all the possible complications, increased risk of surgical intervention and the other stresses involved in having a multiple birth, it is perhaps not surprising that there is an increased risk of depression (Spillman 1993, Thorpe et al 1991).

The health professionals caring for the mother should recognize the signs that depression is developing. It is helpful if there is continuity of care by a known midwife and a health visitor who has been introduced to the family before the babies are born. If the babies are still in hospital, it is still important for the mother to receive visits from her midwife and health visitor at home.

## Bereavement

Mortality rates for multiple births have long been established as significantly higher than those of singletons, with twins about 5 times, and triplets about 10 times, more likely to die within the first year of life (MacFarlane & Mugford 2000) (Fig. 59.6).

The higher incidence of preterm delivery and the associated complications are the main reason for the increased death rates. The loss of all the babies in a multiple pregnancy is tragic and the grief of the parents is usually fully recognized, but the situation is more complex when one twin or triplet dies. Parents then have to cope with grieving for the dead baby (or babies if two triplets die) at the same time as caring for the survivor. Professionals, as well as family and friends, can fail to realize that the grief is just as great when one baby dies, and the joy of having a healthy child will not diminish the depth of the emotions or compensate for the loss. Parents may be regarded as ungrateful for the survivor, particularly if one twin dies during pregnancy or delivery or shortly after birth. They may need help to fully acknowledge their feelings and should be given information and support and offered counselling, which should be ongoing, as soon as the death is confirmed. The loss of status of being parents of twins, triplets or more must not be underestimated. They will continue to be parents of however many children are born and this should always be acknowledged (Bryan 1986).

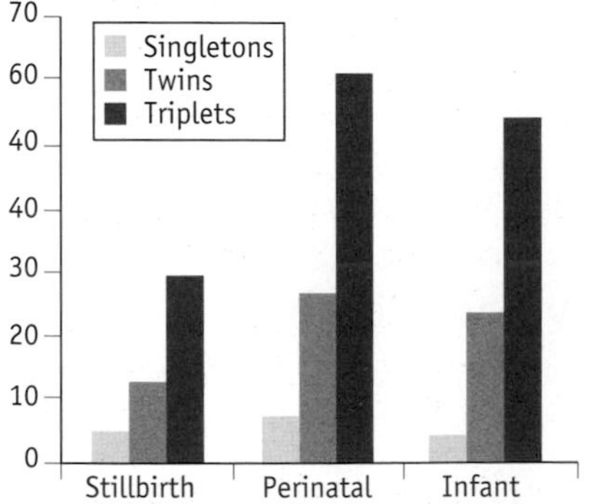


**Figure 59.6** Mortality in multiple births, England and Wales, 2005, per 1000 births *(Source: ONS London.)*

Encouragement should be given to the parents to talk about the confusing, contradictory feelings they may have and to think and talk about their dead baby, as this will allow the mourning process to take place (Lewis 1979, Lewis & Bryan 1988).

If the babies are dichorionic, same-sex twins (triplets), the parents should be given the option for DNA testing so they will know the zygosity of their babies.

Each case must be treated individually, and the information and care required will vary in some ways, depending upon when the baby died. The different situations and recommendations for the care of these families is given in detail in the section on bereavement in the Multiple Births Foundation *Guidelines for professionals* (Bryan & Hallett 1997).

**Reflective activity 59.3**

Find out what services are available nationally and locally to support bereaved parents of twins or more.

## Disability

The risk of disability is greater with multiple births. The chance of a triplet pregnancy resulting in a baby with cerebral palsy is 47 times greater, and for a twin pregnancy 8 times greater, than that of a singleton pregnancy (Petterson et al 1990). Caring for one child with a disability and another who is healthy brings many challenges, especially with twins. Often, the healthy child has just as many problems and may imagine that he or she caused the problem or resent the attention paid to the other child. Many potential emotional and behavioural problems may be avoided if the family are supported and advised appropriately as early as possible.

### Multifetal pregnancy reduction

Multifetal pregnancy reduction may be offered to parents who conceive triplets or more on the basis that reduction to two or even one fetus provides a better chance of the healthy survival of each baby. The procedure is usually carried out between the 10th and 12th weeks of pregnancy; the most common method is to inject potassium chloride into the fetal thorax. When parents are presented with this immensely difficult decision, they must be provided with information about the risks and consequences of the procedure and offered counselling so that they consider the implications fully before making a final choice (see Ch. 28).

### Selective feticide

If one of the babies in a multiple pregnancy has a serious abnormality, the same clinical procedure as described for multifetal pregnancy reduction may be used. Again, the parents will need very detailed information about the risks and counselling before making their final decision. As the dead baby will remain in the uterus until the delivery, the midwife has an important role to play in acknowledging the bereavement and supporting the mother through this very emotional time before and after the birth.

## Planning ahead

It is important that good family planning advice is offered to the parents following a multiple birth. Genetic counselling may be needed for those who have lost a baby. Follow-up of survivors should be arranged, especially when the infants are monozygous or have experienced neonatal complications.

**KEY POINTS**

- Multiple birth families have special needs. Midwives should be prepared for the additional and different management, information and support needed to ensure the best outcomes for the whole family.
- The incidence of multiple births is increasing because of the wider availability of infertility treatments.
- It is important to determine chorionicity and zygosity accurately.
- Risk management is an important part of care.
- Obtaining adequate support throughout childbirth and beyond is essential.
- Established voluntary networks are an important source of support.

## REFERENCES


Baldwin VJ: *Pathology of multiple pregnancy*, New York, 1994, Springer-Verlag.

Barrett JFR: Management of labour in multiple pregnancies. In Kilby M, Baker P, Critchley H, et al, editors: *Multiple pregnancy*, London, 2006, RCOG, pp 223–233.

Botting B, Macfarlane AJ, Price FV: *Three, four & more: a study of triplets and higher order births*, London, 1990, HMSO.

Bowman E, Doyle LW, Murton LJ, et al: Increased mortality of preterm infants transferred between tertiary perinatal centres, *British Medical Journal* 297(6656):1098–1100, 1988.

Bryan EM: The death of a newborn twin. How can support for the parents be improved? *Acta Geneticae Medicae et Gemellologiae* 35(1–2):115–118, 1986.

Bryan EM, Hallett F: *Guidelines for professionals: bereavement*, London, 1997, The Multiple Births Foundation.

Bryan EM, Hallett F: *Guidelines for professionals: twins and triplets: the first five years and beyond*, London, 2001, The Multiple Births Foundation.

Bryan EM, Denton J, Hallett F: *Guidelines for professionals: multiple pregnancy*, London, 1997, The Multiple Births Foundation.

Carlin A, Neilson JP: Twin clinics: a model for antenatal care in multiple gestations. In Kilby M, Baker P, Critchley H, et al, editors: *Multiple pregnancy*, London, 2006, RCOG, pp 121–137.

Clarke JP, Roman JD: A review of 19 sets of triplets, *Australian and New Zealand Journal of Obstetrics and Gynaecology* 134(1):50–53, 1994.

Chitayat D, Hall J: Genetic aspects of twinning. In Kilby M, Baker P, Critchley H, et al, editors: *Multiple pregnancy*, London, 2006, RCOG, pp 89–94.

Collins J, Graves G: The economic consequences of multiple gestation pregnancy in assisted conception cycles, *Human Fertility* 3(4):275–283, 2000.

Davies ME: Managing multiple births, supporting parents, *Modern Midwife* 5(11):10–14, 1995.

Davies ME, Denton J: *Feeding twins, triplets and more*, London, 1999, The Multiple Births Foundation.

Denton J, Bryan EM: Prenatal preparation for parenting twins, triplets or more: the social aspect. In Whittle M, Ward RH, editors: *Multiple pregnancy*, London, 1995, RCOG, pp 119–128.

Derom R, Derom C, Vlietnick R: The risk of monozygotic twinning. In Blickstein I, Keith LG, editors: *Iatrogenic multiple pregnancy, clinical implications*, New York, 2001, Parthenon, pp 9–19.

Fisk NM: The scientific basis of feto-fetal transfusion syndrome and its treatment. In Humphrey WR, Whittle M, editors: *Multiple pregnancy*, London, 1995, RCOG, pp 235–250.

Fisk NM, Bryan EM: Routine prenatal determination of chorionicity in multiple gestation: a plea to the obstetrician, *British Journal of Obstetrics and Gynaecology* 100(11):975–977, 1993.

Fuducia A: Breastfeeding three babies at once, *Twins, Triplets and More* 6(3):10–11, 1995.

Khunda S: Locked twins, *Obstetrics and Gynecology* 39(3):453–459, 1972.

Kurinczuk J: Epidemiology of multiple pregnancy: changing effects of assisted conception. In Kilby M, Baker P, Critchley H, et al, editors: *Multiple pregnancy*, London, 2006, RCOG, pp 121–137.

Landy HJ, Nies BM: The vanishing twin. In Keith L, Papiernik E, Keith D, et al, editors: *Multiple pregnancy, epidemiology, gestation, and perinatal outcome*, New York, 1995, Parthenon, pp 59.

Lewis E: Mourning by the family after a still birth or neonatal death, *Archives of Disease in Childhood* 54(4):303–306, 1979.

Lewis E, Bryan EM: Management of perinatal loss of a twin, *British Medical Journal* 297(6659):1321–1323, 1988.

Lipitz S, Reichman B, Uval J: A prospective comparison of the outcome of triplet pregnancies managed expectantly or by multifetal reduction to twins, *American Journal of Obstetrics and Gynecology* 170(3):874–879, 1994.

MacFarlane AJ, Mugford M: *Birth counts: statistics of pregnancy and childbirth*, Norwich, 2000, The Stationery Office.

MacGillivray I, Campbell DM: Management of twin pregnancies. In MacGillivray I, Campbell DM, Thompson B, editors: *Twinning and twins*, Chichester, 1988, John Wiley, pp 111–139.

Moore TR, Gale S, Benirschke K: Perinatal outcome of forty nine pregnancies complicated by acardiac twinning, *American Journal of Obstetrics and Gynecology* 163(3):907–912, 1990.

Papiernik E: Costs of multiple pregnancies. In Harvey D, Bryan EM, editors: *The stress of multiple births*, London, 1991, The Multiple Births Foundation, pp 22–34.

Pasquini L, Wimalasundera RC, Fichera A, et al: High perinatal survival in monoamniotic twins by prophylactic sulindac, intensive ultrasound surveillance, and Cesarean delivery at 32 weeks, *Ultrasound in Obstetrics & Gynecology* 28(5):681–687, 2006.

Perlman EJ, Stetton G, Tuckmuller CM, et al: Sexual discordance in monozygotic twins, *American Journal of Medical Genetics* 37(4):551–557, 1990.

Petterson B, Stanley F, Henderson D: Cerebral palsy in multiple births in Western Australia, *American Journal of Medical Genetics* 37(3):346–351, 1990.

Pons JC, Mayenga JM, Plu G, et al: Management of triplet pregnancy, *Acta Geneticae Medicae et Gemellologiae* 37(1):99–103, 1988.

Salha O, Sharma V, Dada T, et al: The influence of donated gametes on the incidence of hypertensive disorders of pregnancy, *Human Reproduction* 14(9):2268–2273, 1999.

Spillman JR: *The role of birthweight in maternal–twin relationships*, MSc Thesis, Cranfield, 1984, Cranfield Institute of Technology.

Spillman JR: Expecting a multiple birth: some emotional aspects, *British Journal for Nurses in Child Health* 1(10):298–299, 1986.

Spillman JR: Perinatal loss in multiple pregnancy. In Proceedings: 23rd International Congress of Midwives, vol IV, Vancouver Canada, 1993, pp 1776–1785.

Steinberg LH, Hurley VA, Desmedt E, et al: Acute polyhydramnios in twin pregnancies, *Australian and New Zealand Journal of Obstetrics and Gynaecology* 30(3):196–200, 1990.

Theroux R: Multiple birth: a unique parenting experience, *Journal of Perinatal and Neonatal Nursing* 3(1):35–45, 1989.

Thompson B, Pritchard C, Corney G: Perinatal mortality in twins by zygosity and placentation. Paper given at the 4th Congress of International Society of Twin Studies, London, 1983.

Thorpe K, Golding J, Macgillivray I, et al: Comparison of prevalence of depression in mothers of twins and mothers of singletons, *British Medical Journal* 302(6781):875–878, 1991.

# Chapter 60

# Pre-term labour

Nicola Wales

## LEARNING OUTCOMES

After reading this chapter, you will be able to:

- identify the factors associated with preterm labour and birth
- highlight the implications of risk factors and the possibilities of risk assessment
- discuss the available tocolytic drugs, including associated risks
- critically explore midwifery management of preterm labour and birth
- discuss the implications of preterm birth for the baby, and the family.

## INTRODUCTION

Labour is defined as preterm when it occurs before the end of the 37th week of pregnancy. Babies are described in terms of either birthweight or gestational age. Infants delivered less than 37 completed weeks from the first day of the last menstrual period are referred to as *preterm*, irrespective of weight, while infants weighing less than 2500 g are classified as of *low birthweight*. Babies may be both preterm and of low birthweight.

Recent advances in neonatal care have resulted in the survival of very small and immature infants and these classifications have been expanded: *very low birthweight infants* (VLBW) are defined as those weighing less than 1500 g at birth and *extremely low birthweight infants* (ELBW) as less than 1000 g at birth. Some authorities add a further category which describes infants weighing 750 g or less: these may be referred to as *incredibly low birthweight* (ILBW) (Amon 1999).

It is important to differentiate between the low birth weight preterm infant and the baby whose birthweight is low because of intrauterine growth restriction, as each group has different needs and problems after birth.

The incidence of preterm delivery as a proportion of all births is around 7% in the UK, translating into roughly 50,000 babies every year. Rates of preterm delivery increase with increasing gestational age, up to 37 weeks, with less than a quarter occurring before 32 weeks. Preterm birth is directly responsible for 75–90% of all neonatal deaths not due to lethal congenital malformations and is a major cause of both short-term and long-term neonatal morbidity (Amon 1999).

## AETIOLOGY

Preterm birth may occur as a result of any of the following situations:

- *Elective preterm delivery*: This may be undertaken as a result of severe pre-eclampsia, maternal renal disease or severe intrauterine growth restriction. In developed countries, iatrogenic delivery is responsible for almost half of the births between 28 and 35 weeks; mostly due to hypertensive and pre-eclamptic disease (Steer 2005).
- *Premature rupture of the membranes*: This is an antecedent in about 20% of cases of preterm birth.
- *Complicated emergency delivery*: Complications include placental abruption, eclampsia, rhesus isoimmunization, maternal infection and prolapsed

cord. This group accounts for about 25% of preterm births.

- *Uncomplicated spontaneous preterm labour of unknown cause*: This is the largest group, accounting for up to 40% of preterm births.

## Risk factors

A number of risk factors have been associated with preterm labour and these may be related to maternal or fetal circumstances. Identification of the higher-risk woman may, in theory, make intervention and prevention easier. However, many of the factors are interlinked and it is difficult to disentangle the effects of discrete risks, such as drug abuse, from the pattern of deprivation which often accompanies it (Amon 1999, El Bastawissi et al 2000, Minakami et al 2000, Schieve et al 2000, Shah & Bracken 2000, Shumway et al 1999).

### Biological/medical factors

- Age less than 16 years or more than 35 years
- Low weight for height
- Chronic medical conditions, such as diabetes or renal disorders
- Infections, such as urinary tract infections.

### Reproductive history

- History of previous preterm birth – a history of more than two preterm deliveries increases the risk by 70%
- Bleeding in previous pregnancy
- Uterine abnormality, such as bicornuate, unicornuate or didelphic uterus (see Ch. 58), which increases the risk of preterm birth to 19%.

### Current pregnancy

- Poor nutrition – especially if the pre-pregnancy body mass index (BMI) was low, i.e. less than 19.8
- Bleeding
- Retained intrauterine contraceptive device
- Abdominal surgery
- Infections, especially pyelonephritis
- Genital tract infection, especially non-specific vaginitis, bacterial vaginosis, chlamydia, *Ureaplasma urealyticum* and group B haemolytic *Streptococcus*. This latter organism is carried by 5% of women and is associated with preterm prelabour rupture of the membranes. Amnionitis resulting from genital tract infection may stimulate the local release of prostaglandin $E_2$ and $F_{2a}$: this may cause labour to begin. Evidence of infection is common in preterm labour occurring before 30 weeks' gestation. This association seems to weaken with advancing gestation (Goldenberg et al 2000).
- Multiple pregnancy: the risk of preterm birth is nine times higher for a multifetal pregnancy compared with a singleton pregnancy
- Polyhydramnios
- Fetal malformation
- Rhesus disease
- Fetal death
- Violence – including verbal abuse – may cause a fourfold increase in preterm labour
- Hypertensive disease.

### Socioeconomic

- Poverty and social deprivation
- Employment that involves hard physical work
- Psychological – psychological distress is associated with preterm delivery.

### Cultural/behavioural

- Cigarette, alcohol or drug use
- Short inter-pregnancy interval
- Late antenatal booking
- Poor attendance for antenatal care.

The pathophysiology of spontaneous preterm labour is poorly understood. It seems most likely that uterine contractions begin as a result of the interplay of several factors. Infection appears to be a factor in about 30% of preterm labours (Amon 1999).

**Reflective activity 60.1**

What information on preterm labour do you provide to women during the pregnancy? Consider how you would advise a woman to understand her normal physiology, that is, differentiating between Braxton Hicks and the contractions of preterm labour.

## PREDICTION AND PREVENTION OF PRETERM LABOUR

Several methods have been used to try to identify women at risk of preterm labour, though prediction is difficult and may not be effective in preventing preterm birth. Formal *risk-scoring* systems have been used, based on the factors described above. This method has relatively poor predictive value for spontaneous preterm labour, especially for primigravid women; a low score may induce a false sense of security (Amon 1999). However, it may be more useful where it is possible to identify factors relating to past obstetric history and current events.

*Regular pelvic examination*: The difficulty with digital examination of the cervix is the lack of consistency between examinations and examiner, though it may reveal signs of cervical changes that may herald the onset of labour. However, this procedure may of itself introduce infection and has a low predictive value for women at risk of preterm birth (Colombo 2002, Enkin et al 2000).

*Ultrasonographic measurement of cervical length* may be an accurate predictive tool in high-risk women. Funnelling of the internal cervical os may indicate impending preterm labour; however, there is no cervical length *below which* all women deliver prematurely and no cervical length *above which* none of the women deliver early. The only conclusion that can be made is an increased risk for early delivery with a shortened cervix (Colombo 2002).

*Fetal fibronectin tests* may predict the onset of preterm labour (Lockwood et al 1991). Fetal fibronectin is a component of the extracellular matrix, secreted by the anchoring trophoblastic villi. Although its presence in vaginal secretions is a normal finding in the first half of pregnancy, concentrations greater than 50 ng/mL after 22 weeks' gestation are indicative of chorio-decidual disruption (Amon 1999).

If preterm labour is imminent, there is separation of maternal and fetal tissue at the chorio-decidual junction, leading to leakage of fibronectin. However, false positive results can occur, which means that some women may be subjected to unnecessary interventions. The test should be carried out every 2 weeks from 24 weeks' gestation and cannot be used in the presence of vaginal bleeding or rupture of the membranes, as both blood and amniotic fluid contain fibronectin.

*Vaginal pH monitoring* may be useful, as a rise in pH often indicates the presence of infection, which may precipitate labour.

*Fetal breathing movements* cease before preterm labour commences, and although this may not occur in every case, it is a reasonably reliable indicator of imminent preterm delivery (Amon 1999, Castle & Turnbull 1983). However, the time and resources required to screen large populations of at-risk women may make this unattractive as a screening procedure.

Prevention of preterm birth is dependent upon preventing uterine activity and/or cervical dilatation. In the past, *bedrest* was advocated as a preventive measure, though now has been shown to be ineffective, and it may actually increase the risk for deep vein thrombosis (Enkin et al 2000, Kovacevich et al 2000). Antibiotic therapy has been used in the management of women at risk of preterm labour, though there is no powerful evidence to support the routine use of antibiotics where the membranes are intact. A large randomized study of *metronidazole* treatment for asymptomatic bacterial vaginosis also failed to demonstrate any reduction in the incidence of preterm labour (Carey et al 2000, Enkin et al 2000, King & Flenardy 2000).

*Prophylactic cervical cerclage* may be helpful where there is a recognized cervical weakness, such as may follow previous second trimester abortions or cone biopsy, or where there is a diethylstilbestrol-related abnormality of uterine structure. It is also sometimes employed in the management of multifetal pregnancy (Silver & Ware Branch 1999, Smith-Levitin et al 1999). The usefulness of cervical suture in women who do not have a cervical weakness is not proven.

The technique involves the insertion of a strong, non-absorbable suture such as Mersilene tape or Mersilk 4 around the cervix at the level of the internal os. This keeps the cervical canal closed. The procedure is carried out under general anaesthesia. The suture is removed at 39 weeks' gestation or when labour commences.

The role of *social support* in preventing preterm birth has been examined and does not appear to have any influence on physical outcomes, although it may improve psychological wellbeing (Enkin et al 2000, Oakley 1989).

## PRETERM PRELABOUR RUPTURE OF THE MEMBRANES

Spontaneous rupture of the membranes before 37 weeks' gestation and before labour commences is termed preterm prelabour rupture. The cause may be unclear but it is associated with maternal smoking, vaginal bleeding in the second trimester, cervical incompetence and genital tract infection, especially group B haemolytic *Streptococcus*, *Chlamydia trachomatis* and bacterial vaginosis (Walkinshaw 1995).

If preterm rupture of the membranes occurs at home, the midwife must contact the doctor and arrange for the woman to be admitted to a hospital with a neonatal unit. On admission of the woman to hospital, the midwife should assess the maternal and fetal condition, noting any uterine activity. A speculum examination is carried out to visualize the cervix. A pool of amniotic fluid may be seen in the posterior fornix. A cervical swab is taken and sent for microscopy and culture. Digital vaginal examination should be avoided in order to reduce the risk of ascending infection.

Steroids such as *dexamethasone* 12 mg or *betamethasone* 12 mg may be prescribed (both can be used but betamethasone is preferred) and will be administered intramuscularly in two doses 12 hours apart. This accelerates surfactant production in the fetal lungs and reduces the risk of respiratory distress syndrome (hyaline membrane disease) to the neonate. These drugs are effective after 24 hours and for up to 7 days, and of most benefit between 24 and 32 weeks' gestation.

The woman's temperature and pulse should be recorded at least twice daily, as chorioamnionitis occurs in at least 20% of cases of preterm rupture of the membranes. Blood may be taken to estimate the white cell count and for serum screening for C-reactive protein. This is a globulin of hepatic origin which rises in the acute phase of any infection. A single measurement of more than 30–40 mg/L or consecutive values of more than 20 mg/L indicate infection (Walkinshaw 1995). If there is evidence of infection or vaginal colonization, antibiotic therapy may improve perinatal outcome.

The midwife should monitor the fetal condition and observe the state of any liquor draining. Abnormal signs, such as pyrexia, tachycardia, uterine tenderness or offensive liquor, or fetal signs, such as abnormal fetal heart patterns or alterations in fetal activity should be reported to the obstetrician. If the woman's condition is stable after 48 hours following the membrane rupture, she may be offered the option of going home. She will be asked to observe for signs of chorioamnionitis by twice-daily temperature measurements and observation of any vaginal loss and requested to return to the hospital for regular assessments (RCOG 2006a).

## MANAGEMENT OF PRETERM LABOUR

Preterm labour may be difficult to recognize but documented uterine contractions (2 in 10), documented cervical changes, cervical effacement of 80%, or cervical dilatation of 2 cm or more are accepted as diagnostic (Amon 1999). The midwife should be aware of the likelihood of preterm labour in any woman who complains of the following prior to 37 weeks' gestation:

- menstrual-like cramps
- signs of urinary tract infection, frequency and/or pain on passing urine
- backache
- pink vaginal secretions
- diarrhoea
- pelvic pressure or increased vaginal discharge (Amon 1999).

If a possible premature labour begins at home, the midwife must arrange for the woman to be admitted to a hospital with an appropriate level of neonatal unit. On admission, she should be made comfortable and the fetus should be continuously monitored. Plans for the management of labour and its implications should be discussed with the couple in language that they understand, enabling time for questions to be asked, and the information assimilated. The neonatal unit should be informed and a member of the neonatal unit staff should visit the parents to discuss the proposed management of the baby at delivery. It is essential that accurate information is available regarding number of fetuses, estimated gestation, estimated fetal weight and presentation.

If the gestation is 35 weeks or more, labour will probably be allowed to continue, as most babies of this age make good progress if given appropriate care after birth. Below 35 weeks, tocolytic drugs may be used if both mother and fetus are in good condition, with no signs of intrauterine infection, vaginal bleeding or rupture of the membranes.

**Reflective activity 60.2**

Find and read the local guidelines in your unit for the care of women with threatened preterm labour. Does it include meeting the neonatologist and neonatal unit staff? Do you understand your unit's transfer policy, so you can help and prepare the women and families?

### Tocolytic drugs

Tocolytic agents are used to suppress uterine activity in an attempt to 'buy' the fetus more 'growing time' in utero. Between 23 and 26 weeks, each day gained improves the survival prospects for the infant and allows steroid-induced lung maturation to take place. Using tocolytic agents may enhance the chance of a transfer to a neonatal intensive care unit if required.

Although it may be possible to prolong the pregnancy, no medication has been found to be universally effective and all have adverse side-effects (Gyetvai et al 1999).

The group of drugs historically most commonly used is the beta-adrenergic agonists, such as *ritodrine hydrochloride (Yutopar)*, *salbutamol (Ventolin, Salbuvent)* and *terbutaline (Bricanyl)* (RCOG 2002a). However, beta-adrenergic agonists have unpleasant and sometimes severe adverse effects.

Present evidence indicates that if a tocolytic drug is to be used, ritodrine is no longer the best choice. *Atosiban* or *nifedipine* are preferable as they have fewer adverse effects with comparable effectiveness. Atosiban is licensed for this usage in the UK but nifedipine is not (RCOG 2002a). Atosiban (Tractocile) is a synthetic peptide which acts as an oxytocin competitor (Ferring Pharmaceuticals 2000). This has a specific action which inhibits uterine contractions by blocking myometrial oxytocin receptors.

In comparative trials with ritodrine, salbutamol and terbutaline, atosiban was associated with fewer maternal adverse effects such as nausea, vomiting, headache, tachycardia, hypotension and palpitations (Worldwide Atosiban versus Beta-agonists Study Group 2001).

The drug is given as an initial intravenous bolus of 6.75 mg, followed by a high-dose 'loading infusion' of 18 mg/hour for 3 hours. This is followed by a low-dose intravenous infusion of 6 mg/hour for up to 45 hours (Ferring Pharmaceuticals 2000). During administration of the bolus dose, transient nausea, vomiting, palpitations and headache may occur and the midwife must continue to monitor maternal and fetal condition closely. Any apparent adverse reaction must be reported to the doctor and the hospital pharmacist.

Nifedipine has the advantage of oral use and it is cheaper than atosiban. However, it has yet to be licensed in the UK for use as a tocolytic agent. Nifedipine is a calcium channel blocker which reduces muscle contraction by controlling the influx of calcium across the plasma membrane. Nifedipine is given orally, with a loading dose of 10–40 mg in the first hour, then 60–160 mg (slow release) daily until 34 weeks (Papatsonis et al 2000). However, at present, the balance of evidence indicates that atosiban is as effective as nifedipine and more effective than beta-adrenergic agonists and is safer than both (Lamont 2008).

Prostaglandin synthesis inhibitors, such as indometacin, may be used to arrest preterm labour. Maternal side-effects include nausea, vomiting, diarrhoea, dizziness and headaches. Long-term use may cause fetal effects, such as constriction of the ductus arteriosus, right-sided heart failure and fetal death. Contraindications are maternal infection, bleeding disorders, renal disease and peptic ulcers (Amon 1999).

Finally, glyceryl trinitrate (GTN) skin patches have been used as a method of suppressing preterm labour (Duckitt & Thornton 2002). There is yet insufficient evidence for any conclusions about its effectiveness compared with other tocolytics.

## Corticosteroids

A Cochrane meta-analysis of 18 randomized trials indicates that antenatal corticosteroid therapy reduces the incidence of respiratory distress syndrome (RDS) (see Ch. 45), neonatal death and intraventricular haemorrhage (Crowley 2002). Both dexamethasone and betamethasone can be used, but betamethasone is the steroid of choice (RCOG 2002a). Although a single course may be helpful in preventing neonatal respiratory disease, there is some doubt about the value of repeated courses (RCOG 2004).

There is also some evidence that repeated exposure to corticosteroids has deleterious effects. Measurable adrenal suppression has been found in women. Infants tend to be of lower than expected birthweight and (where corticosteroid therapy is continued after birth) there is an increased incidence of cerebral palsy. Corticosteroids should not be used where there is evidence of chorioamnionitis or tuberculosis (Helal et al 2000, Shinwell et al 2000). The use of antenatal corticosteroids in pregnancies complicated by maternal diabetes mellitus is presently recommended, but a significant reduction in rates of RDS has not been demonstrated. If commenced, inpatient supervision by an experienced diabetic/obstetric team is essential to regulate diabetic control (RCOG 2004).

## Monitoring

In all cases where drugs are used to suppress uterine activity, maternal and fetal condition must be closely observed. Continuous monitoring of uterine contractions and of the fetal heart rate should be carried out and recordings of maternal pulse and blood pressure made every 15 minutes. Side-effects of the drugs must also be recorded. If the dilatation of the os uteri reaches 4 cm or more or the membranes rupture, it is unlikely that the attempt to prevent labour progressing will be successful.

## Labour and delivery

If the labour progresses despite attempts to control it, the midwife must inform both an obstetrician and a paediatrician. Continuous monitoring of the uterine contractions and fetal heart are carried out and all tocolytic drugs are stopped. Fetal hypoxia due to cord compression may occur, particularly if the membranes have ruptured before the onset of labour. Amnio-infusion has been used to reduce cord compression following oligohydramnios, but this remains a contentious and relatively unevaluated technique (Enkin et al 2000).

It is essential that an accurate assessment of fetal presentation is made; many fetuses present by the breech prior to 34 weeks' gestation. An ultrasound scan may be helpful if the presentation is difficult to define.

There is little evidence that elective caesarean section produces better long-term outcomes for the baby (Grant 2000). Routine caesarean section for the delivery of preterm breech presentation is not advised (RCOG 2006b). Care must be exercised in the choice and timing of drugs given for pain relief. Epidural anaesthesia or the inhalation of nitrous oxide and oxygen are the preferred methods of pain relief as they have no adverse effect on the fetus. Analgesic drugs, especially morphine and its derivatives, should be given as sparingly as possible and avoided altogether within 3–4 hours of delivery, as they may severely depress the fetal respiratory centre. The midwife should be aware that recent use of tocolytic drugs may increase the risk of uterine atony during and following the third stage of labour.

A paediatrician should be present at delivery. Because of the poor ossification of the fetal skull, the infant is at risk of intracranial injury. However, there is no evidence in favour of routine elective episiotomy for the delivery of a preterm infant. The midwife should be guided by the circumstances of each particular birth. Equally, there is no evidence that elective forceps delivery reduces trauma (Enkin et al 2000). Ventouse delivery should be avoided because of the risk of vascular rupture and subsequent haemorrhage in an immature infant (Edebiri 1999).

The paediatrician will resuscitate the baby should it be necessary. The child should be given an injection of *phytomenadione* (Konakion) 0.5–1 mg IM (dosage depends on birthweight) to lessen any risk of haemorrhage. When the mother has seen and held her baby, the baby is transferred to the neonatal unit.

The midwife has a multifaceted role in caring for the woman, her baby and family during preterm labour and delivery. The first is the educative role in ensuring that the woman is in optimum health during pregnancy and that any deviations from the norm are identified and reported by the woman. The midwife provides the continuity and support through the stress of admission and preterm labour, ensuring that the woman and her family are both fully informed and as prepared as possible for the birth.

Preterm delivery is extremely stressful for the parents. The birth often comes as a shock and parents may be psychologically unprepared for a baby's arrival. Any feelings of joy are quickly submerged by fears for the child's health. Both parents need time to discuss the event and its implications with the midwife. This will include fears about immediate events and also about long-term prospects: there is significant morbidity, mortality and developmental delay in infants born weighing less than 750 g (Agustines et al 2000). The parents may also experience the grief of dashed expectations, both of the expected birth experience and of the healthy term baby. Again, the midwife can prepare the mother and her family for the normality of these feelings and assist them in coming to terms with the reality of preterm birth, and help them to develop their relationship with this new baby.

Colostrum and breast milk confer significant benefits to the preterm infant (Hodge & Puntis 2000) and the mother should be encouraged to breastfeed or express as soon as is possible. She will need a great deal of support from the midwife in establishing and maintaining lactation for her preterm baby.

The financial burden may be considerable if the infant is transferred to another hospital and the parents have to travel long distances to visit. In addition to this, there may be the needs of older children to consider. The midwife should not underestimate the stress which preterm birth causes to all the family. Viewing the preterm neonate and the family in context will assist the midwife in understanding and supporting the family appropriately.

**Reflective activity 60.3**

Consider the management of preterm labour and birth in your unit. Identify one midwifery strategy which could be implemented to improve either the experience or outcome of preterm birth.

**KEY POINTS**

- Preterm birth continues to be a major cause of perinatal death and morbidity.
- The pathophysiology of preterm birth is unclear and individual aetiology may include a range of interrelated factors.
- The midwife must be aware of the associated factors in order to provide optimum care for women at higher risk.

## REFERENCES


Agustines LA, Lin YG, Rumneu PJ, et al: Outcomes of extremely low-birth weight infants between 500 and 750g, *American Journal of Obstetrics and Gynecology* 182(5):1113–1116, 2000.

Amon E: Premature labour. In Reece E, Hobbins J, editors: *Medicine of the fetus and mother*, Philadelphia, 1999, Lippincott-Raven.

Carey J, Klebanoff M, Hauth J, et al: Metronidazole to prevent preterm delivery in pregnant women with asymptomatic bacterial vaginosis, *New England Journal of Medicine* 342(8):534–540, 2000.

Castle B, Turnbull A: The presence or absence of fetal breathing movements predicts the outcome of preterm labour, *The Lancet* ii(8348):471–472, 1983.

Colombo D: Predicting spontaneous preterm birth, *British Medical Journal* 325(7359):289–290, 2002.

Crowley P: Prophylactic corticosteroids for preterm birth, *Cochrane Database of Systematic Reviews* (4):CD000065, 2002.

Duckitt K, Thornton S: Nitric oxide donors for the treatment of preterm labour, *Cochrane Database of Systematic Reviews* (3):CD002860, 2002.

Edebiri A: Is the vacuum safe for preterm vaginal delivery? *Journal of Maternal-Fetal Medicine* 8(5):234–235, 1999.

El Bastawissi A, Williams M, Riley D, et al: Amniotic fluid interleukin-6 and preterm delivery: a review, *Obstetrics and Gynecology* 95(6 Pt 2):1056–1064, 2000.

Enkin M, Keirse MJNC, Neilson J, et al: *A guide to effective care in pregnancy and childbirth*, Oxford, 2000, Oxford University Press.

Ferring Pharmaceuticals: *Tractocile resource pack*, Langley, 2000, Ferring Pharmaceuticals.

Goldenberg R, Hauth J, Andrews W: Intrauterine infection and preterm delivery, *New England Journal of Medicine* 342(20):1500–1507, 2000.

Grant A: Elective versus selective caesarean section for delivery of the small baby, *Cochrane Database of Systematic Reviews* (2):CD000078, 2000.

Gyetvai K, Hannah M, Hodnett E, et al: Tocolytics for preterm labor: a systematic review, *Obstetrics and Gynecology* 94(5 Pt 2) 869–877, 1999.

Helal K, Gordon M, Lightener C, et al: Adrenal suppression induced by betamethasone in women at risk of premature delivery, *Obstetrics and Gynecology* 96(2):287–290, 2000.

Hodge D, Puntis J: The use of expressed breast milk for the premature newborn, *Clinical Nutrition* 19(2):75–77, 2000.

King J, Flenardy V: Antibiotics for preterm labour with intact membranes, *Cochrane Database of Systematic Reviews* (2):CD000246, 2000.

Kovacevich G, Gaich S, Lavin J, et al: The prevalence of thromboembolic events among women with extended bed rest prescribed as part of the treatment for premature labor or preterm premature rupture of membranes, *American Journal of Obstetrics and Gynecology* 182(5):1089–1092, 2000.

Lamont R: The choice of a tocolytic for the treatment of preterm labor: a critical evaluation of nifedipine versus atosiban. In *Expert Opinion on Investigational Drugs Online*. www.informapharmascience.com/doi/abs/10.1517/13543784.16.6.843. 2008. Accessed December 22, 2008.

Lockwood C, Senyei A, Dishe M, et al: Fetal fibronectin in cervical and vaginal secretions as a predictor of preterm delivery, *New England Journal of Medicine* 325(10):669–674, 1991.

Minakami H, Kosuge S, Fujiwara H, et al: Risk of premature birth in multifetal pregnancy, *Twin Research* 3(1):2–6, 2000.

Oakley A: Can social support influence pregnancy outcome? *British Journal of Obstetrics and Gynaecology* 96(3):260–262, 1989.

Papatsonis D, Kok J, Van Geijn H, et al: Neonatal effects of nifedipine and ritodrine for preterm labor, *Obstetrics and Gynecology* 95(4):477–481, 2000.

Royal College of Obstetricians and Gynaecologists (RCOG): *Tocolytic drugs for women in preterm labour*, Green top guidelines, London, 2002a, RCOG.

Royal College of Obstetricians and Gynaecologists (RCOG): *Intrauterine infection and perinatal brain injury*, Scientific Advisory Committee Opinion Paper 3, London, 2002b, RCOG.

Royal College of Obstetricians and Gynaecologists (RCOG): *Antenatal corticosteroids to prevent respiratory distress syndrome*, Green top guidelines no. 7, London, 2004, RCOG.

Royal College of Obstetricians and Gynaecologists (RCOG): *Preterm prelabour rupture of membranes*, Green top guidelines, London, 2006a, RCOG.

Royal College of Obstetricians and Gynaecologists (RCOG): *The management of breech presentation*, Green top guidelines, London, 2006b, RCOG.

Schieve L, Cogswell M, Scanlon K, et al: Pre-pregnancy body mass index and pregnancy weight gain: associations with preterm delivery, *Obstetrics and Gynecology* 96(2):194–200, 2000.

Shah N, Bracken M: A systematic review and meta-analysis of prospective studies on the association between maternal cigarette smoking and preterm delivery, *American Journal of Obstetrics and Gynecology* 182(2):465–472, 2000.

Shinwell E, Karplus M, Reich D, et al: Early postnatal dexamethasone treatment and increased incidence of cerebral palsy, *Archives of Disease in Childhood Fetal and Neonatal Edition* 83(3):F177–F181, 2000.

Shumway J, O'Campo P, Gielen A, et al: Preterm labor, placental abruption and premature rupture of membranes in relation to maternal violence or verbal abuse, *Journal of Maternal-Fetal Medicine* 8(3):76–80, 1999.

Silver R, Ware Branch D: Sporadic and recurrent pregnancy loss. In Reece E, Hobbins J, editors: *Medicine of the fetus and mother*, Philadelphia, 1999, Lippincott-Raven.

Smith-Levitin M, Skupski D, Chervenak F: Multifetal pregnancies: epidemiology, clinical characteristics and management. In Reece E, Hobbins J, editors: *Medicine of the fetus and mother*, Philadelphia, 1999, Lippincott-Raven.

Steer P: The epidemiology of preterm labour, *British Journal of Obstetrics and Gynaecology* 112(Suppl 1):1–3, 2005.

Walkinshaw S: Preterm labour and delivery of the preterm infant. In Chamberlain G, editor: *Turnbull's obstetrics*, London, 1995, Churchill Livingstone.

Worldwide Atosiban versus Beta-agonists Study Group: Effectiveness and safety of the oxytocin antagonist atosiban versus beta-adrenergic agonists in the treatment of preterm labour, *British Journal of Obstetrics and Gynaecology* 108(2):133–142, 2001.

Chapter |61|

# Procedures in obstetrics

Stephanie Meakin

## LEARNING OUTCOMES

After reading this chapter, you will be able to:

- reflect upon your own practice to assess any aspects that may influence operative delivery rates
- explore local protocols, policies and guidelines that may have the potential to impact on the increasing operative delivery rates
- examine the information given to women regarding their choices in labour and delivery
- ensure that appropriate and effective care is provided for women experiencing instrumental and operative deliveries
- ensure that the most appropriate and relevant post-delivery care is provided for both mother and baby.

## INTRODUCTION

A baby may enter the world spontaneously through the mother's vagina, with only the occasional need for guidance from attendants, by operative means with the use of forceps, vacuum extraction, or by caesarean section. Yet rates for normal birth have seemingly fallen over the previous two decades. The Healthcare Commission review of the maternity services (Healthcare Commission 2008) revealed normal birth rates in maternity units are as low as between 32% and 40%. Whilst there are some areas where home births are increasing and despite admirable drives by a small number of celebrities, many midwives and various pressure groups, instrumental delivery rates continue to increase annually along with caesarean sections. It might be considered that, soon, spontaneous vaginal delivery will no longer be the accepted normal route.

The following chapter explores some of the issues for midwives within the trends of increasing operative deliveries, including the impact that this can have on women's and children's health. The sections on instrumental and caesarean style deliveries will begin with the morbidity associated with them. Indications for each type of delivery will be listed, followed by a brief exploration of aspects of care given to the woman in labour that may have the potential to increase the need for an instrumental or an operative delivery. The midwife's role in providing the most effective and appropriate care for any woman undergoing an instrumental or an operative delivery will be discussed.

## OPERATIVE VAGINAL DELIVERIES

Forceps and ventouse extraction have the potential to safely remove the infant and mother from a hazardous situation (Dennen & Hayashi 2005), and even to save lives. Taking this into consideration, however, the increase in their use has an impact on the health of women and their babies. Highest rates of trauma are consistently observed with operative procedures, with short-term and long-term morbidity.

### Neonatal complications

After any instrumental vaginal delivery, the baby may suffer hypoxia, have lower Apgar scores and require appropriate resuscitation. Facial or scalp abrasions or bruising are common. A cephalhaematoma may develop because of friction between the fetal head and pelvis or forceps blade, as well as from the suction of the ventouse cup. There may be an increase in jaundice due to reabsorption of haemoglobin associated with this bruising (Dennen & Hayashi 2005). Facial palsy, which is usually temporary, may occur owing to the compression of the facial nerve which runs anteriorly to the ear, by the forceps blade. Intracranial trauma and haemorrhage is higher amongst infants delivered by vacuum extraction, forceps or caesarean section (Towner et al 1999). In more rare circumstances, tentorial tears and rupture of the great vein of Galen may occur, leading to bleeding and compression of the brainstem. Skull fractures are usually linear but occasionally a depressed fracture can result in a subarachnoid haemorrhage. Kielland's forceps can cause unexplained convulsions. Retinal haemorrhages are more common in vacuum extraction deliveries (Vacca 1996). The most serious complication to occur is that of subgaleal haemorrhage.

### Maternal complications

The most common injuries to the genital tract are cervical, vaginal and perineal tears, haematomas and rectal lacerations (see Ch. 40). Bladder or urethral injury may occur, causing urinary retention and even the formation of a fistula. Perineal pain due to bruising, oedema, trauma and episiotomy can impair sexual function and infant feeding. Pelvic floor disorders and long-term pelvic floor morbidity are strongly associated with instrumental delivery (Bahl et al 2005). There is an increased risk of haemorrhage (Walsh 2000). A rare complication is that the cervix and lower segment of the uterus may be damaged.

The psychological effects of instrumental delivery may include fear and anxiety in relation to subsequent pregnancy, and feelings of failure, inadequacy and disappointment. Both forceps and ventouse-assisted deliveries were found to be predictive factors of acute trauma symptoms and post-traumatic stress disorder as a result of women's birth experiences (Creedy et al 2000). Jolly et al (1999) concluded that caesarean section and vaginal instrumental birth are associated with voluntary and involuntary infertility as many mothers may be left with fearful feelings about future childbirth: 13% more of women who had a caesarean section and 6% more of those who had instrumental births had not had a second child compared with those following normal birth.

**Reflective activity 61.1**

Owing to the maternal and neonatal morbidity associated with instrumental deliveries, it appears appropriate for all midwives to reflect in and on their own practice to ensure that aspects of care for women in normal labour are not increasing the possibility of operative deliveries. Take time to explore your beliefs regarding the points for midwifery practice below. Each time you care for a woman who requires an instrumental delivery or an emergency caesarean section, reflect upon the course of her labour to assess whether there were any aspects of her care that may have contributed to the outcome. Record your thoughts for future reference.

## Key aspects of midwifery practice

Some critical consideration of aspects of care may enable the midwife to plan care to ensure the woman's comfort and safety and also to reduce the need for intervention and augmentation. This has wide-ranging implications for the quality of care and for effective use of both human and other resources within the service. It is also crucial that the midwife work in partnership with the woman to ensure that she is informed and fully prepared for the labour and birth.

### Policies

Blanket policies to treat prolonged labour and 'failure to progress' should be examined as there is much literature available to explore long-held beliefs of the definition of the duration and progress of labour. Even in 1973, when medicalization was really taking control of childbirth, Studd (1973) questioned the arbitrary application of time limits on labour considering the confusion over the diagnosis of the onset of active labour. Yet this confusion remains and time limits for stages of labour remain in place.

### Position for labour and delivery

An upright position, preferably mobile, assists the woman to feel in control, can reduce her distress and help her to adopt comfortable positions more easily. During a review of trials for The Cochrane Library, Gupta & Nikoderm (2001) highlighted that adopting upright positions in labour appeared to reduce the number of assisted deliveries and fewer abnormal fetal heart rate patterns were noted (see Chs 36 and 37).

### Diet, fasting and nutrition

Fasting women throughout a normal labour can add to exhaustion, as labour is a time of great energy demand and it is estimated that a labouring woman may require 800–1100 kcal/hour (Ludka & Roberts 1993). Whilst women adapt to a small rise of ketones in labour, blood pH can be reduced in starving women and result in ketoacidosis. Even as far back as the 1960s, Mark (1961) discovered that uterine activity was influenced by environmental pH and that myometrial cells spontaneously contract with increased alkalinity, preferably between 7.8 and 7.1. Ketones that build up may also cross the placenta, and if there is an accumulation in the fetus, this can affect fetal wellbeing and fetal activity (Swift 1991).

### Supportive presence during labour

A Cochrane review highlights that the presence of an appropriate support person throughout labour is associated with a decreased incidence of epidural anaesthesia, dystocia and instrumental deliveries (Hodnett 2001).

### Amniotomy and Syntocinon

Amniotomy can increase the requirement for instrumental delivery and caesarean section (Johnson et al 1997). It is recognized that amniotomy causes fetal heart abnormalities owing to cord and head compression, which then increases the risk of interventions. It can inhibit the rotation of some malpositions – for example, occipitoposterior positions – which may predispose to delay. There is an increase in pain during contractions, which may, in turn, increase the demand for epidural analgesia. Syntocinon reduces the oxygen supply to the baby's brain. The fetus may then display signs of fetal distress, increasing the need to dramatically shorten the labour (O'Regan 1998).

### Pain relief

Epidurals are associated with a substantially increased use of assisted vaginal delivery (Mander 1994). Epidurals increase the length of the first and second stages, often affecting the efficacy of contractions, increasing the need for Syntocinon (Page 2000).

## Indications for the use of assisted vaginal delivery

The following short list is not absolute but meant to give a general idea of the most common indications for the use of forceps or vacuum extraction during the second stage of labour:

- when a shortening of the second stage of labour is required, most frequently due to maternal distress/exhaustion
- fetal jeopardy
- to spare the mother muscular effort, as is necessary in medically significant indications including cardiopulmonary or vascular conditions.

## Contraindications to instrumental delivery

- Unengaged head
- Malpresentation (face/brow)
- Inability to define position
- Fetal macrosomia (>4–4.5 kg estimated weight, especially in maternal diabetes)
- Inexperienced operator.

## If an instrumental delivery is necessary

The woman and her companion are likely to be extremely apprehensive once the need for an instrumental delivery is recommended. When the midwife has summoned the appropriate personnel, who will preferably include a senior obstetrician, a paediatrician and another person who can assist with assembling equipment, there will be several strangers in the room. Midwives then have to prioritize the care they give and, where possible, involve other members of the team to assist the doctors rather than leave the woman's side. Midwives must remember that they remain the woman's advocate and must be present to explain all the procedures, support, encourage and ensure that there is a respectful environment within the delivery room. There should be little discussion in the room that does not include the woman.

### Procedure

- Prior to the procedure, consent should be obtained from the woman. This will require full but simple explanation and rationale of the procedures being provided to the woman, which may require the presence of a translator.
- An abdominal examination is performed to check lie, presentation, position and descent of the fetus and that uterine contractions are satisfactory.
- Adequate analgesia/anaesthesia must be considered.

Prior to the delivery, the mother is helped into the lithotomy position. The midwife must ensure that the woman is covered with a sheet as much as possible and for as long as possible, to protect her dignity. Both legs are flexed simultaneously and gently onto the abdomen, and the feet moved to the outer sides of the supports and placed in the leg rests or stirrups together to avoid *sacroiliac strain*. To prevent obstruction of venous return and possible thrombosis by pressure, care is taken to ensure that the legs are fully abducted. Once the mother is correctly positioned, the foot part of the bed is lowered and the mother's buttocks lifted to the edge of the bed. The operator can now proceed.

- The bladder is emptied by means of a catheter.
- A vaginal examination is performed to ensure that the cervix is fully dilated and that the membranes are ruptured, the position and station of the fetal head is defined, the degree of moulding is ascertained and there is a final check that there is no presence of cephalopelvic disproportion.

- Checks are made that necessary equipment is present, correct and in good working condition.
- A paediatrician should be in attendance for the delivery (where possible).
- Checks are made that neonatal resuscitation equipment is available, clean and in good working order (see Ch. 45). The resuscitaire, including the overhead heater, should be switched on.

### Ventouse vs forceps

Debate exists over the preferred instrument for vaginal delivery once it is believed to be necessary. There are two methods for instrumental delivery: forceps and vacuum (ventouse) extraction. A Cochrane systematic review of nine randomized controlled studies involving 2849 primiparous and multiparous women compared vacuum extractions with forceps. Ventouse appears to be significantly more likely to fail at achieving a vaginal delivery, but is less likely to produce maternal trauma and less likely to be associated with severe perineal pain. However, it does produce increased rates of cephalhaematoma, retinal haemorrhages and low Apgar scores at 5 minutes. There appeared no difference in long-term outcome between the two instruments (Johanson & Menon 2000).

## Forceps

Forceps were first described in 400 BC by Hippocrates to extract dead fetuses. From a birthroom scene on a marble relief, it would appear that forceps were also used in Roman times, but in modern history the use of forceps as an aid to vaginal delivery has been known only since their invention by the Chamberlen family in the 1600s (Pearson 1981). The family tried to keep the nature of their instruments a secret, as these forceps offered a practical possibility of live births from obstructed labours and were a source of fame and money to those who used them.

Since the introduction of forceps, many attempts have been made to improve the efficacy and safety of the instrument for specific obstetrical situations and the shortcomings of current forceps design is acknowledged. In fact, the blades of some designs were designed for delivery of the long ovoid moulded head, which was a common shape adapted from prolonged labour. As a result of present-day care, this shape is less frequently seen and the head is less moulded and more spherical (Hibbard 1989).

Forceps may be used in two ways: *to exert traction without rotation*; and to correct malposition, for example, occipito-posterior position, *by rotation prior to traction*. Rotation is rarely performed now owing to the trauma to the mother and the baby (Figs 61.1 and 61.2). There are definitive texts available (see website) which outline the procedures for forceps delivery, but here it would appear more pertinent to discuss certain principles for all types of the delivery.

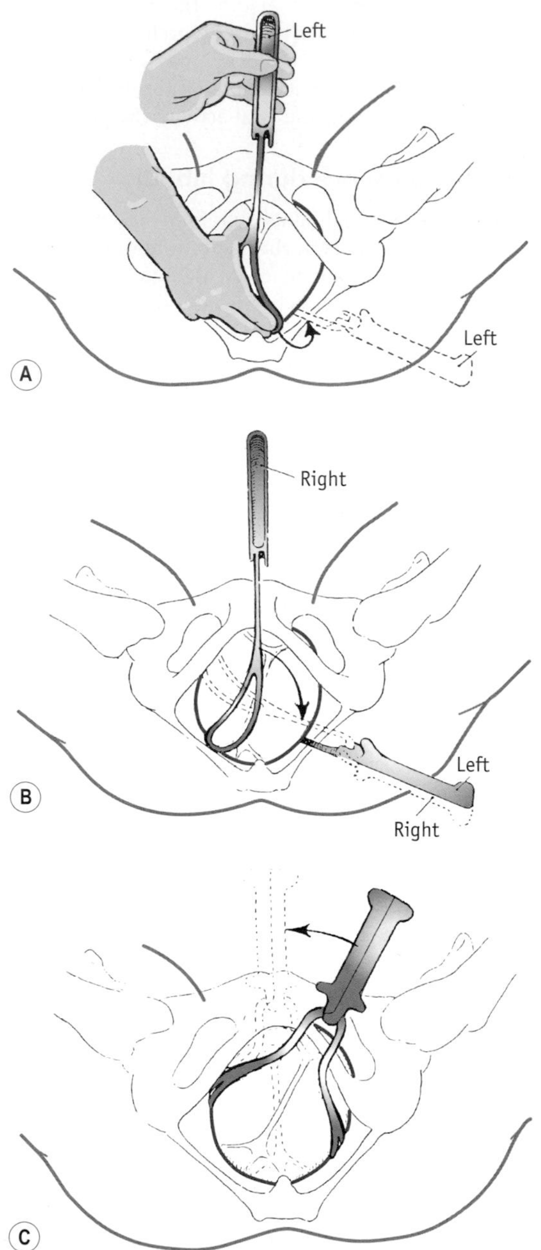


**Figure 61.1** Forceps application. *(From Dennen & Hayashi 1999)*

## Vacuum extraction

Vacuum extraction is a method of instrumental delivery which involves the use of a vacuum device as a traction instrument to assist delivery. The technique was developed from early work by Young, a Royal Navy surgeon in 1705, and Simpson in the 1840s (Chamberlain 1989). The

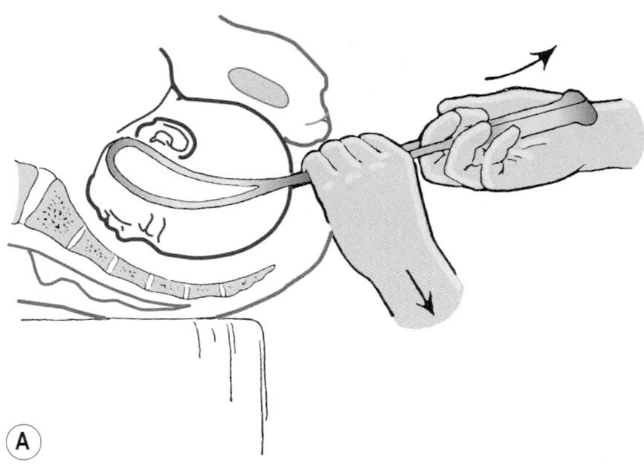

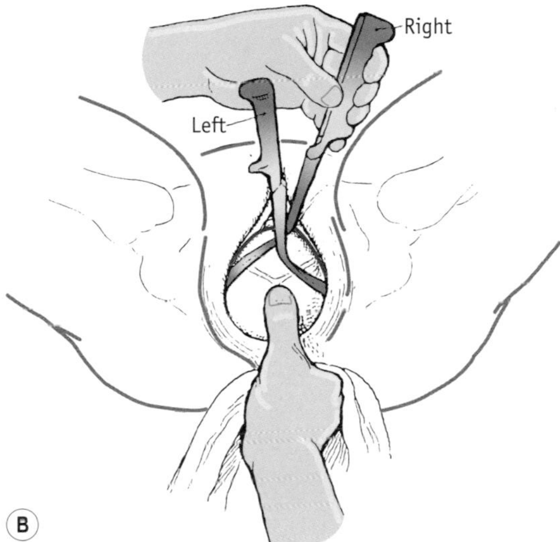


**Figure 61.2** **A.** Traction. **B.** Removal of forceps. *(From Dennen & Hayashi 1999)*

modern version was developed by Malmstrom in the 1950s.

The vacuum extractor or ventouse consists of a cup made of metal or soft material, such as silicone rubber, a traction device and a vacuum system providing negative pressure, by which the cup is attached to the fetal scalp. For equipment and procedure, see Figure 61.3.

The cups were originally metal, but the softer caps which have been available since the early 1980s are proving more popular. Previously, the metal cup formed a 'chignon', but now the soft cup relies on covering a larger surface area in order to develop sufficient traction, and this has led to less scalp trauma.

Contraindications specific to ventouse and in addition to those listed above for all instrumental deliveries are:

- malpresentations; for example, face, brow, breech
- preterm labour at less than 36 weeks' gestation
- suspected fetal coagulopathy.

**Reflective activity 61.2**

Reflect on the last instrumental delivery that you attended. Consider whether you felt that you adequately prepared:

- the woman
- her partner
- the equipment.

Looking through the information here, what would you have done differently?

## Postnatal care

At delivery, if the baby's condition permits, he or she should be given to the mother immediately. If resuscitation is required, then as soon as the condition is satisfactory, the baby should be given to the mother with relevant explanation for any necessary procedures that were undertaken. If the baby is transferred to the neonatal intensive care unit, then the parents must be kept informed of the baby's condition and taken to visit as soon as possible. Once the doctors have left, the midwife should ensure that the parents have a quiet and protected time to recover and develop a relationship with their baby.

Postnatal observations will be as for any delivery, but particular attention should be paid to pain from perineal trauma, urinary output in case any damage has occurred to the bladder, and signs of postpartum haemorrhage due to uterine atony and trauma. Particular requirements may include analgesia and assistance with feeding owing to discomfort. It is also important to observe the neonate for any sign of trauma, and ensure that a thorough, careful examination is carried out, with appropriate referral should any deviations from the normal be noted. Owing to the possible link discussed earlier with acute trauma symptoms and post-traumatic stress disorder, there must be an opportunity for the midwife to review with the woman, her experience, and discuss any concerns regarding the intervention and the procedure with the parents. It is also an appropriate time to ensure that the woman is assured that she did not 'fail'.

# CAESAREAN SECTION

Caesarean section is the delivery of the fetus, placenta and membranes through a surgical incision in the abdominal wall and uterus. There are two types of caesarean section:

- *Lower segment caesarean section* (LSCS) is most frequently performed through a suprapubic

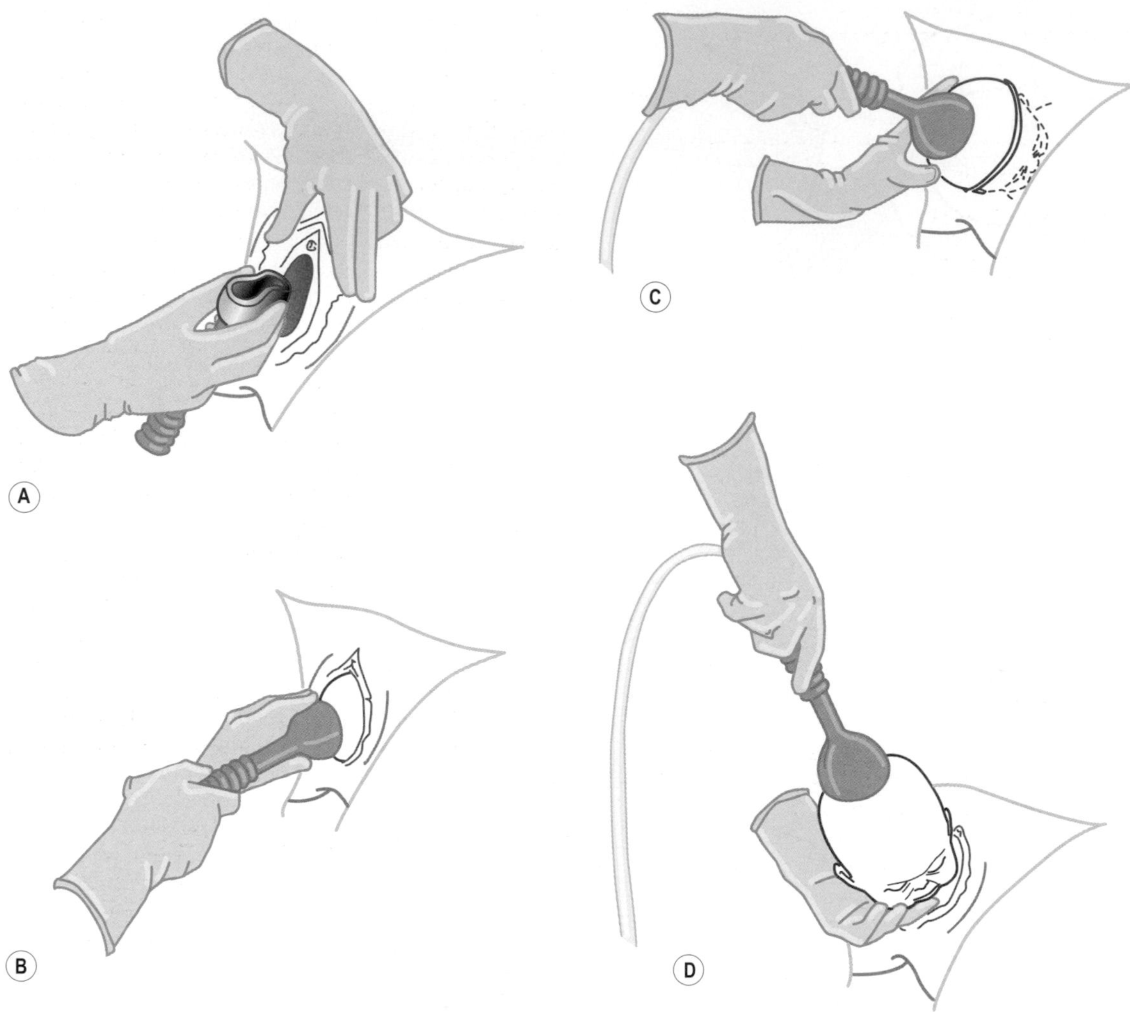


**Figure 61.3** Application and delivery with ventouse. *(From Dennen & Hayashi 1999)*

(Pfannenstiel) transverse incision. This is the method of choice as there is a low incidence of wound dehiscence togther with an excellent cosmetic appearance (Dickinson 2005). Occasionally, a midline vertical incision proves necessary, as it allows rapid access and can be enlarged without difficulty.

- *Classical upper segment caesarean section* involves a longitudinal incision in the upper uterine segment and is rarely performed, because of the higher risk of scar rupture in a subsequent pregnancy (incidence 2.2%). It may be used in the case of a major degree of placenta praevia, cervical carcinoma, lower segment uterine myomas, or for the delivery of preterm infants prior to the 28th week when the lower uterine segment has not fully formed (Crichton et al 1991).

The increasing caesarean section rate in the UK is attributed to a variety of causes in varying sources of literature. These include delivery of preterm infants now likely to survive with good neonatal care, avoidance of litigation, lack of staff on maternity units, maternal request, increased medicalization of childbirth, increased induction rate, and individual obstetrician's preferences in their practice. The Sentinel study also illustrates that the caesarean rate is raised in older women, black African or Caribbean women, previous caesarean section, and breech presentation and multiple pregnancy (Thomas & Parenjothy 2001) (Table 61.1). It was suggested that in all of these categories, there may be an increased risk of complications requiring such intervention.

Caesarean section is a major surgical procedure and, in a small number of cases, it can save both neonatal and

**Table 61.1 Indications for caesarean section**

| Indications | Caesarean section rate |
|---|---|
| Fetal distress/abnormal CTG | 22% |
| Failure to progress/induction | 20.4% |
| Previous caesarean section | 13.8% |
| Breech position | 10.8% |
| Maternal request | 7.3% |
| Malpresentations | 3.4% |
| Placenta praevia/bleeding | 2.2% |
| Pre-eclampsia/eclampsia/HELLP | 2.3% |
| Multiple pregnancy | 1.2% |
| (Thomas & Parenjothy 2001) | |

maternal lives, improve outcome for some babies who may have undergone extended labour, and reduce the potential risks of infection associated with some vaginal deliveries (Duff 2000). Nevertheless, though the caesarean section rates have significantly increased, maternal and neonatal mortality do not appear to be decreasing and, indeed, neonatal and maternal morbidity is increasing. Hillan (2000) realized from available figures that 9–15% of women delivered by caesarean section suffer serious maternal morbidity, whilst another 65% did not feel fully recovered until 3 months after caesarean section.

There is a plethora of literature highlighting the morbidity and the increased risk of mortality associated with caesarean section. Physical effects range from tiredness, backache, sleeping difficulties and depression, to wound and urinary tract infection (Hillan 2000). There is an increased risk of haemorrhage, thromboembolism, peripartum hysterectomy, future miscarriages, ectopic pregnancies, placenta abruptio and praevia, and reduced fertility (Wagner 2000). Some mothers experience a sense of loss or failure because they have been unable to deliver their baby vaginally. Psychological effects of caesarean section include extreme disappointment, intense anxiety, and a sense of inadequacy and failure, and may include acute trauma symptoms or post-traumatic stress disorder as previously associated with instrumental delivery (Creedy et al 2000). There appears little difference between emergency or elective surgery.

## Risks of caesarean section to the fetus

Owing to maternal cardiovascular changes, especially with spinal anaesthesia, low Apgar scores and relative fetal acidosis may occur. Later, respiratory distress may develop, which is usually due to transient tachypnoea of the newborn (see Chs 41 and 45), the incidence being four times greater in babies delivered by elective caesarean section than in those who are delivered vaginally. This is thought to be due to the lack of catecholamines being produced by the mother, which would normally cross the placenta and 'switch off' the production of lung fluid by the fetal lung pneumocytes. It was thought that at birth there was an excess of up to 30 mL of fluid which may not have been absorbed by the lymphocytes, or by 'vaginal squeezing' as would happen during a vaginal birth, and therefore the neonate needs to cry lustily at birth to assist the absorption of this excess lung fluid (Strang 1991). However, it is now thought that there is only about 35% of this fluid at term, and that it is absorbed through the lymphatics and changes in the pulmonary blood flow (Blackburn 2007), and that the vaginal squeeze has a minor effect on fluid clearance.

Annibale et al (1995) concluded in their study that abdominal delivery following an uncomplicated pregnancy remains a risk factor for adverse neonatal outcome. During a conference in 1999 entitled *The rising caesarean section rate: a public health issue*, a neonatologist came to the conclusion that babies should only be born by caesarean section if they are very large, in a difficult position or known to have a mother with a serious viral condition such as HIV (Duff 2000).

## Indications for caesarean section

Examples of some indications for caesarean section include the following:

- hypertensive disorders, for example, pre-eclampsia and eclampsia
- fetal distress
- failure or delay to progress in labour
- malpresentations, such as breech, brow or shoulder presentations, but a breech presentation may be delivered vaginally if there is no suspected cephalopelvic disproportion or other complications
- previous or predicted shoulder dystocia
- prolapse of the umbilical cord in the first stage of labour
- antepartum haemorrhage due to severe abruption or placenta praevia
- major cephalopelvic disproportion
- severe intrauterine growth restriction
- severe rhesus isoimmunization
- active herpes genitalis
- maternal HIV infection
- previous vaginal reconstruction surgery
- pelvic tumours, for example, cervical myomas (fibroids)
- fetal abnormality, for example, hydrocephalus, gastroschisis.

### Implications for midwifery practice

Whilst the majority of the list above appears appropriate for caesarean section, there is an increase of caesarean section due to 'failure to progress' and fetal distress. It would be advantageous now to revisit the areas discussed earlier in relation to instrumental delivery as they are also relevant to caesarean section. Additional points to be considered include:

- Early amniotomy is associated with an increased risk of caesarean section (Segal et al 1999).
- The use of continuous electronic fetal monitoring during labour can lead to an increase in caesarean sections and instrumental delivery. Thacker & Stroup (2000) reviewed the effects of routine electronic fetal monitoring during labour compared with intermittent auscultation. The review included 58,855 women in 10 clinical trials, and showed that there was no change in perinatal deaths or neonatal unit admissions and there was no evidence that cerebral palsy was reduced.

**Reflective activity 61.3**

How do you normally gauge whether a woman is in the active stage of labour? Is this normally by examination or by maternal behaviour? If you were unable to examine the woman, how would you measure her progress?

### Midwife's role

Whether surgery is an emergency or elective procedure, the midwife should ensure that the woman understands the reasons for surgery and that a written consent form is obtained for the operation.

A sample of venous blood must be collected for full blood count, haemoglobin level and cross-matching. The woman should be dressed in a theatre gown and wearing identification labels. Antiembolic (TED) stockings should be applied. It is preferable that the woman is not wearing any make-up to ensure that the anaesthetist can observe her colour, that jewellery is taped or removed for safety reasons because of the use of diathermy during the procedure, and that her pubic area has been shaved, removing as little as absolutely necessary for the incision.

#### *In theatre*

Along with the usual theatre staff, a paediatrician will be present for each case and the midwife will usually assist at the resuscitaire after receiving the baby at delivery. It is preferable that the anaesthetist can meet, examine and discuss any procedures with the woman prior to the surgery, although this may not be possible in emergency circumstances. The anaesthetist will be fully involved with the woman once in theatre but the midwife should remain with her and her partner as support for both of them. Operating theatres can be quite frightening areas to be in. The fetal heart will still require frequent auscultation, and this must be recorded.

## Anaesthesia

General anaesthesia in obstetric women is fraught with difficulties. One of the complications which may occur during anaesthesia is acid aspiration syndrome, which may be reduced through cricoid pressure during intubation (see website for more detailed information). The problems also include raised maternal intragastric pressure; acidity of gastric contents; aortocaval occlusion if the supine position is employed; the adverse effects on the fetus of the drugs used, or of maternal hypoxia or hypotension; placental insufficiency; and intrapartum fetal hypoxia. These problems are exacerbated in the case of preterm infants, or in the woman whose condition is poor, that is, if she is eclamptic.

Intubation in the pregnant woman may be difficult because of the posture of the neck in pregnancy or laryngeal oedema in cases of pregnancy-induced hypertension.

To minimize the risk of supine hypotensive syndrome, the operating table is tilted laterally, or the woman is wedged at a lateral tilt until the infant is delivered. A foot cushion is usually employed to elevate the legs from the table to avoid venous stasis in the calf muscles; other means, such as TED stockings, should be used to avoid the risk of venous thrombosis. The bladder will be emptied and a catheter inserted which will remain in place during the procedure. The fetal heart will be listened to prior to surgery.

### Spinal (subarachnoid) and epidural anaesthesia

Many caesarean sections are now performed under epidural or spinal, rather than general, anaesthesia (see Ch. 38). This removes the risks associated with general anaesthesia and enables the mother to see and hold her baby at birth. It is reported that this method is superior in facilitating the mother–baby relationship. The partner may be present so that he can be supportive to the mother and share in the experience.

This text is inappropriate for discussion of either epidural or spinal anaesthesia in depth and the reader is recommended to visit anaesthesia textbooks to explore the technicalities further.

## Immediate postoperative care

If the woman is awake, the midwife should ensure that the baby is shown to her as soon as possible. If the baby does not require resuscitation following delivery, opportunity for the mother to hold and touch her baby as soon as possible should be actively encouraged (see below).

In the immediate postoperative recovery period, regardless of the method of anaesthesia, pulse, blood pressure, respirations, colour, state of consciousness, vaginal loss, wound dressing, catheter and wound drainage are observed, as appropriate. If the woman has had a general anaesthetic, extubation is performed. This involves removal of the endotracheal tube once reflexes have returned, suction is carried out and the operating table is tilted head down. Vigilance at this stage is important as the woman may not be fully conscious and inhalation of gastric contents may still occur. The woman is placed on her side to maintain the airway, assist drainage of secretions and prevent airway obstruction by the tongue.

Infusion of intravenous fluids is monitored and recorded on the anaesthetic sheet. An analgesic may be administered for pain relief. When the woman's postoperative condition is satisfactory, the anaesthetist will give permission for her to be discharged to the care of the ward staff. Instructions and details of the surgery and anaesthetic are recorded in the notes and given to the receiving midwife.

## Maternal–infant attachment

The baby is received by the midwife and any resuscitative measures are carried out by a paediatrician, or by a midwife skilled in neonatal resuscitation. However, if the mother is conscious and the baby appears well at birth, the baby should be given to the mother immediately. There are many maternity units now that actively encourage breastfeeding in the theatre if the mother wishes it, and skin-to-skin contact if it is safe and convenient so to do. A preterm or ill baby will be admitted to the neonatal unit for special or intensive care. The parents will naturally be very anxious if their baby requires such care and should be encouraged to visit as soon as possible. The neonatal unit staff often take photographs of the baby to give to the parents when visiting is difficult.

## Record keeping

Accurate and contemporaneous records are made of all observations and treatments. The midwife responsible for the care of mother and baby will give a detailed handover report to the ward midwife. This report will include the condition of the mother and the baby at birth, including the care and any treatment given before transfer to the ward or, in the case of a sick or preterm baby, to the neonatal unit. This information will enable all staff involved with the mother and baby during the early postnatal period to give appropriate care and support.

## Postnatal observations

There is a high risk of postpartum haemorrhage, adding to the amount of blood lost during the operation. The uterus may not contract effectively and there is the very serious complication of the unsuspected continuation of intraperitoneal bleeding after the operation. The following observations and care routines are guidelines only, but denote safe and best practice:

- *Pulse and blood pressure*: These should be checked every 15 minutes for the first 2 hours, then every 30 minutes for the next 2 hours, reducing to hourly for 2 hours, 2-hourly for 2 days, then 4-hourly for 3 days.
- *Temperature*: This should be recorded twice daily for the first 3 days, then daily, because of the frequency of infection following caesarean section. Other symptoms of infection vary according to the virulence of the organisms involved. A mild uterine infection would present on about the 3rd postnatal day with a raised temperature and pulse rate, subinvolution of the uterus, and profuse red, offensive lochia. If untreated, it may cause peritonitis, and the danger signs, for which the midwife should be constantly alert, include a rising pulse rate, pyrexia, vomiting, and abdominal pain and distension.
- *Intravenous line*: It should be ensured that this is patent and effective whilst it is in situ to assist with fluid administration until the woman maintains her own fluid balance and provide an emergency line should there be a haemorrhage.
- *Vaginal loss*: Check for excessive bleeding and wound loss on the dressing at each observation.
- *Pain relief*: Adequate relief must be offered frequently, acknowledging that the woman has undergone major abdominal surgery. Initially, pain relief may be administered in the form of intramuscular opiates, for example, morphia, but later, suppositories or oral analgesics will be given, as required, within prescribed limits.
- *Nutritional intake*: Oral fluids are offered soon after the operation. A light diet can be commenced when the woman feels ready to eat, unless the surgeon requests that food is withheld until bowel sounds are heard, usually if the bowel has been handled excessively during surgery. Intravenous fluids are then maintained until bowel sounds are heard and the woman has begun to eat. *Paralytic ileus* frequently accompanies peritonitis and is recognized by an inability to pass flatus or have the bowels open because the bowel has become paralysed. This is a very serious complication. Antibiotic drugs are given to overcome the infection. Because the absorption of fluids and nutrients from the paralysed intestinal tract is disrupted, fluids, electrolytes and glucose are given intravenously until the condition is resolved. Aspiration of the stomach with a Ryle's tube is

necessary until the paralytic ileus recovers and the mother is able to take fluids by mouth without vomiting.

- *Urinary output*: A urinary catheter, if in situ, is removed as per the surgeon's recommendations. However, even without a catheter, fluid balance should be observed for the first 3 days as the woman may be actually passing urine but not in significant amounts, leaving a residual amount in the bladder.
- *Activity:* Antiembolic stockings, early ambulation, and active and passive leg exercises are encouraged to help reduce the incidence of deep vein thrombosis. There is always a possibility of pulmonary embolism whenever a laparotomy has been performed. Collapse and even sudden death may occur from this serious complication, often between the 10th and 14th postoperative days.
- *Hygiene*: A bed bath and a vulval toilet are still enjoyed by women following a caesarean section. They should have an opportunity to clean their teeth and put on fresh and light clothing. The dressing is usually removed on the following day and the woman is assisted with a shower and afterwards shown how to dry the wound. She will be encouraged to shower daily when she can manage safely alone.
- *Wound care*: This includes inspection and, if a drain is present, it is shortened and removed according to the doctor's instructions. If clips or non-absorbable skin sutures have been used, they too will be removed at a time directed by the surgeon, usually about the 5th postoperative day. If possible, the woman should be encouraged to expose the wound to the fresh air to dry the wound and assist with healing when she is resting.
- *Positioning*: With a painful abdominal wound, a mother will require help in finding a comfortable position in which to breastfeed her baby. The midwife can suggest that she tries lying on her side in bed with her baby alongside her, or on a pillow tucked under her arm, with the baby's trunk and feet under her arm, rather than lying across her abdomen. Although early contact and involvement in the care of her baby is encouraged, a caesarean section is a major abdominal operation and the mother will require more help and support during the first few postoperative days, and again when she is transferred home.
- *Transfer home*: Following caesarean section, most women are ready to go home on the 5th postoperative day to the care of their community midwife. An earlier discharge may not always be appropriate, as some women may not have any support at home and may have other children to care for, and are sometimes in inadequate housing.
- *Contraception*: This will be discussed before discharge and advice given, if required, about the provision of services and appropriate methods.
- *Psychological support*: This may be necessary because of the findings discussed earlier of acute trauma symptoms and post-traumatic stress disorder. Discussion regarding the reasons for the operation and the procedures is necessary.

### Trial of scar – vaginal birth after caesarean section (VBAC)

There are many different rates of successful vaginal birth reported after caesarean section. Dickinson (2005) gave the results of two studies undertaken in the last decade: one, by Flamm, included 5022 women and revealed a 75% vaginal birth rate; the other was by Miller, who reviewed 12,707 trials of labour and reported an 82% successful vaginal birth rate. The indication for the previous caesarean section should, of course, come into consideration.

There is no evidence to support the policy of some hospitals that these women should have an intravenous cannula sited and continuous electronic fetal monitoring once labour has commenced. There is also debate regarding place of birth, some opting for home birth and others in hospital. This has to be considered individually with each woman. As in all labours, close observations of maternal and fetal condition are made, especially noting any tenderness or pain over the caesarean scar. The other signs that may occur include signs of abnormal uterine action, signs of maternal haemorrhage and acute fetal bradycardia. (For cervical cerclage, please see website.)

## CONCLUSION

The number of normal physiological births appears to be decreasing in the UK, whilst figures for caesarean section and instrumental deliveries are rising, with increasing neonatal and maternal morbidity and static mortality (Thomas & Parenjothy 2001). This rise may cause an eroding of the midwife's role, skills and knowledge, with an associated lack of confidence in the ability of midwives to care for physiological birth. In this climate, midwives should reflect upon their own practice and make continuous professional and practice development part of their work. Nevertheless, there are still a significant number of women who will require an operative-style delivery and they require the midwife's unique skills and understanding in addition to 'normal' postnatal care. Midwives must ensure that they provide appropriate and relevant care tailored to each individual woman to minimize the associated morbidity.

## KEY POINTS

- The potential morbidity and mortality risk to the woman and the neonate of any operative delivery must be balanced by the value of these procedures in bringing the woman and baby at risk to safety.
- There are several aspects of the care provided by midwives and their colleagues which may reduce the need for intervention and augmentation, such as positioning, nutrition and the presence of a supportive person.
- It is important that midwives are familiar with caring for women who may require anaesthesia or instrumental delivery.
- The midwife must consider strategies for ensuring adequate preparation for the woman and her partner for all possibilities, and work to ensure that whatever intervention may be needed they will feel positive, empowered and supported throughout.

## REFERENCES


Annibale D, Hulsey T, Wagner C: Comparative neonatal morbidity of abdominal and vaginal deliveries after uncomplicated pregnancies, *Archives of Pediatrics and Adolescent Medicine* 149(8):862–867, 1995.

Bahl R, Strachan B, Murphy D: Pelvic floor morbidity at three years after instrumental delivery and caesarean section in the second stage of labour and the impact of a subsequent delivery, *American Journal of Obstetrics and Gynaecology* 192(3):789–794, 2005.

Blackburn ST: *Maternal, fetal and neonatal physiology – a clinical perspective*, ed 3, Philadelphia, 2007, WB Saunders.

Chamberlain G: The vacuum extractor. In Turnbull A, Chamberlain G, editors: *Obstetrics*, London, 1989, Churchill Livingstone.

Creedy D, Shochet I, Horsfall J: Childbirth and the development of acute trauma symptoms: incidence and contributing factors, *Birth* 27(2):104–111, 2000.

Crichton SM, Pierce JM, Stanton SL: Complications of caesarean section. In Studd JWW, editor: Progress in obstetrics and gynaecology, vol 9, Edinburgh, 1991, Churchill Livingstone.

Dennen PC, Hayashi R: Assisted vaginal delivery. In James DK, Steer PJ, Weiner CP, et al, editors: *High risk pregnancy: management options*, London, 2005, WB Saunders.

Dickinson JE: Cesarean section. In James DK, Steer PJ, Weiner CP, et al, editors: *High risk pregnancy: management options*, London, 2005, WB Saunders.

Duff E: Risks of caesarean section: who is sneezing, who is catching the cold? *MIDIRS Midwifery Digest* 10(1):73–74, 2000.

Gupta JK, Nikodem VC: Women's position during the second stage of labour, *The Cochrane Library*, Issue 1, Oxford, 2001, Update Software.

Healthcare Commission: *Towards better births. review of maternity services in England*, Lonndon, 2008, Commission for Healthcare Audit and Inspection.

Hibbard BM: Forceps delivery. In Turnbull A, Chamberlain G, editors: *Obstetrics*, London, 1989, Churchill Livingstone.

Hillan E: The aftermath of caesarean delivery, *MIDIRS Midwifery Digest* 10(1):70–72, 2000.

Hodnett ED: Caregiver support for women during childbirth (Cochrane Review), *The Cochrane Library*, Issue 1, Oxford, 2001, Update Software.

Johanson R, Menon B: Vacuum extraction versus forceps for assisted vaginal delivery (Cochrane Review), *The Cochrane Library*, Issue 1, Oxford, 2000, Update Software.

Johnson N, Lilford R, Guthrie K, et al: Randomised trial comparing a policy of early with selective amniotomy in uncomplicated labour at term, *British Journal of Obstetrics and Gynaecology* 104(3):340–346, 1997.

Jolly J, Walker J, Bhabra K: Subsequent obstetric performance related to primary mode of delivery, *British Journal of Obstetrics and Gynaecology* 106(3):227–232, 1999.

Ludka LM, Roberts C: Eating and drinking in labour: a literature review, *Journal of Nurse-Midwifery* 38(4):199–207, 1993.

Mander R: Epidural analgesia 2: research basis, *British Journal of Midwifery* 2(1):12–16, 1994.

Mark R: Dependence of uterine muscle contractions on pH with reference to prolonged labour, *Journal of Obstetrics and Gynaecology* 68:584, 1961.

O'Regan M: Active management of labour, *AIMS Journal* 10(2):1–7, 1998.

Page L: *The new midwifery: science and sensitivity*, London, 2000, Churchill Livingstone.

Pearson JF: A short history of the obstetric forceps, *Maternal and Child Health* 6(May):198–204, 1981.

Segal D, Sheiner E, Yohai D, et al: Early amniotomy – high risk factor for cesarean section, *European Journal of Obstetrics and Gynecology and Reproductive Biology* 86(2):145–149, 1999.

Strang LB: Fetal lung fluid secretion and reabsorption, *Physiological Reviews* 71:991–1016, 1991.

Studd J: Partograms and nomograms of cervical dilatation in management of primigravid labour, *British Medical Journal* 4(5890):451–455, 1973.

Swift L: Labour and fasting, *Nursing Times* 87(48):64–65, 1991.

Teng FY, Sayre JW: Vacuum extraction: does duration predict scalp injury? *Obstetrics and Gynecology* 89(2):281–285, 1997.

Thacker S, Stroup D: Continuous electronic heart rate monitoring for fetal assessment during labour, *The Cochrane Library*, Issue 3, Oxford, 2000, Update Software.

Thomas J, Parenjothy S: *The National Sentinel Caesarean Section Audit*, London, 2001, RCOG.

Towner D, Castro M, Eby-Wilkens E, et al: Effects of mode of delivery in nulliparous women on neonatal intracranial injury, *New England Journal of Medicine* 342(23):1709–1714, 1999.

Vacca A: Birth by vacuum extraction: neonatal outcome, *Journal of Paediatrics and Child Health* 32(3):204–206, 1996.

Wagner M: Choosing caesarean section, *The Lancet* 356(9242):1677–1680, 2000.

Walsh D: Evidence-based practice. Part 4: Fetal monitoring should be controlled, *British Journal of Midwifery* 8(8):511–516, 2000.

Chapter |62|

# Induction of labour and post-term pregnancy

Pat McGeown

**LEARNING OUTCOMES**

After reading this chapter, you will be able to:

- discuss the indications and contraindications for induction of labour
- review the efficacy of the common methods used
- evaluate the management of post-term pregnancy
- consider the impact and attitudes toward induction of labour.

## INDUCTION OF LABOUR

Induction of labour is when labour is artificially initiated before spontaneous onset occurs. It has been described as being 'one of the most drastic ways of intervening in the natural process of pregnancy and childbirth' (Enkin et al 2000:375). It may also affect the birth experience itself, as it can be less efficient and more painful than spontaneous labour. In addition, it increases the risk of further medical intervention.

In 2005–06 in NHS units in England, the incidence was 20.2%, with less than two-thirds of women delivering spontaneously. Where delivery was induced by drugs, whether or not surgical induction was also attempted, about 15% had instrumental deliveries and 23% emergency caesareans (Richardson & Mmata 2007). Despite this, it is common practice in modern maternity units in the UK.

Indications for induction of labour mainly relate to increased risk of fetal and/or maternal compromise if delivery is delayed. The risks and benefits and any possible consequences should be carefully considered and discussed with the woman prior to its commencement. Induction of labour should only be contemplated when a vaginal birth is feasible (National Collaborating Centres for Women's and Children's Health [NCC-WCH] 2008a)

### Maternal indications

**Hypertension:** Hypertensive disorders are one of the principal indications for induction, and timely intervention may become necessary to avoid serious maternal morbidity and perinatal compromise (Ch. 56).

**Diabetes:** Diabetes is associated with increased risk of maternal and perinatal mortality and morbidity. The NCC-WCH *Diabetes in pregnancy* guideline (2008b) recommends elective delivery or induction of labour after 38 weeks' gestation to reduce the risk of stillbirth and fetal macrosomia.

**Other medical conditions:** Pre-existing renal, cardiac or other medical disease can deteriorate as pregnancy progresses, and induction may be indicated in some of these pregnancies (Ch. 55).

**Reflective activity 62.1**

Find out the induction rate in your local maternity unit and compare it with other regional and national rates. Analyse and reflect upon the rationale for any variability between the rates.

**Prelabour rupture of the membranes:** Preterm, prelabour rupture of the membranes (PPROM) occurs before the onset of regular uterine contractions and before 37 weeks (Ch. 60). The two main risks of PPROM are preterm birth and infectious morbidity due to ascending intrauterine infection. PPROM occurs in only 2% of births but is responsible for around 40% of all preterm births (Douvas et al 1984, Maxwell 1993, Merenstein & Weisman 1996). Unless there are additional obstetric indications, such as infection or fetal compromise, induction of labour is not indicated before 34 weeks (NCC-WCH 2008a).

At 37 weeks or after, induction is known as *prelabour rupture of membranes* at term (PROM). PROM occurs in 8% of all term pregnancies (Dare et al 2006). Complications include: maternal and neonatal infection, prolapsed cord, increased risk of caesarean section and a low 5-minute Apgar score. Induction of labour may reduce the numbers of babies admitted to neonatal units and increase maternal satisfaction (Dare et al 2006).

Women with PROM should be offered either immediate induction or expectant management. National guidance recommends that induction of labour is appropriate 24 hours after PROM (NCC-WCH 2007).

**Maternal request:** Induction of labour may be requested by women for social or emotional reasons. For example, partner being posted abroad with armed services or increased anxiety or stress which may or may not be directly associated with the pregnancy. Induction should not be routinely offered, but in exceptional circumstances it may be considered at or after 40 weeks (NCC-WCH 2008a).

**Poor obstetric history:** Induction is sometimes undertaken to alleviate the anxiety and stress associated with subsequent pregnancies following previous adverse outcome, although it may have no clinical relevance to the current pregnancy. However, it is not indicated where there is a history of precipitate labour (NCC-WCH 2008a).

## Fetal indications

**Fetal growth restriction:** Induction may be indicated if there is evidence of diminished fetal wellbeing caused by uteroplacental insufficiency, which is often characterized by intrauterine growth restriction, abnormal fetal movements and/or abnormal fetal umbilical blood flow detected by Doppler ultrasound. However, induction is not indicated if the fetus is severely growth restricted (NCC-WCH 2008a). As the fetus is likely to become severely compromised in labour, a caesarean section is the preferred method of elective delivery.

**Macrosomia:** Macrosomia not associated with diabetes has been an indication to induce labour in order to avoid difficult delivery, shoulder dystocia and their consequences. However, accurate diagnosis of estimated fetal weight remains problematic. The evidence suggests that there is little benefit in induction for suspected fetal macrosomia (Irion & Boulvain 1998).

**Fetal death:** When fetal death has occurred with no other apparent obstetric or medical complications, there are no overwhelming benefits or risks of induction of labour over expectant care. The woman should be allowed to choose the best option for her and her family. If, however, there is evidence of ruptured membranes, infection or bleeding, immediate induction is indicated (NCC-WCH 2008a).

**Rhesus isoimmunization:** Induction of labour is an optional management for established isoimmunization when the fetus is considered sufficiently mature, is not too severely affected and can be effectively treated after birth (Enkin et al 2000).

**Fetal anomaly:** Labour may be induced to terminate pregnancy if the fetus has a lethal abnormality or a malformation likely to result in significant handicap. It may also be useful when the baby would benefit from planned early surgery.

## Contraindications

Contraindications for induction of labour are the same as for vaginal delivery. If the woman cannot have a safe vaginal delivery, induction of labour should not be considered.

**Placenta praevia:** There is almost no indication for vaginal birth when the fetus has reached a viable age, because of the risks of maternal and fetal haemorrhage, cord accidents and malpresentations (Enkin et al 2000).

**Cephalopelvic disproportion:** Proven cephalopelvic disproportion may be a contraindication for induction of labour. However, it is rarely possible to make an accurate diagnosis except in cases of known altered anatomy, for example, severe contracture or pelvic fractures. The literature shows that successful vaginal birth occurs in over 50% of caesarean sections for disproportion, dystocia or failure to progress (Paterson & Saunders 1991, Rosen & Dickinson 1990, Rosen et al 1991).

**Oblique or transverse lie in labour:** These are absolute contraindications because of the risks of cord prolapse and obstruction.

**Severe fetal compromise:** In this situation, the fetus is unlikely to tolerate the stress of labour, and caesarean section is the safest option.

## Methods

Induction is usually timed for when it will be most successful, that is, near the onset of spontaneous labour. But there are situations when it will be necessary to intervene before term to reduce the risk of fetal and/or maternal compromise. Corticosteroids should be administered to a woman who will deliver before 36 weeks to promote fetal pulmonary maturity and thereby reduce the risk of mortality, respiratory distress syndrome and intraventricular haemorrhage in preterm infants (RCOG 2006).

Methods used to induce labour mainly aim to replicate the physiological processes that naturally occur in spontaneous labour. However, mechanisms that control this complex process are not clearly understood, limiting available methods for the purpose. Current methods available attempt to stimulate cervical ripening and uterine contractions.

## Cervical ripening

The success of induction and subsequent length of labour are primarily determined by the state of the cervix at the time of induction. An 'unripe' or unfavourable cervix fails to dilate adequately and results in high failure rates (Enkin et al 2000). Prior to induction, the state of the cervix is assessed using a score based on that originally proposed by Bishop (1964). Five qualities are rated (see Table 62.1):

- cervical dilatation
- cervical consistency
- length of cervix
- position of the cervix
- station of the presenting part.

When the total score is greater than 8, the cervix is said to be favourable (NCC-WCH 2008a).

### *Risks of cervical ripening*

Cervical ripening is the first step to inducing labour; it should not be attempted unless the aim is to bring pregnancy to an end. The complications that can arise include:

- intrauterine infection
- uterine hyperstimulation
- fetal heart rate abnormalities
- maternal discomfort and inconvenience.

Intrauterine infection is mainly associated with invasive techniques, such as mechanical devices and extra amniotic procedures. Iatrogenic uterine hyperstimulation and fetal heart rate abnormalities during the cervical ripening period can lead to emergency caesarean section with its associated morbidity (Ch. 61). Failure to produce any significant change in cervical favourability may lead to delivery by caesarean. The consequences of initiating any procedure with its sequelae should always be considered and discussed in full with the woman prior to its commencement.

**Table 62.1 Modified Bishop's scoring system**

| Feature for assessment | Score | | | |
|---|---|---|---|---|
| | 0 | 1 | 2 | 3 |
| Dilatation of cervix (cm) | <1 | 1–2 | 2–4 | >4 |
| Consistency of cervix | Firm | Medium | Soft | – |
| Length of cervix (cm) | 4 | 2–4 | 1–2 | <1 |
| Position of cervix | Posterior | Mid | Anterior | – |
| Station in cm relative to ischial spines | −3 | −2 | −1/0 | +1/+2 |

## Membranes sweeping

Sweeping or stripping the membranes from the lower uterine segment at term has traditionally been used to induce labour in the hope that amniotomy or oxytocic drugs may be avoided. It involves placing a finger inside the cervix and making a circular, sweeping action to separate the membranes from the cervix. The theory behind this method is that localized prostaglandin production is increased (Mitchell et al 1977).

Boulvain and colleagues (2005) found that membrane sweeping reduced the time from intervention to spontaneous onset of labour or birth by a mean of 3 days. It also reduced the incidence of prolonged pregnancy if performed from 38 to 40 weeks and thereby reduced the need for formal induction of labour. However, the reviewers felt there is little justification to undertake the procedure routinely prior to 40 weeks' gestation.

Sweeping the membranes was not associated with an increase in maternal or neonatal infection or premature rupture of the membranes, but one trial (Boulvain et al 1998) reported increased maternal discomfort during and after the procedure with both vaginal bleeding and painful contractions not leading to the onset of labour during the 24 hours following the intervention.

National guidance recommends that all women with uncomplicated pregnancies at 40 or more weeks should be offered sweeping of the membranes prior to formal methods of induction. Repeated sweeping of the membranes at 41 weeks may also be performed where labour does not commence spontaneously. The NCC-WCH guideline (2008a:61) also states that 'membrane sweeping is an integral part of preventing prolonged pregnancy' and should be be routinely discussed at the 38-week antenatal visit.

## Prostaglandin

Prostaglandin ($PGE_2$) has been used since the late 1960s for cervical ripening and induction of labour in a variety of different preparations and doses. In the UK, vaginal prostaglandin is one of the most commonly used induction agents. It is more likely than either placebo or no treatment to start labour and to avoid the need for induction with oxytocin (Enkin et al 2000). Vaginal $PGE_2$ is associated with improved cervical status, reduced need for oxytocin augmentation and meconium staining. With a favourable cervix, it improves the successful vaginal delivery rate within 24 hours (NCC-WCH 2008a).

Vaginal $PGE_2$ in tablet or gel preparations, is the recommended method of induction of labour irrespective of cervical favourability or membrane status. Controlled-release pessary may be more appropriate when the cervix is unfavourable, to reduce the need for repeated doses of single-dose preparations (NCC-WCH 2008a). The recommended cycle for single vaginal dose preparations is one dose followed by a second dose 6 hours later if not in established labour (two doses maximum).

The associated complications of prostaglandin administration include:

- maternal gastrointestinal side-effects
- maternal pyrexia from the effect on the thermoregulating centre in the brain
- uterine hyperstimulation with or without fetal heart rate abnormalities (Enkin et al 2000).

There is also the risk of an 'unjustified' induction of labour because of the ready availability of prostaglandin.

## Oxytocin

Oxytocin is the commonest induction agent used worldwide. Intravenous infusion is the licensed method of administration most commonly used to augment labour as well as a method of induction.

Concerns over achieving a minimal effective dose are related to the serious complication of excessive uterine contractions. Excessively frequent (*hyperstimulation/tachysystole*) or prolonged contractions (*hypertonus*) may cause fetal hypoxia due to compromised placental circulation.

Uterine rupture is a rare but life-threatening consequence of uterine hypercontractility. The suggested management for uterine hyperstimulation is to stop the oxytocin, as the short half-life of the drug will reduce the degree of fetal compromise, dependent upon fetal reserve. Tocolytics are also recommended (NCC-WCH 2008a).

The antidiuretic effect of oxytocin can lead to water retention and hyponatraemia with serious associated maternal sequelae, although this is preventable with strict fluid management and minimal infusion volume.

There is also evidence that the incidence of neonatal hyperbilirubinaemia is increased with the use of oxytocin (Enkin et al 2000).

## Amniotomy

Amniotomy is the deliberate artificial rupture of the amniotic membranes. More than any other method of induction, amniotomy implies a firm commitment to delivery (Enkin et al 2000).

During a vaginal examination the clinician digitally identifies the cervical os and membranes, piercing the forewaters using a specially designed plastic 'Amnihook' (EMS Medical Group). Less commonly, surgical steel forceps are used. Artificial rupture of the hindwaters was previously undertaken using the S-shaped metal Drew Smythe catheter; this is now rarely used in the UK, though it may have a place in countries where resources are limited.

Amniotomy is usually used with intravenous oxytocin; however, evidence of their effectiveness and safety is lacking (Howarth & Botha 2001). National guidance indicates they should not be used as a primary method of induction unless vaginal $PGE_2$ is contraindicated (NCC-WCH 2008a).

Evidence from clinical trials (Bricker & Luckas 2000) shows that women who receive oxytocin at the time of amniotomy are more likely to be delivered within 24 hours, less likely to have a caesarean section or forceps delivery, require less analgesia and sustain lower rates of postpartum haemorrhage than those who do not receive oxytocin. Less depressed Apgar scores are also found. This method is not without certain risks.

Potential hazards of amniotomy include:

- ascending intrauterine infection, including mother-to-child vertical transmission of HIV infection
- early decelerations of the fetal heart rate
- umbilical cord prolapse
- bleeding from the cervix, fetal vessels in the membranes (vasa praevia) or the placental site.

## Other methods

Other methods for cervical ripening or inducing labour have been used but are not currently recommended for routine use. Other medical methods appear effective but require further rigorous evaluation. Natural methods of cervical ripening and induction of labour that allow women to have greater control over the induction process are inexpensive and are perceived as being less medicalized. However, further research is required to establish the safety and efficacy of certain methods. They should not be used when induction of labour is considered necessary for the safety of the mother or baby. Table 62.2 gives an overview of the various medical and natural methods and agents.

**Reflective activity 62.2**

You may have cared for a woman requesting induction of labour for no obvious medical indication. Reflect upon the advice and/or information given to her. Consider the reasons why some women request induction of labour.

How do healthcare professionals respond to such requests?

How do you feel about (a) the woman and (b) the caregivers? Discuss this issue with a colleague(s).

Table 62.2 Other methods and agents for inducing labour

| Method/Agent | Recommendation | Reference |
|---|---|---|
| Misoprostol | Only use for induction of labour for intrauterine fetal death | NCC-WCH 2008b |
| Mifepristone (RU 486) | There is insufficient information available from clinical trials to support the use of mifepristone to induce labour<br>Only use for induction of labour for intrauterine fetal death | Neilson 2000<br>NCC-WCH 2008b |
| Castor oil, bath +/– enema | Not recommended Insufficient evidence and has uncomfortable side-effects | Kelly et al 2001 |
| Breast stimulation | Appears beneficial in initiating labour by 72 hours and reducing postpartum haemorrhage rates<br>Should not be used in high-risk women. Requires further research | Kavanagh et al 2005 |
| Sexual intercourse | Role uncertain – linked to prostaglandins in semen<br>Not recommended | Kavanagh et al 2001<br>NCC-WCH 2008b |
| Acupuncture | Requires further research to determine efficacy<br>Not recommended | Smith & Crowther 2004<br>NCC-WCH 2008b |
| Homeopathy | Requires further research to determine efficacy<br>Not recommended | Smith, 2003<br>NCC-WCH 2008b |
| Herbal supplements | Not recommended<br>Requires further research to determine efficacy | NCC-WCH 2008b |

## POST-TERM PREGNANCY

Post-term pregnancy is defined as a pregnancy continuing for more than 42 weeks or greater than 294 days (International Federation of Gynecology and Obstetrics [FIGO] 1980). The reported incidence is between 5% and 10% (Olesen et al 2003). Previous prolonged pregnancy increases the incidence of subsequent prolonged pregnancy two- to threefold and daughters of mothers who have had prolonged pregnancy have an increased incidence (Mogren et al 1999).

Epidemiological studies indicate that there is increased risk to both the mother and, particularly, the baby as pregnancy progresses beyond 40 weeks (Gülmezoglu et al 2006). However, the incidence of congenital malformation in babies born post-term is higher and data should be adjusted to account for life-threatening anomalies. Perinatal death occurs mainly during the intrapartum and neonatal periods and not during the pregnancy. Meconium aspiration syndrome is a common feature and the incidence of neonatal seizures is increased two to five times in babies born after 41 weeks (Enkin et al 2000).

### Accurate dating

Post-term pregnancy and social factors account for approximately 70% of inductions (Thomason 1999). The traditional method of establishing the due date is by the last menstrual period (LMP) following Naegele's rule. However, inaccuracies in maternal recollection of LMP (Geirsson & Busby-Earle 1991) and the wide variance in the distribution of ovulation and conception dates (Guerrero & Florez 1969) introduce substantial error when using LMP as the principal tool for dating. In developed countries, ultrasound scanning is now routinely used. Dating by ultrasound scan alone has been shown to be a more accurate predictor of the birth date than dating by LMP alone or with a 14, 10 or 7 day adjustment 'rule' (Mongelli et al 1996). Current guidance recommends early ultrasound scan to assess gestational age to ensure consistency of approach and reduce the number of inductions of labour for perceived post-term pregnancy (NCC-WCH 2008c).

### Associated features of post-term pregnancy

#### *Uteroplacental insufficiency*

A tenaciously held but mistaken belief is that the placenta ages as pregnancy progresses. No morphological feature of the term placenta can be considered as a manifestation of ageing (Fox 1979, Larsen et al 1995); indeed, fresh villous growth and continuing DNA synthesis have been demonstrated in the placenta at term (Fox 1978, Sands & Dobbing 1985). However, the fetoplacental circulation decreases after 35 weeks of pregnancy (Lingman & Marsel 1986) and Doppler studies show varied and numerous fetal circulatory modifications in the post-term fetus (Vetter 1998).

Calcification in the term and especially the post-term placenta is a frequent clinical observation in normal pregnancy; it is also seen on ultrasound scanning (Gudmundsson & Laurini 1998).

Some studies have shown a gradual deterioration in placental function in the post-term pregnancy, associated with chronic progressive uteroplacental insufficiency, which is thought by some to 'mimic a mild fetal growth restriction' (Battaglia et al 1995).

### *Fetal behaviour*

This also changes in normal post-term pregnancy. Van de Pas and colleagues (1994) found that the increasingly 'wakeful' fetal heart rate (FHR) pattern could imitate an abnormal pattern that might lead to intervention. However, further studies are required to evaluate the usefulness of assessment of fetal behavioural states in differentiating the at-risk fetus from normal.

### *Oligohydramnios*

Amniotic fluid volume diminishes in post-term pregnancies, thereby limiting the cushioning effect on the umbilical cord and fetus. Cord compression during uterine contractions may lead to fetal heart rate abnormalities. Meconium staining of the amniotic fluid is also associated with a decreased volume (Crowley et al 1984), which in turn may lead to meconium aspiration syndrome in the baby (Katz & Bowes 1992). This often has a significant influence on the care and management of labour and the newborn.

### *Fetal macrosomia*

In the absence of uteroplacental insufficiency, fetal growth continues, though at a reduced rate after 38 weeks' gestation (Boyd et al 1988, Gruenwald 1967). Babies born at 42 completed weeks are three to seven times more likely to weigh over 4000 g than those delivered before 41 completed weeks (Fabre et al 1998). Macrosomia increases the risk of dysfunctional labour, shoulder dystocia, brachial plexus injury and clavicular fracture in the baby and subsequent morbidity to the woman as a result of intervention. However, ultrasound estimation of fetal weight is more difficult and less accurate near term and induction of labour for suspected macrosomia does not alter the incidence of neonatal or maternal morbidity (Irion & Boulvain 1998).

### *Post-maturity syndrome*

This condition affects babies born post-dates. Gibb (1985) first described the features of the postmature infant. Such infants are alert and appear mature, but have a decreased amount of soft tissue mass, particularly subcutaneous fat; their body length is increased in relation to body weight; and the skin may hang loosely on the extremities and is often dry and peeling. There is an absence of vernix and lanugo, although they often have abundant scalp hair. The fingernails and toenails are long. The nails and umbilical cord may be stained with meconium passed in utero.

It is also associated with oligohydramnios (Clement et al 1987), with similar features to those seen in the growth-restricted infant. Knox Ritchie (1992) describes this syndrome as an expression of chronic fetal malnutrition which is not confined to post-term pregnancy. However, as few as 10% of post-term pregnancies are complicated by this syndrome (Resnik 1994).

## Management of post-term pregnancy

The recommended alternatives available to clinicians when caring for women with confirmed post-term pregnancy are:

- membrane sweeping from 40 weeks
- expectant management with increased antenatal surveillance of fetal wellbeing from 42 weeks
- active induction of labour from 41 weeks (NCC-WCH 2008a).

Thus, interventionalist methods are to be offered before the pregnancy is strictly post-term, that is, 42 completed weeks or more.

**Membrane sweeping:** This has been discussed earlier in the chapter (see p. 853).

**Expectant management with increased surveillance:** From 42 weeks, women who decide not to be induced and await spontaneous labour should be offered twice-weekly cardiotocography (CTG) and ultrasound estimation of maximum amniotic pool depth (NCC-WCH 2008a). However, there are limitations of antenatal CTG as a predictive tool for fetal wellbeing and a tendency for it to provide false reassurance (Pattison & McCowan 1999). Indeed, some suggest that antepartum surveillance in pregnancies where the risk of adverse outcome is very low may actually cause rather than prevent morbidity (Alfirevic et al 1997).

The importance of the self-monitoring of patterns of fetal movements as an ongoing surveillance tool should not be forgotten and should be reiterated to all women.

**Active induction of labour from 41 weeks:** Women should be offered formal induction of labour from 41 weeks to avoid the risks of post-term pregnancy (NCC-WCH 2008a). Gülmezoglu and colleagues (2006) conclude that a policy of routine induction of labour after 41 weeks reduces the risk of perinatal death and meconium aspiration syndrome in normally formed babies, whilst having other comparable maternal and fetal outcomes.

Management of otherwise uncomplicated prolonged pregnancy has standardized in the UK since publication of the *Induction of labour* guideline (RCOG 2001). The evidence confirms that both induction of labour and expectant management remain valid options and ultimately the woman should choose whichever pathway is best suited to her and her family.

### Economic considerations

Cost-effectiveness and clinical governance dominate processes that evaluate financial calculations about patient management. The National Collaborating Centre's (NCC-WCH 2008a) recent cost–benefit analysis of induction of labour versus expectant management concluded that offering induction of labour from 41 weeks is the most cost-effective and beneficial strategy. It demonstrated that the overall health benefits of induction from 41 weeks outweighed any additional cost.

## WOMEN'S VIEWS

Available research suggests that women prefer induction of labour to expectant management when pregnancy is prolonged (Out et al 1986, Roberts & Young 1991). Sarkar (1997) has confirmed that women have significantly high levels of anxiety when pregnancy extends beyond the expected date.

Redshaw and colleagues (2007) sought women's views of maternity care and found that although 30% of women did not feel they had had a say in their labour being induced, they believed it to be necessary for the health and wellbeing of themselves and the baby. Another survey established that 48% of women wanted more information about induction (Singh & Newburn 2000). The data suggested that women receiving maternity care in the UK were unable to make informed choices or give informed consent regarding induction of labour.

## MIDWIFERY CARE

The decision to pre-empt the spontaneous onset of labour needs to be made in a climate of honest interchange of information, with the benefits and risks of induction explained by the obstetrician and midwife, so that an informed choice may be made. It is the responsibility of the clinicians involved to ensure women are given evidence-based information, where it is available, to make the most appropriate decision for them.

Women and their partners are likely to experience a range of emotions when faced with induction of labour. However, involving the woman and her partner in decision making is likely to increase their feelings of control over what happens. An individual plan of care can then be made and documented in the woman's notes.

**Reflective activity 62.3**

Review your unit's guideline for induction of labour and assess if it reflects the principles of the national guideline. Where there are any inconsistencies, evaluate whether they are supported with valid evidence.

### Planning for induction

Consideration needs to be given regarding timing and setting of the procedure for women with complicated pregnancies and clear indications for induction. Discussions and decisions should be undertaken at Consultant level. Liaison with the antenatal ward, delivery suite, neonatal unit and other specialist services, if appropriate, may be required to communicate any relevant details, and ensure availability of beds and appropriate staff.

The midwife providing care for a woman with a normal pregnancy will need to consider the appropriate time for referral to an obstetrician in the event of the pregnancy becoming post-term. Adjustment of the expected date of delivery should not occur on the day a woman presents to discuss management options for supposed prolonged pregnancy.

### Location and timing of induction of labour

Women who decide to have membrane sweeping from 40 weeks to reduce the risk of post-term pregnancy may receive care in the community but it is important they have access to advice and assessment if required.

There is much discussion about the efficacy of undertaking more formal induction of labour in an outpatient setting. National guidance supports induction in an outpatient setting provided that there are safety and support procedures in place whilst continuously auditing (NCC-WCH 2008a). Unfortunately, the guidance does not define the rigorous procedures that are required to offer this service which achieves greater satisfaction for women and has the potential to reduce the numbers of antenatal admissions (Biem et al 2003, Neale & Pachulski 2002, Sciscione 2001).

It is recommended that planned induction of labour in an inpatient setting should be carried out in the morning, owing to increased maternal satisfaction (Dodd et al 2006) and the potential to reduce the length of stay in hospital (NCC-WCH 2008a).

### Care during induction of labour

Options for management and care during induction and labour are dependent upon accessibility, availability and informed choice whilst promoting safety for both the mother and the baby. The NCC-WCH (2008a) *Induction of labour* guideline makes several recommendations about management:

Wherever induction of labour is carried out, facilities should be available for continuous electronic fetal heart rate and uterine contraction monitoring.

Before induction of labour is carried out, the Bishop score should be assessed and recorded, and a normal fetal heart rate pattern should be confirmed using electronic fetal monitoring. After administration of vaginal $PGE_2$, it is advised that the woman lies down for 30–60 minutes to aid absorption. When contractions begin, fetal wellbeing should be assessed with continuous electronic fetal monitoring. Once the cardiotocogram is confirmed as normal, intermittent auscultation should be used unless there are clear indications for continuous electronic fetal monitoring as described in *Intrapartum care* guideline (NCC-WCH 2007).

If the fetal heart rate is abnormal after administration of vaginal $PGE_2$, recommendations on management of fetal compromise in *Intrapartum care* (NCC-WCH 2007) should be followed.

The Bishop score should be reassessed 6 hours after vaginal $PGE_2$ tablet or gel insertion, or 24 hours after vaginal $PGE_2$ controlled-release pessary insertion, to monitor progress.

If a woman returns home after insertion of vaginal $PGE_2$ tablet or gel, she should be asked to contact her obstetrician/midwife:

- when contractions begin, or
- if she has had no contractions after 6 hours.

Once active labour is established, maternal and fetal monitoring should be carried out as described in *Intrapartum care* (NCC-WCH 2007).

(Adapted from NCC-WCH 2008a:72–73)

## Recommendations on pain relief during induction of labour

*Women being offered induction of labour should be informed that induced labour is likely to be more painful than spontaneous labour and be advised of the various pain relief options available to them, with the risks and benefits explained. The range includes natural/alternative methods, positions, mobility and aids, encouraging coping strategies, simple analgesics, and epidural analgesia. The opportunity to labour in water is also recommended for pain relief.*

(Adapted from NCC-WCH 2008a:75)

These guidelines provide basic requirements for the safety of mother and baby. However, they do not consider the woman's physical, cultural, emotional or psychological needs, which remain to be addressed. These topics are considered in Chapters 12, 35 and 36.

## KEY POINTS

- Accurate dating of pregnancy is essential to avoid unnecessary induction of labour.
- Membrane sweeping should be offered after 40 and 41 weeks.
- Vaginal prostaglandin is the preferred induction agent.
- Expectant management and induction of labour are both valid options for management of post-term pregnancy.
- Midwives need to be up-to-date with current management of induction and post-term pregnancy.

## REFERENCES


Alfirevic Z, Luckas M, Walkinshaw SA, et al: A randomised comparison between amniotic fluid index and maximum pool depth in the monitoring of post-term pregnancy, *British Journal of Obstetrics and Gynaecology* 104(2):207–211, 1997.

Battaglia C, Artini PG, Ballestri M, et al: Hemodynamic, hematological and hemorrhological evaluation of post-term pregnancy, *Acta Obstetricia et Gynecologica Scandinavica* 74(5):336–340, 1995.

Biem SR, Turnell RW, Olatunbosun O: A randomized controlled trial of outpatient versus inpatient labour induction with vaginal controlled release prostaglandin-E2: effectiveness and satisfaction, *Journal of Obstetrics and Gynaecology Canada* 25(1):23–31, 2003.

Bishop EH: Pelvic scoring for elective induction, *Obstetrics and Gynecology* 24:266–268, 1964.

Boyd ME, Usher RH, McClean FH, et al: Obstetric consequences of postmaturity, *American Journal of Obstetrics and Gynecology* 158(2):343–348, 1988.

Boulvain M, Fraser W, Marcoux S, et al: Does sweeping of the membranes reduce the need for formal induction of labour? A randomised controlled trial, *British Journal Obstetetrics and Gynaecology* 105(1):34–40, 1998.

Boulvain M, Stan C, Irion O: Membrane sweeping for induction of labour, *Cochrane Database of Systematic Reviews* (1):CD000451, 2005.

Bricker L, Luckas M: Amniotomy alone for induction of labour, *Cochrane Database of Systematic Reviews* (4):CD002862, 2000.

Clement D, Schifrin BS, Kates RB: Acute oligohydramnios in postdate pregnancy, *American Journal of Obstetrics and Gynecology* 157(4 Pt 1):884–886, 1987.

Crowley P, O'Herlihy C, Boylan P: The value of ultrasound measurement of amniotic fluid volume in the management of prolonged pregnancies, *British Journal of Obstetrics and Gynaecology* 91(5): 444–448, 1984.

Dare MR, Middleton P, Crowther CA, et al: Planned early birth versus expectant management (waiting) for prelabour rupture of membranes at term (37 weeks or more), *Cochrane Database of Systematic Reviews* (1):CD005302, 2006.

Dodd JM, Crowther CA, Robinson JS: Morning compared with evening induction of labor: a nested randomized controlled trial, *Obstetrics and Gynecology* 108(2):350–360, 2006.

Douvas SG, Brewer JMJ, McKay ML, et al: Treatment of preterm rupture of the membranes, *Journal of Reproductive Medicine* 29(10):741–744, 1984.

Enkin M, Keirse MJNC, Neilson J, et al: *A guide to effective care in pregnancy and childbirth*, ed 3, Oxford, 2000, Oxford University Press.

Fabre E, Gonzalez de Aguero R, de Augustin JL, et al: Macrosomia: concept and epidemiology. In Kurjak A, editor: Textbook of perinatal medicine, vol 2, London, 1998, Parthenon, pp 1273–1289.

Fox H: *Pathology of the placenta*, London, 1978, WH Saunders.

Fox H: The placenta as a model for organ ageing. In Beaconsfield P, Villee C, editors: *Placenta – a neglected experimental animal*, Oxford, 1979, Pergamon, pp 351–378.

Geirsson RT, Busby-Earle RMC: Certain dates may not provide a reliable estimate of gestational age, *British Journal of Obstetrics and Gynaecology* 98(1):108–109, 1991.

Gibb D: Prolonged pregnancy. In Studd J, editor: *The management of labour*, London, 1985, Blackwell Scientific.

Gruenwald P: Growth of the human fetus. In McLaren A, editor: Advances in reproductive physiology, vol 2, London, 1967, Logos, pp 279–309.

Gudmundsson S, Laurini RN: Placental haemodynamics and morphological evaluation. In Kurjak A, editor: Textbook of perinatal medicine, vol 2, London, 1998, Parthenon, pp 1273–1289.

Guerrero R, Florez PE: The duration of pregnancy, *The Lancet* 2(7614):268–269, 1969.

Gülmezoglu AM, Crowther CA, Middleton P: Induction of labour for improving birth outcomes for women at or beyond term, *Cochrane Database of Systematic Reviews* (4):CD004945, 2006.

Howarth GR, Botha DJ: Amniotomy plus intravenous oxytocin for induction of labour, *Cochrane Database of Systematic Reviews* (3):CD003250, 2001.

International Federation of Gynecology and Obstetrics (FIGO): International classification of disease update, *International Journal of Gynecology and Obstetrics* 17:634–640, 1980.

Irion O, Boulvain M: Induction of labour for suspected fetal macrosomia, *Cochrane Database of Systematic Reviews* (2):CD000938, 1998.

Katz VL, Bowes WA: Meconium aspiration syndrome: reflections on a murky subject, *American Journal of Obstetrics and Gynecology* 166(6):171–183, 1992.

Kavanagh J, Kelly AJ, Thomas J: Sexual intercourse for cervical ripening and induction of labour, *Cochrane Database of Systematic Reviews* (2):CD003093, 2001.

Kavanagh J, Kelly AJ, Thomas J: Breast stimulation for cervical ripening and induction of labour, *Cochrane Database of Systematic Reviews* (3):CD003392, 2005.

Kelly AJ, Kavanagh J, Thomas J: Castor oil, bath and/or enema for cervical priming and induction of labour, *Cochrane Database of Systematic Reviews* (2):CD003099, 2001.

Knox Ritchie JW: Obstetrics for the neonatologist. In Roberton NRC, editor: *Textbook of neonatology*, ed 2, London, 1992, Churchill Livingstone, pp 83–119.

Larsen LG, Clausen HV, Anderson B, et al: A stereologic study of postmature placentas fixed by dual perfusion, *American Journal of Obstetrics and Gynecology* 172(2 Pt 1):500–507, 1995.

Lingman G, Marsel K: Fetal central blood circulation in the third trimester of normal pregnancy. Longitudinal study. 1. Aortic and umbilical blood flow, *Early Human Development* 13(2):137–150, 1986.

Maxwell GL: Preterm premature rupture of membranes, *Obstetrical & Gynecological Survey* 48(8):576–583, 1993.

Merenstein GB, Weisman LE: Premature rupture of the membranes: neonatal consequences, *Seminars in Perinatology* 20(5):375–380, 1996.

Mitchell MD, Klint APF, Bibby J, et al: Rapid increases in plasma prostaglandin concentrations after vaginal examination and amniotomy, *British Medical Journal* 2(6096):1183–1185, 1977.

Mogren I, Stenlund H, Hogberg U: Recurrence of prolonged pregnancy, *International Journal of Epidemiology* 28(2):253–257, 1999.

Mongelli M, Wilcox M, Gardosi J: Estimating the date of confinement: ultrasonographic biometry versus certain menstrual dates, *American Journal of Obstetrics and Gynecology* 174(1):278–281, 1996.

National Collaborating Centre for Women's and Children's Health (NCC-WCH): *Intrapartum care: care of healthy women and their babies during childbirth*, London, 2007, RCOG.

National Collaborating Centre for Women's and Children's Health (NCC-WCH): *Induction of labour*, London, 2008a, RCOG.

National Collaborating Centre for Women's and Children's Health (NCC-WCH): *Diabetes in pregnancy: management of diabetes and its complications from preconception to the postnatal period*, London, 2008b, RCOG.

National Collaborating Centre for Women's and Children's Health (NCC-WCH): *Antenatal care: routine care of the healthy pregnant woman*, London, 2008c, RCOG.

Neale E, Pachulski A: Outpatient cervical ripening prior to induction of labour, *Journal of Obstetrics and Gynaecology* 22(6):634–635, 2002.

Neilson JP: Mifepristone for induction of labour, *Cochrane Database of Systematic Reviews* (4):CD002865, 2000.

Olesen AW, Westergaard JG, Olsen J: Perinatal and maternal complications related to postterm delivery: a national register-based study, 1978–1993, *American Journal of Obstetrics and Gynecology* 189(1):222–227, 2003.

Out JJ, Vierhout ME, Verhage F, et al: Characteristics and motives of women choosing elective induction of labour, *Journal of Psychosomatic Research* 30(3):375–380, 1986.

Paterson CM, Saunders AJ: Mode of delivery after one caesarean section: audit of current practice in a health region, *British Medical Journal* 303(6806):818–821, 1991.

Pattison N, McCowan L: Cardiotocography for antepartum fetal assessment, *Cochrane Database of Systematic Reviews* (1):CD001068, 1999.

Redshaw M, Rowe R, Hockley C, et al: *Recorded delivery: a national survey of women's experience of maternity care 2006*, Oxford, 2007, National Perinatal Epidemiology Unit, University of Oxford.

Resnik R: Post-term pregnancy. In Creasy RK, Resnik R, editors: *Maternal-fetal medicine: principles and practice*, ed 3, London, 1994, WB Saunders, pp 521–526.

Richardson A, Mmata C: *NHS maternity statistics, England: 2005–06*, London, 2007, The Information Centre for Health and Social Care.

Roberts LJ, Young KR: The management of prolonged pregnancy – an analysis of women's attitudes before and after term, *British Journal of Obstetrics and Gynaecology* 98(11):1102–1106, 1991.

Rosen MG, Dickinson JC: Vaginal birth after cesarean: a meta-analysis of indicators for success, *Obstetrics and Gynecology* 76(5 Pt 1):865–869, 1990.

Rosen MG, Dickinson JC, Westhoff CL: Vaginal birth after cesarean: a meta-analysis of morbidity and mortality, *Obstetrics and Gynecology* 77(3):465–470, 1991.

Royal College of Obstetricians and Gynaecologists (RCOG): *Induction of labour: evidence-based clinical guideline No. 9*, London, 2001, RCOG.

Royal College of Obstetricians and Gynaecologists (RCOG): *Green top guideline 44. Preterm prelabour rupture of membranes*, London, 2006, RCOG.

Sands J, Dobbing J: Continuing growth and development of the third-trimester human placenta, *Placenta* 6(1):13–22, 1985.

Sarkar PK: Anxiety in women who go postdates, *Contemporary Reviews in Obstetrics and Gynecology* 9(2):107–111, 1997.

Sciscione AC: Transcervical Foley catheter for preinduction cervical ripening in an outpatient versus inpatient setting, *Obstetrics and Gynecology* 98(5 Pt 1):751–756, 2001.

Singh D, Newburn M: *Access to maternity information and support*, London, 2000, NCT Publications.

Smith CA: Homoeopathy for induction of labour, *Cochrane Database of Systematic Reviews* (4):CD003399, 2003.

Smith CA, Crowther CA: Acupuncture for induction of labour, *Cochrane Database of Systematic Reviews* (1):CD002962, 2004.

Thomason JS: Elective induction of labour. Why, when and how? *Obstetrician and Gynaecologist* 1(1):20–25, 1999.

Van de Pas M, Nijhuis JG, Jongsma HW: Fetal behaviour in uncomplicated pregnancies after 41 weeks of gestation, *Early Human Development* 40(1):29–38, 1994.

Vetter K: Doppler velocimetry in late normal pregnancy: fetal arterial circulation. In Kurjak A, editor: Textbook of perinatal medicine, vol 1, London, 1998, Parthenon, pp 427–432.

Chapter | 63 |

# Rhythmic variations of labour

*Sarah Church and Tracey Hodgson*

**LEARNING OUTCOMES**

After reading this chapter, you will be able to:

- identify the factors that contribute to prolonged labour
- recognize altered patterns of uterine action and understand how this may contribute to a prolonged or precipitate labour
- discuss the midwife's role in the prevention, care and management of altered patterns of uterine action.

## INTRODUCTION

This chapter looks at prolonged labour and explores the issues that surround altered uterine action; prevention, diagnosis, management and associated problems. To maximize learning, it is anticipated that the reader has a working knowledge of the underlying physiology, care and management of normal labour (Chs 35–37).

In normal labour, the uterine contractions become progressively longer, stronger, and increase in frequency, causing the complete effacement and progressive dilatation of the os uteri in the first stage, steady delivery of the baby in the second stage, and expulsion of the placenta and membranes and the control of haemorrhage to complete the third stage of labour (Ch. 35).

Altered uterine action can occur at any stage of labour and is often attributed to an abnormal pattern of uterine contractility, resulting in slow or rapid progress. Vigilant observation and assessment of a woman in labour is therefore paramount in the prevention, detection and diagnosis of altered uterine action. Unfortunately, there is no way to predict the kind of labour progression (in terms of dilatation and descent) that a given contractile pattern will produce – that is, the quality of contractions can give little information about the course of labour. In this context, the value of antenatal education in preparing the woman and her partner for labour and the possibility of a non-perfect labour is important. Since abnormal uterine action may be *inefficient* or *over-efficient*, a useful tool to assess the progress of labour is the partogram.

## The partogram

The partogram is an observation chart that may be used to facilitate assessment of the progress of labour, including maternal and fetal wellbeing (Ch. 37). Historically, progress is measured by linear progression along a prescribed time scale, whereby a curve of cervical dilatation is measured in centimetres plotted against time in hours (Friedman 1955), and descent of the head abdominally. Over the years, modifications to the partogram have occurred, resulting in the introduction of *alert* and *action* lines. Originally, the action line was 2 hours to the right of the alert line, and augmentation instituted at this time (Fig. 63.1). Once labour is confirmed as in the active phase, cervical dilatation is expected to progress at <2 cm dilatation in 4 hours (NICE 2008). Albers (2007) supports this as a realistic expectation; she goes on to say that for some women, progress may be as little as 0.3 cm per hour. Clearly this demonstrates that partograms are only a tool and the progress of labour should not be assessed upon cervical effacement and dilation alone, without the assessment of the descent of the presenting part abdominally. Behaviour is shown to be a key part in normal progression alongside one-to-one care by a midwife.

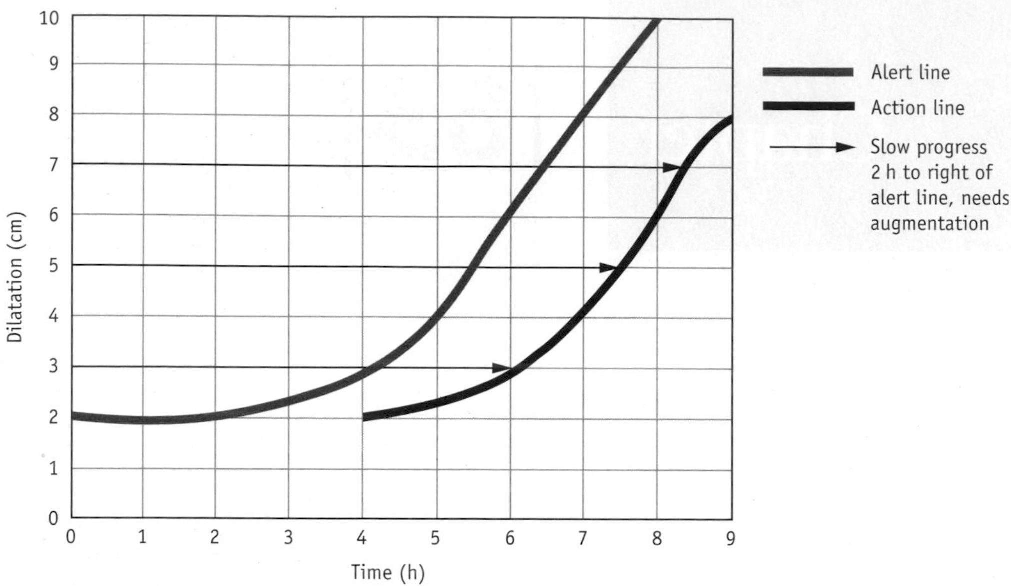


**Figure 63.1** Normogram/partogram of the cervimetric progress commencing at 2 cm dilatation. 'Alert' line outlines normal progress. 'Action' line indicates when augmentation should be instituted. *(After Studd 1973)*

To maximize use, NICE (2008) recommends that, if a partogram is used, it should record all of the following observations:

- fetal heart rate every 15 minutes (after a contraction)
- half-hourly assessment of length, strength and frequency of contractions
- 4-hourly blood pressure and temperature
- vaginal examination offered 4-hourly
- frequency of bladder emptying (bladder fullness can cause delay in progress at any stage of labour).
- ongoing consideration of the woman's emotional and psychological needs.

Further research and education is warranted to review the current mindset of women, midwives and obstetricians.

**Reflective activity 63.1**

Review your local trust partogram or labour assessment chart in relation to the NICE guidelines for intrapartum care (NICE 2008).

What supportive evidence is acknowledged to justify its use?

How could it be improved?

## PROLONGED LABOUR

Prolonged labour is described as a clinical presentation of labour which has exceeded the expected time limits. This is owing to an alteration in uterine contractility that is considered to interfere with the normal progress of labour. Furthermore, it is viewed as a deviation in normal progress of labour indicated by cervical dilatation or in the descent of the presenting part.

The term 'prolonged labour' is difficult to define, since it is dependent upon the actual time at which labour is presumed to have begun; therefore, accurate history is essential. Enkin et al (2000) suggest that the most frequently used marker for the onset of labour for women choosing a hospital birth is the time of admission. Since this is an arbitrary measurement, it can lead to an inaccurate diagnosis of the onset of labour. The presumed failure of the cervix to dilate within a given time limit based on the inaccurate diagnosis of labour, may result in the use of inappropriate intervention, preventing the woman from following her own labour pattern.

The majority of women whose labours are prolonged are primigravidae, with *inefficient uterine action* being the most common cause (El-Hamamy & Arulkumaran 2005). The birth of the first child alters the birth canal and subsequent deliveries are usually easier, since the mother has the potential benefits of experience and belief in herself.

### Causes of prolonged labour

- Inefficient uterine action
- Cephalopelvic disproportion
- Occipitoposterior position
- Malpresentation of the fetus

- Macrosomia – infants weighing above 90th centile for gestational age
- Cervical dystocia
- Maternal obesity (Ramsey et al 2006).

Any one of these factors, or a combination of them, may cause prolonged labour, which remains a major cause of maternal death and infant morbidity in developing countries (Berhane & Hogberg 1999).

The provision of appropriate midwifery care is crucial to the early diagnosis of underlying problems, which, if undetected, may create potential hazards to the mother and fetus. Midwifery care should be focused on the following areas:

- *Prevention of maternal dehydration.* Dehydration can result in ketosis and excessive tiredness (Micklewright & Champion 2002), causing maternal distress and physical exhaustion (Ch. 36). A rise in temperature, pulse and blood pressure, dehydration, oliguria and ketosis is accompanied by vomiting. Psychologically, the woman becomes demoralized and restless and her pain threshold is lowered.
- *Regular emptying of bladder and/or rectum.* A full bladder and/or rectum can impede progress by delaying descent and cause potential damage to maternal structures.

## Dangers to the mother

- *Risk of intrauterine infection*: owing to the early rupture of membranes and increased intervention, there is a greater risk of infection, which can be transmitted to the fetus.
- *An obstructed labour*: caused by undetected cephalopelvic disproportion
- *Ruptured uterus*: caused by undetected cephalopelvic disproportion
- *Increased risk of operative intervention, anaesthesia and postpartum haemorrhage*: owing to the inability of the uterus to contract strongly and rhythmically.
- *Psychological trauma*: caused by the cumulative effects of interventions in labour and at delivery.

## Dangers to the fetus

Prolonged labour is associated with fetal acidosis and intrauterine hypoxia, which can result in meconium aspiration and may lead to perinatal death (MCHRC 2000).

## Overview of midwifery management

If the principles in management of labour care are followed, it should alert the midwife to the development of a prolonged labour and, therefore, the subsequent action necessary. The following points are particularly relevant:

- The midwife should carefully assess the woman's physical and psychological condition, reporting any deviations from normal to an obstetrician, whilst maintaining accurate and contemporaneous records (NMC 2004). Continuous fetal heart monitoring may be required (NICE 2008), although intermittent auscultation may be appropriate to encourage mobility if only an amniotomy has been performed.
- One-to-one support (DH 2007) for the woman and her partner is crucial to facilitate assessment of progress, aid good communication and enhance informed consent.
- The use of water during labour is important as a means of encouraging the woman to return to her normal labour pattern. Water has been shown to ease pain, lessen anxiety and induce relaxation, resulting in a reduction in the use of epidural anaesthesia (Ch. 38) (Cluett et al 2004).
- Adequate management of pain may help reduce anxiety and provide an opportunity for the body to return to natural rhythms. It is thought that high maternal anxiety interferes with normal uterine activity (Haddad et al 1985), and the value of providing sufficient information to meet women's individual needs during preparation for childbirth has been recognized.
- Enabling women to mobilize, as well as to eat and drink, should be considered in the first instance (Champion & McCormick 2002), rather than use of medical intervention, to treat non-existent dystocia.
- The midwife should act as an advocate for the woman as required and work collaboratively with members of the multidisciplinary team (NMC 2008).

## Principles of the active management of labour

The principles of the active management of labour centre on actions taken to promote the continuance of regular effective contractions resulting in a shorter labour. Since O'Driscoll implemented this approach in 1968 (O'Driscoll et al 2003), the policy of active management has been modified along the years to accommodate opposition to the management.

The focus should be placed on the following:

1. Education:
   - Preparation for labour
2. Promote effective uterine action:
   - Accurate diagnosis of labour
   - Regular monitoring of labour
   - Appropriate use of amniotomy
   - Appropriate use of oxytocin
3. Care in labour:
   - Adequte hydration and pain relief
   - Close surveillance of mother and fetus

- Companion in labour to provide one-to-one support.

Active management of labour is not normally applied to women in labour with twins or malpresentations. Augmentation should be used with extreme caution in multigravidae and women with uterine scars, because of the risk of uterine rupture (Lewis 2007). To appreciate the implications of active management, an understanding of amniotomy and use of oxytocin is required.

## Amniotomy

Amniotomy is a procedure in which the amniotic membranes are ruptured. Whilst amniotomy has been used as a means of accelerating labour in normal labour, a recently published Cochrane review of 14 studies calls into question the use of amniotomy for this purpose. Smyth et al (2007) conclude that the current evidence does not support the use of routine amniotomy in normally progressing labours or in labours which have become prolonged.

The underlying physiology that instigates contractions is the increase in prostaglandin release and the pressure from the fetal head upon the cervix, which is associated with the increase in pain and the use of epidural anaesthesia (Smyth et al 2007). The benefits of intact membranes are the maintenance of an even hydrostatic pressure to the whole fetal surface during labour and a reduced likelihood of infection. Fetal hypoxia is therefore less likely because retraction of the placental site, and thus impairment of the uteroplacental circulation, will not occur. Accurate assessment of established labour and justification of amniotomy must be carefully addressed. The woman needs to retain control and make informed choices even when deviation from normal progress occurs (DH 2007).

## Augmentation with oxytocin

If augmentation with oxytocin is required, vigilant midwifery care is essential. The use of oxytocin in the active management of labour varies. Although it is rare for a primigravid uterus to rupture, in a multigravida, oxytocin should be used with extreme caution after obstructed labour has been excluded. In these situations, a multidisciplinary approach to care is required.

### *Use of oxytocin*

- Oxytocin is administered intravenously using an infusion pump and titrated according to local policies.
- The midwife carefully observes uterine action, ensuring that the uterus relaxes adequately between contractions and there are no signs of hyperstimulation or fetal distress.
- If uterine hyperstimulation or fetal distress occurs, the oxytocin infusion should be turned off immediately. In addition to being referred to an obstetrician (NMC 2004), the woman should be encouraged to adopt the left lateral position and oxygen should be administered via a facemask. NB: Oxygen should not be administered for long periods as it is thought it may be detrimental to the fetus. This is an area requiring further research (NICE 2008).
- If intravenous fluids are necessary, oral fluids may be restricted and a drug to reduce gastric aspiration syndrome (such as *ranitidine*) should be administered in case of the need for a general anaesthetic.
- After delivery, the infusion is usually continued for 1 hour to reduce the risk of postpartum haemorrhage.

**Reflective activity 63.2**

Consider the action of Syntocinon, indications and contraindications for its use and possible side-effects.

Check your answers using the *British National Formulary* (BNF).

## Management of a prolonged second stage of labour

It is important to consider that prolonged labour can occur at any stage and the progress of the first stage may influence the management of the second and third stages. Historically, time limits have been imposed on the length of the second stage; however, it is now considered good practice to assess each woman on an individual basis, ensuring that maternal and fetal observations remain within normal limits.

The main causes of delay in the second stage of labour are inefficient uterine action, maternal obesity, full bladder or rectum, a rigid perineum, and, rarely, a contracted pelvic outlet.

Fetal causes include a persistent occipitoposterior position, deep transverse arrest, malpresentations, fetal macrosomia and fetal abnormality, such as hydrocephaly.

If progress is slow and the woman is able to and wishes to adopt an upright position, the midwife should support this, as it is believed that the direct pressure of the presenting part against the posterior wall of the vagina stimulates the release of oxytocin (Ferguson's reflex; see Chs 35 and 37) and thereby enhances the urge to bear down. As in the first stage of labour, meticulous observations continue during the second stage. The obstetrician must be informed if there appears to be lack of progress or if fetal or maternal distress develops.

### Midwifery management of the third stage of labour following a prolonged first and/or second stage

Invariably, if the first and second stages of labour have progressed normally, the third stage will too. However, the midwife must remain observant. If problems have occurred during the labour, active management will be the method of choice because of the associated risks. Women at greater risk of complications of prolonged third stage are those who have had inadequate contractions or have developed a constriction ring, a full bladder or morbidly adhered placenta.

In addition to active management of the third stage of labour with oxytocic drugs, the midwife should be vigilant, avoid 'fiddling' with the uterus and ensure that the bladder is empty. Alternative strategies may be used, which include the encouragement of skin-to-skin contact between mother and infant (Ashmore 2001), change of maternal position, and breastfeeding, which may stimulate the uterus to contract by the release of oxytocin. In some instances, oxytocin may have to be administered intravenously by infusion, if contractions are inadequate or absent or the above management has failed.

### The psychological aspects of prolonged labour

The psychological needs of women who undergo a prolonged or augmented labour focus on the level of pain experienced resulting from increased intervention and the knowledge of an associated risk of an emergency caesarean section or instrumental delivery. In a recent study where women reported a negative birth experience following a prolonged labour, feelings of immense pain and deep negative emotions during labour were common (Nystedt et al 2005). Inadequate pain relief made women feel more anxious, out of control, and fearful. These feelings are associated with the risk of developing trauma symptoms following delivery. Women who negatively appraise their birth experience may be at risk of a difficult postnatal recovery, in which their transition to motherhood and their interaction with their babies may be interrupted (Fenwick et al 2003) (Ch. 69). In situations where women encounter a negative birth experience with their first child, Gottvall & Waldenstrom (2002), suggest that they are more likely to delay a second pregnancy and have fewer subsequent children.

Good communication is essential to allay unnecessary anxiety and to enable women and their partners to understand what is happening, to feel involved in all discussions and make decisions regarding their care. Maintaining control during a long and protracted labour can be facilitated by good midwifery support, in which the need for pain relief is regularly assessed with options discussed. After delivery, discussion between the woman and the midwife who cared for her in labour should take place at a suitable time. This can help the woman to come to terms with the events of her labour and raise her self-esteem.

**Reflective activity 63.3**

To complete this activity, you will need access to your local database.

What is the normal delivery rate in your unit?

How long is the average length of labour for primigravid and multigravid women?

How many women had their labours augmented with: (a) amniotomy; (b) amniotomy with intravenous oxytocin?

Of these, how many women had: (a) normal deliveries; (b) instrumental deliveries; (c) caesarean section?

## OVER-EFFICIENT UTERINE ACTION (PRECIPITATE LABOUR)

Labour is sometimes very rapid with intense frequent contractions, and delivery occurs within an hour (Stables 2010). This is more common in the multiparous woman and is usually caused by a minimal resistance of the maternal soft tissues. The first stage of labour may occur almost without pain and only when the head is about to be born does the woman become aware of it. The mother may sustain lacerations of the cervix and perineum and is at risk of postpartum haemorrhage. Fetal complications include hypoxia as a result of intense frequent contractions, and intracranial haemorrhage may occur as a result of rapid descent through the birth canal. Other dangers include injuries sustained as a result of being delivered in an unsuitable place or falling to the ground. If the woman has a history of precipitate births, it is advisable for her to have a delivery pack at home and for local midwives to be made aware of her history and address.

## TONIC UTERINE ACTION

### Definition

This is a rare condition in which the uterus increases powerful contractions to overcome an obstruction; eventually, one long contraction is maintained. It is synonymous with severe acute pain accompanied by rapid deterioration in maternal condition and intrauterine death due to cessation of oxygen delivery to the fetus.

### Midwifery management

The midwife's role is to administer oxygen while summoning emergency medical and midwifery aid to resuscitate the mother, as immediate delivery is required to prevent a ruptured uterus. The management is usually by caesarean section. Caution must be taken not to confuse tonic uterine action with tetanic uterine action, which occurs as a result of uterine hyperstimulation, caused usually by injudicious use of oxytocics. If oxytocin is being administered intravenously, the infusion should be stopped. Encourage the woman to adopt the left lateral position to enhance uteroplacental blood flow, and inform the obstetrician.

## CERVICAL DYSTOCIA

This is when the uterus contracts normally but the cervix fails to dilate. Its occurrence is rare but diagnosis is important to prevent maternal and fetal distress. The cervix might efface but fails to dilate; the woman may have a history of cervical surgery or congenital abnormality of the cervix. It is important that this condition is excluded prior to the use of oxytocin, because of the associated risk of uterine rupture. Vaginal delivery is therefore impossible and a caesarean section is performed.

## SUMMARY

Good midwifery care, including the accurate diagnosis of established labour, prevention of maternal dehydration, and good communication skills, may prevent the development of prolonged labour. However, if prolonged labour occurs, the midwife needs to remember the importance of vigilance and accurate record-keeping. Working in partnership with the woman and liaising with relevant healthcare professionals is essential.

Sensitive and empathetic midwifery care is also required to support women experiencing precipitate delivery, and in the careful planning of future births. In either situation, the midwife should recognize the potential need for an opportunity for the woman to discuss her labour experiences.

### KEY POINTS

- An accurate assessment of the onset of labour should be made, to minimize the introduction of unnecessary intervention.
- Collaboration and cooperation between the woman, midwife and obstetrician are essential.
- The midwife should remain vigilant throughout labour and recognize that prolonged labour can occur at any stage and the progress of the first stage may influence the management of the second and third stages.

## REFERENCES


Albers L: The evidence for physiologic management of the active phase of the first stage of labor, *Journal of Midwifery & Women's Health* 52(3):207–215, 2007.

Ashmore S: Implementing skin to skin contact in the immediate postnatal period, *MIDIRS Midwifery Digest* 11(2):247–250, 2001.

Berhane Y, Hogberg U: Prolonged labour in rural Ethiopia: a community based study, *African Journal of Reproductive Health* 3(2):33–39, 1999.

Champion P, McCormick C: Putting the evidence into practice. In Champion P, McCormick C, editors: *Eating and drinking in labour*, Oxford, 2002, Books For Midwives, pp 124–136.

Cluett ER, Pickering R, Getliffe K, et al: Randomised controlled trial of labouring in water compared with standard of augmentation for management of dystocia in first stage of labour, *British Medical Journal* 328(314):1–6, 2004.

Department of Health (DH): *Maternity matters: choice, access and continuity of care in a safe service*, London, 2007, DH.

El-Hamamy E, Arulkumaran S: Poor progress of labour, *Current Obstetrics and Gynaecology* 15(1):1–8, 2005.

Enkin M, Keirse MJNC, Neilson J, et al: Prolonged labour. In *A guide to effective care in pregnancy and childbirth*, Oxford, 2000, Oxford University Press, pp 332–340.

Fenwick J, Gamble J, Mawson J: Women's experiences of Caesarean section and vaginal birth after Caesarean: a Birthrites initiative, *International Journal of Nursing Practice* 9(1) 10–17, 2003.

Friedman EA: Primigravid labor – a graphicostatistical analysis, *Obstetrics and Gynecology* 6:567–589, 1955.

Gottvall K, Waldenstrom U: Does a traumatic birth experience have an impact on future reproduction? *British Journal of Obstetrics and Gynaecology* 109(3):254–260, 2002.

Haddad PF, Morris NF, Spielberger CD: Anxiety in pregnancy and its relation to use of oxytocin and analgesia in labour, *Journal of Obstetrics and Gynaecology* 6(2):77–81, 1985.

Lewis G, editor: The Confidential Enquiry into Maternal and ChildHealth (CEMACH). Saving mothers' lives: reviewing maternal deaths to make motherhood safer – 2003–2005. The Seventh Report on Confidential Enquiries into Maternal Deaths in the United Kingdom, London, 2007, CEMACH.

Maternal and Child Health Research Consortium (MCHRC): *Confidential Enquiry into Stillbirths and Deaths in Infancy: 7th Annual Report*, London, 2000, MCHRC.

Micklewright A, Champion P: Labouring over food: the dietician's view. In Champion P, McCormick C, editors: *Eating and drinking in labour*, Oxford, 2002, Books For Midwives, pp 29–45.

National Institute for Health and Clinical Excellence (NICE): *Intrapartum care: care of healthy women and their babies during childbirth, CG 55*, London, 2008, NICE.

Nursing and Midwifery Council (NMC): *Midwives rules and standards*, London, 2004, NMC.

Nursing and Midwifery Council (NMC): *The code. Standards of conduct, performance and ethics for nurses and midwives*, London, 2008, NMC.

Nystedt A, Hogberg U, Lundman B: The negative birth experience of prolonged labour: a case-referent study, *Journal of Clinical Nursing* 14(5):579–586, 2005.

O'Driscoll K, Meagher D, Robson M: *Active management of labour*, ed 4, London, 2003, Mosby.

Ramsey JE, Greer I, Sattar N: Obesity and reproduction, *British Medical Journal* 333(7579):1159–1162, 2006.

Smyth RMD, Alldred SK, Markham C: Amniotomy for shortening spontaneous labour, *Cochrane Database of Systematic Reviews* (4): CD006167, 2007.

Stables D, Rankin J: Abnormalities of uterine action and onset of labour. In *Physiology in childbearing with anatomy and related biosciences*, ed 3, London, 2010, Elsevier.

Studd J: Partograms and normograms of cervical dilatation in management of primigravid labour, *British Medical Journal* 4(5890):451–455, 1973.

Chapter |64|

# Malpositions and malpresentations

*Paul Lewis*

## LEARNING OUTCOMES

After reading this chapter, you will be able to:

- have an understanding of the factors which predispose to malpositions and malpresentations of the fetus
- recognize features of malpositions and malpresentations and, where necessary, take appropriate action
- consider the management and care to facilitate normality, ensuring a safe and positive experience for the woman and baby
- use appropriate sources of evidence to support safe, effective and women-centred practice
- understand the complex, controversial and uncertain state of knowledge that surrounds the management of malpositions and malpresentations and use this to inform your clinical judgements; appropriately advising and supporting women in their choices of care.

## INTRODUCTION

This chapter considers the recognition, management and care of the fetus when it presents in an occipitoposterior (OP) position, by the breech, face or brow and when an oblique or transverse lie results in a shoulder presentation. Compound presentation is also discussed.

Malposition and malpresentations of the fetus can occur in both pregnancy and labour. The midwife has a key role in identifying these, using best evidence to inform and support the mother and effective skills to undertake safe management and care. With associated higher rates of maternal and perinatal morbidity and mortality, it is essential that careful attention be given to the diagnosis of malposition and malpresentations in order to maximize fetal outcomes (Baxley 2001, Cheng & Hannah 1993, Hannah et al 2000, Pritchard & MacDonald 1980).

While primarily a practitioner of the 'normal', the midwife must be fully conversant with the problems and practicalities that both malposition and malpresentations can present. In such circumstances, skills are often tested to the limit and the midwife's ability to gain the confidence of the woman and to work effectively with the wider healthcare team is paramount in achieving a safe and successful outcome for both mother and baby (ALSO 2003). In dealing with malpositions and malpresentations of the fetus, the midwife needs to be knowledgeable about the latest evidence or lack of it, that will help to inform a woman's decisions in relation to her care and provide her with the options available (Evans 2007).

This may be difficult and, in spite of the evidence, some women may choose a path, for personal, cultural or religious reasons, that is not in keeping with the recommended evidence or accepted institutional practices. Nevertheless, it is a woman's right to choose for herself and the midwife needs to ensure that in such circumstances, the woman continues to receive the relevant information, advice and support necessary. In achieving this, the midwife should consult with her supervisor of midwives and, with the woman's permission, share the proposed plan of care with her and the lead obstetrician. All discussions with the woman must be clearly documented in her maternity notes and accurately reflect the advice given, the options available and choices she has made.

## IDENTIFYING MALPOSITIONS AND MALPRESENTATIONS OF THE FETUS

Midwives must be able to employ a range of skills to assist them in identifying the fetus in:

*Malpositions* (where the occiput is in one or other posterior quadrant of the pelvis):

- deflexed attitude such as an occipitoposterior (OP) position.

*Malpresentations* (any presentation other than vertex):

- extended attitude:
  - face
  - brow
- breech presentation
- shoulder presentation/oblique lie.

These require midwives to take a detailed history, keenly observe the woman's body and behaviours, and carry out a considered and careful clinical examination. Above all, they must be able to draw the findings together in order to analyse and make sense of them. From this, the midwife can then make a diagnosis, upon which discussions with the woman, clinical decisions and further professional judgements will be based.

## INCIDENCE

The incidence of malpositions and malpresentations varies according to lifestyle, gestation and parity, as well as the condition of the mother and fetus. The midwife needs to consider the likelihood and the reasons why these presentations might occur as part of the assessment, diagnosis and plan of the woman's care.

It is essential that the midwife recognize that a malposition is the commonest cause of non-engagement of the fetal head at term in a primigravida. It is the commonest cause of prolonged labour and mechanical difficulties associated with the birth. Persistent OP position was a significant factor in caesarean section and instrumental deliveries with less than half of the OP labours ending in a spontaneous birth of the baby (Fitzpatrick et al 2001).

## CLINICAL ASSESSMENT

In identifying malpositions and malpresentations, the midwife should take into account the gestational age of the fetus, the woman's parity, and any history that might suggest the likelihood of such anomalies or abnormalities. The clinical skills of abdominal and vaginal assessment that the midwife may perform as part of a woman's antenatal and intrapartum care, are central to the recognition of the presentation, engagement, attitude, lie and position of the fetus. Underlying this is the need to be fully conversant with the anatomy of the maternal pelvis, the engaging diameter of the fetal presentations, and the implications of these for the birthing process.

## MALPOSITION OF THE OCCIPUT

The fetus is in an occipitoposterior position (OPP) when the fetal occiput lies adjacent to the sacroiliac joint and occupies either the left or right posterior quadrants of the mother's pelvis with the brow directed anteriorly.

Occipitoposterior positions occur in approximately 10–25% of pregnancies during the early stage of labour and in 10–15% during the active phase, most of which end normally (Gardberg & Tuppurainen 1994a).

**Causes** of OPP include the following:

- *Modern lifestyle of less physical activity and poor posture* has increased the risk of OPP. With some positional changes/movement, many fetuses can be persuaded to change their position before labour begins, but midwives need to consider different strategies to support mother and fetus if the baby remains in an OPP (Sutton 2000).
- *Use of epidural anaesthesia* (Saunders et al 1989, Thorp et al 1993): the anaesthesia reduces the tone of the pelvic floor muscles and resistance to the presenting part. This causes failure of the vertex to rotate, increasing the chance of persistent OPP, asynclitism and transverse arrest of the fetal head. In one study (Gardberg et al 1998), persistent OPP at birth primarily resulted from a malrotation rather than the absence of rotation.
- *Android pelvis*: the narrow forepelvis forces the fetal head to adjust and take up a posterior position in order to enter the pelvic brim.
- *Anthropoid pelvis*: may also lead to a persistent OPP.
- *Pendulous abdomen or a flat sacrum.*
- *Anterior placenta* is also associated with an OPP towards term (Gardberg & Tuppurainen 1994b).

Sutton and Scott (1996) highlighted the use of *optimal fetal positioning* (see website) in helping women to increase their chances of normal childbirth. Other work suggests that such strategies for reducing persistent OPP at birth may be more complex (Hunter et al 2007) (see website).

Occipitoposterior positions (Fig. 64.1) throw a heavy responsibility on the midwife, but being overly pessimistic does little to help the mother. Where the labour is progressing satisfactorily, the outcome is likely to be spontaneous rotation to an anterior position followed by a normal vertex delivery.

While malpositions can and do resolve, the midwife should be aware of the potential for delay and the

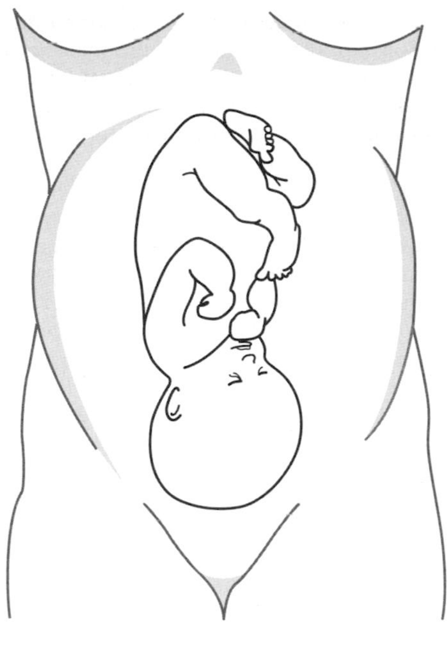


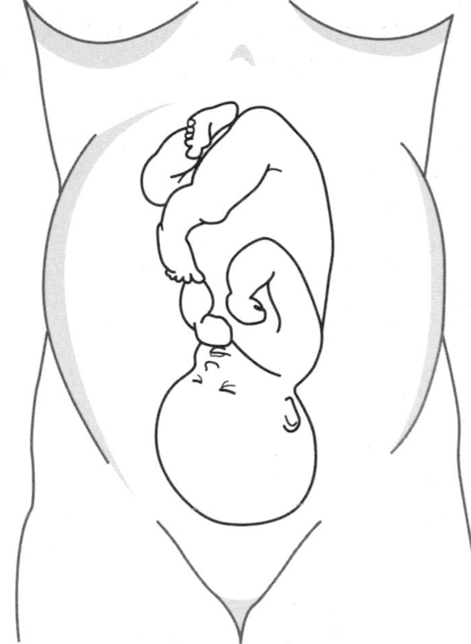


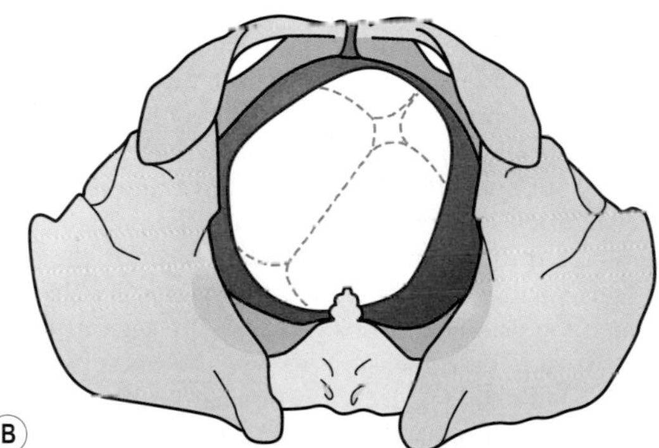


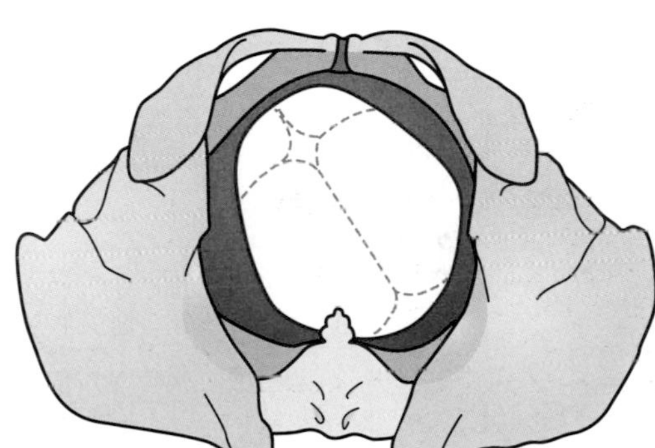

**Figure 64.1** Occipitoposterior positions. **A.** Abdominal findings – the anterior shoulders are well out from the midline or fetal limbs are easily palpable. This may cause a misdiagnosis of multiple pregnancy. **B.** Vaginal findings – on vaginal examination, the anterior fontanelle is easily felt and recognized by its shape and size.

possibility of adverse outcomes that may arise when the labour is prolonged or the OPP persists.

*Slow progress* should alert midwives to the possibility of abnormal labour and they must be vigilant to promptly recognize any complications that may arise and call for assistance. They should be ready to act and make decisive professional judgements when indicated by the maternal or fetal condition, poor progress of labour, or the mother's psychological state and frame of mind. In the presence of an obstetric urgency or emergency, such as deep transverse arrest (DTA) or cord prolapse, the midwife must seek immediate medical assistance.

In caring for a woman in prolonged labour, the midwife has the exacting task of maintaining a close watch on the progress she is making, attending to her physical care and providing the encouragement, reassurance and emotional support that the woman needs.

The midwife also needs to be aware of the altered mechanism of a fetus in a posterior position, during which the fetus tends to be in a deflexed attitude, with the anterior fontanelle immediately over the internal cervical os. The fetal spine is towards the forward curve of the maternal lumbar spine, so that the fetus finds it difficult or impossible to adopt a flexed position. As the fetal spine straightens, the fetus tends to 'square' the shoulders and raise the chin from the chest, resulting in a deflexed, erect 'military' attitude of the fetal head, as shown in Figure 64.2.

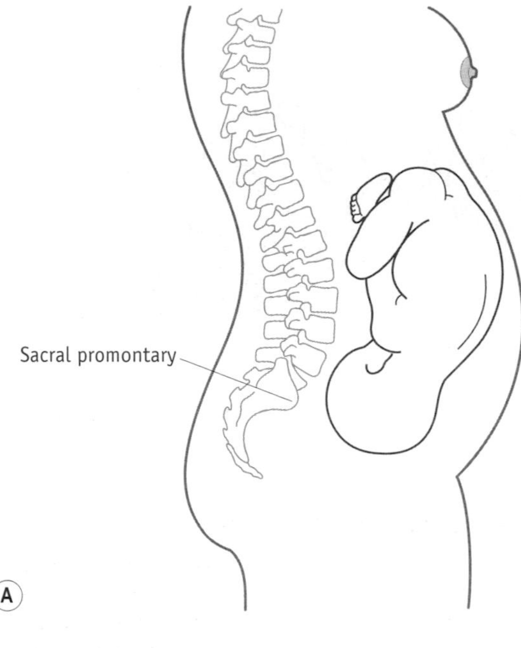


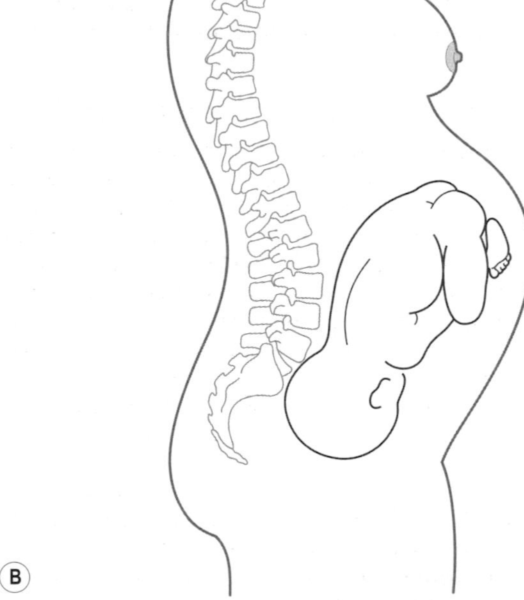


**Figure 64.2** The 'military' posture of the fetus in an occipitoposterior position. **A.** Well-flexed fetus. **B.** OP position. Deflexed with straight spine and wider engaging diameter.

Such movements bring the fetal head into a more difficult relationship with the inlet of the maternal pelvis. Misaligned above the pelvic brim, the fetal head is slow to engage as its larger diameters present. This ill-fitting presentation may also result in early rupture of the membranes and the danger of cord prolapse.

There is a *loss of fetal axis pressure*, contractions are not effectively stimulated and descent is delayed. This can lead to slow, uneven cervical dilatation and prolonged labour. In the process of birth, the engaging diameter of the fetal head is reduced, with that at right angles being elongated. In an occipitoposterior position, the fetal head is compressed in unfavourable diameters, resulting in '*sugar loaf*' moulding, creating a greater risk of damage to the tentorium cerebelli and the likelihood of intracranial haemorrhage. With a persistent occipitoposterior position, these wider diameters may also result in increased trauma to the woman's vagina and perineum.

## Diagnosis of the occipitoposterior position

### During pregnancy

The diagnosis is often made by abdominal examination. On inspection, the abdomen appears flattened, or slightly depressed, below the umbilicus (see Fig. 64.3). On palpation, the fetal head is commonly high. If the fetus is almost occipitolateral, the deflexed head may feel large, because the occipitofrontal diameter is palpated.

The occiput and brow may be felt at the same level at the pelvic inlet, while the fetal back can be palpated out in the flank. If the occiput is markedly posterior, the high head feels small, as the bitemporal diameter is palpated; movements of the fetal limbs can often be seen or easily felt and it may be impossible to feel the back (see Fig. 64.1). The fetal heart sounds can be heard in the midline just below the umbilicus. If the heart sounds are audible in one flank, it suggests that the fetal back is directed towards that side.

### During labour

The diagnosis may be made by abdominal examination, though as labour advances, the head may become flexed and engaged. The cephalic prominence of the sinciput can be felt above the pubic bone and on the opposite side to the fetal back. The midwife should be alert whenever the cephalic prominence is felt on the same side as the fetal back and should consider the possibility of a face or brow presentation and seek to exclude these. A deflexed head prior to or in the process of engagement in the maternal pelvis can become extended to a brow, or hyperextended to a face presentation. 'Coupling' of contractions is associated with

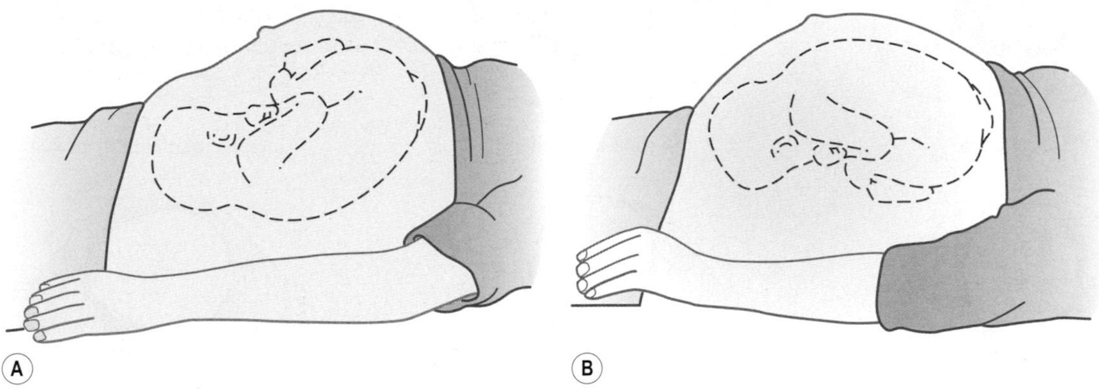


**Figure 64.3** Abdominal contour: **A.** when the fetus is in the occipitoposterior position, compared to **B.** the more rounded contour of the occipitoanterior position.

occipitoposterior positions (ALSO 2003). The midwife may identify this phenomenon when she palpates the mother's abdomen or else on the tocograph tracing if electronic fetal monitoring is in progress.

On vaginal examination the findings depend on the degree of flexion of the fetal head. Palpation of the anterior fontanelle is usually diagnostic of an occipitoposterior position. When the head is partially or well flexed, the anterior fontanelle is felt towards the front of the pelvis, while occasionally the posterior fontanelle is just within reach at the back. With a deflexed head, the anterior fontanelle is almost central and, unless obscured by caput, easily recognizable by its size and shape.

## Progress in labour

The progress of labour will depend upon the regularity and strength of uterine contractions and the *degree of flexion* of the fetal head. The shape of the maternal pelvis and the maternal position may be significant in determining how the fetus negotiates the pelvic inlet, cavity and outlet.

### Flexion of the fetal head

If the head is flexed, labour will probably be completely normal. The engaging diameter is the suboccipitofrontal (10 cm). The occiput reaches the pelvic floor and rotates anteriorly through three-eighths of a circle and the baby is born with the occiput anteriorly (Fig. 64.4).

When the head remains deflexed, it tends to remain high or is slow to engage. Labour is slow to become established, with hypotonic and irregular uterine contractions. However, flexion may improve, and once the head becomes flexed, labour usually accelerates and continues normally, with a long internal rotation and an occipito-anterior birth (Fig. 64.4A).

### Deflexion of the fetal head

The midwife needs to be fully conversant with the mechanism of the persistent occipitoposterior position and how this translates into what the woman experiences. If the head remains deflexed, labour is likely to be prolonged and painful, with backache a prominent characteristic. The outcome is then dependent on the size, shape and dimensions of the pelvis in relation to those of the fetal skull.

### Persistent occipitoposterior position (POP)

The mechanism is that the lie is longitudinal, presentation vertex and attitude deflexed – the engaging diameter is the occipitofrontal and measures 11.5 cm. The position may be either right or left occipitoposterior and the presenting part is the anterior aspect of the right (ROP) or left (LOP) parietal bone. Descent takes place with deficient flexion and the biparietal diameter of the fetal head is held up on the sacrocotyloid diameter of the maternal pelvis, so that the sinciput becomes the leading part. When the sinciput meets the resistance of the pelvic floor, it rotates forward one-eighth of a circle (Fig. 64.4C). The sinciput passes under the pubic arch and the occiput into the hollow of the sacrum. With good contractions, spontaneous delivery ensues and, with flexion, the occiput sweeps the maternal perineum and, once the glabellar is visible, the brow and face are delivered by extension. The rest of the mechanism follows that of a normal, vertex presentation (see Ch. 37). This is called *persistent occipitoposterior position* or *'face-to-pubes'* delivery and is often associated with an anthropoid pelvis (Fig. 64.4C).

### Deep transverse arrest (DTA)

DTA (Fig. 64.4B) may occur if the head remains deflexed. The fetal head may attempt a long rotation, but because

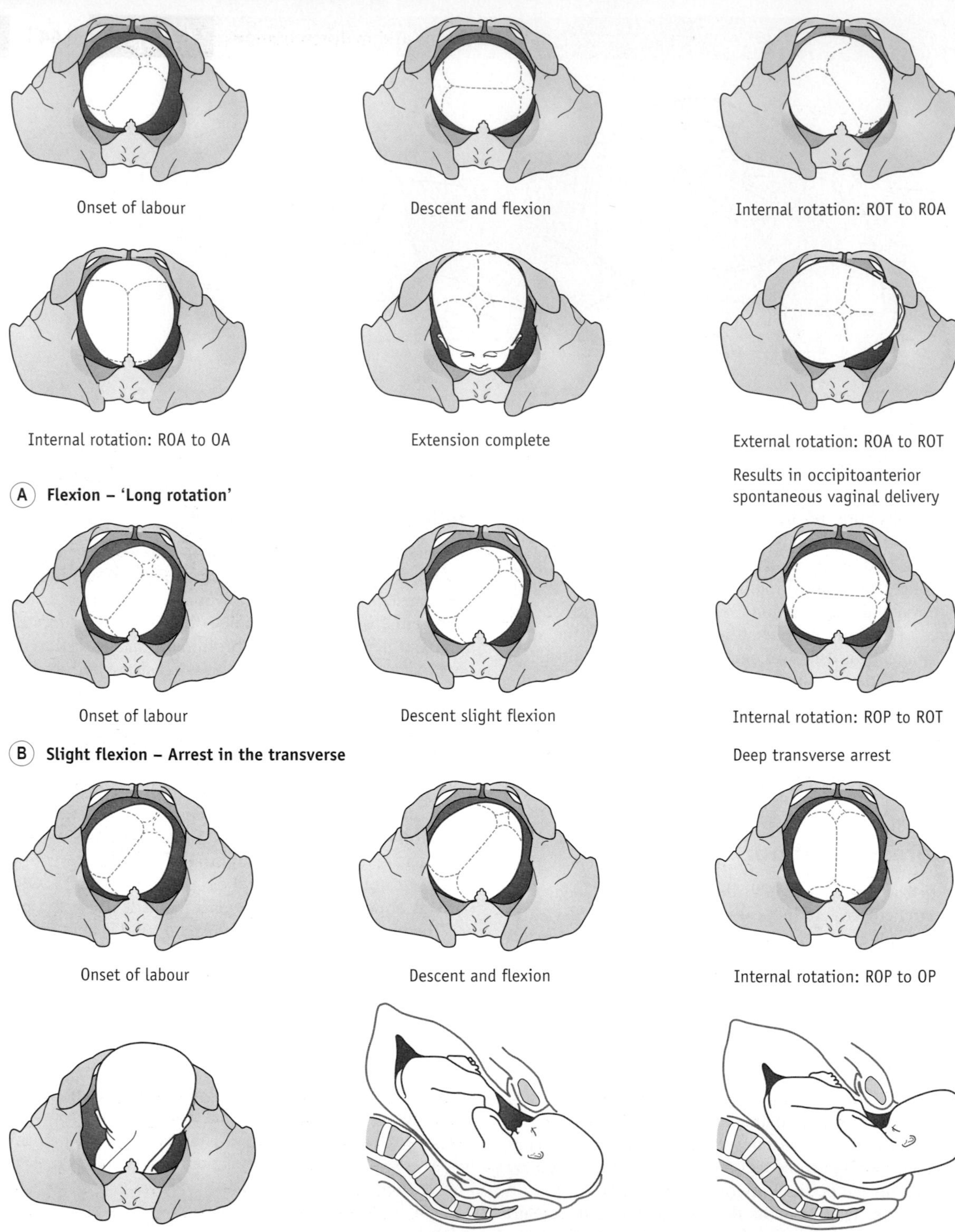


**Figure 64.4** Possible outcomes of an occipitoposterior position. The fetal head enters the pelvis with the occiput posteriorly.

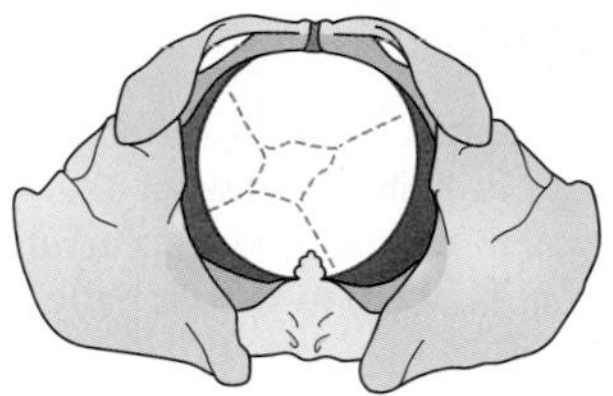

No mechanism for delivery

(D) **Slight flexion – Brow presentation**

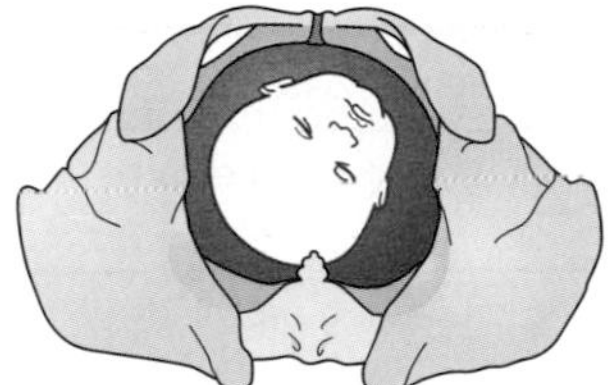

LMA: onset of labour

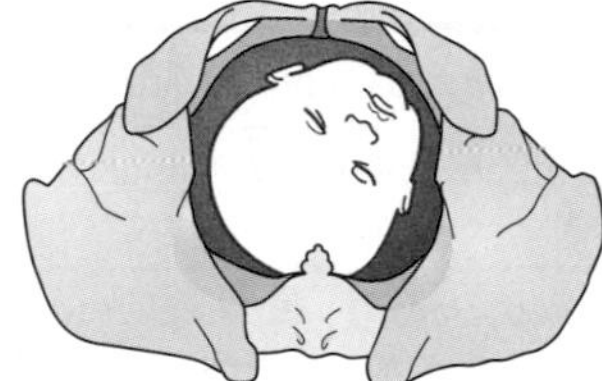

Extension and descent

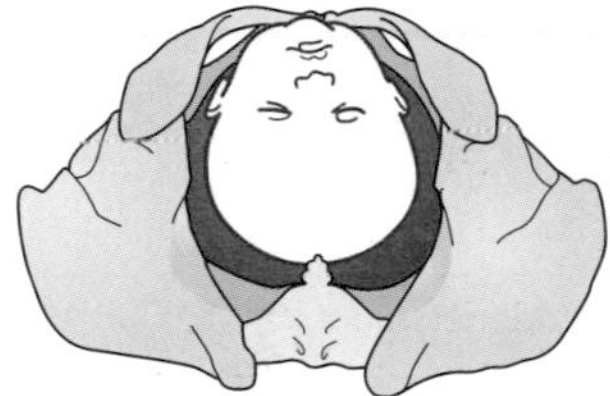

Internal rotation: LMA to MA

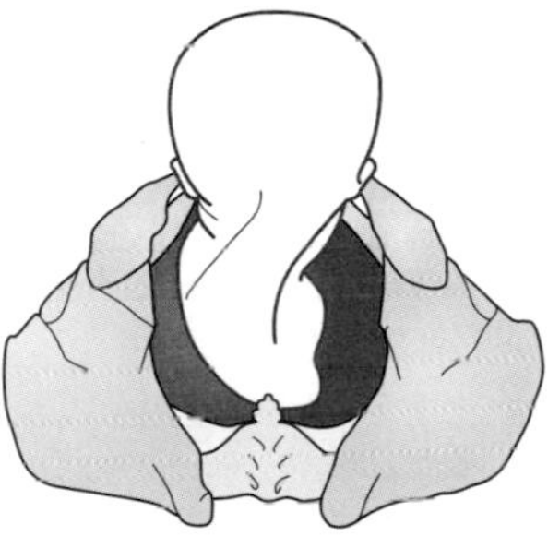

Flexion

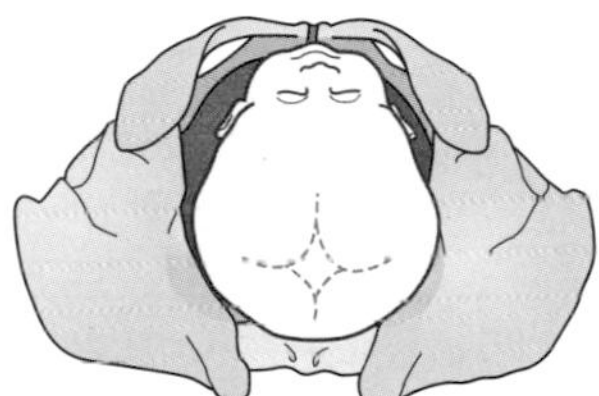

Extension

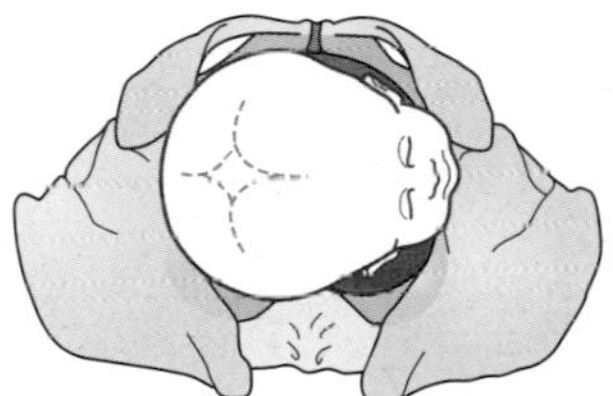

External rotation: LMA to LMT

(E) **Extension – face presentation**

**Figure 64.4** *(continued)*

of wider diameters and prominence of the ischial spines, it can become caught in the transverse diameter of the obstetric outlet, between the ischial spines.

DTA should be suspected if there is delay in the second stage of labour. On vaginal examination, the sagittal suture is found in the transverse diameter of the pelvis with a fontanelle at each end, close to the ischial spines. In such circumstances, appropriately skilled midwifery or medical assistance should be obtained and, with the use of vacuum extraction (ventouse), the fetal head may be rotated to an anterior position and delivered. Manual rotation of the occiput may also be considered. The midwife should be knowledgeable about this procedure (NMC 2008), and needs to explain the procedure fully to the woman, obtaining informed consent (see website). This should not delay summoning additional assistance.

Occasionally, caesarean section is necessary to deliver the fetus in an occipitoposterior position. This is likely when complications such as cord prolapse and fetal distress occur, or when true cephalopelvic disproportion is diagnosed.

## Extension of the fetal head

It is possible that the fetal head may either be in a slightly extended position, or may adopt this as labour progresses, resulting in a *brow* presentation (Fig. 64.4D). Unless the fetus is particularly small or preterm, then it is unlikely that it will be born vaginally. Full extension of the fetal head may lead to a face presentation, which, if mento-anterior, may deliver vaginally (Fig. 64.4E).

## Complications of OPP

Midwives need to carefully consider complications that might arise (Table 64.1) and be fully aware of what action should be taken to prevent or minimize these occurring in their management and care of a woman whose baby is in an occipitoposterior position.

**Table 64.1 Complications of occipitoposterior (OP) position**

| Complication | Reason |
|---|---|
| Early rupture of the membranes | Poorly fitting presenting part and uneven pressure on the forewaters |
| Cord prolapse | As with any ill-fitting presenting part, the membranes tend to rupture early and the cord may prolapse |
| Prolonged labour | This is associated with a deflexed head, poorly fitting presenting part and misaligned fetal axis pressure. A slightly contracted pelvis may compound this. Hypotonic and inefficient or over-efficient uterine contractions may result. In such circumstances, the development of either fetal or maternal distress is more likely and operative intervention and anaesthesia are often necessary. Postpartum haemorrhage is therefore an added risk |
| Retention of urine | This may occur with prolonged labour and the pressure on the urethra that results from the wider diameters of the OP position |
| Premature expulsive effort | The wider diameter of the OP position results in pressure on the sacral nerves and the woman may feel the need to push before full dilatation of the cervix. Early distension of the perineum and dilatation of the anus can also occur while the head is still high |
| Infection | This is more likely because of early rupture of the membranes, especially if labour is prolonged, and can be compounded by an increased number of vaginal assessments |
| Trauma to the mother's soft tissues | The risk of trauma is increased with the wider diameter of the OP position. When this is persistent, the biparietal diameter and large occiput distend the maternal perineum. Instrumental delivery may also increase the risk of maternal trauma |
| Post-traumatic stress disorder or postnatal depression | Prolonged, difficult, painful and traumatic labour might result in mental ill-health. This can be exacerbated when the mother has no control over events and is not involved in decision-making. This, together with maternal exhaustion and an unsettled baby, may lead to difficulty in maternal–infant bonding |
| Maternal exhaustion | In prolonged labour, maternal exhaustion may follow the birth |
| Unsettled or difficult-to-feed infant | In an OP position and a prolonged labour, the baby's head will have been compressed in an unnatural angle, resulting in discomfort and pain |
| Fetal intracranial haemorrhage | Upward moulding of the fetal skull may lead to stretching and damage of the tentorium cerebelli and consequent tearing of the great vein of Galen, resulting in haemorrhage and intracranial damage |
| Increased perinatal mortality and morbidity | This might result from cord prolapse, prolonged labour, instrumental delivery, infection and intracranial haemorrhage, and is increased because of hypoxia and birth trauma |

## Care in labour

When caring for a woman in labour whose baby is in an occipitoposterior position, the following aspects of care are paramount:

- communication and support
- one-to-one care
- general comfort and pain relief
- ambulation and position
- assessment of progress
- effective assessment of maternal and fetal wellbeing
- appropriate and decisive clinical decisions
- appropriate referral when necessary
- accurate and detailed record-keeping
- careful debriefing following the birth of the baby.

# MALPRESENTATIONS OF THE FETUS

*Malpresentation* refers to the orientation of the fetus and may be diagnosed during pregnancy or in labour. Any presentation other than vertex is termed a malpresentation and this therefore includes *breech*, *face*, *brow* and *shoulder*. When midwives encounter a malpresentation of the fetus, they will draw upon similar knowledge and many of the skills they use in the care and management of women whose babies were in an occipitoposterior position.

In all malpresentations there is commonly an ill-fitting presenting part: often associated with early rupture of the membranes because of uneven pressure on the bag of forewaters. This results in an increased risk of cord prolapse. An ill-fitting presenting part is also associated with poor uterine action and slower cervical dilatation, and therefore labour may be prolonged with the concomitant risk of infection and operative intervention.

## Breech presentation

A breech presentation occurs when the fetal buttocks lie lowermost in the maternal uterus and the fetal head occupies the fundus. The lie is longitudinal, the denominator is the sacrum and the presenting diameter is the bitrochanteric, which measures 10 cm.

Breech presentation is common before 37 weeks' gestation, with a suggested incidence of 15% at 29–32 weeks' gestation reducing to 3–4% at term (Hannah et al 2000, MIDIRS 2008). One fetus in four will present by the breech at some stage in pregnancy. In preterm labour it is not surprising to find the breech presenting and these infants comprise a quarter of all babies born by the breech. However, by the 34th week of pregnancy, the majority will have turned to a vertex presentation.

### Types

Four types of breech presentation are described (Fig. 64.5). They are determined by the way in which the fetal legs are flexed or extended, and these have implications for the birth.

- *Flexed* or *complete* breech: the fetus sits with the thighs and knees flexed with the feet close to the buttocks. This is more common in multigravidae.
- *Extended* or *frank* breech: the fetal thighs are flexed, the legs are extended at the knees and lie alongside the trunk, with the feet near the fetal head. This is the commonnest type of breech presentation and occurs most frequently in primigravidae towards term. This is because their usually firm uterine and abdominal muscles allow only limited fetal movement and the fetus is therefore unable to flex its legs and turn to a cephalic presentation.
- *Footling presentation:* one or both feet present below the fetal buttocks, with hips and knees extended. This relatively rare type of breech presentation is more likely to occur when the fetus is preterm. A foot may occasionally be felt at the level of the buttocks and might be confused with a footling presentation. Usually, as labour advances, it slips behind the buttocks, returning to an obvious flexed breech position.
- *Knee presentation:* one or both knees present below the fetal buttocks, with one or both hips extended and the knees flexed. This is the least common of all types of breech presentation.

There is a higher perinatal mortality and morbidity rate with breech presentation, which is largely due to prematurity and congenital abnormalities of the fetus, as well as birth asphyxia and birth trauma (Cheng & Hannah 1993, Hannah et al 2000). The clinical setting, failure to respond to delay and lack of clinical experience may also contribute to poorer outcomes (Kotaska et al 2009).

In providing care, the midwife needs to be conversant with the latest developments surrounding the management and optimal mode of delivery. While the outcomes of the 'Term Breech Trial' have dominated the discourse around the mode and management of breech births (Hannah et al 2000) and significantly influenced practice in the United Kingdom and abroad, the evidence is at best uncertain, conflicting and contradictory (Glezerman 2006, Goffinet et al 2006, Hofmeyr & Hannah 2003, Kotaska 2004, Kotaska et al 2009, Van Idderkinge 2007, Waites 2003, Whyte et al 2004).

However, as Shennan & Bewley (2001) point out, the need to provide expertise in vaginal breech delivery will not disappear. Some women present too late, even when a policy of planned caesarean section is in place, and some women will reject the choice of a planned caesarean section and choose to have a vaginal breech birth in either the hospital or home setting because of personal, cultural or religious reasons.

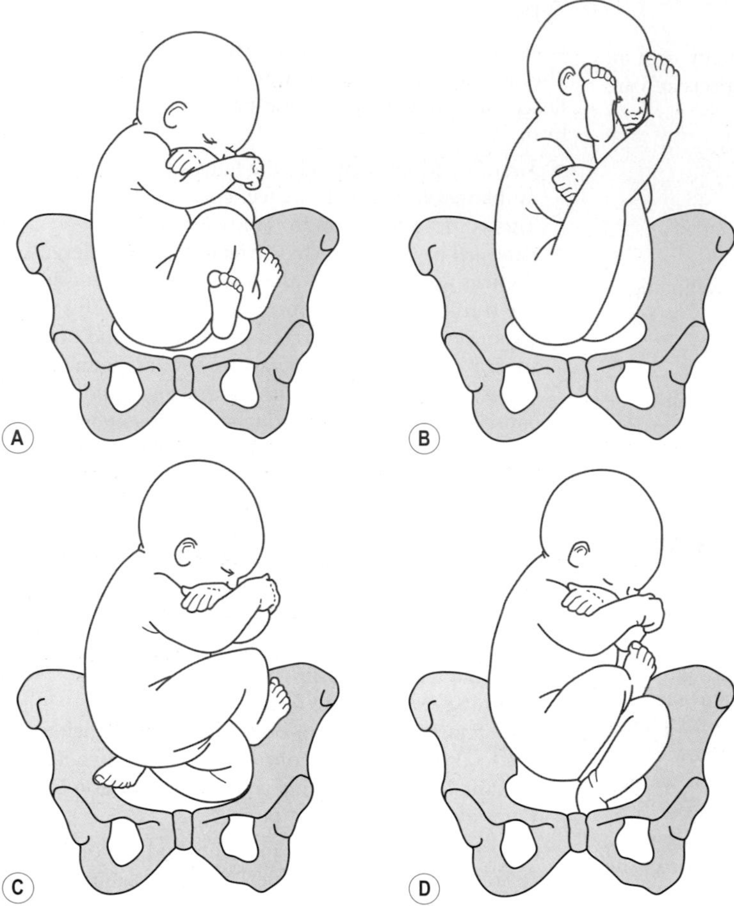


**Figure 64.5** Types of breech presentation. **A.** Flexed. **B.** Extended. **C.** Knee. **D.** Footling.

## Causes

The fetus may adopt the breech position for a variety of reasons, though the true cause is often unknown. Waites (2003) found that in most cases no single cause can be identified, and it may result from a random occurrence (Bartlett & Okun 1994). The most common cause is likely to be a *'benign error of orientation'* in which the fetus sits in the breech for no known cause and without any obvious abnormalities. Other causes include:

- abnormal size and shape of the pelvis
- uterine causes: placenta or fibroids occupying the lower uterine segment
- abnormal liquor volume
- multiple pregnancy
- maternal conditions or fetal abnormalities resulting in poor postural tone
- congenital anomalies: incidence known to be two to three times higher in those fetuses that present by the breech (Lauszus et al 1992).

See Table 64.2.

## Diagnosis during pregnancy

The midwife needs to be alert to the gestational age of the fetus but should not be unduly concerned prior to 36 weeks' gestation. A history of a previous breech presentation may be significant, and if the breech persists, then referral to an obstetrician should be made and the likely cause identified.

The woman may give a history of discomfort under the ribs due to the presence of the hard fetal head or describe fetal movements in the lower pole of the uterus. Her description of her baby's movements and how she feels can be valuable elements in the diagnosis of a breech presentation (Banks 2000).

*Abdominal examination* usually allows the diagnosis to be confirmed. It may be difficult to distinguish between a breech and a vertex presentation and a high index of suspicion is an asset for diagnosis (ALSO 2003).

The method of conducting the abdominal examination may have consequences for detecting a breech

**Table 64.2 Causes of breech presentation**

| | |
|---|---|
| Primigravidae | Firm abdominal and uterine muscles may prevent flexion of the fetal legs, especially when they are already extended. |
| Uterine anomalies | Bicornuate uterus may restrict fetal movement.<br>Previous breech birth may also be strongly associated with a uterine anomaly. |
| Oligohydramnios | Reduced liquor volume restricts the ability of the fetus to turn in the uterus. The condition may also be associated with fetal anomalies and fetal compromise. |
| Placental location | Placenta praevia may prevent the fetal head from fitting into the lower uterine segment and entering the pelvis.<br>A placenta situated in one or other cornua of the uterus reduces the breadth of space in the upper segment and can lead to a breech presentation. |
| Uterine fibroids | These can interfere with fetal activity or when situated in the lower uterine segment can prevent the fetal head from entering the lower pole of the uterus. |
| A contracted pelvis | The fetal head is unable to enter the pelvic brim. |
| Fetal anomalies such as trisomy 21 and hydrocephalus | These can lead to fetal hypotonia in which the lack of movement, reduced or restricted fetal activity makes it difficult for the fetus to turn.<br>Hydrocephalus can prevent the fetal head engaging in the pelvis. |
| Multiple pregnancy | There is usually insufficient space to turn. Twins may present vertex and breech and, as such, spontaneous version is unlikely. |
| Maternal alcohol or drug abuse | May lead to fetal hypotonia in which the lack of movement, reduced or restricted fetal activity makes it difficult for the fetus to turn. |
| Grande multiparity | Lax abdominal and uterine muscles allow movement and may lead to an unstable lie. |
| Polyhydramnios | Overdistension of the uterus enables the fetus to be more mobile. |
| Prematurity | Increased incidence at earlier gestation.<br>Smaller fetus with greater space within the uterus to adopt a breech position. |
| Impaired fetal growth, short umbilical cord and fetal death | Compromised fetus may result in decreased fetal activity.<br>May be associated with fetal or maternal conditions having an adverse effect on the fetus, which results in reduced or restricted fetal mobility. |

presentation or finding a ballottable fetal head in the uterine fundus.

Although inspection of the maternal abdomen usually reveals nothing that indicates a breech presentation, occasionally fetal movements can be seen in the lower pole. On palpation the presenting part feels firm but less hard and less rounded than the head. The diagnosis is usually made by feeling the hard, round and ballottable head in the fundus of the uterus.

Over time, the sequence in which *Leopold manoeuvres* (see website) have been applied during abdominal palpation have changed, with identification of the lie often taking place before palpation of the presenting part. In such circumstances, especially at term, the uterus might be stimulated, increasing tone or even stimulating a contraction. This results in the presenting part feeling hard, and the fetal head, if in the uterine fundus, becomes fixed and more difficult to ballot. As a consequence, breech presentations can be missed.

A primigravida with an extended breech may simulate a cephalic presentation. The woman's firm abdominal muscles brace the extended legs and compress the breech, allowing it to enter deep into the pelvis. The presenting part may be out of reach of the midwife's palpating fingers and can be mistaken for the deeply engaged head. The baby's feet, lying under the chin, make ballottement more difficult. If the placenta is situated on the anterior uterine wall, identification of the fetal head is further obscured.

Fetal heart sounds, classically heard above the umbilicus in breech presentations, may be heard at maximum intensity in an extended breech where the heart sounds are commonly heard in a vertex presentation: halfway between the superior anterior iliac spine and the maternal umbilicus.

Ultrasound imaging is helpful in:

- confirming presentation
- identification of fetal attitude
- fetal weight and liquor volume estimation
- confirmation or ruling out possible abnormalities
- confirmation of those women with breech presentation after 36 weeks' gestation, for which external cephalic version (ECV) should be offered (RCOG 2006a, Vause et al 1997).

*Vaginal examination* may be carried out by the midwife or obstetrician to exclude a deeply engaged head and confirm breech presentation. If the head is deeply engaged, the shoulders palpate just above the pelvic brim and are sometimes difficult to distinguish from the breech. On vaginal examination, an extended breech has a hard, compressed presenting part similar to a cephalic presentation, and the cleft of the buttocks may imitate the line of the sagittal suture.

Midwives should be aware of these deceptive findings and unless certain that the presentation is vertex, should be cautious. If in doubt or convinced that the presentation is breech after 36 weeks' gestation, they should seek confirmation by ultrasound examination, informing the woman of the findings. Where a breech presentation exists, the midwife should discuss the evidence and implications and, as appropriate, refer to a senior obstetric colleague.

## Diagnosis during labour

In labour the presenting part may initially be high. On vaginal examination the breech feels soft and irregular and no sutures or fontanelles are palpable. The hard sacrum and the anus should be felt and it is important to distinguish the breech from a face presentation.

The midwife will note that in a breech presentation the landmarks of the fetal ischial tuberosities are on either side of the fetal anus and form a straight line. This differs from a face presentation, in which the fetal mouth and malar prominences form a triangle (ALSO 2003).

Fresh, 'toothpaste like', thick meconium may be found on the examining finger and is diagnostic of a breech presentation. The fetal genitalia are soft and not easily recognized because they become oedematous.

In a flexed breech, the feet may be palpable alongside the buttocks, but these usually fall back behind the presenting part as labour advances. On vaginal examination, the features of the foot that distinguish it from a hand are: shorter digits, larger size but limited range of movements of the big toe, and the presence of a heel.

## Associated risks

Breech presentation carries increased risks to a healthy mother and fetus from either a complicated vaginal delivery or caesarean section (Cheng & Hannah 1993, Hofmeyr 1991, Kotaska et al 2009, Van Idderkinge 2007). A high incidence of childhood handicap following breech presentation has also been identified and found to be similar in those infants delivered after a trial of labour and following an elective caesarean section (Danielian et al 1996). Poor outcomes following vaginal breech delivery, therefore, might result from some underlying condition causing breech presentation rather than damage during delivery (Hofmeyr & Hannah 2003). A study following up the 'Term Breech Trial', found no differences in long-term neonatal morbidity between babies born by vaginal birth and those born by caesarean section (Whyte et al 2004).

## Care and management – pregnancy

The midwife who diagnoses a breech presentation should, depending on the woman's preferences, either refer her to a senior obstetrician or discuss the case with her Supervisor of Midwives. The midwife must inform the woman as to her options of care and these, together with the mother's choices, should be clearly documented in her maternity record.

The three options she will need to consider are:

- planned ECV
- spontaneous or assisted vaginal breech birth
- planned caesarean section (MIDIRS 2008).

### Spontaneous cephalic version of the breech

While the vast majority of breech presentations will have turned to the vertex by term – 57% of pregnancies after 32 weeks' gestation and 25% after 36 weeks' gestation (Westgren et al 1985) – it occurs with diminishing frequency as pregnancy advances.

The use of alternative approaches and techniques to promote spontaneous cephalic version has been widely reported, though the effectiveness of these has yet to be confirmed. There is insufficient evidence from well-controlled trials to support the use of postural management in converting breech to cephalic presentations (Hofmeyr & Kulier 2000). *Moxibustion* – used in traditional Chinese medicine to encourage fetal activity and version of the fetus in breech presentations (Budd 2000, Cardini & Weixin 1998) – was found, in a systematic review (Coyle et al 2005), to have insufficient evidence to support its use to correct breech presentation.

*External cephalic version (ECV)* is strongly advocated (RCOG 2006a) and well evaluated (Collins et al 2007, Hofmeyr & Kulier 1996a) (see website). The procedure is considered both safe and effective, reducing the chance for breech presentation at birth and caesarean section. Tocolysis is also associated with fewer failures of ECV (Hofmeyr & Gyte 2004). ECV should be offered to all women with an uncomplicated breech presentation at term. This role could be undertaken by appropriately trained and supported midwives and obstetric colleagues, and could significantly reduce the incidence of breech presentation (Taylor & Robson 2003).

## Mechanism of vaginal breech delivery

Although caesarean section is increasingly considered as the optimal mode of delivery for the breech presentation (Hannah et al 2000), women may still choose to have a vaginal breech birth or may present in advanced labour with an undiagnosed breech. Midwives must be fully conversant with the management and mechanisms of breech presentation and be able to orientate themselves to the position that the mother adopts in labour (RCM 2008).

There are six positions in breech presentation. The denominator is the sacrum, and its relationship to the maternal pelvis determines the position. The positions are the same as the vertex presentations, substituting the sacrum for the occiput (Fig. 64.6):

1. *Left sacroanterior position (LSA):* The sacrum points to the left iliopectineal eminence, and the abdomen and legs are directed towards the right sacroiliac joint. The left buttock is anterior and the bitrochanteric diameter is in the left oblique diameter. The natal cleft is in the right oblique diameter. A caput may form on the left buttock and on the genitals.
2. *Left sacrolateral (LSL):* The sacrum is towards the left side of the pelvis.
3. *Left sacroposterior (LSP):* The sacrum points to the left sacroiliac joint, and the abdomen towards the right iliopectineal eminence.
4. *Right sacroanterior position (RSA):* The sacrum points to the right iliopectineal eminence, and the abdomen is directed towards the left sacroiliac joint. The right buttock is anterior and the bitrochanteric diameter is in the right oblique diameter. The natal cleft is in the left oblique diameter. A caput may form on the right buttock and on the genitals.
5. *Right sacrolateral (RSL):* The sacrum is towards the right side of the pelvis.
6. *Right sacroposterior (RSP):* The sacrum points to the right sacroiliac joint, and the abdomen towards the left iliopectineal eminence.

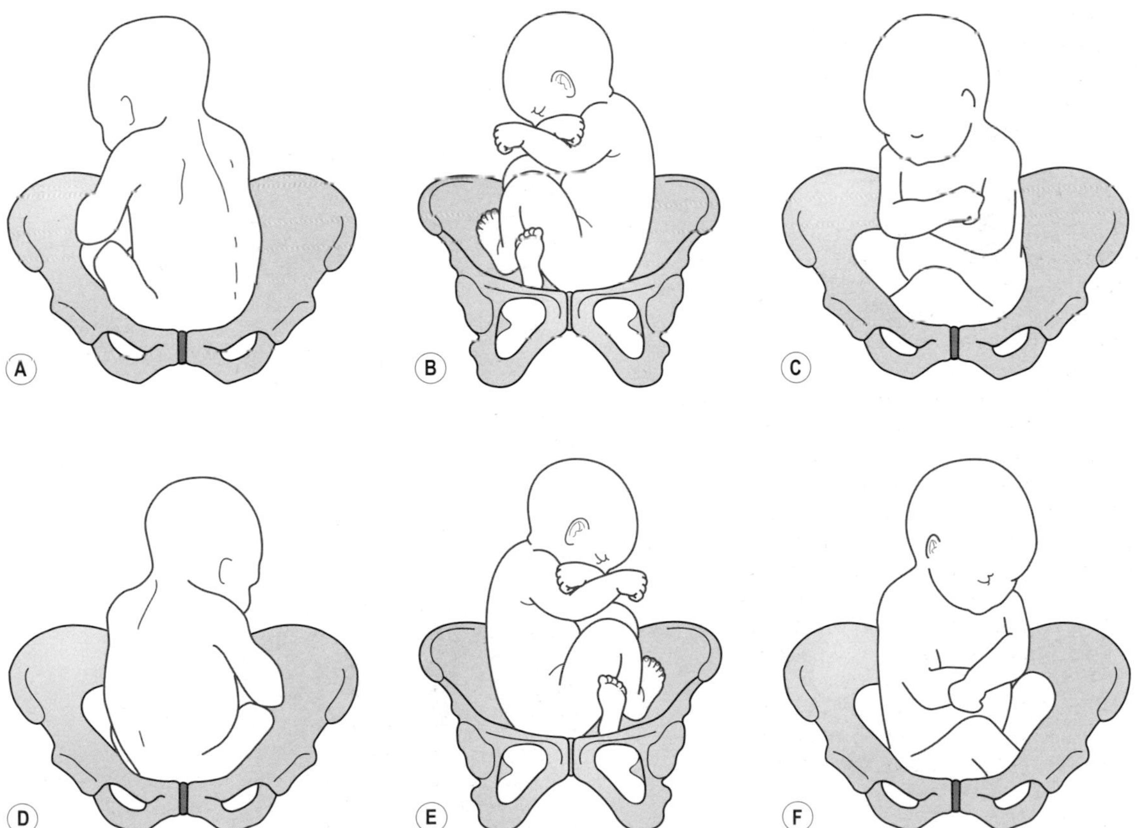


**Figure 64.6** Breech positions. **A.** Left sacroanterior (LSA). **B.** Left sacrolateral (LSL). **C.** Left sacroposterior (LSP). **D.** Right sacroanterior (RSA). **E.** Right sacrolateral (RSL). **F.** Right sacroposterior (RSP).

The fetus may be positioned in a direct anterior or posterior position.

With the breech in either the left or right sacroanterior position and good contractions, there is descent. The mechanism of the right sacroanterior position is illustrated in Figure 64.7. The fetus engages with the bitrochanteric diameter (10 cm) in the right oblique diameter of the pelvic brim and descends into the pelvic cavity.

With further contractions, the anterior buttock meets the resistance of the pelvic floor and rotates forwards through one-eighth of a circle (45 degrees) and comes to lie behind the symphysis pubis. The bitrochanteric diameter now lies in the anteroposterior diameter of the outlet. Lateral flexion of the trunk allows the continued descent of the buttocks along the curve of the birth canal (Fig. 64.8). The anterior buttock normally passes under the symphysis pubis and 'rumps', followed by the posterior buttock, which sweeps over the perineum.

With the birth of the buttocks the shoulders descend into the pelvis with the bisacromial diameter (11 cm) in the right oblique diameter of the brim. Internal rotation of the shoulders through one-eighth of a circle brings the anterior shoulder behind the symphysis. The right (anterior) shoulder and arm escape under the symphysis and the left (posterior) shoulder and arm pass over the perineum (Fig. 64.9).

The flexed head engages with the suboccipitobregmatic (9.5 cm) or suboccipitofrontal diameter (10 cm) lying in the right oblique or transverse diameter of the brim. Internal rotation of the head carries the occiput behind the symphysis. The face now lies in the hollow of the sacrum. External rotation of the buttocks and shoulders is

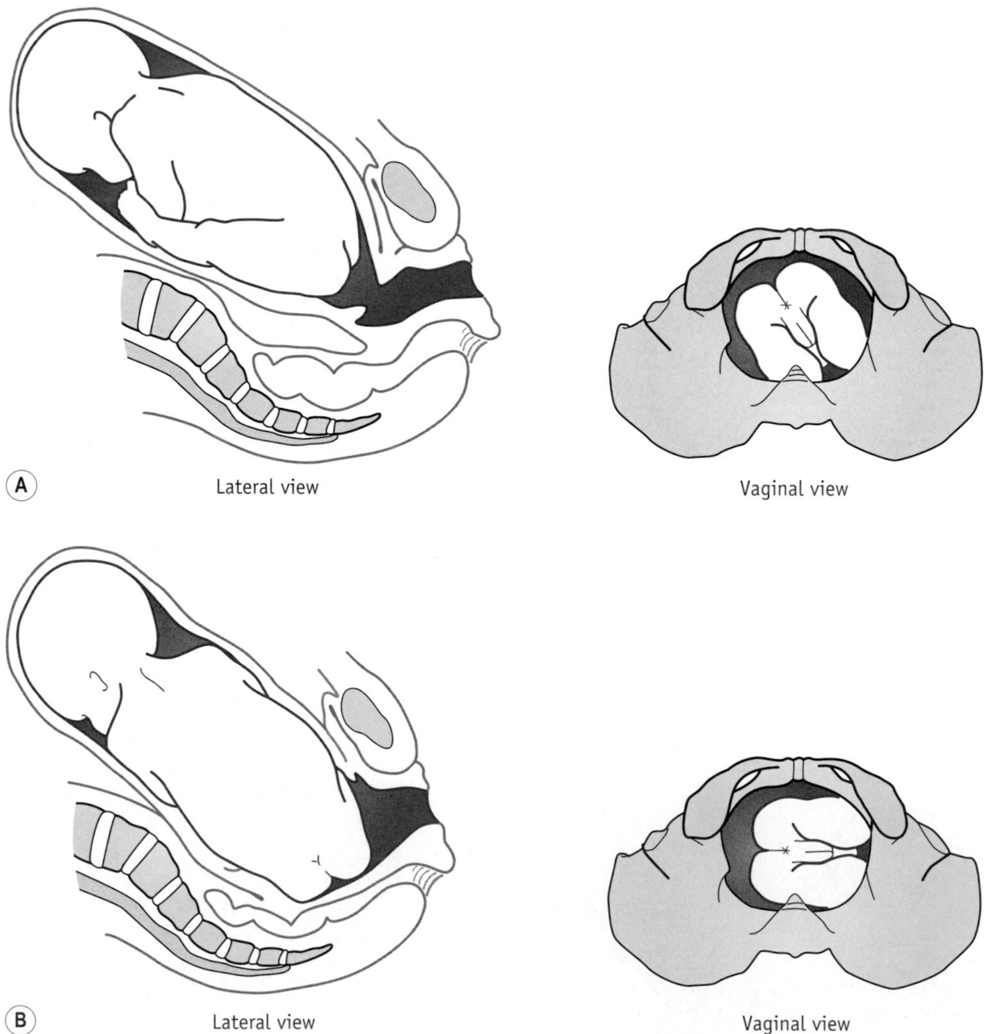


**Figure 64.7** Right sacroanterior position. **A.** Onset of labour. **B.** Descent and internal rotation of the buttocks.

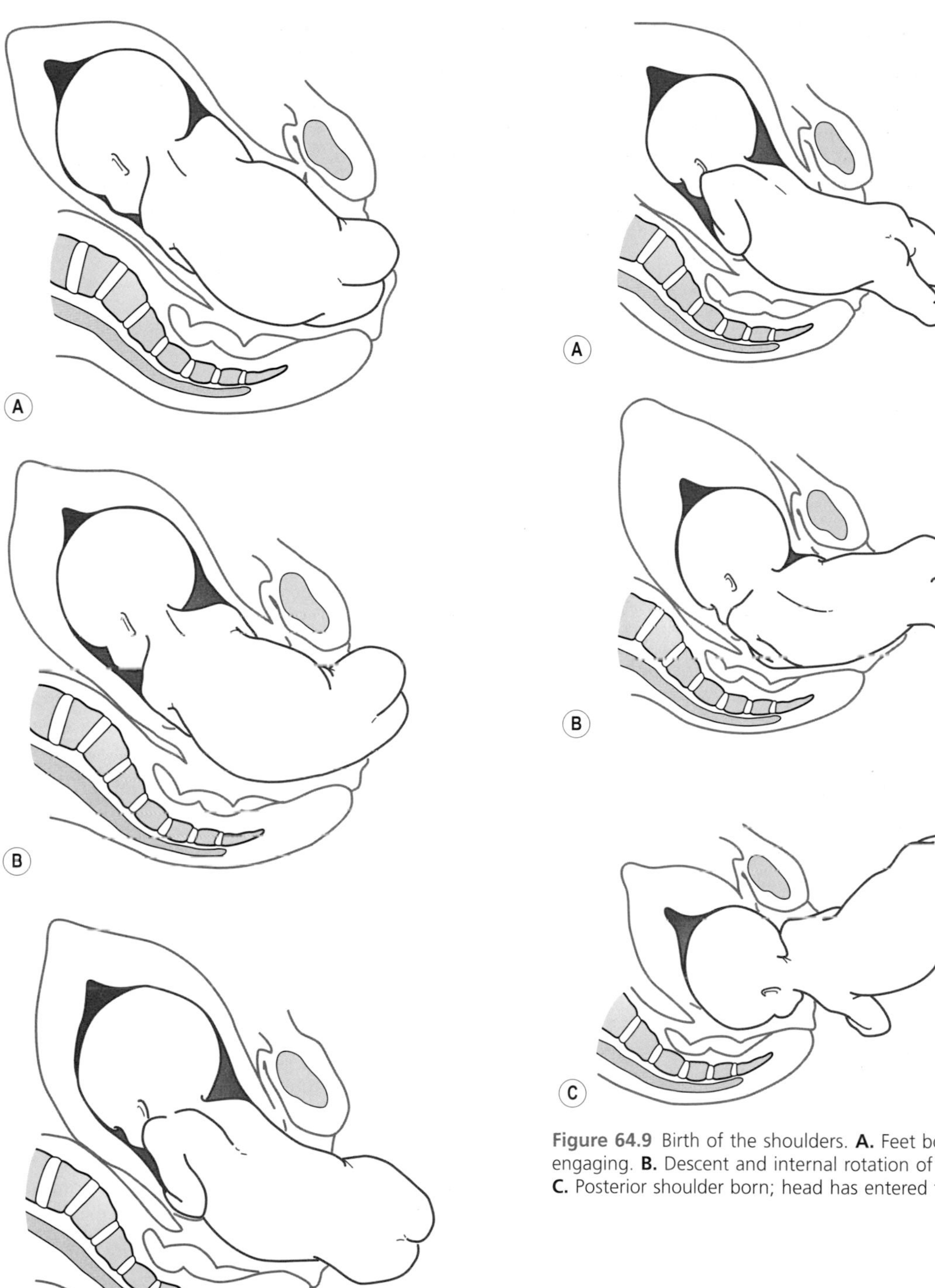


Figure 64.9 Birth of the shoulders. **A.** Feet born, shoulders engaging. **B.** Descent and internal rotation of shoulders. **C.** Posterior shoulder born; head has entered the pelvis.

Figure 64.8 Birth of the buttocks. **A.** Breech crowning or 'rumping'. **B.** Birth of posterior buttock. **C.** Birth of anterior buttock.

produced by the internal rotation of the head. The back of the baby's head and body now face in the same direction as the mother's abdomen.

It is essential that the back of the fetus orientates in the same direction as the mother's abdomen, and if it does not, it is gently assisted to do so. The chin, face, vertex and occiput are born over the perineum by a movement of flexion to complete the delivery (Fig. 64.10).

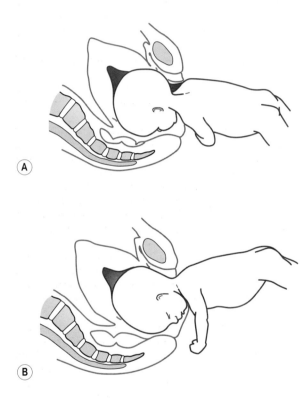

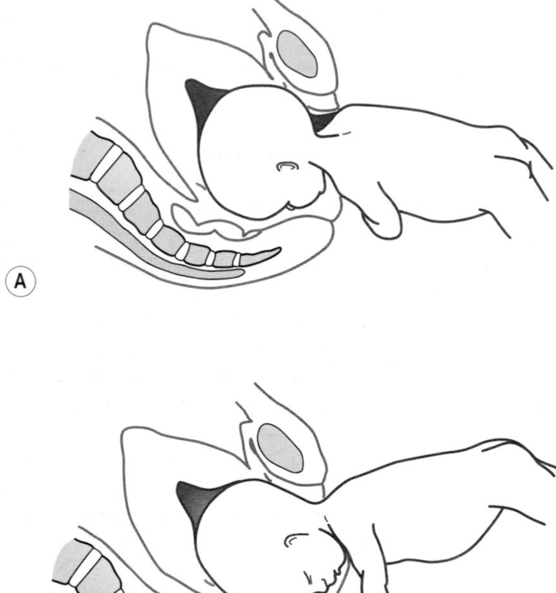


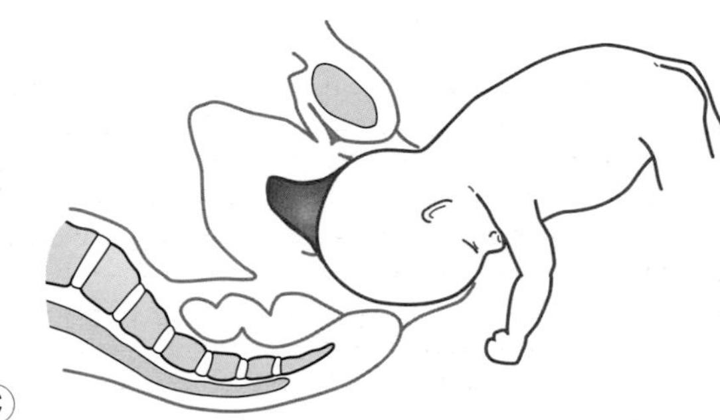


**Figure 64.10** Birth of the head. **A.** Anterior shoulder born; descent of the head. **B.** Internal rotation and beginning flexion of the head. **C.** Flexion of the head complete.

## Management of breech labour

When a woman chooses to have a vaginal breech birth, the midwife needs to ensure that she does so from an informed position. A careful history should be taken to ensure that there are no medical or obstetric contraindications for vaginal breech birth and that both woman and baby are in good health.

If possible, a detailed ultrasound scan should be carried out to:

- confirm a singleton pregnancy
- exclude obvious fetal abnormality
- estimate fetal weight and attitude
- determine placental position
- assess liquor volume.

A thorough clinical assessment of pelvic capacity should be performed. Today, pelvimetry to measure maternal pelvic diameters for safe delivery is deemed unnecessary, with good progress in labour being indicative of adequate fetal–pelvic proportions (Kotaska et al 2009).

Even when labour is established, consideration should be given to performing an ECV in an attempt to alter the presentation of the fetus to cephalic. While it is preferable for a vaginal breech labour to be conducted in hospital and under the supervision of an experienced obstetrician or midwife, this may not always be possible; maternal choice, as well as unexpected and rapid delivery, sometimes prevents transfer to hospital. Supervisors of midwives also have a role in facilitating the woman's admission to hospital and in supporting those midwives with the relevant skill to accompany her if requested to do so by the mother.

### *First stage of labour*

This differs little from that of normal labour. If the breech is not engaged, as is probable in a flexed breech, there is a risk of early rupture of the membranes and prolapse of the umbilical cord. The midwife must be vigilant and immediately exclude the possibility of cord prolapse when the membranes rupture. Where the breech is engaged, the legs are probably extended and the risk of cord prolapse reduced.

The value of upright positions, ambulation and support in labour are equally pertinent to women labouring with a breech presentation. The midwife provides continued support and continuity, carefully monitoring the progress of labour and the condition of the woman and fetus. A close working relationship with the wider maternity care team is also essential, and while the experienced midwife may conduct the breech delivery, the support of a senior obstetrician should be readily available if necessary.

Because of the associated risk in breech presentation, continuous monitoring of the fetal heart should be offered and recommended in breech labour (NICE 2007, RCOG 2006b). Some women who pursue a vaginal birth may reject this evidence, and opt for intermittent monitoring. In such circumstances, observations on the maternal condition and progress in labour should be carried out in keeping with the recommended guidelines for intermittent monitoring (NICE 2007).

In most cases, the first stage of labour progresses normally. Augmentation may be required should uterine action be hypotonic. This must be done with extreme caution – in some units, breech presentation may be considered a contraindication for augmentation. There is no evidence that epidural anaesthesia is essential, and its use depends upon the wishes and needs of the woman.

Occasionally, the breech may begin to descend through the cervix before the cervical os is fully dilated and this gives the woman a desire to push. Although uncommon, the buttocks may then descend easily, but the larger head cannot pass through the incompletely dilated cervix and dangerous delay results. The use of epidural anaesthesia makes this less likely as the woman does not experience the premature urge to push; however, a large retrospective study on breech presentation found that epidurals were associated with a longer duration of labour, increased need for augmentation and a significantly higher caesarean section rate in the second stage (Chadha et al 1992).

### *Second stage of labour*

When full dilatation of the cervical os has been confirmed, the mother may adopt a semi-recumbent, all-fours, upright or supported squatting position aiding expulsive efforts and the descent of the fetus.

Standing positions for the birth should be treated with caution because of an association with premature separation of the placenta. Midwives experienced in the management of breech birth advocate women adopting an all-fours or a forward-leaning 'prayer position' for the birth (Cronk 2005, Evans 2005).

Where an obstetrician is conducting the delivery, the woman is usually in the lithotomy position. The woman can mobilize prior to the onset of the second stage and lithotomy may be delayed until the breech is visible.

The midwife should ensure that appropriate and experienced help is at hand and that a paediatrician and senior obstetrician are present or readily available and that an anaesthetist can be quickly in attendance in case operative intervention suddenly becomes necessary.

If the fetal breech and body descend well, then it is likely that spontaneous breech delivery will occur with little assistance from the midwife or obstetrician. This is more common in multigravidae or when the fetus is small and preterm.

## Assisted breech delivery

A medically managed vaginal breech birth employs techniques to assist the delivery with the woman predominantly in the lithotomy position. The bladder is emptied prior to delivery. When the posterior buttock distends the perineum, the perineum is infiltrated with local anaesthetic (unless an epidural anaesthetic or a pudendal block is employed) and an episiotomy is performed. The posterior buttock then emerges and the breech advances more quickly.

As the trunk descends, the back will rotate anteriorly, allowing the fetal shoulder to enter the maternal pelvis in the transverse or oblique diameter of the inlet. Traction on the fetus **is not a part** of British practice, as this can give rise to extension of the head and nuchal displacement of the arms. There should be no interference and, increasingly, obstetricians, like midwives, apply the rule of '*hands off the breech*' and will try to avoid unnecessary manipulations.

Once the umbilicus is visible, previous practice dictated gently pulling down a loop of the umbilical cord to relieve any tension. This is *no longer* advocated. At this stage, compression of the cord is likely and time is an imperative.

From the complete delivery of the buttocks, some authorities advocate that the baby should be delivered within 15 minutes. Some believe that in vaginal breech birth, there may be benefits from rapid delivery of the baby to prevent progressive acidosis. This needs to be weighed against the potential trauma of a quick delivery. To date, there is insufficient evidence to evaluate the effects of expedited vaginal breech birth (Hofmeyr & Kulier 1996b).

If the fetal legs do not deliver spontaneously, inserting the index finger behind the thigh to flex the knee and abduct the leg may gently disengage them. However, if the practitioner is prepared to wait, they will usually deliver as the trunk descends.

With the next contraction, the shoulder blades appear; the arms, which are normally flexed across the chest, will usually slip out on their own and the shoulders are born in the anteroposterior diameter of the pelvic outlet. The head at this stage is entering the transverse or oblique diameter of the pelvic inlet. Some authorities advocate that from complete delivery of the baby's body until full delivery of the head, no more than 5 minutes should elapse.

At this stage, a number of manoeuvres may be used to facilitate the delivery of the head. If all is proceeding well, spontaneous, but controlled, delivery may be used when the head is at the pelvic outlet. Midwives who assist women to give birth using a forward-leaning position, use the analogy of 'getting the woman to move from a Christian prayer position to a Muslim prayer position' as this aids release of the head, facilitating its delivery. It has been observed that when the fetus begins to draw up its knees, the fetal head also flexes. If the woman then moves forward as described above, her pelvis rotates over the fetal head, causing its spontaneous release (Evans & Cronk, personal communication, 2002).

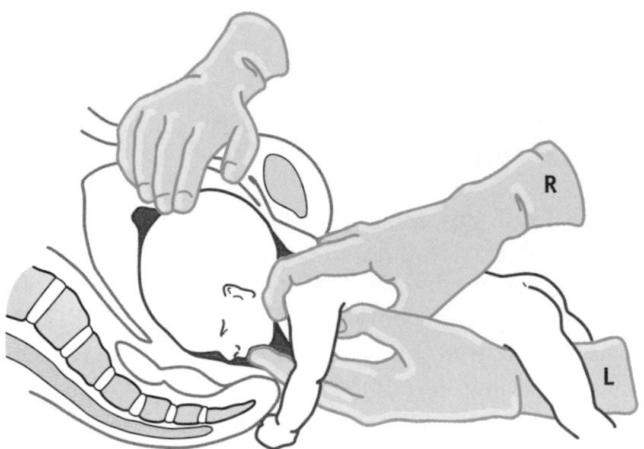


**Figure 64.11** Mauriceau–Smellie–Veit manoeuvre.

Alternatively, the Mauriceau-Smellie-Veit or Burns–Marshall manoeuvre may be used.

*Mauriceau–Smellie–Veit manoeuvre* is an effective method of delivering the fetal head, and the underlying principle is that of *'flexion before traction'* (Fig. 64.11). It offers good control of the head and may also be used when there is delay in the descent of the head.

The manoeuvre involves a combination of jaw flexion and shoulder traction and can be used for any breech delivery, but is of particular value when the fetal head is extended and forceps may be difficult to apply.

The practitioner supports the baby with the legs straddling their left arm (Fig. 64.11); three fingers slide into the vagina, feeling for the baby's cheekbones (malar bones). Originally, the middle finger was inserted into the baby's mouth in order to maximize traction but this is not recommended as it can result in dislocation of the jaw (ALSO 2003). Instead, the ring and index fingers rest on the cheekbones while the middle finger applies pressure to the chin.

The index and ring fingers of the practitioner's right hand are hooked over the baby's shoulders, to apply traction, while the middle finger presses on the occiput to aid flexion. An assistant may apply suprapubic pressure if needed.

As gently as possible, the baby's head is flexed and aided through the pelvic cavity to the outlet, after which the trunk is raised to bring the mouth into view. The air passages are then cleared and the birth of the head completed in the usual way.

*Burns–Marshall manoeuvre* is a medical procedure. Once the body is born, the baby is allowed to hang by his own weight for a few moments to facilitate descent and flexion of the head. When the nape of the neck and hairline come into view, the head is ready to be delivered (Fig. 64.12). Grasping the baby by the ankles and using slight traction, the practitioner directs the trunk upwards in a wide arc over the woman's abdomen.

The perineum should then be depressed with the fingers to expose the mouth of the fetus and allow it to be cleared of any blood or mucus, enabling the baby to breathe freely.

The birth of the head then proceeds very slowly to avoid any sudden release of pressure that might give rise to an intracranial haemorrhage. To avoid this danger, Wrigley's or Neville-Barnes forceps may be applied to the aftercoming head, which allows careful control of the speed with which the head is born.

**Reflective activity 64.1**

Using a manikin or doll and pelvis, rehearse the mechanisms of a breech presentation, and the different manoeuvres that can be used (Mauriceau– Smellie–Veit; Lövset's manoeuvres).

## Complications of vaginal breech delivery

### Extended arms

If the baby's arms are not flexed across the chest, they are likely to be stretched up alongside the head. It is not possible for head and arms to enter the pelvis together, so the arms must come first and then the head. This is best achieved by *Lövset's manoeuvre,* shown in Figure 64.13. With the baby in a right sacrolateral position, the manoeuvre depends on the fact that the posterior shoulder is below the sacral promontory and anterior shoulder above the symphysis pubis.

The practitioner grasps the baby's thighs with thumbs over the sacrum, and, being careful to avoid pressure above the pelvic girdle, which could cause abdominal injury, pulls the baby gently downwards, at the same time turning him, back upwards, through a half circle (180 degrees). The former posterior shoulder now becomes anterior and is released under the symphysis pubis, while at the same time; the other shoulder is brought into the pelvic cavity. The baby is then turned back through a half circle in the opposite direction and the other arm is released in the same way.

This procedure does not require an anaesthetic, can be carried out by a midwife, and, correctly performed, is safe and successful, even in cases where the baby has one arm at the back of the neck (nuchal displacement).

### Extended head

After the birth of the shoulders, the baby is allowed to hang from the vagina to facilitate descent and flexion of the head. If the neck and hairline are not visible within a few seconds, the most likely reason is extension of the

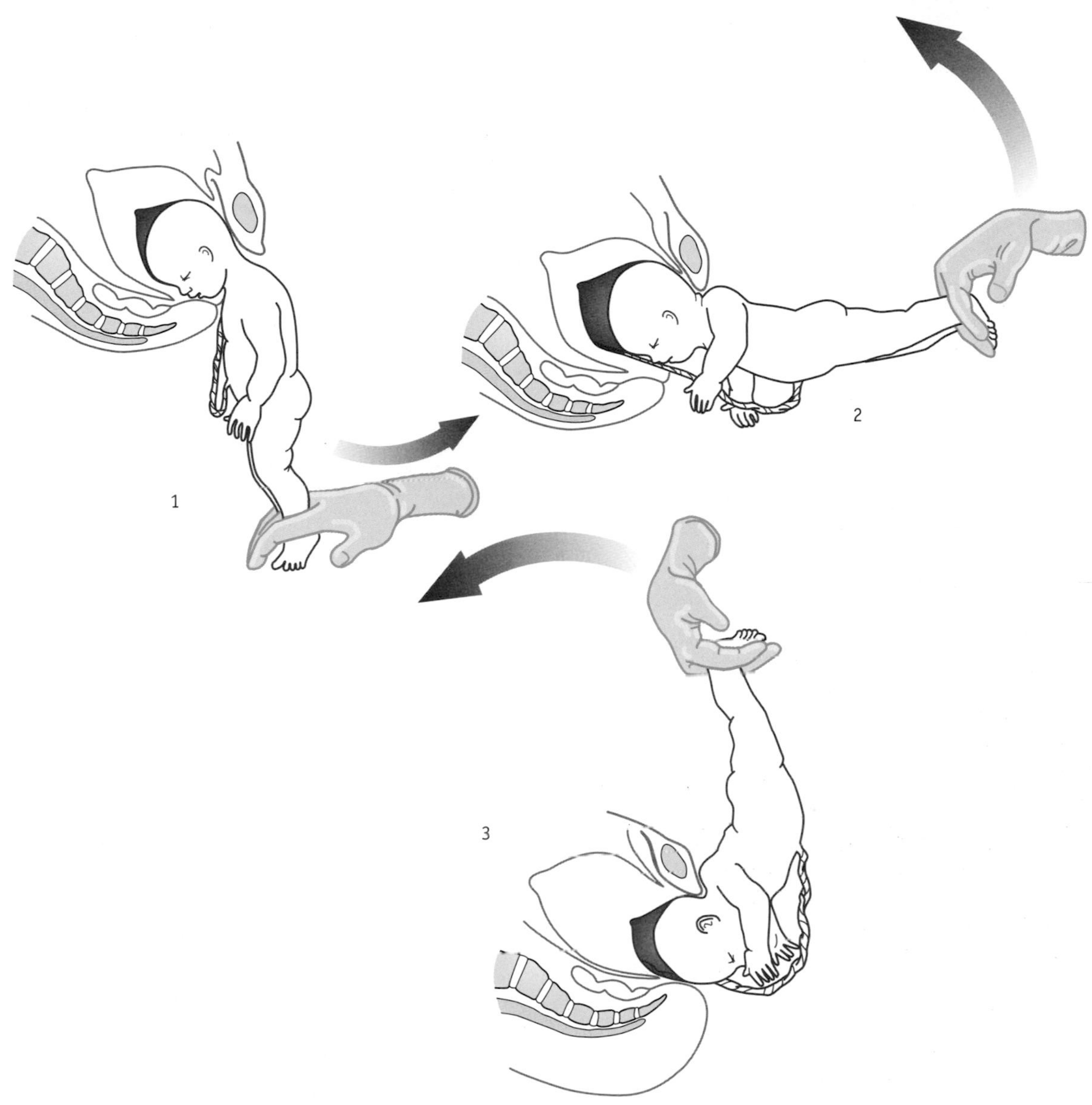


**Figure 64.12** Burns–Marshall manoeuvre.

head. The head may be delivered by the Mauriceau-Smellie–Veit manoeuvre, described above.

### *Entrapment of the fetal head*

This is an extremely rare but dangerous situation in the term breech. It occurs when the breech is delivered and the cervix is not fully dilated and traps the fetal head. In this situation, the midwife must call for urgent medical assistance. The obstetrician will try to release the head from the cervix, but mortality and morbidity rates are high. Although more commonly used in shoulder dystocia, McRobert's manoeuvre (see Ch. 66) has been used as a means to facilitate release of the fetal head (Shushan & Younis 1992).

It is possible, for a variety of reasons, for a midwife to be faced with an unexpected and emergency breech delivery. In community practice, the midwife should, with the mother's consent, make every effort to transfer her into hospital. When labour is not advancing very quickly, this is usually possible.

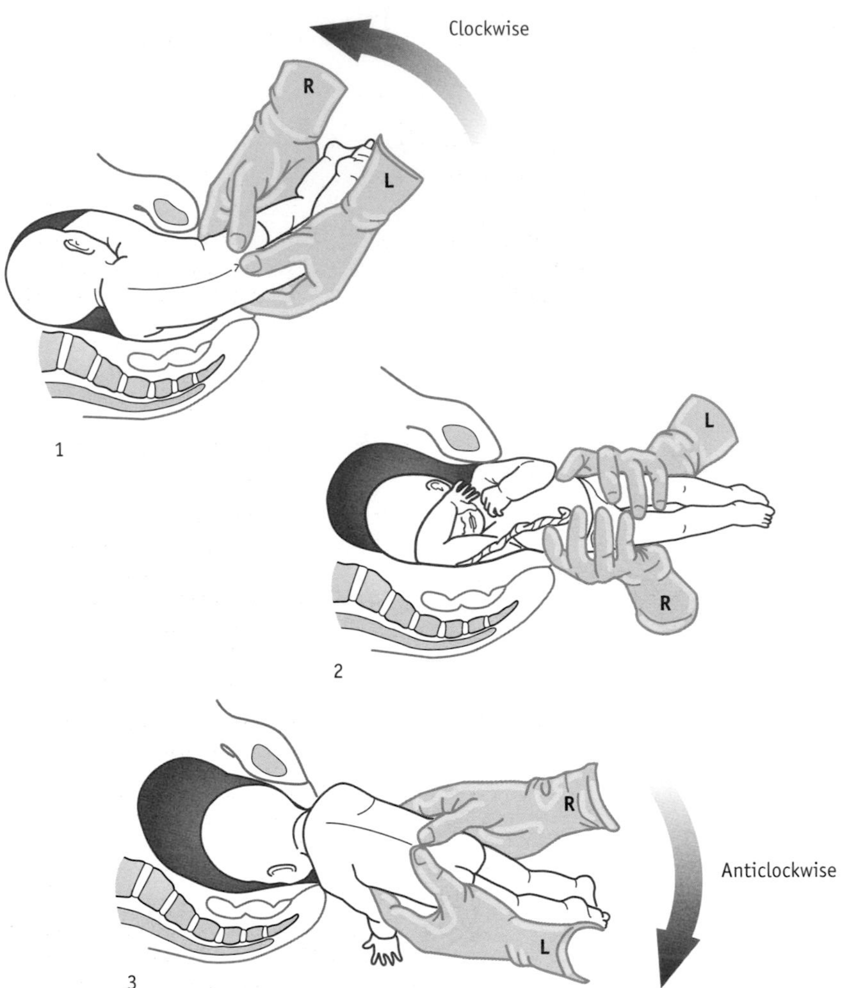


**Figure 64.13** Lövset's manoeuvre.

If the labour is progressing rapidly, however, delivery may be imminent and the risks of transfer considerable. If the contractions are strong and effective, there is every chance that the breech will deliver easily, though the midwife should call for skilled help as unexpected complications may still occur. The midwife's management of the breech birth is as described above.

## Face presentation

Face presentation occurs when the head and neck are hyperextended but the limbs flexed, so that the fetus lies in the uterus in a curious S-shaped attitude with the occiput against its shoulder blades and the face directly over the internal os (Fig. 64.14). The presenting portion is between the orbital ridges and the chin, with the latter being the denominator (Chitra & Marino 2010). Face presentation is uncommon, and occurs in 1 of every 600–800 live births, averaging about 0.2% of live births.

*Primary face presentation* is present before the onset of labour and causative factors are similar to those leading to general malpresentation and those that prevent head flexion or favour extension (Chitra & Marino 2010), including:

- *anencephaly* – where there is no vertex to present
- tumours of the fetal neck preventing flexion of the head
- excessive tone in the fetal extensor muscles may cause extended attitude, then face presentation (may persist for a few days after birth).

*Secondary face presentations* develop in labour. Causes include:

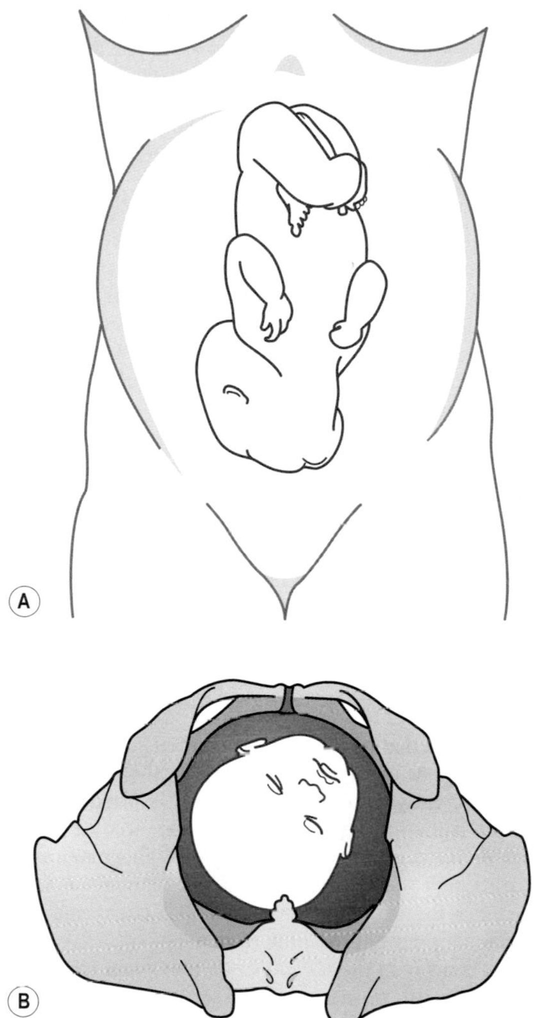


Figure 64.14 Anterior face presentation. **A.** Abdominal view. **B.** Vaginal view.

- deflexed occipitoposterior position – the biparietal diameter has difficulty in passing the sacrocotyloid diameter of the maternal pelvis; the bitemporal diameter descends more quickly, the head extends and the face presents
- uterine obliquity (uterus tilted sideways) – the force of uterine contractions may be directed towards the front of the head, so that the head extends as it enters the pelvis
- more likely to occur in a flat pelvis
- uterus laxity
- prematurity
- polyhydramnios
- multiple pregnancy
- no obvious reason.

**Table 64.3 Complications that may occur with a face presentation**

| Complication | Reason |
|---|---|
| Cord prolapse | Ill-fitting presenting part and early rupture of the membranes. |
| Obstructed labour | The face does not mould and therefore cannot overcome minor degrees of cephalopelvic disproportion.<br>A persistent posterior face presentation leads to obstructed labour. |
| Emergency operative delivery | As a result of obstructive labour or fetal distress. |
| Severe perineal trauma | Wider diameters: although the presenting diameter is the submentobregmatic at 9.5 cm, it is the submentovertical of 11.5 cm that distends the vagina and perineum.<br>Risk of operative delivery. |
| Intracranial haemorrhage | Anoxia and abnormal moulding of the fetal skull. |
| Facial bruising and oedema | The inability of the face to mould and injury to the soft tissue. |

The presenting diameters of the face presentation are to some degree favourable (i.e. 9.5 cm); however, the initial reason for the fetus adopting this position, the risk of the fetus being in a mentoposterior position, and the reduced ability of the facial bones to mould, carry additional risks to the fetus (see Table 64.3).

## Identification in pregnancy

Face presentation is not easily diagnosed in pregnancy, but should be suspected if a deep groove is felt between the fetal head and back and when the cephalic prominence and the fetal back are palpated on the same side.

If heart sounds are heard through the anterior chest wall on the side where the limbs are palpated, these may seem unusually loud and clear when the position is mentoanterior (MA). In mentoposterior (MP) positions, the fetal heart sounds are more difficult to hear.

When face presentation is suspected, ultrasound should be used to confirm the clinical diagnosis.

During labour, the high presenting part may give rise to suspicion. The diagnosis can be made on vaginal examination, when gentle palpation will reveal the orbital ridges and the gums within the mouth. Occasionally, the fetus will further help the diagnosis by sucking the examining finger.

Once a face presentation is diagnosed, it is essential to determine the position of the chin, whether it is anterior or posterior. A *posterior face presentation*, unless it rotates to an anterior position, will lead to obstructed labour. When the midwife diagnoses a face presentation, a senior obstetrician should be informed as soon as possible. If the chin is lateral or posterior, the urgency of the situation must be stressed.

As labour progresses, it becomes increasingly difficult to distinguish facial landmarks on vaginal examination because the face becomes oedematous. Vaginal examinations must be carried out with great care to avoid trauma to the eyes.

**Reflective activity 64.2**

Using a manikin and doll that presents by the face, explore how the contours feel on vaginal examination. Alter the position from anterior to posterior and examine again. Attempt to feel and describe the difference.

## Mechanisms

The lie is longitudinal, the presentation is the face, the denominator is the chin and the attitude is hyperextended. The engaging diameter is submentobregmatic (9.5 cm). There are six positions in which the face may present (Fig. 64.15).

1. *Right mentoposterior* (RMP) is an extension of an LOA. The chin points to the right sacroiliac joint.
2. *Left mentoposterior* (LMP) is an extension of an ROA. The chin points to the left sacroiliac joint.
3. *Right mentolateral* (RML) is an extension of an LOL. The chin is directed towards the right side of the pelvis.
4. *Left mentolateral* (LML) is an extension of an ROL. The chin is directed towards the left side of the pelvis.
5. *Right mentoanterior* (RMA) is an extension of an LOP. The chin points to the right iliopectineal eminence.
6. *Left mentoanterior* (LMA) is an extension of an ROP. The chin points to the left iliopectineal eminence.

Face presentation develops before the head is engaged in the pelvis. The mentum is anterior in 60–80% of cases; transverse in 10–12%; and posterior in 20–25%, with most rotating to the anterior (Chitra & Morino 2010).

In a mentoanterior position, the extended head enters the brim of the pelvis with the face presenting. The chin points to the iliopectineal eminence, and the sinciput to the opposite sacroiliac joint (Fig. 64.16).

The submentobregmatic diameter (9.5 cm) engages and the face descends into the pelvis. The chin, being the lowest part, meets the resistance of the pelvic floor and rotates through one-eighth of a circle to escape under the pubic arch. The face appears at the vulval outlet (Fig. 64.17). Further uterine contractions drive the vertex and occiput over the perineum, and thus, by a movement of flexion, the head is born. Restitution and external rotation take place.

*A face presentation can only be born spontaneously if the chin is anterior*. There is no mechanism by which the chin can be born when it lies at the back of the pelvis. The neck is too short to span the length of the sacrum and is already at the point of maximum extension, and obstructed labour occurs. Spontaneous rotation of the head from the mentolateral or mentoposterior to the mentoanterior position can, and occasionally does, take place, and spontaneous delivery may then occur. See Figure 64.18.

In a face presentation with the chin to the front, an adequate pelvis, a healthy fetus and good contractions, the labour will usually progress normally, with a vaginal delivery rate of 60–70%. However, in spite of this, in developed countries in the 21st century there is a lower threshold to move to caesarean section when face presentation is identified.

## Management

In a mentoanterior position, labour often proceeds normally, though, as in any malpresentation, the membranes may rupture early, prolapse of the cord is possible, and labour is sometimes prolonged. In the second stage, normal delivery is anticipated, aided by an episiotomy, since, although the submentobregmatic diameter is only 9.5 cm, it is the submentovertical of 11.5 cm which distends the perineum at the time of delivery.

If there is delay in the second stage, the obstetrician will apply forceps. If normal delivery occurs, extension is maintained by applying pressure on the sinciput until the chin has escaped under the symphysis pubis; the head is then flexed to allow the vertex and occiput to sweep the perineum.

At birth, the baby is usually in good condition, although the eyelids and lips will be grossly oedematous and the face congested. The bruising and unsightly appearance can cause the mother considerable alarm and anxiety. The midwife should warn her what to expect and describe how the baby might look. The mother should be reassured that the bruising and oedema will subside within a few days and suckling, which at first may be difficult, is usually normal in 48 hours.

# Brow presentation

Brow presentation (Fig. 64.19) is the least common presentation. The head is midway between flexion and extension, with the mentovertical diameter of 13.5 cm attempting unsuccessfully to enter the transverse diameter

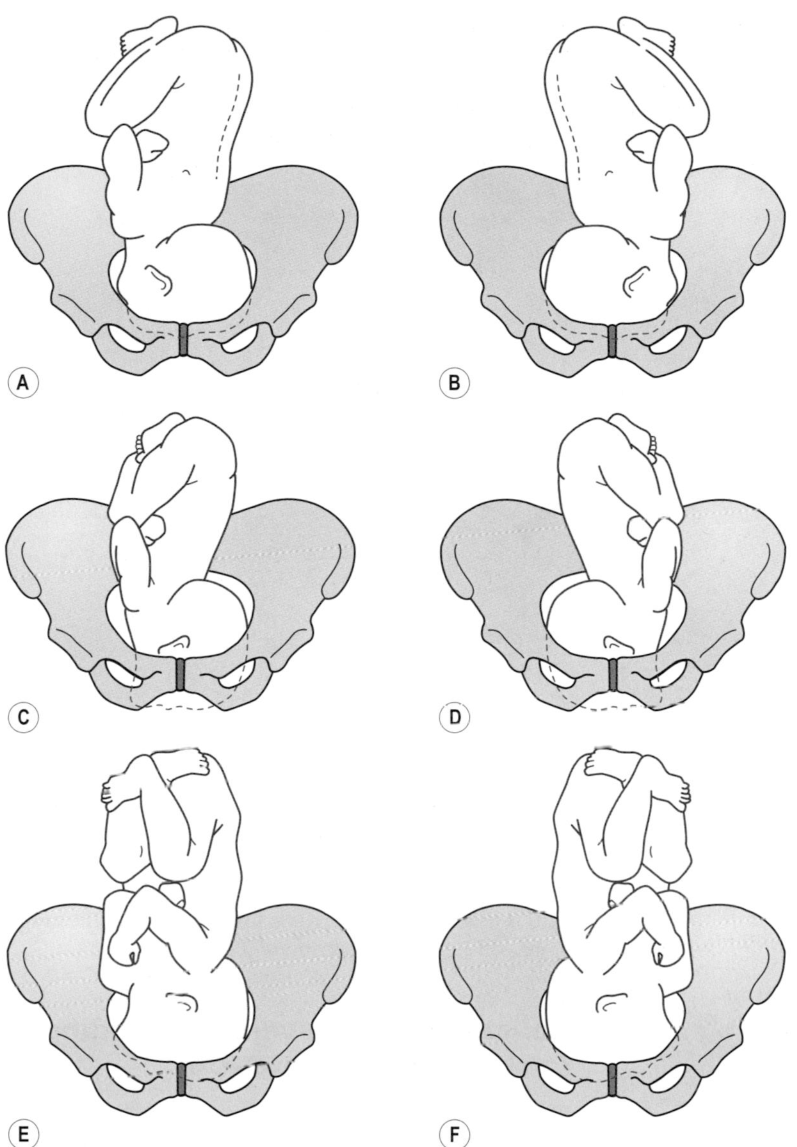


Figure 64.15 Face presentations. **A.** Right mentoposterior. **B.** Left mentoposterior. **C.** Right mentolateral. **D.** Left mentolateral. **E.** Right mentoanterior. **F.** Left mentoanterior.

of the pelvic brim. A small head might enter a large pelvis only to be arrested in the cavity.

The incidence varies from 1 in 500 to 1 in 1400 deliveries. Brow presentation may be encountered early in labour but is usually a transitional state and converts to a vertex presentation after the fetal neck flexes. Occasionally, further extension may occur, resulting in a face presentation.

The causes are, with the exception of anencephaly, the same as in face presentation, and include (Chitra & Marino 2010):

- cephalopelvic disproportion
- fetal prematurity
- increasing parity.

These account for more than 60% of cases of persistent brow presentation.

Brow presentation, undiscovered and untreated, will lead to obstructed labour, uterine rupture, and raised perinatal and maternal morbidity and mortality.

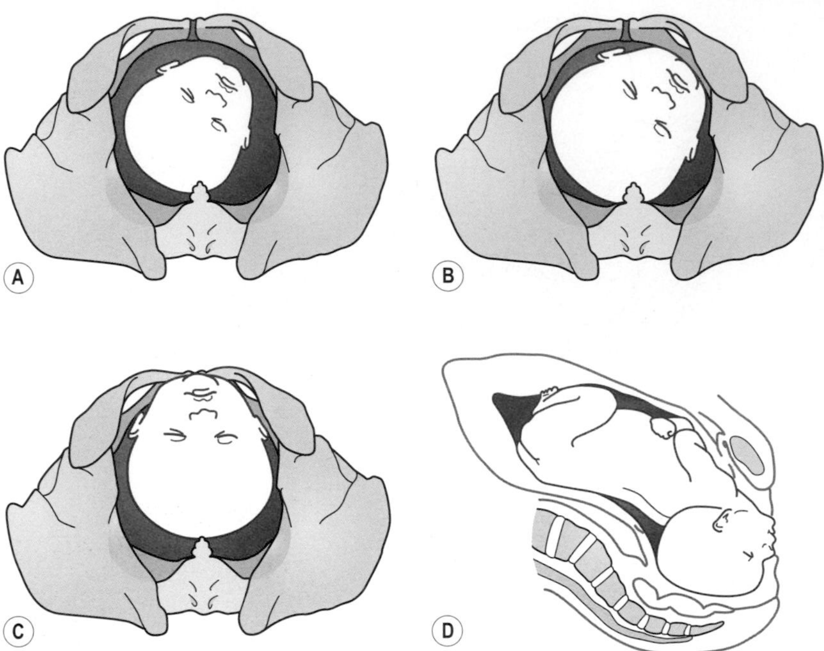


**Figure 64.16** Mechanism of labour of anterior face presentation. **A.** LMA – onset of labour. **B.** Extension and descent. **C.** Vaginal view. **D.** Lateral view.

### Identification

On abdominal examination, the head is high and the presenting diameter unusually large. As with face presentation, a groove may be felt between the occiput and the back, and the cephalic prominence will be on the same side as the fetal back.

On vaginal examination, the presenting part may be too high to identify. If the brow is within reach, the orbital ridges may be felt on one side and the anterior fontanelle on the other. The diagnosis should be confirmed by ultrasound.

### Management

In brow presentation, three outcomes are possible. The brow may:

- convert to a vertex presentation
- convert to a face presentation, or
- remain as a persistent brow presentation.

The midwife must immediately call an obstetrician if a brow presentation is suspected or diagnosed in labour, and a woman at home should be alerted to the situation and its dangers and transferred into hospital.

As in all malpresentations, the membranes are likely to rupture early and there is a risk of cord prolapse; thus, a vaginal examination should be made as soon as the membranes rupture, to exclude this.

If a brow presentation is diagnosed early in labour, it may convert to a face presentation becoming fully extended or it may flex to a vertex presentation and deliver normally. If the brow presentation persists, however, and the fetus is a normal size, it will be impossible to deliver vaginally and a caesarean section will be performed.

## Oblique and transverse lie leading to shoulder presentation

A shoulder presentation occurs as a result of a transverse or an oblique lie (Fig. 64.20). Shoulder presentation is not uncommon and is only problematic if the fetus is not cephalic by 36 weeks' gestation. At term, an unstable or transverse lie presents a considerable risk to both mother and fetus, with cord prolapse being 20 times more common than with a flexed vertex presentation (Baxley 2001). If uncorrected, shoulder presentation will result in obstructed labour, and unless the lie is corrected, a caesarean section is the only mode of delivery.

Causes of an unstable lie and shoulder presentation are:

- laxity of the uterine and abdominal muscles (most frequent with high parity)
- placenta praevia (if a woman has a persistent oblique lie, even without sentinel bleeding, placenta praevia should be considered as a possible cause).

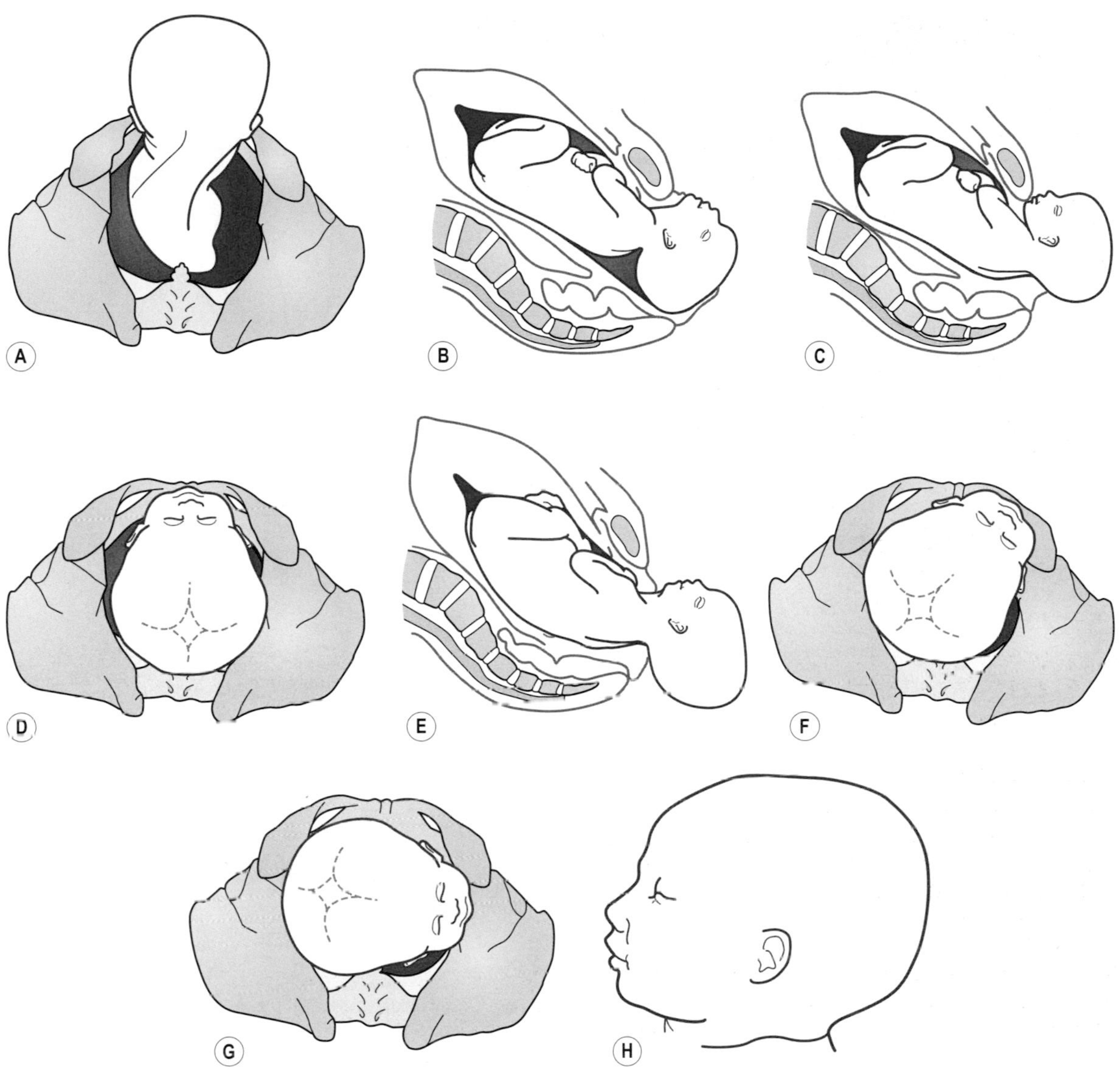


**Figure 64.17** Mechanism of labour of anterior face presentation – birth of the face. **A.** Flexion. **B.** Flexion beginning. **C.** Flexion complete. **D.** Vaginal view. **E.** Lateral view. **F.** Restitution – MA to LMA. **G.** External rotation – LMA to LMT. **H.** Moulding.

Contributory factors are:

- multiple pregnancy
- polyhydramnios
- uterine abnormality
- contracted pelvis
- occasionally a large uterine fibroid
- an overdistended bladder may displace the presenting part and cause a transient oblique lie.

## Identification

Abdominal examination and continuity are key to making the diagnosis of an oblique, transverse or unstable lie and therefore the presence of a shoulder presentation. The abnormal lie is easily diagnosed in pregnancy from the shape of the uterus, which appears too broad, with the fetal poles felt on either side of the abdomen, while the fundus is unusually low. Palpation will reveal the fetal

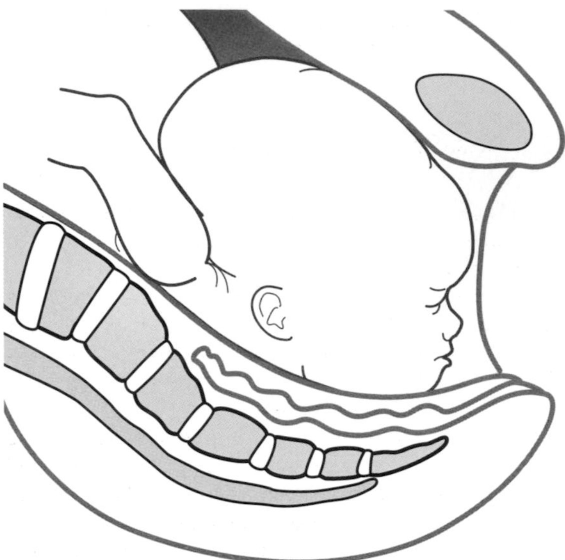

Figure 64.18 Obstructed labour with fetus in the mentoposterior position.

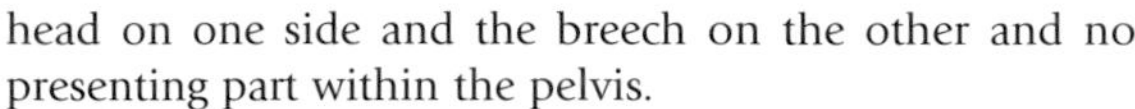

head on one side and the breech on the other and no presenting part within the pelvis.

In an oblique lie, the fetal head, or breech, is found in one or other iliac fossa. If a non-longitudinal lie is found after the 36–37th week of pregnancy, an obstetrician must be informed. Ultrasound may be used to confirm the diagnosis, identify the presentation and detect the possible cause.

## Management

As pregnancy advances, a non-longitudinal lie tends to revert to longitudinal and stabilize; however, if this does not occur, after 36 weeks' gestation, the obstetrician will attempt to correct the lie by external version to a longitudinal lie and cephalic presentation. At term, labour may then be induced while the lie remains longitudinal and the presentation cephalic.

The likelihood of reversion to an oblique or transverse lie is high. The attendant risk is that the membranes may rupture and the cord or arm prolapse; or labour may commence before the lie is corrected. Often the woman is admitted to hospital for observation.

Ultrasound examination should exclude placenta praevia, and fetal or uterine abnormalities. A vaginal examination may be made to detect any pelvic abnormality such as a contracted pelvis. In labour, the lie is closely monitored and, if necessary, gentle lateral pressure may be applied to the uterus to help maintain a longitudinal lie.

Once labour is established and the fetal head enters the pelvis, the membranes can be ruptured. Labour should

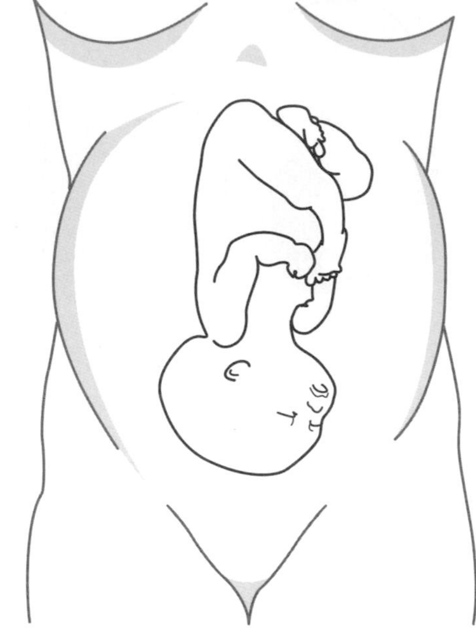


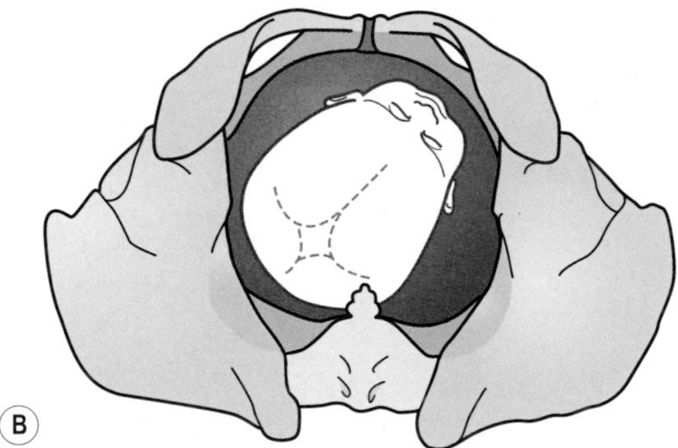


Figure 64.19 Brow presentation. **A.** Abdominal view. **B.** Vaginal view.

then progress normally. In cases where the woman has a poor obstetric history, or if complications occur in labour, there is likely to be early recourse to caesarean section as the safest mode of delivery.

If undetected or inadequately monitored, an unstable lie in labour is a serious obstetric emergency. With contractions, the fetal shoulder will be forced down into the pelvis, the membranes are likely to rupture, and the cord and/or the fetal arm may prolapse.

The midwife should recognize shoulder presentation during abdominal examination. Once placenta praevia has been excluded, vaginal examination can be carried out, and the fetal ribs or the hand may be felt. On detecting an unstable lie or shoulder presentation, the midwife must immediately inform an obstetrician, and if in the

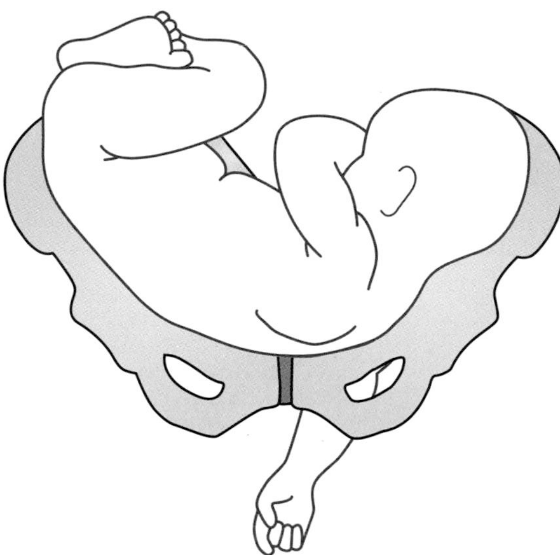

**Figure 64.20** Shoulder presentation, with prolapse of one arm.

community, rapidly transfer the woman to hospital. Turning the woman onto all fours is of value in displacing the shoulder and reducing the mother's urge to push. Where an arm or cord prolapses, this manoeuvre is **essential** (see Ch. 67). If the lie is uncorrected, caesarean section will be necessary and it may well be the safest mode of delivery even when the fetus has died.

## Compound presentation

Compound presentation is a presentation in which a hand or foot lies alongside the head. Very rarely, both a hand and a foot come down. This tends to occur when the fetus is small and the pelvis large or when there is any condition preventing the descent of the head into the pelvis. Lower abdominal pain and a lack of fundal dominance is often noted. The pain experienced by the mother is best dealt with through effleurage, where the midwife applies light circular stroking movements to massage the mother's lower abdomen. Compound presentation is only of significance in advanced labour when the membranes have ruptured. Usually, the presenting limb will recede as the presenting part descends. Labour usually ends in a normal or a low instrumental delivery, but where the compound presentation persists, there is an increased risk to the mother of vaginal and perineal trauma.

## CONCLUSION

It is important that the midwife is knowledgeable about contemporary care and management of malpositions and malpresentations, and is able to impart this information to the woman in a realistic and accessible manner. Good preparation for labour and birth, and different strategies which might be required, should be discussed prior to labour if possible, and a plan agreed and documented, involving the whole maternity care team.

The midwife's primary role is to monitor, support and enhance the experience of the pregnancy and birth, and where there are deviations from normal, make quick and appropriate referral. Midwives should be familiar with the mechanisms of malpositions and malpresentation and the manoeuvres which they may use in facilitating birth. It is important to inspire confidence in the mother, but midwives must also have confidence in themselves and in their ability to support the woman in her choice of birth and to manage this effectively when a malposition or malpresentation occurs.

### KEY POINTS

- Malpositions and malpresentations of the fetus may increase the risks of fetal and neonatal morbidity and mortality.
- The midwife should be able to identify women and babies at risk of malpositions and malpresentations through effective clinical assessment, and take appropriate and timely action.
- The midwife should ensure that the woman and her partner feel prepared, supported and enabled to make informed choices.
- Effective communication and teamwork are crucial in the provision of safe and appropriate care to women and their babies.
- Manoeuvres and other skills based on anatomical, physiological and evidence-based principles should be practised by those providing care to women and their babies, on a regular basis.

## REFERENCES


Advanced Life Support in Obstetrics (ALSO): *Advanced support in obstetrics manual*, ed 4, Kansas City, 2003, American Academy of Family Physicians.

Banks M: *Breech birth – woman wise*, New Zealand, 2000, Birthspirit Books.

Bartlett DJ, Okun NB: Breech presentation: a random event or an explanable phenomenon? *Developmental Medicine and Child Neurology* 36(9):833–838, 1994.

Baxley EG: Malpresentations and malpositions. In Ratcliffe SD, Baxley

EG, Byrd JE, et al, editors: *Family practice obstetrics*, ed 2, Philadelphia, 2001, Hanley & Belfus.

Budd S: Moxibustion for breech presentation, *Complementary Therapies in Nursing and Midwifery* 6(4):176–179, 2000.

Cardini F, Weixin H: Moxibustion for correction of breech presentation; a randomised control trial, *Journal of the American Medical Association* 280(18):1580–1584, 1998.

Chadha YC, Mahmood TA, Dick MJ, et al: Breech delivery and epidural anaesthesia, *British Journal of Obstetrics and Gynaecology* 99(2):96–100, 1992.

Cheng M, Hannah M: Breech delivery at term: a critical review of the literature, *Obstetrics and Gynecology* 82(4):605–618, 1993.

Chitra MI, Marino T: *Face and brow presentation* (website). http://emedicine.medscape.com/article/262341-overview. 2010. Accessed April 2010.

Collins S, Ellaway P, Harrington D, et al: The complications of external cephalic version: results from 805 consecutive attempts, *British Journal of Obstetrics and Gynaecology* 114(5):636–638, 2007.

Coyle ME, Smith CA, Peat B: Cephalic version by moxibustion for breech presentation, *Cochrane Database of Systematic Reviews* (2):CD003928, 2005.

Cronk M: Hands off that breech! *Aims Journal* 17(1):3–4, 2005.

Danielian PJ, Wang J, Hall MH: Long term outcome by method of delivery of fetuses in breech presentation at term: population based follow up, *British Medical Journal* 312(7044):1451–1453, 1996.

Evans J: *Breech birth: what are my options?* London, 2005, AIMS Publications.

Evans J: First do no harm, *The Practising Midwife* 10(8):22–23, 2007.

Fitzpatrick M, McQuillian K, O'Herlihy C: Influence of persistent occiput posterior position on delivery outcomes, *Obstetrics and Gynecology* 98(6):1027–1031, 2001.

Gardberg M, Tuppurainen M: Persistent occiput posterior presentation – a clinical problem, *Acta Obstetrica Gynecologica Scandinavia* 73(1):45–47, 1994a.

Gardberg M, Tuppurainen M: Anterior placental location predisposes for occiput posterior presentation near term, *Acta Obstetrica Gynecolgica Scandinavia* 73(2):151–152, 1994b.

Gardberg M, Laakkonen E, Salevaara M: Intrapartum sonography and persistent occiput posterior position: a study of 408 deliveries, *Obstetrics and Gynecology* 91(5 Pt 1):746–749, 1998.

Glezerman M: Five years to the term breech trial: the rise and fall of a randomized controlled trial, *American Journal of Obstetrics and Gynecology* 194(1):20–25, 2006.

Goffinet F, Carayol M, Foidart JM, et al: Is planned vaginal delivery for breech presentation at term still an option? Results of an observational prospective study in France and Belgium, *American Journal of Obstetrics and Gynecology* 194(4):1002–1011, 2006.

Hannah ME, Hannah WJ, Hewson SA, et al; Term Breech Trial Collaborative Group: Planned caesarean section versus planned vaginal birth for breech presentation at term: a randomised multicentre trial, *Lancet* 356(9239):1375–1383, 2000.

Hofmeyr GJ: External cephalic version at term: how high are the stakes? *British Journal of Obstetrics and Gynaecology* 98(1):1–3, 1991.

Hofmeyr GJ, Hannah ME: Planned caesarean section for term breech delivery, *Cochrane Database of Systematic Reviews* 2003, Issue 2. (Art. No.: CD000166. DOI: 10.1002/14651858.CD000166)

Hofmeyr GJ, Gyte G: Interventions to help external cephalic version for breech presentation at term, *Cochrane Database of Systematic Reviews* (1):CD000184, 2004.

Hofmeyr GJ, Kulier R: External cephalic version for breech presentation at term, *Cochrane Database of Systematic Reviews* (1):CD000083, 1996a.

Hofmeyr GJ, Kulier R: Expedited versus conservative approaches for vaginal delivery in breech presentation, *Cochrane Database of Systematic Reviews* (1):CD000082, 1996b.

Hofmeyr GJ, Kulier R: Cephalic version by postural management for breech presentation, *Cochrane Database of Systematic Reviews* (3):CD000051, 2000.

Hunter S, Hofmeyr GJ, Kulier R: Hands and knees posture in late pregnancy or labour for fetal malposition (lateral or posterior), *Cochrane Database of Systematic Reviews* (4):CD001063, 2007.

Kotaska A: Inappropriate use of randomised trials to evaluate complex phenomena: case study of vaginal breech delivery, *British Medical Journal* 329:1039–1042, 2004.

Kotaska A, Menticoglou S, Gagnon R, et al, Maternal Fetal Medicine Committee, Society of Obstetricians and Gynaecologists of Canada: Vaginal delivery of breech presentation, *Journal of Obstetrics and Gynaecology Canada* 31(6):557–566, 2009.

Lauszus FF, Petersen A, Praest J: Strategy for delivery in breech presentation. A retrospective study, *Ugeskrift for Laeger* 154(3):123–126, 1992.

Midwives Information and Resource Service (MIDIRS): *Breech presentation options for care*, Informed Choice Leaflet No. 9, Bristol, 2008, MIDIRS.

National Institute for Health and Clinical Excellence (NICE): *Intrapartum care: management and care to women in labour*, London, 2007, NICE.

Nursing and Midwifery Council (NMC): *Code of professional conduct*, London, 2002, NMC.

Nursing and Midwifery Council (NMC): *Midwives rules and standards*, London, 2004 (reissued 2010 with minor amendment), NMC.

Pritchard JA, MacDonald PC: Dystocia caused by abnormalities in presentation, position, or development of the fetus. In Pritchard JA, MacDonald PC, editors: *Williams obstetrics*, Norwalk, CT, 1980, Appleton-Century-Crofts, pp 787–796.

Royal College of Midwives (RCM): *Brown Study Series Number 6: Breech presentation*, London, 2008, RCM.

Royal College of Obstetricians and Gynaecologists (RCOG): *External cephalic version and reducing the incidence of breech presentation* (Green-top Guideline No. 20b) (website). www.rcog.org.uk/files/rcog-corp/uploaded-files/GT20aExternalCephalica2006.pdf. 2006a. Accessed April 2010.

Royal College of Obstetricians and Gynaecologists (RCOG): *The management of breech presentation* (Green-top Guideline No. 20a) (website). www.rcog.org.uk/files/rcog-corp/uploaded-files/GT20bManagement_ofBreechPresentation.pdf. 2006b. Accessed April 2010.

Saunders NJ, Spiby H, Gilbert L, et al: Oxytocin infusion during second stage of labour in primiparous women using epidural analgesia, *British Medical Journal* 299(6713):1423–1426, 1989.

Shennan A, Bewley S: How to manage term breech deliveries (Editorial), *British Medical Journal* 323(7307):244–245, 2001.

Shushan A, Younis JS: McRoberts manoeuvre for the management of the aftercoming head in breech delivery, *Gynecologic and Obstetric Investigation* 34(3):188–189, 1992.

Sutton J: Occipito-posterior positioning and some ideas about how to change it, *The Practising Midwife* 3(6):20–22, 2000.

Sutton J, Scott P: *Understanding and teaching optimal foetal positioning,* New Zealand, 1996, Tauranga.

Taylor P, Robson S: External cephalic version – a new midwifery role, *British Journal of Midwifery* 11(4):207–210, 2003.

Thorp JA, Hu DH, Albin RM, et al: The effects of intrapartum epidural analgesia on nulliparous labour: a randomised, controlled prospective trial, *American Journal of Obstetrics and Gynecology* 169(4):851–858, 1993.

Van Idderkinge B: Planned vaginal breech delivery: should this be the mode of choice? *Obstetrics and Gynaecology* 9(3):171–176, 2007.

Vause S, Hornbuckle J, Thornton JG: Palpation or ultrasound for detecting breech babies? (Editorial), *British Journal of Midwifery* 5(6):318–319, 1997.

Waites B: Self-help and alternative therapies for turning breech babies. In Waites B, editor: *Breech birth,* London, 2003, Free Association Books, pp 67–78.

Westgren M, Edvall H, Nordstrom E, et al: Spontaneous cephalic version of breech presentation in the last trimester, *British Journal of Obstetrics and Gynaecology* 92(1):19–22, 1985.

Whyte H, Hannah M, Saigal S: Outcomes of children at two years after planned cesarean birth vs planned vaginal birth for breech presentation at term: the international randomised Term Breech Trial, *American Journal of Obstetrics and Gynecology* 191(3):864–871, 2004.

Chapter |65|

# Disproportion, obstructed labour and uterine rupture

*Margaret Brock*

## LEARNING OUTCOMES

By the end of the chapter, the reader should be:

- aware of the principles of antenatal pelvic assessment
- able to recognize cephalopelvic disproportion (CPD)
- able to recognize signs of obstructed labour
- aware of the hazards of obstructed labour
- able to recognize predisposing factors for ruptured uterus
- aware of sites of occurrence of ruptured uterus.

## CEPHALOPELVIC DISPROPORTION

Cephalopelvic disproportion (CPD) is failure of the fetal head to descend through the pelvis despite the presence of efficient uterine contractions and moulding of the fetal head. It occurs when the presenting diameter of the fetal head is larger than the diameters of the maternal pelvis through which it has to pass. Malpresentations, malpositions, pelvic tumours and fetal abnormalities which prevent the head descending through the pelvis are viewed as *obstruction* rather than as causes of cephalopelvic disproportion.

The head is the largest part of the fetus and once it has passed through the brim of the pelvis (see Ch. 24) the rest of the fetus should pass through without difficulty (but always remain mindful of shoulder dystocia). The probability is that the cavity and outlet are also of adequate dimensions to accommodate the passage of a normal fetus. However, in practice, there can be cephalopelvic disproportion at the cavity or outlet of the pelvis too. The reader should bear in mind the different types of pelves (see Ch. 24) and how these may influence the way the fetal head negotiates its passage through the bony canal.

During the last 2 or 3 weeks of pregnancy it will sometimes be found that the head is not engaged. The most common reason for non-engagement is an occipitoposterior position of the fetal head. The deflexed head results in a larger presenting diameter (the occipitofrontal diameter of which is 11.5 cm). In labour, however, the head usually flexes, and descends into the pelvis.

### Diagnosis

The possibility of disproportion should be considered if there is a history of:

- medical conditions such as rickets or osteomalacia which could adversely affect the size and shape of the pelvis
- spinal deformities such as scoliosis
- pelvic fractures or injuries which may have altered the normal shape and dimensions of the pelvis
- obstetric complications such as previous prolonged labour, difficult birth, caesarean section or perinatal death.

The possibility of cephalopelvic disproportion might also be considered from the collective assessment of:

- the woman's stature – particularly if less than 150 cm
- size of fetus if unduly large
- the woman's body mass index (BMI).

Regarding the above points, Hofmeyr (2004) suggests uncertainty as to the use of maternal height as a predictor for CPD. Whilst it is difficult to assess the size of the fetus accurately by palpation, with experience it is possible to determine whether the fetus is unduly large for the duration of the pregnancy. Despite improvements in ultrasound technology, and more accurate estimation of fetal size, Hofmeyr (2004) questions the value of this practice. Technology is no substitute for the expert midwifery skills required to obtain an accurate medical and obstetric history, or for midwives developing the clinical expertise to assess fetal and pelvic size and interpret the idiosyncratic combinations of all the above findings and take appropriate action. Finally, of note, is an increasing body of evidence pointing to the association of raised BMI and cephalopelvic disproportion (Roman et al 2008).

The possibility is that the presence of disproportion is much greater in a primigravida than in a multigravida who has had a history of previous normal deliveries, though it can never be ruled out, since the size of the fetus may have been smaller in previous pregnancies. Worthy of mention here is that disproportion resulting from excessive fetal size may be controlled by good management of maternal diabetes, a predisposing factor in macrosomia.

**Reflective activity 65.1**

Consider what midwifery skills and strategies could be employed that may enhance/encourage flexion and descent of the fetal head through the pelvis.

### X-ray pelvimetry

In recent years, the benefit of X-ray and magnetic resonance imaging (MRI) pelvimetry has been questioned (Zaretsky et al 2005). Ikhena et al (1999) point out that there are no agreed measurements considered satisfactory to allow vaginal birth, and, in addition, pelvimetry may serve to increase the caesarean section rate. Furthermore, Pattinson (1998) concludes that even in situations of anticipated cephalopelvic disproportion, women do better if allowed to labour. The evaluation of the progress of labour is considered a far more accurate indicator of cephalopelvic disproportion (Chhabra et al 2000, Impey & O'Herlihy 1998). Hence, there are only rare situations where pelvimetry is indicated (for example, history of fractured pelvis).

From these examinations and assessments, the mother will fall into one of three categories:

1. No disproportion is evident and spontaneous labour and vaginal birth can be awaited.
2. There is a slight degree of disproportion which may be overcome successfully in labour. Providing there are no other complications, the woman is admitted to hospital for a trial of labour.
3. There is evidence of disproportion, either because the pelvis is small or abnormal in shape or because the fetus is unusually large. Vaginal birth is out of the question and caesarean section is necessary.

## Dangers

If cephalopelvic disproportion is not detected, it will lead to obstructed labour, which may result in a ruptured uterus and in maternal and fetal death.

## Trial of labour

A trial of labour is an ordinary labour conducted in hospital when there is a minor degree of cephalopelvic disproportion. The aim is to ascertain if the contractions of labour will flex and mould the fetal head sufficiently to make it engage and descend through the pelvis. If the head engages, labour is likely to continue normally. The purpose is to give maximum opportunity for the woman to benefit from a vaginal birth within the parameters of fetal and maternal safety. A successful trial of labour prevents unnecessary operative intervention and the associated risks of increased morbidity and mortality, including psychological problems. It also influences the management of future labours, in that if the woman delivers safely vaginally, this is likely to be the pattern in the future.

It is considered that all primigravidae with a non-engaged head are undergoing a trial of labour. With careful selection in the antenatal period and using an upright position in labour, or active management of labour to ensure effective uterine action, most will experience a normal birth. A hands–knees posture may be of benefit to encourage anterior rotation of the lateral or posterior head positions in the pelvis (Lewis et al 2002).

### Conditions necessary in labour when a minor degree of cephalopelvic disproportion is suspected

The presentation must be *cephalic (including occipitoposterior position)*. **The midwife should be conscientious in excluding a brow presentation, which would contraindicate a trial of labour**. Similarly, a trial of labour is not carried out in breech presentations. Further to this, there should be no major degree of cephalopelvic disproportion. The woman should be *young* and *healthy* with an uncomplicated medical and obstetric history. There should be *no complications* of pregnancy such as hypertension or antepartum haemorrhage and the pregnancy must not be postmature, otherwise the fetal head may not mould satisfactorily. There is strong evidence to suggest that it is safe to conduct a trial of labour with a transverse lower segment uterine scar, providing there is careful management and monitoring in labour (Brill & Windrim 2003).

## Management

Labour should take place in an obstetric unit where there are both the facilities and the personnel available for electronic monitoring and any interventions that may be required to achieve a safe outcome in labour for both mother and baby. Good preparation of the woman and her partner before the onset of labour is essential to gain their understanding of the situation and their cooperation in labour. When faced with obstetric emergencies and the need to minimize morbidity and mortality, available options/choices may be diminished. However, women and their partners can still experience a sense of control through the sharing of information and in the decision-making process.

During labour the mother is encouraged to be ambulant because an upright position promotes flexion and descent of the head, cervical dilatation and the maintenance of contractions (Lewis et al 2002). Continuous electronic monitoring of the fetal heart and uterine contractions is recommended.

Progress is assessed by:

- the efficiency of uterine contractions
- abdominal palpation to determine progressive descent of the fetal head
- vaginal examination to note descent and position of the head, effacement of the cervix and dilatation of the os uteri.

All observations and findings of examinations are plotted on a partogram (see Ch. 36). This facilitates rapid recognition of any delay in cervical dilatation and descent of the head and indicates when action should be taken to aid progress. Once labour is established, cervical dilatation of less than 1 cm per hour over a 2-hour period is often regarded as delayed progress (Enkin et al 2000), though there may be local specific protocols for a trial of labour.

If progress is found to be slow due to inefficient uterine action, active management of labour may be undertaken, after careful assessment by an obstetrician. Oxytocic drugs can be used to overcome active phase arrest that is unrelated to cephalopelvic disproportion (Foley et al 2004). Otherwise a diagnosis of cephalopelvic disproportion may be made in cases when the real problem is inefficient uterine action. The use of oxytocin in a trial of labour may be viewed as controversial because of the risk of uterine rupture. However, there is support for its use, provided that continuous electronic cardiotocography is carried out and facilities for the management of any emergencies are readily available (ACOG 2004). Having said that, an increase in the incidence of ruptured uterus is associated with the overuse of Syntocinon. It should be stressed that active management would never be undertaken if more than a minor degree of cephalopelvic disproportion was suspected – emphasizing selective and judicious use of oxytocin.

Conditions necessary for the use of oxytocin in a trial of labour can be summarized thus:

- expert midwifery care to monitor uterine activity both by abdominal palpation and by skilled interpretation of the cardiotocograph trace
- continuous electronic cardiotocography
- close surveillance of fetal and maternal wellbeing
- avoidance of hyperstimulation of uterine activity by oxytocin and, in the absence of significant progress, a limited period of use.

If uterine hyperstimulation or fetal distress occurs, the oxytocin is immediately stopped and the obstetrician informed. If progress in labour does not improve with the use of oxytocin for a limited period, caesarean section is indicated.

If contractions are ineffective, no 'trial' is possible. Oxytocic drugs may therefore be used to augment labour, as described above. If, with effective contractions, the head fails to engage, a caesarean section will need to be considered.

However, Sunday-Adeoye et al (2004) suggest (as an alternative to caesarean section) that symphysiotomy is worthy of consideration in the management of cephalopelvic disproportion in selected cases:

- to facilitate a ventouse extraction when the os uteri is fully dilated – forceps delivery is contraindicated following a symphysiotomy because of the risk of injury to the bladder and to the thinned lower segment of the uterus
- when operative intervention is best avoided, due to lack of facilities, particular hazards or cultural preferences.

Symphysiotomy is associated with minimal morbidity in expert hands. Equally, it should be contrasted with the risks of caesarean section performed in less than optimal circumstances and the future risk of scar rupture. Symphysiotomy is rarely carried out in the UK because caesarean section is considered safe and is more culturally acceptable.

# OBSTRUCTED LABOUR

Obstructed labour will occur in any case in which there is an insuperable barrier to the passage of the fetus through the birth canal, in spite of good uterine contractions.

## Causes

Obstructed labour may occur if:

- the maternal pelvis is grossly contracted, probably owing to rickets, osteomalacia or severe injury
- the available space in the pelvis is occupied by a large tumour, for example a fibroid or an ovarian cyst

- the fetus is unusually large or abnormal with a condition such as hydrocephalus
- malpositions or malpresentations, such as shoulder, brow and persistent mentoposterior face presentations, occur
- cephalopelvic disproportion is unrecognized.

It is important to distinguish clearly between *delay in labour*, known as *active phase arrest* (delay occuring beyond 3–4 cm dilatation and progress at a rate of 0.5 cm/hour or less), when progress is slow, probably because the uterine contractions are not sufficiently strong, but delivery is possible; and *obstruction*, when there is no progress in spite of good uterine contractions, because vaginal birth is mechanically impossible.

## Signs and symptoms

Obstructed labour should be suspected if there is little or no progress in labour despite good uterine contractions. On examination, the presenting part remains high and the cervix dilates slowly, and because the presenting part remains high, the cervix is therefore not well applied. Recognition of the condition at this stage will prevent serious complications.

If the condition is allowed to continue, the contractions become longer, stronger and more frequent in an effort to overcome the obstruction, until, eventually, tonic contractions occur. Uterine exhaustion may occur, especially in primigravidae, when the contractions cease for a while and then restart with renewed vigour. The mother is in severe and continuous pain, greatly distressed and looks very anxious and ill. The temperature is raised, the pulse is rapid; the woman may be vomiting and showing signs of dehydration with reduced urinary output. When the abdomen is inspected, the uterus appears closely moulded around the fetus, the liquor amnii having drained away. On palpation, the presentation remains high and the uterus is continuously hard instead of contracting intermittently. In advanced obstructed labour, an oblique ridge may actually be seen running across the abdomen. This is *Bandl's retraction ring* (see website for Fig. 65.1) and denotes a marked difference in thickness between the tonically retracted upper uterine segment and the dangerously thinned lower segment, which is now in imminent danger of rupturing. The continuous retraction soon cuts off the fetal oxygen supply, resulting in fetal demise. The woman herself is in grave danger of dying from exhaustion or from rupture of the uterus. On vaginal examination, the vagina may feel hot and dry and the presenting part remains high. A large caput succedaneum will be present and, if the presentation is cephalic, there will be excessive moulding.

## Morbidity and mortality associated with obstructed labour

Morbidity and mortality associated with obstructed labour are greatly increased in cases where the condition is not recognized at an early stage, and where there is delay in referral and perhaps inadequate facilities and trained personnel to cope with such an emergency. When obstructed labour is prolonged, the presenting part is impacted against the soft tissues of the pelvis, causing ischaemic vascular injury and ensuing tissue necrosis resulting in either vesico- or rectovaginal fistula formation. Fistulae can be up to 2 cm long and 2.5 cm wide and carry with them a wide spectrum of both physical and social trauma (Miller et al 2005).

According to Chhabra et al (2000), obstructed labour and its sequelae is mainly a problem in certain well-defined geographical regions in Africa and the Indian subcontinent. These authors emphasize the value of the use of a partogram to aid early recognition of delay in labour and to initiate prompt referral.

## Prevention

By good antenatal care and close observation in early labour, the causes of obstructed labour can be recognized and treatment instituted before obstruction occurs. Thus, an ovarian cyst is removed during pregnancy; a caesarean section is planned in late pregnancy for conditions such as cephalopelvic disproportion; a transverse lie is corrected at the onset of labour, or earlier, and safe birth is achieved.

**Reflective activity 65.2**

Outline the factors that would alert you to the possibility of obstructed labour.

## Management

If obstruction occurs later in labour, for instance when the fetal head extends to a brow presentation or to a posterior face presentation, immediate caesarean section is performed. In the second stage of labour, early recognition of deep transverse arrest (see Ch. 64) is essential so that the woman can be safely delivered with ventouse or forceps once the fetal head has been rotated.

There is rarely a place in modern obstetrics for destructive operations, such as craniotomy and cleidotomy, in cases of obstructed labour, because of the risk of trauma to the overstretched and thinned lower uterine segment and to other parts of the birth canal. There is also the profound psychological trauma to the parents to be considered when such procedures are undertaken. Maharaj & Moodley (2002), however, suggest that there remains a limited place for destructive operations in developing countries in carefully selected cases which present late with obstructed labour, an intrauterine death and advanced intrauterine sepsis.

## UTERINE RUPTURE

Rupture of the uterus is a serious obstetric emergency which can result in fetal and/or maternal death (see website for figures). One such case was reported in the latest CEMACH report (Lewis 2007).

The true incidence of ruptured uterus is difficult to determine from the medical literature because authors have different interpretations of what constitutes a ruptured uterus. Some only include a complete rupture, whereas others do not distinguish between complete and incomplete ruptures. The incidence of ruptured uterus is higher in parts of the world where ante- and intrapartum care are deficient and obstructed labour is a more frequent occurrence. Mesleh et al (1999) suggest this occurs up to 10 times more often in developing countries than in developed countries.

### Causes

Ziadeh et al (1996) conclude that the most common contributing factor to uterine rupture in developing countries is obstructed labour, whereas rupture of previous uterine scars is the most common cause in developed countries (possibly constituting 70% of reported uterine ruptures [Mesleh et al 1999]). The latter is undoubtedly influenced by the rising caesarean section rates and the corresponding increase in vaginal birth after caesarean (VBAC). It should be noted that there is a 77% success rate of vaginal birth and a high degree of maternal and neonatal safety associated with VBAC (Kwee et al 2007, Turner et al 2006). The VBAC success rate, in turn, is possibly influenced by improved intrapartum care, assisted by established guidelines and policies.

#### Scar rupture

This can result from previous uterine surgery, usually caesarean section. A classical scar (a longitudinal scar in the body of the uterus) is particularly likely to rupture (Caughey et al 1999) (see website for Figs 65.2 and 65.3). The most likely time for rupture to occur is in late pregnancy or in labour. Because of the high risk of uterine rupture following a classical uterine incision, an elective caesarean section is usually planned in a subsequent pregnancy at about 38 weeks' gestation.

The incidence of uterine rupture following a lower segment caesarean section (most frequently in labour) is 0.22–1.5% (Kwee et al 2007, Turner et al 2006).

Other causes of scarring of the uterus include surgery for conditions such as evacuation of the uterus or fibroids, and some investigations, for example hysteroscopy. During these procedures, trauma or perforation, which is not always recognized, may lead to a scarred uterus, which can result in rupture, usually at the fundus, in a subsequent pregnancy (Hockstein 2000).

#### Traumatic rupture

Traumatic (and often iatrogenic) rupture is caused by:

- misuse of oxytocic drugs and prostaglandins
- use of instruments
- intrauterine manipulations.

Because of the increased maternal and fetal morbidity and mortality associated with high- or mid-cavity forceps deliveries, caesarean section is now considered a preferable mode of delivery. Similarly, intrauterine manipulations to correct unstable lie or malpresentation, such as a shoulder presentation, carry a risk of uterine rupture. The risks are increased when manipulations are attempted when there is scarring; in cases of prolonged or obstructed labour, because of the excessive thinning of the lower uterine segment; and also when the integrity of the uterus is suspect, as in grande multigravidae.

A dominating predisposing risk factor for ruptured uterus highlighted in the literature is the misuse of oxytocic drugs and uterine stimulants such as prostaglandins (Grossetti et al 2007, Kayani & Alfirevic 2005, Lewis 2007). Great care must be exercised in the use of oxytocic drugs for inducing or augmenting labour, especially in multiparous women because hypertonic contractions are more easily stimulated. There is also an increased risk of uterine rupture in those with an intrauterine fetal death if high levels of oxytocic drugs are administered because the effects on the fetus do not have to be considered.

#### Spontaneous rupture

This may occur as a result of very strong uterine contractions (not induced or augmented by the use of oxytocic drugs) (see website for Fig. 65.4). The cause of spontaneous rupture is not always clear. Abruptio placentae can increase the risk, because of disruption and distension of the uterine wall. The risk is further increased when oxytocic drugs are used to stimulate uterine action. Although spontaneous rupture of the primigravid uterus is rare, several authors cite examples of this occurrence (Mesleh et al 1999, Walsh & Baxi 2007).

### Types of uterine rupture

**Complete or true rupture:** This involves the full thickness of the uterine wall and pelvic peritoneum. Ripley (1999) describes it as a sudden, acute event associated with pain and blood loss and a raised maternal and fetal morbidity. It is most commonly associated with spontaneous or traumatic rupture of an unscarred uterus.

**Incomplete rupture:** This involves the myometrium but not the pelvic peritoneum, which remains intact. It may also be called *occult* or *silent rupture*, or sometimes *dehiscence* or *uterine window*. Incomplete rupture is more frequently associated with a previous lower segment caesarean section scar and tends to present with less violent and dramatic signs and symptoms, possibly owing to the avascular nature of the scar tissue.

## Sites of uterine rupture

**The unscarred uterus:** Longitudinal tears appear to be more common in ruptures in the unscarred uterus. Many cases in the literature describe a cervical tear which extends longitudinally into the lower uterine segment, either anteriorly or posteriorly, resulting in serious haemorrhage because of the poor retraction there (Eden et al 1986, Golan et al 1980). It may further extend into the vascular upper uterine segment, thereby increasing morbidity and mortality. In some cases, a rupture may occur in the upper uterine segment only. Ruptures in the unscarred uterus are usually complete and tend to be more extensive and therefore associated with higher maternal and fetal morbidity and mortality rates (Mesleh et al 1999).

**The scarred uterus:** In these cases, the rupture is usually through the scar. The risk of scar rupture in a subsequent pregnancy following a longitudinal incision in the upper uterine segment (that is, a classical caesarean section) is estimated to be 4–12% (Caughey et al 1999). In a pregnancy following a previous lower segment caesarean section, the risk of rupture is 1.22–1.5%.

Although the rupture usually follows the line of the scar, Golan et al (1980) cite cases of transverse rupture into the posterior lower uterine segment and vertical lower segment ruptures.

## Signs and symptoms

Complete rupture of the uterus often presents as an acute event with dramatic maternal collapse. The mother usually complains of severe and constant abdominal pain, followed by a marked reduction or cessation of uterine contractions, and vaginal bleeding. The fetus may be palpated in the abdomen separately from the uterus, and fetal distress followed by intrauterine death is usual.

An incomplete rupture is far less dramatic and often difficult to diagnose. Sometimes it is diagnosed after the birth or at caesarean section (Ripley 1999). The mother may complain of constant abdominal pain and her contractions may slow or cease. Although abdominal pain and/or scar tenderness are regarded as classical signs, these symptoms do not present in many cases. A rise in maternal pulse rate and the cessation of fetal heart sounds or significant change (variable/late decelerations or bradycardia) were identified by Sakka et al (1998) and Ayres et al (2001) as the most common clinical features of impending rupture. Vaginal bleeding may also occur. There is a gradual deterioration in the mother's condition. If the rupture is diagnosed early and delivery is expedited, the fetus might survive.

## Management

All obstetric units must have a written protocol for this emergency and staff familiar with the management of sudden unexpected haemorrhage. The initial management will depend on the maternal and fetal condition. If the mother is in a state of shock, she is urgently resuscitated and prepared for immediate surgery, either caesarean section or, if the rupture is suspected after delivery, laparotomy. A blood transfusion will be necessary for severe haemorrhage and/or shock. Once the baby is delivered and the obstetrician has identified the type, location and extent of the rupture, the appropriate treatment can be instituted.

The surgical options are:

- simple repair of the rupture – the treatment of choice whenever possible (Lim et al 2005, Mesleh et al 1999)
- uterine and internal hypogastric artery ligation to control haemorrhage
- hysterectomy.

## Aftercare

It is essential that mothers and their partners who have experienced such traumatic complications in childbirth receive adequate support and a clear explanation of the events from their obstetrician and midwife during the postnatal period. Some mothers suffer long-term psychological problems after a traumatic birth experience – Leeds & Hargreaves (2008) align it to post-traumatic stress disorder. The opportunity to debrief and the provision of good support from midwife, doctor and family may help to prevent these additional problems. The circumstances may be even more complex if the baby has died and the parents require an approach which facilitates the grieving process. On occasion, the midwife will realize that the mother needs specialist help which is beyond her capabilities and referral for appropriate professional counselling or treatment may be required. Midwives themselves often benefit from the opportunity to debrief after caring for a woman who has experienced such traumatic complications in childbirth.

**Reflective activity 65.3**

Consider how a midwife could present the evidence to enable a woman to make her decision to plan a home birth after a previous caesarean section.

How might a supervisor of midwives contribute constructively to support the woman and the midwife in the above scenario?

## CONCLUSION

The advent of risk management strategies in most maternity units has resulted in a system of follow-up in situations of less than optimal clinical outcomes. This encourages a structured examination of critical events aimed *not* to apportion blame, but rather to identify aspects of care that went well, along with things that have been learnt and areas for improvement and change, thereby improving standards of care.

**KEY POINTS**

- The use of a partogram aids recognition of obstructed labour.
- There is a 77% chance of successful vaginal birth with VBAC.
- Look for the 'big picture' when assessing for CPD, obstructed labour and uterine rupture.
- *Any* scars on the uterus may rupture during labour, and the likelihood increases when oxytocin and prostaglandins are used.
- Sharing information and decisions made with parents is of crucial importance.

## REFERENCES


American College of Obstetrics and Gynecology (ACOG): Practice Bulletin. Dystocia and augmentation of labor, *International Journal of Gynaecology and Obstetrics* 85(3):315–324, 2004.

Ayres AW, Johnson TRB, Hayashi R: Characteristics of fetal heart rate tracings prior to uterine rupture, *Journal of Gynecology and Obstetrics* 74(3):235–240, 2001.

Brill Y, Windrim R: Vaginal birth after Caesarean section: review of antenatal predictors of success, *Journal of Obstetrics and Gynaecology Canada* 25(4):275–286, 2003.

Caughey A, Shipp T, Repke J, et al: Rate of uterine rupture during a trial of labor in women with one or two prior caesarian deliveries, *American Journal of Obstetrics and Gynecology* 181(4):872–876, 1999.

Chhabra S, Gandhi D, Jaiswal M: Obstructed labour – a preventable entity, *Journal of Obstetrics and Gynaecology* 20(2):151–153, 2000.

Eden RD, Parker RT, Gall SA: Rupture of the pregnant uterus: a 53 year review, *Obstetrics and Gynecology* 68(5):671–674, 1986.

Enkin MW, Keirse MJNC, Neilson J, et al: *A guide to effective care in pregnancy and childbirth*, Oxford, 2000, Oxford University Press.

Foley ME, Alarab M, Daley L, et al: The continuing effectiveness of active management of first labor, despite a doubling in overall nulliparous cesarean delivery, *American Journal of Obstetrics and Gynecology* 191(3):891–895, 2004.

Golan A, Sandbank O, Rubin A: Rupture of the pregnant uterus, *Obstetrics and Gynecology* 56(5):549–554, 1980.

Grossetti E, Vardon D, Creveuil C, et al: Rupture of the scarred uterus, *Acta Obstetricia et Gynecologica Scandinavica* 86(5):572–578, 2007.

Hockstein S: Spontaneous uterine rupture in the early third trimester after laparoscopically assisted myomectomy, *Journal of Reproductive Medicine* 45(2):139–141, 2000.

Hofmeyr GJ: Obstructed labor: using better technologies to reduce mortality, *International Journal of Gynecology and Obstetrics* 85(suppl. 1):S62–S72, 2004.

Ikhena SE, Halligan AWF, Naftalin NJ: Has pelivimetry a role in current obstetric practice? *Journal of Obstetrics and Gynaecology* 9(5):463–466, 1999.

Impey L, O'Herlihy C: First delivery after caesarean delivery for strictly defined cephalopelvic disproportion, *Obstetrics and Gynecology* 92(5):799–802, 1998.

Kayani SI, Alfirevic Z: Uterine rupture after induction of labour in women with previous caesarean section, *British Journal of Obstetrics and Gynaecology* 112(4):451–455, 2005.

Kwee A, Bots MI, Vissser GH, et al: Obstetric management and outcome of pregnancy in women with a history of caesarean section in the Netherlands, *European Journal of Obstetrics, Gynecology, and Reproductive Biology* 132(2):171–176, 2007.

Leeds L, Hargreaves I: Psychological consequences of childbirth, *Journal of Reproductive and Infant Psychology* 26(2):108–122, 2008.

Lewis G, editor: *The Confidential Enquiry into Maternal and Child Health (CEMACH). Saving mothers' lives: reviewing maternal deaths to make motherhood safer – 2003–2005. Seventh Report on Confidential Enquiries into Maternal Deaths in the United Kingdom*, London, 2007, RCOG.

Lewis L, Webster J, Carter A, et al: Maternal positions and mobility during first stage labour (Cochrane Protocol), *Cochrane Database of Systematic Reviews*, Issue 4, 2002.

Lim AC, Kwee A, Bruinse HW: Pregnancy after uterine rupture – a report of 5 cases and a review of the literature, *Obstetrical and Gynecological Survey* 60(9):613–617, 2005.

Maharaj D, Moodley J: Symphysiotomy and fetal destructive operations, *Best Practice & Research. Obstetrics & Gynaecology* 16(1):117–131, 2002.

Mesleh R, Kurdi A, Algwiser A, et al: Intrapartum rupture of the gravid uterus, *Saudi Medical Journal* 20(7):531–535, 1999.

Miller S, Lester F, Webster M, et al: Obstetric fistula: a preventable tragedy, *Journal of Midwifery & Women's Health* 50(4):286–294, 2005.

Pattinson RC: Pelvimetry for cephalic presentations (Cochrane Review). In *The Cochrane Library*, Issue 3, Oxford, 1998, Update Software.

Ripley D: Uterine emergencies – atony, inversion and rupture, *Obstetrics and Gynecology Clinics of North America* 26(3):419–433, 1999.

Roman H, Goffinet F, Hulsey TF, et al: Maternal body mass index at delivery and risk of caesarean due to dystocia in low risk pregnancies, *Acta Obstetricia et Gynecologica Scandinavica* 87(2):163–170, 2008.

Sakka M, Hamsho A, Khan L: Rupture of the pregnant uterus – a 21 year review, *International Journal of Gynaecology and Obstetrics* 63(2):105–108, 1998.

Sunday-Adeoye IM, Okonta P, Twomey D: Symphysiotomy at the Mater Misericordiae Hospital Afikpo, Ebonyi State of Nigeria (1982–1999): a review of 1013 cases, *Journal of Obstetrics and Gynaecology* 24(5):525–529, 2004.

Turner MJA, Agnew G, Langan H: Uterine rupture and labour after a previous low transverse caesarean section, *British Journal of Obstetrics and Gynaecology* 113(6):729–732, 2006.

Walsh CA, Baxi LV: Rupture of the primigravid uterus: a review of the literature, *Obstetrical and Gynecological Survey* 62(5):327–334, 2007.

Zaretsky MV, Alexander JM, McIntire DD, et al: Magnetic resonance imaging pelvimetry and the prediction of labor dystocia, *Obstetrics and Gynecology* 106(5):919–926, 2005.

Ziadeh S, Zakaria M, Sunna E: Obstetric uterine rupture in North Jordan, *Journal of Obstetrics and Gynaecology Research* 22(3):209–213, 1996.

Chapter |66|

# Shoulder dystocia

Terri Coates

## LEARNING OUTCOMES

After reading this chapter, you will be able to:

- identify risk factors for shoulder dystocia
- describe shoulder dystocia and be able to recognize the signs which suggest it
- demonstrate a series of manoeuvres that are likely to be effective in resolving shoulder dystocia
- identify which manoeuvres are not likely to be effective in this emergency situation
- state which manoeuvres are likely to cause harm if undertaken
- anticipate the consequences of shoulder dystocia for the mother and the infant
- perform or participate in a locally agreed drill or procedure for shoulder dystocia
- provide support and information to women and their families during and after a case of shoulder dystocia.

## INTRODUCTION

Shoulder dystocia is an obstetric emergency with a potentially catastrophic outcome. It refers to deliveries where manoeuvres other than gentle downward traction are needed to complete the delivery of the anterior shoulder (Resnik 1980).

## MECHANISM

In a normal labour the shoulders enter the pelvic brim in the oblique or transverse diameter. (For a complete description of the normal mechanism of labour, see Ch. 37.) In shoulder dystocia there is an arrest of the normal mechanism of labour as the shoulders attempt to enter the pelvis in the anteroposterior diameter of the pelvic brim. The diameter of the fetal shoulders or bisacromial diameter is 12.4 cm and should fit comfortably through the widest diameter of the pelvic brim. Shoulders are sufficiently flexible to allow those of even a large baby to negotiate the pelvis.

There is no current agreement on a definition for shoulder dystocia. Smeltzer (1986) suggests that shoulder dystocia is a failure of the shoulders to spontaneously traverse the pelvis after the fetal head has been delivered.

Some or all of the following will alert midwives to suspect that shoulder dystocia has occurred:

- difficulty with delivery of the face and chin
- head remaining tightly applied to the vulva or even retracting (*turtle sign*)
- failure of restitution of the head
- failure of the shoulders to descend (RCOG 2005).

The *turtle sign* is caused by reverse traction from the shoulders. The anterior shoulder is wedged onto the symphysis pubis and the posterior shoulder may still be above the pelvic brim (Fig. 66.1). Pulling to deliver the anterior shoulder is likely to impede delivery by wedging the

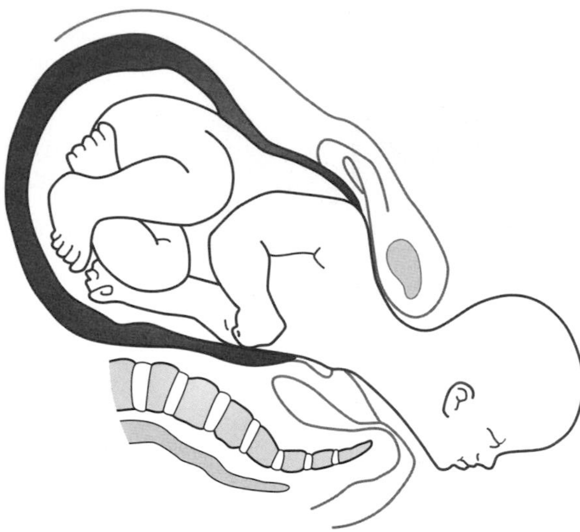

Figure 66.1 Shoulder dystocia.

infant's anterior shoulder more firmly onto the symphysis pubis and can cause damage to the brachial plexus (see Fig. 66.10).

The midwife must recognize shoulder dystocia and summon help immediately from midwifery, obstetric, paediatric and anaesthetist colleagues, as the outcome for both mother and infant is potentially very serious.

The midwife's anxiety is likely to be communicated to the mother even if little is said. The midwife should remain calm and in control of the situation, and maintain communication with the mother and her partner.

## INCIDENCE AND RISK

The incidence of shoulder dystocia is around 0.6% at term, but the risk increases to 1.3% by 42 weeks' gestation (Johnstone & Meyerscough 1998, RCOG 2005). However, a lack of agreement over the definition affects the number of cases reported (Johnstone & Myerscough 1998).

The risk of shoulder dystocia rises with increasing birthweight and length of gestation, birth order and maternal age (Acker et al 1986, Gross et al 1987, Johnstone & Myerscough 1998). Johnstone & Myerscough (1998) point out that half of all babies with shoulder dystocia weigh less than 4 kg and are not considered to be large, and only 4% of large babies suffer shoulder dystocia.

Mortimore & McNabb (1998) suggested that some practitioners may use the term shoulder dystocia to describe any general difficulty with the delivery of the shoulders. If RCOG (2005) diagnostic criteria for shoulder dystocia cannot be fulfilled, then 'difficulty with delivery of the shoulders' should be recorded to avoid overdiagnosis (Mahran et al 2008).

### Identification of risk factors

Ideally, all potential cases of shoulder dystocia would be identified antenatally; the associated maternal and neonatal morbidity and mortality could then be prevented. The sensitivity of single predictive risk factors is poor. At present, midwives and obstetricians can do no more than anticipate the problem by identifying those factors which give a strong index of suspicion.

Maternal obesity is a frequently occurring factor associated with shoulder dystocia (maternal BMI >30 at booking, or weight at delivery >90 kg) (RCOG 2005). The greater the maternal weight, the higher the risk (Athukorala et al 2007).

Maternal diabetes and gestational diabetes are associated with asymmetrical fetal growth. The body and particularly the shoulders are larger than in babies of mothers who are not diabetic (Acker et al 1985).

Spellacy et al (1985) studied the data from 33,545 deliveries and concluded that women with either insulin-dependent or gestational diabetes are more likely to deliver a macrosomic infant and are therefore at a higher risk of a delivery complicated by shoulder dystocia.

Fetal macrosomia is the strongest independent risk factor for shoulder dystocia (Athukorala et al 2007). Infants of non-diabetic mothers who have birthweights of 4000–4449 g have a 10% risk of shoulder dystocia, while infants of the same weight born to diabetic mothers have a 31% risk of developing shoulder dystocia, because of their asymmetrical growth (Acker et al 1985, Spellacy et al 1985).

A previous delivery complicated by shoulder dystocia is a predictive risk factor, with a recurrence rate of around 10% for subsequent deliveries (Olugbile & Mascarenhas 2000, Smith et al 1994).

### Use of ultrasound to predict the macrosomic fetus

Ultrasonic estimation of fetal weight is widely used, as it is objective and can be reproduced (Combs et al 1993). However, Chauhan et al (1992) suggest that ultrasonic diagnosis of the large infant is generally no more accurate than clinical estimation and that if a woman has had a baby before, her own estimate is likely to be as good as an ultrasound measurement. Elective induction for infants diagnosed as macrosomic on ultrasound scan increases the risk of caesarean section and does not prevent shoulder dystocia (Hall 1996, RCOG 2005).

In spite of the inadequacy of ultrasound estimation of fetal weight, it is currently used along with clinical judgement to assess the safest method of delivery, especially for the postmature, large for gestational age or suspected macrosomic fetus.

### Prediction of impending shoulder dystocia

Most labours preceding shoulder dystocia are normal (McFarland et al 1995). In some cases the first hint of trouble the midwife may experience during a delivery is the slow extension of the baby's head and then the chin remaining tight against the mother's perineum (Coates 1995). In spite of current technology, shoulder dystocia usually occurs unexpectedly (RCOG 2005).

Unfortunately, the absence of risk factors cannot be relied upon to exclude the possibility of shoulder dystocia. It is therefore important that the midwife has a sound knowledge of the interaction between the physiology and mechanism of labour and the manoeuvres that may be used to complete the delivery in the shortest time possible. This is to ensure the best outcome for the mother and her infant. All members of the labour ward team should be familiar with the agreed protocol, and 'drills' should be practised on a regular basis by all grades of staff (Draycott et al 2008, MCHRC 1998).

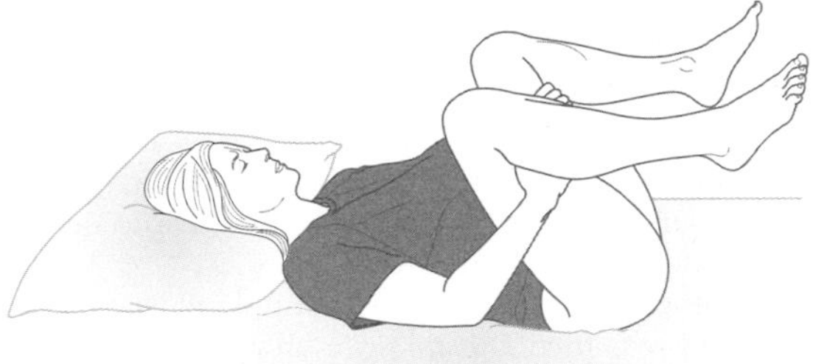

Figure 66.2 McRoberts' manoeuvre.

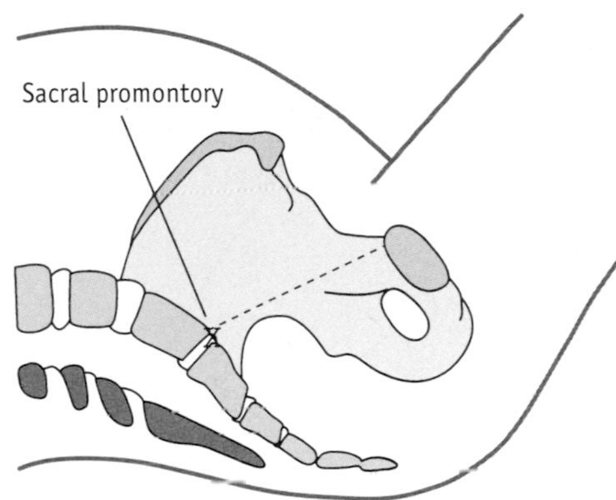


Figure 66.3 Diagram to show brim of pelvis in dorsal position.

## MANOEUVRES FOR MANAGEMENT OF SHOULDER DYSTOCIA

The following descriptions of manoeuvres are arranged from the simple, requiring only movement of the mother, to the complex, where direct manipulation of the baby is required. These manoeuvres cannot really be learned or fully understood by reading alone and it is suggested that the reader works through the manoeuvres using a doll and pelvis or phantom.

### McRoberts' manoeuvre

This is the first choice of manoeuvre in most circumstances as it has been proven to be safe and effective. The manoeuvre (Fig. 66.2) requires the mother to lie flat on her back (or with a slight lateral tilt to prevent supine hypotension), then she is assisted into an exaggerated knee–chest position (Gonik et al 1983).

Once the mother has adopted this position, the midwife should be able to proceed with a normal delivery of the shoulders. Smeltzer (1986) suggests that this manoeuvre:

1. rotates the symphysis pubis superiorly by approximately 8 cm
2. elevates the anterior shoulder
3. pushes the posterior shoulder over the sacrum
4. flexes the fetal spine
5. straightens maternal lordosis
6. opens the pelvic inlet to its maximum
7. brings the inlet perpendicular to the maximum expulsive force
8. removes weight-bearing forces from the sacrum, and
9. removes the sacral promontory as a point of obstruction (Figs 66.3 and 66.4).

This was supported by later radiological studies (Gherman et al 2000).

Maternal and fetal models were used by Gonik et al (1989) to assess the forces used to extract the fetal shoulders. The McRoberts' manoeuvre was compared with the lithotomy position and consistently required less force to remove the shoulders.

RCOG (2005) advocates the use of the McRoberts' manoeuvre as a first step if shoulder dystocia is diagnosed, and, if the manoeuvre is unsuccessful at the first attempt, to try it a second time before attempting other manoeuvres.

### All-fours position

When there is a minor degree of shoulder dystocia, movement of the mother can dislodge the obstruction so the shoulders can negotiate the pelvis normally; assisting the mother into an *all-fours position* can work in this way.

The all-fours position (Fig. 66.5) also can be used to optimize the space in the sacral curve for the midwife to undertake the direct or rotational manoeuvres as described below. Generally, this position, which acts as an 'upside-down McRoberts' position' carries the same positive effects as above, and will allow the posterior shoulder to deliver first (Macdonald & Day-Stirk 1995).

If a mother is already on all fours and shoulder dystocia is encountered, then the midwife should assist her to move into the McRoberts' position. If this is not possible, then direct manoeuvres can be undertaken whilst the all-fours position is maintained.

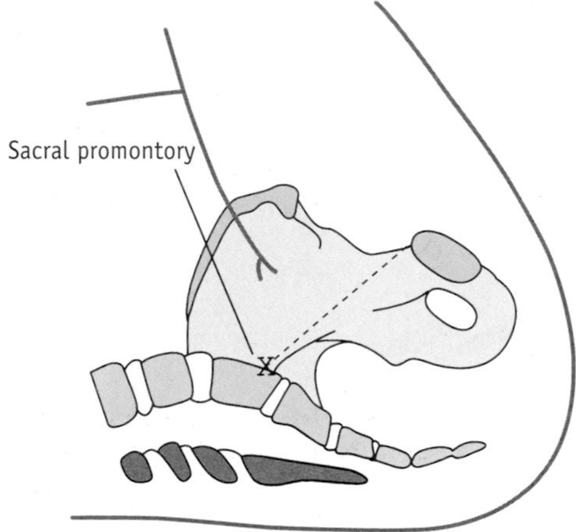


**Figure 66.4** Diagram to show brim of pelvis in McRoberts' position.

The all-fours position can only be used if the woman is willing and able to manoeuvre onto her knees, and is not suitable for women who have a dense epidural block. Whilst the woman is in the all-fours position it is difficult to maintain eye contact and the midwife must ensure that good clear verbal contact is maintained. It is a useful position for a larger or overweight woman, who may find it difficult to adopt the McRoberts' position.

> **Reflective activity 66.1**
>
> Using role play, with one of you 'playing' the woman and one the midwife, work with a colleague and try:
>
> - assisting a woman from the lithotomy position into:
>   - the McRoberts' position
>   - the all-fours position
> - assisting a woman from a semi-recumbent position into:
>   - the McRoberts' position.
>
> Practise the instructions that you might have to give to a mother moving from one position to another. Consider how easy/difficult it was getting into these different positions, and how you could prepare women antenatally for such an emergency.

## Suprapubic pressure

The application of suprapubic pressure is intended to adduct and then displace the anterior shoulder away from the symphysis pubis and so allow it to enter the pelvis in an oblique diameter (Fig. 66.6). Pressure is applied by either the midwife or assistant, using the flat of the hand

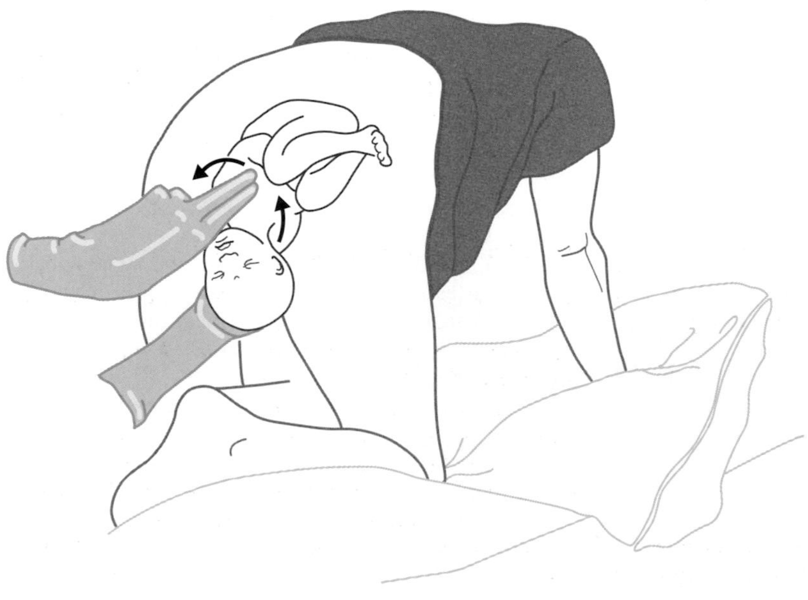

**Figure 66.5** Wood's manoeuvre with the woman in the all-fours position.

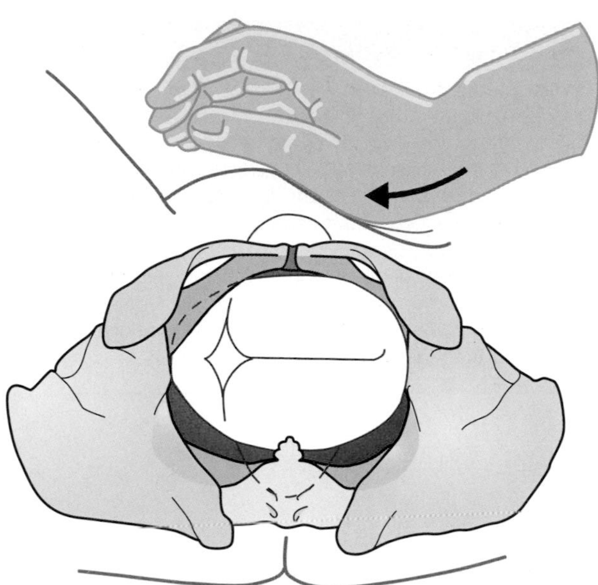

**Figure 66.6** Diagram to illustrate the use and direction of suprapubic pressure when the back is on the woman's left.

against the baby's back in the direction that the baby is facing.

Suprapubic pressure can be used on its own or with other non-invasive manoeuvres, such as the McRoberts' or all-fours manoeuvre. It may also be used with the Rubin manoeuvre or the Woods' manoeuvre (see below).

Non-invasive procedures have been shown to be effective in up to 69/76 (91%) of cases of shoulder dystocia (Luria et al 1994). However, if the non-invasive manoeuvres described have been unsuccessful, then direct rotational manoeuvres are required. It is at this stage that extra analgesia or anaesthesia may be required. Meanwhile, the midwife should not delay attempting to complete the delivery.

## Episiotomy

Shoulder dystocia is a bony dystocia and as such is not greatly affected by soft tissue. An episiotomy may prevent injury to the mother's pelvic floor and perineum during any direct manipulation of the fetus and/or accommodate the midwife's or obstetrician's hand whilst undertaking direct rotational manoeuvres.

## Woods' manoeuvre and Rubin manoeuvre

### Woods' manoeuvre

To undertake the Woods' or the Rubin manoeuvre, the midwife should assist the woman into the lithotomy position with her buttocks well over the edge of the bed so that there is no restriction to the sacrum or coccyx during the manoeuvre. If this is not possible, in a home confinement for instance, then the McRoberts' or all-fours position should be used. These are practical positions for undertaking further manoeuvres and remove restrictions to the sacrum and coccyx that are present when the mother is in the dorsal or semi-recumbent position.

The method Woods (1943) used to relieve shoulder dystocia involves applying one hand to the mother's abdomen, putting firm but gentle pressure onto the fetal buttocks, and inserting as much of the hand as is necessary into the vagina to locate the anterior surface of the posterior shoulder (clavicle). The shoulder is then rotated through 180 degrees in the direction of the fetal back (Fig. 66.5), which actually causes an abduction (see website) of the fetal shoulders.

This rotation may dislodge the anterior shoulder and enable the posterior shoulder to enter the pelvic brim. The posterior shoulder becomes the anterior following the rotation, and may be delivered by normal downward traction and the delivery completed.

### Rubin manoeuvre

Rubin (1964) emphasized the importance of having both of the infant's shoulders adducted, and presented measurements to demonstrate that in this position the circumference of the baby's body is less than if the shoulders were abducted. To achieve the Rubin manoeuvre, a hand must be inserted into the vagina as far as is necessary to locate a shoulder. Then, working from behind the fetus, the shoulders are pushed into the oblique diameter (see website). Once the shoulders are in the oblique diameter and free of the symphysis pubis, then delivery can be completed (Fig. 66.7).

O'Leary (2009) suggests that both the Woods' and Rubin manoeuvres may be more successful if they are used in conjunction with gentle but firm suprapubic pressure in the direction that facilitates the vaginal rotation (see Fig. 66.6).

## Delivery of the posterior arm

The technique is to insert a hand into the vagina along the curve of the sacrum and locate the posterior arm or hand. The fetal arm should then be swept over the chest and delivered (Fig. 66.8).

If this manoeuvre fails once the posterior arm has been delivered, the fetus may be rotated using either the Woods' or Rubin manoeuvre so that the shoulder and arm that have been delivered are rotated to the anterior position, thus unlocking the obstruction (this is similar to the Burns–Marshall manoeuvre as described in Chapter 64).

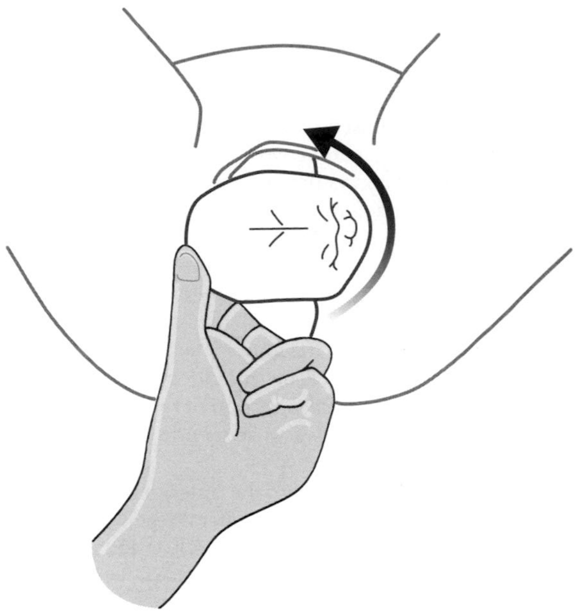

**Figure 66.7** Rubin manoeuvre: the shoulders are adducted as the shoulder is rotated anteriorly.

## Zavanelli manoeuvre

The Zavanelli manoeuvre is a revolutionary concept (Sandberg 1985). Unlike the other manoeuvres described, it reverses the whole mechanism of delivery. Cephalic replacement is followed by a caesarean section. Whilst it is unlikely that a midwife would ever need to undertake this manoeuvre, it may be a last resort if practising in a remote area away from immediate obstetric support.

To carry out the manoeuvre, the fetal head is returned to the pre-restitution position of either direct occipito-anterior or direct occipitoposterior. The head is then manually flexed and returned to the vagina (Sandberg 1985) (Fig. 66.9). Delivery is then completed by caesarean section.

The role of the midwife in such circumstances would normally be to support the mother, monitor and record the condition of both the mother and the fetus, and ensure that all the personnel necessary are called to deal with this obstetric emergency.

Sandberg (1985:482) suggests that the Zavanelli manoeuvre 'must occupy the bottom priority until its virtue and applicability ... can be confirmed'. The Zavanelli manoeuvre must remain the last resort; however, it has proved to be a life-saving procedure. Midwives should understand the mechanisms of the Zavanelli manoeuvre and hope that they will never need to use it.

**Reflective activity 66.2**

When you believe that you are familiar with the manoeuvres, use a doll and pelvis to reinforce your knowledge of the pelvic angles achieved with each manoeuvre. Try to undertake the direct manoeuvres with the pelvis in the correct position for an all-fours delivery. Ask a colleague to hold the pelvis in the correct position for you whilst you try to undertake the manoeuvres and note the different degrees of force which may be used.

Use the mnemonics in Boxes 66.3 and 66.4 if you find that they help you, or make up your own mnemonic to memorize the sequences of the manoeuvres.

# OTHER PROCEDURES

## Symphysiotomy

Surgical separation of the symphysis pubis to enlarge the pelvis for delivery has been proven clinically useful for cephalopelvic disproportion but is associated with high maternal morbidity. Although symphysiotomy has been used for the relief of shoulder dystocia, the few cases reported reveal high maternal morbidity (Broekman et al 1994).

## Cleidotomy

A clavicle can fracture spontaneously during a normal delivery of a normal-weight infant or a delivery complicated by shoulder dystocia. Deliberate fracture of the clavicle is a difficult procedure, especially in a large, mature fetus. O'Leary (1992:78) points out that although clavicular fracture is often mentioned, 'its use has never been substantiated' to resolve shoulder dystocia.

## Fundal pressure

Fundal pressure together with traction provides the worst outcome for brachial plexus injury (Gross et al 1987). Fundal pressure will further impact the shoulder or shoulders and impede progress, can damage the brachial plexus and has also been associated with uterine rupture and maternal death (O'Leary 2009). Fundal pressure has also been implicated in uterine rupture, and thus maternal morbidity and mortality. It is therefore a practice which **should not** be used (RCOG 2005).

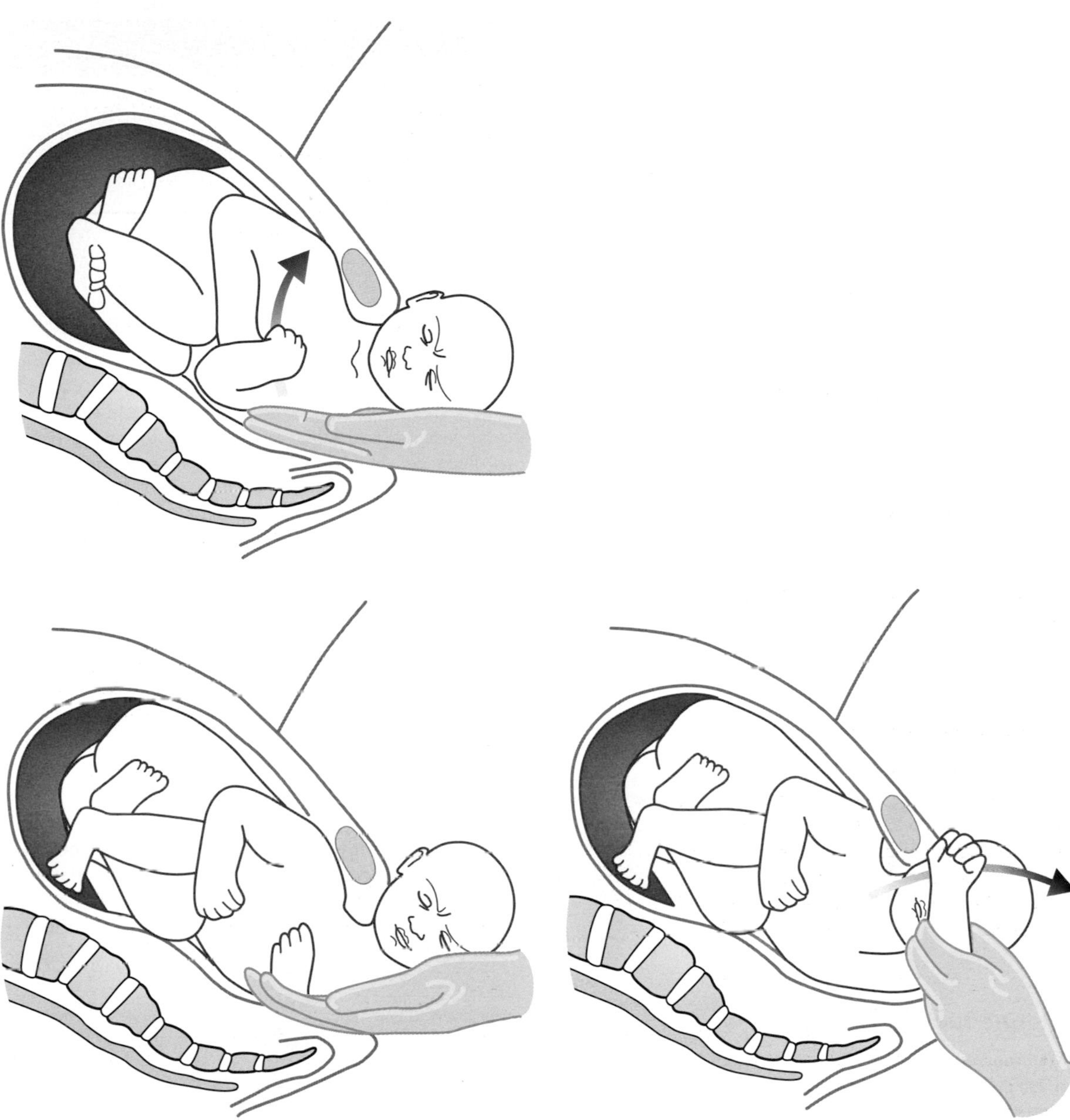

Figure 66.8 Delivery of the posterior arm.

## MATERNAL OUTCOME

Shoulder dystocia is associated with a higher risk of physical and psychological morbidity and mortality for mother and baby:

- potential for physical and psychological trauma to mother
- possibility of uterine rupture from fundal pressure
- postpartum haemorrhage (PPH) and/or shock
- soft tissue damage – cervix and vagina
- infection
- postnatal depression
- the loss of the perfect birth and the perfect baby
- possible problems with maternal–infant interaction.

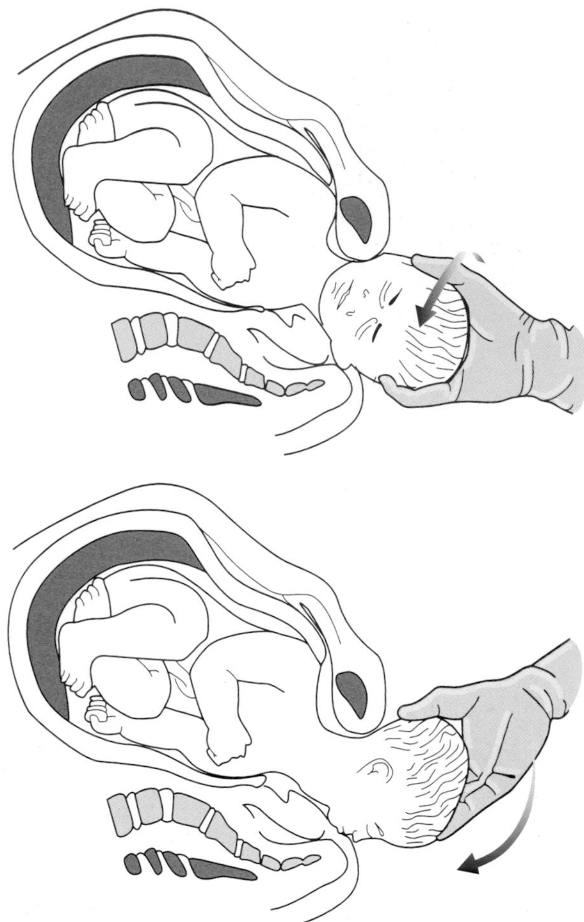

Figure 66.9 Zavanelli manoeuvre.

## Uterine rupture

Maternal deaths associated with shoulder dystocia have been caused by the use of fundal pressure resulting in uterine rupture and from haemorrhage during delivery or immediately postpartum (RCOG 2005).

## Postpartum haemorrhage and/or shock

Benedetti & Gabbe (1978) described maternal morbidity from shoulder dystocia as considerable: in their study, 68% of cases had an estimated blood loss of more than 1000 mL. Others have recorded extensive vaginal, cervical and perineal lacerations, uterine rupture and vaginal haematoma as sequelae to shoulder dystocia (Gross et al 1987).

It is wise to anticipate postpartum haemorrhage if shoulder dystocia is encountered.

**Box 66.1 Calling for help (hospital)**

- Senior midwifery colleagues
- Senior obstetrician
- Senior paediatrician/neonatologist
- Anaesthetist

## Soft tissue damage – cervix and vagina

Soft tissue damage may include vulval haematoma and minor and major lacerations. As these may cause a significant degree of blood loss, the midwife should examine the cervix, vagina and labia very carefully following delivery to diagnose any lacerations and take appropriate action (see Ch. 40).

## Infection

Increased vaginal examinations, and manoeuvres are likely to increase the risk of infection for the woman. This may be exacerbated by soft tissue damage and blood loss.

## The loss of the perfect birth and the perfect baby

Women will have had plans and expectations for the birth of the baby. It may be difficult for the woman to come to terms with the reality of a shoulder dystocia birth and its sequelae. As with any traumatic experience, the mother and her partner may wish to discuss the events surrounding the delivery. This is discussed further in Chapter 70.

# BIRTH INJURY AND FETAL OUTCOMES

The most obvious and immediate consequence for the infant whose birth has been complicated by shoulder dystocia is asphyxia (MCHRC 1998, RCOG 2005).

Airway protective reflexes are reduced by asphyxia. Midwives should therefore prepare for the reception of an asphyxiated baby, and must call for a paediatrician to attend the delivery (Box 66.1). (Resuscitation of the newborn is described in Chapter 45.)

Careful examination of the newborn is always important but is imperative following a traumatic delivery (see also Ch. 41). The most commonly reported injuries following deliveries complicated by shoulder dystocia involve the brachial plexus.

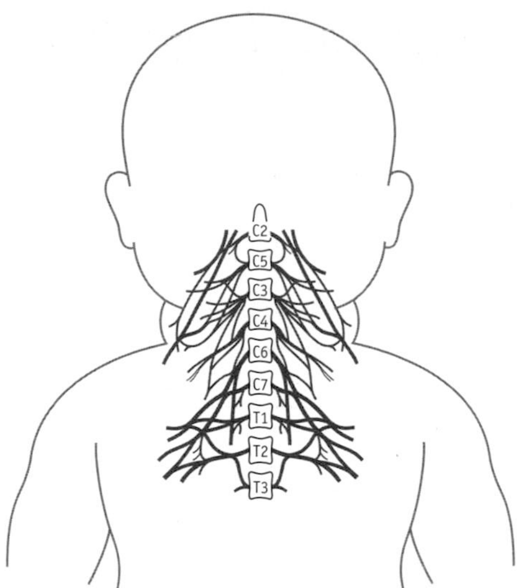


**Figure 66.10** The brachial plexus of the neonate.

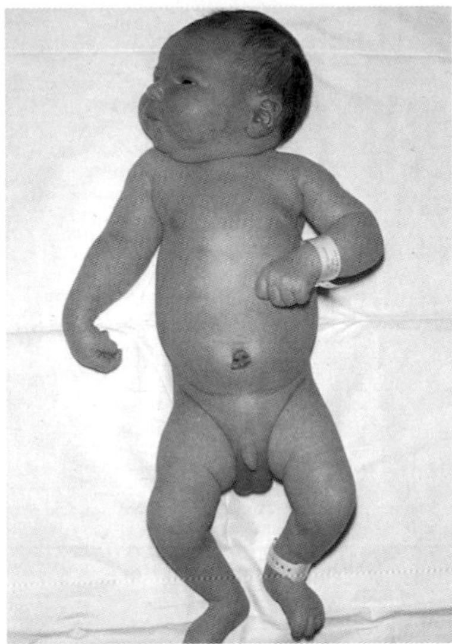

**Figure 66.11** Erb's palsy. *(From Beischer et al 1997.)*

## Brachial plexus injury

The prevalence of congenital brachial palsy (CBP) is 1:2300 of all live births; 64% of CBP is associated with shoulder dystocia, compared with the normal population risk of 0.2–1% (RCPCH 2000). Whilst many brachial plexus injuries are associated with shoulder dystocia, high birthweight and assisted delivery, around 7.5% of cases have no associated risks reported (RCPCH 2000). There is no reliable method of predicting risk of either shoulder dystocia or brachial plexus injuries.

Erb's palsy is the most commonly reported brachial plexus injury following shoulder dystocia. This is the result of damage to the nerve roots C5–6 (Fig. 66.10). The arm on the affected side lies in the classical 'waiter's tip' position (Fig. 66.11).

Following delivery, if the baby has a flaccid arm or an unequal Moro reflex (see Ch. 41), then the midwife must suspect a brachial plexus injury and inform a senior paediatrician. Serious conditions are associated with congenital brachial plexus injury, such as cervical cord injury and cerebral injury, and these will require urgent treatment.

There are four degrees of injury to the brachial plexus:

1. *Stretch injury*. Injury depends on the degree of stretch. Further damage is caused by compression due to swelling and bruising. This is the least severe injury; recovery may be complete within 6–18 months.
2. *Rupture*. The nerve is torn, perhaps in several places, and may require surgery to restore function.
3. *Neuroma*. Scar tissue that develops following injury.
4. *Avulsion*. Nerves are pulled or torn from the spinal cord. This is the most severe injury and is likely to require several stages of surgery to restore nerves, and may require muscle graft and tendon transfer.

Diagnosis may be complex as there may be a combination of injuries.

### Treatment for congenital brachial plexus injury

The baby will be referred to a physiotherapist and the parents will be taught how to maintain the affected arm in a natural position until any bruising or swelling resolves. The physiotherapist will then teach the parents a series of exercises for the affected arm.

Physiotherapy is used to maximize the use of the arm to prevent muscle contracture. Motion exercises develop strength and flexibility, and tactile stimulation is used to improve sensory awareness. It is important to keep the joints supple for the best outcome. However, these exercises are time consuming, and parents will require support and encouragement, in addition to as much information as is available concerning their baby's condition. Parents should be referred to support groups (see website for contact addresses).

Most congenital brachial plexus injuries resolve within 6–12 months; those that have not resolved may need surgery to improve function.

## Bony injury

Shoulder dystocia and high birthweight are considered risk factors for clavicular fractures. Clavicular fractures can also be unpredictable and unavoidable, and may occur in

**Box 66.2 Injuries associated with shoulder dystocia**

- Sternomastoid tumour
- Congenital brachial palsy (CBP)
- Horner's syndrome
- Paralysed hemidiaphragm
- Facial palsy
- Phrenic nerve palsy
- Fractured clavicle
- Fractured humerus
- Shoulder dislocation
- Bruising
- Cerebral palsy

2–4% of normal births (Roberts et al 1995). The baby may be in considerable pain and on examination an irregularity may be felt over the site of the fracture. However, if the fracture is not displaced, an irregularity may only be felt over the site of the fracture several days after birth as a callus forms as part of the healing process. The callus will resolve within a couple of months. If a midwife suspects that a clavicle has been fractured, a paediatrician must examine the baby. The paediatrician may order X-rays to confirm the diagnosis and to rule out other bony injury. An analgesic, such as paracetamol in a paediataric dosage, may be prescribed if the baby appears to be suffering any discomfort.

The humerus may have also been damaged following shoulder dystocia, especially if the posterior arm has to be delivered to release the impaction. Both arms should be examined carefully after delivery, and in the first weeks following delivery, to exclude bony injury and monitor CBP.

Careful examination of the newborn must be undertaken following any delivery, and special attention taken following a traumatic delivery, to exclude any injury not immediately apparent (see Box 66.2).

## NOTES AND RECORD-KEEPING

There are many events in midwifery that happen with alarming rapidity (NMC 2007) and as such are difficult to record contemporaneously. Accurate records are vital for all deliveries and especially following any emergency situation. The midwife must take care to record all events in chronological order. The important or main events in a case of shoulder dystocia are:

- time of delivery of the head
- position of the baby's head after restitution
- position of the woman before and during birth
- time assistance was summoned
- time of each manoeuvre
- time and duration of traction
- episiotomy and when this was performed
- effect of each manoeuvre used
- time assistance arrived
- time of delivery of the body
- Apgar score and condition of the baby
- results of the examination following birth
- information provided to parents at and after the birth (RCM 2000).

**Box 66.3 The HELPERR mnemonic**

H Help – call for help
E Episiotomy
L Legs hyperflexed (McRoberts' position)
P Pressure suprapubically
E Enter the vagina
R Remove the posterior arm
R Roll the woman onto her hands and knees

(ALSO 2000)

## EDUCATION, TRAINING AND DEVELOPMENT

Regular scenario training or 'drills' and thorough knowledge of local procedure for shoulder dystocia are recommended (Draycott et al 2008, MCHRC 1998). Most maternity units have instituted such educational and development strategies and have demonstrated improved staff performance and outcome.

The Advanced Life Support in Obstetrics (ALSO) training has been a useful means of gathering multidisciplinary groups together to practise emergency skills in a safe environment, and for the emergency of shoulder dystocia (Sokol et al 2003) has promoted the HELPERR mnemonic (see Box 66.3). Other mnemonics are in use (see Box 66.4).

If a mnemonic is in use, it should be underpinned by a clear evidence-based rationale and should be clearly understood by the whole team.

The nature of shoulder dystocia as a comparatively rare but serious emergency means that some practitioners may never have the experience of dealing with it, or may never observe a case before they have to deal with it as lead practitioner. It is therefore vital that following an incident of shoulder dystocia (and any other emergency) there is a

**Box 66.4 The SLEEP mnemonic**

S Shout for help
L Legs hyperflexed
E External suprapubic pressure
E Enter vagina to perform Woods' screw manoeuvre
P Posterior arm removal

(Etches & Klein 1995)

forum to discuss the individual case and its management in a systematic and critically reflective way. This will highlight elements of good practice and communication, and identify areas that require additional attention. This forum should be multidisciplinary, and should at its heart have a non-blame and development principle (DH 2000).

**Reflective activity 66.3**

Review your local protocols and clinical guidelines. Are these up-to-date and evidence based? Is there a regular shoulder dystocia drill carried out locally? You may wish to work with colleagues to plan a regular drill as recommended by CESDI (MCHRC 1998) and the RCOG (2005) involving a range of colleagues, to practise the manoeuvres and management. Ensure that there is an opportunity to reflect together after the sessions.

## CONCLUSION

Shoulder dystocia is a rare but serious complication of labour. Midwives should commit to memory a series of manoeuvres that have been proven to be effective and be aware of those manoeuvres that are ineffective or dangerous. Current knowledge of labour ward protocol or procedure is necessary for all members of the labour ward staff. All members of staff who may be involved in such an emergency should take part in practice 'drills' on the labour ward (MCHRC 1998, RCOG 2005, RCM 2000).

Permanent damage is rare. Babies who do suffer brachial plexus injury should be swiftly referred to a specialist centre, and parents provided with appropriate support and information to help them care for their child. The psychological impact of such a traumatic birth should be considered by the care team, and opportunities provided for debriefing and for further counselling, should this be necessary.

**KEY POINTS**

- Shoulder dystocia is an emergency and midwives should prepare for the unexpected, be involved in 'drills' and ensure that local procedures are manageable.
- If shoulder dystocia occurs, help should be summoned immediately.
- The most simple and non-invasive manoeuvres should be attempted, progressing to the direct and rotational manoeuvres as needed.
- Careful examination of the newborn must be carried out to exclude injuries not immediately obvious at birth. Any deviations from the norm should be investigated and specialist referral organized, ensuring parents are fully informed throughout.
- Full and accurate records must be maintained.
- Reflection and discussion with the mother and partner and all those involved in the delivery is essential.

## REFERENCES


Acker DB, Sachs BP, Friedman EA: Risk factors for shoulder dystocia, *Obstetrics and Gynecology* 66(6):762–768, 1985.

Acker DB, Sachs BP, Friedman EA: Risk factors for shoulder dystocia in the average weight infant, *Obstetrics and Gynecology* 67(5):614–618, 1986.

Advanced Life Support in Obstetrics (ALSO): *Advanced Life Support in Obstetrics provider course syllabus*, ed 4, Leawood, Kan, 2000, American Academy of Family Physicians.

Athukorala C, Crowther CA, Willson K, et al: Women with gestational diabetes mellitus in the ACHOSIS trial: risk factors for shoulder dystocia, *Australian and New Zealand Journal of Obstetrics and Gynaecology* 47(1):37–41, 2007.

Beischer N, Mackay E, Colditz P: *Obstetrics and the newborn*, London, 1997, WB Saunders.

Benedetti TJ, Gabbe SG: Shoulder dystocia a complication of fetal macrosomia and prolonged second stage of labour with mid pelvic operative delivery, *Obstetrics and Gynecology* 52(5):526–529, 1978.

Broekman AMW, Smith YG, van Dessel T: (1994) Shoulder dystocia and symphysiotomy: a case report, *European Journal of Obstetrics, Gynecology, and Reproductive Biology* 53(2):142–143.

Chauhan SP, Lutton PM, Bailey KJ, et al: Intrapartum clinical, sonographic, and parous patients' estimates of newborn birth weight, *Obstetrics and Gynecology* 79(6):956–958, 1992.

Coates T: Shoulder dystocia. In Alexander J, Levy V, Roch S, editors: Midwifery practice, Vol. 5, London, 1995, Macmillan.

Combs AC, Singh NB, Khoury JS: Elective induction versus spontaneous labour after sonographic diagnosis of fetal macrosomia, *Obstetrics and Gynecology* 81(4):492–496, 1993.

Department of Health (DH): *An organisation with a memory: report of an expert group on learning from adverse events in the NHS*, London, 2000, DH.

Draycott TJ, Crofts JF, Ash JP, et al: Improving neonatal outcome through practical shoulder dystocia training, *Obstetrics and Gynecology* 112(1):14–20, 2008.

Etches D, Klein M: 'SLEEP' a mnemonic to use in shoulder dystocia, *Accoucheur* 2(2):1–2, 1995.

Gherman RB, Tramont J, Muffley P, et al: Analysis of McRoberts' manoeuvre by X-ray pelvimetry, *Obstetrics and Gynecology* 95(1):43–47, 2000.

Gonik B, Stringer CA, Held B: An alternate manoeuvre for management of shoulder dystocia, *American Journal of Obstetrics and Gynecology* 145(7):882–883, 1983.

Gonik B, Allen R, Sorab J: Objective evaluation of the shoulder dystocia phenomenon: effect of maternal pelvic orientation on force reduction, *Obstetrics and Gynecology* 74(1):44–48, 1989.

Gross SJ, Shime J, Forrine D: Shoulder dystocia: predictors and outcome. A five year review, *American Journal of Obstetrics and Gynecology* 56(2):336–344, 1987.

Hall MH: Guessing the weight of the baby, *British Journal of Obstetrics and Gynaecology* 103(8):734–736, 1996.

Johnstone FD, Myerscough PR: Shoulder dystocia, *British Journal of Obstetrics and Gynaecology* 105(8):811–815, 1998.

Luria S, BenArie A, Hagay Z: The ABC of shoulder dystocia management, *Asia-Oceania Journal of Obstetrics and Gynaecology* 20(2):195–197, 1994.

Macdonald SE, Day-Stirk F: A midwife's perspective (shoulder dystocia), *Clinical Risk* 1(2):61–65, 1995.

McFarland M, Hod M, Piper JM, et al: Are labor abnormalities more common in shoulder dystocia? *American Journal of Obstetrics and Gynecology* 173(4):1211–1214, 1995.

Mahran MA, Sayed AT, Imoh-Ita F: Avoiding over diagnosis of shoulder dystocia, *Journal of Obstetrics and Gynaecology* 28(2):173–176, 2008.

Maternal and Child Health Research Consortium (MCHRC): *Confidential Enquiry into Stillbirth and Deaths in Infancy: 5th Annual Report*, London, 1998, MCHRC.

Mortimore VR, McNabb M: A six year retrospective analysis of shoulder dystocia and delivery of the shoulders, *Midwifery* 14(3):162–173, 1998.

Nursing and Midwifery Council (NMC): *Guidelines for records and record keeping*, London, 2007, NMC.

O'Leary JA, editor: Shoulder dystocia and birth injury: prevention and treatment, New Jersey, 2009, Humana Press.

Olugbile A, Mascarenhas L: Review of shoulder dystocia at the Birmingham Women's Hospital, *Journal of Obstetrics and Gynaecology* 20(3):267–270, 2000.

Resnik R: Management of shoulder girdle dystocia, *Clinical Obstetrics and Gynecology* 23(2):559–564, 1980.

Roberts SW, Hernandez C, Maberry MC, et al: Obstetric clavicular fracture: the enigma of normal birth, *Obstetrics and Gynecology* 86(6):978–981, 1995.

Royal College of Midwives (RCM): Clinical risk management. Paper 2: Shoulder dystocia, *RCM Midwives Journal* 3(11):348–351, 2000.

Royal College of Obstetricians and Gynaecologists (RCOG): Shoulder dystocia. RCOG Guideline No. 42, London, 2005, RCOG.

Royal College of Paediatrics and Child Health (RCPCH): *British Paediatric Surveillance Unit 14th Annual Report 1999–2000*, London, 2000, BPSU.

Rubin A: Management of shoulder dystocia, *Journal of the American Medical Association* 189(11):835–837, 1964.

Sandberg EC: The Zavanelli maneuver: a potentially revolutionary method for the resolution of shoulder dystocia, *American Journal of Obstetrics and Gynecology* 152(4):479–484, 1985.

Smeltzer JS: Prevention and management of shoulder dystocia, *Clinical Obstetrics and Gynecology* 29(2):299–308, 1986.

Sokol RJ, Blackwell SC; American College of Obstetricians and Gynecologists (ACOG) Committee on Practice Bulletins-Gynecology, ACOG practice bulletin: shoulder dystocia. Number 40, November 2002, *International Journal of Gynecology and Obstetrics* 80(1):87–92, 2003.

Smith RB, Lane C, Pearson JF: Shoulder dystocia: what happens at the next delivery? *British Journal of Obstetrics and Gynaecology* 101(8):713–715, 1994.

Spellacy WN, Miller S, Winegar A, et al: Macrosomia, maternal characteristics and infant complications, *Obstetrics and Gynecology* 66(2):158–161, 1985.

Woods CE: A principle of physics as applicable to shoulder delivery, *American Journal of Obstetrics and Gynecology* 45:796–805, 1943.

Chapter |67|

# Presentation and prolapse of the umbilical cord

Patricia Lindsay

### LEARNING OUTCOMES

After reading this chapter, you will be able to:

- differentiate between presentation and prolapse of the umbilical cord
- identify situations when this emergency might occur
- discuss the midwife's management of cord presentation and prolapse
- discuss the possible consequences to the woman and the infant.

## INTRODUCTION

In approximately 0.1–0.6% of births, the umbilical cord descends below the presenting part (RCOG 2008). The cord vessels may become occluded by pressure of the descending presenting part, potentially resulting in irreversible brain damage, stillbirth or neonatal death. There are three variants:

- *Cord presentation* occurs when a loop of cord lies below the presenting part of the fetus (Fig. 67.1), the membranes being intact.
- *Cord prolapse* occurs when the membranes rupture and the cord descends below the presenting part (Fig. 67.2).
- *Occult cord presentation* occurs when a loop of cord lies beside, rather than before, the presenting part. This will not be felt on vaginal examination but may cause unexplained fetal distress in labour, characterized in the early stages by deep early decelerations of the fetal heart. When confronted with a case of unexplained fetal distress, the midwife should consider the possibility of cord compression (Chakravarti et al 2004).

## CAUSES

Presentation and prolapse of the umbilical cord may occur in any situation which results in a poorly fitting presenting part: normally, the well-flexed fetal head enters the pelvis in late pregnancy or early labour, fitting snugly, to prevent the descent of the cord.

### Risk factors

- An unusually long umbilical cord
- A high presenting part, for any reason
- Malpresentations, such as shoulder and breech presentations, especially a flexed or footling breech
- Transverse, oblique or unstable lie
- Prematurity or low birthweight <2500 g
- Multiparity
- Malpositions, such as occipitoposterior positions
- Polyhydramnios
- Artificial rupture of the membranes, if the presenting part is ill-fitting or high
- Multiple births, especially the second fetus of twins
- Internal podalic version
- Malformation or contracture of the pelvis and cephalopelvic disproportion, as these are associated with a high presenting part
- Fetal congenital anomaly

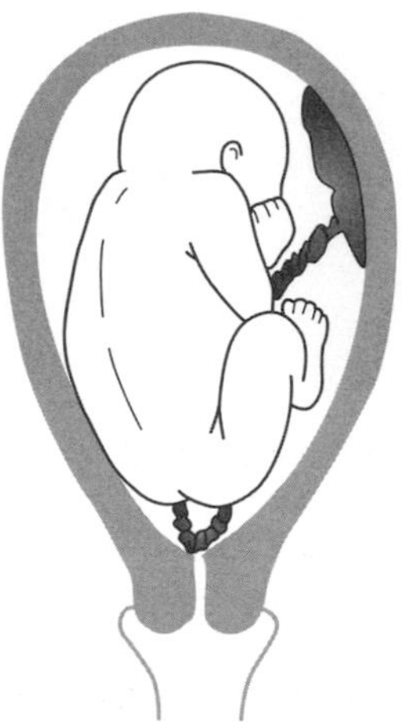

**Figure 67.1** Cord presentation.

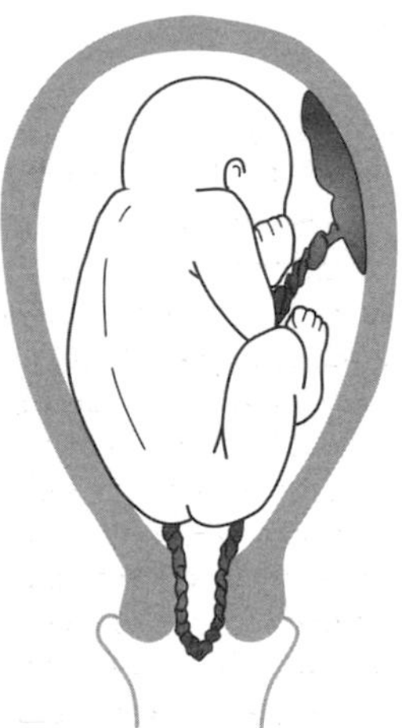

**Figure 67.2** Cord prolapse.

- Fibroids or placenta praevia, because they occupy space in the pelvis
- External cephalic version
- Male fetus
- True knot in the cord

(Dilbaz et al 2006, Kahana et al 2004, RCOG 2008, Sheiner et al 2004).

## DIAGNOSIS

Vaginal examination may reveal a cord presentation, the cord being palpated through the fetal membranes. Pulsation, synchronous with the fetal heart, may be felt. If the presenting part is high, the cord may float away from the examining fingers. Uterine arterial pulsation will be felt in the vaginal fornices, synchronous with the maternal pulse.

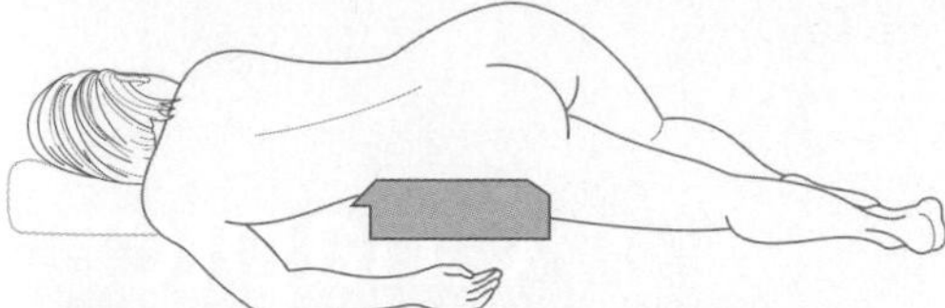

**Figure 67.3** Exaggerated Sims' position. (© Boyle M. Emergencies Around Childbirth, Oxford: Radcliffe Medical Press 2002. Reproduced with permission of the copyright holder)

Therefore, the midwife should auscultate the fetal heart and simultaneously take the maternal pulse if she is unsure of the source of pulsation. If a cord presentation is suspected, the midwife must aim to keep the membranes intact and should attempt to reduce any cord compression by placing the mother in an exaggerated Sims' position with the hips and buttocks elevated by a wedge or pillows (Squire 2002) (Fig. 67.3). Medical assistance should be called at once and the midwife must stay with the woman. Elevating the maternal pelvis may encourage the umbilical cord to move, but if the cord presentation persists, the fetus will be delivered by caesarean section.

When the membranes rupture, the fetal heart must be auscultated and a vaginal examination made in order to diagnose cord prolapse. The risk of cord prolapse should be borne in mind whenever there is a high head, malpresentation or malposition, polyhydramnios or multiple pregnancy. The prolapsed cord may be palpated in the cervical canal, in the vagina or may be visible at the vulva. The midwife should assess cervical dilatation and the descent of the presenting part, as management of this condition depends upon the stage of labour.

## DANGERS

Umbilical cord prolapse has a perinatal mortality rate of 50% (Dilbaz et al 2006). There may also be considerable morbidity from hypoxic-ischaemic encephalopathy and cerebral palsy (RCOG 2008).

The main risks to the fetus are:

- hypoxia when the cord is compressed between the presenting part and the maternal pelvis
- cooling, drying or handling the cord, which may cause the umbilical vessels to go into spasm and affect blood supply to the fetus.

The prognosis for the fetus depends upon prompt recognition of the prolapse and speedy delivery.

The main risks for the mother are:

- operative delivery and anaesthesia (including the risk of Mendelson's syndrome if general anaesthesia is used)

- haemorrhage
- sepsis
- psychological trauma and potential impact on the mother–child relationship.

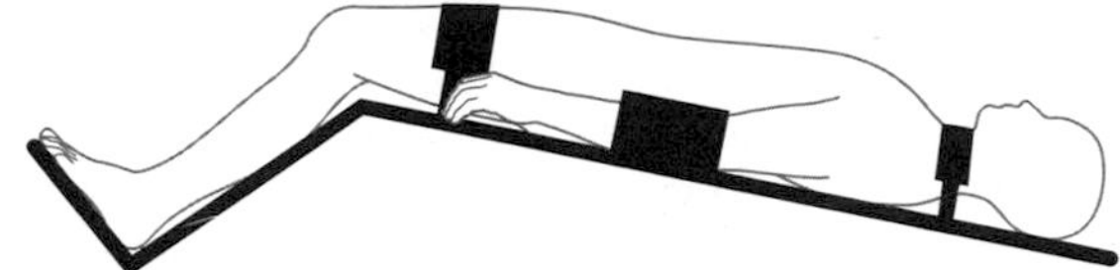

Figure 67.4 The Trendelenburg position. *(Adapted from Kumar 1998, with permission of Elsevier Ltd.)*

## MANAGEMENT OF CORD PROLAPSE

The management will depend upon the stage of labour and whether the fetus is alive or dead.

### Key points

- Call medical assistance urgently.
- Remain with the woman.
- Relieve pressure on the cord.
- Improve fetal oxygenation.
- Expedite delivery.
- Keep a clear, accurate and contemporaneous record.

Absence of both cord pulsation and fetal heart are suggestive of fetal death, but this should be confirmed by ultrasound scan. If fetal death is confirmed, labour will proceed without intervention, as a caesarean section would not be performed for a dead baby. If the fetus is known or suspected to be alive, the treatment is immediate delivery, which may be instrumental or by caesarean section. The midwife must attempt to keep the fetus in good condition until delivery is effected.

### Prelabour and first stage

Obstetric, anaesthetic and paediatric assistance is summoned urgently and the time that the prolapse was detected is noted.

If this emergency occurs at home, the midwife should call the paramedic ambulance service at once.

Meanwhile, the midwife must manage the emergency and conserve the fetal condition:

- Explain the situation to the woman and her partner.
- Attempt to relieve pressure on the cord by moving the woman into the knee–chest position or the exaggerated Sims' position.
- Elevate the foot of the bed if possible.
- Insert two fingers into the vagina and push up the presenting part to further relieve cord compression. This must be maintained until the obstetrician is ready to deliver the baby.
- Stop the Syntocinon infusion if this is in progress.
- Administer oxygen by close-fitting facemask and reservoir at a rate of up to 15 L/min (Thurlow & Kinsella 2002). However, this treatment can only be of benefit if there is still some fetoplacental circulation; the midwife must make every effort to ensure that cord compression is relieved and the fetoplacental circulation maintained.

There is insufficient evidence to recommend the practice of umbilical cord replacement (funic reduction) in managing cord prolapse (RCOG 2008).

The obstetrician may prescribe an intravenous infusion of a tocolytic drug such as terbutaline to arrest uterine contractions.

### Bladder filling

An effective alternative to digital pressure to displace the presenting part is bladder filling, especially if there may be a delay between the cord prolapse and delivery, such as may occur in the community (Houghton 2006, RCOG 2008). Either the foot of the bed should be elevated to provide a head-down tilt or the woman placed in the Trendelenburg position (Fig. 67.4). A 16G self-retaining (Foley) catheter is passed into the bladder. Sterile normal saline (0.9%) is instilled, using a bag for intravenous infusion and an intravenous fluid administration set connected to the catheter. This procedure has been shown to dislodge the fetal head to 2 cm above the ischial spines and should relieve pressure on the umbilical cord. The amount of fluid required is assessed by the degree of elevation of the presenting part but would probably be a *minimum* of 500 mL. The fetal condition should be continuously monitored and response to this intervention assessed (Katz et al 1988, RCOG 2008, Runnebaum & Katz 1999). Once the bladder has been filled, the woman's position should be altered to achieve a lateral tilt and avoid supine hypotension, which would exacerbate the fetal hypoxia. It is unsafe to attempt an ambulance transfer of a woman in the knee–chest position, and the left lateral position should be used (RCOG 2008).

The urinary catheter is secured by filling the self-retaining balloon and remains in situ until the woman is in theatre and the obstetric surgeon requests that the bladder is drained. Delivery will be by caesarean section, preferably under regional anaesthesia (RCOG 2008).

### Second stage

If the cervix is fully dilated and there is no evidence of cephalopelvic disproportion or malpresentation, an immediate instrumental delivery is performed. Late in second stage, the midwife should make an episiotomy and encourage the woman's expulsive efforts in order to effect a quick delivery. Caesarean section may be the preferred mode of delivery even in second stage if there is evidence of malpresentation which would require correction or if the presentation is breech with the buttocks high in the pelvis.

**Reflective activity 67.1**

Locate and read your local policy for management of umbilical cord presentation and prolapse. What instructions does it give with regard to midwifery management of such incidents at home and in the community?

### Psychological care

The midwife should remember that the woman and her partner are likely to be confused and frightened by the sudden nature of the emergency and the speed with which delivery is effected. This has implications for informed consent in this situation.

Careful explanations should be given as soon as the midwife is aware of the possibility of cord presentation or prolapse. Even if the outcome is good, feelings of powerlessness may cause the couple to feel resentful or angry. The midwife should ensure that she makes the time to discuss the events with them.

**Reflective activity 67.2**

What are the possible emotional/psychological consequences for the woman and her family following prolapse of the umbilical cord? If you have cared for a woman who has experienced this, reflect on what you observed in her, and her interaction with the baby. What were her perceptions of what happened and how did these match with the 'professional' perceptions of events? If there are radical differences, why would this be?

## CONCLUSION

Prolapse of the umbilical cord threatens the life of the fetus. The midwife must be aware of potential high-risk situations and be able to take the appropriate action when this emergency is suspected or detected. The psychological and support needs of the woman and her partner must not be forgotten in the haste to save the life of the baby. The safe management of this emergency demands a high level of clinical and interpersonal skills from the midwife.

**Reflective activity 67.3**

Consider what you have read and the previous activities you have done. Has your understanding of this emergency changed? What are the key points of management for you in your particular sphere of practice?

**KEY POINTS**

- Umbilical cord presentation and prolapse happen relatively infrequently.
- They are often unexpected occurrences but there is an association with particular conditions.
- The midwife is often the professional who makes the diagnosis.
- The outcome is likely to be poor for the baby if action is not swift and effective.
- The midwife must be aware of those women who are at higher risk and know what emergency action to take in the event of cord presentation or prolapse.
- Accurate record-keeping is vital, particularly with regard to times and action taken.
- Psychological care and 'debriefing' after the event are essential for the woman and her family.

## REFERENCES


Boyle M: *Emergencies around childbirth*, Oxford, 2002, Radcliffe Medical.

Chakravarti S, Gupta K, Datta S: Malposition, malpresentations and cord prolapse. In Arulkumaran S, Sivanesaratnam V, Chatterjee A, et al, editors: *Essentials of obstetrics*, Tunbridge Wells, 2004, Anshan.

Dilbaz B, Ozturkoglu E, Dilbaz S, et al: Risk factors and perinatal outcomes associated with umbilical cord prolapse, *Archives of Gynecology and Obstetrics* 274(2):104–107, 2006.

Houghton G: Bladder filling: an effective technique for managing cord prolapse, *British Journal of Midwifery* 14(2):88–89, 2006.

Kahana B, Sheiner E, Levy A, et al: Umbilical cord prolapse and perinatal outcomes, *International Journal of Gynecology and Obstetrics* 84(2):127–132, 2004.

Katz Z, Shohan Z, Lancet M, et al: Management of labor with umbilical cord prolapse: a 5 year study, *Obstetrics and Gynecology* 72(2):278–281, 1988.

Kumar B: *Working in the Operating Department*, London, 1998, Churchill Livingstone.

Royal College of Obstetricians and Gynaecologists (RCOG): *Umbilical cord prolapse – green top guideline no.*

*50*, London, 2008, Royal College of Obstetricians and Gynaecologists, London.

Runnebaum I, Katz M: Intrauterine resuscitation by rapid urinary bladder instillation in a case of occult prolapse of an excessively long umbilical cord, *European Journal of Obstetrics, Gynecology, and Reproductive Biology* 84(1):101–102, 1999.

Sheiner E, Levy A, Katz M, et al: Gender does matter in perinatal medicine, *Fetal Diagnosis and Therapy* 19(4):366–369, 2004.

Squire C: Shoulder dystocia and umbilical cord prolapse. In Boyle M, editor: *Emergencies around childbirth*, Oxford, 2002, Radcliffe Medical.

Thurlow J, Kinsella S: Intrauterine resuscitation: active management of fetal distress, *International Journal of Obstetric Anesthesia* 11(2):105–116, 2002.

Chapter |68|

# Complications of the third stage of labour

Luisa Acosta

## LEARNING OUTCOMES

After reading this chapter, you will be able to:

- understand the reason why complications arise in the third stage of labour
- discuss the midwife's management in emergency situations
- outline further treatments which may be necessary
- discuss the implications of these complications for women and their partners.

## POSTPARTUM HAEMORRHAGE

Postpartum haemorrhage (PPH) is a significant cause of maternal mortality and morbidity (Knight et al 2008, Lewis 2007). It may happen without warning after any delivery. The only professional in attendance for the majority of births is the midwife, whose prompt action may spare the mother dangerous blood loss and save her life. It is essential that midwives have a thorough understanding of this subject. Maternity services must have a policy for management of PPH so that all members of the multidisciplinary team work together and attend regular 'fire drills' to ensure quick and appropriate responses (Lewis 2007).

### Definition

PPH is defined as excessive bleeding from the genital tract occurring any time from the birth of the baby to the end of the puerperium.

- *Primary PPH* occurs in the first 24 hours. This is the most common and most dangerous type, complicating approximately 6% of all births (Carroli et al 2008).
- *Secondary PPH* occurs after 24 hours and before the end of the puerperium, and affects approximately 2% of deliveries (Alexander et al 2002).

Primary PPH is often defined by the estimated blood loss. Traditionally, a loss of 500 mL or more has been regarded as a PPH (WHO 1990), yet this may be considered as a normal physiological blood loss if a woman is not anaemic (Rogers & Chang 2008).

Estimating blood loss after birth is notoriously difficult. Bleeding may be hidden; and if visible, it is likely to be underestimated (Prasertcharoensuk et al 2000, Toledo et al 2007). However, regular clinical simulations may improve blood loss estimation (Bose et al 2006).

Hence, defining PPH by estimating blood loss may have little clinical usefulness, and, therefore, the word *'excessive'* is used to mean any amount which adversely affects the mother.

When estimating blood loss to define PPH, Coker & Oliver (2006) propose that if blood loss is estimated as 500 to 1000 mL and there are no clinical signs of maternal compromise, staff should be alerted to monitor the woman and be ready for possible action. Should the estimated blood loss be above 1000 mL or the mother shows any sign of compromise, then prompt action must be taken to resuscitate and arrest bleeding. The Royal College of Obstetricians and Gynaecologists (2009) have used these principles to define minor and major PPH. The guidelines suggest that with a minor PPH (a blood loss of 500 to 1000 mL, with no maternal compromise) basic measures need to be undertaken, and when a major PPH is diagnosed (a blood loss of over 1000 mL or clinical shock present) a full obstetric protocol must be followed (see website).

### Causes

PPH may arise from the placental site or from a genital tract laceration, and may be classified by using the '4 Ts' (see website) (Anderson & Etches 2007):

*Tone* – uterine atony
*Trauma* – genital tract lacerations, haematomas, ruptured or inverted uterus
*Tissue* – retained placenta, placental products and blood clots
*Thrombin* – blood coagulation disorders.

## PPH from uterine atony

The immediate cause of primary placental site PPH is failure of the uterus to contract and retract adequately. As there is a placental circulation of approximately 600 mL/min at term (Blackburn 2007), if the uterine arteries are not ligated by the muscle fibres surrounding them, blood loss can be rapid and dangerous. This may occur because the myometrium is atonic, or because retained placental tissue prevents effective uterine contraction.

### Prediction and risk factors

It is not possible to predict a PPH accurately, but the risk is increased in certain circumstances:

- *Previous PPH or retained placenta.*
- *Multiple pregnancy, polyhydramnios and fetal macrosomia*: All may cause uterine over-distension, leading to poor retraction. In multiple pregnancy, there is a larger placental site, which is more likely to encroach upon the poorly retractile lower uterine segment, thus increasing the risk of haemorrhage.
- *Anaemia* may affect the ability to withstand haemorrhage.
- *Antepartum haemorrhage* from placenta praevia or abruptio placentae may subsequently result in PPH. With placenta praevia the retractile ability of the lower uterine segment is deficient and therefore control of bleeding from the placental site is poor. A Couvelaire uterus may occur in severe, concealed placental abruption and the damaged muscle fibres fail to contract and retract effectively (Fig. 68.1). Women who have had an antepartum haemorrhage may be anaemic, increasing the threat from PPH.
- *Prolonged labour*: If contractions were weak or uncoordinated during labour, it may continue into the third stage. The uterus will fail to contract and retract effectively. Occasionally, prolonged labour, because of mechanical difficulty, may lead to uterine exhaustion and atony.

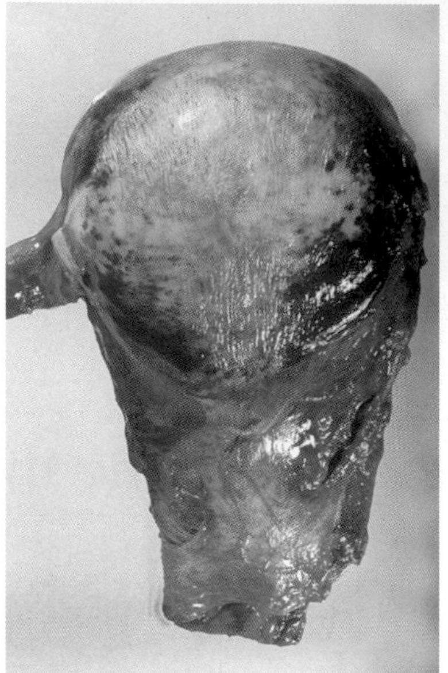

**Figure 68.1** Couvelaire uterus. *(From Beischer et al 1997.)*

- *Previous caesarean section and caesarean section.*
- *Pre-eclampsia/hypertensive disease in pregnancy*: Both increase the risk of induction and operative deliveries. Coagulopathy is also a potential complication of hypertensive disease, and some drugs used to prevent seizures may contribute to uterine atony.
- *General anaesthesia*: Uterine atony may occur if anaesthesia is prolonged, and is especially likely if halogenated anaesthetic agents are used.
- *Fibroids:* May interfere with efficient contraction and retraction.
- *Mismanagement of the third stage of labour*: Unnecessary massaging, squeezing or otherwise 'fiddling' with the uterus can disrupt the rhythm of myometrial activity, causing only partial separation of the placenta.
- *Retained placenta and blood clots*: Unless the uterus is empty, it cannot retract completely.
- *Tocolytic drugs*: Drugs given to suppress uterine activity in preterm labour may cause atony in the third stage should labour progress.
- *Induced or augmented labours:* Uterine inefficiency necessitating the use of oxytocics may contribute to PPH.
- *Inversion of the uterus:* Any degree of uterine inversion will interfere with efficient contraction and retraction.
- *Chorioamnionitis.*
- *Grand multiparity* has been associated with PPH, but high parity on its own is not considered to be a risk (Page 2006). Women who have borne several children are more likely to have a history of risk factors. Iron stores, in particular, may be depleted

when there are short inter-pregnancy intervals. Thereby, a comparatively small blood loss may produce signs of underperfusion.

- *Disseminated intravascular coagulation* may occur secondarily to other major problems, including concealed abruptio placentae, amniotic fluid embolus, severe pre-eclampsia and eclampsia. It can also follow prolonged retention of a dead fetus in utero.
- *Medical disorders* such as idiopathic thrombocytopenia and inherited coagulopathies, such as von Willebrand's disease also increase the risk of both primary and secondary PPH (Chi & Kadir 2007).

## Prophylaxis

### *Pregnancy*

Preventing PPH begins at the initial booking interview when midwives will identify women at higher risk. Any woman whose history suggests that she is at risk should be booked for a hospital birth where immediate and effective treatment can be provided. Conditions such as anaemia should be treated with iron and folic acid supplements. In severe cases, intramuscular iron or even blood transfusion may be required to raise the haemoglobin levels prior to delivery.

### *Labour*

During labour, careful management will reduce the likelihood of PPH. For women at risk:

- An intravenous cannula is inserted and blood samples are taken.
- Haemoglobin level is estimated and the blood group confirmed.
- Serum is saved, thereby speeding up the process of cross-matching donor blood, should it become necessary.

The midwife will monitor the progress of labour and avoid dehydration and exhaustion. An obstetrician should be called for signs of prolonged labour (Ch. 63). An oxytocin infusion may be required which should be maintained for at least 1 hour after the end of the third stage. The bladder should be kept empty, as a full bladder may impede efficient uterine action.

Correct management of the third stage of labour is crucial. The midwife should discuss the management of the third stage with the woman, preferably before labour commences. Active management of the third stage is associated with reduction in PPH (Prendiville et al 2000). The use of fundal massage following the delivery of the placenta is recommended to reduce the risk of PPH (Hofmeyr et al 2008). Breastfeeding or nipple stimulation will also help the uterus to contract, though it is not an effective treatment for PPH. *Ergometrine maleate* 500 mcg should be available. Accurate estimation of blood loss and timely observation of vital signs will enable early detection and prompt treatment.

The National Institute for Health and Clinical Excellence (NICE) (2005) guidelines suggest that women at risk of haemorrhage during or following caesarean section may be offered intra-operative blood cell salvage (see website). Guidelines for women who refuse blood transfusion have been recommended by a previous Confidential Enquiry into Maternal and Child Health (CEMACH) report (Lewis 2004) (see website).

## Treatment

The principles of management are:

- arrest bleeding
- resuscitate the mother
- replace fluids.

Units vary in the management of PPH, especially with pharmacological protocols (Winter et al 2007). This may be due to limited research on the specific treatment combinations for PPH. Midwives should follow their hospital guidelines as appropriate.

### *Before delivery of the placenta*

Prolonged brisk bleeding prior to the delivery of the placenta should alert the midwife to take action. Skilled medical assistance should be summoned immediately, whilst the midwife must remain with the mother for support and commence treatment. If at home, the midwife should deliver the placenta, if possible, before transferring the woman to hospital.

The degree of uterine contraction should be assessed. If the fundus feels soft, the first consideration is to stimulate uterine contraction and give an oxytocic drug. *Oxytocin* 10 international units (iu) may be given intramuscularly, causing the uterus to contract within 2.5 minutes. *Syntometrine* (oxytocin 5 iu and ergometrine 500 mcg) should be avoided if there is a history of hypertension. There is also some evidence that ergometrine may cause the placenta to become entrapped (Begley 1990, Cotter et al 2001, Hammar et al 1990), thus exacerbating the bleeding.

The bladder should be empty before another attempt is made to deliver the placenta with controlled cord traction and the genital tract should be inspected to exclude traumatic haemorrhage.

If the placenta cannot be delivered, prepare for the doctor to perform a manual removal of the placenta and membranes under anaesthetic. Retained placenta is discussed later.

### *After delivery of the placenta*

The following principles should be applied when a minor PPH is diagnosed. The order in which the actions are to be taken may vary and where possible actions should be taken simultaneously:

- *Call for assistance.*
- *'Rub up' a contraction*: Massaging the uterus will usually stimulate a contraction and expel any blood clots (Fig. 68.2).

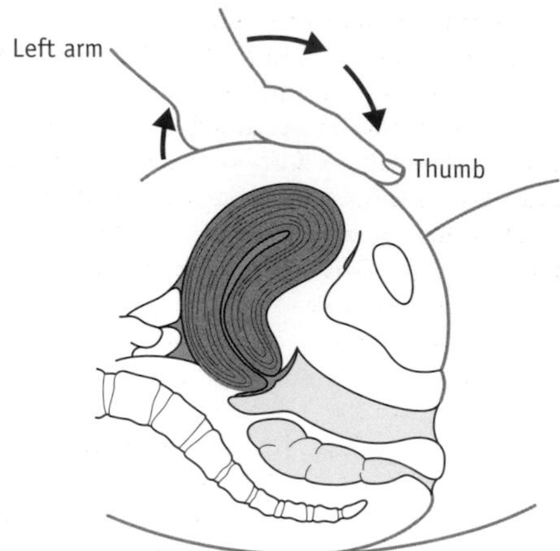


The left hand is cupped over the uterus ( ) and massages it with a firm circular motion in a clockwise direction

**Figure 68.2** 'Rubbing up' a contraction. The left hand is cupped over the uterus and massages it with a firm circular motion in a clockwise direction. *(From Boyle (2002) Radcliffe Publishers, with permission.)*

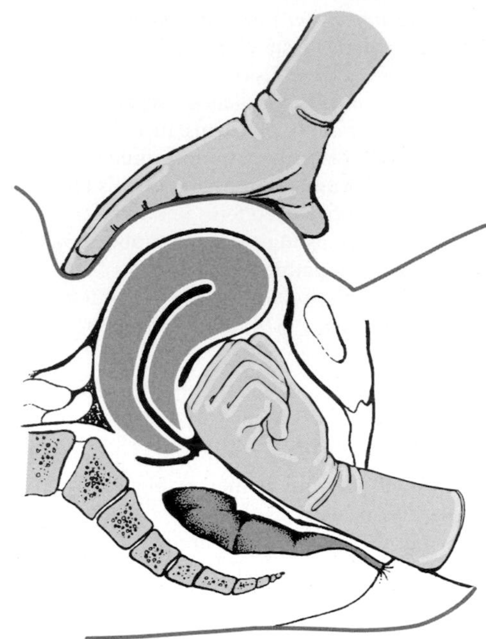

**Figure 68.3** Internal bimanual compression of the uterus.

- *Give oxytocic drug*: Drug protocols vary. The drugs of first choice for uterine atony are oxytocin and ergometrine (Mousa & Alfirevic 2007). The following may be considered:
  - Intramuscular Syntometrine.
  - Intravenous or intramuscular injection of oxytocin 5–10 iu followed by ergometrine 250–500 mcg. This may be given intramuscularly or, cautiously, intravenously in the absence of hypertension. No more than two doses of ergometrine may be administered (Joint Formulary Committee 2008).
  - An intravenous infusion of 40 iu of oxytocin in 500 mL of normal saline over 4 hours should be commenced.
- Ensure the bladder is empty. Passing a catheter is useful, as a full bladder can impede uterine contraction and retraction.
- Intravenous access is needed to obtain blood samples and an infusion needs to be commenced to replace fluids if not already done.

It is essential that these steps are taken as soon as the midwife suspects that the uterus is failing to contract and bleeding is unusually heavy. In most cases they are effective if used in good time. Delay will result in further blood loss and the woman's condition can deteriorate rapidly.

The placenta and membranes are examined to ensure that they are complete. If not, an exploration and evacuation of the uterus is carried out by an obstetrician under anaesthesia.

With PPH, the midwife should not elevate the foot of the bed as this encourages blood to pool within the uterine cavity, which would hinder uterine contraction and retraction. The woman's legs may be elevated on pillows, taking care to avoid undue pressure on the calves, which would predispose to venous thrombosis.

### Further measures

If bleeding continues despite the above treatment, compression of the uterus or main abdominal vessels may be needed.

#### *Internal bimanual compression* (Fig. 68.3)

A fist is made with the right hand and introduced into the vagina. It is then pushed up towards the anterior vaginal fornix. The left hand dips down behind the uterus and pulls it forwards towards the symphysis. The hands are pushed together, compressing the uterus and placental site. The pressure is maintained until the uterus contracts and remains retracted.

#### *External bimanual compression*

The left hand dips down behind the uterus; the right hand is pressed flat on the abdominal wall; the uterus is compressed and, simultaneously, pulled upwards in the abdomen. This compresses the bleeding area while the pulling up of the uterus straightens the kinked uterine veins, allowing free drainage, relieving the congestion and decreasing the bleeding.

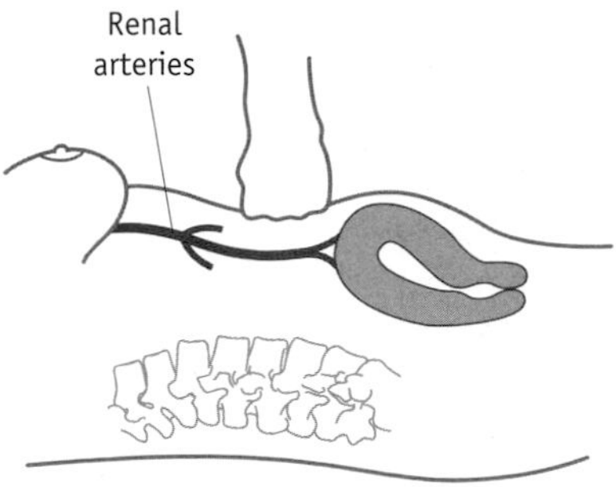


Figure 68.4 Abdominal aortic compression.

### *Abdominal aortic compression*

This has been used as a short-term emergency measure to control severe haemorrhage while awaiting emergency assistance. The midwife places a fist above the fundus and below the level of the renal arteries. Pressure is directed towards the spine in order to compress the aorta and reduce blood flow to the uterus (Fig. 68.4). Adequacy of compression can be assessed by checking for the absence of femoral pulses (Keogh & Tsokos 1997).

Once bleeding is controlled, uterine contraction is maintained by an intravenous infusion solution of 40 iu of Syntocinon in 500 mL of normal saline at 10 iu per hour. A blood transfusion may be required. If the bleeding persists or recurs, an exploration of the genital tract under general anaesthesia may be required.

**Reflective activity 68.1**

Find out how emergency transfer of a woman from her home to hospital is managed in your area.

## Massive obstetric haemorrhage

This is a life-threatening event, characterized by severe maternal compromise. A blood loss of 1000 to 1500 mL or more, or any lesser amount which causes a sustained fall in systolic blood pressure, constitutes a 'massive obstetric haemorrhage'.

In addition to the measures taken above for a minor PPH, the following should be done:

- The multidisciplinary protocol or 'drill' for managing severe haemorrhage should be initiated at once. The team should include the midwife caring for the woman and key senior staff, including midwives, obstetricians, haematologists and anaesthetists. Portering staff should be available for transfer of specimens for laboratory analysis. One member of staff should take responsibility for documenting all care given during the emergency.
- Maternal resuscitation should begin immediately, including oxygen therapy.
- Intravenous access with two large-bore (at least 16G) cannulae and a *central venous pressure* line are inserted.
- Blood samples are taken for full blood count, cross-matching and clotting studies. At least six units of cross-matched blood are requested.
- Two litres of crystalloid may initially be infused. This should be followed by colloid, which is more efficient in expanding the intravascular volume (Plaat 2008). All maternity units should keep at least two units of emergency group O Rhesus-negative blood in the blood fridge. This may be used while awaiting cross-matched supplies. Blood should be passed through a warming device and infused as rapidly as possible.
- In addition to *oxytocin* and *ergometrine*, the following drugs may be considered if the uterus remains atonic:
  - *Carboprost (Hemabate)* 250 mcg may be administered by deep intramuscular injection and can be repeated every 15 minutes, up to eight doses (maximum dosage of 2 mg) (Joint Formulary Committee 2008). It may also be injected directly into the myometrium.
  - *Misoprostol* (800 mg) may be given rectally. However, there is limited evidence that it reduces blood loss from PPH when used alongside other oxytocics (Hofmeyr & Gülmezoglu 2008).
- Early transfer to theatre is advised if bleeding persists. An *anti-shock garment* may be useful to shunt blood from the extremities to the vital organs whilst the woman is awaiting surgical procedures (Miller et al 2008).

### *Surgical procedures*

- *Uterine packing or tamponade*: This may be attempted prior to laparotomy. The hydrostatic balloon catheter – for example, the 'Rusch' balloon – is now more popular than uterine packing. The balloon is inflated with sterile normal saline, taking the shape of the uterus, and applying pressure to the placental site (Howell & Irani 2007).
- *Compression sutures*: These are absorbable sutures which are inserted through the thickness of both uterine walls to compress the uterus. An example of this is the B-Lynch suture (B-Lynch et al 1997) (Fig. 68. 5).
- *Pelvic vessel ligation*: If other methods fail, arterial ligation will be necessary. This may involve the internal iliac artery, ovarian artery or uterine artery.
- *Hysterectomy*: Every attempt to conserve the uterus will be made, but if these measures fail to control the bleeding, a hysterectomy is necessary to save the woman's life.

### *Radiological procedures*

- *Uterine artery embolization*: This can be performed before laparotomy if the woman is stable enough and facilities for interventional radiology are present. The procedure is done by femoral artery puncture, where the catheter is guided to the site and the vessel is

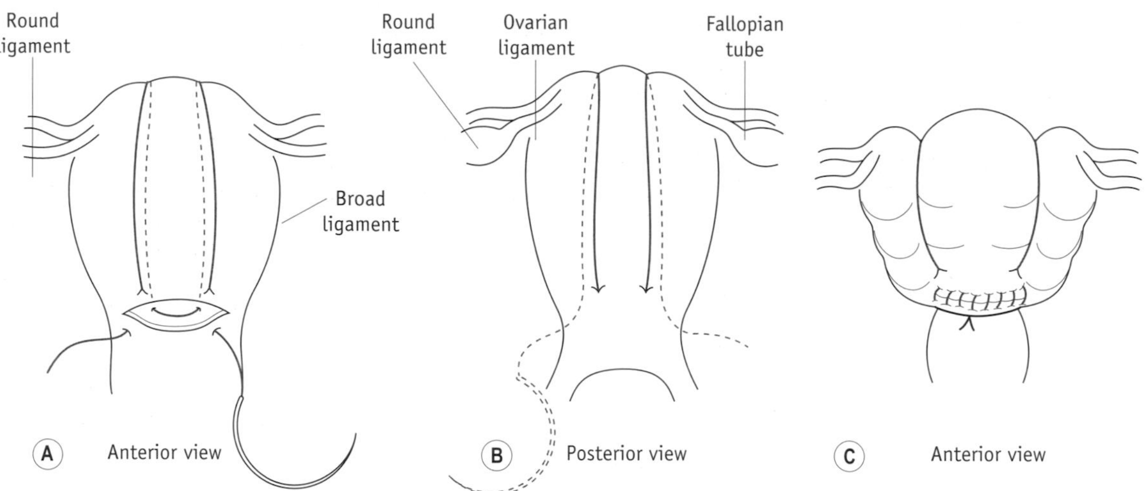


**Figure 68.5** B-Lynch suture in the uterus: **A.** anterior and **B.** posterior views showing the application of the suture; **C.** the anatomical appearance after competent application. *(Reprinted from B-Lynch et al 1997, with permission. Illustrations by Mr Philip Wilson FMAA RMIP.)*

embolized with gelatin sponge. The success rate of this procedure is about 70–100% (Winograd 2008).

- *Internal iliac balloon catheter*: These can be inserted via the femoral artery for women who are at high risk. Should haemorrhage occur, the balloon can be inflated to control bleeding.

## Observations

The mother's general condition is assessed continuously. It is important to palpate the fundus repeatedly to ensure that it remains well contracted and to observe the amount and nature of the blood loss. Her pulse, blood pressure and oxygen saturations are recorded every 15 minutes until her condition is satisfactory. A fluid balance chart is maintained to record the fluid intake and urinary output. A catheter, attached to a urometer, is needed and urine output is recorded hourly. Central venous pressure should be measured when it is necessary to give large volumes of fluid intravenously, to avoid overtransfusion.

Elevating the woman's legs may help to maintain core circulation. Oxygen is given by facemask and sedation may be required. The mother needs to be kept dry and comfortable.

The woman may need to be transferred to an intensive care unit.

## Disseminated intravascular coagulation (DIC)

DIC is a coagulopathy which results in steady, persistent oozing of blood even though there is adequate uterine contraction and retraction (see Ch. 58). Blood does not clot, venepuncture sites may ooze, and petechiae may appear. DIC occurs as a result of severe haemorrhage, when supplies of circulating fibrinogen and other blood clotting factors become depleted and the coagulation system fails. Hypoxia which accompanies major haemorrhage may cause the local release of thromboplastin from the damaged tissue, triggering the formation of microthrombi all round the body. This further exhausts the circulating coagulation factors. The thrombi will block capillaries, thus causing more tissue damage and release of thromboplastin.

As the condition worsens, blood levels of fibrin degradation products (FDPs) rise. These are toxic to the myometrium and will interfere with efficient uterine contraction and retraction, thus exacerbating haemorrhage. If DIC is allowed to progress, the condition will become uncontrollable and maternal death may ensue.

At every delivery, the midwife should note whether the blood is clotting and whether the clot is firm or friable. Absent or unstable clot formation along with results from clotting studies are an indication of DIC. Treatment must be prompt and the midwife should call for medical assistance and the on-call haematologist immediately.

Once the underlying cause and hypovolaemia are treated, blood products, such as red cells, fresh frozen plasma and platelets, are used to replace clotting factors. In some cases, *cryoprecipitate* is administered. NICE (2007) recommends the use of intravenous *tranexamic acid* and *recombinant factor VIIa* if clotting factors are normal, under the direction of a consultant haematologist.

## Traumatic PPH

Approximately 10% of cases of PPH arise from a laceration of the genital tract (Anderson & Etches 2007). Occasionally, these are perineal tears or episiotomies. Lacerations involving the labia or clitoris often bleed freely. Deep lacerations of the vaginal walls, cervix and, exceptionally, lower uterine segment will produce severe haemorrhage. This is much more likely to complicate a difficult instrumental delivery, or may follow a rapid labour. Uterine rupture may occur in obstructed labour or if a scar ruptures.

Superficial bleeding points can be easily seen and treated by direct pressure. A laceration of the cervix is suspected if the bleeding begins immediately following the birth and continues steadily though the uterus is well contracted. It may be temporarily controlled by digital pressure or by applying a sponge or arterial pressure forceps. An obstetrician must be summoned and the laceration sutured. Tears to the upper part of the vagina, the cervix or the uterus are sutured under anaesthesia. In cases of severe haemorrhage from a ruptured uterus, it may be necessary to perform a hysterectomy.

A *vulval haematoma* may cause a PPH. This can occur following perineal repair with inadequate haemostasis or where there has been damage to vulval varicosities. There may be no obvious trauma and the perineum is intact (Baskett et al 2007). It appears as a localized swelling, usually one-sided, which looks tense and shiny. The pain may be severe and there may be signs of shock. A surprisingly large amount of blood may be present. The midwife must call for medical assistance and intravenous access must be secured, as replacement fluids may be needed. The haematoma should be drained under anaesthesia. Attention to perineal hygiene and pain relief is essential.

## Following PPH

The mother may suffer from chronic iron-deficiency anaemia unless adequate treatment is instituted during the puerperium. She is more likely to develop puerperal sepsis and lactation may be poor. In severe and prolonged shock, the woman may develop anuria due to tubular necrosis. Another serious complication is anterior pituitary necrosis. If the mother survives, she will suffer from Sheehan's syndrome, where lactation will not occur, owing to deficient prolactin secretion. Atrophy of the breasts and genital organs will follow.

The midwife should make the opportunity to discuss events with the couple. The sudden nature of the emergency often means that explanations given at the time are brief and hurried. The midwife should give them time to ask questions and can advise them about the likely causes and how future births may be managed.

# PROLONGED THIRD STAGE

The risk of PPH is linked with a prolonged third stage of labour. The third stage is considered prolonged when it exceeds 30 minutes with active management, and up to 1 hour with physiological management (NICE 2007). The risk of PPH increases significantly with time, possibly doubling after 10 minutes (Magann et al 2005).

The incidence of retained placenta is approximately 3.3% (Weeks 2008). A retained placenta may be partially or completely separated but trapped in the cervix or lower uterine segment. In this situation, bleeding will occur from the placental site. If the retained placenta is completely adherent to the uterine wall, there may be no bleeding.

## Causes

The following may cause delay in the third stage by interfering with the descent and expulsion of a separated placenta:

- *Full bladder.*
- *Constriction ring*: a localized spasm of uterine muscle just above the lower segment – this is unusual.

Other causes matching those of PPH:

- *Inadequate uterine contraction and retraction:* This prevents detachment and may follow prolonged labour (Ch. 63) (notably the second stage) or when there is an overdistended uterus (Magann et al 2008).
- *Uterine abnormality:* More likely if the uterus contains a fibroid (Berck & Baxi 1999). A bicornuate or subseptate uterus may also be a cause, as the uterine contour is irregular.
- *Older maternal age* (Magann et al 2008).
- *Chorioamnionitis* (Magann et al 2008).
- *Induced and preterm labour* (Adelusi et al 1997).
- *Multiparity* (Adelusi et al 1997).
- *Previous retained placenta* (Adelusi et al 1997).
- *History of uterine surgery* (Adelusi et al 1997).
- *Mismanagement* of the third stage, and fundal 'fiddling'.

### Morbid adherence of the placenta

This occurs when the placental villi penetrate deeper than the decidua basalis. A combination of previous caesarean section and current placenta praevia are high-risk factors for abnormal trophoblastic penetration.

There are three types of abnormally adherent placenta:

- *Placenta accreta:* The decidua basalis is deficient and the chorionic villi adhere to the myometrium.
- *Placenta increta:* The villi deeply invade the myometrium.

- *Placenta percreta:* The villi have penetrated the myometrium as far as the serous coat of the uterus. Involvement of adjacent structures may occur. This type is very rare.

The area of adherence may be focal, partial or total. Cases of focal or partial adhesion may be successfully treated by manual removal of the placenta, possibly followed by curettage. Attempts to remove a placenta percreta are likely to result in uterine perforation and haemorrhage. The obstetrician may perform a hysterectomy or may leave the placenta in place to be reabsorbed.

## Management

After catheterizing the bladder, an attempt is made to deliver the placenta and membranes. Ultrasound may help to establish the position and adherence of the placenta. Nitroglycerine is effective in treating a trapped placenta by causing uterine relaxation (Bullarbo et al 2005). If an adherent placenta is suspected, oxytocin 20 iu in 20 mL saline injected via the umbilical vein following proximal cord clamping is recommended (Carroli & Bergel 2001). The NICE (2007:44) care pathway gives the management of retained placenta.

If these measures fail, manual removal of the placenta may be carried out under anaesthesia (Fig. 68.6). Blood is taken for cross-matching, and an intravenous infusion is commenced because there is a risk of severe haemorrhage occurring during the procedure.

Following manual removal of the placenta, uterine contraction is achieved by intravenous uterotonic drugs. If bleeding recurs or continues, bimanual compression may be required. Antibiotics are given, as manual removal is a highly invasive procedure with a risk of puerperal sepsis.

Though the activities of a midwife include the manual removal of placenta in an emergency (NMC 2004), in the developed world it is unlikely that the midwife would be required to undertake this.

The midwife must carefully monitor the woman's condition in the postnatal period and refer her for medical attention if signs of uterine infection appear. The woman should be advised to have future births in hospital, as the risk of recurrence is high.

## ACUTE UTERINE INVERSION

This is a rare but serious complication of the third stage of labour, where the uterus is partly or completely turned inside out (Fig. 68.7). The condition is associated with profound shock, and may also be associated with haemorrhage if the placenta has become separated from the uterus.

- *First degree inversion:* The fundus is inverted but does not pass through the cervix.
- *Second degree inversion:* The inverted fundus protrudes through the cervix and lies in the vagina.
- *Third degree inversion:* The uterus is completely inverted and the fundus appears outside the vulva.

### Causes

- *Mismanagement of the third stage of labour:* This is the most common cause, and results from either pressure on the fundus or from traction on the cord when the

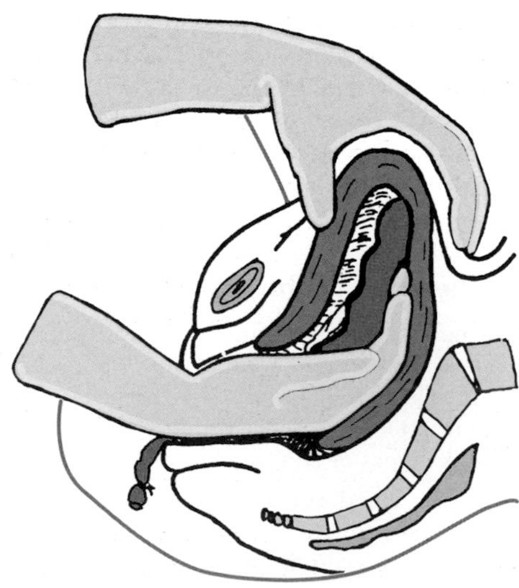

**Figure 68.6** Manual removal of placenta.

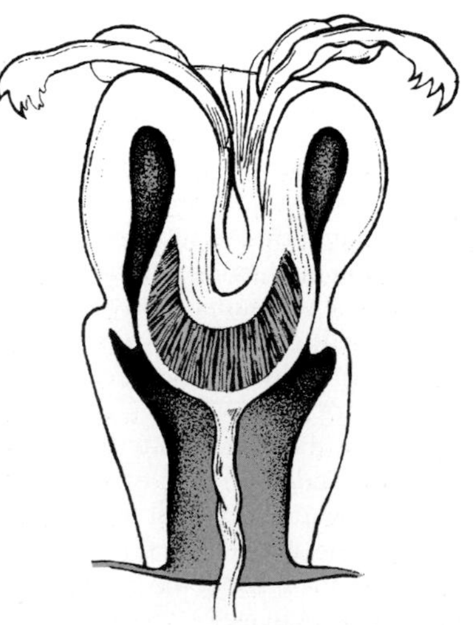

**Figure 68.7** Inversion of the gravid uterus.

uterus is relaxed. It is particularly likely to occur when the placenta is situated in the uterine fundus.

- *Short cord.*
- *Manual removal of placenta:* Inversion of the uterus may occur if the operator's hand is quickly withdrawn from the uterus while the other hand is still applying fundal pressure.
- *Precipitate delivery*: Especially if the woman is in an upright position.
- *Spontaneous inversion*: Occasionally, the cause is unknown. It may result from uterine atony and a sudden increase in the intra-abdominal pressure such as occurs during coughing or straining.

### Diagnosis

Minor degrees of uterine inversion may not be recognized if there is only a slight indentation of the fundus. The woman may complain of pain and lochia will probably be heavy.

If the inversion is more serious, the woman will complain of severe pain and, on palpation, a hollow will be felt in the fundus of the uterus. Haemorrhage will occur if the placenta has separated.

If there is a complete inversion, the uterus will not be palpable in the abdomen and the inverted fundus will be visible at the vulva. The woman will complain of severe lower abdominal pain and may report a sensation of prolapse or 'something coming down'. Neurogenic shock occurs owing to traction on the infundibulopelvic and round ligaments and compression of the ovaries (Calder 2000).

### Management

Uterotonic drugs, if in progress, must be stopped. Where possible, the uterus should be replaced immediately, as maternal shock will increase and may become irreversible. Vascular congestion and oedema of the uterus may occur, making replacement more difficult the longer it is delayed. If immediate replacement is not possible and the uterus is outside the vulva, it should be gently replaced inside the vagina, if possible. Rough or prolonged digital manipulation will increase the accompanying vasovagal shock. The foot of the bed should be raised in order to alleviate shock by reducing traction on the infundibulopelvic ligaments. Intravenous access is required to take blood for cross-matching and clotting studies, and to commence intravenous fluid replacement. Catheterization is needed and intramuscular opiates are recommended. If the placenta is still attached, it **must not** be removed (Evans & B-Lynch 2006) as torrential haemorrhage may result. The woman must be transferred to theatre immediately.

In theatre, the uterus is replaced either manually or by the hydrostatic method under anaesthetic. The part of the uterus which inverted last is replaced first and the fundus last. A hand is placed on the abdomen to give counter pressure, otherwise the uterus may be pushed up too high. Drugs may be given to relax the cervical ring.

If this is unsuccessful, the hydrostatic method, as described by O'Sullivan (1945), is carried out. Once the obstetrician replaces the uterus in the vagina, warm normal saline is infused into the vagina via a rubber tube. This is held in place and the introitus sealed by the other hand. A ventouse cup attached to a giving set may also be used to produce a good seal (Ogueh & Ayida 1997). A better seal is produced when the woman lies with her legs together. The pressure exerted by the fluid distends the vagina and effects replacement of the uterus without aggravating the shock.

If other interventions fail, surgical correction via laparotomy is performed. Following replacement of the uterus, intravenous oxytocics are needed to ensure that the uterus contracts and bleeding is controlled. Further treatment for shock may then be required. If the mother survives, she may suffer from anuria and Sheehan's syndrome as a result of shock. As the risk of puerperal sepsis is high, antibiotic cover is required.

The woman should be seen by the obstetrician 6–8 weeks after delivery in order to exclude chronic uterine inversion. The midwife should encourage the woman to carry out her postnatal exercises; referral to an obstetric physiotherapist may be helpful if the abdominal and pelvic floor muscle tone is particularly poor. As this condition may recur, the woman should be advised to give birth in hospital if she becomes pregnant again (Calder 2000).

## SHOCK

Shock is a condition in which the circulatory system cannot maintain sufficient perfusion to the vital organs (WHO 2003). Cellular oxygen and nutritional requirements are not met and metabolic waste cannot be removed. The ensuing hypotension and reduced tissue perfusion may result in irreversible organ damage or death. Shock is classified according to its cause:

- *Hypovolaemic shock* occurs when the circulating blood volume is too low to meet tissue requirements. It is associated with severe obstetric haemorrhage and may follow coagulopathy, such as that associated with amniotic fluid embolism.
- *Cardiogenic shock*: Cardiac output is reduced due to heart failure. In maternity, it more commonly occurs as a result of pulmonary embolism, congenital cardiac defects, acquired valvular disease or severe anaemia.
- *Neurogenic shock* occurs as a result of an insult to the central nervous system. It is associated with uterine inversion, regional anaesthesia and aspiration of gastric contents.

- *Septic shock* (toxic shock, bacterial shock) occurs as a result of severe generalized infection.
- *Anaphylactic shock* occurs as a result of an adverse drug reaction.

The latter three categories of shock are also known as *distributive shock*, which is characterized by peripheral circulatory abnormalities. The effects of shock may be exacerbated by pain, dehydration and exhaustion. The midwife is more likely to come across hypovolaemic shock.

## Signs of deterioration

Most childbearing women are healthy and are unlikely to suffer harm provided that blood loss does not exceed the physiological volume expansion which occurs in pregnancy. However, after losing more than 35% of the total circulating volume, clinical signs of hypovolaemia will appear (Grady 2007). Midwives must be alert for changes in the condition of any woman in their care.

Initially, the signs of hypovolaemic shock are less obvious than those of the other forms of shock, and it is therefore more difficult to detect. The following signs indicate deepening shock which will affect all body organs and systems:

- *Heart rate*: In the early stages of shock, the pulse will remain normal. As the heart rate rises, the volume grows weaker until the rapid thready pulse of severe haemorrhage is noted. Tachycardia reflects the cardiac response to underperfusion of the vital organs. Above 100 beats per minute is considered abnormal. However, even though most women become tachycardiac, a *paradoxical* bradycardia can occur, which may be misleading (Grady 2007).
- *Blood pressure*: Though the mother is losing blood, for some time the compensatory mechanisms in her body will keep her blood pressure normal. Peripheral, splanchnic and renal vasoconstriction ensure that vital organs, such as the heart and brain, continue to be perfused. Once 30–40% of the blood volume is lost, the blood pressure will fall (Cockings & Waldmann 2006). If the systolic pressure falls below 90 mmHg or it falls by 30 mmHg, there is cause for concern and by this time the woman will already be in the late stages of shock.
- *Increasing pallor of the skin*: The skin becomes cold and sweaty. The lips become bluish and mucous membranes blanched. Perfusion of the skin decreases. Capillary refill time is assessed by pressing a fingernail for 5 seconds. The colour should return in 2 seconds (Baskett et al 2007).
- *Temperature*: Falls to a subnormal level.
- *Respiration*: Initially tachypnoea occurs, but as the shock deepens, breathing becomes deep and sighing.
- *Urinary output*: Output decreases, followed by anuria.
- *Altered mental state*: In early shock, restlessness and anxiety may occur. The woman may experience thirst, nausea or faintness. Later, as perfusion of the brain decreases, she may become confused and finally lose consciousness after 50% of her blood volume has been lost (Baskett et al 2007).
- *Metabolic acidosis*: A late sign occurring after cellular metabolism becomes deranged, following reduced tissue perfusion and cellular hypoxia. Cell death is irreversible and the woman will be close to death at this stage (Baskett et al 2007).

The latest CEMACH report recommends that all obstetric units develop an 'early warning scoring system' to aid in the timely identification, referral and treatment of women who develop complications that may lead to severe illness (Lewis 2007) (see website for reference of example).

## Treatment

The midwife must closely observe the woman's condition and call for obstetric assistance at the first sign of a rising pulse rate. Urgent resuscitation will be needed (airway, breathing, circulation). Once achieved, and the source identified and taken care of, the principles underlying treatment are as follows:

- *Fluid replacement*: Two large-bore (at least 16G) intravenous cannulae are sited. Blood is taken and cross-matching requested: at least six units of blood will be required. In the meantime, the circulating blood volume must be restored and maintained. Crystalloids are good short-term intravascular volume expanders. Up to 2–3 litres of Ringer's lactate or Hartmann's solution can be given to initiate fluid replacement. Colloids, such as Haemacell and Gelofusine, may then be given. Colloids will remain in the intravascular space for longer. However, colloid may rarely cause anaphylaxis. Packed red blood cells are given for their oxygen-carrying capacity. Fresh frozen plasma will be given in between units of packed cells. All fluids should be warmed prior to administration.
- *Other means of maintaining the circulation*: If there is persistent hypotension after fluid replacement, inotropic drugs may be used. These increase myocardial contractility and are effective in maintaining cardiac output. Vasopressor agents such as noradrenaline (norepinephrine) may be useful, especially in cases of septic shock where fluid volume replacement alone is insufficient to maintain blood pressure. These drugs are used with caution as pulmonary and renal vasoconstriction can occur. In an emergency situation, raising the woman's legs may assist in maintaining core circulation.

- *Monitoring:* Accurate volume replacement is essential to save the woman's life and cannot be safely managed without central venous monitoring. There should be no delay in inserting a central venous pressure line. The heart rate should be monitored continuously by electrocardiograph and a pulse oximeter applied. Blood is taken for estimation of plasma gases, haemoglobin, clotting studies, urea and electrolytes. The patency of the woman's airway is monitored and her position adjusted to allow adequate ventilation and lung expansion. Intubation may be necessary. The midwife must watch carefully for any signs of cyanosis. Frequent records of pulse, blood pressure, respiratory rate, oxygen saturations, blood loss, urine output and level of consciousness are maintained.
- *Oxygen* should be administered. The rate may be adjusted according to results of blood gas estimation or pulse oximetry.
- *Pain relief,* such as intramuscular morphine, may be given to relieve pain. The mother should be kept as quiet and undisturbed as possible.
- *Avoiding hypothermia:* Rapid warming, however, may be dangerous. The cold, pale skin is evidence that the body's compensatory mechanism is working. Superficial capillaries and arterioles are constricted and blood is diverted to the vital organs. Overwarming the skin until it is flushed may undo this compensatory mechanism and deepen the shock.
- The woman should be transferred to a high dependency or intensive care unit as soon as possible.

## Septic shock

This is cardiovascular collapse due to septicaemia. Bacterial toxins are released, resulting in marked vasodilation. Blood collects in the capillary bed rather than returning to the heart. Cardiac output is reduced and peripheral failure ensues, resulting in tissue destruction, especially in the kidneys. Septic shock may follow puerperal uterine infection, septic abortion, intra-amniotic infection and urinary tract infection.

### Signs

These are similar to other types of shock. However, there is earlier and more marked hypotension, tachycardia, tachypnoea and altered mental state due to metabolic acidosis. The woman may have pyrexia, along with hot, dry flushed skin. In the late stages of shock she will become hypothermic with cold clammy skin. Uterine infection may be accompanied by acute abdominal tenderness and scanty malodorous lochia. Multiple organ failure, adult respiratory distress syndrome and DIC may develop. Mortality can be high unless appropriate measures are instituted rapidly (Lewis 2007).

### Management

This is similar to other types of shock. Additionally, the midwife must call for early medical assistance if there is any evidence of infection. If at home, the woman should be admitted to a hospital which has high dependency or intensive care facilities.

A midstream specimen of urine, high vaginal swab, wound swab and blood cultures are sent for bacterial investigation. Serum lactate, blood gases and clotting factors are measured.

A woman suffering with septic shock will need an intensive regimen of intravenous antibiotics, and any products of conception must be removed from the uterus. The midwife should pay attention to the woman's personal hygiene and general comfort.

**Reflective activity 68.2**

Visit your local delivery unit and obstetric theatres and find out where the drugs and intravenous fluids required for management of haemorrhage and shock are kept.

## AMNIOTIC FLUID EMBOLISM

Amniotic fluid embolism (AFE) is thought to be an acute anaphylactic-type response to amniotic fluid, fetal hair and debris in the maternal circulation. It is unpredictable and unpreventable, and occurs closer to term, during labour or delivery. Signs of AFE may also appear immediately after childbirth (Clarke et al 1995), although this is rare. The incidence in the UK is 1.8 per 100,000 maternities, with a mortality rate of 24% (Knight et al 2008) to 37% (Tuffnell 2005). Symptoms occur within minutes of the event and most deaths occur within 1 hour of the event. All cases of AFE are reported to the United Kingdom Obstetric Surveillance System (UKOSS) (see website).

Risk factors include older, multiparous women, and cases where the physical barriers between the maternal and fetal circulation are mechanically disrupted (Abenhaim et al 2008). This includes caesarean section, artificial rupture of membranes, induction of labour, placental abruption, placenta praevia, uterine rupture and instrumental delivery. It may also be associated with multiple pregnancy or follow polyhydramnios.

In the above cases, the intra-amniotic pressure is increased and when the membranes rupture, amniotic fluid may be forced into the maternal circulation via the endocervical veins or the placental bed. Signs of fetal hypoxia commonly precede or accompany AFE (Thomson & Greer 2000).

Diagnosis is difficult but the UK (Knight et al 2008) and the US (Clarke et al 1995) AFE registries recommend that the following criteria must be present for a diagnosis to be made:

- Acute hypotension or cardiac arrest
- Acute hypoxia
- Coagulopathy
- The onset of the above must be during labour or within 30 minutes of delivery, and in the absence of any other explanation for the symptoms.

In the UK, an autopsy confirming the presence of fetal squames or hair in the lungs is also accepted (Knight et al 2008). However, women who have fetal material in their circulatory system do not necessarily develop AFE.

Symptoms may include:

- hypotension
- fetal distress
- pulmonary oedema or acute respiratory distress
- cardiovascular collapse
- cyanosis
- dyspnoea
- seizures
- anxiety.

If the woman survives the initial event, the thromboplastin-like effects of amniotic fluid will cause a coagulopathy and she may subsequently die from coagulation failure. As the presence of intravascular amniotic fluid depresses myometrial activity, the uterus may become atonic and this will compound the haemorrhage due to coagulopathy (Clark 1990).

The midwife must immediately call for medical assistance and commence cardiopulmonary resuscitation. High concentrations of oxygen should be administered. An intravenous infusion is commenced and a central venous pressure line is inserted. Intubation and mechanical ventilation may be needed. A caesarean section will be carried out as quickly as possible. The aim is not simply to salvage the fetus but also because adequate and effective resuscitation of the mother is better achieved when the uterus is empty.

**Reflective activity 68.3**

If you attend a woman following a major complication in the third stage of labour, talk to her afterwards about her perception of the experience.

## CONCLUSION

The third stage is the most dangerous part of labour for the woman. Complications can arise with little warning. As the senior professional present at the majority of births in the UK, it is usually the midwife who has the responsibility for identifying the problem and beginning emergency treatment. Midwives must be aware of potential dangers, observe for signs of impending problems and know how to respond appropriately, as well as keep accurate records. Long-term consequences may be physical or psychological. The emotional needs of the parents must be addressed once the emergency is over. Parents will probably need to talk through the events with the midwife. The emergency often results in separation from the baby, which will cause distress. Breastfeeding may be more difficult to establish and the woman's long-term relationships both with her baby and her partner may suffer.

Adequate emotional support should be available for the midwife and a discussion with the Supervisor of Midwives may be helpful.

### KEY POINTS

- The third stage is the most dangerous part of labour for the woman.
- PPH is still a major cause of maternal death in the UK.
- Complications may arise without warning and the woman's condition can deteriorate rapidly.
- Effective management of blood loss and shock is crucial.
- Accurate assessment and rapid response to emergencies may save the woman's life.
- The midwife needs to be able to monitor the woman's condition, refer appropriately and work collaboratively, to ensure safe and effective care at this time.

## REFERENCES

Abenhaim HA, Azonday L, Kramer MS, et al: Incidence and risk factors of amniotic fluid embolisms: a population-based study on 3 million births in the United States, *American Journal of Obstetrics and Gynecology* 199(1):49–52, 2008.

Adelusi B, Soltan M, Chowdhury N, et al: Risk of retained placenta: multivariate approach, *Acta Obstetricia et Gynecologica Scandinavica* 76(5):414–418, 1997.

Alexander J, Thomas P, Sanghera J: Treatments for secondary postpartum haemorrhage (Systematic Review), *Cochrane Database of Systematic Reviews* (1):CD 002867, 2002.

Anderson JM, Etches D: Prevention and management of postpartum hemorrhage, *American Family Physician* 75(6):875–882, 2007.

Baskett TF, Calder AA, Arulkumaran S: *Munro Kerr's operative obstetrics*, ed 11, London, 2007, Elsevier.

Begley CM: A comparison of 'active' versus 'physiological' management of the third stage of labour, *Midwifery* 6(1):3–17, 1990.

Beischer N, Mackay E, Colditz P: *Obstetrics and the newborn*, London, 1997, Baillière Tindall.

Berck D, Baxi L: Benign tumours in pregnancy. In Reece E, Hobbins J, editors: *Medicine of the fetus and mother*, Philadelphia, 1999, Lippincott-Raven.

Blackburn ST: *Maternal, fetal and neonatal physiology*, ed 3, St Louis, 2007, Saunders Elsevier.

B-Lynch C, Coker A, Lawal A, et al: The B-Lynch surgical technique for the control of massive postpartum haemorrhage: an alternative to hysterectomy? Five cases reported, *British Journal of Obstetrics and Gynaecology* 104(3):372–375, 1997.

Bose P, Regan F, Paterson-Brown S: Improving the accuracy of estimated blood loss at obstetric haemorrhage using clinical reconstructions, *British Journal of Obstetrics and Gynaecology* 113(8):919–924, 2006.

Boyle M: *Emergencies around childbirth: a handbook for midwives*, Oxon, 2002, Radcliffe Medical Press, Chapter 10, p 123, figure 10.2.

Bullarbo M, Tjugum J, Ekerhovd E: Sublingual nitroglycerin for management of retained placenta, *International Journal of Gynecology and Obstetrics* 91(3):228–232, 2005.

Calder A: Emergencies in operative obstetrics, *Baillière's Best Practice Research Clinical Obstetrics and Gynaecology* 14(1):43–55, 2000.

Carroli G, Bergel E: Umbilical vein injection for management of retained placenta (Cochrane Review), *Cochrane Database of Systematic Reviews* (4):CD001337, 2001.

Carroli G, Cuesta C, Abalos E, et al: Epidemiology of postpartum haemorrhage: a systematic review, *Best Practice and Research in Obstetrics and Gynaecology* 22(6):999–1012, 2008.

Chi C, Kadir RA: Management of women with inherited bleeding disorders in pregnancy, *The Obstetrician and Gynaecologist* 9(1):27–33, 2007.

Clark SL: New concepts of amniotic fluid embolism: a review, *Obstetrical and Gynecological Survey* 45(6):360–368, 1990.

Clarke SL, Hankins GD, Dudley DA, et al: Amniotic fluid embolism: analysis of the national registry, *American Journal of Obstetrics and Gynecology* 172(4):1158–1167, 1995.

Cockings JGL, Waldmann CS: Assessing and replenishing lost volume. In B-Lynch C, Keith LG, Lalonde AB, et al, editors: *A textbook of postpartum hemorrhage: a comprehensive guide to evaluation, management and surgical intervention*, Duncow, 2006, Sapiens, pp 45–54.

Coker A, Oliver R: Definitions and classifications. In B-Lynch C, Keith LG, Lalonde AB, et al, editors: *A textbook of postpartum hemorrhage: a comprehensive guide to evaluation, management and surgical intervention*, Duncow, 2006, Sapiens, pp 11–16.

Cotter A, Ness A, Toledo J: Prophylactic oxytocin for the third stage of labour, *Cochrane Database of Systematic Reviews* (4):CD001808, 2001.

Evans DG, B-Lynch C: Obstetric trauma. In B-Lynch C, Keith LG, Lalonde AB, et al, editors: *A textbook of postpartum hemorrhage: a comprehensive guide to evaluation, management and surgical intervention*, Duncow, 2006, Sapiens, pp 70–79.

Grady K: Shock. In Grady K, Howell C, Cox C, editors: *Managing Obstetric Emergencies and Trauma. The MOET Course Manual*, London, 2007, Advanced Life Support Group and Royal College of Obstetricians and Gynaecologists, pp 96–104.

Hammar M, Boström K, Borgvall B, et al: Comparison between the influence of methylergometrine and oxytocin on the incidence of retained placenta in the third stage of labour, *Gynaecologic and Obstetric Investigation* 30(2):91–93, 1990.

Hofmeyr GJ, Gülmezoglu AM: Misoprostol for the prevention and treatment of postpartum haemorrhage, *Best Practice and Research Clinical Obstetrics and Gynaecology* 22(6):1025–1041, 2008.

Hofmeyr GJ, Abdel-Aleem H, Abdel-Aleem MA: Uterine massage for preventing postpartum haemorrhage (Cochrane Review), *Cochrane Database of Systematic Reviews* (3):CD006431, 2008.

Howell C, Irani S: (2007) Massive obstetric haemorrhage. In Grady K, Howell C, Cox C, editors: *Managing Obstetric Emergencies and Trauma. The MOET Course Manual*, London, 2007, Advanced Life Support Group and Royal College of Obstetricians and Gynaecologists, pp 171–194.

Joint Formulary Committee: *British National Formulary*, ed 56, London, 2008, British Medical Association and Royal Pharmaceutical Society of Great Britain.

Keogh J, Tsokos N: Aortic compression in massive postpartum haemorrhage – an old but lifesaving technique, *Australian and New Zealand Journal of Obstetrics and Gynaecology* 37(2):237–238, 1997.

Knight M, Kurinczuk JJ, Spark P, et al: *United Kingdom Obstetric Surveillance System (UKOSS) Annual Report*, Oxford, 2008, National Perinatal Epidemiology Unit.

Lewis G, editor: The Confidential Enquiry into Maternal and Child Health (CEMACH). Why mothers die. The Sixth Report of the Confidential Enquiries into Maternal Deaths in the United Kingdom 2000–2002, London, 2004, Royal College of Obstetricians and Gynaecologists.

Lewis G, editor: The Confidential Enquiry into Maternal and Child Health (CEMACH). Saving mothers' lives: reviewing maternal deaths to make motherhood safer – 2003–2005. The Seventh Report on Confidential Enquiries into Maternal Deaths in the United Kingdom, London, 2007, CEMACH.

Magann EF, Evans F, Chauhan SP, et al: The length of the third stage of labor and the risk of postpartum hemorrhage, *Obstetrics and Gynecology* 105(2):290–293, 2005.

Magann EF, Doherty DA, Briery CM, et al: Obstetric characteristics for a prolonged third stage of labor and risk for postpartum hemorrhage, *Gynecologic and Obstetric Investigation* 65(3):201–205, 2008.

Miller S, Martin HB, Morris JL: Anti-shock garment in postpartum haemorrhage, *Best Practice and Research Clinical Obstetrics and Gynaecology* 22(6):1057–1074, 2008.

Mousa HA, Alfirevic Z: Treatment for postpartum haemorrhage (Systematic Review), *Cochrane Database of Systematic Reviews* (1):CD003249, 2007.

National Institute for Health and Clinical Excellence (NICE): *Intraoperative blood cell salvage in obstetrics. Interventional procedure guidance 144*, London, 2005, NICE.

National Institute for Health and Clinical Excellence (NICE): *Intrapartum care. Care of healthy women and their babies during childbirth. Clinical Guideline*, London, 2007, NICE.

Nursing and Midwifery Council (NMC): *Midwives rules and standards*, London, 2004, NMC.

Ogueh O, Ayida G: Acute uterine inversion: a new technique of hydrostatic replacement, *British Journal of Obstetrics and Gynaecology* 104(8):951–952, 1997.

O'Sullivan JV: Acute inversion of the uterus, *British Medical Journal* 2(1):282–283, 1945.

Page L: Being with Jane in Childbirth: putting science and sensitivity into practice. In Page L, editor: *The new midwifery: science and sensitivity in practice*, Philadelphia, 2006, Churchill Livingstone, pp 359–376.

Plaat F: Anaesthetic issues related to postpartum haemorrhage (excluding antishock garments), *Best Practice and Research Clinical Obstetrics and Gynaecology* 22(6):1043–1056, 2008.

Prasertcharoensuk W, Swadpanich U, Lumbiganon P: Accuracy of the blood loss estimation in the third stage of labour, *International Journal of Gynecology and Obstetrics* 71(1):69–70, 2000.

Prendiville WJ, Elbourne D, McDonald S: Active versus expectant management in the third stage of labour (Cochrane Review), *Cochrane Database of Systemic Reviews* (3):CD000007, 2000.

Rogers MS, Chang AM: Postpartum haemorrhage and other problems of the third stage. In James DK, Steer PJ, Weiner CP, et al, editors: *High risk pregnancy: management options*, ed 3, Philadelphia, 2008, Saunders Elsevier, pp 1559–1582.

The Royal College of Obstetricians and Gynaecologists: *Prevention and management of postpartum haemorrhage*. Green-top Guideline No. 52, London, 2009, RCOG.

Thomson A, Greer I: Non-haemorrhagic obstetric shock, *Baillière's Clinical Obstetrics and Gynaecology* 14(1):19–41, 2000.

Toledo P, McCarthy RJ, Hewlett BJ, et al: The accuracy of blood loss estimation after simulated vaginal delivery, *Anesthesia & Analgesia* 105(6):1736–1740, 2007.

Tuffnell DJ: United Kingdom amniotic fluid embolism register, *British Journal of Obstetrics and Gynaecology* 112(12):1625–1629, 2005.

Weeks AD: The retained placenta, *Best Practice and Research Clinical Obstetrics and Gynaecology* 22(6):1103–1117, 2008.

Winograd RH: Uterine artery embolization for postpartum hemorrhage, *Best Practice and Research Clinical Obstetrics and Gynaecology* 22(6):1119–1132, 2008.

Winter C, Macfarlane A, Deneux-Tharaux C, et al: Variations in policies for management of the third stage of labour and the immediate management of postpartum haemorrhage in Europe, *British Journal of Obstetrics and Gynaecology* 114(7):845–854, 2007.

World Health Organization (WHO): *The prevention and management of postpartum haemorrhage. Report of a Technical Working Group, Geneva 3–6, July 6, 1989*, Geneva, 1990, WHO.

World Health Organization (WHO): *Shock. Managing complications in pregnancy and childbirth. A guide for midwives and doctors (MCPC)*, Geneva, 2003, WHO.

Chapter |69|

# Maternal mental health and psychological problems

Kathryn Gutteridge

## LEARNING OUTCOMES

After reading this chapter, you will:

- appreciate the global context of women's mental health across all cultures and economies
- understand the range of mental health problems that present during pregnancy and childbirth
- appreciate the impact of pregnancy, childbirth and transition to parenting on women's mental health and psychological wellbeing
- understand the importance of early detection of mental illness, and know how to contribute effectively to treatment and management of minor and major disorders
- appreciate the value of working collaboratively within the wider multidisciplinary team within each professional boundary
- confidently offer advice and support to women and be aware of the sources of help and support available locally and nationally.

## INTRODUCTION

This chapter offers a comprehensive overview of the psychological and mental health problems that pregnant and childbearing women may encounter. Pregnancy is a time associated with joy and happiness. The reality, however, is that for many women, pregnancy will, in fact, cause a recurrence of impaired mental health, increase otherwise controlled anxiety problems or be the precursor of a primary illness. Pregnancy is more often described as a life crisis and a time where there is a huge shift in the emotional and psychological balances in a woman's life. In some ways the emotional ebb and flow mask the real issues that women are trying to deal with and society often considers these emotional changes as the pregnancy norm.

There is recognition that despite improvements in the understanding, detection and treatment of pregnancy-related mental health disorders, many women will not seek help and try to cope with their illness, hiding their unhappiness from their caregivers and family. Women still fear discrimination and long-term repercussions if they reveal a previous emotional disturbance or psychiatric illness (MIND 2001, Robinson 2002). This remains the case despite the fact that one in four people will experience mental health problems at some time during their lifetime. Up to 50% of all women are thought to have suffered some form of emotional disturbance during their lives and the risk is much higher amongst women who are socially excluded (MIND 2001).

## A GLOBAL PERSPECTIVE OF WOMEN'S MENTAL HEALTH

In western society there is greater awareness of mental wellbeing and illness; however, it remains by and large a poorly understood aspect of healthcare.

Depression is a serious public health issue and it is estimated by the World Health Organization to be the greatest burden of disease and cause of premature death worldwide by 2020 (WHO 2000). In this authoritative report, WHO propose that women are twice as likely as men to be diagnosed with depression and that violence and self-inflicted injuries will also feature as a characteristic of women's mental health.

Saltman (1991) identified that one of the reasons for the high rates of women's psychological and mental morbidity is the focus on mortality. Whilst mortality overall is reduced, there has been little progress in the understanding and redressing of factors that contribute to mental illness. Another primary concern in understanding the mental wellbeing of women is suicide and its determinants (DH 1999). In global studies of women in their peak reproductive years, ages 15–44, it was shown that suicide was second only to tuberculosis as a cause of death. Murray & Lopez (1996) found that in 1990, 180,000 women in China alone committed suicide and 87,000 women in India died by self-immolation.

Further research has shown that there are strong inverse relationships with poverty, social position, ethnic background, marital support and access to healthcare (Bartley & Owen 1996). Being a participant in decisions about healthcare and life choices has a significant impact upon psychological and mental wellbeing, during and outside of pregnancy; a sense of control is critical to wellness.

Health and social behaviours may have an impact upon wellbeing, with tobacco usage and drug and alcohol misuse being common in women with anxiety and depressive disorders (DH 2003). Understanding the dependency that such behaviours provoke is critical for midwives to support positive pregnancy outcomes.

Whilst it would be easy to believe that in the western world higher stress levels might indicate a higher predilection for mental health disorders, there is substantial evidence that developing societies are also at risk. The most common cause in the underdeveloped and Third World populace is the impact of unstable governments and social structures giving rise to conflict and violence.

## VIOLENCE AGAINST WOMEN

Whether by their intimate partners or men not known to them, violence is probably the most prevalent and certainly the most representative gender-based cause of depression in women. In studies of the effect upon women in war-torn communities, it was revealed that rape, torture and murder were by far the most common weapon in the entrapment and subjugation of women and their children (WHO 2000). The impact of these crimes leads to a range of mental health illnesses; depression, self-harm and trauma.

Violence and abuse of women consistently features in mental health and physical morbidity. Abusive behaviour, particularly in an intimate relationship, has a detrimental impact on the woman; fear, lack of freedom, humiliation and threat of harm all contribute to deny women's Human Rights (WHO 1997) (Ch. 23).

Women are more likely than men to suffer abuse throughout their lifetime, particularly rape, sexual assault and child sexual abuse. Research has consistently shown that between 20% and 30% of women have been sexually abused as a child, compared with 10% of male children (DH 2003). This report indicates that 1 in 10 women have experienced some form of sexual victimization, including rape, and that 'strangers' are only responsible for 8% of rapes. Sexual abuse particularly experienced as a child has considerable significance for childbearing women, physically during the birth and psychologically throughout childbirth and parenting (Gutteridge 2001).

It would appear that societal influences, largely gender based, have negative influences on the psychological/mental wellbeing of women. Mental health cannot be explained through biomedical determinants alone and it is naive to see women's mental health only through a framework of reproductive perspective. This explanation is understandable since, globally, women's health is often influenced by fertility and childbearing. Understanding the impact of pregnancy and childbearing on women's mental wellbeing with its application across all cultures is significant to developing approaches suitable for women and their families.

## PREGNANCY, CHILDBIRTH AND MENTAL HEALTH

There is an increased risk of mental illness associated with childbirth, mostly in the postpartum period, but problems may also be present before or during pregnancy. Many of the factors associated with postnatal mental illness, such as lack of a confiding relationship, lack of support, marital tension, socioeconomic problems and a previous psychiatric history, are present during pregnancy (O'Hara & Zekoski 1988, O'Hara et al 1991, Romito 1989) and so depression may occur both in pregnancy and in the postpartum period (Evans et al 2001, Green & Murray 1994, Watson et al 1984). There appears to be a positive correlation between women who lack positive maternal role models and the development of anxiety-based depressive disorders during pregnancy and the postnatal period (Gutteridge, unpublished data, 1998).

Whilst there is deepening awareness of postnatal depression and psychotic illness following childbirth, there is relatively little published work on the incidence of, and morbidity associated with, *antenatal* depression. This is despite the fact that depressed mood in pregnancy has been associated with poor attendance at antenatal clinics, substance misuse, low birthweight and preterm labour (Hedegaard et al 1993, Pagel et al 1990). Whereas it was once thought that pregnancy was a protective factor against depression, Watson et al (1984) found that in 24%

of cases of detected postnatal depression, symptoms were present during pregnancy.

There is now clear evidence that psychopathological symptoms in pregnancy have physiological consequences for the fetus (Teixeira et al 1999). A cohort study of depressed mood during pregnancy and after childbirth concluded that research and clinical efforts towards recognizing and treating antenatal depression must be improved (Evans et al 2001). The Confidential Enquiry into Maternal Deaths (Lewis 2004) recommends better detection and management of psychiatric disorders antenatally, to reduce the mortality rate. Services must be designed to meet the needs of all women, and a crucial part of the service should address the mental health needs of women.

## WHO IS 'AT RISK'?

Many women experience mixed reactions to their pregnancy, with transient feelings of anxiety and fear; they should be reassured that this is normal and be encouraged to discuss these feelings openly (Ch. 12). The incidence of detected mental illness in the first trimester of pregnancy is thought to be as high as 15%, with only 5% of these women having suffered from previous episodes of mental illness. In the second and third trimesters of pregnancy, the incidence of new episodes of mental illness is less, only about 5%.

The majority of episodes of new mental illness during pregnancy are minor conditions or neuroses. The commonest condition is depressive neurosis with anxiety, but phobic anxiety states and obsessive–compulsive disorders may also occur. In most cases, these neurotic mental illnesses resolve by the second trimester of pregnancy and there seems to be no added risk of these women developing postnatal depression.

The outlook is different for those women who begin their pregnancies with *chronic* neurotic conditions. Their illness is likely to continue throughout pregnancy and may be exacerbated during the third trimester into the puerperium.

Minor mental illness is more likely to occur in the first trimester of pregnancy in women who have marked neurotic traits in the premorbid personality. It also tends to occur in women who have a history of neurotic disorders and in those with social problems, such as marital tension. Other predisposing factors include a history of previous abortion and the possibility of the present pregnancy being terminated (Wilson et al 1996). Women with a poor obstetric history or those who have undergone extensive infertility treatment may exhibit signs of increased anxiety in early pregnancy.

The onset of minor mental illness later in pregnancy, usually during the third trimester, is less common than in the first trimester. When it occurs at this stage in pregnancy, however, the risk of the woman developing postnatal depression is increased (Forman et al 2000).

Major mental illnesses include *bipolar disorder, severe depression* and *schizophrenia*. The risk of a woman developing a new episode of one of these conditions in pregnancy is lower than at other times in her life. When women with a history of major mental illness become pregnant, there is no particular increase in the risk of a relapse during pregnancy if they are well stabilized and their illness is in remission. Although the risk of major mental illness is reduced in pregnancy, it is greatly increased in the first 3 months after delivery.

## THE MIDWIFE'S ROLE IN THE ANTENATAL PERIOD

There is growing emphasis on the development of the public health role of the midwife, with promotion of mental wellbeing representing an area where the midwife can make a valuable contribution (DH 2007). The midwife has a responsibility to provide holistic care, meeting the physical, psychological and emotional needs of all women. There should be an emphasis on promoting emotional and psychological wellbeing for all women, not just those perceived to be at risk. Ideally, all women should be treated with sensitivity during pregnancy and enabled during meetings with the midwife to reveal and discuss any issues that may predispose them to impaired mental health.

A midwife has a special relationship in a woman's lifetime; s/he has a privileged position in which s/he is able to ask direct and intrusive questions regarding a woman's fertility and sexual history. This is a trusting and a confiding relationship in which the midwife begins to feature strongly in a woman's life history (Ch. 12), entrusting her body to the midwife and allowing her to care for her developing fetus.

Kirkham (2000) acknowledges the exclusivity of this relationship and identifies themes such as trust, friendship, purpose and the place of self within this dynamic context (Ch. 12). In no other professional relationship is there such a potential for influencing change than between midwife and childbearing woman.

Some women will live within a culture where there is no recognition of minor depressive illness or anxiety states (Wilson et al 1996). Any attempt to enquire whether the woman is symptomatic may be restricted by other family members who associate impaired mental health only with major psychotic illness to which there is shame and stigma attached (Oates 2001). The midwife should recognize that presentations of ongoing minor physical disorders and concerns about the pregnancy may be the only way the woman can express her feelings. To ensure that all women receive adequate support and help, independent, trained interpreters should be available for women whose first language is not English and every attempt must be made to see the woman unaccompanied.

## Assessment

Taking a comprehensive history at the beginning of pregnancy is vital to assess risk, review and plan care around any deterioration of mental and psychological health. Emotional lability during pregnancy is expected; however, the midwife should make ongoing assessments throughout. NICE (2007:6) recommend a universal and continuous enquiry approach:

### FIRST HEALTH CONTACT VISIT

At a woman's first contact with services in both the antenatal and postnatal periods, healthcare professionals (including midwives, obstetricians, health visitors and GPs) should ask questions about:

- past or present severe mental illness, including schizophrenia, bipolar disorder, psychosis in the postnatal period and severe depression
- previous treatment by a psychiatrist/specialist mental health team, including inpatient care
- family history of perinatal mental illness.

Other specific predictors, such as poor relationships with her partner, should not be used for the routine prediction of the development of a mental disorder.

### ONGOING SCREENING

At a woman's first contact with primary care, during her booking visit and postnatally (usually at 4 to 6 weeks and 3 to 4 months), healthcare professionals (including midwives, obstetricians, health visitors and GPs) should ask two questions to identify possible depression.

- During the past month, have you often been bothered by feeling down, depressed or hopeless?
- During the past month, have you often been bothered by having little interest or pleasure in doing things?

A third question should be considered if the woman answers 'yes' to both of the initial questions.

- Is this something you feel you need or want help with?

Although NICE (2007) do not specifically advise against using screening tools such as the Edinburgh Postnatal Screening Scale (EPDS) (see below) or the Hospital Anxiety and Depression Scale (HADS) or the Patient Health Questionnaire-9 (PHQ-9), caution is advised (see website). Assessment tools should only be used as part of a subsequent evaluation for the routine monitoring of outcomes and only by appropriately trained health professionals (NICE 2007).

It is essential that an accurate history is taken and any reported current or past mental illness is adequately investigated and assessed. This should be done with extreme sensitivity to eradicate any fears the woman may have of discrimination (Robinson 2002). If the woman is under the care of a GP, psychiatrist, community psychiatric nurse or psychologist, attempts should be made to work collaboratively within this team to ensure the woman's whole needs are met.

The majority of minor illnesses will resolve spontaneously by the second trimester of pregnancy. The woman will require support, counselling, reassurance and information communicated in a caring, intelligible way. Psychotropic drugs are rarely necessary or prescribed at this stage of pregnancy. Instead, therapy to help the woman relax and reduce her anxiety seems to be effective. Midwives may be involved in counselling and supporting these women and teaching relaxation techniques. Sometimes a social worker is also required to help tackle social issues which may be the cause of the problem.

Women with a history of single episodes of major mental illness in the past but who have been well for some time are usually advised by their psychiatrist to stop their medication before conception and remain off the medication particularly in the first trimester (NICE 2007). An assessment should be made by a specialist service, usually consisting of a perinatal psychiatrist and specialist midwife/mental health nurse.

Whilst there is no significant risk of relapse during pregnancy for this group of women, there is a marked risk of developing a puerperal psychosis during the first 3 months after delivery (Cox 1986). Measures should be put in place to monitor and assess for deterioration postnatally (Bick et al 2002). This should be in collaboration with specialist perinatal psychiatric services.

## RISK OF SUICIDE

The Confidential Enquiry into Maternal Deaths (Lewis 2004 & 2007) using the Office for National Statistics (ONS) linkage data indicates that suicide is the current leading cause of maternal death (indirect category). There is a misconception that women who live within socially deprived situations suffer a greater risk of mental health problems; in contrast, CEMACH highlighted that the following characteristics were risk indicators:

- white, older woman
- married and living in comfortable circumstances
- in her second or subsequent pregnancy
- generally well educated
- working in the caring or health industry

- has a history of a mental health disorder
- has a baby under 3 months old
- is in contact with or receiving treatment from psychiatric services
- likely to die violently.

Therefore, the suicide profile of childbearing women is significantly disparate to that of the non-pregnant population. The risk of deterioration is significantly elevated in the last trimester of pregnancy and the first 12 weeks postpartum, when both suicide and infanticide should be considered. Though rare, most cases of infanticide where there is evidence of serious maternal mental illness will be associated with a suicide attempt or successful suicide (Marks & Kumar 1993).

CEMACE (previously CEMACH) recommend that women with a history of severe depression or psychotic disorder be referred to a specialist perinatal mental health team and an appropriate care plan developed, aiming to support the woman through pregnancy and minimize the risk of severe postnatal disorder (Oates 2004). Where a woman is under the care of a psychiatrist when pregnancy is diagnosed, there should be careful liaison between the obstetrician, midwife and mental health team to ensure that the woman's care is seamless and holistic, and that appropriate management plans are made to maximize the outcome for mother and baby. This is especially relevant when deciding upon the woman's ongoing and future drug regimen. Additionally, Oates (2000) recommends care is best delivered under the auspices of a managed network approach, whereby those women who are at greatest risk of relapse receive care from specialist service providers.

## COMMON MATERNAL MENTAL HEALTH DISORDERS

### Generalized anxiety disorder (GAD)

This is a condition where excessive anxiety is experienced on most days. Symptoms are described as: a fast heart rate, palpitations, feeling sick, tremor, sweating, dry mouth, chest pain, headaches, nausea, tachypnoea. GAD develops in about 1 in 50 people at some stage in life. Slightly more women are affected than men and usually it first develops in the early 20s. The most effective treatment is considered to be *cognitive behavioural therapy* (CBT).

#### *Advice and care*

- Referral to GP and/or mental health services if anxiety is affecting daily life.
- May stop medication and refer to start CBT.
- May need to change to a safer drug, if the decision is to maintain medication.

### Panic disorder

This is an anxiety disorder and is characterized by unexpected and repeated episodes of intense fear accompanied by physical symptoms that may include chest pain, heart palpitations, shortness of breath, dizziness, or abdominal distress.

#### *Advice and care*

- Refer to GP or mental health services.
- If symptoms are managed by medication, may stop medication and start CBT.
- May switch to a safer drug, if the decision is to maintain medication.

### Obsessive–compulsive disorder (OCD)

OCD is a common mental health condition that affects 2% of the population. It is characterized by obsessive thoughts that cause anxiety. This leads to rituals or repetitive actions. Examples of compulsions include excessive hand washing, cleaning, counting, checking, touching, arranging, hoarding, measuring, excessive neatness, and repeating tasks or actions (NICE 2005a).

OCD has two main features:

- experiencing frequent, disturbing, unwanted thoughts that result in fears, and compulsions
- acts or rituals carried out in response to fears caused by the obsessions.

#### *Advice and care*

- Refer to specialist mental health services for management of symptoms.
- If taking medication alone, may stop the medication and start psychological therapy.
- If not taking medication, psychological therapy should be considered before drug treatment.

### Post-traumatic stress disorder (PTSD)

This is a normal reaction to an extraordinary event where the individual experiences intense terror and fears for his or her life. It is reported from survivors of road/air accidents, military combat, physical, emotional and sexual abuse, terrorist attacks, hostage situations and being diagnosed with a life-threatening illness (NICE 2005b). Childbirth is now recognized as a situation that may trigger a PTSD response and this might not have been recognized from past pregnancies but may present in a subsequent pregnancy. PTSD symptoms include flashbacks and nightmares, avoidance, numbing of emotions and hyperarousal.

#### *Advice and care*

- Recognize that childbirth has the potential to induce trauma symptoms.

- There is no convincing evidence for drug treatments for PTSD in any patients, so psychological treatments are preferred. The favoured therapies in this situation are NLP (neuro-linguistic programming) and EMDR (eye movement desensitization and reprocessing).

## Bipolar disorder

The prevalence of bipolar disorder at the onset of pregnancy has not been estimated and there are no age-related data for childbearing women (Lewis 2004). Estimates would suggest that it is likely that approximately 2 per 1000 pregnancies occur in women with chronic schizophrenia and approximately the same number in women with pre-existing bipolar disorder. These women are likely to be in contact with secondary psychiatric services (Wilson et al 1996).

There are a growing number of women with pre-existing psychotic and affective disorders who will suffer a relapse in their illness during or after pregnancy. It is estimated that 2 per 1000 live births will fall into this category (Wilson et al 1996).

### *Advice and care*

- Early referral to specialist perinatal mental health services.
- If a woman with bipolar disorder has an unplanned pregnancy and is stopping lithium as prophylactic medication, an antipsychotic should be offered.
- If a pregnant woman with bipolar disorder is stable on an antipsychotic and likely to relapse without medication, she should be maintained on the antipsychotic, and monitored for weight gain and diabetes.
- If a pregnant woman who is not taking medication develops acute mania, medication is considered. The dose should be kept as low as possible and monitored carefully.
- If moderate to severe depressive symptoms occur in pregnant women with bipolar disorder, psychological treatment (CBT) should be considered.
- Use combined medication and structured psychological treatments for severe depressive symptoms.
- A multi-professional approach should be used to manage the complex symptoms, treatment programmes and achieve best outcomes.
- Fetal medicine obstetric services and neonatology should be involved with fetal screening and management of the baby following birth.

## Schizophrenia

There are no data for the prevalence of schizophrenia in women of reproductive age group. General figures suggests that around 1 in every 100 people are affected. It affects men and women equally and seems to be more common in city areas and in some minority ethnic groups. It is rare before the age of 15, but can start at any time after this, most often between the ages of 15 and 35. Estimates would suggest it is likely that approximately 2 per 1000 pregnancies occur in women with chronic schizophrenia. Schizophrenia is characterized by hallucinations, hearing voices, delusions, loss of insight and depression. Suicide is common in people diagnosed with schizophrenia.

### *Advice and care*

- Early referral to specialist perinatal mental health services.
- Women with schizophrenia who are planning a pregnancy or who are pregnant should be treated according to the NICE clinical guideline on schizophrenia (NICE 2002).
- If the woman is taking an atypical antipsychotic drug, consideration should be given to switching to a low-dose typical antipsychotic, such as haloperidol, chlorpromazine or trifluoperazine.
- If breastfeeding, treat according to NICE (2002) clinical guidance for schizophrenia, except that women receiving depot medication should be advised that their infants may show extrapyramidal symptoms several months after administration of the depot. These are usually self-limiting.
- A multi-professional approach should be used to manage these complex symptoms, treatment programmes and achieve best outcomes.
- Fetal medicine obstetric services and neonatology should be involved with fetal screening and management of the baby following birth.
- Child protection and social service support may be required to support parenting.

## Self-harm

Self-harm, also known as *self-injury*, is a common behaviour and is more likely to affect young women than men; up to 10% of 14–16-year-olds have self-harmed. A prevalence is noted among young ethnic females and other discriminated groups. It is a way of coping with extreme emotional distress and is secretive in its manifestation. Some expressions of self-harm are: cutting, gouging, burning, scratching, purging, eating disorders and hair pulling (NICE 2004a).

### *Advice and care*

- Referral to specialist mental health services.
- Identification of the type of self-harm and risk assessment of current frequency of self-harming behaviours.
- Offer support throughout pregnancy.
- Consider child protection and social service support if self-injury escalates.

## Eating disorders

These are characterized by a fear of being fat and out of control with food, which ultimately has a detrimental impact on the health of the individual. Girls and women are 10 times more likely than boys and men to suffer from anorexia or bulimia. Prevalence is estimated to be about 1 in 150 girls. Women with bulimia nervosa are prone to unplanned pregnancy, in part because vomiting reduces the efficacy of oral contraceptives. Some of the effects of eating disorders are:

- reduced stomach capacity
- tired, weak and temperature changes
- metabolism slows down
- constipation
- stunted height
- brittle bones (which break easily)
- failure to get pregnant
- liver damage
- dental problems, particularly in bulimia
- hair loss
- death in extreme cases – anorexia nervosa has the highest death rate of any psychological disorder.

### *Advice and care*

- A woman with anorexia nervosa who is planning a pregnancy, has an unplanned pregnancy or is breastfeeding should be treated in reference to guidance (NICE 2004b).
- If a woman who is taking medication for bulimia nervosa is planning a pregnancy or is pregnant, healthcare professionals should consider gradually stopping the medication.
- Referral for specialist treatment should be considered.
- Midwifery support and education about dietary needs should be provided throughout pregnancy.
- Refer to consultant obstetrician if BMI is below 19.
- Referral to nutritionist or dietician.

### *Substance misuse*

It is increasingly evident since the global growth of social drug consumption and the incidence of substance abuse that the general mental health of the population has suffered. Mental diagnoses such as bipolar disorder and personality disorders are increasing; theories suggest that social drug use is one of the main reasons and therefore this factor will increase the number of women at risk presenting during pregnancy.

There is good evidence to suggest that during the postnatal period all women are at increased risk of developing a mental illness and for those women who are already diagnosed with a severe mental illness, rates of relapse increase profoundly and they will therefore require specialist services (Lewis 2007).

### *Advice and care*

- Booking history should enquire about all drug and alcohol usage.
- If there is illicit drug usage, refer to specialist drug and alcohol team.
- Refer to social services and consider child protection programme of support.
- Maintain close contact and work as part of the multidisciplinary team.
- If drug usage is controlled, a plan of care for birth and immediate postnatal care should be shared with the team.
- If drug usage is uncontrolled and dismissed, then a child protection plan should be initiated and baby will need observation for neonatal abstinence syndrome.
- Breastfeeding is not necessarily excluded and may be the best form of managing neonatal abstinence programmes.

These conditions are not exclusive and constitute a range of problems with which women may present when pregnant. The midwife's role must be to recognize the problems, risk assess the woman's current mental wellbeing and refer to the appropriate health professional or specialist service; the midwife must continue to work within the multidisciplinary team whilst continuing to offer support and guidance to the woman so that she receives normal midwifery care throughout her childbearing experience.

**Reflective activity 69.1**

Consider how you might respond when a woman with bipolar disorder books early in her pregnancy at your antenatal clinic. (See website for points you may consider.)

## FEAR, TRAUMA IN LABOUR AND BIRTH

Some women find childbirth a fulfilling experience, but for others it is the most traumatic experience of their life (Niven 1992). The anticipation and unpredictability of birth can cause women anxiety and in some cases extreme distress. In most cases apprehension is normal; however, if the worry is all-consuming and the woman overwhelmed by these emotions, she is more likely to experience heightened pain levels and discomfort.

The experiences of labour and birth for those women who have longstanding fear of hospitals and associated procedures, such as needle phobia, are likely to be more difficult. In these situations it is important that the midwife understands and helps the woman plan her care around these anxieties to avoid further trauma.

Women who have experienced traumatic life events are much more likely to have issues with control and pain. Examples of this are women who were abused as children, survivors of rape/sexual abuse, and women who have experienced violent relationships (Gutteridge 2001).

There is increasing awareness that events around the time of birth can seriously affect a woman's mental and pyschopathological wellbeing (Laing 2001, Pantlen & Rohde 2001). Women have reported experiencing intense fear, helplessness and a loss of control when recalling their birth experiences. One study found that women who suffered an adverse birth experience were likely to develop trauma symptoms associated with post-traumatic stress disorder (Creedy et al 2000), described as 'extreme psychological distress following exposure to a traumatic and threatening experience' (Lyons 1998:93).

## Midwife's role

A detailed history should be taken for all women and risks identified in relation to pre-existing mental health problems and psychological disorders. Monitoring of mood and anxiety levels throughout pregnancy is by using the questions recommended by NICE (2007). A discussion should take place with the woman to identify the source of her concerns and a plan formulated for the birth which should be acceptable to her. This must be communicated to the maternity team and documented clearly so that when a woman comes into hospital she does not have to negotiate with her caregivers (Bloom 2002). Problems may arise where there is doubt about a woman's capacity to consent to or refuse treatment. Where a woman's capacity is questioned, a supervisor of midwives should be involved and appropriate legal advice should be sought (see Ch. 9). The primary aim should always be to act in the woman's best interests and as her advocate.

Support during labour is vital; this could be the woman's birthing partner but should also consist of continuous midwifery input and support. Throughout the birth it is important that the woman understands and is kept informed; she should be asked for consent prior to any procedures. Following the birth it is important to consider the woman's reaction to the event and any signs of emotional distress noted and documented. Postnatal debriefing following a 'difficult' birth is generally discouraged although explanations about procedures and events may be a natural part of the woman's way of coming to terms with the birth (NICE 2007). However, there is a growing body of opinion that women would benefit from a form of postnatal debriefing to help reduce the psychological morbidity experienced by many women following pregnancy and childbirth (Lavender & Walkinshaw 1998, Pantlen & Rohde 2001).

If the woman's reaction and anxieties appear to be severe, she should be referred to specialist psychiatric services for an assessment and possible treatment. It is important that the midwife works together with any other health professionals in supporting the woman and her baby during recovery.

# POSTNATAL PERIOD

The reported incidence of depression after childbirth is between 10% and 15% of women (Cox et al 1993, Kumar & Robson 1984), but, when questioned, many midwives and women report a higher incidence. The actual cause of depressive illness following childbirth is unknown but is thought to be multifactorial, a combination of biological, psychological and social factors. Rarer forms of psychiatric illness, such as psychoses, affect even fewer women but are dramatic in effect and impact.

Biological reasons include genetic make-up, gynaecological and obstetric problems (Stein et al 1989), parity and maternal age, the hormonal changes which occur in the early puerperium, and the appearance and behaviour of the baby. The mother may experience a reactive depression if her baby dies or is born with a congenital abnormality, particularly if previously undiagnosed. Psychological factors may include the woman's early relationship with her parents, personality development, acceptance of her sexuality and the ability to accept dependence (Cox 1986). Women who display anxious or obsessional traits in their personality, or appear too controlled and compliant have a greater risk of developing postnatal depression. Another symptom is *anomie*, which is a painful feeling of inability to experience love or pleasure. These mothers often feel that they do not or cannot love their babies but their baby is obviously lovingly handled and cared for by the mother.

### Detection and recognition

The previous psychiatric history of the woman (and her family) has been found to be a risk factor in many cases. The consistent finding of epidemiological studies carried out to date is that the major factors of aetiological importance are psychosocial in nature (Murray & Cooper 1997). The occurrence of stressful life events and lack of personal support from family, partner or friends have consistently been found to raise the risk of postnatal depression (Levy & Kline 1994, Stein et al 1989).

The midwife has the opportunity to assess mood changes and adaptation to parenthood, often knowing the woman before the birth. This relationship is vital and the information the midwife has will often be the first step in identifying a problem. There are tools that may assist in confirming the presence of depressive and anxiety symptoms that may be used to confirm the midwife's suspicions. Using questions recommended by NICE (2007) at every contact visit is important. If the midwife has confidence in her skills to use other assessment tools, there are several commonly used.

### *Edinburgh Postnatal Depression Scale*

The Edinburgh Postnatal Depression Scale (EDPS) has been developed for the diagnosis of postnatal depression (Cox & Holden 1994) (see website). It is a simple, self-rating, 10-item scale which was designed to be used at about 6 weeks postpartum, but can also be used at other times, including the antenatal period, for high-risk women (Clement 1995). Scores for individual items range from 0 to 3 according to severity, and the total score is the sum of the scores for the individual items. Women who score 12 or more on the scale are likely to be suffering from depressive illness. Referral for further assessment and treatment should then be offered. Initially the midwife's responsibility is to detect the symptoms, and refer the woman for specialist support.

Because of the difficulties associated with detecting postnatal depression within other cultures, a Punjabi version of the EPDS has been developed which has proved to be successful in trials to date (Clifford et al 1999).

Where midwives have been trained to deliver evidence-based postnatal advice and support, based upon the woman's description of symptoms, rates of postnatal depression have been shown to be reduced (MacArthur et al 2002). Women at risk of postnatal depression will require particularly close observation in the postnatal period.

## Postnatal conditions

### Emotional changes during childbirth

Pregnancy is a time that both women and health professionals accept as emotionally labile. The change of hormones in early pregnancy and again after the birth gives way to emotional ebb and flow, with some women more prone than others. However, it is fair to say that some degree of emotional instability is normal and should be explained as such to women and their families.

#### *Advice and care*

- Reassurance and support through family and friends or external measures, such as family support worker, Homestart or other support groups.
- Antenatal support from Parent Education, National Childbirth Trust and local women's support groups.

### Postpartum blues or 'baby blues'

It is important to distinguish between the normal mood and emotional changes that occur following the birth, known as 'baby blues' which is a period of tearfulness and mood lability. This transition lasts a matter of days and affects more than 50–80% of all women, especially primigravida (Romito 1989). The condition typically presents between 2 and 4 days after birth and symptoms include tearfulness, irritability, mood instability, headache, tiredness and oversensitivity (Hannah et al 1992). The woman needs the opportunity to talk about her feelings, and her physical discomfort, which should reduce, as the condition frequently coincides with breast discomfort. In most cases the condition is self-limiting but studies have found that women who suffer from this condition are more likely to go on to develop postnatal depression (Beck et al 1992, O'Hara & Zekoski 1988, O'Hara et al 1991).

#### *Advice and care*

- Rest and extra support.
- Generally requires no treatment but reassurance and support.
- Distinguish between transient mood changes and clinical signs of puerperal psychosis.

### Postnatal depression

This is considered to be any non-psychotic depressive illness of mild to moderate severity within the first year following childbirth. Prevalence rates range between 10% and 28% and it affects women from all cultures, ethnic backgrounds and socioeconomic groups. However, for many women, up to 75%, their illness will begin in the antenatal period and may go undetected. Some features of postnatal depression are low mood, poor sleep pattern, loss of appetite, tearfulness, anxiety, sense of failure, guilt, shame and isolation. The most common time for detection is around 4–6 weeks postnatally (Cox et al 1993). Early recognition is critical for effective intervention measures and reducing morbidity. The response to treatment and prognosis is good if detection and support is initiated early.

#### *Advice and care*

- Treatment may consist of pharmacological methods, such as antidepressants, depending upon presenting symptoms and other medication.
- Other forms of psychotherapeutic treatments may be appropriate, such as cognitive behavioural therapy, interpersonal psychotherapy, guided self-help and non-directive counselling in the woman's home.
- Exercise and other forms of positive self-nurture, such as yoga and relaxation, are also helpful.
- Social services intervention and child protection referral may be necessary if illness is severe with risk to self and baby.

### Post-traumatic stress disorder (PTSD)

PTSD is an adjustment, anxiety or dissociative disorder following exposure to a traumatic event, either as a victim or witness (real or perceived). Whilst PTSD in the general population is better acknowledged, there remains some scepticism around its incidence and childbirth.

Although it is difficult to imagine that such an extreme reaction can be caused by childbirth, a normal life event, it is the perception of the woman that is the critical denominator. Some of the triggers that may precipitate a stress reaction have been identified as:

- vaginal examination
- catheterization
- assisted birth – forceps or ventouse delivery
- theatre delivery
- separation – baby taken to NICU
- breastfeeding.

The trauma experienced during childbirth has many causative factors that are entirely perceptual for the individual woman; however, the work of Kendall-Tackett & Kaufman-Kantor (1993) identified that there are significant outcomes that will occur:

- *Physical trauma*: performing an episiotomy or other invasive procedure may result in physical harm/ trauma and therefore the woman's perception could be feelings of mutilation.
- *Stigma*: the woman feels blemished or marked in some way because of an aspect of her birth experience – this might be a scar of some sort or indwelling catheter.
- *Betrayal*: the woman perceives herself to have been let down or abused by the health professionals associated with her delivery.
- *Powerlessness*: maternal perceptions relating to lack of, or loss of, control, which often is central to birth-related trauma.

The *ICD-10 classification of mental and behavioural disorders* (WHO 1992) stipulates that trauma symptoms should include re-experiencing of the event(s) by flashbacks and/ or nightmares. The individual may also be hypervigilant and experience physical and emotional 'numbing'; avoidance of triggers that may cause distress is common. Symptoms often present after weeks and may persist for years, if not recognized and treated, followed by depression and suicide attempts.

### Advice and care

- Early recognition of symptoms and behaviours following birth.
- Allow woman to talk about her experiences.
- Refer to specialist services if symptoms are intrusive and limiting.
- Information about support – Birth Trauma Association.
- Provide ongoing multidisciplinary support.
- Social services intervention and child protection referral may be necessary if illness is severe with risk to self and baby.

## Puerperal psychosis

This is regarded as a serious mental illness during the perinatal period, consistently affecting 2 per 1000 women. It is a psychotic illness and requires immediate psychiatric intervention and expert support. Severe episodes of the 'baby blues' may lead to postnatal depression, and untreated depression may develop into a major depressive psychosis (Cox 1986).

Characteristics of the illness are rapid onset (usually within the first postnatal week), hallucinations, mood swings, loss of contact with reality, intrusive thought processes and loss of inhibitions (Kendell et al 1987).

One explanation for the development of puerperal psychosis is the major change which occurs in the levels of the steroid hormones at this time, especially the drop in oestrogen (Wieck 1989). It is thought that high-risk patients develop a hypersensitivity of the *central* $D_2$ receptors and that this may be related to the effect of the drop in the oestrogen level on the dopamine system. Another theory is that the condition is related to the fall in progesterone levels which occurs after delivery (Dalton 1985).

Psychosocial and obstetric factors are also thought to be possible causes of puerperal psychosis. Those who appear to be at higher risk include:

- primiparae who have had major obstetric problems, including caesarean section
- those from the higher socioeconomic groups
- those who are older than average at the birth of their first child, are married, and have a relatively long interval from marriage to the birth of their first child
- those who have had a major life event shortly before or after the birth of their child.

### Advice and care

- Antenatal risk assessment is critical; a family history of perinatal mental illness increases the risk.
- Risk of suicide and infanticide is high, so a careful and timely response is critical to best outcomes.
- Need to exclude organic illness, such as sepsis (which could make the woman febrile and confused).
- Treatment consists of medication, hospitalization with baby into specialist mother and baby services and, sometimes, electroconvulsive treatment.
- Prognosis is usually good, with complete recovery; however, risk of recurrence is increased for future pregnancies.
- Social services intervention and child protection referral may be necessary if illness is severe with risk to self and baby.
- Ongoing support may be necessary from specialist services following hospital discharge to monitor wellbeing.

**Reflective activity 69.2**

You are preparing to transfer home a woman who had her baby by emergency caesarean section 3 days ago. She appears agitated, unsettled and is reluctant to care for her baby. On further communication she appears disturbed, unable to hold eye contact and finds it difficult to answer your questions. Some of her responses to your questions concern you. See the website for points you may consider.

## MEDICATION DURING PREGNANCY AND BREASTFEEDING

To minimize the risk of harm to the fetus or infant, drugs should be prescribed cautiously for women who are planning a pregnancy, pregnant or breastfeeding. As a result, the thresholds for non-drug treatments, particularly psychological treatments, are likely to be lower than those set in NICE clinical guidelines on specific mental disorders, and prompt and timely access to treatments should be ensured if they are to be of benefit.

Discussions about treatment options with a woman with a mental disorder who is pregnant or breastfeeding should cover:

- the risk of relapse or deterioration in symptoms and the woman's ability to cope with untreated or sub-threshold symptoms
- severity of previous episodes, response to treatment, and the woman's preference
- the possibility that stopping a drug with known teratogenic risk after pregnancy has been confirmed may not remove the risk of malformations
- the risks from stopping medication abruptly
- the need for prompt treatment because of the potential impact of an untreated mental disorder on the fetus or infant
- the increased risk of harm associated with drug treatments during pregnancy and the postnatal period, including the risk in overdose
- treatment options that would enable the woman to breastfeed if she wishes, rather than recommending she does not breastfeed.

When prescribing a drug for a woman with a mental disorder who is planning a pregnancy, pregnant or breastfeeding, prescribers should:

- choose drugs with lower risk profiles for the mother and the fetus or infant
- start at the lowest effective dose, and slowly increase it; this is particularly important where the risks may be dose related
- use monotherapy in preference to combination treatments
- consider additional precautions for preterm, low birthweight or sick infants.

> *Stopping any medication that is prescribed for a mental illness should be managed by a medical practitioner and preferably a psychiatrist; the risk to the woman may outweigh any fetal benefit. Acute withdrawal and rapid deterioration is likely with tragic consequences.*
>
> (NICE 2007)

## CONCLUSION

All women must be cared for with sensitivity, and encouraged to explore their own feelings in a safe and supported way. They should be confident that their care will be non-prejudiced and that there will be no stigma associated with disclosure of previous mental illness. Adequate resources must be made available to ensure the woman receives the care appropriate to her needs. There is a growing recognition amongst midwives of the value of self-reflection. Midwives caring for women with profound emotional disturbances may reflect on their own life experiences, identifying a personal need for support.

Initially midwives should be encouraged to discuss any areas of difficulty with their supervisor of midwives, but ultimately they will only be able to offer holistic woman-centred care if they are emotionally well themselves (Ch. 12). It is essential that employers recognize the potential stress midwives may be under when caring for women with profound problems and ensure that an adequate level of non-judgemental support exists for staff as well as for women using the service (Hammett 1997).

### KEY POINTS

- It is important that midwives assess and monitor women's mental health during pregnancy and childbirth.
- Mental health problems may be experienced prior to, during or after the physiological and socio-psychological impact of pregnancy and childbirth.
- Midwives can support and prepare women should they experience minor or major mental health problems.
- Collaborative working and effective referral are crucial in supporting and managing women who experience mental health difficulties, and their families.
- Midwives need to be aware of the potential impact of mental health problems on the family and wider society.

## REFERENCES


Bartley M, Owen C: Relation between socioeconomic status, employment and health during economic change, *British Medical Journal* 313(7055):445–449, 1996.

Beck C, Reynolds MA, Rutowski P: Maternity blues and postpartum depression, *Journal of Obstetric, Gynecologic and Neonatal Nursing* 21(4):287–293, 1992.

Bick D, MacArthur C, Knowles H, et al: *Postnatal care: evidence and guidelines for management*, Edinburgh, 2002, Harcourt, pp 129–146.

Bloom J: Midwifery and perinatal mental health care provision, *British Journal of Midwifery* 9(6):385–388, 2002.

Clement S: 'Listening visits' in pregnancy: a strategy for preventing postnatal depression? *Midwifery* 11(2):75–80, 1995.

Clifford C, Day A, Cox J, et al: A cross-cultural analysis of the use of the Edinburgh Post-Natal Depression Scale (EPDS) in health visiting practice, *Journal of Advanced Nursing* 30(3):655–664, 1999.

Cox J: *Postnatal depression. A guide for health professionals*, Edinburgh, 1986, Churchill Livingstone.

Cox J, Holden J, editors: *Perinatal psychiatry*, London, 1994, Gaskell.

Cox J, Murray D, Chapman G: A controlled study of the onset, duration and prevalence of postnatal depression, *British Journal of Psychiatry* 163(1):27–31, 1993.

Creedy DK, Shochet IM, Horsfall J: Childbirth and the development of acute trauma symptoms: incidence and contributing factors, *Birth* 27(2):104–108, 2000.

Dalton K: Progesterone prophylaxis used successfully in postnatal depression, *The Practitioner* 229:507–508, 1985.

Department of Health (DH): *National service framework for mental health: modern standards and service models for mental health*, London, 1999, DH.

Department of Health (DH): *Mainstreaming gender and women's mental health: implementation guidance*, London, 2003, DH.

Department of Health (DH): *Maternity matters: choice, access and continuity of care in a safe service*, London, 2007, DH.

Evans J, Heron J, Oke S, et al: Cohort study of depressed mood during pregnancy and after childbirth, *British Medical Journal* 323(7307):257–260, 2001.

Forman DN, Videbech P, Hedegaard MD, et al: Postpartum depression: identification of women at risk, *British Journal of Obstetrics and Gynaecology* 107(10):1210–1217, 2000.

Green JM, Murray D: The use of the Edinburgh Postnatal Depression Scale in research to explore the relationship between antenatal and postnatal dysphoria. In Cox JL, Holden JM, editors: *Perinatal psychiatry: use and misuse of the Edinburgh Postnatal Depression Scale*, London, 1994, Gaskell.

Gutteridge KEA: Failing women: the impact of sexual abuse on childbirth, *British Journal of Midwifery* 9(5):312–315, 2001.

Hammett PL: Midwives and debriefing. In Kirkham MJ, Perkins ER, editors: *Reflections on midwifery*, London, 1997, Baillière Tindall, pp 135–159.

Hannah P, Adams D, Lee A, et al: Links between early post-partum mood and post-natal depression, *British Journal of Psychiatry* 160(6):777–780, 1992.

Hedegaard M, Henriksen TB, Sabroe S, et al: Psychological distress in pregnancy and preterm delivery, *British Medical Journal* 307(6898):234–239, 1993.

Kendall-Tackett K, Kaufman-Kantor G: *Postpartum depression: a comprehensive approach for nurses*, Newbury Park, CA, 1993, Sage.

Kendell RE, Chalmers JC, Platz C: Epidemiology of puerperal psychoses, *British Journal of Psychiatry* 150:662–673, 1987.

Kirkham M, editor: *The mother–midwife relationship*, Hampshire, 2000, Palgrave MacMillan.

Kumar R, Robson K: A prospective study of emotional disorders in childbearing women, *British Journal of Psychiatry* 144(1):35–47, 1984.

Laing KG: Post-traumatic stress disorder: myth or reality? *British Journal of Midwifery* 9(7):447–451, 2001.

Lavender T, Walkinshaw SA: Can midwives reduce postpartum psychological morbidity? A randomized trial, *Birth* 25(4):215–219, 1998.

Levy V, Kline P: Perinatal depression: a factor analysis, *British Journal of Midwifery* 2(4):154–159, 1994.

Lewis G, editor: *Why mothers die. The Sixth Report of the Confidential Enquiries into Maternal Deaths in the United Kingdom 2000–2002*, London, 2004, RCOG.

Lewis G, editor: *Saving mothers' lives: reviewing maternal deaths to make motherhood safer – 2003–2005. The Seventh Report on Confidential Enquiries into Maternal Deaths in the United Kingdom*, London, 2007, CEMACH.

Lyons S: A prospective study of post traumatic stress symptoms one month following child birth in a group of 42 first-time mothers, *Journal of Infant and Reproductive Psychology* 16(2/3):91–105, 1998.

MacArthur C, Winter HR, Bick DE, et al: Effects of redesigned community postnatal care on women's health 4 months after birth: a cluster randomised controlled trial, *The Lancet* 359(9304):378–385, 2002.

Marks MN, Kumar R: Infanticide in England and Wales, *Medicine Science and the Law* 33(4):329–339, 1993.

MIND: *Understanding postnatal depression*, London, 2001, Mind Publications.

Murray JL, Lopez AD: *The global burden of disease: a comprehensive assessment of mortality and disability from diseases, injuries and risk factors in 1990 and projected to 2020. Summary*, Boston, 1996, Harvard School of Public Health/World Health Organization.

Murray L, Cooper P: Effects of postnatal depression on infant development, *Archives of Disease in Childhood* 77(2):99–101, 1997.

NICE: *CG1 Schizophrenia – core interventions in the treatment and management of schizophrenia in primary and secondary care*, London, 2002, NICE.

NICE: *CG16 Self-harm: the short-term physical and psychological management and secondary prevention of self-harm in primary and secondary care*, London, 2004a, NICE.

NICE: *CG9 Eating disorders: core interventions in the treatment and management of anorexia nervosa, bulimia nervosa and related eating disorders*, London, 2004b, NICE.

NICE: *CG31 Obsessive compulsive disorder: core interventions in the treatment of obsessive compulsive disorder and body dysmorphic disorder*, London, 2005a, NICE.

NICE: *Post-traumatic stress disorder (PTSD): the management of PTSD in adults and children in primary and secondary care*, London, 2005b, NICE.

NICE: *CG45 Antenatal and postnatal mental health – treatment and service provision*, London, 2007, NICE.

Niven C: *Psychological care for families: before, during and after birth*, Oxford, 1992, Butterworth-Heinmann.

Oates M: *Perinatal maternal mental health services (Council Report CR88)*, London, 2000, Royal College of Psychiatrists.

Oates M: Deaths from psychiatric causes. In Lewis G, editor: *Why mothers die 1997–99: Fifth Report of the Confidential Enquiries into Maternal Deaths in the United Kingdom*, London, 2001, RCOG, pp 165–187.

Oates M: Deaths from psychiatric causes. In Lewis G, editor: *Why mothers die 2000–2002: The Sixth Report of the Confidential Enquiries into Maternal Deaths in the United Kingdom*, London, 2004, RCOG.

O'Hara MW, Zekoski EM: Postpartum depression: a comprehensive review. In Kumar R, Brockington IF, editors: *Motherhood and mental illness*, vol. 2, London, 1988, Wright, pp 17–63.

O'Hara MW, Schlechte JA, Lewis DA: Prospective study of postpartum blues, *Archives of General Psychiatry* 48(9):801–806, 1991.

Pagel MD, Smilkstein G, Regen H, et al: Psychosocial influences on new born outcomes: a controlled prospective study, *Social Science & Medicine* 30(5):597–604, 1990.

Pantlen A, Rohde A: Psychological effects of traumatic deliveries, *Zentralblatt fur Gynakologie* 123(1):42–47, 2001.

Robinson J: The perils of psychiatric records, *British Journal of Midwifery* 10(3):173, 2002.

Romito P: Unhappiness after childbirth. In Chalmers I, Enkin M, Keirse MJNC, editors: *Effective care in pregnancy and childbirth*, Oxford, 1989, Oxford University Press.

Saltman D: *Women and health: an introduction*, Sydney, 1991, Harcourt Brace Jovanovich.

Stein A, Cooper PJ, Campbell EA, et al: Social adversity and perinatal complications: their relation to postnatal depression, *British Medical Journal* 171(29):1073–1074, 1989.

Teixeira JMA, Fisk NM, Glover V: Association between maternal anxiety in pregnancy and increased uterine artery resistance index: cohort based study, *British Medical Journal* 318(7177):153–157, 1999.

Watson JP, Elliott SA, Rugg AJ, et al: Psychiatric disorder in pregnancy and the first postnatal year, *British Journal of Psychiatry* 144(5):453–462, 1984.

Wieck JP: Endocrine aspects of postnatal depression, *Baillière's Clinical Obstetrics and Gynaecology* 3(4):857–877, 1989.

Wilson LM, Reid AJ, Midmer DK, et al: Antenatal psychosocial risk factors associated with adverse postnatal family outcomes, *Canadian Medical Association* 154(6):785–799, 1996.

World Health Organization (WHO): *The ICD-10 classification of mental and behavioural disorders*, Geneva, 1992, WHO.

World Health Organization (WHO): *Violence against women: a priority health issue*, Geneva, 1997, WHO.

World Health Organization (WHO): *Women's mental health – an evidence based review*, Geneva, 2000, WHO.

Chapter |70|

# Grief and bereavement

Jenni Thomas OBE

## LEARNING OUTCOMES

After reading this chapter, you will be able to:

- understand the complexities of the grieving process and how this may manifest in different women, their partners and families
- consider the needs of women, their partners and families who are suffering a bereavement around childbirth
- develop practice strategies which will increase the support to families and which facilitate the positive preservation of memories
- explore your own attitudes to death and bereavement and consider how these might affect the care provided to families and colleagues.

*And can it be that in a world so full and busy, the loss of one weak creature makes a void in any heart, so wide and deep that nothing but the width and depth of vast eternity can fill it up!*

(Charles Dickens, *Dombey and Son*)

With better antenatal care and advances in technology, childbirth is now relatively safe, and the birth of a child is usually a cause for celebration and joy rather than as in Dickens' time, when childbirth itself held significant dangers for mother and baby (see Fig. 70.1). Sadly, even now, some babies do die – there were 3603 stillbirths and 2380 neonatal deaths recorded in England, Wales and Northern Ireland in 2006 (Lewis 2007, ONS 2006). In addition, it is estimated that 20% of confirmed pregnancies end in miscarriage before 20 weeks' gestation.

Death is a part of life and therefore inevitable, but the death of a baby before, at, or shortly after birth, because of miscarriage, termination for fetal abnormality, stillbirth or neonatal death, is unexpected and against the natural order of things. It is unique, incomprehensible and unlike any other death. When an adult or a child dies, family members have memories to draw upon and a life to remember, but when a baby dies, parents grieve the lack of memories and any future with their child. For most parents the death of a baby is a significant and painful experience, regardless of the cause or gestational age. Parents depend on those in the health service, including midwives, to care for them and offer relevant information to guide them in the choices they have to make in this time of crisis.

It has only been in the last 15–25 years that the importance of grieving in achieving a healthy long-term outcome has been recognized. Research at the Tavistock Clinic in London has shown that, following stillbirth, bereaved mothers may suffer lifelong repercussions, including hypochondria, phobias and disturbances in relationships (Lewis & Bourne 1989). Appropriate professional help and support throughout the period are essential. Recognizing and responding to the parents' feelings, sensing what they need and helping them to make informed choices are the challenges for professionals involved in caring for these parents before, during and after the birth of their baby (Schott et al 2007).

There is no right way to grieve, no set way of managing these difficult situations, and the midwife needs to learn through involvement with grieving families. The insights and suggestions for practice made in this chapter are based on what parents have taught professionals through sharing their particular needs.

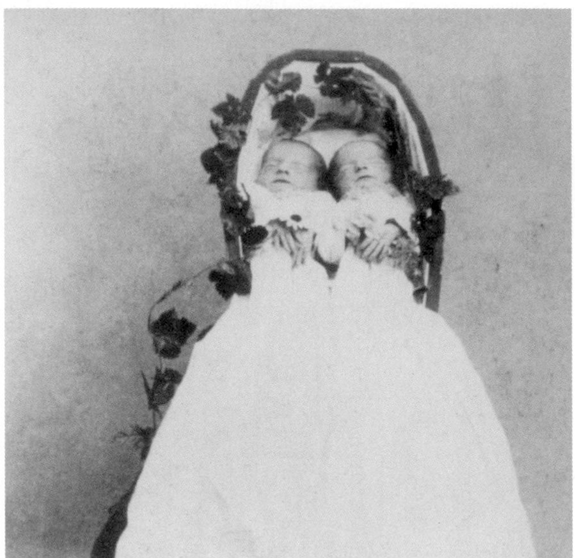

**Figure 70.1** Twins in casket at home, 1890.

## THERAPEUTIC USE OF OURSELVES

As individuals we naturally tend to turn away from looking at painful things, yet it is only in looking at ourselves that we can grow and ultimately help others. When a baby dies at or soon after birth, the exposure to the parents' grief, sadness and pain may remind us of our own previous losses. Midwives themselves may have experienced pregnancy loss, or had difficulty in achieving motherhood, and this can impact on their feelings and experience of caring for women and families who also lose babies (Bewley 2010).

The process of helping is an active one, requiring a willingness to become involved, to share in the painful process, be congruent, express concern but remain separate, enabling the provision of sensitive care. This requires a high degree of self-awareness and recognition of our own feelings. This can be assisted by reflecting on previous life experiences that have been difficult – hurts experienced, broken relationships and other situations that have involved loss. This increases understanding of why we react in certain ways, our own limitations and when professionally we are likely to need support. As carers, if we are able to acknowledge and appropriately express our own anger, fear, sadness and embarrassment, other people's emotions can be accepted more easily.

Interactions with people who are profoundly distressed engender feelings of inadequacy and helplessness, and this is in contrast to the normal healthcare role of helping 'make people feel better and remove pain'. In bereavement, people cannot be made better – in contrast, healing occurs when people are able to feel and express their painful feelings.

When caring for bereaved families, the caregiver's feelings often mirror those of the family – anger, sadness, confusion, a sense of failure. Management that recognizes and acknowledges the value of staff's contributions in this work and their need for support helps to build individuals' self-esteem in times of stress. Having access to a professional offering support or counselling based in the hospital can be as valuable for staff as it is for parents.

## LOOKING AFTER OURSELVES AS PROFESSIONALS

Emotions are also felt physically and we carry them in different parts of our body – tension can be felt in the muscles of the shoulder, grief and sadness perhaps in the muscles around the neck, heart and stomach. Knowing which parts of our body are affected in times of stress, enables identification of ways of releasing these trapped emotions. Relaxation, vigorous exercise, listening to music, counselling or perhaps watching a comedy programme on television and seeking support are therapeutic outlets.

When people feel unable to deal with their own emotions, they develop protective strategies, such as distancing themselves from other people's emotions, appearing unaffected and detached or conversely becoming very busy in order to avoid their emotional pain. They may develop negative feelings about themselves and their work and see themselves as failures. This can manifest itself as anger or resentment, which can colour family and professional relationships. Some of the warning signs of feeling depleted include experiencing chronic exhaustion, frequently feeling upset, difficulties in eating or sleeping or engaging with people; developing headaches or backaches; having nightmares; feeling worthless and pessimistic; avoiding contact with others; arriving late for work and leaving early.

### Support and training for midwives working in partnership with families

Caring for distressed parents is difficult and demanding, and requires staff who are in a working environment that considers their needs and values them as individuals. Where appropriate support mechanisms are in place, midwifery teams are able to provide the best possible care to families. Bereaved parents are deeply grateful and remember the care they received throughout their lives (see website).

Bereavement skills training and support should be an intrinsic part of maternity care, whatever the setting (Schott et al 2007). Using counselling and listening skills is an essential part of the professional's role and requires training, enabling midwives to care effectively when managing the death of a baby.

It is important that the midwife is aware of:

- policies relevant to different areas of care
- different choices available for parents
- suppporting and developing student midwives' skills in bereavement
- the need for different members of staff to be involved in providing bereavement care
- the psychological and professional needs of colleagues
- the value of debriefing/reflective sessions, as a support, development and sharing grood practice process
- support available from the Supervisor of Midwives.

When staff do take the time to talk about their needs, their feelings, their reactions to situations and to understand their strengths and limitations, then working with families in grief is special and rewarding.

## UNDERSTANDING LOSS AND GRIEF

> *If bereavement is what's happened to you, grief is how you feel, and mourning is what you do.*
>
> (Dr Richard Wilson, Consultant Paediatrician)

There are many theories explaining the grieving process, including Bowlby's (1980) attachment theory, Kubler-Ross (1970) and Parkes' (1972) series of predictable grief reactions which make up stages or phases of the grief response; and Worden's (1991) 'tasks of mourning'.

**Reflective activity 70.1**

Review your knowledge of the stages and tasks of the grieving process. Think of a hurt or loss that you have experienced. What were some of the feelings that you experienced associated with that loss? What help did you need?

Consider the behaviour of the last person you cared for who was coping with a death or loss – perhaps a woman who had a baby with a congenital abnormality. Did the person experience any of the recognized tasks in the process of mourning? Did the person move in and out of various tasks?

Which behaviour did you find hardest to manage as a practitioner?

These tasks of mourning are useful as a framework for understanding the grieving response following the death of a baby. Worden (1991) stresses that mourning, defined as the emotional process that occurs after a loss, is an essential and necessarily painful healing process. As with healing after physical injury, the process can be delayed or go wrong. The midwife has a significant part to play in helping parents begin to accomplish in particular the first two of the following tasks:

1. Accept the reality of the loss.
2. Work through to the pain of grief.
3. Adjust to an environment in which the deceased is missing.
4. Emotionally relocate the deceased and move on with life.

### Accepting the reality of the loss

Initially, the parents are unlikely to believe the bad news and will be in a state of shock and denial, even when a death has been anticipated. Some bereaved parents cry uncontrollably, become hysterical or collapse, whereas others feel faint or numb and display few signs of emotion, appearing very controlled, calm and detached. The initial shock may last for hours or several days. This natural reaction is a form of emotional protection that disappears as parents gradually take in the full impact of events. Each experience of grief is unique and previous losses may also complicate the reaction to this current bereavement.

Parents may initially be unable to acknowledge what has happened and may manage by denying the reality. These parents need time and help to do what is right for them. It is not helpful for professionals to collude with denial and unreality, for example by avoiding talking about the dead baby, somehow making the child's death seem less important – not showing or fully acknowledging its significance.

Midwives can help enable parents to gradually face reality. Being sensitive to parents' needs, discussing what other parents have valued, offering choices, such as seeing and holding their dead baby, being involved as much as possible in the preparations for the funeral, and observing rituals and traditions, all help to make what has happened real. Families from different faiths need support for the mourning rituals appropriate to their culture (Thomas 2001, Schott et al 2007, CBC 2007d).

### Working through to the pain of grief

As denial and numbness gradually subside, the bereaved parents usually experience the full impact of what has happened. Intensely painful feelings may last many weeks or months. This normal reaction to an abnormal event can be overwhelming as they think about what could have been and what the future now holds. Bereaved mothers are often incapable of thinking about anything or anybody else and are consumed with their child, themselves and how they feel. Painful reminders get in the way and are all around them. Innocent comments may get misinterpreted and cause distress and irritability. Susan Hill (1990), a writer and bereaved mother, eloquently described her extreme sensitivity after the death of her baby Imogen as 'like having one skin less', and appreciated the professionals who treated her gently.

It is normal to feel extremely sad, guilty, angry and resentful. Many parents struggle with guilty feelings about some aspect of their baby's death, especially if they were initially ambivalent about becoming parents. Mothers may think about their behaviours or actions taken which they may blame for causing the death of their baby, such as running for a bus or carrying heavy shopping. These punishing thoughts can intrude into all aspects of their life.

Feelings of anger are often unexpected and hard to manage. The father or mother may feel anger for the loss of control that death brings; their anger can be directed at the medical and midwifery team for not recognizing the problem sooner, for not keeping their baby alive; anger at a God who allowed it to happen; and possibly anger towards their baby for not living and leaving them. Sometimes, unexpected resentment towards a family member or their partner adds to this exhausting and painful time.

Grief is not a mental illness, although sleeplessness, anxiety, fear, anger and a preoccupation with self can all add up to a feeling of 'going mad'. These feelings are normal, and when experienced and expressed, slowly become less intrusive and frequent. Talking or writing about difficult experiences with someone who is interested and willing to listen is one of the healing ways to express grief. Attempts to cut short these emotions rarely help in the long term and may cause deep-seated problems in the years ahead. If grief is denied, or anger and guilt persist to the exclusion of other feelings over a number of months, help may be needed from someone trained in counselling.

## Adjusting to an environment in which the deceased is missing

However short a time the parents had to get to know their baby, both during pregnancy and after the birth, facing a future without this child in the family is a difficult and painful process. Nothing can fill the aching void their baby has left and each day of life brings constant reminders of their baby's absence. The future seems uncertain and frightening, while a tremendous effort is required to carry on as normal.

Grief is exhausting. It may take many months before the mother, particularly, is able to focus less on the sad events surrounding the death and regain some of her interest in life. Parents may also revisit the feelings of loss at what would have been significant milestones in their child's life, such as expected date of birth, anniversaries and birthdays.

## Emotionally relocating the deceased and moving on with life

This involves moving on to a different and new way of life without their child, whilst remembering and holding on to precious memories. It is a process of reinvesting in life again alongside the knowledge that their baby will not be forgotten. This can often feel like a betrayal and is perhaps more difficult than generally recognized.

When parents are able to move on with their lives together, there is a sense of putting the distress aside and looking to the future, whilst recalling memories of their baby and finding comfort and pleasure in these memories. It is a way of making life meaningful again and gaining back some control, so that the bereaved parents are not continually ambushed by memories of the death and trapped by painful feelings.

## The importance of the loss

When a baby lives only a short time or dies before birth, because of miscarriage, termination for fetal anomaly or stillbirth, a common assumption is that the loss is not as significant. Pregnancy is a time of anticipation and many parents, particularly mothers, develop a strong bond with their baby long before it is born (Fig. 70.2). When a baby dies, parents grieve for all they had hoped and the lost opportunity of getting to know their child in a future they had planned together.

This grief response may be seen in families when a baby is born with a disability, who may experience the same feelings of loss of the healthy baby they were expecting and anger at the extinction of their hopes and plans. For some parents, the need for a caesarean section can result

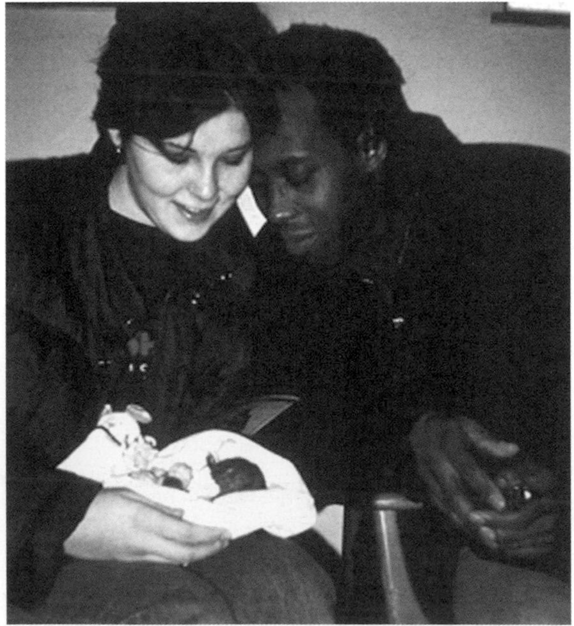

**Figure 70.2** Claire and Joseph with daughter Ellie, who died at birth.

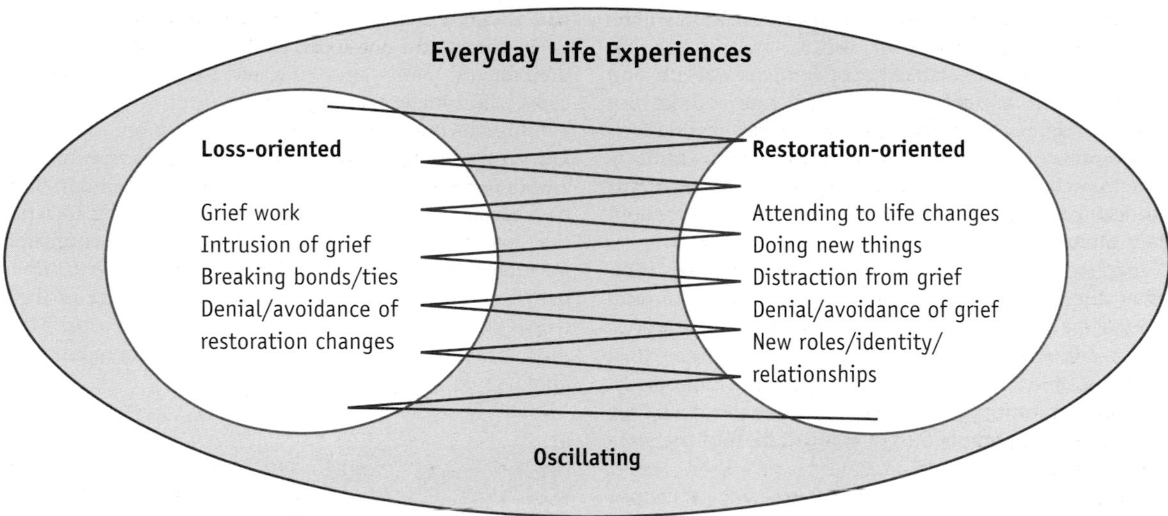


**Figure 70.3** A dual process model of coping with loss. *(From Stroebe and Schut, 1999, with permission.)*

in a sense of failure and a reaction of grief for a different birth expectation.

A Stillbirth and Neonatal Death Society (SANDS) teardrop sticker placed on the mother's notes after a baby's death alerts all professionals to the parents' immediate and long-term need for sensitivity. At initial booking, it is important for the midwife to identify women who have had previous losses – miscarriage, stillbirth or neonatal death – and discuss the implications for the current pregnancy. This requires opening up a potentially painful subject; however, the midwife needs to be aware that this discussion allows the dead child to be acknowledged and their existence as an individual valued.

The midwife can also help prepare the woman for reactions and feelings that she might experience during the pregnancy and birth of this baby, which might include mixed feelings at the birth, and high levels of anxiety concerning the baby's wellbeing and survival (Caelli et al 1999, Hunfeld et al 1997). The healthcare team can be alert to this mother's needs, and ensure that support systems are available during the pregnancy and puerperium (Thomas 2001, Schott et al 2007). Bereaved mothers may be inclined to develop postnatal depression, particularly in cases of complicated grief.

## DIFFERENT PARENTAL RESPONSES IN BEREAVEMENT

Grief is solitary – even when a couple are grieving, each parent can feel alone in his or her grief, and normal patterns in relationships may become disrupted. As a father's and mother's needs are different, they may find they are unable to communicate with one another, to express the awfulness of their feelings. Women naturally tend to be more loss-oriented and focus on their loss and the emotions they are experiencing. They need memories and to constantly recall, be reminded of and talk about their baby who has died. Men are generally more restoration-oriented – they want things to return to normal and prefer to look to the future. Although they feel the loss, it is a loss not to be acknowledged (Puddifoot & Johnson 1997) and this response may be interpreted by their partner, and others, as being uncaring and less interested in their baby. The dual process model of grieving (Stroebe & Schut 1999) illustrates the way bereaved people engage in both loss-oriented and restoration oriented grieving behaviour and oscillate in healthy grieving between the two behaviours (Fig. 70.3).

The midwife needs to assist the couple to understand the different perspectives and ways of dealing with grief, so that they are able to support each other through this period (see website).

### Supporting parents

Women and men say that the most supportive care is when professionals are able to help and encourage parents to 'parent' (CBT 2003a, 2003c, CBC 2007a), to be involved with their baby before and after death.

Both parents need support and both need information, though it should be remembered that it is often difficult for distressed parents to absorb and understand what they are told. It is useful to ask the parents to explain to you what they have understood. They may want more information about their baby's condition or to know more about the reason for their baby's death, and so any help the midwife can provide in obtaining this information will be welcomed (Schott et al 2007).

Parents appreciate staff who offer them warmth and understanding, are able to show they care and are not afraid to express their own emotions. In expressing feelings, professionals act as role models and tears are unlikely to be viewed negatively if genuinely felt. However, parents need support and should not have to be concerned about their midwife's feelings or experiences of grief.

*Touching* is the most basic form of comfort and communication. This may be a hand on the arm, or an arm around the parent's shoulder. Parents need the opportunity to talk about how they feel with someone they trust and if possible to be able to express their emotions openly. It is not helpful for parents to be told how they feel; only they can know. Parents do not want to be told the stage of grief they are seen to be at.

Often midwives spend many hours with a couple. Talking about everyday things, offering opportunities for normal conversation, can be useful, as well as being quiet and recognizing that just being there and being available to the parents is valuable. Self-aware midwives can be intuitive and trust their own instincts when interacting with parents; listening carefully is the key.

It is important to talk to both parents and acknowledge that both parents are grieving. It is helpful to provide information to parents who may want to do the practical things that have to be done, together.

All staff – hospital and community midwife, doctor, chaplain, counsellor and social worker, support staff and, later, GP and health visitor – need to adopt a team approach with everyone being aware of the procedures to follow when a bereavement occurs. Good team relationships are essential to provide the best possible care to bereaved parents.

## BREAKING BAD NEWS

> *The worst bit for me was knowing something was going wrong but no one actually told me.*
>
> (Bereaved mother)

Whether their baby's death is anticipated or occurs suddenly, parents value the support of caring professional staff. Parents remember the way they are told bad news and the words, actions and attitudes of the professionals involved. This places a heavy burden on the professional who has the responsibility of telling parents such sad information. Explaining bad news involves both parents together whenever possible, and should take place in a private and appropriate room. Parents appreciate honesty and a genuinely caring approach by the professional in such a situation. Clear, unambiguous information needs to be sensitively given, in a way that uses language the parents understand. An interpreter needs to be present when parents do not speak or understand English. Children in the family must not be used to translate and convey information to parents.

Information may have to be repeated more than once. Questions should be answered as honestly as possible and allowances should be made for parents to respond in their own time. Offering time and actively listening to what they have to say avoids parents being left with confusing information. Parents remember when you refer to their baby by name and acknowledge the significance of their baby's death. Saying that you are sorry that their baby has died does not mean anyone did anything that requires an apology.

## THE SCAN – THE DIAGNOSIS

The ultrasonographer may be the first person to know that something is wrong. When an appointment is made for a scan, the parents need to be clearly told and understand that the scan is being performed to detect any problem that their baby may have and that a partner or friend may accompany the mother.

When the scan reveals an abnormality or that their baby has died, the sonographer present needs initially to explain to the parents that there is reason for concern. These situations require the presence of a doctor as soon as possible to confirm a possible diagnosis and future course of action. The mother and father should be offered an opportunity to see the scan of their baby while the doctor explains honestly and sensitively what is wrong. All staff need to be familiar with the unit policy to be followed in such a crisis. When further tests are necessary, these need to be carried out as soon as possible and the reliability of these tests and any risks involved carefully explained.

Parents are likely to be in shock and the couple need privacy and time to absorb what they have been told and their options. Keeping a scan photograph in the mother's notes for collection at a later date is helpful. It is the responsibility of the midwife looking after these parents to inform them that the community team and their GP will receive all the relevant information. This liaison between the hospital and the community is vital for parents when leaving the hospital.

**Reflective activity 70.2**

What system does your unit/service have in place to ensure effective communication when managing a pregnancy loss or the death of a baby? How do you personally ensure that a death has been appropriately communicated to colleagues in the community including midwives, GP and health visitors?

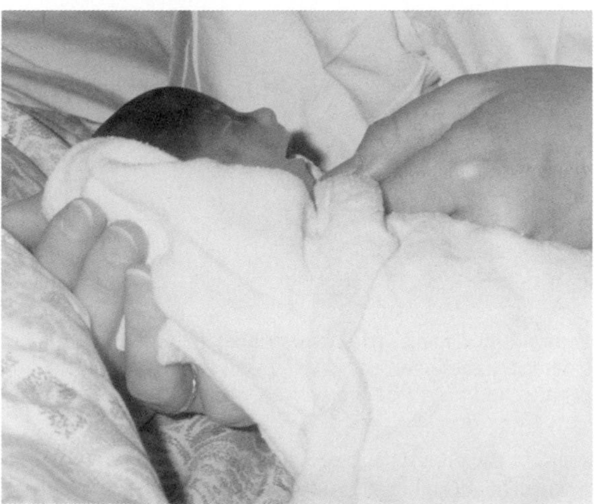

**Figure 70.4** Rose Elizabeth at 21 weeks' gestation being held by her father. (By kind permission of the parents, and not to be reproduced without permission.)

## MISCARRIAGE

Miscarriage is the loss of a pregnancy before 24 weeks' gestation. For many people the miscarriage of their baby at any gestation in pregnancy is a devastating experience (Fig. 70.4) and especially so when couples have previously experienced infertility or an ectopic pregnancy. Pregnancy and the feelings associated with becoming parents are unique. Parents find phrases used by professionals such as 'blighted ovum', 'missed abortion' or 'non-viable fetus' unhelpful, meaningless and hurtful. During the second trimester, most parents-to-be acknowledge openly that they are expecting a baby and a miscarriage may be experienced as the stillbirth of their baby. There are no set rules to follow in caring for people at such sensitive times and staff need to recognize and respond to parents' very varied feelings, trying to sense what each individual needs. Hospitals are now being asked to offer parents a form of certificate acknowledging the birth of their baby at less than 24 weeks' gestation should the baby be born with no signs of life (Stillbirth and Neonatal Death Society – SANDS).

## TERMINATION DUE TO ANOMALY

When informed about an anomaly detected in pregnancy, parents in distress may make decisions in haste which they later regret. Staff should encourage parents not to hurry decisions, to acknowledge how difficult it is for them at this time and suggest they take time together, preferably at home, before making any final decisions. Parents need clear, unbiased information, in understandable language, about their baby's condition and the options available to them, including information about the mode of delivery. Providing written information before any decisions are made is crucial. A leaflet from the organization ARC (Antenatal Results and Choices) is useful to parents. Some choose to continue with their pregnancy and need support to do what is right for them, whether their baby will have significant problems or will not live. Whatever the outcome, their choice will affect the rest of their lives and their decision will involve grieving for the baby they had been expecting.

When parents have made a decision to end the pregnancy, they may not feel able to experience or express any attachment to their baby. The grief of these parents is complicated and the guilt often profound, as they have taken the responsibility for ending the life of their child; for some parents, their attachment is as significant as if their baby had survived. It is important for staff not to be judgemental and to offer as much emotional support as is needed. The decision made by parents is no indication of the amount of love they have for their baby.

## LABOUR WHEN A BABY HAS DIED OR IS NOT EXPECTED TO LIVE

> *A baby who has issued forth from its mother after the 24th week of pregnancy and has not at any time after being completely expelled from its mother's body breathed or shown any signs of life is a stillborn baby.*
>
> (NMC 2004:42)

Hospitals can be impersonal, frightening places and the sensitive care offered by a midwife is crucial. Providing an atmosphere in which parents are able to trust the professional caring for them is enhanced by having a suitable, comfortable and private bereavement room. The entire team needs to know when bereaved people are admitted to the unit.

On meeting these parents, the midwife needs to immediately acknowledge the situation and say how sorry he or she is, then to spend time listening to parents, building a relationship and responding to their varied needs and feelings. Not all parents realize that the labour and delivery of their baby will need to be physically the same as giving birth to a live baby. This realization may be hard to comprehend and may cause anger and disbelief.

> *To find myself carrying death and, even worse, being told I had to give birth to death, was the most horrific scenario.*
>
> (Bereaved mother)

## Practical considerations

> *The silence in the delivery room was deafening. This was the reality – this was death at birth.*
>
> (Bereaved mother)

The mother who is expecting a stillbirth or late miscarriage requires significant psychological support, but the principles of care during labour for this woman are similar to those for a woman expecting a live birth.

In situations where a baby has died in utero, the mother may request a substantial amount of pain relief, not being aware that later on, the birth of her baby may be a time she wishes she could fully remember. Experiencing the labour enables a mother to begin to face the reality of giving birth to her baby.

Discussing a birth plan and having some control in a situation where parents feel powerless is psychologically valuable. These choices provide important memories on which to focus in the process of grieving.

> *I didn't have any control over the situation at all and I don't think either of us really knew what was happening until well after.*
>
> (Bereaved mother)

The woman may be in a state of shock, and therefore it is preferable to provide good continuity of care, and the midwife providing that care should be aware of the possibility that information may not be as easily understood, and that this information needs to be simple and accessible, and may need to be repeated.

This woman may be at an increased risk of complications, such as inefficient uterine action, infection, and disseminated intravascular coagulation (DIC), and therefore the care provided must include monitoring of maternal observations and wellbeing, and scrupulous attention to asepsis during examinations. The midwife needs to be aware that the woman is often so immersed in her grief that she will pay scant attention to what she may be physically experiencing.

Having a general anaesthetic for an emergency caesarean section creates what is a potentially complicated grief reaction. These mothers need additional help in facing the reality of what has happened: that their baby, who they will have no recollection of having, has in fact died (Fig. 70.5).

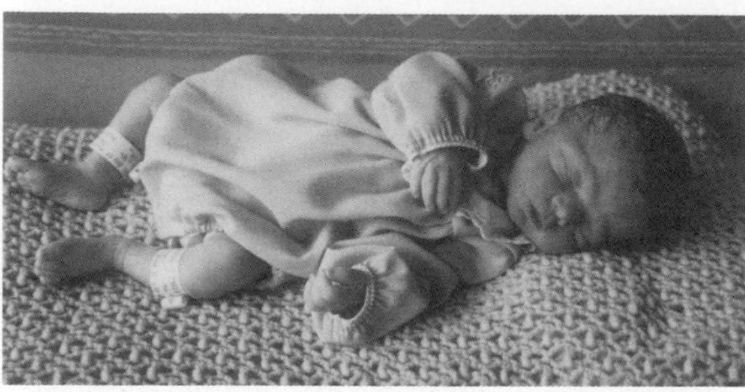

**Figure 70.5** Charlie, who was stillborn following an emergency caesarean section. (By kind permission of the parents, and not to be reproduced without permission.)

## UNEXPECTED DEATH OF A BABY AT OR SOON AFTER BIRTH

When there is serious cause for concern in labour or at delivery, it is essential that the parents are informed immediately of what is suspected and that a doctor is asked to speak to the parents and provide confirmation of the prognosis. The designated midwife needs to be present, to provide additional support to parents and clarify any information as needed.

In this situation, practitioners themselves may experience trauma and guilt and need to have time, opportunity and support for reflection and review.

## Neonatal death

Following the birth of a baby who is not expected to live, parents need to be honestly informed and given time to gradually absorb the painful information. They need reassurance that nothing more can be done for their child and helped to be involved in any decision regarding their baby. When a decision is made to withdraw active treatment, it is vital that it is made with the parents, and that they are provided with whatever time is necessary to make these difficult choices (McHaffie 2001). The availability of a bereavement room in the hours leading to a change from intensive to palliative care will provide parents with the privacy, time and space they need with their child (Fig. 70.6). Some parents prefer to be alone; however they need to know when and where staff can be contacted.

### Spending time with their baby

Initially some parents may actually fear seeing their dead baby; they may be afraid that it will make them more attached and therefore make saying goodbye even harder. For some parents, this will be their first experience of death, and they may be frightened of what their baby will look or feel like. Frequently parents are unable to accept fully what has happened and may manage by denying the reality. There is no need for parents to make any decisions in a hurry. Time and understanding are required with grieving parents, as their denial is a form of emotional protection and with time it will lessen. It is useful for the midwife to explain to the parents that other parents have also felt concerned about seeing or holding their baby, and have later valued the time they have had with their baby. NICE

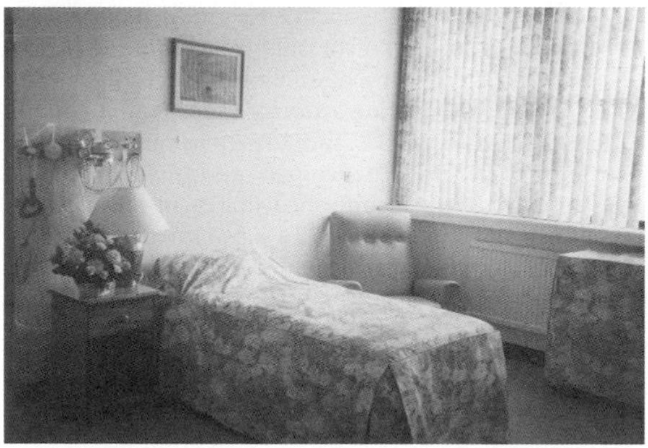

Figure 70.6 The bereavement room adjacent to the delivery suite at Wycombe General Hospital.

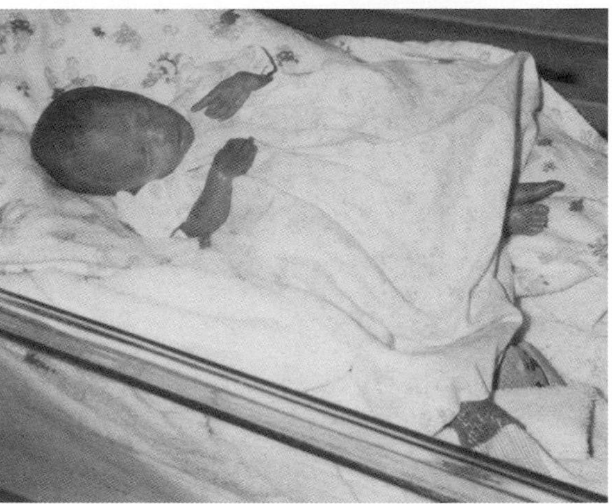

Figure 70.7 Sophie's parents appreciated being able to see her little feet and choose her dress themselves. (By kind permission of the parents, and not to be reproduced without permission.)

guidelines highlighted 'the findings of (Hughes et al 2002) which suggest that women should not be encouraged to hold their dead baby if they do not wish to' (NICE 2007:196). This statement has been challenged by leading organizations, including SANDS and the Royal College of Midwives (RCM), and leading workers within perinatal bereavement (Schott & Henley 2009) as being open to misinterpretation and running the risk of denying many parents an important experience. This guidance is being reviewed. What the guidelines should underline for professionals is the importance of preparing and supporting parents to make an informed choice at this crucial time, and that this will be individual to each family.

These hours after the birth are immensely valuable. Nothing in life can prepare parents for such a tragedy and observing the staff's tenderness and interactions with their baby will remain in the parents' memories for a lifetime.

## Washing and dressing the baby after death

This may be the one opportunity parents have to choose clothes for their child (Fig. 70.7). Staff can make a difference by providing information enabling parents to make choices, including:

- Would the parents like to wash and dress their baby themselves on their own?
- Would they prefer to watch their baby being washed and dressed by a member of staff?
- Do they have clothes they would like to dress their baby in?

It should be unit policy to have a selection of baby clothes from which parents can choose to dress their baby and later keep when they return home. In the future, parents will treasure everything that gives them a sense of their baby. Clothes their baby has worn are best left unwashed, as initially the smell of the clothes will provide parents with a tangible reminder of their baby.

## The importance of memories

Midwifery and neonatal staff who help parents to get to know their baby in the brief time they have together provide a source of precious memories, which will be vitally important in the months ahead (Schott & Henley 2001). Some units now offer parents a memory folder and memory box which can be used to store any special mementoes of their baby. This can include photographs, their baby's name-band, foot and hand prints, a lock of hair, a page where words can be written by anyone who knew the parents and baby, a blessing or naming card, letters and perhaps the clothes their baby wore, the anniversary cards and gifts that people choose to collect and keep for the future.

## The value of photographs

For many people, scan and camera photographs of their baby who has died are immensely important. These parents will be interested in what their baby looked like and will value pictures that clearly show details – their baby's profile, the tiny hands and feet, and perhaps sensitively taken pictures of their baby naked. These photographs help parents to face the reality of what has happened, provide evidence they had a baby and that their child died. Parents may like to know they can have a photograph of themselves holding their baby, a family picture with their other children or the grandparents, or with midwives who cared for them. When a twin dies, taking care and time to photograph the live twin and the dead twin together (Fig. 70.8) is something parents may not naturally consider and yet may so value in what can be a complicated grief process in the years ahead. Later in

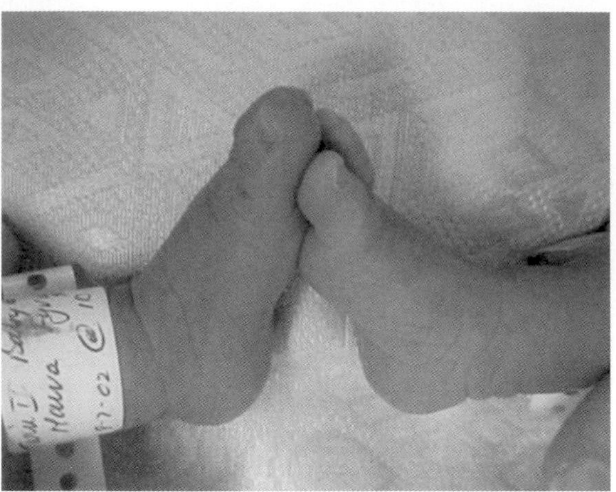

**Figure 70.8** Twins, Christopher and Jessica: Christopher died before he was born. Their parents e-mailed this photograph to announce the birth of their twins. (By kind permission of the parents, and not to be reproduced without permission.)

life the surviving twin may well be interested to know about the sibling who died and to know that his or her twin was acknowledged and mourned – parents in multiple birth and death situations have a great deal to manage and can find this information helpful. A photographic memory guide providing information and practical guidance is available for families and professionals (CBC 2007b, CBC 2007c).

## THE POSTNATAL PERIOD

Physically, the woman requires a high standard of postnatal care, including psychological support, physical assessment, and educational elements of ensuring the woman understands the normal physiological process of the puerperium, and what can be considered normal.

The midwife needs to discuss with the woman where she wishes to be cared for whilst in hospital. The choice is usually between a rapid discharge home, a single room in the antenatal and/or postnatal ward, or on the gynaecology ward. Previous research and experience suggests that some women may wish to have contact with other mothers and babies, while some would wish to be in their home environment, and some may actually feel abandoned after being sent to the gynaecology ward (Hughes 1987). Thinking that a woman can be 'protected' against the sounds of a crying baby may be too simplistic a view.

Wherever the woman is cared for, continuity of carer must be an aim, and the same principles of keeping information simple and accessible should be retained. A difficulty which many women experience and find especially hard will be when a few days after the delivery, the breasts fill with milk, which is a tangible reminder that there was to be a baby to suckle. Previously, bromocriptine has been prescribed to suppress lactation; however, recent concerns with women experiencing serious cardiovascular complications, including stroke and hypertension, has led to reluctance to use this. The woman needs firstly to be told that this may happen, informed that pain relief can be prescribed, and advised to wear a supportive brassiere. For some women, homeopathic remedies may be useful: one study indicated that jasmine flowers were effective (Shrivastav et al 1988).

## POSTMORTEM EXAMINATION (AUTOPSY)

All staff should receive appropriate training in how to sensitively discuss consent for a hospital postmortem with parents. Although a doctor may request and provide information for written postmortem consent, it is often the midwife to whom parents turn for further information, clarification and support, and all midwives must understand the ethical, legal and emotional responsibilities involved (HTA 2006). Obtaining parents' consent should be seen as a continuing process, not limited to the signing of a form.

Key principles to highlight with parents (see website) are as follows:

- The postmortem may provide information as to the cause of their baby's death – this information is important for the future.
- It may not fully ascertain the cause, but may exclude some factors as potential causes.
- It will not affect their baby's face or limbs.
- It will be carried out respectfully and with care.
- Tissue blocks and slides obtained will be kept in medical records. If used for research or education, further consent would be sought (HTA 2006). This should be explained, as parents need to clearly understand the difference.

Graphic details about the postmortem examination may be too overwhelming for some parents, and they need to be offered the opportunity to choose how much or how little information they would like and given time to consider their decision and ask any questions. Sensitive and caring communication is essential in this situation, to ensure consent is a process and is properly sought. It is important that parents feel in control, understand what they are consenting to and have the right to say what happens during and after the postmortem examination (see website).

It is important that the consultant involved in the baby's death meets with the parents and discusses the findings of the postmortem within 4–6 weeks of the death. Many parents value an opportunity to talk to the pathologist before or after the examination.

### Coroner's postmortem

In the event of a sudden or unexplained death, a coroner's postmortem is legally required and in this situation the parents' permission is not requested. The parents' need for time, information and sensitive support is vital. The coroner is responsible for informing parents if organs and/or tissue have been retained to ascertain the cause of death. The length of time an organ will be retained and when it will be returned to the body prior to burial or cremation should be discussed. It is crucial that parents are informed that, with their consent, tissue blocks and slides may be kept as part of the medical record. Parents need to understand that while enquiries into the cause of their baby's death are underway, the death cannot be registered and so final funeral arrangements cannot be made. Normally, however, when an inquest is required, it is held very soon after the death and the funeral need not be delayed. Information regarding a coroner's postmortem and whether an inquest is needed should be available for parents in written format (INQUEST 2003).

### Organ donation

Parents will not necessarily consider asking about heart valve or other tissue or organ donation. They will rely on and appreciate – the professionals who care for them to provide them with information to make informed choices; it is therefore important that information is informed by circumstances when organ donation is possible and in particular that a cause of death is known. Parents who are not asked may wonder why and later may even resent this lack of information.

Parents need to have clear information and explanations from the donor team in their particular region, and would need to be aware that heart valve donation (usually referred to as tissue donation), carried out up to 48 hours after the death of a term baby, may require a large part of the heart to be retained. If a donation from their baby is to be used, blood samples will need to be taken from the mother, father and baby to test for HIV, hepatitis B and C and syphilis.

## RESPECTING PARENTS

As soon as possible after their baby's death, a visit from a senior doctor, accompanied by their midwives, is valuable for parents and provides acknowledgement of the importance of their baby's existence. They will need time with a designated person who can help them with the practical arrangements, to understand what steps to take, legal requirements, what the hospital can and cannot arrange and choices about the funeral. Providing written information, devised in consultation with families, is useful so parents can refer back to it as necessary whilst in hospital and also at home.

## SPIRITUAL NEEDS

All cultures have rituals and traditions that are followed in a major life event, and these provide an opportunity to honour the importance of what has happened and help reality to be faced. When religions and cultures are different from our own, a lack of knowledge and understanding of specific spiritual needs may leave professionals feeling even more helpless, and families dissatisfied (Arshad et al 2003). Asking parents what they would like, offering them time to explore what is important for them, will be invaluable. Some parents who never go to church may find comfort in a visit from the Hospital Chaplain, a blessing or baptism for their baby, while others may like a visit arranged with their own religious leader. Many hospitals today keep a Book of Remembrance in which parents may make an entry, either soon after the birth or at a later date.

Other parents who have a deep faith may choose not to have a religious ceremony. It is best to refrain from talking about your personal beliefs with bereaved families, but to be open to what may be appropriate for and a comfort to them. This illustrates the need for the midwife to be knowledgeable about different cultures and religions and their rituals, but not to make assumptions about what parents from a particular group will wish to do following a bereavement (Schott et al 2007, CBT 2003b, CBC 2007d).

## INVOLVING BROTHERS AND SISTERS

It can be difficult for professionals to raise with parents that they may need to consider the involvement of their other children when a baby brother or sister has died. Children can arouse strong feelings in adults. For midwives, they may evoke memories of their own childhood, their own children, or perhaps the children they had hoped to have. Professional staff increasingly recognize the importance of work with adults, but children and their emotions have often been ignored.

When a baby dies, parents may be reluctant to involve their other children. They themselves are grieving, feeling helpless and overwhelmed and may be uncertain about their own ability to regain control. It is natural for them to want to protect their children from painful situations and it can be helpful if they are told this is a normal reaction. However, this stance may leave the siblings confused, unprotected from their fantasies and unsupported in their feelings.

### Communicating with siblings

The decision is not whether or not to talk to children, but who will do the talking, when and how, as it is impossible for parents not to communicate with children. They read body language, overhear conversations and notice changes in routine. Momentous situations in a family cause changes, and children quickly sense when something serious is happening. They require clear, simple, truthful and often repeated but brief explanations about what has happened, and what may happen next. Although the children will not have known the baby and so are unlikely to be deeply grieving for their brother or sister, they will be affected by the grief of their parents.

Children do not need protecting from their feelings, but support in them. Young siblings will not grieve in the same way as older children and often express themselves through play, drawing or with friends.

## Children's reactions and understanding

Children have a shorter concentration span than adults and cannot tolerate intense emotions for very long. This does not mean that they are not sometimes upset and sad. Few children under the age of 5 will understand the permanence of death. They think in literal, concrete terms and therefore metaphors or euphemisms such as 'lost' or 'gone away' are confusing. Children need adults to say the words 'has died' or 'is dead'. By 6 years of age, most children begin to understand death as permanent and that it can happen to them.

### Preparation before the death

Whenever possible, it is helpful if parents prepare their other children when their baby sibling is not expected to live, giving honest information appropriate to their children's age. Children need to understand that most sick babies in the hospital get better and go home, but sadly sometimes babies die. It is important not to overwhelm children with information but to be guided by them and to answer their questions honestly.

### Preparation after the death

Most children who have been carefully prepared and have chosen to see their dead baby brother or sister are not afraid and generally gain an understanding of death and what has happened (Fig. 70.9). What children do not know or are not told about, they often make up and their fantasies are usually worse than the reality. Sometimes they experience feelings of guilt, especially if they were not looking forward to a new sibling. They need to be reassured that the baby's death had nothing to do with their thoughts or actions, and that their parents love them and life will not always be so sad.

Parents may be concerned that frightening memories of a dead baby will leave their children with upsetting images – this is unlikely, especially when the children have been prepared for what to expect (Fig. 70.10). Children respond well to factual explanations of death and having information such as: 'When people die it means their body doesn't work any more.' It is useful to explain that the baby may feel cold to touch and that the skin may be mottled and the baby's lips or skin may be blue. It is not helpful to liken death to sleeping because people who are asleep are not dead and their bodies work very well (CBT 2003c, CBC 2007e).

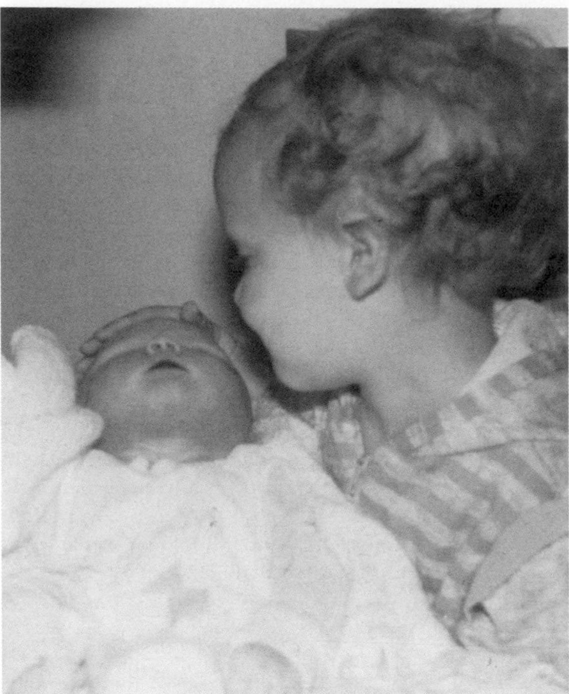

**Figure 70.9** Naomi holding her baby sister Katie after she died. (By kind permission of the parents, and not to be reproduced without permission.)

### Attending the funeral

Although some parents and grandparents feel that children need to be protected from being present at the funeral, children themselves usually say that they find it helpful to be there. They need to be prepared for and included in the family's rituals of mourning. To be excluded from these events can widen the gap between the grieving parents and the child. However, a child who is frightened about attending a funeral should not be pressured or forced to do so. Some other way can be found for the child to say goodbye – such as putting a letter or flowers in the coffin, lighting a candle, saying a prayer or visiting the grave.

If children want to attend the funeral, thought needs to be given to the support that will be required. They need to know what will happen and be given the opportunity to ask questions. They may like to take an active part in the service by choosing a favourite song, poem or reading. It is often a good idea for the children to be cared for by an adult who is close to them during the service, to relieve the parents at such an emotional time.

### How professionals can help

It is important for staff to make a direct offer of help to families and ensure there is time to discuss parents' worries and anxieties. However, parents are individuals and not

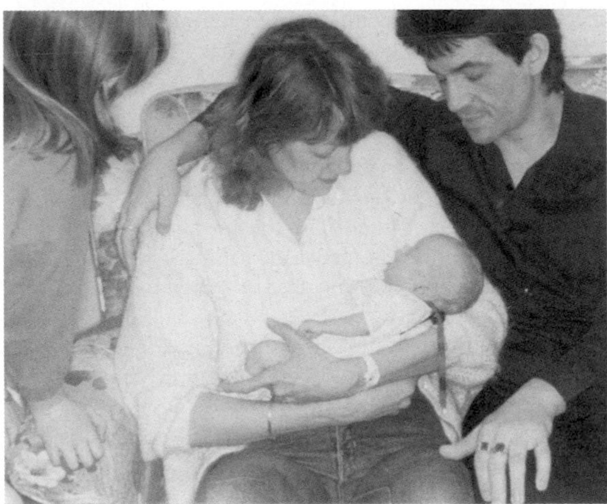

Figure 70.10 Baby Rikki with parents Jane and Adrian and sister Jaycee, who, with her younger sister Donna, helped to bath him after his death. (By kind permission of the parents, and not to be reproduced without permission.)

all of them will feel able to involve their children directly or tell them about the death immediately. Different cultures will have different ways of dealing with death, and sensitivity is paramount when offering parents information so that they can make informed choices, for example, a photograph to take home to the children of their brother or sister who has died. It is helpful for staff to explain to parents that they may meet resistance from grandparents and others who did not receive this care years ago.

Professionals can suggest children might like to have something special for themselves – perhaps a footprint on coloured paper they have chosen or a photograph of them with their baby brother or sister. Children are helped if they are allowed to share in and create memories.

## FAMILY AND FRIENDS

Grandparents too will be grieving and perhaps feeling guilty that they are still alive when their grandchild has died. They will grieve for their grandchild and for the sadness of their son or daughter. They may be a main source of comfort to the grieving parents in the months ahead and are more able to share this grief with the parents if they have been involved from the start. Other family members and friends may experience similar feelings of grief and unhappiness for the bereaved parents.

Involvement of a close family friend can also be supportive, particularly if for whatever reason a mother is having to face bereavement on her own without a partner. It is important to have someone to share the few memories of a baby's brief existence and to help when taking decisions such as funeral arrangements.

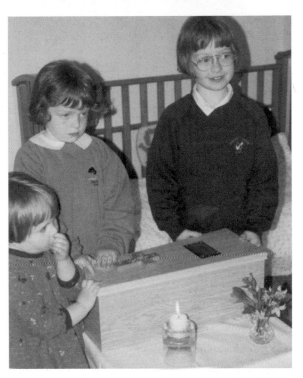

Figure 70.11 Colette, Elizabeth Ann and Eugenie with their brother Benedict's coffin at home before his funeral.

## TAKING A BABY HOME

Parents appreciate information about taking their baby home with them before the funeral – this can usually be arranged with the local funeral director (CBC 2007f, CBT 2003d). Hospitals are large and impersonal and parents may prefer the family to have the opportunity to see their baby and say goodbye in familiar surroundings (Fig. 70.11). When there is a coroner's postmortem, permission must be sought from the coroner (CBT 2003e, CBC 2007g).

### Leaving hospital

When parents leave the hospital, where possible, a member of staff should walk with them out to their car or taxi. It is crucial that community staff are aware of the baby's death and parents know who to contact once at home. Hospital policies need to be clear and enhance liaison between hospital and home in order to provide continuity of care for bereaved parents.

Making an appointment for the parents to visit the consultant again, and perhaps the midwife who cared for them, within 6 weeks, for a follow-up bereavement visit is useful. They can share again what happened at their baby's death or maybe have explained anything they did not understand in crisis. This time can be a valuable way of finding out what support the parents have or may need.

## REGISTRATION OF THE DEATH

Legally, when a baby is *born dead before 24 weeks' gestation* there is no birth certificate or need for registration. However, if the parents choose to have their baby buried or cremated, they will need written confirmation of the birth from the doctor or midwife attending the delivery. Some units issue a form/certificate to record that the parents are taking their baby's body, and this is formally recommended as best practice. This certificate also serves to recognize the baby's existence and can become an important memento.

*After 24 weeks' gestation*, when a baby is stillborn, the doctor or midwife who attended the delivery gives the parents a Medical Certificate of Stillbirth and should explain that the stillbirth of their baby must be registered by either or both parents at the registry office within 42 days.

When a baby is born alive, *regardless of gestational age*, and then dies within 28 days of birth, by law a doctor must confirm the death and provide a medical certificate to enable both the birth and death to be registered within 5 days of the death.

When parents are married, either or both can register, but when parents are unmarried, the registration needs to be done by the mother. The baby's father should accompany her if he wishes his name to appear on their baby's certificate.

## RESPECTFUL DISPOSAL

Parents of babies born dead before 24 weeks' gestation who choose to arrange a burial or cremation for their baby themselves, may need help with planning a ceremony, which can be held in the hospital chapel, in a church, or at the crematorium or cemetery (DH 2005, RCN 2001). Parents do not generally know about how to manage this and may welcome the suggestion if it is made to them. Other parents may prefer not to be involved in the arrangements themselves but will want to be reassured that the hospital will treat their baby's body with respect (RCN 2001).

All parents need information about the options available to them. An information sheet with the relevant costs and considerations is valuable, as also is plenty of time, ensuring parents are not rushed and are able to make informed choices.

## THE MONTHS AHEAD

In order to begin to heal the pain of a traumatic loss, parents need to find a way to express their feelings and to communicate these feelings to a caring supportive person. Parents continue to grieve for their baby throughout their lives. They know they can never replace the baby who has died – grieving is about remembering, not forgetting. But it is the very absence of memories that makes grieving so hard when a baby dies. Parents are likely to feel a bond with the staff who cared for them and their baby. Appropriate care needs to be available in the months following the death on the unit. Parents need to know how to access support no matter how long it is since their baby died (Jennings 2001).

In a busy unit it is not always possible for professional staff to give parents as much time as they need, both at the time of the death and on return. A designated bereavement counsellor is in a position to support the parents and the staff. Using counselling skills and working as a counsellor are two different tasks. Being a counsellor requires a professional qualification, and is a skilled task for which aptitude, training and experience are necessary. It can only happen if the client has asked for counselling.

Bereavement counselling takes time and is best offered as a home or hospital visit after the baby's death. The crucial times appear to be 3 and 6 weeks after the death and also 3, 6 and 12 months. Parents say that just knowing that as a couple, they can see a counsellor, perhaps once a month, helps them to manage their feelings and relationship. The bereavement counselling session gives them permission to talk about their feelings and their relationship and helps them to recognize that it is normal to grieve.

## RETURN VISIT TO THE HOSPITAL UNIT

Some parents want to come back to the unit to see the midwife in the antenatal clinic or to see the person who cared for them and their baby. The opportunity to talk through what happened at the time of their baby's death, particularly if the mother had a general anaesthetic, can be very valuable. Ideally, a time should be arranged so that when parents arrive on the unit someone expects them and they have a clear idea how long the member of staff can spend with them. Parents may want to return around the first anniversary of their baby's death, and it is useful to be aware of this.

## SUPPORT AGENCIES

There are a number of voluntary organizations (see website for Additional resources) which offer support to bereaved families in the form of helplines, parent support groups and resources for grieving families. Most parents will also welcome information about the local support groups. These agencies, such as SANDS and the Child Bereavement

Charity (formerly the Child Bereavement Trust), now the Child Bereavement Charity (CBC) are sources of information and support, and are also involved in developing literature and resources for bereaved parents and professionals (see website).

**Reflective activity 70.3**

Gather information about facilities, protocols, information leaflets and booklets that are available in your unit for women and their families who have lost a baby, or are facing perinatal bereavement. Review the material so that you are aware of the content, and where to get further information on:

- local support agencies/groups available to bereaved parents in your area
- useful contact numbers centred on bereavement support
- information available for parents – leaflets, websites, etc.

Review local support groups and make sure you have contact details in your personal resource file.

## CONCLUSION

The essence of working with bereaved families is to respect their wishes and feelings whatever they may be; to offer them as much time as they need to talk about what has happened; to really listen to what they have to say; to ensure they have as much information as they want and that they have understood it; to answer their questions honestly; and to make sure they have someone to contact for support in the future.

The Chief Medical Officer's recommendation that all NHS trusts should provide support and advice to families at the time of bereavement highlighted the need for the role of bereavement advisor and recognized the need for training in all aspects of dealing with grieving families (CMO 2001). The Child Bereavement Charity (CBC) (originally the Child Bereavement Trust set up in 1994) has developed an audit model for the monitoring and evaluation of bereavement services (CBT 2003f, CBC 2007h).

Midwives have to balance caring for the complex needs that the mother and her family have, which must include a consideration for physical, social, psychological and spiritual needs, at a time when she requires a high level of sensitive and skilled care (Thomas 2001). This balance requires significant self-knowledge and an ability to be truly 'with woman' through her pain and sadness, in order to support and guide her through this period. An awareness of their own needs and those of their healthcare colleagues is also imperative in ensuring a strong and supportive team.

Working with grieving parents can be difficult and emotionally draining, but knowing that the family have been helped through one of the worst periods of their lives, by what was said or done making a difference, can be immensely rewarding.

## KEY POINTS

- Grief is a normal reaction to an abnormal event and the midwife's role is to identify and continually assess what parents need and help them to make informed choices.
- The way midwives manage their own emotions has a direct influence on how they manage to help others express themselves; this requires effective support systems to be in place to support them in their interactions with grieving parents.
- Seeing and spending time with their dead baby helps parents to face the reality of what has happened and creates precious memories. Most children who have been included and have chosen to see their dead sibling are not afraid and have a better understanding of what has happened.
- It is essential for staff to recognize the process of consent and always obtain written informed consent from parents for the postmortem examination of their baby and for the retention of any tissue, blocks or slides.
- NHS trusts need to take into account the recommendations of the CMO for the role of bereavement advisor.
- Effective support needs to extend beyond the death on the unit into the community.

## REFERENCES


Arshad M, Horsfall A, Yasin R: Pregnancy loss and the Holy Qu'ran, *British Journal of Midwifery* 12(8):481–484, 2003.

Bewley C: Midwives and failed motherhood: working with midwives who have experienced their own reproductive or pregnancy related loss, *MIDIRS* 20(1):7–10, 2010.

Bowlby J: *Attachment and loss. Volume 3. Loss, sadness and depression*, Harmondsworth, 1980, Penguin.

Caelli K, Downie J, Knox M: Through grief to healthy parenthood: facilitating the journey through a family pregnancy support programme, *Birth Issues* 8(3):85–90, 1999.

Chief Medical Officer (CMO): *The removal, retention and use of human organs and tissue*, London, 2001, DH.

Child Bereavement Charity (CBC): *Best practice guidance for the care of a family when their baby dies in the maternity unit*, High Wycombe, 2007a, CBC.

Child Bereavement Charity (CBC): *Best practice guidance for the taking of photographs following the death of a baby*, High Wycombe, 2007b, CBC.

Child Bereavement Charity (CBC): *Guidance for professionals: a photographic memory*, High Wycombe, 2007c, CBC. (First published by the Child Bereavement Trust in 2003.)

Child Bereavement Charity (CBC): *Best practice guidance regarding cultural and religious issues at the time of a baby or child's death*, High Wycombe, 2007d, CBC.

Child Bereavement Charity (CBC): *Best practice guidance for the care of siblings following the death of a brother or sister*, High Wycombe, 2007e, CBC.

Child Bereavement Charity (CBC): *Best practice guidance for families who wish to take their baby home after death*, High Wycombe, 2007f, CBC.

Child Bereavement Charity (CBC): *What happens in a post mortem examination*, High Wycombe, 2007g, CBC.

Child Bereavement Charity (CBC): *A bereavement audit model: auditing your work in bereavement support*, High Wycombe, 2007h, CBC. Available: http://www.childbereavement.org.uk/files/images/12.pdf

Child Bereavement Trust (CBT): *Best practice guidance for the care of a family when their baby dies in the maternity unit*, High Wycombe, 2003a, CBT.

Child Bereavement Trust (CBT): *Best practice guidance regarding cultural and religious issues at the time of a baby or child's death*, High Wycombe, 2003b, CBT.

Child Bereavement Trust (CBT): *Information series: The death of a baby or child; When a baby dies (for parents); Understanding bereaved children and young people*, High Wycombe, 2003c, CBT.

Child Bereavement Trust (CBT): *Best practice guidance for families who wish to take their baby home after death*, High Wycombe, 2003d, CBT.

Child Bereavement Trust (CBT): *What happens in a post mortem examination*, High Wycombe, 2003e, CBT.

Child Bereavement Trust (CBT): *A bereavement audit model: auditing your work in bereavement support*, High Wycombe, 2003f, CBT.

Department of Health (DH): *When a patient dies: advice on developing bereavement services in the NHS*, London, 2005, DH.

Henley A, Kohner N: *When a baby dies: the experience of late miscarriage, stillbirth and neonatal death*, London, 2001, Routledge.

Hill S: *Family*, London, 1990, Penguin.

Hughes P, Turton P, Hopper E, et al: Assessment of guidelines for good practice in psychosocial care of mothers after stillbirth: a cohort study, *Lancet* 360:114–118, 2002.

Hughes P: The management of bereaved mothers: what is best? *Midwives Chronicle* 100(1195):226–229, 1987.

Human Tissue Authority (HTA): *Code of Practice – Post mortem examination* (website). www.hta.gov.uk/guidance/codes_of_practice.cfm. 2006.

Hunfeld JAM, Taselaar-Kloos AKG, Agterberg G, et al: Trait anxiety, negative emotions, and the mothers' adaptation to an infant born subsequent to late pregnancy loss: a case-control study, *Prenatal Diagnosis* 17(9):843–851, 1997.

INQUEST: *An information pack for families, friends and advisors*, London, 2003, INQUEST.

Jennings P: *The first two years experience of child bereavement support posts. Evaluation of the Department of Health project*, High Wycombe, 2001, CBT.

Kohner N, Thomas J: *Grieving after the death of your baby [for parents]*, High Wycombe, 1995, Child Bereavement Charity.

Lewis G, editor: *The Confidential Enquiry into Maternal and Child Health (CEMACH). Saving mothers' lives: reviewing maternal deaths to make motherhood safer – 2003–2005. The Seventh Report on Confidential Enquiries into Maternal Deaths in the United Kingdom*, London, 2007, CEMACH.

Kubler-Ross E: *On death and dying*, London, 1970, Tavistock.

Lewis E, Bourne S: Perinatal death, *Baillière's Clinical Obstetrics and Gynaecology* 3(4):935–953, 1989.

McHaffie HE: *Crucial decisions at the beginning of life. Parents' experiences of treatment withdrawal from infants*, Oxford, 2001, Radcliffe Medical.

NICE: *NICE Guideline 45. Antenatal and postnatal mental health* (website) http://guidance.nice.org.uk/CG45. 2007.

Nursing and Midwifery Council (NMC): *Midwives rules and standards*, London, 2004, NMC.

Office for National Statistics (ONS): Series DH3 Mortality statistics: childhood, infant and perinatal, *Health Statistics Quarterly* 3:62–69, 2006.

Parkes CM: *Bereavement: studies of grief in adult life*, Harmondsworth, 1972, Penguin.

Puddifoot JE, Johnson MP: The legitimacy of grieving: the partner's experience at miscarriage, *Social Science & Medicine* 45(6):837–845, 1997. .

Royal College of Nursing (RCN): *Sensitive disposal of all fetal remains*, London, 2001, RCN.

Schott J, Henley A, Kohner N: *Pregnancy loss and the death of a baby: guidelines for professionals*, ed 3, London, 2007, Stillbirth and Neonatal Death Society (SANDS).

Schott J, Henley A: After a stillbirth – offering choices, creating memories, *British Journal of Midwifery* 17(12):798–800, 2009.

Shrivastav P, George K, Balasubramaniam N, et al: Suppression of puerperal lactation using jasmine flowers (*Jasminum sambac*), *Australian and New Zealand Journal of Obstetrics and Gynaecology* 28(1):68–71, 1988.

Stroebe MS, Schut H: The dual process model of coping with bereavement: rationale and descriptions, *Death Studies* 23(3):197–224, 1999.

Thomas J: The death of a baby: guidance for professionals in hospital and community, *Journal of Neonatal Nursing* 7(5):167–170, 2001.

Thomas J, Chalmers A: Working with families and loss: the therapeutic use of ourselves, *Infant* 1(6), 2005. http://www.infantgrapevine.co.uk/pdf/inf_006_fal.pdf accessed September 2010.

Thomas J, Williams B: *When our baby died* (DVD). Available from the Child Bereavement Charity (CBC).

Thomas J, Williams B: *Death at birth* (DVD). Available from the Child Bereavement Charity (CBC).

Worden JW: *Grief counselling and grief therapy*, London, 1991, Routledge.

*N.B. The Child Bereavement Trust, founded by Jenni Thomas in 1994, became the Child Bereavement Charity in 2006, and many of the publications have since been republished under CBC.*

# Part 10

# The future

Chapter |71|

# Midwifery for the 21st century

*Julia Magill-Cuerden*

## LEARNING OUTCOMES

After reading this chapter you will be able to:

- reflect upon future developments in midwifery in order to practise with confidence in providing women with optimum care, in a changing climate during the present century
- recognize the sources that may be utilized to ensure that knowledge, skills and practice are not static but adapt to changing societal, cultural and political circumstances in delivery of midwifery care
- be aware of the quality enhancement required in maternity services to keep birth normal and also to ensure safe and effective practice that meet the needs of women and their families
- consider the future of midwifery practice and the significance of the Millennium Development Goals (MDGs) in promoting the health and wellbeing of women and families worldwide
- consider the multi-professional context within which midwives work in healthcare services and how to work effectively and autonomously with others within their professional boundaries
- reflect on their place as a midwife in 21st century midwifery.

## INTRODUCTION

The first chapter of this book states 'It is midwives who make their profession, what it is today and what it will be tomorrow, globally.' This final chapter will briefly address challenges that may face midwives in the 21st century in order to maintain their roles within the midwifery profession and maternity service. (Supporting information is on the website, which, therefore, is not referred to within the chapter.)

## THE FUTURE

If midwives wish to have their role recognized, they must be clear of their role and its professional boundaries. Where overlaps in responsibilities occur in caring for women and families when working within the multi-professional environment, agreeing distinct pathways for the role of the midwife is essential. Where multiple providers are offering support and care in health and social care, then, ideally, a choice should be made for a key worker from one group who can build the best relationship. The essential element, here, is to ensure good channels of communication between all healthcare providers. In many cases, the midwife is most likely to provide continuity to the woman during the pregnancy and childbirth period.

In responding to new disease patterns, changes in society and public expectations, it is opportune to consider how midwives may work flexibly and broaden their remit within the public health agenda to meet the needs of society (DH 1999, 2001b, UN 2001). Altering economic climates will also demand new ways of working to provide an effective and efficient midwifery service that utilizes support where necessary.

Though many resources for this book and the website have drawn upon midwifery in UK literature, messages for midwives working with women throughout the world are similar. In countries where the midwifery profession is established, women have optimum opportunity to birth in ways that suit them. The aim must be to provide trained midwives for all women all over the world, as this is proven to impact on quality of maternity care, and reduction in mortality and morbidity (WHO 2004).

## Clinical care

Providing women with choices and enabling families to make decisions in their care is government policy in the UK (DH 2007a). A recent review of women's maternity care experiences demonstrates diversity in experiences that women receive in the UK; however, the report notes that midwives are in a powerful position to influence the care that women receive (Redshaw et al 2007). Women's voices and views need to be heard antenatally, in labour, and during the postnatal and neonatal care periods, so that clinical care takes place in non-threatening spaces, and always with the ability to respond to emergencies.

Features of practice environments will include:

- provision of unbiased information that meets the needs of individuals
- ensuring mutuality through knowledge-sharing in partnership through communication with women as a way forward to promoting women's decision-making (NHS Scotland 2009) and their feelings of their own control
- promotion of normality in all processes of birth and its environment with the option of working with women to accomplish as normal a birth as possible (RCM 2009a)
- direct communication with, and referral between, medical and midwifery teams
- pathways for rapid access to emergency care, to medical facilities and other interventions as necessary
- ensuring communication in complex cases (RCOG RCA RCM RCP 2007) and, as professionals and women may not share the same language and knowledge base, to review ways of mediating understandings
- development for all midwives of their leadership qualities to articulate for women in their care, recognizing their individual wishes
- education and training of midwives to develop knowledge and skills to practise with autonomy and recognize when to liaise with other agencies (Reid 2007). All midwives need to continuously develop their knowledge and skills.

Clinical care may need to be offered flexibly to ensure that women's societal and cultural needs are accommodated within provision of best evidence for practice. With increasing medical advances midwives need to balance sound knowledge of normalization of birthing processes with appropriate use of science and technology in clinical care. Advances are increasingly enabling women with complex medical conditions to become fertile and give birth. This brings higher levels of complexity in caring. The aim is to ensure optimum health outcomes for mother and baby with reduction of morbidity and mortality.

## Working with women

Women want clear unbiased advice, offered in simple lay terms, that does not indicate a professional's individual view, but gives the options and implications of a choice of action to tailor this to their individual circumstances. This is not an easy task for each professional who has a mantle of their own prejudices and biases that need to be set aside. The Darzi report (DH 2007b) indicates that professionals must provide a personalized service that gives control to women and families.

Women may find advice contradictory and confusing, therefore, current information could be improved (Healthcare Commission 2008). This often means listening to women and confirming that they understand the implications of advice (Redshaw et al 2007). Building partnerships with women and working with their organizations, such as the Association for Improvement of the Maternity Services (AIMS; http://www.aims.org.uk/) and the National Childbirth Trust (NCT), and local groups, will assist in providing a service where their needs are met.

If women do not like what is offered, they may take their own decision for their birth, as shown by the movement for *free birthing* (Cooper & Clarke 2008). Care must be equitable for all women and families regardless of their individual circumstances (DH 2007a).

The influence of a trained midwife present at birth has been shown to effect a reduced morbidity and mortality rate for both mother and baby (WHO 2004). In this century, an aim would be to see education, training and registration for midwives in all countries of the world. The caveat is that as midwives become qualified, the costs of midwifery service may rise, thus there may be those who work in affiliation with midwives. Clear parameters and boundaries will be necessary to ensure that it is midwives who provide skilled care to women through the pregnancy and childbirth continuum. Their responsibility is to be knowledgeable, know their limitations and how to harness appropriate multi-professional help when needed. This would be the aim to ensure safer birth. To see a fulfilment of this aim for safer birth and to reduce inequalities in birth means continuing training and lifelong learning for all midwives, including professional updating that recognizes the value of normalization of birth where possible. This includes changing behaviours and attitudes that have become reliant on interventions, however minor.

## A multi-social and multicultural society

Inevitably, with changes in living styles and social family structures, economic uncertainty, and with differing cultures in our society, the demands are for professionals to adapt and manage change in caring for women and families with diverse needs whilst ensuring equality of provision (DH 2008). One group in the UK who require specific midwifery support are those who live in deprived circumstances, or have special social needs.

Whilst there have always been people who have lived by travelling, now, with easier modes of travel enabling crossing of national boundaries, different populations and societies are migrating, some willingly, for their own interests and economics, but others enforced, as political migrants, with an emergence of a varied multicultural society. These people may require high levels of health interventions and lack the language and knowledge to seek their own health needs. The first health encounter for many is the maternity service. Thus, the midwife may be the first person to identify those in different groups at risk of special needs, and has an opportunity for taking a broad health review to identify health concerns. A social and health needs assessment may divulge specific problems for subsequent care.

Some who may require particular attention are:

- teenagers and vulnerable women who are unsupported
- families where young men are to become fathers
- adoptive parents and those who have had fertility treatment
- women who wish for care outside health service expectations
- families with disabled members
- asylum seekers and refugee women
- homeless women
- those with alternative lifestyles or those who are socially deprived
- those with mental health problems
- those dependent upon drugs, alcohol or smoking
- women who seek pregnancy outside normal expectations of fertility or with complex medical conditions.

Whatever their circumstances, a midwife will need to identify their individual choices for care and overcome any language problems with advice for appropriate actions. It is the midwife who becomes a mediator and pivot between the health agencies in providing flexibility and continuity in care.

## GOVERNANCE

Whilst clinical governance and its structures are discussed in Chapter 7, midwives have a responsibility to determine their own governance to meet women's needs. This means their involvement in decision-making for themselves, collaborating with women and in their maternity services policy development, to influence the way in which they are governed. In essence, they will be political at local levels. For example, it is good practice to discuss national publications multi-professionally and collaborate and communicate through structures in the labour ward and maternity units (RCOG RCA RCM RCP 2007, RCOG 2008) prior to decisions for implementation.

### Management structures meeting the needs of women

A management structure for a maternity unit is planned so that efficient services deliver quality effectively and meet the needs of women (RCM 2009b). Quality is measured by criteria and standards but may also be perceived in different ways by those who receive care. Strategy development is a measure of quality of a maternity service and is a multi-professional activity requiring involvement of all the teams involved (RCOG 2008). Furthermore, involving women in a maternity unit decision-making assists creating a culture where women-centred care is recognized (Proctor 1998).

### Midwives as leaders

Key leaders within the profession promote midwifery and maternity services within national and local organizations (DH 2002). These people negotiate on behalf of the midwifery service but each midwife requires demonstrable leadership skills. It is essential for all midwives to have the confidence to:

- practise within a changing environment, recognizing when to be flexible to meet service needs
- articulate the needs of women and families
- ensure delivery of service and care is appropriate to the working climate
- influence the women's health agenda
- contribute to organizations' standard-setting, policy-making and development of guidelines
- use evidence appropriately, ensuring that it is tailored to the individual needs of women and families
- take a lead on key activities that promote midwifery care.

### Supervision of midwives: action imperatives

Supervision is a statutory responsibility which provides a mechanism for support and guidance to every midwife practising in the UK. It supports the health service governance agenda; the standards of practice and training of midwives; and seeks to represent the views of women and ensure that their requirements for care within safety parameters are met. One legal requirement overseen by supervision of midwives is maintenance of records for professional practice (NMC 2009). Developing records that may be shared with women and understood by them without using arcane language is essential for involvement of women in their care. With public recognition of their rights under legislation, the importance of record-keeping that women understand cannot be understated.

## Organizations of learning

The health service environment can promote an organization of learning which is responsive to the needs of its clients (Wilkinson et al 2004). This environment is one that actively supports multi-professional education and training sessions and has an effective review system for staff that actively develops its staff (Timpson 1998). It learns from critical review and involves staff and women in the process (Healthcare Commission 2007).

## Continuing professional development

A basic training in midwifery is not adequate to equip a midwife with the knowledge and skills required for life (DES 1997). Whilst an initial programme provides a platform for building a future career, continuous learning will be essential to provide midwifery care in different and flexible ways in changing environments (DES 1997, DH 2001a). Consolidation of an initial training in midwifery is essential to practise confidently. As the way women birth will not change, technology, new knowledge and changes in society will demand future midwives who can practise flexibly in any environment, offering individualized care (DH 2001b).

Midwives need to be able to:

- learn from incidents and mistakes
- lack defensiveness, reflecting and permitting people to see where there is a fault
- regularly commit to education, training and development through active reflection
- use technology competently to share information with women
- question the status quo to create new ways of caring for women
- contribute through innovation and creativity to developing a dynamic and appropriate maternity service.

## Communication and relationships

With so many variations in the way we communicate and differences between professional cultures and communication across societies, it is not surprising that situations often present with often unimagined difficulties, especially where there is hurry, stress or a lack of attention. Our society is not trained to listen, increasingly with use of information technology (IT). Therefore, in order to relate to women, we need to train ourselves to listen, to communicate and to recognize cues from women as they will pick up non-verbal messages from the midwife (Kirkham 2000).

## Quality enhancement structures

The prime concern for women and families is the outcome of a healthy mother and child. The effects on families of childbirth are little researched and the impact of long-term effects of maternity care on family relationships requires exploration. We have little knowledge of the long-term impact of interventions and minor trauma on the mother/child relationships and family dynamics. Therefore, reducing any risk of complications or problems is important in providing care. Being prepared for an eventuality and possible emergencies, ensuring systems are in place to reduce delays, and efficient management are essential. This includes midwives being aware of their own limitations and having an intuitive sense of situations. In view of this, corporate maternity unit policies will be in place for risk reduction for maternal and infant mortality and morbidity. Risk management includes reducing mortality and morbidity through:

- risk reduction
- reporting
- analysis
- statistical analysis of outcome figures in pregnancy, labour and postnatal care.

The institutional figures may be compared to those at national level but the implications for individual midwives are that they constantly undertake reflection and self-review of their own engagement with areas of risk and reduction of safety at birth to improve practices. A balance needs to be set between women's choices and perceived risks by a professional as we all have different views of what is meant by the term 'risk'. Whilst the concept of risk may be considered a measurement of safety, each person has different notions of what is acceptable to them.

# TECHNOLOGY AND HEALTH

Possibilities for advancing technology applications will filter into every aspect of childbirth with opportunities emerging for individual access to data and resources that have not hitherto been imagined. For example, in the less developed world it may be possible to use a telephone to access advice direct, on how to deal with emergencies or undertake surgery remotely or to have regular updates on evidence relayed through internet or telephone connection. Whilst technical equipment may assist in detection and prevention of problems, a responsibility will be to ensure data protection for all personnel and care taken with all electronic records that may be accessed. All technology applications must be used ethically in care of women.

Midwives will need to exploit the current systems in such ways as setting up health libraries for immediate access to evidence support in home birth and this could be on a palm-held machine.

**Reflective activity 71.1**

What kind of technology would you wish to see implemented to promote normal birth? Remember that ideally birth would have minimum technology present in the practical care of the mothers.

## THE MIDWIFE WITH GLOBAL VISION

The introductory chapter indicates the need to work toward the Millennium Development Goals (UN 2001, 2008). The impact of midwifery care on the health of a nation is little understood. Recognizing the work of a midwife in all countries of the world is a WHO priority in the Safe Motherhood Initiatve (Maternity Worldwide; WHO 2004). Midwives now have opportunities to learn from each other in different countries to discover how midwifery may be adapted to the needs of women in differing societies, for example, through organizations such as the International Confederation of Midwives (ICM; http://www.internationalmidwives.org/). Preventing morbidity and mortality are key objectives. Unless current trends of mortalities are reduced, women and families will continue to be at risk. In all countries, reducing morbidity from the effects of childbirth is equally important. We do not know what impact good midwifery care has on family life, with little evidence of the impact of the role of the midwife and maternity care for women's future relationships with their children.

We all take a responsibility in the changes taking place within the environment, and promoting normal birth is one way of conserving naturalness in our society. An active approach towards reducing climate change that affects the many lives of vulnerable societies requires a new way of thinking in all maternity units to conserve and reduce energy consumption. It is suspected that the MGD for 2015 will not be met (Homer et al 2009) and that climate change is affecting the health and welfare of society (Costello & White 2001, Costello et al 2009); therefore, the onus for making changes that reduce environmental effects is a responsibility for all the midwifery society.

**Reflective activity 71.2**

Think of one aspect of midwifery care where you could implement a measure to reduce the carbon footprint in the maternity unit and make savings for the environment.

## CONCLUSION

The vision of the future of midwifery is in the hands of midwives. It is they who will articulate their views for themselves and for women, to policy-makers. Midwives need to listen to organizations for women and cultural groups who act on behalf of women. Social divides between rich and poor will make it essential that midwives hone their skills to recognize those most at risk, using preventive action to mitigate the risks that are life-endangering. A global economy, with global information technology (IT) and increasing advances in digitization, will mean new modes of working and ways of communicating with women internationally, especially in building upon evidence. Midwifery will always link between basics of practice using a sound knowledge base and practical skills and advances in new forms of care. Thus, in the 21st century, midwives in all parts of the world will become increasingly skilled through their own professional development. In retaining separateness as a profession but engaging with other professions collaboratively and exploiting advantages in technology to support essential midwifery practice, vision, integrity and flexibility will be essential attributes for all in readiness to face the future.

### KEY POINTS

- Midwives, in conjunction with women, will need to create their own vision of their role and the midwifery services.
- Each midwife will need to achieve leadership skills, to articulate for women and to ensure that midwifery practice responds to societal needs.
- Midwifery will need to be socially and culturally responsive to ensure that the psychological and physical individual needs of women, their babies and families are met.
- Midwives will recognize the governance agenda and professional responsibility and ensure accountability in actions when practising autonomously.
- Collaboration and partnership with women and multi-professionals and agencies in all aspects of care, identifying a lead professional, will be essential to provide comprehensive maternity care.
- Utilization of technology and digitization has the propensity to transform communication in all parts of the world and thus the ways in which midwives practise. This needs to be incorporated into providing care that retains normality but supports improved care for those at risk.
- The WHO Millennium Development Goals pertain to all countries of the world and thus midwives have responsibility to be aware of their international role in caring for women and children.

## REFERENCES


Costello A, White H: Reducing inequalities in child health, *Archives of Disease in Childhood* 84(2):98–102, 2001.

Costello A, Abbas M, Allen A, et al: Managing the health effects of climate change: Lancet and University College London Institute for Global Health Commission, *Lancet* 373(9676):1693–1733, 2009.

Cooper T, Clarke P: Birthing alone: a concern for midwives, *Midwives* August/September issue:33–34, 2008.

Department of Education and Science (DES): *National Committee of Inquiry into Higher Education (NCIHE) (Dearing Report): Higher education in the learning society*, London, 1997, Department of Education and Science.

Department of Health (DH): *Working together – learning together: a framework for lifelong learning for the NHS*, London, 2001a, DH.

Department of Health (DH): *Making a difference – the nursing, midwifery and health visiting contribution. The Midwifery Action Plan*, London, 2001b, DH.

Department of Health (DH): *Shifting the balance of power: the next steps*, London, 2002, DH.

Department of Health (DH): *Maternity matters: choice access and continuity of care in a safe service*, London, 2007a, DH.

Department of Health (DH): *Our NHS our future (The Darzi report)*, London, 2007b, DH.

Department of Health (DH): *Making the difference: the pacesetters beginner's guide to service improvement for diversity and equality and diversity in the NHS*, London, 2008, DH.

Healthcare Commission: *Towards better births: a review of maternity services in England*, London, 2007, Healthcare Commission.

Healthcare Commission: *Women's experiences of maternity care in the NHS in England* (website). www.cqc.org.uk/_db/_documents/Maternity_services_survey_report.pdf. 2008.

Homer CS, Hanna E, McMichael AJ: Climate change threatens the achievement of the Millennium Development Goal for maternal health, *Midwifery* 25(6):606–612, 2009.

Kirkham M: *The midwife-mother relationship*, Basingstoke, 2000, Macmillan.

Maternity Worldwide: *Safe motherhood* (website). www.maternityworldwide.org/pages/safe-motherhood-initiative.html. Accessed July 2010.

National Childbirth Trust: *Working in partnership* (website) www.nctpregnancyandbabycare.com/professional/partnership. 2010.

NHS Scotland: *Enabling partnerships: sharing knowledge for a mutual NHS national strategy for NHS Scotland Knowledge Services – final consultation* (website). www.nes.scot.nhs.uk/initiatives/news/items/default.asp?id=708. 2009.

Nursing and Midwifery Council (NMC): *Record keeping guidance for nurses and midwives*, London, 2009, NMC.

Proctor S: What determines quality in maternity care: comparing perception of childbearing women and midwives, *Birth* 25(2):85–93, 1998.

Redshaw M, Rowe R, Hockley C, et al: *Recorded delivery: a national survey of women's experience of maternity care*, Oxford, 2007, National Perinatal Epidemiology Unit (NPEU).

Reid L, editor: *Midwifery: freedom to practise: an exploration of midwifery practice*, Edinburgh, 2007, Churchill Livingstone.

Royal College of Midwives (RCM): *Normal birth campaign* (website). www.rcmnormalbirth.org.uk/. 2009a.

Royal College of Midwives (RCM): *Guidance Paper: Staffing Standard in Midwifery Services* (website). www.rcm.org.uk/college/standards-and-practice/guidance-papers/. 2009b.

Royal College of Obstetricians and Gynaecologists (RCOG): *Standards for maternity care*, London, 2008, RCOG.

Royal College of Obstetricians (RCOG), Royal College of Anaesthetists (RCA), Royal College of Midwives (RCM), Royal College of Paediatrics and Child Health (RCP): *Safer childbirth: minimum standards for the organisation and delivery of care in labour*, London, 2007, RCOG.

Timpson J: The NHS as a learning organization: aspirations beyond the rainbow, *Journal of Nursing Management* 6(5):261–272, 1998.

United Nations (UN): *Road map towards the implementation of the United Nations Millennium Development Goals (MDG)* (website), 2001. http://www.un.org/documents/ga/docs/56/a56326. Accessed November 2010.

United Nations (UN): *United Nations Millennium Development Goals* (website), 2008. http://www.un.org/millenniumgoals. Accessed August 5 2008.

Wilkinson J, Rushmer R, Davies H: Clinical governance and the learning organization, *Journal of Nursing Management* 12(2):105–112, 2004.

World Health Organization (WHO): *Making pregnancy safer: the critical role of the skilled attendant: a joint statement by WHO, ICM and FIGO*, Geneva, 2004, WHO Regional Office.

# Index

Page numbers followed by "f" indicate figures, "t" indicate tables, and "b" indicate boxes.

## B

## C

## D

# E

## F

## G

## H

## J



## K



## L

## M

## N

## O

## P

## Q



## R

## S

## T

## V